W0193027

Pharmaceutical Product Development

Other Books by Dr. N.K. Jain

- Advances in Controlled and Novel Drug Delivery
- Controlled and Novel Drug Delivery
- Health Education and Community Pharmacy, 2nd ed.
- Pharmaceutical Arithmetic, 2nd ed.
- Progress in Controlled and Novel Drug Delivery Systems

Pharmaceutical Product Development

Third Edition

Edited by

N.K. Jain PhD
Emeritus Fellow (UGC)
Rajiv Gandhi Technical University, Bhopal

Formerly
Lecturer in Pharmacy, Holkar College, Indore
Reader in Pharmaceutical Technology, MS University, Baroda
Professor and Principal, College of Pharmacy, Nasik
Principal, College of Pharmacy, New Delhi
Visiting Professor, Dubai Pharmacy College, Dubai (UAE)
Professor of Pharmaceutics, Dr Hari Singh Gour University
(formerly University of Saugor), Sagar

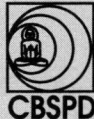

CBSPD

CBS Publishers & Distributors Pvt Ltd

New Delhi • Bengaluru • Chennai • Kochi • Kolkata • Lucknow • Mumbai
Hyderabad • Jharkhand • Nagpur • Patna • Pune • Uttarakhand

Disclaimer

Science and technology are constantly changing fields. New research and experience broaden the scope of information and knowledge. The author have tried their best in giving information available to them while preparing the material for this book. Although, all efforts have been made to ensure optimum accuracy of the material, yet it is quite possible some errors might have been left uncorrected. The publisher, the printer and the author will not be held responsible for any inadvertent errors, or inaccuracies.

Pharmaceutical Product Development

Third Edition

ISBN: 978-93-86827-56-2

First Edition: 2006
Reprint: 2007, 2008, 2010
Second Edition: 2011
Reprint: 2013, 2017
Third Edition: 2018
Reprint: 2024

All rights reserved. No part of this book may be reproduced or transmitted in any form or by any means, electronic or mechanical, including photocopying, recording, or any information storage and retrieval system without permission, in writing, from the author and the publisher.

Published by Satish Kumar Jain and Produced by Varun Jain for

CBS Publishers & Distributors Pvt Ltd

4819/XI Prahlad Street, 24 Ansari Road, Daryaganj, New Delhi 110 002, India
Ph: 011-23289259, 23266861   Website: www.cbspd.com
                                    e-mail: delhi@cbspd.com
Corporate Office: 204 FIE, Industrial Area, Patparganj, Delhi 110 092
Ph: 011-4934 4934   Fax: 011-4934 4935   e-mail: publishing@cbspd.com; publicity@cbspd.com

Branches

• **Bengaluru:** Seema House 2975, 17th Cross, K.R. Road, Banasankari 2nd Stage, Bengaluru 560 070, Karnataka, India
  Ph: +91-80-26771678/79   Fax: +91-80-26771680   e-mail: bangalore@cbspd.com
• **Chennai:** 7, Subbaraya Street, Shenoy Nagar, Chennai 600 030, Tamil Nadu, India
  Ph: +91-44-26680620, 26681266   Fax: +91-44-42032115   e-mail: chennai@cbspd.com
• **Kochi:** 42/1325, 1326, Power House Road, Opp KSEB, Power House, Ernakulam 682 018, Kerala, India
  Ph: +91-484-4059061-65   Fax: +91-484-4059065   e-mail: kochi@cbspd.com
• **Kolkata:** 147, Hind Ceramics Compound, 1st Floor, Nilgunj Road, Belghoria, Kolkata-700056
  West Bengal, India
  Ph: 033-25633055, 033-25633056   e-mail: kolkata@cbspd.com
• **Lucknow:** Basement, Khushnuma Complex, 7-Meerabai Marg (Behind Jawahar Bhawan), Lucknow 226001, India
  Ph: 0522-4000032   e-mail: tiwari.lucknow@cbspd.com
• **Mumbai:** PWD Shed. Gala no. 25/26, Ramchandra Bhatt Marg, Next to JJ Hospital Gate no. 2, Opp. Union Bank of India Noorbaug
  Mumbai-400009, Maharashtra, India
  Ph: 022-66661880/89   e-mail: mumbai@cbspd.com

Representatives

• **Hyderabad**   0-9885175004   • **Jharkhand**   0-9811541605   • **Nagpur**   0-8692091830
• **Patna**   0-9334159340   • **Pune**   0-9664372571   • **Uttarakhand**   0-9716462459

Printed at Chaman Enterprises, Daryaganj, Delhi, India

Preface to the Third Edition

Pharmaceutical Product Development is a dynamic as well as most sought after topic in pharmaceutical industry and hence warrants updating from time to time. Three editions of this book in a span of one decade from 2006 to 2016 is the testimony to its popularity.

Four new chapters included in the third edition are (9) Vaginal Drug Delivery Systems, (12) Drug Release Kinetic Modelling of Extended Release Drug Delivery Systems, (13) *In Vitro/In Vivo* Correlations (IVIVC) as a Vital Tool in Pharmaceutical Product Development and Federal Biowaivers, and (14) Quality by Design (QbD) and its Role in Pharma Product Development.

Remaining chapters have been thoroughly revised to provide the latest information to the readers.

I wish to acknowledge all the contributors for the timely revision of their respective chapters and the feedback from all corners.

Special thanks are due to the publisher M/s CBS Publishers & Distributors Pvt. Ltd., for their sincerity and timely publication of this third edition.

Hope the revised and expanded edition shall be of greater avail to students, faculty members, scientists and researchers in academia and industry.

Bhopal, 2018   **Prof. N.K. Jain**

List of Contributors

Dr. Naveen Ahuja
Principal Scientist, Pharma Research (QbD)
Lupin Ltd, Nande, Pune - 412115, India
E-mail: anaveen76@gmail.com

Mr. Sarwar Beg
UGC Meritorious Research Fellow
University Institute of Pharmaceutical Sciences
Panjab University, Chandigarh - 160014, India
E-mail: sarwar.beg@gmail.com

Dr. Sanjay P. Boldhane
Sr. General Manager
Formulation Development, Micro Labs Ltd.
Micro Advanced Research Centre
Singasandra Post, Bengaluru - 560068, India
E-mail: sanjayboldhane@hotmail.com

Professor Bhupinder Singh Bhoop
Chairperson, University Institute of Pharmaceutical
Sciences (UIPS), Coordinator, UGC-Centre of
Excellence in Applications of Nanomaterials
Nanoparticles & Nanocomposites
Panjab University, Chandigarh - 160014, India
E-mail: bsbhoop@yahoo.com

Dr. Virendra Gajbhiye
Scientist in 'Nanomedicine', Nanobioscience
Group, Agharkar Research Institute
Pune - 411004, India
E-mail: cme_virendra@yahoo.co.in

Dr. Babita Garg
DST Women Scientist
University Institute of Pharmaceutical Sciences
Panjab University
Chandigarh - 160014, India
E-mail: garg_babita02@yahoo.co.in

Dr. Umesh Gupta
Assistant Professor
Department of Pharmacy
School of Chemical Sciences and Pharmacy Central
University of Rajasthan
Bandarsindri, Ajmer - 305817, India
E-mail: umeshgupta175@gmail.com
umeshgupta@curaj.ac.in

Mr. Atul Jain
Research Fellow
UGC-Centre of Excellence in Nano Biomedical
Applications, Panjab University
Chandigarh - 160014, India
E-mail: atuljaindops@gmail.com

Professor N.K. Jain
Emeritus Fellow (U.G.C.)
School of Pharmaceutical Sciences
Rajiv Gandhi Technical University
Bhopal - 462036, India
E-mail: dr.jnarendr@gmail.com

Dr. Sanjay Jain
London, UK E12 6UF
E-mail: sanghi_s@yahoo.com

Dr. Subheet Kumar Jain
Professor and Head
Department of Pharmaceutical Sciences
Guru Nanak Dev University
Amritsar - 143005, India
E-mail: subheetjain@rediffmail.com

Dr. Vikas Jain
Assistant Professor, JSS College of Pharmacy
Jagadguru Sri Shivarathreeshwara University
Mysore - 570015, India
E-mail: jainvk@hotmail.com

Dr. Kour Chand Jindal
Head, R&D, Boehringer Ingelheim
14, Blackburn Road, East Tamaki
Auckland 2013, New Zealand
E-mail: Kour.jindal@merial.com

Dr. Rishi Kapil
Assistant Manager
Formulation Development
Mylan R&D Center
Hyderabad - 502325, India
E-mail: kapilrishi@ymail.com

Professor O.P. Katare
Director Research
Formerly Chairperson & Dean
UGC Center for Advanced Studies
University Institute of Pharmaceutical Sciences
Panjab University
Chandigarh - 160014, India
E-mail: drkatare@yahoo.com; katare@pu.ac.in

Ms. Harneet Kaur
University Institute of Pharmaceutical Sciences
Panjab University
Chandigarh - 160014, India
E-mail: harneetk07@gmail.com

Ms. Lakhvir Kaur
SRF (DST-INSPIRE)
Department of Pharmaceutical Sciences
Guru Nanak Dev University,
Amritsar - 143005, India
E-mail: lakhvir86@gmail.com

Ms. Ranjot Kaur
UGC Meritorious Research Fellow
University Institute of Pharmaceutical Sciences
Panjab University
Chandigarh - 160014, India
Commonwealth Split-Site Scholar
University of Central Lancashire, Preston, UK
E-mail: ranjotkaur92@gmail.com

Ms. Ripandeep Kaur
Research Fellow
UGC Centre of Excellence in Nano Biomedical
Applications
Panjab University, Chandigarh - 160014, India
E-mail: ripandeep111@gmail.com

Ms. Sandeep Kaur
University Institute of Pharmaceutical Sciences
Panjab University, Chandigarh - 160014, India
E-mail: mannsandy898@gmail.com

Ms. Rajneet Kaur Khurana
UGC Meritorious Research Fellow
University Institute of Pharmaceutical Sciences
Panjab University, Chandigarh - 160 014, India
E-mail: khurana.neeti@gmail.com

Dr. Rajendra Kumar
Scientific Assistant
UGC Centre of Excellence in Nano Biomedical
Applications
Panjab University, Chandigarh - 160014, India
E-mail: rajendra.bits@hotmail.com

Dr. Rajiv Kumar
Principal Scientist
Pharma Research Foundations R&D
Lupin Limited (Research Park)
Pune - 412115, India
E-mail: rajivkhurana@lupin.com

Dr. R Kumria
Ind-Swift Ltd., Parwanoo, India
E-mail: kumaria_r@yahoo.com

Ms. Shikha Lohan
Research Fellow
UGC Centre of Excellence in Nano Biomedical
Applications
Panjab University
Chandigarh - 160014, India
E-mail: lohanshikha@rediffmail.com

Mr. Jitender Madan
Pharmaceutics Division
Hygia Institute of Pharmaceutical Education and
Research, Ghazipur, Balram, Ghaila Road,
Lucknow - 226001, India
E-mail: madanjitender@gmail.com

Mr. Mohit Mahajan
Department of Pharmaceutical Sciences
Guru Nanak Dev University
Amritsar - 143005, India
E-mail: m.mahajan86@gmail.com

Dr. Prabhat Ranjan Mishra
Principal Scientist & Associate Professor (AcSIR)
Pharmaceutics Division
Central Drug Research Institute
Lucknow - 226031, India
E-mail: prabhat_mishra@cdri.res.in
        mishrapr@hotmail.com

Professor Ambikanandan Misra
Faculty of Pharmacy
The Maharaja Sayajirao University of Baroda
Kalabhavan Campus, Vadodara - 390001, India
E-mail: misraan@hotmail.com

Dr. Manoj Nahar
Senior Manager, Product Development
Sentiss Research Center
261 Udyog Vihar, Phase IV
Gurgaon - 122001, India
E-mail: mnjnahar@gmail.com

Mr. Pradip Nirbhavane
Research Scholar
University Institute of Pharmaceutical Sciences
(UIPS)
Panjab University, Chandigarh - 160014, India
E-mail: pradeep_niper@yahoo.in

Dr. Harvinder Popli
Professor & Dean, Delhi Pharmaceutical Sciences
and Research University
Pushp Vihar, Sector III, New Delhi - 110017, India
E-mail: popli.harvinder@gmail.com

Dr. Vure Prasad
VP FRD, Vichrow Laboratories Limited
Jeedimetla, Hyderabad - 500055, India
E-mail: vureprasad@gmail.com

Mr. Nikhil Sahajpal
Research Scholar
Department of Pharmaceutical Sciences
Guru Nanak Dev University,
Amritsar - 143005, India
E-mail: nikkhilsehajpal@gmail.com

Mr. Sumant Saini
UGC Meritorious Research Fellow
University Institute of Pharmaceutical Sciences
Panjab University
Chandigarh - 160014, India
E-mail: sumantarya15@gmail.com

Mr. Premjeet Singh Sandhu
Research Fellow
UGC Centre of Excellence in Nano Biomedical
Applications
Panjab University, Chandigarh - 160014, India
E-mail: premjeetsandhu27@gmail.com

Dr. Amita Sarwal
Assistant Professor
University Institute of Pharmaceutical Sciences
Panjab University, Chandigarh - 160014, India
E-mail: sarwalamita@gmail.com

Mr. Sumit Sharma
Research Scholar
University Institute of Pharmaceutical Sciences
Panjab University
Chandigarh - 160014, India
E-mail: sumit.ssharma17@gmail.com

Professor Saranjit Singh
Professor and Head
Department of Pharmaceutical Analysis
National Institute of Pharmaceutical Education and
Research (NIPER)
Sector 67, S.A.S. Nagar - 160 062, India
E-mail: ssingh@niper.ac.in

Professor V.R. Sinha
University Institute of Pharmaceutical Sciences
Panjab University, Chandigarh - 160014, India
E-mail: vr_sinha@yahoo.com

Professor Naazneen Surti
Babaria Institute of Pharmacy
BITS Edu Campus, Vadodara - 391240, India
E-mail: naazsurti@hotmail.com

Ms. Teenu
DST Inspire Research Fellow
University Institute of Pharmaceutical Sciences
Panjab University, Chandigarh - 160014, India
E-mail: teenu88sharma@gmail.com

Professor A.K. Tiwari
Department of Pharmaceutical Sciences and
Drug Research, Punjabi University
Patiala - 147002, India
E-mail: aktiwary2@rediffmail.com

Dr. Sonia Trehan
General Manager Industrial Projects
Center for Dermal Research (CDR) & Laboratory
for Drug Delivery (LDD)
NJ Center for Biomaterials
Life Sciences Building, Rutgers
The State University of New Jersey
Piscataway, NJ - 08854
E-mail: trehans@dls.rutgers.edu

Contents

Pharmaceutical Product Development

Umesh Gupta and N.K. Jain

PHARMACEUTICAL PRODUCTS AND DEMAND

Product is an article, which a customer obtains in exchange of another article (usually money) to satisfy his own needs. Thus, cars and computers, bread and biscuits, shirts and trousers, pens and notebooks are all products as they cater to different needs of the customers.

A single product can be available from different manufacturers under different trade names (brands) to satisfy the requirements of different individuals those have different needs. Some individuals look for economy products whereas for some others costly brands symbolize their social status. The first group would prefer economic brands while other expensive. The socioeconomic need is just one of the factors responsible for brand selection. The other factors involved are gender, age, profession etc.

The term 'pharmaceutical product' covers a wide spectrum of materials, ranging from drugs to surgical and diagnostic instruments and in broad sense more commonly known as drugs or medicines, are a fundamental component of the health system. It is essential that such products and their uses are assured to be safe, effective and rational.

The scope of the present discussion is limited to drugs. One unique feature of the pharmaceutical marketing is indirectness, i.e., the manufacturers do not market their products (apart from OTC products) to end users (patients) but to intermediate users (doctors) who recommend (prescribe) them to end-users. A few pharmaceutical products are tabulated in Table 1.1.

In its crude sense, product development is the process of satisfying the needs of the customers. For example, the need of faster mathematical calculations is satisfied by calculators. The need for speedy transport is satisfied by vehicles. Bread and butter, noodles, and corn flakes make readymade food available to the customers and do well in markets where life moves in faster lane. Similarly, the need of curing diseases is met by drugs.

Product development is a multi-step process as shown in Fig. 1.1. As the schematic shows, the needs act as trigger for ideas; ideas are converted in to concepts, and concepts ultimately take shape of product in research and development section of any organization. The product

Table 1.1. Pharmaceutical products			
Drug	**Category**	**Brand**	**Manufacturer**
Chloroquine	Anti-malarial	Lariago, Malaquin, Resochin	Ipca, PCI, Bayer
Primaquine	Anti-malarial	Malarid, Primaline, PMQ-Inga	Ipca, Unicure, Inga
Doxorubicin	Anti-cancer	Adrim, Doxorubin	Dabur, Khandelwal
Methotrexate	Anti-cancer	Zexate, Oncotrex, Tevatrex	Dabur, Sun Pharma, SPPL
Zidovudine	Anti-HIV	Retrovir, Zidovir, Ziv	Burroughs Wellcome, Cipla, Samarth
Stavudine	Anti-HIV	Stavir, Stag	Cipla, Genix
Chlorpromazine	Anti-psychotic	Megatil, Clozine	Intas, Pil

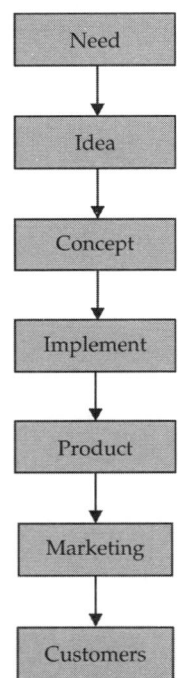

Fig. 1.1. The process of product development.

that meets the quality requirements is marketed and finally reaches the end user through sales and distribution chain. We shall now discuss the steps involved in product development one by one and try to explain the terms with the help of simple questions.

Need: What customers require?

The key to company growth is to create more value for customers; means better satisfying the customer's regular needs, so, it is integral part to identify the customer need for survive in the market. Needs are personality dependent and personality is influenced by socioeconomic surrounding of an individual and factors like age, gender, profession etc. For example, the need of a salesman is a vehicle for speedy travel. A banking clerk may also need a vehicle but his priority is a calculator for calculations.

Need is a constant changing phenomenon. A product that satisfies a customer at one point of time may not satisfy him every time. To explain this we continue with the example of salesman. At early stages of his career he desires for a sturdy vehicle with a good mileage, e.g., a motorcycle. After a few years in profession as he reaches some hierarchical position in middle management, he feels more comfortable with a small utility vehicle (SUV), Maruti Alto (MUL), for example. It becomes more suitable option for him as a SUV can take care of a small family keeping economy at hand. With his progress in profession, he shifts from SUV to large utility vehicle (LUV), Accent (Hyundai), and so on.

Myths about the customer's need

Top management and even employees hold some of the mistaken beliefs. These beliefs are a key reason that is why a company struggles to innovate. These myths (Fig. 1.2) have survived for decades because company defines the customer need, traditionally.

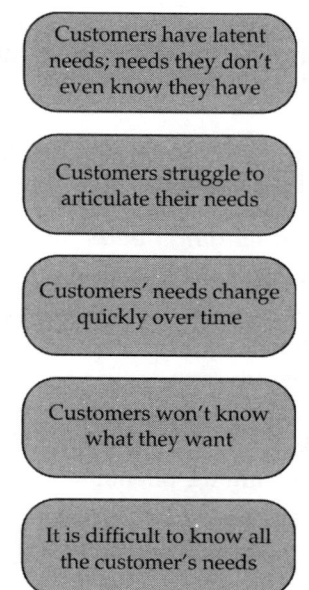

Fig. 1.2. Myths about the customer's need.

Idea: What one can do to satisfy the needs? Needs trigger ideas!

There was always a need for faster, effective and convenient communication. This need triggered the idea of developing a device which would keep the individual in connection with the rest of the world, 24 hours a day, 7 days a week. This idea took shape of a mobile phone with 'stay connected' as the most effective slogan.

Today, the need of a pollution free vehicle, which consumes very little of fuel is utmost. Idea is to make modifications in the existing vehicle design to make them eco-friendly and reduce their fuel consumption. Imagine a step ahead and the idea of non-conventional energy as fuel comes to mind. We should not be surprised that this idea got translated into a vehicle, which runs on solar energy.

Concept: How can it be done?

For conversion of an idea into a concept sound technical skills are required. It is essentially a process of putting the thoughts into reality. The research and development department of any organization shoulders this responsibility.

Product: Is the need satisfied?

Technical excellence alone is not sufficient to make the product successful. Marketability and commercial viability of a product depend on how the customer views it. Ultimate success of the product lies in customer's satisfaction.

The basic strategies behind a new product development by a pharmaceutical manufacturer can be summarized under six key features:

1. **Time-to-market:** This involves an orientation to getting a product to market fastest. This is typical of companies involved with rapidly changing technology or products with rapidly changing fashion. Pursuit of this strategy will typically lead to trade-offs in optimizing product performance, cost and reliability. It is designed to improve the patient compliance as well as to satisfy the need of patients.

2. **Low product cost:** Focusing on developing the lowest cost or highest value product is the prime concern of a pharmaceutical company. This orientation typically will require additional time and development cost to optimize product cost and the manufacturing process.

3. **Low development cost:** This orientation focuses on minimizing development cost or developing pharmaceutical products within a constrained budget. While this orientation is not as common as the other orientations, it occurs when companies are developing pharmaceutical products under contract for other parties, where a company has severely constrained financial resources. This strategy is somewhat compatible with time-to-market, but involves trade-offs with product performance, innovation, cost and reliability.

4. **Quality, reliability, robustness:** This strategy focuses on assuring high levels of product quality, reliability and robustness.

This orientation is typical of industries requiring high quality because of the significant costs to correct a problem e.g. the need for high levels of reliability, or where there are significant safety issues (e.g., medical devices, pharmaceuticals). This orientation requires added time and cost for planning, testing, analysis and regulatory approvals.

5. **Product performance, technology and innovation:** This strategy focuses on having the highest level of product performance to the patient, or the highest level of product innovation in terms of activity and compliance.

6. **Service, responsiveness and flexibility:** This strategy focuses on providing a high level of service in terms of stock and proper supply of the medicine to the hospitals as well as medical shopkeepers, being very responsive to patient's requirements as part of development, and maintaining flexibility to respond to new demands based on the performance of the existing pharmaceutical products. This orientation requires additional resources (and their related costs) to provide this service and responsiveness.

Pharmaceutical context

The need for the treatment of the diseases might have existed since the dawn of civilization. Drugs were available but not without side effects. Paul Ehrlich dreamed of a 'magic bullet' that would selectively act at the site of action. This idea triggered many scientists to work on targeted drug delivery devices. The entire pharmaceutical world is optimistic of making the targeted delivery of the drug a reality product. Similarly, need to make a patient compliant and more effective dosage form triggered development of once a day products (Cifran OD., Ranbaxy). The need to relieve the pain quickly and that too in a more convenient manner led to the development of mouth dissolving tablets (Toroxx MT; Nimulid MD). The elderly and the children find it difficult to swallow a tablet. The need to develop a tablet that would be easily swallowed by patients of this group was satisfied by dispersible tablets.

What is the need for new product development (NPD)?

Constantly changing needs

It is essential to consider all the features while developing new product like; a company should identify all the features that are offered by all its major competitors and second one is to identify important features/benefits used in making purchase decisions. As stated earlier, need is a constantly changing phenomenon. A product which satisfies all or maximum needs of a customer at one point of time may prove inadequate some other time. A black and white TV used to satisfy the entertainment need of the customer in the past. The expectations of the customer then raised and development of color TV became a necessity for television companies. As the time progressed the companies had to introduce advanced features in their products. That's how Golden Eye Technology (LG) and advanced sound technology (Bazooka, Videocon) were launched; thin, sleek, flat TV with blue ray being the ultra-modern. A continuous introduction of higher antibiotics exemplifies the same process in pharmaceutical industry. An indiscriminate use of existing antibiotics reduces their effectiveness due to development of resistance. In order to satisfy the demand of an effective antibiotic (and to maintain their market share) the pharmaceutical industries keep developing higher and newer generations of antibiotics. Today we have a long series of antibiotics like fluoroquinolones (from norfloxacin to gatifloxacin), cephalosporins (first-to-fourth generation). Needs for drug delivery systems also have been changing over the period of time. Pills were most primitive of the oral drug delivery systems. There was, however, always a need for more effective and sophisticated oral dosage form. Formulation of controlled or sustained release dosage form favors the minimization of dosing frequency. When it was realized that a few drugs degrade in acidic environment, the need to avoid the release of such drugs in stomach surfaced. That was satisfied with enteric-coated tablets. Advances in pharmacokinetics demonstrated that the drug effectiveness could be enhanced by maintaining its steady plasma concentration. This generated the need of a drug delivery system, which would give the said effect. As a consequence sustained release tablets were developed.

In general, the life cycle of a pharmaceutical product can be observed at different stages according to Fig. 1.3.

Shortened product life cycle

Sony used to enjoy a three years lead time on its new products before they were extensively copied by the competitors. Now the competitors are copying the new products within six months of their launch, hardly leaving any time for Sony to recoup its investment.

A classic example of this in Indian pharmaceutical industry was the launch of Sildenafil citrate. Companies saw a very potential market for Indian version of Viagra. The first Indian brand was launched with a bang, but it took not even a month for other about 20 companies to launch their brands of Sildenafil citrate thus putting a very steep competition to 'first in India' brand.

Image build-up

Constant and continuous pumping of new products in market helps the company to build-up its image. Such company is viewed as a very active company constantly working on product improvement for customer satisfaction. Company can present itself as a thinking machine with a bountiful of innovative ideas.

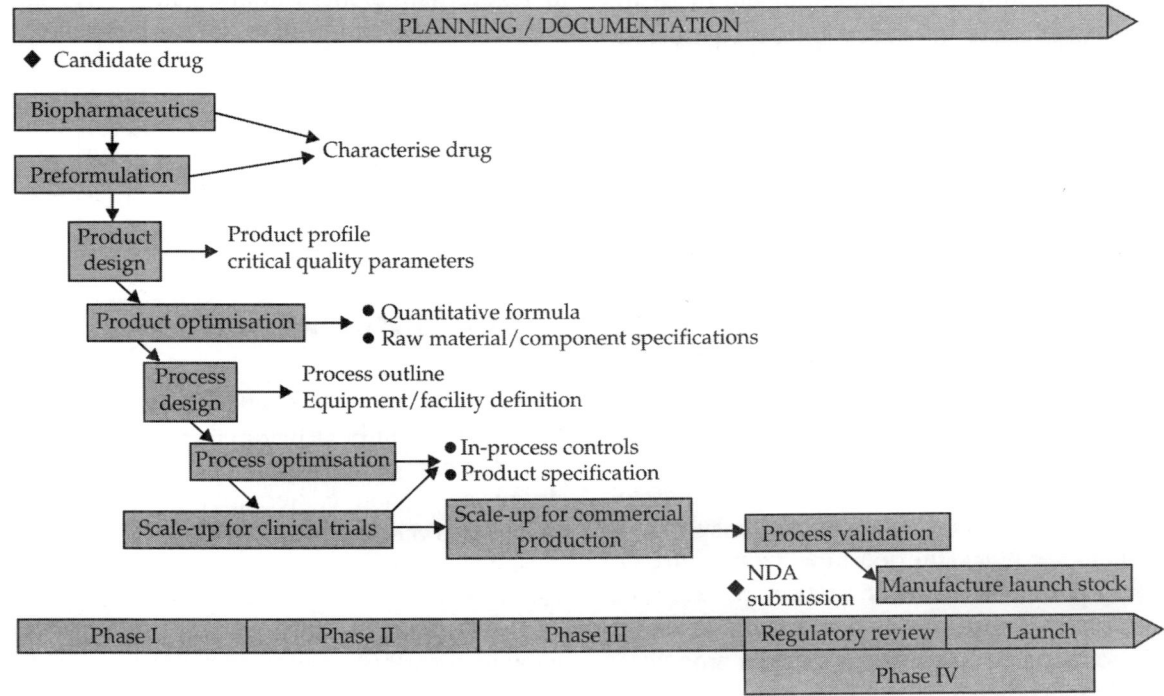

Fig. 1.3. Sequential steps in the development of new pharmaceutical product.

What are the obstacles in NPD?

- **Shortage of important new product ideas in certain areas:** There may be few ways to improve some basic products such as steel, detergents etc.
- **Fragmented markets:** Keen competition is leading to market fragmentation. Companies have to aim their new products at similar segments and this means lower sales and profits for each product.
- **Social and governmental constraints:** New products have to satisfy public criteria such as consumer safety and ecological compatibility. Government requirements have slowed down innovation, e.g., in pharmaceutical industry, and have complicated product design and advertising decisions in industries such as chemicals, automobiles, industrial equipments and toys.
- **Costliness of the NPD process:** The discovery and creation of new product (drug, for example) is time consuming and costly process. It is estimated that every new drug takes 12 to 15 years to develop, at a cost of over $ 800 million. High probability of failures makes it financially a very risky proposition.
- **Faster development time:** Many competitors are likely to conceive the same idea at the same time and the swiftest one often emerges to be the victorious. Alert companies have to compress the development time by using CAD and advanced manufacturing techniques, joint partners, early concept tests and advanced market planning.
- **Challenges to identify appropriate user:** There are obstacles to identifying appropriate users from broad range of people, many of them are not identified in advance. Further, obstacles are found in the division of responsibilities within organizations that are set up to develop and market such products.
- **Financial crisis:** Many companies may have novel ideas but can't raise/generate appropriate funds actually needed for the new product development.
- **Short product life cycle:** Shortened life cycle has left the companies with less time for recapturing their investment. This effect has already been discussed.

TYPES OF PRODUCTS

Breakthrough products

These are 'new to world' products. They create new markets like AIDS vaccine, which is presently in various phases of clinical trial, could be the most awaited breakthrough product. Other future products, which could be included in the list, are malaria vaccine, cancer treatment products etc.

Incremental products

Incremental products are just the extension of existing products. They are launched in familiar markets where the company has a certain reputation. Iodex ointment is available in the market for decades. GlaxoSmithKline launched Iodex spray as incremental product, similarly, Volini® spray was launched as incremental product of Volini gel. Pharmaceutical market is flooded with incremental products (Table 1.2). All the product line extensions and the combination products fall under this category.

Pharmaceutical new products

Discovery of a new drug, however, is a very costly and time-consuming process. High probability of failures makes it even more risky. Development of new formulation of an existing drug is an economic alternative of introduction of new product in market (Fig. 1.4). A third option is to discover new indications or optimization of the existing formulations. Analgesic and antipyretic properties of aspirin were already known. Its effectiveness in reversing the lipid blockade in blood vessels made companies to position it against atherosclerosis.

Table 1.2. Incremental products (product line and combination products)

Product family	Product line	Specifications/Contents	Manufacturer
Nimulid	Nimulid	Nimesulide tablets (100 mg)	Panacia
	Nimulid-Sp	Nimesulide + Serratiopeptidase	
	Nimulid-MD	Mouth dissolving tablet	
	Nimulid-MD KID	Mouth dissolving tablet for paediatrics	
	Nimulid-MR	Nimesulide + Tizanidine	
	Nimulid-DS	Double strength Nimesulide tablets (200 mg)	
	Nimulid-Nugel	Nimesulide gel	
	Nimulid-HF	Nimesulide + Paracetamol	

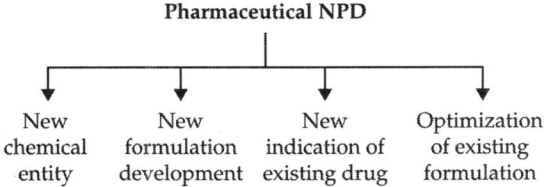

Fig. 1.4. The pharmaceutical new products.

PHARMACEUTICAL NEW PRODUCT DEVELOPMENT

The process of pharmaceutical new product development can be explained with the help of following figure (Fig. 1.5). The figure explains different departments involved in development of a new pharmaceutical product highlighting their respective contributions. Out of all the steps only preformulation is dealt with here comprehensively. Most of the remaining steps are covered in separate chapters of this book.

Preformulation

Early part of 1960s witnessed a considerable advancement in the fields of analytical techniques, pharmacokinetics and biopharmaceutics. The first development made it possible to detect a large number of stability and drug-excipient incompatibility related problems; whereas later two indicated poor bioavailability issues, which, till then, were ill-understood. Nearly, about the same time, the companies started many synthetic programs. As a result

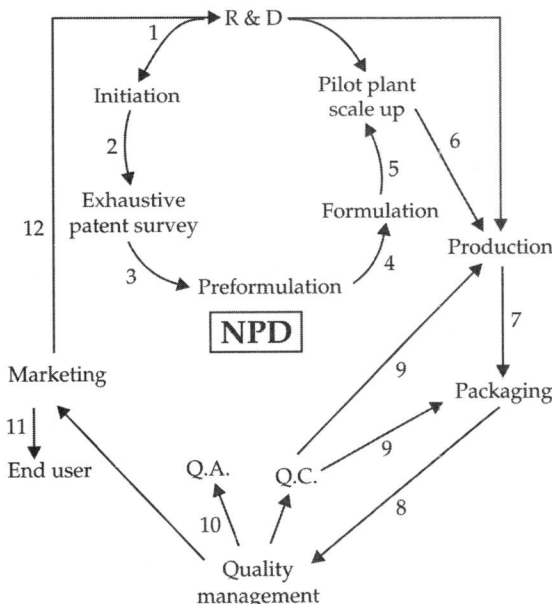

Fig. 1.5. The departments involved in and their contributions towards NPD. (1) Based on marketing feedback initiates the project. (2 & 3) Initial feasibility search and patent survey are followed by preformulation. (4) Generates background information necessary in future steps. (5) Generates a formula that could be developed into a product with desired specifications. (6) Transforms a laboratory curiosity into a product suitable for large scale manufacturing. (7) Manufactures a product. (8) Packaging ensures product stability and enhances aesthetic value. (9) Analyses product at every step for its quality. (10) Ensures consistent product quality. (11) Markets and distributes products to end users. (12) Feedback to R&D on market opportunities.

promising drug molecules started becoming available in quick succession and formulation scientists were faced with the tasks of rapid formulation. It was realized that if, keeping in mind the subsequent needs, a few physico-chemical properties of the new drug are investigated prior to the formulation; an efficient, elegant formulation development is relatively easier. This was the period, probably, when concept of preformulation started evolving. It eventually has become part of official require-ment of new drug approvals (NDAs).

Preformulation is the first learning phase or prior step of formulation development for a new drug molecule. It involves generating infor-mation regarding physicochemical properties of the drug, its interactions with the excipients, stability profile both in solid and solution state and preliminary *in vivo* properties. A detailed understanding of the properties of the drug substance is essential to minimize formulation problems in later stages of drug development, reduce drug development costs, and decrease the product's time to market (i.e., from drug substance to drug product). The motives of preformulation studies are to choose the correct form of the drug substance, evaluate its physical properties, and generate a thorough under-standing of the material's stability under the conditions that will lead to development of an optimal drug delivery system. Information gathered during preformulation is of immense importance for the development of a stable dosage form. Preformulation study begins at the point after biological screening, when a decision is made for further development of compound in clinical trials (CT). The fact that the quantity of the drug available at this early stage is often very limited (normally in milligrams) makes the job of the preformulation scientist even tougher. Thus, it becomes important to decide the priorities and selectively determine only those preformulation parameters, which affect drug performance, and dosage form development,

which are meaningful. Before beginning the formal preformulation programme the pre-formulation scientist must consider a few factors, which include:

1. The amount of drug available.
2. The physicochemical properties of the drug already known.
3. Therapeutic category and anticipated dose of the compound.
4. The development schedules.
5. The nature of information a formulator should have or would like to have.

Goals of preformulation study

1. To establish the necessary physicochemical parameters of a new drug substance.
2. To establish the compatibility with common excipients.
3. To determine the kinetic rate profile, and
4. To establish its physical characteristics

A typical preformulation design is given in Table 1.3 and briefly discussed below. After these considerations a preformulation scientist can take up the actual studies.

UV spectroscopy

The first requirement of any preformulation study is the development of a simple analytical method for quantitative estimation in subsequent steps. Most of drugs have aromatic rings and/or double bonds as a part of their structure and absorb light in UV range. UV spectroscopy, being a fairly accurate and simple method, is a preferred estimation technique at early preformulation stages. The absorption coefficient (equation 1) of the drug can be determined by formula

$$E_1' = \frac{AF}{X} \qquad \dots(1)$$

where A = absorbance, F = dilution factor, and X = weight of drug (mg).

It is now possible to determine concentration of drug in any solution by measuring absorbance.

Table 1.3. Preformulation drug characterization in a structured programme

Test	Method/Function characterization
Fundamental	
1. UV spectroscopy	Simple assay
2. Solubility	Phase solubility/purity
Aqueous	Intrinsic and pH effects
pKa	Solubility control
	Salt formation
Salts	Solubility, hygroscopicity and stability
Solvents	Vehicles and extraction
K o/w	Lipophilicity, structure activity
Dissolution	Biopharmacy
3. Melting point	DSC-polymorphism, hydrates and solvates
4. Assay development	UV, HPLC and TLC
5. Stability	
In solution	Thermal, hydrolysis, pH
In solid state	Oxidation, photolysis and metal ion
Derived	
1. Microscopy	Particle size and morphology
2. Bulk density	Tablet and capsule formulation
3. Flow properties	Tablet and capsule formulation
4. Compression properties	Aid/excipient choice
5. Excipient compatibility	Preliminary screen by DSC, confirmation by TLC

$$C = \frac{AF}{E_1'} \text{ mg/ml} \qquad \ldots(2)$$

Once the quantitative analytical method is established, the preformulation parameters are investigated in desired order.

Intrinsic solubility (C_0) and dissociation constant (pKa)

For a newly discovered molecule/drug to become an active drug it must traverse through number of physiologic barriers, both aqueous and non-aqueous; these barriers exist to protect our body from the noxious agents that can be toxic. The system by which nature chose to protect us is based on the solubility of compounds. A compound highly soluble in water or highly insoluble in water would not be able to penetrate the deeper tissues and thus rendered ineffective. Neutral compounds without any polarizable centers often prove to be inert pharmacologically; for example, fluorinated hydrocarbons, such as perfluorodecalin, which is a hexane structure with full fluorination. Fluorine is so highly electronegative that it pulls the electrons from the parent structure, making it an inert compound. Interactions at the site of action are often electrically driven and as a result, it is more likely that we will discover a compound that has weak acid or base properties as an active entity. This necessitates studies that would yield information on how well the compound will distribute throughout the body tissues and the lipophilic/hydrophilic balance of the molecular structure becomes the focus of studies at an early stage in preformulation. Compounds that ionize in the aqueous phase are rendered water-soluble because they can polarize the medium and can create solute-solvent electrostatic bonding to increase their solubility. The ionization of a compound depends on the strength of binding of the ionizable group to the core of the molecule, a property that is determined by the value of the dissociation constant; once ionized, the molecule acquires new solubility characteristics; when placed between aqueous and non-aqueous phases, the distribution between these two phases, generally called partitioning, will change. It is this partitioning behavior of drugs that makes them useful as drugs; without a significant degree of partitioning between aqueous and non-aqueous phases of body tissues, no molecule can become active. This ionization also determines the quantity of a solute that is eventually contained in a medium, aqueous or non-aqueous, the solubility of compound. So, what starts with dissociation affects both partitioning and the intrinsic solubility (C_0) of the compound, the two most important parameters that will determine if a newly discovered molecule will end up as an active drug or not. These inter-related properties form the very important step in any preformulation evaluation. Equally important is the dissociation constant (pKa) of the drug molecules. Quantitative determination of solubility helps the preformulation scientist to understand the ease with which the formulations for gavage and intravenous injection studies in animals are obtained. The pKa can be used to predict pH modification required to manipulate solubility, choose salts for improved bioavailability, if required, and to improve stability.

Intrinsic solubility (C_0)

The solubility of drug in water, 0.1 N HCl and 0.1 N NaOH is determined. A rise in solubility in acid than water suggests that the drug is a weak base. Drug is weak acid if its solubility in NaOH is more than in water. An increase in solubility in both acid and alkali indicates either amphoteric or Zwittorionic substance whereas no change in solubility indicates non-ionizable neutral molecule.

Intrinsic solubility (true solubility) (C_0) is the solubility due to unionized form of drug. Phase solubility analysis is an efficient method for determination of intrinsic solubility. The drug is added to a fixed volume of solvent in increasing amount. The concentration is determined after equilibrium is attained. A typical phase solubility diagram for a pure substance is shown in Fig. 1.6. Up to point C, all the solute dissolves in solvent, saturation occurs at C while back extrapolation from C to ordinate yields C_0.

However, it is very less likely, at the early stages that the drug is pure. Phase solubility diagram (Fig. 1.7) constructed between solubility vs increasing drug : solvent ratio can be a good estimation of impurity present. The deviation from horizontal (saturation solubility, II) indicates presence of impurities, as they may increase solubility (I) or decrease it (III) with increasing amount.

Solubility determination is generally carried out at two temperatures, 4°C and 37°C. At 4°C water is most dense and poses the greatest

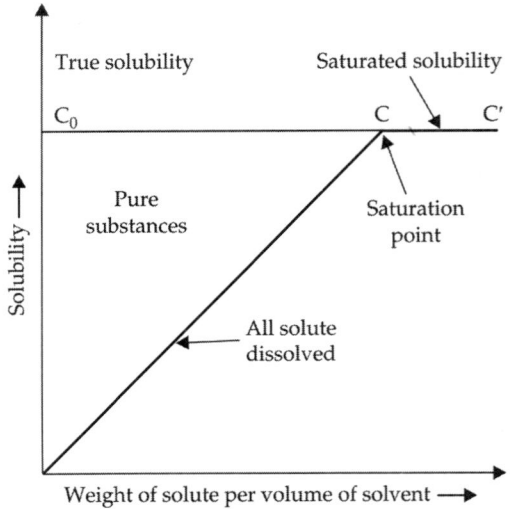

Fig. 1.6. Phase solubility diagram for a pure substance.

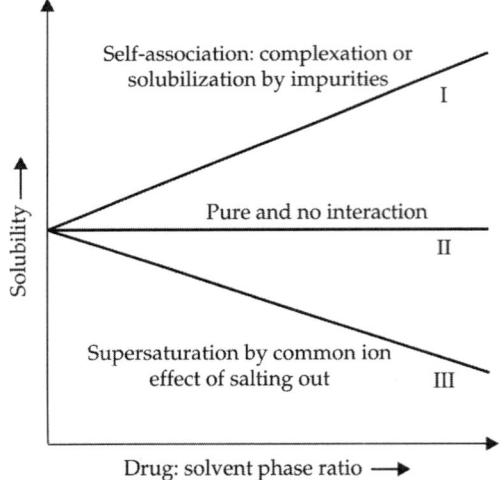

Fig. 1.7. Effect of drug : solvent ratio on solubility when the drug is impure.

challenge to saturated aqueous solubility. 4°C also ensures good stability whereas 37°C simulates body temperature.

Dissociation constant

Many drugs are either weak acids or weak bases i.e. weak electrolytes. Depending upon pH, they exist as ionized or unionised species or both in solution. The relative proportion of ionised and unionised species of drug in solution governs its absorption, along with pH this proportion depends on pKa. Henderson-Hasselbalch equation establishes following correlation among these three factors.

$$pH = pKa + \log\left(\frac{\text{Ionized species}}{\text{Unionized species}}\right)$$

(for acids)   ...(3)

$$pH = pKa + \log\left(\frac{\text{Unionized species}}{\text{Ionized species}}\right)$$

(for bases)   ...(4)

Modified form of Henderson-Hasselbalch equation is more suitable for quantitative determination of pKa.

$$pKa = pH + \log\left(\frac{C_s - C_o}{C_o}\right) \text{ (for bases)} \quad ...(5)$$

$$pKa = pH + \log\left(\frac{C_o}{C_s - C_o}\right) \text{ (for acids)} \quad ...(6)$$

where C_s = saturated solubility, and C_o = intrinsic solubility.

For example, the intrinsic solubility (C_o) of a weak base is 2 mg/ml. The saturated solubility at pH 4 and pH 6 are 14.6 and 2.13 mg/ml, respectively. Then from equation 5

$$pH = 4 + \log\left(\frac{14.6 - 2}{2}\right) = 4.799$$

$$pH = 6 + \log\left(\frac{2.13 - 2}{2}\right) = 4.813$$

Several methods for pKa determination are concisely reported. For compounds with a reasonable solubility (about 0.01 M) acid-base potentiometric titrations can be performed on 100 ml portions using titrants of about 0.1 molarity. Automatic titrimeters are used to measure pH as a function of amount of titrant added. An accurate pKa value can be calculated by measuring the pH at the half neutralization point where pH equals pKa. A difference in UV or Vis absorption by ionized and unionized species, if existing, can also be utilized for determination of pKa.

The pKa values are also temperature-dependent, often in a nonlinear and unpredictable way. Samples measured by potentiometry are, therefore, held at a constant temperature bath and, therefore, pKa value should be quoted at a specific temperature. Often a temperature of 25°C is chosen to reflect room temperature whereas this may be quite different from the body temperature. Percent ionization at different temperatures can be calculated as:

$$\text{Percent ionization} = 1/1 + 10^{(\text{charge (pKa} - \text{pH}))}$$

where charge is +1 for bases and –1 for acids. Percent ionization is 50% when the pH equals pKa (Figs. 1.8 and 1.9). The ionization status of the given acid/base can be determined from the examples given in Figs. 1.7 and 1.8.

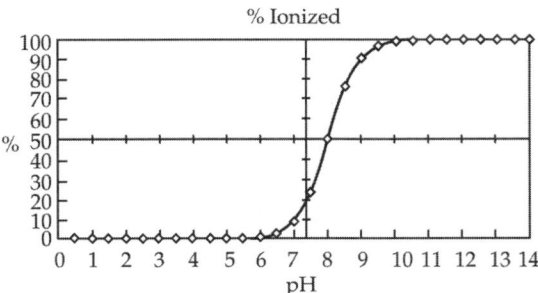

Fig. 1.8. Percent ionization of an acid having the pKa value of 8.0.

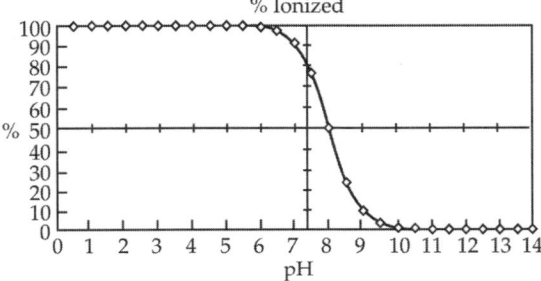

Fig. 1.9. Percent ionization of a base having the pKa value of 8.0.

Salts

The study of above two parameters indicates the need and possibility of making more soluble salts of drug to eliminate solubility related poor bioavailability particularly with solid dosage form.

A salt is the product generated upon the neutralization of an acid or base. Pharmaceutical salts are important in the process of drug development, as converting an acidic or basic drug into a salt via a simple neutralization reaction has the ability to change the physicochemical properties of a drug. Though, multiple options are available for salt formation (Table 1.4), to pick up an appropriate candidate is not an easy job. The selected salt must serve the intended purpose (e.g. improvement in solubility), without affecting stability and bioavailability of drug. The solubility of chlordiazepoxide, a weak base, increases from 2 mg/ml to 165 mg/ml for its strong acid salt, chlordiazepoxide hydrochloride. The interrelation between the different properties and the selection criteria of different salts can be better explained with the help of the Fig. 1.10.

In many cases, salts prepared from strong acids and bases are freely soluble but very hygroscopic and may be responsible for instability of solid dosage form. Accordingly, it is often better to use a weaker acid or base for salt formation provided solubility and biopharmaceutical requirements are not compromised. Besides, this may be advantageous from physiological and pharmaceutics point of view. The pH of injection should be in the range of 3–9 to prevent tissue/vessel damage or pain at the site of injection. Undue alkalinity may attack glass and a propellant acid reaction may corrode aerosol container.

The intended dosage form also influences salt selection, for example, fatty acid salts, which produce low melting oils of free drug, may be used when topical, IM or soft gelatin capsule is the intended dosage form. Thus, dihydrochloride salt of fluphenazine (m.p. 277°C) is used to formulate a tablet, but for IM injection decanoate salt (m.p. 25°C) is used. The observations in Table 1.5 are useful for selection of an appropriate salt.

Table 1.4. Potential pharmaceutical salts

Basic drugs			Acidic drugs		
Anion	pKa (%)	Usage	Cation	pKa (%)	Usage
Hydrochloride	−6.10	43.0	Potassium	16.00	10.8
Sulphate	−3.00, 1.96	7.5	Sodium	14.77	62.0
Tosylate	1.34	0.1	Lithium	13.82	1.6
Mesylate	−1.20	2.0	Calcium	12.90	10.5
Napsylate	0.17	0.3	Magnesium	11.42	1.3
Besylate	0.70	0.3	Diethanolamine	9.65	1.0
Maleate	1.92, 6.23	3.0	Zinc	8.96	3.0
Phosphate	2.15, 7.20, 12.38	3.2	Choline	8.90	0.3
Salicylate	3.00	0.9	Aluminium	5.00	0.7
Tartrate	3.00	3.5	Alternatives	8.8	
Lactate	3.10	0.8			
Citrate	3.13, 4.76, 6.40	3.0			
Benzoate	4.20	0.5			
Succinate	4.21, 5.64	0.4			
Acetate	4.76	1.3			
Alternatives		30.2			

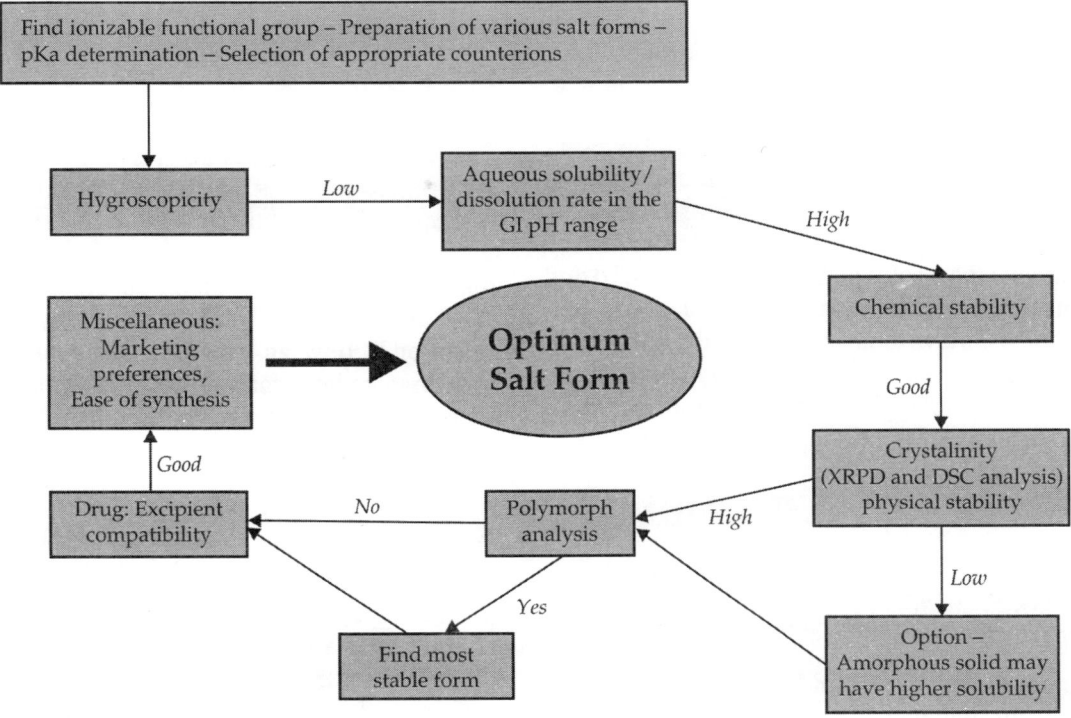

Fig. 1.10. Different interrelated criteria of salt selection.

Solvents

A solvent is a substance that dissolves a solute resulting in a solution. If the drug is found to be poorly soluble in water, or unstable in aqueous solutions, its solubility in co-solvents must be studied. The selection of solvents can be made in anticipation with the intended dosage form. A list of recommended solvents is given in Table 1.6. A quantitative solubility assessment of drug in these solvents/solvent mixtures would help in the subsequent formulation steps.

Partition coefficient

The partition coefficient is a measure of the extent a substance partitions between two phases, generally, an oil phase and an aqueous phase. This ratio is often expressed as log P (logarithm of partition ratio). Both pKa and log P measurements are useful parameters for understanding the behavior of drug molecules at the preformu-

lation stage. The pKa will determine the species of molecules, which is likely to be present at the site of action and how quickly or completely would the species cross a large number of transport barriers in the body, regardless of the route of administration. Factors, such as absorption, excretion, and penetration of the central nervous system (CNS) are also related to the log P value of a drug and in certain cases predictions can be made; these are important in assessing the endogenous toxicity of compounds and their activity.

Partition coefficient is a ratio of the concentration in two immiscible solvents.

Partition coefficient, P =
[Organic or oil phase] / [Aqueous phase]
$$\dots(7)$$

where the values in brackets describe measured concentrations.

$$\log P = \log_{10} (\text{partition coefficient})$$

Table 1.5. Counterion cluster groups to manipulate basic drug salt performance: melting point, solubility, stability, hygroscopicity, processing and organoleptic properties.

	Grouping	T_m (°C)	Application
GROUP A	*Organic acids*		Increase T_m of aromatic bases; processing and stability
	Hydrobromide	—	
	Hydrochloride	—	
	Sulphate	—	
	Nitrate	—	
	Sulphonic acids		
	Methane sulphonate	20	
	Ethane sulphonate	—	
	Benzene sulphonate	43	
	Toluene sulphonate	70	
	[1]Naphthalene-2-sulphonate	124	
	Carboxylic acids		
	Maleate	131	
	Benzoate	122	
	Salicylate	158	
GROUP B	Acetate	16.6	Increase T_m bonds; decrease T_m symmetrical bases and increase Cs
	Malate	100	
	Succinate	185	
	Gluconate	131	
	Glycolate	80	
	Lactate	17	
	Tartrate	205	
	Citrate	153	
	Ascorbate	191	
GROUP C	Hexanoate	−3.4	Reduce T_m producing oils (ion pairing ?) for IM injections, topical or soft gelatin capsules
	Octanoate	16.7	
	Decanoate	31.4	
	Undecylenate	24	
	Dodecyl sulphate (& group D)		
	Oleate	4	
	Stearate (& group D)	69	
GROUP D	*Insoluble salts (suspensions)*		Reduce solubility for taste masking and suspensions
	Napsylate	124	
	5,5′-methylene disalicylate	238	
	Pamoate	280	
	Polystyrene sulphonate (resinate)		
	Bitter taste-masking		
	Saccharinate	229	
	Aspartamate	246	

In practical terms, the uncharged or neutral molecule exists for bases > 2 pKa units above the pKa and for acids > 2 pKa units below the pKa. In practice, the log P will vary according to the conditions under which it is measured and the choice of the partitioning solvent. It is worth noting that this is a logarithmic scale; therefore, log P = 0 means that the compound is equally

Table 1.6. Recommended solvents for preformulation screening			
Solvent	**Dielectric constant (e)**	**Solubility parameters (d)**	**Application**
Water	80	4.4	All
Methanol			
0.1 M HCl (pH 1.10)	32	147	Extraction, separation, dissolution (gastric), extraction of base
0.1 M NaOH (pH 13.1)			Extraction of acid
Buffer (pH 6–7)			Dissolution (intestinal)
Ethanol	24	12.7	Formulation
Propylene glycol	32	12.6	
Glycerol	43	16.5	
PEG 300 or 400	35		

soluble in water and in the partitioning solvent. If the compound has a log P = 5, then the compound is 100,000 times more soluble in the partitioning solvent. A log P = –2 means that the compound is 100 times more soluble in water, that is, it is quite hydrophilic.

Log P values have been studied in approximately 100 organic liquid-water systems. As it is virtually impossible to determine log P in a realistic biological medium, the octanol-water system has been widely adopted as a model of the lipid phase. While there has been much debate about the suitability of this system, it is the most widely used in pharmaceutical studies. Octanol and water are immiscible, but some water does dissolve in octanol in a hydrated state. This hydrated state contains 16 octanol aggregates, with the hydroxyl head groups surrounded by trapped aqueous solution. Lipophilic (unionized) species dissolve in the aliphatic regions. Generally, compounds with log P values between 1 and 3 show good absorption, whereas those with log Ps greater than 6 or less than 3 often have poor transport characteristics. Highly non-polar molecules have a preference to reside in the lipophilic regions of membranes, and highly polar compounds show poor bio-availability because of their inability to penetrate membrane barriers. Thus, there is a parabolic

relationship between log P and transport, that is, candidate drugs that exhibit a balance between these two properties will probably show the best oral bioavailability.

Many solvents have been used as organic phase in determination of partition coefficient (e.g. hexane, CCl_4, $CHCl_3$, C_6H_6, diethyl ether etc.) but the largest data is available with n-octanol. Although, partition coefficient alone cannot provide an understanding of *in vivo* absorption, yet it can give a fair idea of hydrophilic/lipophilic nature of drug. This may be useful in anticipating the drug absorption.

Dissolution

Newly discovered lead compounds that are ultimately formulated into drug delivery systems should be capable of existing either in a molecular dispersion, such as solutions or in an aggregate state, such as tablets, capsules, suspensions, and so on, that are readily rendered into finer state of dispersion and dissolution. Regardless of the stage of aggregation in the final formulation, the active pharmaceutical ingredient (API) must be released from the drug delivery system and as the first step, should be dissolved in an aqueous environment; this will then be followed possibly by one or more transfers across non-aqueous barriers. To determine these factors it is important to study the dissolution properties. Generally, dissolution is the rate determining step (Fig. 1.11) of hydrophobic, poor aqueous soluble drugs like griseofulvin.

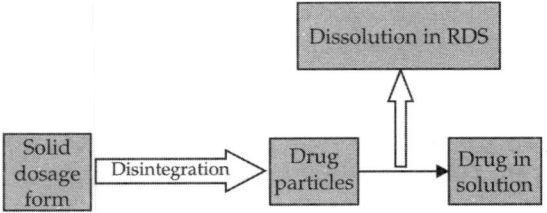

Fig. 1.11. Dissolution as rate determining step (RDS).

If the drug is moderately or poorly soluble, investigation of its dissolution behavior is essential. Often in such cases, the dissolution is slow and absorption may be dissolution rate limited.

The dissolution rate of a solid dosage form is adequately described by the Noyes-Nernst equation.

$$\frac{dc}{dt} = \frac{AD(C_s - C)}{hV} \qquad ...(8)$$

where, dc/dt = dissolution rate, A = surface area of dissolving solid, D = diffusion coefficient, C = solute concentration in bulk medium, h = diffusion layer thickness, V = volume of the dissolution medium, C_s = solute concentration in the diffusion layer.

Under constant experimental conditions C_s is a fixed multiple of solute's equilibrium solubility $[S]$ and can be expressed as:

$$C_s = K_1 [S]$$

where K_1 = constant ≤ 1.

Under sink conditions $C_s \gg C$ and therefore

$$\frac{dc}{dt} = \frac{ADK_1[S]}{hV} \qquad ...(9)$$

During early phase of dissolution, when A and V can be held constant, and under constant temperature and agitation conditions, equation (9) becomes

$$\frac{dc}{dt} = KS \qquad ...(10)$$

where, $K = ADK/hV$ = constant.

Dissolution rate as expressed by equation (10) is called intrinsic dissolution rate (IDR) and is characteristic of each solid compound in given solvent under fixed hydrodynamic conditions. It is generally expressed as mg min^{-1} cm^{-2}. Knowledge of this value helps the pre-formulation scientist in predicting if absorption would be dissolution rate limited.

Compounds with IDR greater than 1 mg min^{-1} cm^{-2} are not likely to present dissolution rate limited absorption problems. Those with rates below 0.1 mg min^{-1} cm^{-2} usually exhibit dissolution rate limited absorption, whereas those with IDR between 0.1 to 1 mg min^{-1} cm^{-2} demand for thorough investigation before any prediction.

Practically, during dissolution, surface area of dissolving solid is uncontrolled as it is undergoing disintegration and degradation. The following method can be used to overcome this difficulty. About 300 mg of drug is compressed slowly in a 13 mm infrared punch and die set (A = 1.33 cm²) to 10 tons, to ensure zero porosity, and a long dwell time to improve compaction. The metal surface in contact should be pre-lubricated with stearic acid using a 5% solution in chloroform. The compressed disc is fixed to the holder of BP rotating basket apparatus using low melting paraffin wax BP and successively dipped so that the top and sides of the disc are coated. The lower circular face of the disc should be cleared of residual wax using a scalpel and carefully scraped to remove any stearic acid transferred from the punch face. The coated disc is rotated at 100 rpm, 2 cm from bottom of a 1 litre flat bottom dissolution flask containing 1 litre of fluid at 37°C. The amount of drug release is then monitored, usually by UV spectroscopy, plotted against time and the slope of the line divided by exposed surface (1.33 cm²) to give IDR in mg min^{-1} cm^{-2}.

Polymorphism

A crystal can exist as more than one polymorph or pseudopolymorph. Polymorphs differ from each other in their physical properties as solubility, melting point, density, crystal shape, optical and electrical properties and vapour pressure.

Polymorphism also influences biopharmaceutical behaviour of the drug. A pure, more soluble B form of chloramphenicol palmitate was more bioavailable after oral administration as compared to less soluble pure A form and their mixtures (Fig. 1.12). Knowledge of polymorphic forms is of importance in preformulation because suspension systems should never be made with a metastable form. Conversely, a metastable form is more soluble than a stable modification, and this can be of advantage in dissolution. Two different polymorphs could exhibit a wide difference in their stability profile. As illustrated by case history of an experimental compound, anhydrous crystalline form, under stress condition, degraded rapidly with a half-life of about 18 weeks. A solvate, however, was essentially stable. The solvate after desolvation by heat generated a new crystal form, which showed most rapid degradation (Fig. 1.13).

Differences in properties of polymorphs make it mandatory for a preformulation scientist

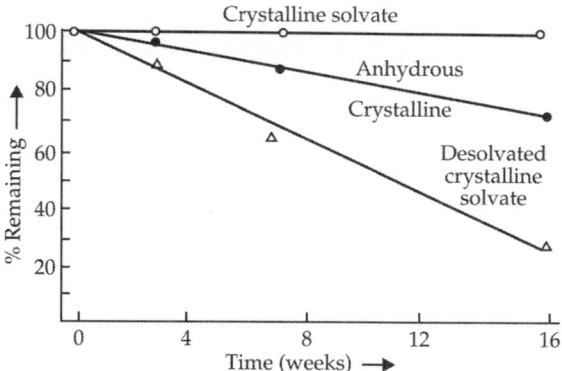

Fig. 1.13. Solid-state decomposition of different polymorphic forms of an experimental compound.

to study this phenomenon in the drug under development. It, thus, becomes essential to identify the internal structure of chemical compound (Fig. 1.14), number of polymorphs and characterize them in view of subsequent developmental steps.

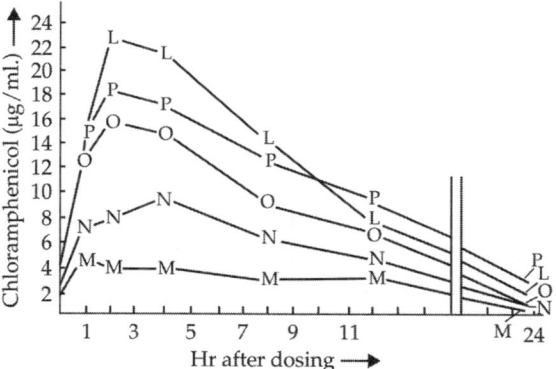

Fig. 1.12. Effect of polymorphism on oral bioavailability of chloramphenicol. M = Polymorph B (0%), N = Polymorph B (25%), O = Polymorph B (50%), P = Polymorph B (75%), L = Polymorph B (100%).

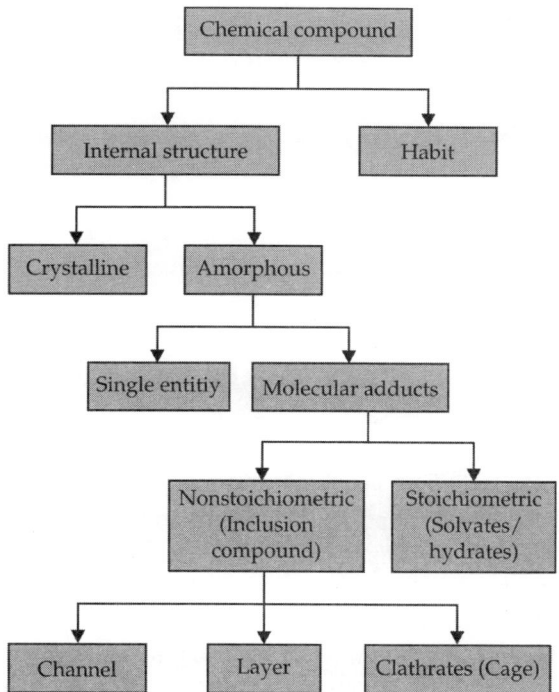

Fig. 1.14. Classification of internal structure of chemical compound.

Pseudopolymorphs (solvates and hydrates) have been confused with true polymorphs and must be identified. Melting the compound dispersed in silicon oil on a hot stage microscope is a good identification technique. Pseudopolymorphs evolve gas (steam/solvent vapour) causing bubbling of the oil near boiling point of water/solvent. Pseudopolymorphs can be discriminated using DSC, as an additional endotherm corresponding to solvent appears provided the heating rate is slow (2°C/min). The technique can be explained with the help of following example (Fig. 1.15).

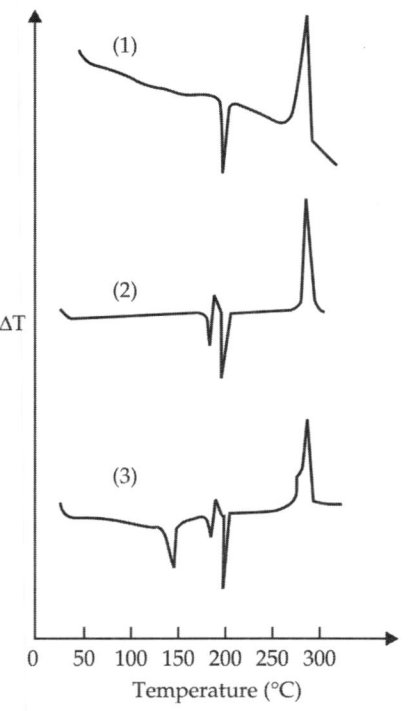

Fig. 1.15. Differential thermograms of polymorphic forms of an experimental compound. (1) Form A; (2) Dioxane solvate; (3) Form B.

The figure shows differential thermograms of 3 forms A, B, C of a compound designated as 1, 2, 3, respectively. Curve 1 shows a melting endotherm at about 195°C followed by decomposition exotherm at 250°–300°C. Curve 2 shows a melting endotherm at 180°C followed by a small endotherm indicating transition to form A, which then melts and decomposes at 190°C and 250°–300°C, respectively. Curve 3 is for dioxane solvate. Endotherm at 140°C is a desolvation endotherm after which B is generated.

Once pseudopolymorphs are identified, focus may be shifted on investigations of true forms. Many polymorphs are obtained by recrystallized solvent manipulation. Typical solvents inducing polymorphic changes are water, methanol, ethanol, acetone and chloroform. Polymorphs can also be prepared by thermal methods, which involve sublimation followed by recrystallization from melt by supercooling.

These different polymorphic forms can be characterized by a variety of techniques. Single-crystal X-ray provides most complete information about solid state but is tedious, time consuming and hence unsuitable for routine use. Powder X-ray diffraction is relatively simple and rapid. X-ray diffraction pattern is unique for each polymorphic form. Amorphous materials do not show any patterns or show one or two broad peaks attributable to the presence of short range molecular arrangements.

A crystalline particle is characterized by definite external and internal structures. 'Crystal habit' describes the external shape of a crystal, whereas polymorphic state refers to the definite arrangement of molecules inside the crystal lattice. Crystallization is invariably employed as the final step for the purification of a solid. The use of different solvents and processing conditions may alter the habit of recrystallized particles, besides modifying the polymorphic state of the solid. Subtle changes in crystal habit at this stage can lead to significant variation in raw-material characteristics. Normal crystal habits of different crystalline materials can be visualized in Fig. 1.16. Furthermore, various indices of dosage form performance, such as particle orientation, flowability, packing, compaction, suspension stability, and dissolution can be altered even in the absence of significantly

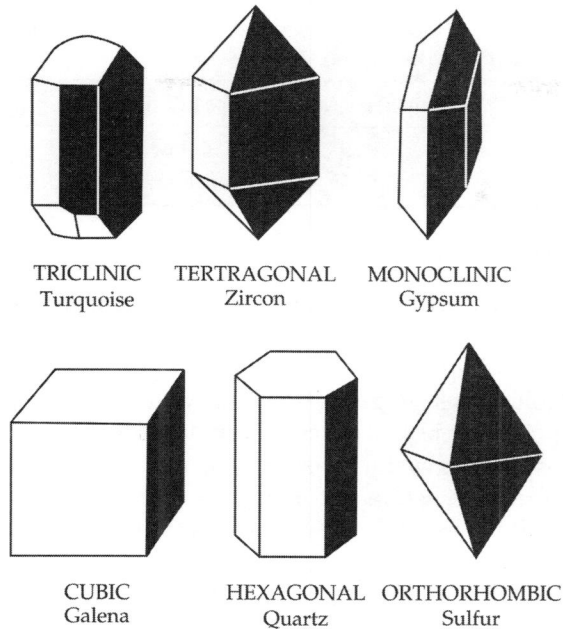

TRICLINIC	TERTRAGONAL	MONOCLINIC
Turquoise	Zircon	Gypsum

CUBIC	HEXAGONAL	ORTHORHOMBIC
Galena	Quartz	Sulfur

Fig. 1.16. Common crystal habits.

altered polymorphic state. These effects are a result of the physical effect of different crystal habits. In addition, changes in crystal habit either accompanied or not by polymorphic transformation during processing or storage, can lead to serious implications of physical stability in dosage forms. Therefore, in order to minimize the variations in raw-material characteristics, to ensure the reproducibility of results during pre-formulation, and to correctly judge the cause of instability and poor performance of a dosage form, it is essential to recognize the importance of changes in crystal surface appearance and habit of pharmaceutical powders.

Particle size, shape and surface area

Particle size (surface area) and shape affect physicochemical and biopharmaceutical properties as well as stability of a drug. Small particles are particularly important in low dose, high potency candidates, since large particle populations are necessary to assure adequate blend homogeneity. Poorly soluble drugs like Griseofulvin show higher dissolution rate and improved bioavailability on micronization. Needle shaped crystals show a poor flow property. Smaller particles are relatively more prone to attack by oxygen, humidity and interact relatively easily with excipients. This shows how important it is to decide on a desired size range and then to maintain and control it.

If particle size of new drug in 100 μm and above, safest practice is to grind it to 10–40 μm. If during further studies it is found that the grinding is not necessary, this step can be omitted.

Particle size determination

Though microscopy is the simplest technique of estimating size ranges and shapes, it is too slow for quantitative determination. The material is best observed as a suspension in non-dissolving fluid. Sieving is a less useful technique at preformulation stage due to lack of bulk material. Instruments based on light scattering (Royco), light blockage (HIAC) and blockage of electrical conductivity path (Coulter counter) are available. The latter is of limited value if most of particles are needle shaped. Andreasen pipette is based on rate difference of sedimentation of different particles, but techniques like this, are relatively seldom used due to their tedious nature.

Surface area determination

Particle size and surface area have an inverse relationship. Surface area is most commonly determined based on Brunauer, Emette, Teller (BET) theory of adsorption. Most substances adsorb a monomolecular layer of gas under certain conditions of partial pressure of gas and temperature. Knowing the monolayer capacity of adsorbent (i.e. quantity of adsorbate that can be accommodated as a monolayer on surface of adsorbent) and the area of adsorbate molecule, the surface area in principle, can be calculated. The adsorption process is carried out with nitrogen (adsorbate) at −195°C, at a partial pressure attainable when nitrogen is in a 30% mixture with an inert gas (helium). The adsorption takes place by virtue of van der Waals forces.

Bulk density

Knowledge of absolute and bulk density of the drug substance is very useful in having some idea as to the size of final dosage form. This is more important for low potency drug, which constitute bulk of the final granulation or tablet. The density of solids also affects their flow properties. Carr's compressibility index and Hausner's ratio can be used to predict the flow property based on density measurement (Tables 1.7 and 1.8).

$$\text{Compressibility index (\%)} = \frac{\left(\dfrac{\text{Tapped}}{\text{density}}\right) - \left(\dfrac{\text{Bulk}}{\text{density}}\right)}{\text{Bulk density}} \times 100$$

...(11)

$$\text{Hausner's ratio} = \frac{\text{Tapped density}}{\text{Bulk density}}$$

...(12)

Compressibility is strictly a misnomer, since no compression is involved and consolidation might be a better term.

Another important parameter for flow property determination is Hausner's ratio (Table 1.8), these predict the flow properties of powder by using inter-particle friction.

Table 1.8. Value of Hausner's ratio and respective flow of powder

Hausner's ratio	Type of flow
< 1.25	Good flow
> 1.25	Poor flow

Flowability

Flowability is intended to determine the ability of divided solids (for example, powders and granules) to flow vertically under defined conditions. A good flowability of powder or granules ensures efficient mixing, uniform dose as well as weight distribution in solid dosage form. Flowability of powder is directly related to its physical property as well as the specific processing conditions in the handling system, intrinsic flow property of drug. Hence, this property must be investigated during pre-formulation studies; especially when the anticipated dose of drug is large. Static angle of repose is a major of flow property of powder (Table 1.7).

The exact value of measured angle of repose depends on the types of method used. The value of angle of repose determined from methods where the powder is poured to form a heap is often distorted by the impact of falling particles. The apparatus shown in Fig. 1.17 is free of this distortion. It consists of a container with a built-in platform. The container is filled with the powder first, which is then drained out from the

Table 1.7. Relationship between flow, angle of repose & consolidation index for powder flow*

Flow	Angle of repose (θ) (degrees)	Consolidation index (%)	Example
Excellent	< 25	5–15	Celutab
Good	25–30	12–16	MCC
Fair to passable	30–40	18–21	Starax-1500
Poor	> 40	23–35	Maize starch
Very poor	33–38	33–40	Mg-Stearate
Very very poor	> 40		

* Addition of glidant should improve flow.

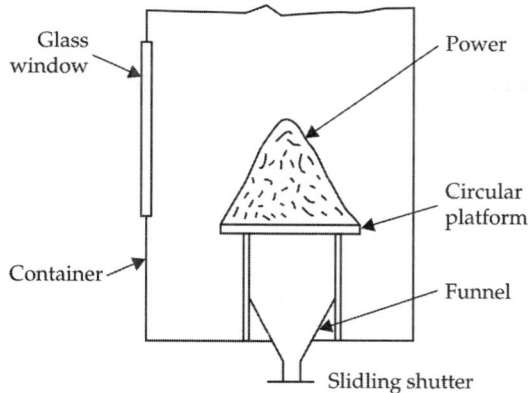

Fig. 1.17. Schematic diagram of the apparatus for measuring angle of repose.

bottom, thus leaving behind heap on the platform. The angle of repose is then measured using cathetometers. A relation between Carr's index and angle of repose is shown in Fig 1.18.

The powder flowability somewhat depends upon its particle size (Table 1.9) hence pre-formulation scientist should ensure the size of particle, which would be potential marker of dissolution as well as bioavailabilty.

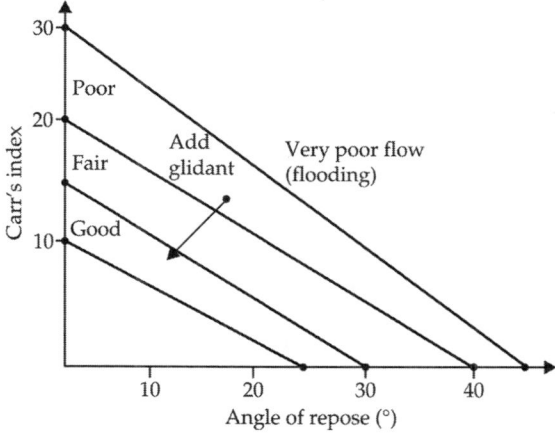

Fig. 1.18. Relationship between flow, angle of repose and Carr's index.

Hygroscopicity

It is the tendency of material to absorb moisture from atmosphere and attain dynamic equilibrium with water in the atmosphere. Hygroscopicity

Table 1.9. Particle size and flow properties

Size of particle (μm)	Flow property
More than 250	Free flowing
Less than 100	Poor flow
Less than 10	Resist flow

may have deleterious effect on the stability of dosage form. It may influence physical properties like flowability and compressibility of powders as well as stability in case of moisture-sensitive API. Preformulation scientist must investigate the rate and extent of moisture uptake by the drug and degree of hygroscopicity. This information might prove useful to decide several factors as nature of granulating solvents, storage conditions, and humidity control during manufacturing operations etc.

Stability indicating assays

The UV method developed during initial stages of preformulation might be useful in determination of some useful preliminary drug properties like quantitative solubility and partition coefficient, but is of limited value when it comes to stability assessment. It is essential to study in detail the stability of drug in solid and solution stage and drug excipient interaction. For this purpose, development of simple and efficient stability indicating assays is required. Though in some cases UV spectroscopy can be used, in general it is not a potent and widely applicable method when stability is concerned or when other compounds (drug or excipient) in analytical sample absorb in UV range. TLC and HPLC in particular, are the widely preferred techniques over UV for stability assessment. TLC is a reliable and sensitive quantitative method for the separation of complex mixtures in stability samples. However, the inherent sensitivity, the great flexibility of choice in mobile phase (solvents ranging from water to hexane), the increasing number of available stationary phases (particularly bonded phases) make HPLC a very efficient analytical technique. Accordingly it is a method of choice in stability indicating investigations.

Stability

Stability of a drug substance or product is defined as the extent to which a product or substance remains within specified limits of identity, strength, quality and purity throughout its intended period of storage and use. Knowledge of inherent stability of drug is important as it is utilized to decide excipients, processing parameters, storage conditions and to predict shelf-life. The objective of the stability study in pre-formulation design is to identify situations, which may pose threat to stability of active agent and help avoid or control them. This objective can be achieved by investigating stability at three fronts:

1. Solid state stability (of drug alone).
2. Compatibility studies (stability in presence of excipients).
3. Solution phase stability.

Solid state stability

The stability of drugs in solid dosage form is most important and common for the study of degradation of drug substance or drug product that are generally decomposed by either first- or zero-order profile. Chemical unstability normally results from either of the following reactions: hydrolysis (solvolysis), oxidation, photolysis and pyrolysis. Chemical structure of the drug is the determinant of susceptibility of drug to either of the above attacks. Esters and lactams, and to lesser extent, amides are prone to solvolysis. Unsaturation or electron rich centres in the structure make the molecule vulnerable for free radical mediated or photo-catalysed oxidation. Physical stability is influenced by physical properties of drug. Amorphous materials are less stable than their crystalline counterparts. Rate of degradation in a series of vitamin A esters was inversely related to their fusion temperature. Denser materials are more stable to ambient stress.

Thus, a thorough knowledge of drug's structure and physical properties is helpful in designing the stress conditions to challenge its suspected weakness in a stability programme. The data obtained under stress conditions can be utilized to predict the stability under normal storage conditions.

Elevated temperature studies

These studies are carried out by accelerating the rate of decomposition, preferably by increasing the temperature of reaction conditions. The elevated temperatures commonly used are 40, 50 and 60°C in conjunction with ambient humidity. The samples stored at highest temperature are observed weekly for physical and chemical changes and compared to an appropriate control (usually a sample stored at 50°C). If a substantial change is seen, samples stored at lower temperatures are examined. If no change is seen after 30 days at 60°C, the stability prognosis is excellent. Corroborative evidence must be obtained by monitoring the samples stored at lower temperatures for longer durations. Data obtained at higher temperatures can be extrapolated using Arrhenius treatment of storage temperatures (Figs. 1.19 and 1.20).

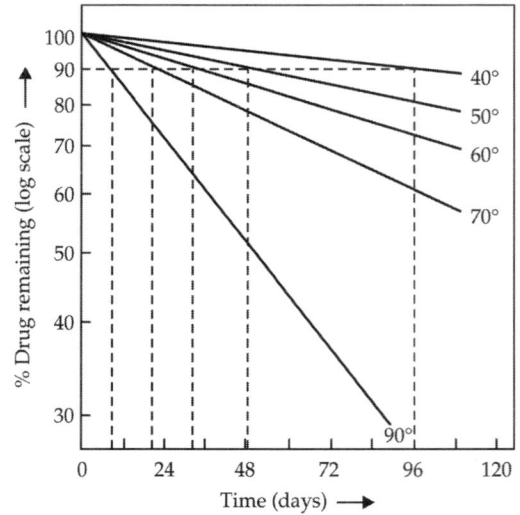

Fig. 1.19. Time in days required for drug potency to fall to 90% of original value.

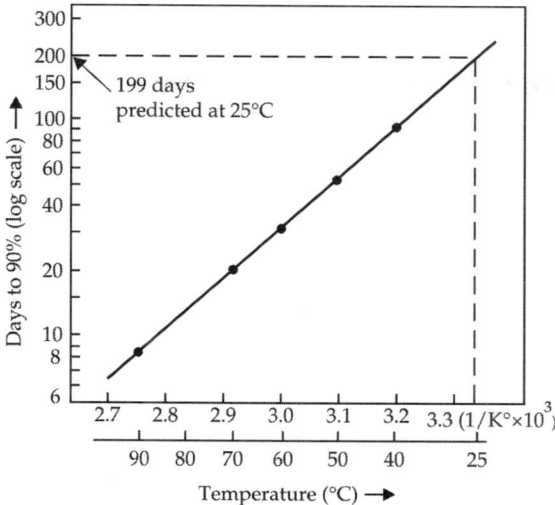

Fig. 1.20. A log plot of t_{90} against reciprocal temperature.

For an in-depth knowledge the readers are advised to refer Chapter 9 on stability testing.

A. Stability under high humidity conditions

Solid drug samples can be exposed to different relative humidity conditions by keeping them in laboratory desiccators containing saturated solutions of various salts. The closed desiccators, in turn, are kept in oven to provide constant temperatures. The preformulation data of this nature are useful in determining if the material should be protected and stored in controlled low humidity environment or if a non-aqueous solvent should be used during formulation.

B. Photolytic stability

In the preformulation study it is important to identify the nature of photosensitivity of the drug because many drugs are prone to fade or darken on exposure to light. Though the extent of degradation is small and limited to the exposed surface area, it presents an aesthetic problem. Exposure of drug to 400 and 900 footcandles of illumination for 4 and 2 week periods, respectively, is adequate to provide some idea of photosensitivity. Resulting data may be useful in determining if an amber colored container is required or if a colour masking dye should be used in formulation.

C. Stability to oxidation

Drug's sensitivity to oxidation can be examined by exposing it to atmosphere of high oxygen tension. Usually, a 40% oxygen atmosphere allows for a rapid evaluation. A shallow layer of drug exposed to a sufficient headspace volume ensures that the system is not oxygen limited. Samples are kept in desiccators equipped with three way stopcocks, which are alternatively evacuated and flooded with desired atmosphere. The process is repeated 3 or 4 times to ensure 100% desired atmosphere. The process is somewhat tedious in that it has to be repeated following each sample withdrawal.

Results may be useful in predicting if an antioxidant is required in the formulations or if the final product should be packaged under inert atmospheric conditions.

D. Compatibility studies

The knowledge of drug-excipient interaction is useful for the formulator to select appropriate excipient. For a new drug or excipient the preformulation scientist has to generate the interaction data. Drug–excipient compatibility study may be performed by physical method, in which drug and excipients are mixed in different proportions in both dry as well as wet conditions. After predetermined storage time all the samples are evaluated for their physical changes like colour, flowability and appearance, if any.

Today, compatibility studies are performed with the help of different thermal techniques like DSC, DTA etc. The described preformulation screening of drug excipient interaction requires only 5 mg of drug in a 50% mixture with the excipient to maximize the likelihood of obscuring an interaction. Mixtures should be examined under nitrogen to eliminate oxidative and pyrolytic effect at a standard heating rate (2, 5 or 10°C/min) on DSC, over a temperature range, which will encompass any thermal changes due to both the drug and the excipient. Thermograms for pure drug and excipients are used as reference. Appearance or disappearance of one or more peaks in thermogram of drug excipient mixtures are considered as indication of interaction. Though interaction can be observed by TLC as well, the rapidity of DSC gives it an edge over TLC. Thermograms of Cephradine and four excipients namely *N*-methyl glucamine, tromethamine, anhydrous sodium carbonate and trisodium phosphate dodeca-hydrate, are shown in Fig. 1.21. Fig. 1.22 shows thermograms for corresponding four mixtures. The 200°C exotherm for cephradine is retained only in thermogram corresponding to its mixture with anhydrous sodium carbonate. This suggests its interaction with all remaining excipients except anhydrous sodium carbonate.

E. Solution phase stability

As compared to the dry form, the degradation is much rapid in solution form and prone to cause

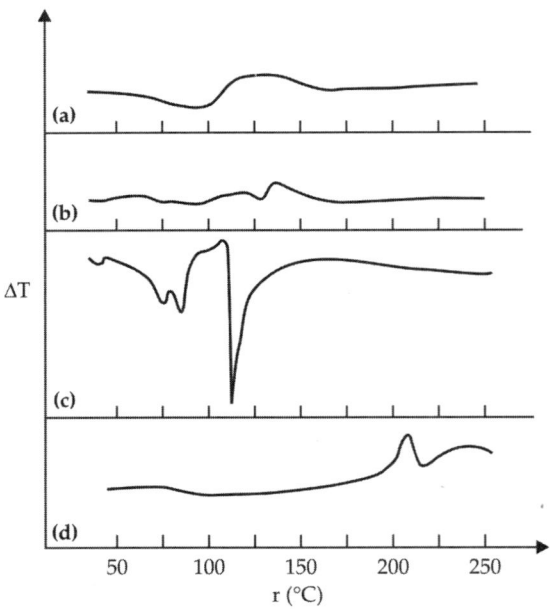

Fig. 1.22. Thermograms of mixtures of cephradine with: (a) *N*-methylglucamine; (b) Tromethamine; (c) Trisodium phosphate dodecahydrate; (d) Anhydrous sodium carbonate.

many challenges related to pH, counter ion of salt, solution components that may be reactive to the exposure of temperature and light. It is important to ascertain that the drug does not degrade when exposed to GI fluids. The pH based stability study, using different simulated GI condition can be designed. Fig. 1.23 shows pH-based degradation of Ampicillin in solution at 35°C. It shows unstability of Ampicillin at extreme pH conditions. A poor solution stability of drug may urge the formulator to choose a less soluble salt form, provided the bioavailability is not compromised. A good example is compa-rative stability profile of salts of erythromycin. Erythromycin is rapidly hydrolysed in acidic environment of stomach ($t_{10\%}$ = 9 sec.). To overcome this problem Erythromycin estolate, a prodrug, was synthesised for use in, both, suspension and capsule dosage form. This not only improved stability but also was absorbed four times more efficiently than formulated free base.

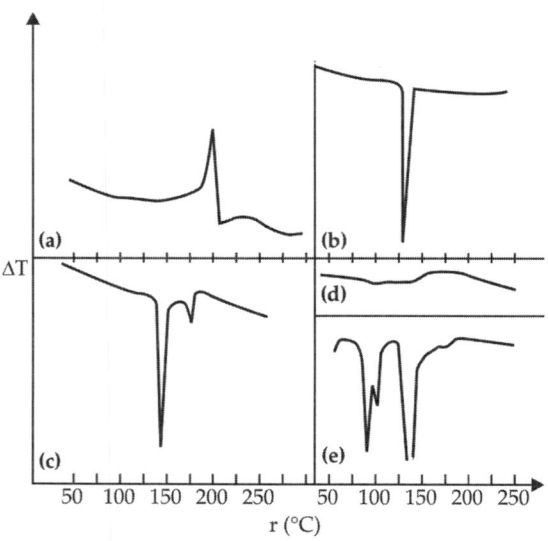

Fig. 1.21. Thermograms of pure materials. (a) Cephra-dine; (b) *N*-methylglucamine; (c) Tromethamine; (d) Anhydrous sodium carbonate; (e) Trisodium phosphate dodecahydrate.

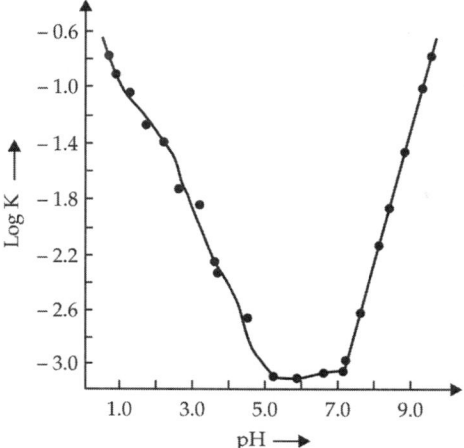

Fig. 1.23. pH based degradation of ampicillin in solution at 35°C. Maximum stability found between pH 5 to pH 7.

F. Absorption behavior

It is essential to test the *in vivo* behavior of new drug for successful formulation of a dosage form for good bioavailability. Partial *in vivo* tests are designed to study pharmacokinetic profile of the drug.

Partial *in vivo* tests can be performed by a number of techniques but everted sac technique is the most commonly used. In this technique, a segment of rat intestine is cut and everted. The ends are tied at both the ends to form a sac with physiological solutions inside (without drug). The sac is then dipped into a buffer solution of drug at 37°C. Oxygen is continuously bubbled into the solution. After specific time, solution in sac is analysed for its drug content.

Rats, dogs, or other species can be used for *in vivo* testing. The animals are divided in test and control groups. Often one set is given drug by parenteral route and the absorption is considered 100%. The oral absorption is then expressed as fraction of total absorption.

CONCLUSION

Active pharmaceutical ingredient (API) is rarely administered solely as a pure chemical substance but almost always given in the form of a dosage form. A dosage form, thus, acts as a vehicle for drug delivery. Dosage form is formulated invariably using drug and excipient(s) in appropriate proportions. Principally, a dosage form is formulated to achieve predictable therapeutic response of the drug included in the formulation.

Preformulation studies, if carried out properly, play a significant role in anticipating the formulation problems. This inter-relationship of preformulation and formulation in context of pharmaceutical product development is expressed in Fig. 1.24. Preformulation helps in indicating the feasibility of the formulation of the desired dosage form, selection of excipients, process variables and storage conditions of the final formulation. It also saves a considerable labour, time and energy and thus makes formulation commercially profitable.

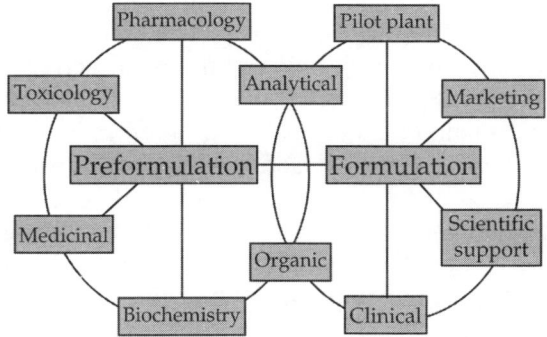

Fig. 1.24. Interrelation between preformulation and formulation.

Development of a formulation suitable for large-scale production with reproducible product quality is a challenge for formulation scientist. The information generated out of exhaustive pre-formulation study certainly provides the necessary platform. Selection of correct excipient(s) in correct proportion(s) is an important step in formulation development. Though excipients are defined as therapeutically inactive agents, which facilitate drug delivery;

it is a well established fact that they may interact with the drug and other excipients in the formulation. The selection of appropriate excipients depends upon the compatibility results, route of administration and the dosage form, as well as the active ingredient and other factors. The interaction may actually reduce the effectiveness of the dosage form instead of enhancing it.

There are a number of dosage forms in which a drug can be formulated. Each dosage form utilizes a different set of excipients. Biocompatibility is the first criterion for selection of excipients. Based on already existing information on compatibility and stability of excipients, those suitable for dosage form under consideration are selected. A few well documented interactions are exemplified below. Incompatibility of lactose and amine drugs in presence of moisture and stearates results in brownish discoloration of tablet and is called as 'Mailard reaction'. Tween 80 interacts to a significant extent with methyl and propyl paraben to form complex. The complexed preservatives lack any antimicrobial activity. Along with the already existing knowledge the information generated through preformulation studies also proves useful. An example of the drug-excipient interaction was already cited in preformulation section of this chapter indicating the compatibility studies of Cephradine with different excipients. Sometimes the excipients have additive effect as well and the additive interactions could be utilized to the profit of the formulation. EDTA, for example, enhances the antibacterial activity of benzalkonium chloride.

Other vitally important factor is the processing parameters. The processing conditions and the time for which the formulation is subjected to a particular process must be defined well at this stage, as this has to be extrapolated during large-scale production. The processing parameters can affect the drug or excipients or both and hence must be carefully controlled. Processing parameters are governed by physicochemical properties of the materials.

The physicochemical characterization during preformulation stage would thus prove useful. The light sensitive drugs like Nifedipine, Omeprazole etc. have to be manufactured in protected light environment. Hygroscopic drugs like Clotrimazole demand for stringent humidity control during formulation. It is difficult to discuss the processing parameters of all different dosage forms at a place as the conditions are quite diversified. Only a few examples of the parameters, which demand attention can be listed as drying temperature, aseptic conditions during injectable preparations, stirring conditions of emulsions and suspensions, rotations of capsule filling machine etc.

Optimization of both the factors mentioned above is essential for batch-to-batch reproducibility of a quality dosage form. Stability of product during shelf-life is an essential requirement of a quality dosage form. Evaluating and confirming stability of formulation developed is an important feature of this stage. Stability of the product must be evaluated keeping in mind the ICH guidelines being discussed in Chapter 10 of this book.

Finally, it must be kept in mind that a quality dosage form is not always a commercially successful one. A product with a predictable and reproducible pharmacological response and excellent stability can be considered a quality product. That is not sufficient, however, for its commercial success. Cost, esthetic value and ease of administration/application are the other factors, which along with two previously discussed ones, influence acceptability of the product to both prescribers and patients. The cost and esthetic value solely depend on the excipients and the formulation process adopted and hence must be given fair attention at the stage of formulation development. Ease of administration/application depends not only on formulation but also on packaging. Though 'first in market' products enjoy the advantage of monopoly for some time, the competitors very quickly catch them up. It becomes very essential for commercial success of the dosage form to add on the properties, which will appeal the end users.

Once a successful formulation is developed its pilot plant scale up studies are planned.

Pilot-plant scale-up techniques

It is a broad term in which pilot-plant (means lab scale) formula is transformed into a viable product by development of liable and practical procedure of manufacture; and scale-up means the art for designing of prototype using the data obtained from the pilot-plant model. During formulation, a satisfactory formulation is designed in R&D department on laboratory scale. An effective, safe and stable formulation must be manufactured on high speed equipments on large scale in a cost-effective manner. The facilities and equipments present on production floor often remotely resemble those present in a R&D laboratory. The responsibility of converting a laboratory curiosity into a successful product is shouldered by pilot-plant scale-up department. This department transforms a formula into a viable robust product by developing a reliable and practical method of manufacturing that effects the orderly transition from laboratory to routine processing in a full scale production facility.

Some industries have pilot-plant department as a section of their R&D setup. In other organizations the formulators who developed the formula themselves take it into production, whereas in some other organizations separate set of personnel handle the responsibility of scale-up. Some companies have scale-up group organizationally separate from R&D. However, there are a few companies who have adopted a composite of both the approaches. Often the formula developed on laboratory scale may demand for the modifications to varying extent in either materials or processing parameters to make it suitable for large-scale production. A scale-up batch is an exactly imitating batch to that of production batch, though of smaller size.

By normal convention, a batch of 1/10th of size of a final batch or minimum 1 lakh units, whichever is more, is considered adequate. The foremost objective is to critically evaluate suitability of formula for large-scale production. It may so happen that one or more of the excipients or their quantities may prove unsuitable for large-scale production. The formula in this case is referred back to formulators.

Selection of most compatible equipments out of all the relevant ones is another important function of scale-up personnel. For example, there are many mills available for reducing the granule size like oscillator granulator, hammer mill, ball mill etc., depending upon the characteristics of unmilled granules, the most suitable mill producing particle size distribution necessary for best performance during compression is selected. During scale-up batch the processing parameters are studied, validated and finalized to produce a product with desired specifications e.g. time of blending, amount of binder and lubricant. Over blending reduces dissolution as the granules get over coated with hydrophobic lubricants. Under mixing, on the other hand, may result in poorly flowing granules. Similarly, compression load and the compression machine rotation speed can also be considered for example. The lower and upper limits of both these parameters are determined, which produce tablets of desired hardness. Records containing detailed description of formulation, equipments, processes and product specifications are generated, which are expected to support GMP in subsequent steps of production. Though different companies call these records by different names e.g. Master Formula Records (MFR), moral behind generating them remains the same and that is ensuring an effective and reproducible process for producing quality product. All the critical features of the process are identified so that as the process is scaled up, it can be adequately monitored to provide assurance that the process is under control, and that the product/

intermediate produced at each level of the scale-up is according to intended specifications. Once a pilot plant batch is satisfactorily prepared the product is released for actual production on large scale on production floor.

The pilot-plant and scale-up techniques are being discussed in Chapter 16 of this book.

Production

Manufacturing in pharmaceutical industry is done in compliance with the current Good Manufacturing Practice (cGMP) regulations. The personnel involved are expected to understand GMP at least as it is applied to their particular area of responsibility. The persons engaged in production department have to take ultimate responsibility of producing a quality product lies with production department. If a product fails, this department is required to find and correct the problem. Depending upon the market demand and production capacity, the production batches are planned. The first three batches are called prospective validation batches. Validation batches confirm that the process parameters are optimum for product specifications required.

Packaging

Pharmaceutical packaging serves as a function of providing protection, identification, information and convenience to encourage compliance with the course of therapy. Packaging of pharmaceutical products is specifically important from its stability point of view. A degraded product may not only lose its potency but also prove hazardous to patients' life. Decision on packaging is, therefore, based on stability profile of the product. Amber coloured bottles, for example, are utilized for light-sensitive products. Ease of administration/application makes the product patient friendly. The applicator supplied with vaginal tablets is a part of its pack and makes the tablet insertion easy. 'Snap-off' ampoules of Voveran (Novartis) also make the product user friendly. Sensur (Grecewell) is a preparation of natural oils,

which the company promotes as a painkiller. It is available in 'Roll on' packs, which facilitate its easy application. Some user friendly kits, the so-called 'compliance kits/packs' are also available, CLO-KIT from Indoco, for example, contains one orange coloured tablet of Chloroquine phosphate, 1 g, and three pink tablets of Chloroquine phosphate, 300 mg each. The patients are instructed to initiate the therapy with orange tablet and continue with pink tablets at 6, 24 and 48 hours. The colour coded pack, thus, helps the patient to understand the dosage regimen properly. Package inserts for patients certainly improve patient compliance.

'Instructions to patients' is an essential part of the pharmaceutical packaging. Instructions like 'For external use only', 'Shake well before use', 'Apply with rubbing', 'Not to be applied on broken skin', etc. help the patients to understand how to use the product. The instructions on storage make it sure that the product is stored properly to ensure the product stability. The expiry date indicates the deadline before which the product is best for use.

Finally, attractive pharmaceutical packs enhance the esthetic value of the product and, in turn, appeal to patient. It also displays an impression to the customers. For further details, the readers are advised to refer to Chapter 15 on Pharmaceutical Packaging in this book.

Quality control/assurance

The quality control department can monitor production process and indicate where the process is deviating from control standards, supply statistical data and constructive comments and help in producing quality product. Both QA/QC are designed to reduce defects and/or errors to identify opportunities for improvements. Thus the job of quality control department is to take samples at every step during production and evaluate them for the desired specifications. Quality assurance, however, is a much broader concept and quality control is only a part of it. Actually this department is responsible for batch-to-batch uniformity and reproducibility of quality products.

Marketing

Marketing the product aggressively is a specialized function. A well-organized, competent marketing team with excellent product knowledge and effective communication skills should be an invaluable asset for any organization, which holds true for pharmaceutical industry as well. The entire promotion of a new product is taken care of by two different sections of marketing department viz. marketing and sales, each having separate responsibility.

Marketing department

A part of marketing department is dedicated to market survey, which taps the market opportunities. Based on their feedback on existing and upcoming opportunities in the market a company takes up the product department projects. Yet another group of personnel is totally involved in promotion of the products. The promotion of a newly developed product is a challenge within itself. Marketing department is involved devising strategies for product promotion, identifying the market segments for promotion, making decision on product positioning, generating promotional material, training the sales personnel on new product and coordinating with sales department with analysis of sales data, taking up customer enquiries, continuously reviving marketing strategies according to situations.

Sales department

This department actually takes up the product to customer. Personnel working in sales (a medical representative in this context) must have excellent product knowledge. In addition, effective communication of unique selling propositions of the product to customer is important. Other functions of the sales department include satisfying the prescriber(s) on his queries, if required in consultation with the marketing section, communicating his views to marketing department, ensuring that the distribution chain is functioning effectively and the product is easily available, keeping an eye on competitors' activity etc. Post-marketing surveillance (PMS) also constitutes an important job of this department. The sales team examines the product stability, acceptability, customer response in initial stages and overall response of the market to the product. With this feedback the product development process can be reevaluated and restructured, if necessary.

SUGGESTED READINGS

- Aguiar, AJ, Kre, J, Kinkel, AW, and Symyn, JC (1967). Effect of polymorphism on chloramphenicol from chloramphenicol palmitate, *J. Pharm. Sci.*, 56: 847.
- Albert, A and Serjeant, EP. **Determination of Ionization Constants**. Chapman and Hall, London, 1971.
- Gregg, SJ and Sing, KSW (1967). **Adsorption, Surface Area, and Porosity**. Academic Press, New York.
- Guillary, K, and Higuchi, T (1962). Solid state stability of some vitamin A compounds, *J. Pharm. Sci.*, 51: 104.
- Mertes, L (Ed.) (1963). **Handbook of Analytical Chemistry**, McGraw-Hill, New York.
- Wadke, DA and Reier, GE (1972). Use of intrinsic dissolution rate to determine thermodynamic parameters associated with phase transition, *J. Pharm. Sci.*, 61: 868.
- Wells, JL (1988). **Pharmaceutical Preformulation: The Physicochemical Properties of Drug Substances**, Ellis Harwood Limited, U.K.
- Jain, NK and Sharma SN (2007). **A Textbook of Professional Pharmacy**, Vallabh Prakashan, New Delhi.
- Niazi, SK (2007). **Handbook of Preformulation: Chemical, Biological, and Botanical Drugs**, Informa Healthcare, New York.
- Banker GS and Rhodes CT (2002). **Modern Pharmaceutics**, Marcel Dekker, Inc., New York.

2

Oral Liquids

Vikas Jain and N.K. Jain

INTRODUCTION

Oral drug delivery is still the most important and most frequently used route of drug administration. However, younger patients suffer from difficulty in swallowing solid tablets. Thus, oral liquid is the most preferred dosage form in pediatric patients. These formulations are primarily employed to enhance the oral bio-availability of a therapeutic agent or eliminate the need for a patient to swallow a tablet or capsule. Liquid formulations offer many advantages over other dosage forms like ease in dosing to ease in administration, and myriad possibilities of innovative drug delivery systems.

One of the most desirable features of liquid formulations is the relatively lesser importance of bioavailability considerations, especially in solution forms, as the drug molecules are already in the dispersed phase, hence can be readily absorbed from gastrointestinal (GI) tract. However, all of the advantages of liquid dosage forms are balanced by many problems in their formulation. These include stability problems, taste masking needs, phase separation, and so forth; compared with traditional solid-state dosage forms, a unique set of considerations is required during the design and formulation of oral liquids.

Oral liquids are intended for oral administration either undiluted or after dilution. They may contain auxiliary substances such as suitable dispersing, emulsifying, suspending, wetting, solubilizing, thickening, stabilizing agents and antimicrobial preservatives. They may also contain suitable sweetening, flavoring and permitted coloring agents.

Oral liquids other than oral emulsions may be supplied as liquids or prepared just before use by dissolving or dispersing granules or powder in the liquid stated on the label. The granules or powder comply with the requirements stated under oral powders. Oral liquids should not be diluted and stored; where, however, the individual formulation directs dilution, the diluted oral liquid should be freshly prepared irrespective of the nature of the diluent. Diluted oral liquids may be less stable physically and chemically than the corresponding undiluted preparation and should be used within the period stated on the label [Indian Pharmacopoeia, 2014].

In order to meet the ever increasing demand of patient population towards ease in administration of medicated preparations the concept of *personalized medicine* has recently been introduced. Numerous investigations focused on the role of metabolizing enzymes and biomarkers in influencing factors on drug metabolism, is an active research field. It could be shown that due to the effects of poor or rapid metabolizing capacities, adapted drug doses are required to ensure a safe and correct therapy. Paediatric and geriatric drug delivery also need individualized dosing, patient adapted drug formulations and delivery devices. Further, some drugs with small therapeutic windows (e.g. Digoxin) need precise dose adaptation, particularly in phases of initial dose titration [Breitkreutz & Boos, 2007; Stegemann et al., 2010]. The present Chapter pertains only to preparations and individualized dosing methodology for delivering oral liquids.

Classification of liquid preparations intended for oral administration

- **Elixirs:** Elixirs are clear, flavored oral liquids containing one or more active ingredients dissolved in a vehicle that usually contains a high proportion of sucrose or a suitable polyhydric alcohol or alcohols and may also contain ethanol (95%) or dilute ethanol.
- **Linctuses:** Linctuses are viscous oral liquids containing one or more active ingredients dissolved in a vehicle that usually contains a high proportion of sucrose, other sugars or a suitable polyhydric alcohol or alcohols. Linctuses are intended for use in the treatment or relief of cough, and are sipped and swallowed slowly without the addition of water.
- **Mixtures:** Mixtures are oral liquids containing one or more active ingredients dissolved, suspended or dispersed in a suitable vehicle. Suspended solids may separate slowly on keeping but are easily redispersed on shaking.
- **Drops:** Oral drops are oral liquids that are intended to be administered in small volumes with the aid of a suitable measuring device such as a dropper.

- **Emulsions:** Oral emulsions are oral liquids containing one or more active ingredients and are stabilized oil-in-water dispersions, either or both phases of which may contain dissolved solids. Solids may also be suspended in oral emulsions. Emulsions may exhibit phase separation but are easily reformed on shaking. The preparation remains sufficiently stable to permit withdrawal of a homogeneous dose.
- **Solutions:** Oral solutions are oral liquids containing one or more active ingredients dissolved in a suitable solvent. It can be further subcategorized in oral rehydration solution and oral colonic lavage solution.
- **Suspensions:** Oral suspensions are oral liquids containing one or more active ingredients suspended in a suitable vehicle. Suspended solids may slowly separate on keeping but are easily redispersed.
- **Syrups:** Syrups are viscous oral liquids that may contain one or more active ingredients in solution. The vehicle usually contains large amounts of sucrose or other sugars to which certain polyhydric alcohols may be added to inhibit crystallization or to modify solubilization, taste and other vehicle properties. Sugarless syrups may contain sweetening agents and thickening agents. Syrups may contain ethanol (95%) as a preservative or as a solvent to incorporate flavoring agents. Antimicrobial agents may also be added to syrups.
- **Tinctures:** Tinctures are alcoholic or hydro-alcoholic solution prepared from vegetable materials or from chemical substances. Tinctures may contain alcohols ranging from 15 to 80%. The alcoholic content protects against microbial growth and keeps alcohol-soluble extractives in solution. Usually tablets/capsules, elixirs, or syrups are preferred over tinctures due to a rather high alcoholic content of later. Parents may also avoid tinctures containing alcohol for their children.
- **Fluid extracts:** These are concentrated alcoholic solutions of animal or vegetable drugs obtained by removal of active

constituent by extraction procedures that may include maceration or percolation.

- **Oromucosal preparations:** Oromucosal preparations are liquid preparations, containing one or more active substances intended for administration to the oral cavity and/or throat to obtain a local or systemic effect. Preparations intended for a local effect may be designed for application to a specific site within the oral cavity such as the gums (gingival preparations) or the throat (oropharyngeal preparations).

Preparations intended for a systemic effect are designed to be absorbed primarily at one or more sites on the oral mucosa (e.g. sublingual preparations). For many oromucosal preparations, it is likely that some proportion of the active substance will be swallowed and may be absorbed via the GI tract. Oromucosal preparations may contain suitable antimicrobial preservatives and other excipients such as dispersing, suspending, thickening, emulsifying, buffering, wetting, solubilizing, stabilizing, flavoring and sweetening agents [British Pharmacopoeia, 2007]. Several categories of preparations for oromucosal use may be distinguished:

- **Gargles:** Gargles are aqueous solutions intended for gargling to obtain a local effect. They are *not to be swallowed*. They are supplied as ready-to-use solutions or concentrated solutions to be diluted. They may also be prepared from powders or tablets to be dissolved in water before use. Gargles may contain excipients to adjust the pH, which, as far as possible, is neutral.

- **Mouthwashes:** Mouthwashes are aqueous solutions intended for use in contact with the mucous membrane of the oral cavity, usually after dilution with water. They are *not to be swallowed*. They are supplied as ready-to-use solutions or concentrated solutions to be diluted. They may also be prepared from powders or tablets to be dissolved in water before use. Mouthwashes may contain excipients to adjust the pH to neutral, as far as possible.

- **Gingival solutions:** Gingival solutions are intended for administration to the gingivae by means of a suitable applicator.

- **Oromucosal solutions and suspensions:** These are liquid preparations intended for administration to the oral cavity by means of a suitable applicator.

- **Oromucosal drops, sprays and sublingual sprays:** These are solutions, emulsions or suspensions intended for local or systemic effect. They are applied by instillation or spraying into the oral cavity or onto a specific part of the oral cavity such as spraying under the tongue (sublingual spray) or into the throat (oropharyngeal spray). A list of commonly used oral liquid preparation is presented in Table 2.1.

REGULATORY CONSIDERATIONS

GMP consideration

Quality, efficacy and safety of a medicinal product have always been a matter of concern for public. GMP is advocated for maintenance of high quality standards in pharmaceutical manufacturing. Government of India included GMP under schedule M of Drug and Cosmetic Act vide G.S.R. 735(E) dated June 24th 1988. The schedule M has again been amended in a major way by the Drugs and Cosmetics (8th amendment) Rules, 2001 w.e.f. December 11th 2001 and embraces Rules 71, 74, 76 and 78 under the Drug and Cosmetics Rules, 1945. GMP includes requirements for factory premises, work space and storage area, health, clothing and sanitation of workers, medical services, sanitation in manufacturing premises, equipment, raw materials, master formula records, batch manufacturing records, manufacturing operations and controls, reprocessing and recovery, product containers and closures, labels and other printed materials, distribution records, records of complaints and adverse reactions, and

Table 2.1. Various oral dosage forms and their marketed products with suppliers

Formulation	Marketed products	Supplier/Manufacturer
Oral solution	Depakene	Abott Laboratories
Oral solution	Cosme	Merck
Oral solution	Uriliser	Martin & Harris
Elixir	Bisolvon sinus – elixir	Boehringer Ingelheim Ltd.
Elixir	Panamax	Sanofi-Aventis
Linctuses	Sudafed dry cough linctus	Superliving Pharmacy
Linctuses	Grilinctus	Franco-Indian
Mixture	Beechamsveno's cough mixture	GlaxoSmithKline
Mixture	AscorilSF	Glenmark
Oral drops	Ebixa oral drops	Lundbeck Ltd.
Oral drops	Clomindrops	Abaris
Oral emulsion	Solubeno oral emulsion	Janssen Animal Health
Oral emulsion	Cremaffin	Abbott Laboratories
Oral suspension	Allegraoral suspension	Sanofi-Aventis
Oral suspension	Zenflox OZ oral suspension	Mankind
Oral suspension	Ancool	Zuventus
Syrup	Duphalac syrup	Solvay Healthcare Ltd.
Syrup	Amycordial	Aimil
Tincture	Calendula tinctures	Naturally Nova Scotia
Gargle	Betadine gargle	Mundipharma
Gargle	Betaseptic gargle	Modi-Mundipharma
Mouthwash	Care antiseptic mouthwash	Thornton & Ross Ltd.
Gingival solution	Paradental gingival solution	Inter-Evrogeneks
Oromucosal solution	Lidocaine oromucosal solution	UCB Pharmaceuticals Ltd.
Oromucosal suspension	Adcortyl in orabase	Bristol-Myers
Oromucosal sprays	Corsodyl sprays	GlaxoSmithKline
Sublingual sprays	Whitelight glutathione spray	Aim Global Inc.
Sublingual sprays	Nitroglycerine lingual spray	Wilshire
Dry syrup	Azee	Cipla
Dry syrup	Kefpod CV 50	Glenmark

the quality control system. Discussion on any pharmaceutical product cannot be completed without GMP considerations. Oral liquids have to comply with the following GMP requirements.

According to **Schedule M 1 (C) – Specific requirement for manufacture of oral liquids** (syrup, elixirs, emulsions and suspension), the layout and design of the manufacturing area shall strive to minimize the risk of cross-contamination and mix-ups. Manufacturing area shall have entry through double door air-lock facility and made fly-proof by use of fly catcher and/or air curtain. The production area shall be cleaned and sanitized at the end of every production process. Equipment design shall be such as to prevent accumulation of residual microbial growth or cross-contamination. The use of glass apparatus shall be minimum.

The chemical and microbiological quality of Purified Water shall be specified and monitored routinely. The microbiological evaluation shall include testing for absence of pathogens and shall not exceed 100 CFU/mL. Care shall be taken to avoid the risk of microbial proliferation with appropriate methods like re-circulation, use of UV treatment, and treatment with heat and sanitizing agent.

Manufacturing personnel shall bear non-fiber shedding clothing to prevent contamination of the product. Materials likely to shed fiber like gunny bags or wooden pallets shall not be carried into the area where products or cleaned containers are exposed. The primary packaging area shall have an air supply filtered through 5 micron filters and temperature shall not exceed 30°C. When the product is not immediately packed, the maximum period of storage and storage conditions shall be specified in the Master formula.

According to USFDA-cGMP guidelines, the primary objective of personnel control is to protect the product from potential contamination from personnel-particulate matter including hair, fibers, and outside dirt', cross-contamination carried on clothing from other processes, microorganisms shed from skin and from the mouth and nose. However, an employer also has a responsibility to protect the employee from unacceptable exposure to the materials being handled, many of which have physiological properties. Where potential exposure is to very potent materials, testing of blood or urine samples may be warranted. Wherever possible, barrier or containment facilities or equipment should be used to protect personnel from extremely hazardous materials. The use of masks or breathing equipment should only be used as the sole precaution in rare circumstances or for less hazardous materials.

Validation

The term *validation* refers to "establishing documented evidence which provides a high degree of assurance that a specific process will consistently produce a product meeting its pre-determined specifications and quality attributes". The other definition of *validation* includes "action of proving, in accordance with the principles of good manufacturing practice, that any procedure, process, equipment, material, activity or system actually leads to the expected results. According to USFDA guideline *validation* is applicable to "any procedure, equipment, material, activity or system" as well as to a process.

Assurance of product quality is derived from careful attention to a number of factors including selection of quality parts and materials, adequate product and process design, control of the process, and in-process and end-product testing. The routine end-product testing alone is not sufficient to assure product quality because many end-product tests have limited sensitivity. In some cases, destructive testing would be required to show that the manufacturing process was adequate, and in other situations end-product testing does not reveal all variations that may occur in the product that may impact on safety and effectiveness. The basic principles of quality assurance have as their goal the production of articles that are fit for their intended use. These principles include (1) quality, safety and effectiveness must be built into the product; (2) quality cannot be tested into the finished product only; and (3) each step of the manufacturing process must be controlled to meet all quality and design specifications of the finished product. Process validation is a key element in assuring that these quality assurance goals are met. It is through careful design and validation of both the process and process controls that a manufacturer can establish a high degree of confidence that all manufactured units from successive lots will be acceptable.

Successfully validating a process may reduce the dependence upon intensive in-process and finished product testing. It should be noted that in almost all cases, end-product testing plays a major role in assuring that quality assurance goals are met; i.e., validation and end-product testing are not mutually exclusive. Current validation topics, particularly insofar as regulatory bodies are concerned, are:

1. Validation of cleaning procedures
2. Validation of equipments and processes
3. Computer systems validation
4. Analytical methods validation

Validation program includes in itself many important characteristics, organized arrangements of which may lead to defined outcomes. Validation program and procedure pertaining to various dosage forms have been discussed in detail in Chapter 20 of this book. The general concept and information discussed in this chapter, to get the product of highest purity and efficacy in various dosage forms is applicable to liquid dosage forms as well.

FORMULATION CONSIDERATIONS

Readers are expected to be familiar with the physicochemical aspects of drugs and formulations, which they might have studied under Physical Pharmacy and Pharmaceutical Technology. A brief discussion of formulation parameters relevant to product development of oral liquids is presented below.

Solubility

Solubility is of utmost importance when developing monophasic oral liquids. The actives and other substances should remain dissolved throughout the life of the product. In order to maintain these characteristics, the drugs must remain in solution at unsaturated concentrations; otherwise, the drug may crystallize because of changes in temperature, by 'seeding' from ingredients, or particulate matter present.

The solubility of a given solute is defined as the maximum concentration to which it can be dissolved in a particular solvent to yield a homogeneous monophasic system. When a

solute dissolves, forces of attraction between the solute and the solvent must overcome intermolecular forces of attraction of the substance. This involves breaking of solute-solute forces and solvent-solvent forces to achieve solute-solvent interaction [Seedher & Bhatia, 2003].

Solubility of a solute in a given solvent is determined at a fixed temperature (normally a little higher than room temperature). For this, a saturated solution of the solute is prepared. The solution is then agitated at a constant temperature, and the amount of drug in solution is determined by chemical analysis of the filtrate. The equilibrium is not achieved until at least two successive samples give the same results. According to a rough estimate up to 40 percent of new chemical entities (NCEs) discovered by pharmaceutical industry, today are poorly soluble, lipophilic compounds. The solubility issues complicating the delivery of these new drugs also affect the delivery of many existing new drugs. The ability to deliver poorly soluble drugs will grow in significance in the coming years as innovator companies rely upon NCEs for a large share of revenue within the pharmaceutical market. Similarly, generic drug manufacturers will need to employ economically efficient methods of delivery (as many low solubility drugs go off-patent) in order to maintain a competitive edge and sufficiently compete as profit margins shrink in this price-sensitive industry. Relative to highly soluble compounds, low drug solubility often manifests itself in a host of *in vivo* consequences, including decreased bioavailability, increased chance of food effect, incomplete release from dosage form and higher patient variability. Many significant *in vitro* formulation obstacles, such as severely limited choices of delivery technologies and, increasingly complex dissolution testing with limited or poor *in vivo-in vitro* correlation, are also encountered. These problems are often sufficient to halt development on many newly synthesized compounds due to solubility issue.

This has motivated the development of new drug delivery technologies to overcome the obstacle of solubilization of poorly soluble drugs through either chemical or mechanical modification of environment surrounding the drug molecule or physically altering the macromolecular characteristics of aggregated drug particles. These technologies include both traditional methods of solubility enhancement such as particle size reduction via comminution or spray drying, addition of surfactants, inclusion in cyclodextrin-drug complexes[Li et al., 1999], and the use of more novel methods such as self-emulsifying systems [Abdalla et al., 2008], micronization via nanoparticles, pH adjustment and salting-in processes [Carstensen, 1989].The amount of active drug dissolved per unit of a solvent or liquid base is a critical parameter subject to many factors including temperature, presence of electrolytes (salting-out effect), complexation with other components, state of crystallinity (such as amorphous), nature of crystals (inclusion or imperfections), hydration, or salvation, and so forth. One of the most important studies conducted on new chemical entities is the solubility characteristics, phase conversion studies, and saturation limits under different conditions [Martin, 2005]. Where the amount of drug is above saturation solubility, equilibrium between the solution (mono-molecular dispersion) is established with un-dissolved particles (often multimolecular dispersions), the direction and extent of which are governed by many physicochemical factors. Because the absorption of drugs takes place only from a monomolecular dispersion (except those instances of pinocytosis, etc.), the equilibrium of the two states is critical to drug absorption. A large number of pH adjusting buffers are used in the liquid products to modify the solubility of drugs as well as to provide the most optimal pH for drug absorption and drug stability. The dielectric constant of the solvent (or composite dispersion phase) is important in determining the solubility. With available values of dielectric constant, for both pure and binary systems, it is easy to project the solubility characteristics of many new drugs.

Another factor determining the solubility of drugs is the *degree of solubilization* in the dispersion phase. *Solubilization* is the process by which the apparent solubility of a poorly water-soluble substance is increased. Solubi-lization techniques include cosolvency, salt formation, prodrug design, complexation, particle size reduction, and the use of surface-active agents (micellization). *Micellization* is defined as spontaneous passage of poorly water-soluble drugs into an aqueous solution of a detergent, the mechanism being entrapment of drug molecules in the micelles of surface-active agent. As a result, many liquid preparations contain surfactants, not only to solubilize but also to "wet" the powders to allow better mixing with liquid phase. Because the critical micelle concentration of surfactants is highly dependent on the presence of other polar or dielectric molecules, the use of surfactants to solubilize drugs requires extensive compatibility studies. The most commonly used solubilizers include polyoxyethylenesorbital fatty acid esters, polyoxyethylenemonoalkyl ethers, sucrose monoesters, lanolin esters and ethers, and so forth.

Many poorly soluble, ionizable drugs can be readily solubilized through salt formation [Agharkar et al., 1976]. Salt forms are regularly selected to serve as self-buffers and enhance the dissolution rates over the cognate conjugate acids and bases by altering pH of the diffusion layer. In fact, salt formation can drastically alter the physicochemical properties of a drug in the solid state, which govern solubility.

Complexation with other components of formulation can give rise to enhanced or reduced solubility [Rasool et al., 1991]. Organic compounds in solution, generally, tend to associate with each other to some extent, but these are weak bonds, and the complex readily disassociates. Where the drug forms a stronger complex, such as with caffeine or other binders, solubility can be extensively altered. Some polyols are known to disrupt complexes, reducing the solubility. Often complexation results in loss of active drug or a preservative used in the system, leading to serious stability problems. Examples of complexation include binding of xanthines, polyvinylpyrrolidone, and others to drugs. The soluble Kollidon products form reversible complexes with many hydrophobic active substances, and clear solutions in water are thus obtained. This may be affected by the molecular weight. The longer the chains or higher the K-value of the Kollidon type are, stronger is the solubility effect, and hence greater the solubility that can be obtained by the active substance. In practice, this effect was mostly exploited for the solubilization of antibiotics in human and veterinary medicine. There are also restrictions on the use of this substance in human parenterals.

Another concept is of **hydrotrophy**, which is defined as an increase in solubility in water caused by the presence of large amounts of additives. It is another type of "solubilization," except that the solubilizing agent is not necessarily a surfactant. The phenomenon is closer to complexation, but the change in solvent characteristics plays a significant role as well [Varagunapandiyan & Gandhi, 2008]. In general, the quantity of other components must be in the range of 20 to 50% to induce hydrotrophy. Sodium salicylate, sodium benzoate, sodium glycinate are few examples of hydrotropic agents. The practical application of hydrotrophy is quite limited in liquid formulations because large amount of additives may be necessary to produce the modest increase in solubility.

Active substances can also be solubilized by Pluronic F-68 (PEO-PPO-PEO triblock copolymer) in addition to the Cremophor and Kollidon products [Rowe et al., 2003; Lin & Kawashima, 1985]. The mechanism is probably based, for the most part, on the principle of hydrophilization. Micelle formation is certainly of minor significance, if it exists at all.

Viscosity

Because the flow of liquid for dispensing and dosing is important, an appropriate control of viscosity is required to prevent the liquid from running and, at the same time, to allow good dosing control. Many thickening agents are available including carboxymethyl cellulose (CMC), methyl cellulose, polyvinylpyrrolidone (PVP), and sugar. Because of the significant opportunities available for interacting with salts and other formulation ingredients, the viscosity control should be studied in the final formulation and over the shelf-life of the product [Ková & Fortelný, 1984].

Particle characteristics

The molecular structure, size and shape of the particles are the most significant characteristics of dispersion. These properties largely depend on chemical and physical nature of the dispersed phase and on the method used to prepare the dispersion. The particle diameter as well as size distribution of the dispersed phase has a profound effect on the properties of the dosage forms, such as appearance, settling rate, stability, re-dispersibility and stability. The particle characteristics can also affect the drug release from the dosage forms that are administered orally.

Variations in lattice energies between amorphous and crystalline forms can significantly influence a drug's aqueous solubility, and increases of several hundredfold were observed for morphine and benzimidazole derivatives [Huang & Tong, 2004]. Furthermore, a substance may exist in more than one crystalline form, such as chloramphenicol, progesterone, sulfathiazole, carbamazepine, cortisone, or prednisolone, to name a few. Polymorphic transformations, routinely observed for pharmaceuticals, are structural differences resulting from different crystal arrangements of molecules in the solid state. Although, thermodynamic differences between polymorphs disappear once dissolved, solid-state disparities in internal crystal structure between polymorphs may yield vastly different physicochemical properties; changes may include melting point, chemical stability, solubility, enthalpy, dissolution rate, and color to name a few.

When suspensions are formulated to provide a stable system, the particle size becomes critical. Flocculated suspensions also require careful particle size control either in the process of manufacturing or in the starting material. Equally important is the crystal habit – the outward appearance of an agglomeration of crystals [Heyd & Dhabar, 1979]. Crystal structure can be altered during the manufacturing process, particularly if the product is subject to temperature cycling, and this can alter the stability of suspensions. Few other particles characteristics to be considered during formulation of suspension have been discussed here in detail.

Aggregation

The aggregation of particles in suspension can be termed aggregation or coagulation. The term 'coagulation' should be used when the forces involved are primarily physical owing to reduction in the repulsive forces at double layer. The term 'flocculation' can be applied to those cases in which weak 'bridging' occurs among the particles. However, since in many pharmaceutical systems the exact nature of the sources is somewhat obscure, we shall restrict ourselves here to term 'aggregation'. By using simple diffusion theory, Von Smoluchowski derived equation for both rapid aggregation (when all particle – particle collisions results in aggregation) and slow aggregation (in which only a fraction of all particle-particle collisions results in aggregation) [Kruyt, 1953]. The pharmaceutical scientists are concerned with slow aggregation, since the aggregation in suspension of drugs is mainly slow. The $t_{1/2}$ time for the initial number of single particles (singlets) in a suspension to decrease by 50% because of aggregation is given by

$$t_{1/2} = \frac{1}{4DRN_0\alpha}$$

where, D is diffusion coefficient of the singlets, R is gas constant, N_0 is initial number of singlets and α is the collision efficiency.

Types of aggregates

The aggregates in a suspension system can be classified according to their morphology. Floccule is an open aggregate system. The structure is rigid and settles quickly to form a high sediment height and is easily redispersible because the particles constituting individual aggregates are sufficiently far apart from one another to preclude caking. A coagule is a closed aggregate formed by surface film bonding. The affinity of surface films for each other is responsible for tenacity of the aggregate not within an individual aggregate, but also surrounding aggregates. Upon sedimentation the aggregates tend to form a single large film bound aggregate, which is difficult, if not impossible to redisperse. The surface films that lead to coagule formation are often surfactants, gases, immiscible liquids and in case of non-aqueous suspensions, water. The third form is dis-aggregated or dispersed form wherein the particles settle as discrete entities. Sedimentation is much slower than the aggregated systems, attains lowest possible sediment height and possesses a high potential for caking.

Crystal growth

The surface free energy for the small particles is greater than for larger particles. In some systems, therefore, small particles will be appreciably more stable than the larger ones. For such systems small fluctuation in the temperature will result in crystal growth as the small particles dissolve with the rise in temperature; and then crystallize at the surface of the existing particles, with a temperature drop. Thus, the larger particles will grow in size at the expense of the smaller particles. The suspension will become coarser as the mean particle size spectrum shift to higher values. Many gums adsorb onto the crystal surfaces and thus can be used to inhibit crystal growth. Freeze – thaw as well as more elevated temperature cycling tests can provide a useful technique for evaluating crystal growth and crystal growth inhibitors.

Sedimentation

The pharmaceutical suspension is destined to settle even though one can slow the processes well within shelf-life times for pharmaceutical products. The rate of settling can be calculated by Stokes' law:

$$v = \frac{2r^2 \Delta \rho g}{9 \eta}$$

where, v = (terminal) velocity, r = radius of the particle, $\Delta \rho$ = the difference in density of the solid dispersed phase and the density of the liquid dispersion medium, g = a constant due to gravity, and η = viscosity of the liquid.

According to Stokes' law the rate of sedimentation can be retarded most effectively by controlling the particle diameter (radius) and viscosity of the medium. However, Stokes' law is applicable only to dilute systems (solid content < 2%). To take into consideration the concentrated systems, Higuchi [1958] developed an equation with fewer limitations. He considered settling phenomenon to be equivalent to movement of liquid medium through the bed of dispersed phase.

Wetting

By definition, a suspension is essentially an incompatible system, but to exist at all, it requires some degree of compatibility, and good wetting of suspended material is important in achieving this. Hydrophobic (lyophobic) solids do not easily get wet with the liquid due to non-existent liquid solid affinity. The liquid has difficulty in displacing the air or other substances surrounding the solids and there exists an *angle of contact* (θ) between liquid and solid. *Angle of*

contact results from an equilibrium involving three interfacial tensions, first at solid and liquid phase interface, second at liquid and vapor phase interface and third at solid and vapor phase interface. These materials are very difficult to disperse and frequently float on the surface of the fluid owing to poor wetting or presence of air pockets.

Hydrophilic solids are, however, readily wet by liquid media, and usually can be incorporated into suspensions without the use of a wetting agent. Surfactants are frequently used as wetting agents. They act by decreasing the solid-liquid interfacial tension. The hydrocarbon chain of a surfactant gets preferentially adsorbed on hydrophobic surface, whereas, polar groups remain directed towards aqueous phase.

Hydrophilic polymers such as sodium CMC, and water insoluble hydrophilic materials such as bentonite, aluminium-magnesium silicates and colloidal silica, either alone or in combination are also used. These agents also have a type and concentration dependent viscosity building effect. At higher concentration they may lead to undesirable gelling effect. A number of techniques are available for selection of wetting agent. Hiestand [1964] suggested use of a narrow lyophobic trough, one end of which holds the solid powder while a solution of the wetting agent is placed in the other end. The relative rate of penetration of different agents can then be directly observed; the better agents show the faster rate. Another technique involves measuring the relative ability of solution of different wetting agents to carry powder through a gauze as the solutions are dropped on to gauze supporting the powder. The better wetters are able to fraction more effectively as vehicles and carry more powder through the gauze than the poor wetters.

The wettability of a solid by non-aqueous solvent can be determined by a few methods developed by paint industry. Methods like wet point method and *flow point method* can be used in pharmaceutical industry as well. '*Wet point method*' measures the amount of vehicle needed to just wet all of the powder. Reduction of wet point by an additive indicates initial surface wetting by that agent in the powder vehicle combination. *Flow point* measures the amount of vehicle needed to produce pourability. The wet point method involves incorporating the additive in the powder by rubbing the mixture on a glass plate with a spatula. The vehicle is then added drop-wise and worked thoroughly through the mass after each addition. The end point is reached when just enough vehicle has been added to form a coherent mass that does not break or separate. The *wet point* is expressed as mL/100 g.

The '*flow point*' is also measured by mixing the additive with the powder but in a beaker rather than on a plate. The vehicle is added and incorporated by thorough mixing. The endpoint is reached when just enough vehicle has been added to permit the mixture to flow from spatula in a uniform stream. The flow point is also expressed as mL/100 g. A similar technique could be applied to aqueous systems. In this analogous method, water is added to a mixture of material to be wetted and various additives to be evaluated.

Emulsification and solubilization

Various pharmaceutical excipients offer several possibilities and mechanisms to solubilize insoluble lipophilic or hydrophobic active substances in an aqueous medium. For micro-emulsions, polyoxyl castor oil derivatives (Cremophor RH 40, Cremophor EL) and poly-ethylene glycol-15-hydroxystearate (Solutol HS 15) act as surface-active solubilizers in water and form the structures of micelles. The micelle that envelops the active substance is so small that it is invisible, or perhaps visible in the form of opalescence. Typical fields of application are oil-soluble vitamins, antimycotics of the miconazole type, mouth disinfectants (e.g., hexiditin), and etherian oils or fragrances. Solutol HS 15 is recommended for parenteral use of this solubilizing system and has been specially developed for this purpose.

The combined effect of various hydrophilic polymers (sodium CMC; HPMC; PVP K30; PEG 6000) and cyclodextrins (ß-cyclodextrin; methyl-ß-CD; HP-ß-CD) on the enhancement of aqueous solubility of naproxen was investigated [Tinwalla et al., 1993]. With regard to the solubilizing effect, the combined use of polymer and CD was always clearly more effective in enhancing the aqueous solubility of Naproxen in comparison with the corresponding drug-polymer or drug-CD binary-systems [Loftsson & Brewster, 1996]. The improvement in solubilizing ability within these water-soluble polymer/drug included CD aggregates requires less CD to solubilize the same amount of drug [Rajewski & Stella, 1996].

Triangular (three-component) phase diagram

A three-component phase diagram has four degrees of freedom: F = 3 − 1 + 2 = 4. These systems are used for determining miscibility/solubility, coacervation regions, gel-forming regions for multicomponent mixtures, etc. To read a 3-phase diagram, each of the three corners of the triangle represent 100% by weight of one of the components and 0% by weight of the other two. If two of the components are known, the third is known by difference. Any combination of the three components is described by a single point on the diagram. Combining different proportions of the three components and observing for an end point (solubility, gel-formation, haziness, etc.), the phase differences can be visualized.

In addition to observing the phase changes in a single plane, the use of stacked ternary phase diagrams enables one to visualize the change using different ratios of one of the components. Constructions like this enable a pharmaceutical scientist to select the best ratios and combi-nations of components for a formulation.

Preservation

Preservatives are an essential part of liquid formulations unless there is sufficient preservative efficacy in the formulation itself, such as due to high sugar content, presence of antimicrobial drugs, or solvents that inhibit growth such as alcohol. An ideal preservative should have a broad spectrum of activity, physical, chemical and microbiological stability, and physiological compatibility. None of the existing preservative satisfies all these requirements and frequently a combination of two or more preservatives is used to achieve the desired antimicrobial effect. In all instances a preservative efficacy challenge is needed to prove adequate protection against the growth of microorganisms during the shelf-life and use of the product (such as in the case of reconstituted powder suspensions).

A large number of approved preservatives are available, including such universal preservatives as parabens, to protect liquid preparations. The admissible levels of preservatives are defined in the Pharmacopoeias. It should be noted that although preservatives provide an essential function, they often cause an unpleasant taste and allergic reactions in some individuals, requiring proper labelling of all products containing preservatives [Zhang et al., 1990].

Appearance and palatability

Although, most drug substances in use today are unpalatable and unattractive in their natural state, their preparations are presented to the patient as colorful, flavorful formulations attractive to the sight, smell, and taste. These qualities, which are the rule rather than the exception, have virtually eliminated the natural reluctance of many patients to take medications exclusively because of disagreeable odor or taste.

There is some psychologic basis to drug therapy, and the odor, taste, and color of a pharmaceutical preparation can play a part. An appropriate drug has its most beneficial effect, when it is accepted and taken properly by the patient. The proper combination of flavor, fragrance, and color in a pharmaceutical product contributes to its acceptance.

The appearance or color of liquid products is often synchronized with the flavors used; for example, green or blue for mint, red for berry, and so forth. Because the amount of dyestuffs allowed in pharmaceutical products is strongly regulated, this presents problems – especially where there is a need to mask features of a preparation. In some instances, solutions are made to "sparkle" by passing them through a filtration process. Often, adsorbents are used in the liquid preparations to remove fine particles, imparting a greater clarity to solutions. Filtration often presents problems, but with the help now available from major filter manufacturers, most problems can be readily solved.

Drugs that are bitter or otherwise unpalatable and administered as oral liquids may be unacceptable, particularly to younger patients. Compliance and therefore efficacy may be compromised unless the product can be made more palatable. Thus, sweeteners, flavors, or taste-masking agents may be present in liquid oral products, in chewable dosage forms, and in effervescent or dispersible tablets that are constituted as liquids prior to use [Roy, 1994].

Finished drug product stability

Drug substances are generally more susceptible to degradation in liquids than in solid dosage forms. As a class of formulations, oral liquids are more complex in composition than parenterals, and more interactions may occur affecting the stability of the product. It is necessary to not only consider the solution stability of the drug, but also the stability of excipients such as colorants, flavors, preservatives, solubilizers, thickening agents, and sweetening agents.

The techniques for predicting the chemical stability of homogeneous drug systems are well defined [Streng 1985; Cartensen 2000]. The formulation chemist should consider both the Ph solubility profile and the pH-stability profile when selecting the optimum pH for formulation of the liquid oral dosage form. Physical instability of liquid formulations involves the formation of precipitates, less-soluble poly-morphs, adsorption of the drug substances onto container surfaces, microbial growth, and changes in product appearance [Shami et al., 1972]. Evaluation of product acceptability is subjective and includes properties such as color, odor, taste, and clarity.

According to the ICH (International Conference on Harmonisation of Technical Requirements for Registration of Pharmaceuticals for Human Use) Guideline for the stability testing, the design of the formal stability studies for the drug product should be based on knowledge of the behavior and properties of the drug substance, results from stability studies on the drug substance, and experience gained from clinical formulation studies. The likely changes on storage and the rationale for the selection of attributes to be tested in the formal stability studies should be stated. Photo-stability testing should be conducted on at least one primary batch of the drug product, if appropriate. Data from stability studies should be provided on atleast three primary batches of the drug product. The primary batches should be of the same formulation and be packaged in the same container closure system proposed for marketing. The manu-facturing process used for primary batches should simulate the process that will be applied to production batches and should provide product that is of the same quality and that meets the same specification as that intended for marketing. Two of the three batches should be at least pilot scale batches; the third one can be smaller, if justified. Where possible, batches of the drug product should be manufactured using different batches of the drug substance. Stability studies should be performed on each individual strength and container size of the drug product

unless bracketing or matrixing are applied. Other supporting data can be provided.

Stability testing should be conducted on the dosage form packaged in the container closure system proposed for marketing (including, as appropriate, any secondary packaging and container label). Any available studies carried out on the drug product outside its immediate container or in other packaging materials can form a useful part of the stress testing of the dosage form or can be considered as supporting information, respectively.

Stability studies should include testing of those attributes of the drug product that are susceptible to change during storage and that are likely to influence quality, safety, or efficacy. The testing should cover, as appropriate, the physical, chemical, biological, and microbiological attributes; preservative content (e.g., antioxidant, antimicrobial preservative); and functionality tests (e.g., for a dose delivery system). Analytical procedures should be fully validated and indicating stability. Whether and to what extent replication should be performed will depend on the results of validation studies. Shelf-life accep-tance criteria should be derived from consi-deration of all available stability information. It may be appropriate to have justifiable differences between the shelf life and the release acceptance criteria based on the stability evaluation and the changes observed on storage. Any differences between the release and shelf-life acceptance criteria for antimicrobial preservative content should be supported by a validated correlation of chemical content and preservative effective-ness demonstrated during drug development on the product in its final formulation (except for preservative concentration) intended for marketing.

Stability studies are necessary to support the storage and shipment of the drug product. These studies are done on packaged as well as on unpackaged drug products. Typically, two types of studies are conducted: *Thermal studies* are done for all products by exposing the drug products to a few temperature cycles (i.e., conducting three cycles where each cycle includes drug products stored at 40°C for 4 days and at 25°C for 3 days). *Freeze-thaw studies* are done especially for liquid products by exposing the drug products to a few temperature cycles (i.e., conducting 3 cycles where each cycle includes drug products stored at –10 to –20°C for 4 days and at 25°C/ambient RH for 3 days).

A single primary stability batch of the drug product should be tested for antimicrobial preservative effectiveness (in addition to preservative content) at the proposed shelf-life for verification purposes, regardless of whether there is a difference between the release and shelf-life acceptance criteria for preservative content.

For long-term studies, frequency of testing should be sufficient to establish the stability profile of the drug product. For products with a proposed shelf-life of at least 12 months, the frequency of testing at the long-term storage condition should normally be every 3 months over the first year, every 6 months over the second year, and annually thereafter during the proposed shelf-life.

At the accelerated storage condition, a minimum of three time points, including the initial and final time points (e.g., 0, 3, and 6 months), from a 6-month study is recommended. Where an expectation (based on development experience) exists that results from accelerated testing are likely to approach significant change criteria, increased testing should be conducted either by adding samples at the final time point or by including a fourth time point in the study design.

When testing at the intermediate storage condition is called for as a result of significant change at the accelerated storage condition, a minimum of four time points, including the initial and final time points (e.g., 0, 6, 9, and12 months) from a 12-month study is recommended. Reduced designs (i.e., matrixing or bracketing), in which the testing frequency is reduced or certain factor combinations are not

tested at all, can be applied if justified. In general, a drug product should be evaluated under storage conditions (with appropriate tolerances) that test its thermal stability and, if applicable, its sensitivity to moisture or potential for solvent loss. The storage conditions and the lengths of studies chosen should be sufficient to cover storage, shipment, and subsequent use. Stability testing of the drug product after constitution or dilution, if applicable, should be conducted to provide information for the labelling on the preparation, storage condition, and in-use period of the constituted or diluted product. This testing should be performed on the constituted or diluted product through the proposed in-use period on primary batches as part of the formal stability studies at initial and final time points; and in case of full shelf-life, long-term data will not be available before submission, at 12 months or at the last time point for which data will be available. In general, this testing need not be repeated on commitment batches.

The long-term testing should cover a minimum of 12 months duration on at least three primary batches at the time of submission and should be continued for a period of time sufficient to cover the proposed shelf-life. Additional data accumulated during the assessment period of the registration application should be submitted to the authorities if requested. Data from the accelerated storage condition and, if appropriate, from the intermediate storage condition can be used to evaluate the effect of short-term excursions outside the label storage conditions (such as might occur during shipping).

Physically stable liquid products are supposed to retain their color, viscosity, clarity, taste, and odor throughout the shelf-life; however, the limits of the specifications for physical attributes are often kept flexible to allow for subjective evaluation criteria often involved and for inevitable, inconsequential, changes in the physical characteristics of these products. Ideally, a freshly prepared product is used as the reference standard; alternately, many companies develop more objective evaluation criteria using instrumental evaluation instead of subjective evaluation. Similar to chemical stability, physical stability can be significantly altered by the packaging type and design; as a result, the New Drug Application (NDA) for every product requires a package interaction description; obviously, final stability data are to be developed in the final package form. Although, glass bottles are fairly resistant to many products, caps and liners are often not. Even the integrity of the caps needs to be evaluated, applying exact torque in closing the bottles intended for stability evaluation; this is important to prevent any cap breakage that might adversely affect stability.

Packaging

Oral liquids may be supplied in multiple dose or single dose containers. Oral emulsions and suspensions should be packed in bottles sufficiently wide-mouthed to facilitate the flow of the contents. They are administered either in volumes such as 5 mL, or multiples of 5 mL, or in small volumes (drops). Each dose of a multiple dose oral liquid is administered by means of a suitable measuring device (usually a dropper) that is usually provided with the container.

Filling of liquid products is governed by their viscosity, surface tension, foam-producing, and compatibility with filling machine components. Liquids are often filled at a higher temperature to allow better flow. In most instances, some type of piston filling and delivery is used to fill bottles, for which proper control of volume is required. The filling can be done on the basis of fixed volume or on the level of fill in the container. The filling can be accomplished through positive pressure or through a vacuum created in the container. If the latter is used, care should be taken not to lose any volatile components through the vacuum process; proper validation is required. Liquid product exposed to environment should be protected and filled under a laminar flow hood where possible. All points

of contact of product to the environment should be similarly protected; however, once the product has been filled and capped, the bottles can be safely taken to an uncontrolled environment. In most instances, either plastic or aluminium caps are applied to bottles. The liners used in the caps should demonstrate full compatibility with the product, including any adhesive used. Proper torque should be applied to ensure a tight seal. Pilfer-evident packaging, where used, must comply with the regulatory requirements.

It is not uncommon for syrups to crystallize out at the edge of the bottles, which the consumer might think a defect. Efforts should be made to formulate products to avoid this type of crystallization; use of sugar-free formulations is becoming more acceptable and offers a good alternate. However, taste masking without using sugar or liquid glucose remains a challenge. Stability testing in final packaged containers should include trial shipment runs as well to ensure that the caps do not come off or leak during the shipment [Indian Pharmacopoeia, 2014].

Storage

Liquids or powders and granules for the preparation of oral liquids should be stored in well-closed containers at temperatures not exceeding 30°C [Indian Pharmacopoeia, 2014].

Labelling

For oral liquids that are supplied as drops, the label states the number of drops per gram of preparation if the dose is stated in drops or the number of drops per milliliter of preparation if the dose is stated in volume. For oral liquids supplied as granules or powder to be constituted before use, the label states that (1) the contents are meant for preparation of an oral liquid; (2) the directions for preparing the oral liquid including the nature and quantity of the liquid to be used; (3) the conditions under which the constituted solution should be stored; (4) the period during which the constituted oral liquid may be expected to remain satisfactory for use when prepared and stored in accordance with the manufacturer's recommendations; and (5) the strength in terms of the active ingredient(s) in a suitable dose-volume of the constituted preparation [Indian Pharmacopoeia, 2014].

Personalized medicines: Needs and approaches

Pharmacists can handle liquid preparations in one of three ways: they may dispense the product in its original container; they may buy the product in bulk and repackage it at the time of dispensation; or they may compound a formulation. Compounding may involve nothing more than mixing two marketed products in the manner indicated on the prescription or may require the incorporation of an active ingredient in a logical and pharmaceutically acceptable manner into aqueous or non-aqueous solvent forming the bulk of the product. Most prescriptions today are dispensed in their original containers. In these cases, the pharmacist depends on the manufacturer to provide a product that is efficacious, pharmaceutically acceptable, and stable when stored under recommended conditions.

Increasing knowledge into personalized medicine has demonstrated the need for individual dosing. Paediatric and geriatric drug delivery also need individualized dosing, patient adapted drug formulations and delivery devices [Breitkreutz & Boos, 2007]. Further, some drugs with small therapeutic windows need precise dosage adjustments. It is obvious that suitable dosage forms are urgently needed enabling the selection and application of individual doses to transfer fundamental knowledge on personalized medicine into daily medical practice. In the best case these dosage forms should be suitable for the complete patient population, starting from young children to the elderly [Standing & Tuleu, 2005; Kearns et al., 2003; Stegemann et al., 2010].

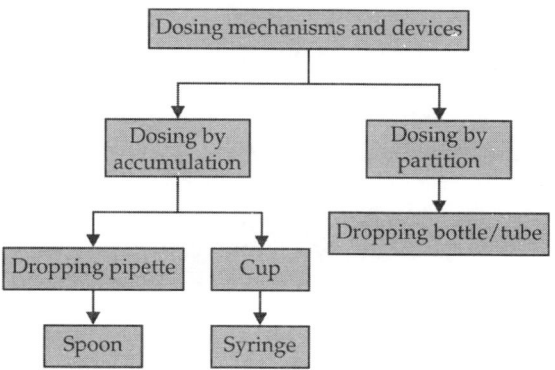

Fig. 2.1. Dosing mechanism and devices under personalized medicine approach.

Liquid drug formulations for oral drug administration are available as solutions, syrups, emulsions or suspensions. Homogeneous liquids like solutions or syrups with completely dissolved APIs show advantages over emulsions and suspensions as they ensure uniform doses when withdrawing single doses out off a multi-dose container. Single-dose containers for oral liquid medications could be sachets or stick-packs, but they are currently not available on the market. Therefore, for accumulating dosing approaches, only dropping bottles and tubes can be considered useful for current need. Partition dosing approaches require measuring or counting tools. It can be distinguished between tools, which are part of the primary packaging such as dropper inlets or dropping tubes and separate dosing devices like dosing spoons, cups, dropping pipettes and oral syringes.

Dosing by accumulation

A dropper inlet in a multi-dose container enables the counting of individual drops from the liquid formulation. Oral droppers may especially useful to administer very small volumes of oral liquids to very young children. Counting errors are a major problem in dosing from dropping bottles. Moreover, adhering to the provided instructions how to hold the package is very important for dose accuracy and consistency [Brown et al.,

2004]. Some bottles must be used vertically, others in a defined angle, e.g. 45°, to ensure the correct volumes of drops and the dosing of the API. Recently introduced dropping tubes ensure higher dose homogeneity as they are designed to deliver precise doses independently from the position or angle of the package during dropping. This is particularly recommended for potent drugs with elevated toxicity risks such as codeine or morphine.

Dosing devices

Dosing devices may be provided with the package or separately purchased. Typical target dose volumes are ≤ 5 mL for children under 5 years and ≤ 10 mL for those of 5 years and older. For liquid dosage forms that require administration with a measuring device, it is important that graduations on the dosing device are clearly visible (e.g. embossed or printed) to enable accurate and precise dosing. In a recently published survey [Griessmann et al., 2007] it became evident that the accomplished dosing devices like dosing spoons and cups are inappropriate to measure correct doses, but oral syringes are much more precise. Graduated dosing cups may be an alternative to dosing spoons or oral syringes, especially if volumes larger than 5 mL are required to be administrated, as they avoid multiple dosing operations.

Dosing cups and spoons are cheap in production, but offers minor dosing flexibility. Dropping pipettes, dropping bottles or tubes and oral syringes are also cheap in production but offer high dose flexibility and are therefore considered more accurate. Out of all available modern dosing options, oral syringes are considered as the best dosing devices. Currently, there is a definite need for the development of novel dosage forms and delivery devices for oral individual drug therapy. Various approaches have been proposed, predominantly in patent literature, but did not reach the market most probably due to financial reasons.

RAW MATERIAL

Raw material specifications are more important in liquid products, as the contaminants can adversely affect the formulation more than in solid dosage form. Also, many features of a liquid product are controlled by including several raw materials such as sweeteners, thickening agents, and so forth; further complicating the matrixing of formulation at the development stage. The microbial quality of raw materials (both solid and liquid) needs to be critically evaluated. It is noteworthy that several raw materials used in liquid products may fall into the "food" category, and even though one is purchasing pharmaceutical-grade material, newly enacted laws in the United States require all foreign manufacturers to make a complete declaration of the composition of materials. Companies are encouraged to revise their specifications based on this additional information, to control the quality of raw materials more tightly.

Vehicles

Aqueous vehicles

Water is the most preferred vehicle because of its lack of toxicity, physiological compatibility and ability to dissolve a wide range of solutes. Potable water is the most economic option. The dissolved salts in potable water, however, may sometimes be undesirable, and lead to incompatibilities with active principals. In these instances purified water is preferred over potable water. Purified water is prepared mainly by techniques such as distillation and ion-exchange. Distillation stills in various shapes and styles are available in a wide capacity range. In ion-exchange method, water is passed through a column of cation- and anion-exchangers. Water obtained in this manner is called de-ionized or de-mineralized water.

Efforts should be made to provide as much microbial-free water as possible; this can be readily achieved by installing a loop system in which the incoming water is first subjected to ultraviolet sterilizer, carbon filter, demineralizer, and a 5-μm filter, and then sent to a heated tank, from where it is passed again through an ultraviolet sterilizer and then a 0.22-μm filter before bringing it into the product; water coming out of the 5-μm filter can be circulated. When using a loop, it is important to establish methods for draining the dead water in the tap and the loop before using it. It must be insured that the flow rate of water does not exceed the sterilizing capacity of the ultraviolet systems installed.

Ion-exchange resins used in the water systems are important for successful maintenance of low bacterial counts. An appropriate example of the mixed resin bed would be Ambergard XE 352 (Rohm & Hass Company) and Amberlite IR-120 (Sigma-Aldrich). The former is a large pore, microreticular, Type 1 quaternary ammonium ion-exchange resin. It is effective for a wide- range of flow rates and for many different bacterial strains. IR-120 is a strongly acidic, cation-exchange resin that balances the chemical equilibrium of the water.

Non-aqueous vehicles

Sometimes it may not be possible to keep the ingredients in aqueous solutions at all temperatures or stability may also be a problem. The use of non-aqueous solvents becomes unavoidable in such situations.

Alcohol and polyhydric alcohols

Ethyl alcohol is the most widely used solvent particularly for external preparations where its rapid evaporation after application gives cooling effect on skin. Industrial methylated spirit contains 5% of methyl alcohol as a denaturant, which makes it too toxic for internal use. Ethanol is used only at lower concentrations as co-solvent with water, orally or parenterally, because of its toxicity.

Polyhydric alcohols like glycols (two OH groups) are rarely used internally due to their toxicity; propylene glycol (CH_3–$CH.OH$–CH_2–

Table 2.2. Some commonly used solvents	
• Purified water	• Water for injection
• Alcohol	• Sterile water for injection
• Glycerin	
• Isopropyl alcohol	• Sterile water for irrigation
• Acacia syrup	
• Aromatic elixir	• Oleic acid
• Aromatic syrup	• Peanut oil
• Cherry syrup	• Corn oil
• Cocoa syrup	• Cottonseed oil
• Orange syrup	• Mineral oil
• Syrup	• Sesame oil

OH) is an exception that is used as a co-solvent with water or glycol. Glycerol, a trihydroxy alcohol, is widely used as a co-solvent with water for oral use.

Other vehicles

Besides commonly used aqueous and non-aqueous vehicles, certain preformulated vehicles can also be used directly in formulation of liquid dosage forms. These include simple syrup, cherry syrup, Ora-Sweet[TM] (Sucrose with glycerin and sorbitol), Ora-Plus[TM] (Purified water, microcrystalline cellulose, sodium CMC, xanthan gum and carrageenan), sorbitol, glycerin and liquid glucose etc. These vehicles can be used in a concentration range of 2–100% according to desired properties of formulations. The vehicles should comply with the reference standard specifications as well as in-house specifications.

Surface-active agents

This part is very crucial in the formulation and product development of all liquid dosage forms. The materials commonly used as surface-active agents can be divided into three categories: naturally occurring and semi synthetic, finely divided solids, and surfactants. In each category, different stabilizing mechanisms are taken advantage of in order to reduce interfacial tension between two phases or to achieve a stable system.

Naturally occurring materials, called hydrophilic colloids, are used to impart viscosity to suspension, solution and to stabilize emulsions i.e. formation of oil in water (o/w) type emulsions. They include polysaccharides (e.g., acacia, tragacanth, agar, pectin, and alginates) and proteins (e.g., gelatin and casein).

Finely divided solid particles have got application mainly in formulation of stable emulsions by preferentially wetting one of the phases. As more solid particles are lodged at the interface, they adhere strongly to each other, forming a stable film at the surface. Examples include clays (e.g., bentonite and magnesium aluminum silicate), colloidal silicone dioxide, aluminum hydroxide, magnesium hydroxide, and carbon black. When clays and aluminum and magnesium hydroxides are preferentially wetted by water, the contact angle is less than 90°, and o/w type emulsions are formed. The most effective wetting liquid makes up the continuous phase, which is dependent on the volume ratio of the two liquids. For example, bentonite forms water in oil (w/o) type emulsions when the oil phase volume is much greater than the aqueous phase.

In surfactant molecules there are two regions (i.e., hydrophilic and hydrophobic). Surfactants are classified into four main categories depending on the nature of the charge carried by the hydrophilic part of the surfactant: anionic, cationic, nonionic, and ampholytic surfactants. Some common examples of surfactants are listed in Table 2.3.

Anionic surfactants are negatively charged in an aqueous solution (i.e., $-COO-$) and widely used because of their economy and performance. Sodium lauryl sulfate, the main component of which is sodium dodecyl sulfate, is highly soluble in water and is commonly used to form o/w emulsions. Reacting an alkali hydroxide with a fatty acid (e.g., oleic acid) can produce alkali metal soaps (e.g., sodium oleate). Careful attention must be paid to the pH of the dispersion medium and the presence of multivalent metals.

Alkali earth metal soaps like calcium oleate produce stable w/o emulsions because of their low water solubility and are produced by reacting oleic acid with calcium hydroxide. Triethanolamine stearate produces stable o/w emulsions *in situ* by reacting triethanolamine in aqueous solution with melted stearic acid at approximately 65°C (e.g., vanishing cream).

Cationic surfactants are positively charged in an aqueous solution (e.g., quaternary ammonium and pyridinium) but are relatively expensive. Because of their bactericidal action, they are widely used for other applications such as preservatives, sterilizing contaminated surfaces, and emulsions.

Non-ionic surfactants consist of a $-(CH_2CH_2O)_nOH$ or $-OH$ as the hydrophilic group and exhibit a variety of hydrophile-lipophile balance (HLB), which stabilize o/w or w/o emulsions. Unlike anionic and cationic surfactants, nonionic surfactants are useful for oral and parenteral formulations because of their low irritation and toxicity. Based on their neutral nature, they are much less sensitive to changes in the pH of the medium and the presence of electrolytes. The best use of nonionic surfactants is to produce an equally balanced HLB of two nonionic surfactants; blend of one hydrophilic and another hydrophobic.

Sorbitan esters (Spans) are the products of the esterification of a sorbitan with a fatty acid. Their hydrophobicity is attributed to the hydroxyl groups of the saturated cyclic ring. They are not soluble in water and used for w/o type emulsions. Polysorbates (Tweens), on the other hand, are soluble in water since the hydroxyl groups of the sorbitan esters adduct a number of ethylene oxides. They are hence used as emulsifying agents for o/w emulsions. In general, both sorbitan esters and polysorbates are used in conjunction to produce a wide range of emulsions. Fatty alcohol polyoxyethylene ethers are condensation products of fatty alcohols with polyethylene glycol, while fatty acid poly-oxyethylene esters are esterification products of

Table 2.3. List of common surface-active agents

Generic name	Brand name	Specifications
Sugar ester, pharma and cosmetic grade	Surfhope D-1616	Non-ionic esters of palmitic acid with sucrose, dispersion and solubilization aid for microemulsions; HLB = 16
Macrogolcetostearyl ether	Simulsol 68 PHA	Polyoxyethylatedcetylstearyl alcohol, hydrophilic surfactant; HLB = 16
Macrogol lauryl ether	Simulsol P 4 PHA	Polyoxyethylated lauryl alcohol, lipophilic surfactant, practically insoluble in water; HLB = 9.7
Macrogol lauryl ether	Simulsol P 23 PHA	Polyoxyethylated lauryl alcohol, hydrophilic surfactant, soluble in water; HLB = 16.9
Macrogololeyl ether	Simulsol 98 PHA	Polyoxyethylatedoleyl alcohol, hydrophilic surfactant, soluble in water; HLB = 15.3
Macrogol glycerol ricinoleate	Simulsol 1285 PHA	Polyoxyl 50 castor oil, solubilizer, co-emulsifier, soluble in water; HLB = 13
Macrogol glycerol hydroxystearate	Simulsol 1292 PHA	Polyoxyl 25 hydrogenated castor oil, solubilizer, co-emulsifier, soluble in water; HLB = 11
Polysorbate 20	Montanox 20	Polyoxyethylatedsorbitanmonolaurate, hydrophilic solubilizer/emulsifier; HLB = 16.7
Polysorbate 60	Montanox 60 PHA	Polyoxyethylatedsorbitanmonostearate, hydrophilic solubilizer/emulsifier; HLB = 14.9
Polysorbate 80	Montanox 80 PHA	Polyoxyethylatedsorbitanmonooleate, hydrophilic solubilizer; HLB = 15
Polysorbate 80	Montanox 80 VG PHA	Polyoxyethylatedsorbitanmonooleate, hydrophilic solubilizer; vegetable origin; HLB = 15.0
Polysorbate 80	Montanox 80 VG DF PPI	Polyoxyethylatedsorbitanmonooleate, hydrophilic solubilizer; vegetable origin, injectable grade; HLB = 15
Sorbitan monolaurate	Montane 20 PHA	Ester of lauric acid and sorbitan; lipophilic emulsifier; HLB = 8.6
Sorbitan monooleate	Montane 80 PHA	Ester of oleic acid and sorbitan; lipophilic emulsifier; HLB = 4.3
Sorbitan trioleate	Montane 85 VG PHA	Triester of oleic acid and sorbitan; lipophilic emulsifier; vegetable origin; HLB = 1.8
Stearoyl macrogol glycerides	Simulsol 165 PHA	PEG-100 stearate and glyceryl stearate; non-ionic, self-emulsifying wax, for use in o/w emulsions; HLB = 11
Alkyl polyglucoside	Montanov 68 PHA	Glucolipid o/w emulsifier, derived entirely from vegetable raw materials

fatty acids with polyethylene glycol. They are soluble in water and used in conjunction with auxiliary emulsifying agents (e.g., cetyl and stearyl alcohols) to give o/w emulsions.

Ampholytic surfactants possess both cationic and anionic groups in the same molecule and are dependent on the pH of the medium. *n-*Dodecyldimethylbetaine and Lecithin are two classical examples.

The selection of a suitable surfactant in right concentration is important. This is because the addition of surfactant to drug systems can, in some instances, enhance the GI absorption and pharmacological activity while inhibit the same in other circumstances. The activity of several preservatives has been found to decrease significantly in the presence of a number of surfactants.

To ensure that optimum concentration of surfactant is chosen, a known weight or volume of surfactant is added to each vial containing solvent. Ensuring adequate temperature control, varying amounts of solubilizates are added to each vial in ascending order of concentration. The maximum concentration of drug, which will form a clear solution with a given concentration of surfactant, can be determined visually or by optical density measurement, and is known as *maximum additive concentration* (MAC). The method is repeated using different amounts of surfactants. A graph then can be constructed of MAC against surfactant concentration, from which optimum amount of solubilizing agent can be chosen for any required amount of drug. The study can be done for several surfactants of interest and most appropriate one can be selected.

Preservatives

Liquid oral preparations are the most likely of all non-sterile pharmaceutical products to be contaminated by microorganisms. Most of these preparations are marketed in a multidose form, enhancing the risk of exposure to microbes upon repeat dosing. The inclusion of sugars and other excipients only enriches the preparation with growth-supporting substrates. The manufacturing process also may contribute to possible microbiological contamination. Therefore, it is essential that liquid preparations be protected against microbiological deterioration by adequate preservation.

Preservatives must fulfill certain criteria for acceptability. The major factors are those of safety and lack of toxicity after oral intake, particularly because liquid medications are often administered to children and the elderly. The literature is replete with reports of various allergic-type reactions to preservatives (parabens, chlorocresol), antioxidants (propyl gallate, metabisulphite), surfactants and solvents [Smith & Dodd, 1982].

There are four major classes of preservatives; acidic, neutral, mercurial and quaternary ammonium compounds. The last three classes find little value in oral liquids but are widely used in ophthalmic, nasal, and parenteral products. Among the acidic group, the most prominent preservatives are phenol, chlorocresol, *o*-phenyl phenol, alkyl esters of *p*-hydroxybenzoic acid, benzoic acid and its salts, boric acid and its salts, and sorbic acid and its salts; neutral preservatives include chlorbutanol, benzyl alcohol, and β-phenylethyl alcohol; mercurial preservatives include thiomersal, phenylmercuric acetate, and nitrate; and nitromersol and quaternary compounds include benzalkonium chloride and cetylpyridinium chloride.

Phenols, due to their characteristic odor and instability in presence of oxygen, are of little use in oral preparations. *p*-Hydroxy benzoic acid esters and salts of benzoic acid and sorbic acid have adequate water solubility and posses both antibacterial and antifungal activity. Frequently, combinations of two or more esters of *p*-hydroxy benzoic acid are used to achieve the desired antimicrobiological effect. Methyl and propyl parabens, for instance, are used in ratio 10 : 1, respectively. Parabens (*p*-hydroxybenzoates) are effective over a wide pH range but are more active in acidic conditions (pH 4–5). Various combinations of methyl and propyl hydroxybenzoate are used to give a total concentration of about 0.1% w/v. Mercurials and quaternary ammonium compounds are subject to a variety of incompatibilities; mercurials are readily reduced to free mercury whereas quaternary compounds are inactivated by a variety of anionic substances. Molecular reactions involving preservatives and commonly used pharmaceutical adjuvants have been observed. For example, it has been shown that Tween 80 interacts to a significant extent with methyl- and propyl-parabens and this preservative-surfactant complex is essentially deprived of any antibacterial activity. A few adverse effects of the preservatives are also documented. The link between benzyl alcohol and neonatal cardiovascular collapse, gasping baby syndrome, is perhaps the most widely publicized adverse reaction related to the use of inert ingredients [Barr & Tice, 1957].

Antimicrobial preservatives

Emulsions are especially prone to attack by fungi and yeasts. Microbial contamination leads not only to pathogenic hazard but also to instability of the preparation. Additives such as polypeptides, carbohydrates, sterols and some surfactants support growth of many types of microorganisms. Commonly used preservatives include quaternary ammonium compounds (benzalkonium chloride and benzathonium chloride) benzoic acid, phenyl mercuric nitrate, phenyl mercuric acetate, parabens etc. Selection of an antimicrobial is a critical step. Generally, a combination of preservatives, one soluble in aqueous phase and the other soluble in oil phase is more effective [Sznitowska et al., 2002]. A combination of water-soluble methyl parabens and oil-soluble propyl parabens constitutes a good example. Another concern during selection is possibility of antimicrobial agent and other ingredient interaction. Parabens, the most widely used antimicrobials in emulsions, get bound to a variety of emulsifying agents. The bound parabens are not available for antimicrobial action. Phenolic preservatives are particularly susceptible to interaction with compounds containing polyoxyethylene groups. Antimicrobial agents may get entrapped into surfactant micelles, which make them less effective.

Complexing agents

There are many types of complexing agents and a partial list can be found in Table 2.4. Complexation relies on relatively weak forces such as London forces, hydrogen bonding and hydrophobic interactions. As the concentration of complexing agent is increased, so is the solubility, up to a point. In some cases, however, the complex can precipitate off solution as the concentration of complexing agent is increased.

Table 2.4. List of common complexing agents

Type	Example
Inorganic	Alkaline metal hydroxide with ammonia
Coordination	Hexaminecobalt(III) chloride
Chelates	EDTA, Ethylene glycol tetra-acetic acid (EGTA)
Metal-olefin	Ferrocene
Inclusion	Choleic acid, cyclodextrins
Molecular complexes	Polymers

Sweetening agents

Sweeteners are indispensable components of many liquid oral dosage forms, especially those containing bitter or other unacceptable tastes. In fact, sweetening agents may comprise large portions of solid content in most liquid oral dosage forms. Sweeteners are often classified as either nutritive (caloric) or non-nutritive (non-caloric). Non-caloric sweetening agents are preferred for diabetic patients, as ingestion does cause increases in systemic glucose concentrations. Some of the most commonly used sweeteners include sucrose, sorbitol, mannitol, liquid glucose, honey molasses, saccharin, Aspartame, Sucralose, and Acesulphame-K.

Sucrose is the most widely used sweetening agent. It is frequently used in conjunction with sorbitol, glycerin and other polyols, which are said to reduce the tendency of sucrose to crystallize out. One of the manifestations of sucrose crystallization is 'cap-locking', which occurs when the product crystallizes on the threads of the bottle and interferes in cap removal.

Artificial sweeteners can be used both in conjunction with sugars and alcohols to enhance the degree of sweetness or on their own in formulation for patients who must restrict their sugar intake. They are also termed as intense sweeteners because they are hundreds, even thousands of times sweeter than sucrose and therefore rarely required at a concentration greater than about 0.2% [Mortensen, 2006].

Saccharin (Sweet'N Low®) was discovered in 1879, and is currently produced from a purified compound found in coal tar. Saccharin is approximately 250 to 500 times sweeter than sugar, but it can have a bitter aftertaste and therefore is normally formulated with sugar. Sodium and calcium salts of saccharin are the most widely used artificial sweeteners. They exhibit high water solubility and are chemically and physically stable over a wide pH range. Saccharin is not metabolized in the digestive tract and is excreted rapidly in the urine. As a result, saccharin does not contribute calories to the diet.

Artificial sweetener, saccharin, is widely used in foods and pharmaceuticals. It is sweet at very low concentrations (equivalent to about 5–10% sugar) but bitter at higher concentrations. Approximately 20% of the population is 'saccharin sensitive'; that is, they perceive saccharin to be bitter even at low concentrations. The artificial sweeteners, Cyclamate and Aspartame, are about 30–200 times as sweet as sugar, but like saccharin, their sweet-bitter profiles are concentration dependent. Aspartame does not have a significant bitter aftertaste when compared to saccharin and has gained in popularity. Monoammoniumglycyrrhizinate has a lingering sweet aftertaste, which can be exploited for taste-masking products with a mildly bitter aftertaste. It is also effective in enhancing chocolate flavor.

Stevia is a South American herb used as a natural sweetener for centuries. The leaves of the *Stevia rebaudiana* plant have a refreshing taste, zero glycemic index and zero calories. It is 200 times sweeter than sugar, and far healthier. Few studies suggest the beneficial effects of stevia in people with hypertension and Type 2 diabetes, but more research is needed to give concluding remarks.

Glycerin is commonly used for its solvent effect on many compounds, as well as its humectant effect. Glycerin is seldom used as a single sweetener in pharmaceuticals because it has a characteristic mouthwarming and burning effect. Some commonly employed sweetening agents in pharmaceutical industry with their important characteristics have been enlisted in Table 2.5.

The choice of incorporation of sweeteners should be made very wisely after considering various adversities associated with each one of them. Sucrose is a very effective sweetener, particularly for liquids dosed to children. Its propensity to cause dental caries and the complications it poses in the management of diabetes may have contributed to its progressive elimination from medicinal products despite its continuing widespread use in foods and confectionery. Sorbitol is another excellent sweetening agent and has been used as a replacement for sucrose in oral liquid products. It has the propensity to cause diarrhea and flatulence, although the effect may only be manifest at high doses. However, there may be additive effects (e.g., if it is formulated with active ingredients that are also associated with GI intolerance, such as antibiotics).

Cyclamate was banned in the United States following reports of carcinogenicity and withdrawal of generally regarded as safe (GRAS) status in 1969. It remains banned despite additional studies to clarify safety and attempts at reinstatement. It remains acceptable in Europe. Saccharin is equally controversial. It also is suspected as being a carcinogen due to cyclohexylamine formation, possibly by gut flora, on ingestion. It was banned as a food additive by the Food and Drug Administration (FDA) in 1977, but has remained available consequent to regular congressional moratoria on the proposed ban. It is not permitted in Canada except for diabetic beverages and foods [Pinco, 1991; Smith & Dodd, 1982].

Aspartame is a newer sweetener but it too may cause angioedema and urticaria. Aspartame intake is known to be dangerous for persons with phenylketonuria, a metabolic disorder that results in dangerously high blood levels of phenylalanine. In addition, aspartame is not

Table 2.5. Sweetening agents

Generic name	Trade name	Functionality
Aspartame	NutraSweet	Amino acid based sweetener (180–200x)
Acesulfam K	Sunett/Sweet One	Sweetener (200x)
Cyclamate sodium	Cyclamate	Sodium Sweetener (30x)
Neohesperidin dihydrochalcone	Neohesperidin DC Natural	High intensity sweetener (1500–2000x)
Saccharin sodium	Sweet'N Low	Sweetener, soluble (500x)
Stevia	NuStevia	Sweetener (200x)
Thaumatin	Thaumatin	Protein-based, natural sweetener (3000x)
Trehalose	Trehalose G	Non-reducing disaccharide; non-hygroscopic, low reactivity; granulation aid, taste-masking
Trehalose	Trehalose SG	Non-reducing disaccharide; non-hygroscopic, low reactivity; stabilizer for lyophilisation
Fructose/Laevulose	Fructofin CFP	Endotoxin free white crystalline powder with a very sweet taste
Sucralose	Splenda	600 times sweeter than sucrose, heat stable, stable over wide pH range
Lactitol	Finlac DC	Monohydrate, non-hygroscopic but very soluble; alternative for sorbitol
Xylitol	Xylitol CM 50	Milled, white crystalline powder grade with very sweet cool taste; marginally hygroscopic at regular storage conditions
D-Xylose	D-Xylose CTR	Fine crystalline powder, also called "wood sugar", it is a natural pentose obtained from the xylan portion of hemicellulose from plant cell walls and fibre; marginally hygroscopic at regular storage conditions
Sorbitol liquid	Syral OD 80 EP	Non-crystallizing aqueous syrup; dry substance 68–72%; Hexitol > 80%

recommended for use in pregnant or lactating women [Magnuson et al., 2007].

Viscosity modifiers

Viscosity builders are used to increase the viscosity of the liquid preparations. An increase in viscosity may be desirable to improve palatability or stability. Agents like polyvinylpyrrolidone, cellulose derivatives (methyl cellulose, propyl cellulose etc.) can be used for this purpose. Viscosity inducing polymers are known to form molecular complexes with a variety of organic and inorganic drugs and hence should be used with caution. Highly viscid solution may resist dilution by gastrointestinal or intestinal fluid and may affect drug release and absorption. Viscosity modifiers mostly utilized nowadays in pharmaceutical preparations have been listed in Table 2.6.

Table 2.6. List of viscosity modifiers

• Acacia	• Carboxymethylcellulose
• Methylcellulose	• Sodium CMC
• Alginic acid	• Colloidal silicon dioxide
• Povidone	• Sodium starch glycolate
• Bentonite	• Iota carrageenan
• Propylene glycol alginate	• Tragacanth
• Carbomer resins	• MCC with sodium CMC
• Sodium alginate	• Xanthan gum

Flavors

The simple use of sweetening agent may not be sufficient to render a product containing a drug with particularly unpleasant taste, palatable. In many cases, therefore, a flavoring agent can be included. The flavoring of pharmaceuticals is of great importance in liquid dosage forms intended for oral use as they mask the disagreeable tastes of drugs. Furthermore, flavoring agents are regularly exploited for taste masking in clinical trials where it is essential for subjects to lack differentiation between placebo and drug-containing formulations. This is particularly useful in pediatric formulations to ensure patient compliance. The inclusion of flavoring agent has an additional advantage of enabling identification of liquid products to be achieved easily.

There are four basic sensations: salty, bitter, sweet, and sour. A combination of efforts is required to mask these tastes. For example, menthol and chloroform act as desensitizing agents; a large number of natural and artificial flavors and their combinations are available to mask the bitterness most often found in organic compounds. Most formulators refer the selection of compatible flavors to companies manufacturing these flavors, as they may allow use of their drug master file (DMF) for the purpose of filing regulatory applications. Some generalizations concerning the selection of a flavoring agent to mask the specific type of taste are given in Table 2.7.

Table 2.7. Taste masking with flavors

Taste	Suitable masking flavor
Salty	Apricot, butterscotch, liquorice, peach, vanilla
Bitter	Anise, chocolate, grapefruit, mint, poison fruit, wild cherry, liquorice, coffee,
Sweet	Vanilla fruits, berries, bubble gum, grape
Sour	Citrus fruits, liquorice, raspberry, lemon, orange, cherry, grapefruit

In some cases there exists a strong association between the use of a product and its flavor or perfume content. For example, products intended for relief of indigestion are often mint flavored. This is because mint has been used for years in such products for its carminative effect. The flavoring industry has many proprietary products purported to have excellent taste-masking properties [Furia, 1971], which have been used with some success. Yet, there are a number of natural and artificial flavors that can be generally described to possess similar taste-masking effects.

Of the many tastes that must be masked in pharmaceuticals, bitterness is most often encountered; to mask it completely is difficult. A tropical fruit has been used for centuries in central Africa to mask the bitter taste of native beers. This so-called 'miracle berry' contains a glycoprotein that transiently and selectively binds to bitter taste buds. Due to stability challenges, attempts to isolate the compound for commercial exploitation have been unsuccessful. Yet, many fruit syrups are relatively stable in pharmaceuticals if formulated with antimicrobial preservative agents. Syrups of cinnamon, orange, citric acid, cherry, cocoa, wild cherry, raspberry, or glycyrrhiza elixir can be used to effectively mask salty and bitter tastes in a number of drug products [Gennaro, 1980].

The extent to which taste masking may be achieved is not usually predictable due to complex interactions of other flavor elements in these products. The degree to which bitterness may be masked by these agents ranks in a descending order: cocoa syrup is most effective, followed by raspberry syrup, cherry, cinnamon, compound sarsaparilla, citric acid, licorice, aromatic elixir, orange, and wild cherry. Sour and metallic tastes in pharmaceuticals also can be reasonably masked. Sour substances containing hydrochloric acid are most effectively neutralized with raspberry and other fruit syrups. Metallic tastes in oral liquid products (e.g., iron) are usually masked by extracts of gurana, a tropical fruit. Gurana flavor is used at concentrations ranging from 0.001 to about 0.5% and may be useful in solid products as well (e.g., chewable tablets and granules).

Flavor enhancers and potentiators

Flavor enhancers are used universally in the food and pharmaceutical industries. Sugar, carboxylic acids (e.g., citric, malic, and tartaric), common salt (NaCl), amino acids, some amino acid derivatives (e.g., monosodium glutamate-MSG), and spices (e.g., peppers) are most often employed. Although, extremely effective with proteins and vegetables, MSG has limited use in pharmaceuticals because it is not a sweetener. Citric acid is most frequently used to enhance taste performance of both liquid and solid pharmaceutical products, as well as a variety of foods. Other acidic agents, such as malic and tartaric acids, are also used for flavor enhancement. In oral liquids, these acids contribute unique and complex organoleptic effects, increasing overall flavor quality. Common salt provides similar effects at its taste threshold level in liquid pharmaceuticals. Vanilla, for example, has a delicate bland flavor, which is effectively enhanced by salt.

Buffers

Changes in pH of a preparation may occur during storage because of degradation of the product, interactions with container components, or dissolution of gases and vapors. To avoid these problems, buffers are added to stabilize pH levels. A suitable buffer system should have adequate buffer capacity to maintain the pH level of the product during storage. It can be based on the pH profile of the drug in solution. Commonly used buffer systems are acetates, citrates, phosphates, and glutamates.

Buffers, if present in solution, resist change in pH of the solution. The choice of a suitable buffer depends on the pH and the buffer capacity required. Most pharmaceutically acceptable buffer systems and the pH range they cover are listed in Table 2.8. The compositions of all physiological and pharmaceutically relevant buffers are available in Indian pharmacopoeia under *Appendix: Buffers and reagents.*

Colors

It is often customary to include a suitable color associated with the flavor to enhance the attractiveness of the product. However, apart from increasing aesthetic value, the colorants may serve a few other purposes as well. Masking

Table 2.8. Buffers and their effective pH ranges

Buffers	Effective pH range
Hydrochloric acid buffer	1.2–2.2
Phosphate buffer	2.0–8.0
Acid phthalate buffer	2.2–4.0
Acetate buffer	2.8–6.0
Neutralised phthalate buffer	4.2–5.8
Citro-phosphate buffer	5.0–7.6
Carbonate buffer	5.8–7.4
Triethanolamine buffer	7.0–9.2
Alkaline borate buffer	8.0–10.0
Glutamate buffer	8.7–10.7
Ammonia buffer	9.5–10.9

of a strongly colored degradation product, which may not affect the therapeutic value of the formulation, is one of them. Easy product identification and differentiation between the similar products are a few others.

It is essential that chosen color is acceptable in the country in which the product is to be sold. A color acceptable in one country may not be acceptable in the other country. In India, Bureau of Indian Standard describes the Indian Standards for edible synthetic colours permitted under the Prevention of Food Adulteration Rules, 1955, Ministry of Health, Government of India. These rules, inter-alia, prescribe: 'All food colours including natural colouring matter and permitted synthetic food colours, and their preparations or mixtures excluding saffron and curcumin shall be sold only under the BIS Certification Mark.'

Further, a single color may have different names in different countries. For example, water-soluble dye amaranth is also known as Bordeaux S, CI Food Red 9, and CI Acid Red 27. It has been allocated the color index number 16185 by the Society of Dyers and Colorists and the American Association of Textile Chemists and Colorists. Under the US Food, Drug and Cosmetics Act it is known as FD and C Red Number 2 and a directive of Council of European Communities has allocated it the reference number E 123.

Both, natural and synthetic colors are available. The former include carotenoids, chlorophylls, anthocyanins; and a miscellaneous group, which includes riboflavins, caramel and extracts of red beetroot. Synthetic or 'coal tar' dyes tend to give brighter colors and are generally more stable than natural materials. Those used for pharmaceutical purpose include, sodium salts of sulphonic acids and therefore they may be incompatible with cationic drugs.

Some of the dyes associated with hyper-sensitivity reactions include azo dyes such as tartrazine (FD&C Yellow 5), FD&C Yellow 6, FD&C Red 36, FD&C Red 17, and triphenyl-methane dyes (FD&C Blue 1 and 2 and Green 3). The first two of these dyes (Yellow 5 and 6) have demonstrated cross-reactivity with Aspirin and Indomethacin. They should be avoided in patients with known allergies to these medications. Quinoline dyes (Yellow 10 and 11) have been linked with contact sensitization. Some xanthene dyes (FD&C Red 3 and Red 22) are potent photo-sensitizers.

Antioxidants

Many drugs in solution are subject to oxidative degradation. Oxidation is defined as a loss of electrons from a compound that results in a change in the oxidation state of the molecule. Such reactions are mediated by free radicals or molecular oxygen, and are often catalyzed by metal ions. Furthermore, oxidation often involves the addition of oxygen (or other electro-negative atoms like halogens) or the removal of hydrogen.

Antioxidants work by consuming oxygen at a faster rate than the rate at which the drug substance reacts with oxygen; and in such cases they will protect the drug substance until they are completely used up. This means that the use of antioxidants imposes a lag time upon the decomposition profile of the drug. Antioxidants may act either as oxidative chain reaction blockers or reducing agents. Sulfites act in a quantitative manner. Once the sulfites are consumed, the oxidation starts. Goncalves et al. [1998] reported the antioxidant activity of 5-aminosalicylic acid in the presence of vitamins C and E of lipid peroxidation. They showed typical S-shaped decomposition curves. Chakrabarti et al. [1993] showed that hamycin (a polyene antifungal antibiotic) can be stabilized by hydroquinone, butylated deoxycholate, and ascorbylpalmitate.

Antioxidants like sodium metabisulphite, ascorbic acid, thioglycerol and cysteine hydro-chloride provide protection primarily in aqueous phases. Oil-soluble antioxidants include lecithin, propyl gallate, ascorbylpalmitate and BHT. BHA, BHT, l-tocopherol and alkyl gallates are particularly popular in pharmaceutical industry. BHA and BHT have a pronounced odour and should be used in low concentrations. Alkyl gallates have bitter taste whereas l-tocopherol is well suited for edible or oil preparation. Some commonly used antioxidants have been enlisted in Table 2.9.

Table 2.9. Commonly used antioxidants	
• 4-Hydroxymethyl-2,6-di-tert-butylphenol	• *l*-Tocopherol
• Acetylcysteine	• Monothioglycerol
• Ascorbic acid	• Propyl gallate
• Ascorbylpalmitate	• Sodium ascorbate
• Butylated hydroxy-anisol (BHA)	• Sodium bisulfite
• Butylated hydroxy-toluene (BHT)	• Sodium formaldehyde
• Gallic acid	• Sodium metabisulfite
• Hypophosphorous acid	• Sulfites
	• Thioglycerol
	• Thiourea

Harmonization of standards

There is great interest in the international harmonization of standards applicable to pharmaceutical excipients. This is because the pharmaceutical industry is multinational, with products sold in markets worldwide, and regulatory approval for these products required in each country. Standards for each drug substance and excipient used in pharmaceuticals are contained in pharmacopeias, or, for new agents, in an application for regulatory approval by the relevant governing authority. The four pharmacopeias with the largest international use are the United States Pharmacopeia–National Formulary (USP–NF), British Pharmacopeia, European Pharmacopeia, and Japanese Pharmacopeia. Uniform standards for excipients in these and other pharmacopeias would facilitate production efficiency, enable the marketing of a single formulation of a product internationally, and enhance regulatory approval of pharmaceutical products worldwide. The goal of harmonization is an ongoing effort by corporate representatives and international regulatory authorities.

FACILITIES AND EQUIPMENTS

The type of product to be manufactured is the deciding factor for the design of facilities and equipments and solely depends on the potential for cross contamination and microbiological contamination. For example, the facilities used for the manufacture of over-the-counter (OTC) oral products might not require the isolation that a steroid or sulfa product would require. However, the concern for contamination remains, and it is important to isolate processes that generate dust (such as those processes occurring before the addition of solvents). The HVAC (heating, ventilation, and air-conditioning) system should be validated just as required for processing of potent drugs. It is advisable not to take any shortcuts in the design of HVAC systems, as it is often very difficult to properly validate a system that is prone to breakdown; in such instances a fully validated protocol would need stress testing – something that may be more expensive than establishing proper HVAC systems in the first place. However, it is also unnecessary to overdo it in designing the facilities, as once the drug is present in a solution form; cross contamination to other products is not a big deal. It is, nevertheless, important to protect the drug from other powder sources (such as by maintaining appropriate pressure differentials in various cubicles).

Equipment should be of sanitary design. This includes sanitary pumps, valves, flow meters, and other equipment that can be easily sanitized. Ball valves, the packing in pumps, and pockets in flow meters have been identified as sources of contamination. To facilitate cleaning and sanitization, manufacturing and filling lines should be identified and detailed in drawings and standard operating procedures (SOPs). Long delivery lines between manufacturing areas and filling areas can be a source of contamination. Special attention should be paid to developing standard operating procedures that clearly establish validated limits for this purpose. Equipment used for batching and mixing of oral solutions and suspensions is relatively basic. These products are generally formulated on a weight basis, with the batching tank on load cells, so that a final volume can be made by weight. Volumetric means, such as using a dipstick or a line on a tank, are not generally as accurate and should be avoided as far as possible. Volumetric means must be properly validated at different temperature conditions in order to eliminate any variation. In most cases, manufacturers assay samples of the bulk solution or suspension before filling. A much greater variability is found with those batches that have been manufactured volumetrically rather than those that have been manufactured by weight.

Fully sanitizable stainless steel #314 or better quality is recommended. Equipment must be cleaned or sterilized; appropriate disinfectants include dilute solutions of hydrogen peroxide, phenol derivatives, and peracetic acid. Equipment lines can be sterilized by using alcohol, boiling water, autoclaving, steam, or dry heat. Where lids are used, due care should be taken as it may be a source of microbial contamination. Operators must conform to all sanitary presentation requirements, including head covering, gloves, and face masks. Use of portable laminar flow hoods to expose ingredients before addition is often desirable.

In most instances the equipments required are mixing tanks equipped with a means of agitation, measuring devices for large and small amounts of solids and liquids, and a filtration system for the final polishing of the solution. In addition, most production facilities are equipped with systems for bulk material handling, such as tote bins and tote bins discharging instruments. Polished stainless steel tanks equipped with heating and cooling jackets in different sizes are available. Tanks used for the compounding of bulk liquids have inbuilt agitation system.

During manufacture the solid is simply added to the solvent in a mixing vessel and the stirring is continued till the dissolution is complete. If the solute is more soluble at elevated temperatures, it may be advantageous to apply the heat to the vessel particularly if the dissolution rate is slow. Care must be taken, however, should any volatile or thermolabile material be present. Size reduction of the solid material to increase the total surface area should also speed-up the process of dissolution.

Solutes present in low concentration, particularly dyes, are often predissolved in small volume of solvent and then added to the bulk. Volatile materials such as flavors and perfumes are, where possible, added to the end of a process and after cooling, if necessary to reduce loss due to evaporation. Finally, it must be ensured that significant amounts of any of the materials are not irreversibly adsorbed onto the filtration medium used for final clarification.

Filling

The basic filling methods comprise of (i) gravimetric, (ii) volumetric, and (iii) constant level liquid filling operations. The latter two are the most frequently used for pharmaceutical liquid filling operation. Filling containers to a given weight (gravimetric filling) is generally limited to large containers or to highly viscous fluids. The process does not lead itself readily to high-speed automatic equipments.

Volumetric filling is usually accomplished by positive displacement piston action. Each filling station is equipped with a measuring piston and a cylinder. The fill accuracy is controlled by close tolerances to which the pistons and cylinders are manufactured. The fill amount is measured by the stroke of the piston, which can be varied to a limited degree on all machines. Major changes in the fill amount usually necessitate changing piston and cylinder assembly. This type of device is capable of accuracy to within fractions of milliliters. There are, however, several problems associated with volume filling. Highly viscous liquid may cause this piston to seize, resulting in either loss in filling accuracy or line break down. On the other hand, thin liquids may flow past the piston; causing uncontrollable dripping from filling spout associated filling inaccuracies. These problems can be controlled to a larger extent by proper engineering of the filling machines. An inherent problem with volumetric filling is often encountered when containers are not dimensionally uniform.

Constant level filling utilizes the containers as a means of controlling the fill of each unit. Adjusting the height to which the container is filled varies the fill amount. Any dimensional variation in the container results in comparable variations in the net filling per unit. The oldest form of constant level filler involves the use of siphon; however, this method of filling is usually slow and is rarely used when high production rates are required. The high speed automatic constant level filling machines in use today are based on siphon principle, with the major modification being the induced pressure differential between the liquid discharge nozzle and the constant level overflow system. The most widely used methods can be broadly classified as vacuum filling, gravity vacuum filling and pressure vacuum filling.

To fill by vacuum a seal must be made between the filling head and the container. The vacuum is then developed within the container, which causes the liquid to flow from bulk liquid tank to container. The liquid level rises until it reaches the vacuum tube, which is positioned at desired constant level. Excess liquid is drawn through the vacuum tube and can be recycled to bulk liquid tank. In gravity vacuum filling, the bulk liquid tanks are a level above the filling stem, so that the driving force for liquid flow results from both, negative pressure in the container and the force of gravity. Similarly, in pressure vacuum filling, a positive pressure is applied to the bulk liquid, which in combination with the vacuum developed in the container, results in the pressure differential that causes rapid filling of even highly viscous liquids. The latter two methods require some valve mechanism that is responsive to presence of container, to open and successively close the valve in the filling system assembly. Vacuum fillers do not require such mechanisms, since a pressure differential to promote liquid flow can only be achieved by vacuum formed when the filling stem forms a seal with the container.

Equipments used for emulsification

Equipments used for emulsification can be divided into four broad categories described as:

A. Mechanical stirrers

Simple top entering propeller mixers are suitable for low viscosity emulsions. If more vigorous agitation is required, or if the preparation has a moderate viscosity, turbine mixers are employed both in laboratory and in production. Paddle mixers, counter rotating blade mixers and planetary mixers are also available for special requirements. The degree of agitation is controlled by the speed of impeller rotation, but the patterns of liquid flow and the resultant efficiency of mixing are controlled by the type of impeller, its position in the container, presence of baffles and the general shape of the container.

B. Ultarsonifiers

The use of ultrasonic energy to produce pharmaceutical emulsions is well known. The dispersion forced through an orifice at modest pressures of 150–350 psi is allowed to collide upon a blade. Due to the pressure, the blade vibrates to produce ultrasonic note, resulting in emulsification.

C. Colloid mills

Colloid mills operate on the principle of high shear, which is normally generated between the rotor and the stator of the mills. Colloid mills are used primarily for the comminution of the solids, dispersion of the suspension of poorly wettable solids and for the preparation of relatively viscous emulsions. The material drawn or pumped through the adjustable gap set between the rotor and the stator is milled or homogenized by physical action and centrifugal force created by high-speed rotation of rotor, which operates within 0.005 to 0.010 inch of stator.

D. Homogenizers

In homogenizer a pump forces dispersion of two liquids under pressure (500–5000 psi) onto a homogenizing valve held in place by a strong spring. The spring compresses under pressure and the dispersion enters the homogenization chamber with intense turbulence and hydraulic pressure, which leads to emulsification. Homogenizers are useful to produce monodisperse emulsions of small globule size (1 nm).

MANUFACTURING DIRECTIONS

Different products are formulated with different manufacturing directions; in some instances, general details are left out that pertain to basic compounding techniques. The order of addition and techniques of adding solutes to a liquid tank can be very important. Flavors are generally added after mixing them first in a smaller volume of the solvent or liquid base and rinsing them with a portion of liquid as well. This also holds true for all other additions, particularly those of smaller quantities of ingredients. Proper mixing is validated; however, unlike solid mixing, where over-mixing may result in segregation, the problems in liquid mixing pertain to air entrapment. Appropriate temperature of the liquid phase is often important to ensure that there is no precipitation of the solute added. Classic examples include use of syrup base, which must be heated to bring it to proper viscosity and to allow proper mixing. Parabens, when used as preservatives, must be dissolved in hot water because the quantity used is small and can be readily lost if complete dissolution is not ensured. In most instances, small quantities of solutes should be predissolved in a smaller quantity of solvent before adding it to the main tank. It is customary to bring the batch to the final volume of weight. The gravimetric adjustments are preferred, as they can be done while taring the vessel. Problems arise when solvents like alcohol are used wherein volume contraction and density are subject to temperature changes. Also, formulations are often presented in a volumetric format and require careful conversion calculation, especially where one or two components are used to compensate for the amount of active used. A schematic representation of common steps with variables and responses during formulation development of oral liquids has been depicted in Fig. 2.2.

PRODUCT DEVELOPMENT

Design of liquid oral solutions involves the combination of ingredients with therapeutically active agents to enhance the acceptability or effectiveness of the product. The formulation of

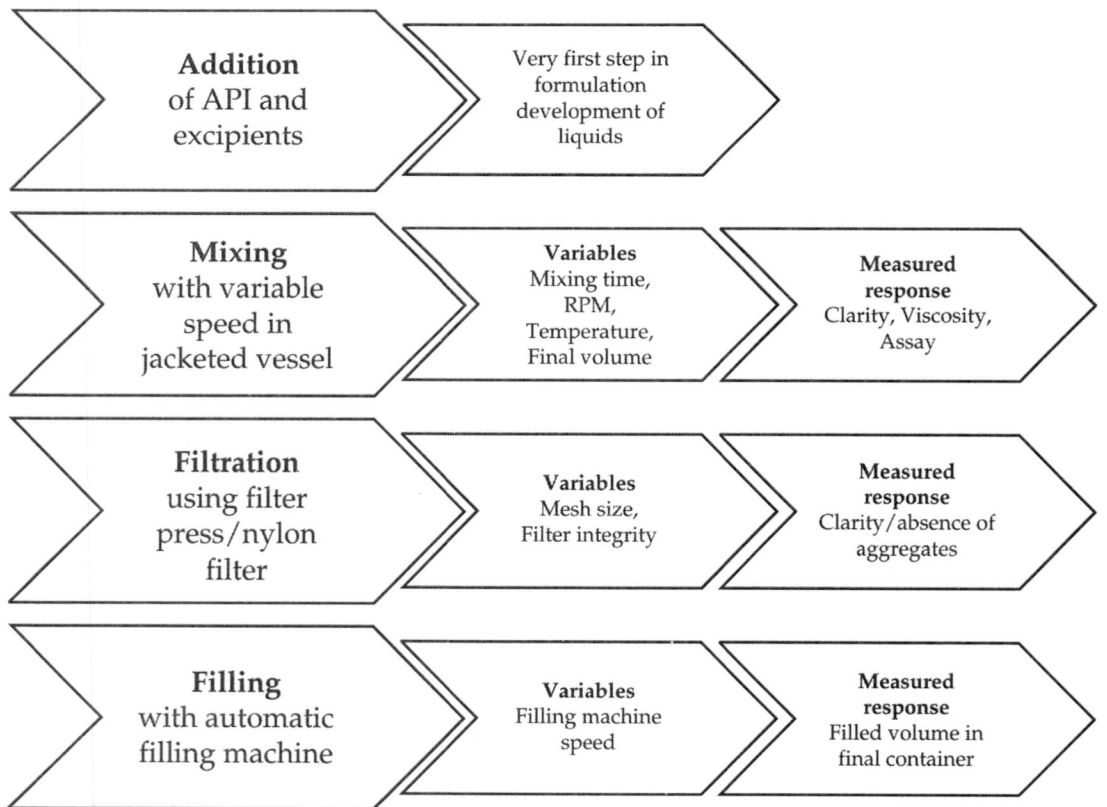

Fig. 2.2. Schematic representation of common steps during product development of liquids.

pharmaceutical liquids requires several considerations: drug concentration, drug solubility, liquid vehicle selection, physical and chemical stability, preservation; and appropriate additives such as buffers, solubilizers, sweetening agents, viscosity-controlling agents, colors, and flavors.

Drug manufacturers attempt to guarantee efficacy by evaluating their products in a scientifically acceptable manner. Thus color, odor, taste, pourability, and homogeneity are important pharmaceutical properties. Hence, the successful design and formulation of liquids, as well as other dosage forms, require both scientific and pharmaceutical acuity [Boylan, 1996].

Solutions/monophasic systems

Formulation of a solution is not less than a challenge due to a few technical problems as instability and low aqueous solubility of a few drugs. Special solubilization techniques are sometimes required and great care has to be taken to maintain pharmaceutical elegance with regard to taste, appearance, and viscosity.

Liquid preparations have a few distinct advantages over more widely used solid dosage forms viz. faster absorption, quicker therapeutic response and its ease to swallow make it more suitable and acceptable for the paediatric and geriatric use. However, disadvantages like inconvenient handling, instability, solubility problem of some drugs, inadequate doses etc., limit their use.

Oral solutions

Oral solutions are usually formulated such that dose of medication remains in convenient volume for administration; as 5 mL (one teaspoonful), 10 mL or 15 mL (one tablespoonful). On the other hand, many solutions used in the paediatric patients are given as drops, utilizing a calibrated dropper usually provided in the product package. Example of Caffeine Citrate Oral Solution is given below.

Caffeine citrate oral solution	
Ingredients	**Quantity**
Caffeine citrate	20.0 g
Citric acid monohydrate	5.0 g
Sodium citrate monohydrate	8.3 g
Purified water, q.s.	1000 mL

Procedure: Dissolve sodium citrate monohydrate and citric acid monohydrate in 90% of purified water. Add specified amount of caffeine in above solution, make up the volume and adjust pH to 4.7.

Dry mixtures for reconstitution

Those drugs, which are not stable in aqueous solution for extended shelf-life period, are formulated as dry powders or granules for reconstitution. These dry formulations contain all the excipients of an oral solution except vehicle. The vehicle for reconstitution is normally provided along with the dry formulation in the final package. Once reconstituted the product remains stable for a period of 7-14 days depending upon preparation, which is a sufficiently long span for patient to complete the dose.

In some instances, preservatives are required to protect the product during use by the patient. It is important to note that the FDA considers this phase of use of product a part of the product development strategy. The manufacturer must ensure label compliance through the use period, as indicated on the package and under the conditions prescribed, such as keeping it in a refrigerator. Whereas the instructions require the product to be stored in a refrigerator, product development should evaluate a wider range of temperatures, as the temperature inside the consumer's refrigerator may not correspond to the official definition of refrigeration. The method of granulation for the powders intended for resuspension before use is a traditional one, as is used in the preparation of uncompressed or even compressed solids; the difference here is obviously the consideration of the effects of stability on reconstitution, which may require addition of stabilizers. In general, the method of granulation requires wet massing, screening, drying, and screening again; fluid bed dryers may be used as well.

Oral rehydration solution

Typical oral rehydration solution (ORS) contains 45 mEq Na^+, 20 mEq K^+, 35 mEq Cl^-, 30 mEq citrate and 25 g of dextrose per liter. These formulations are available in liquid or powder/ packet form for reconstitution. These products should not be mixed with other electrolytes containing liquids such as milk or fruit juices because there is no method available to calculate how much electrolyte the patient actually received. WHO's full formula ORS is usually marketed in factory-produced aluminum-foil packets, or sachets containing exact measurements of salts and a simple sugar. The current standard ORS formula, designed to be mixed with one liter of water, consists of Glucose (20.0 g), Sodium chloride (3.5 g), Potassium chloride (1.5 g), Trisodium citrate dihydrate (2.9 g) (formerly sodium bicarbonate, 2.5 g). Although the standard ORS formula is mixed with one liter of water, commercial products exist, which require different amounts of water, from 200 or 350 mL to one liter. Formula for Magaldrate Dry Powder for Reconstitution is given below.

Oral colonic lavage solution

The traditional way to prepare the bowel for the procedures such as colonoscopy consisted of the administration of clear liquid diets for 24 to 48 hrs. preceding the procedure, the administration of oral laxatives the night before and cleansing enemas 2 to 4 hrs. prior to commencement of the procedure. The drawback is poor patient compliance, and other problems resulting from additive effects of malnutrition and poor oral intake prior to the procedure.

An alternative method involves administration of balanced solution of electrolytes with polyethylene glycol (PEG-3350), reconstituted

Magaldrate dry powder for reconstitution	
Ingredients	**Quantity/Sachet (2 g)**
Magaldrate	800.0 mg
Kollidon CL-M	640.0 mg
Sorbitol, crystalline	200.0 mg
Orange flavor	40.0 mg
Kollidon 90 F	40.0 mg
Coconut flavor	4.0 mg
Banana flavor	4.0 mg
Saccharine sodium	0.80 mg
Purified water q.s.	

Procedure: Granulate mixture of magaldrate, kollidon CL-M, sorbitol and orange flavor with solution of kollidon 90 F, coconut, banana flavor and saccharine sodium in sufficient water and pass through a 0.8-mm sieve to obtain free-flowing granules.

with an isotonic solution having a mildly salty taste. The PEG acts as an osmotic agent within the GI tract and the balanced electrolyte concentration results in virtually no net absorption or secretion of ions. Thus, a large volume of these solutions can be administered without a significant change in water or electrolyte balance. Formula for PEG-3350 Colonic Lavage Solution is given below.

PEG-3350 Colonic lavage solution	
Ingredients	**Quantity**
PEG-3350	236.0 g
Sodium bicarbonate	6.74 g
Potassium chloride	2.97 g
Sodium sulphate	22.74 g
Sodium chloride	5.86 g
Purified water, q.s.	4800.0 mL

Procedure: Dissolve all solid ingredients in required quantity in 80% of the vehicle with continuous stirring and make up final volume with purified water.

Syrups

Syrups are concentrated aqueous preparation of sugar or sugar substitute with or without added flavoring agent and medicinal substances. Syrups containing flavoring agents but not medicinal substance are called non-medicated or flavored vehicles (syrups). Syrups are intended to serve as pleasant tasting vehicles for medicinal substances to be added in extemporaneous compounding of prescriptions or in the preparation of a standard for medicated syrup. Syrups provide a pleasant means of administering a liquid form of a disagreeably tasting drug and administering the drug to children. Formula for Norephedrine Hydrochloride Syrup is given below.

Norephedrine hydrochloride syrup

Ingredients	Quantity
DL-Norephedrine hydrochloride	40.0 mg
Parabens	10.0 mg
Saccharin sodium	50.0 mg
Kollidon 90 F	30.0 mg
Sorbitol solution	500.0 mg
Purified water, q.s.	460.0 mL

Procedure: Dissolve parabens in hot water, add sorbitol to the solution, cool to room temperature, and dissolve other components. Cysteine (0.1-0.5%) could be added as antioxidant to prevent discoloration and flavors can be added to adjust the required taste.

Elixirs

Elixirs are clear, sweetened hydro-alcoholic, usually flavored solutions intended for oral use. They contain less proportion of sugar, and thus are less sweet, less viscous and less efficient in taste masking than syrups. One advantage of elixirs is that they can keep both water- and alcohol-soluble ingredients in solution, and are prepared with ease compared to syrups. The proportion of alcohol and water in an elixir varies and depends on the solubility profile of the components. Elixirs containing 10-12% alcohol are self-preserving. Formula for Codeine Phosphate and Acetaminophen Elixir is given below.

Codeine phosphate and acetaminophen elixir

Ingredients	Quantity
Codeine phosphate	2.4 g
Acetaminophen	24.0 g
Alcohol	48.0 g
Propylene glycol	30.0 g
Citric acid	2.4 g
Sucrose	800.0 g
Sodium benzoate	1.50 g
Saccharin sodium	0.15 g
FD&C yellow No. 6	0.005 g
Flavor	0.20 g
Purified water, q.s.	1000.0 mL

Procedure: Take about 50% of water in a vessel and heat to 90°C, add sodium benzoate and saccharin sodium and mix until dissolved. Next, add sucrose, citric acid and propylene glycol to preformed mixture with constant stirring while maintaining temperature for 30 minutes, and then allow to cool. In another container take about 50 mL of water and add codeine phosphate in it with constant stirring, transfer the content in above mixture. Dissolve color in water and add to above mixture. Finally, dissolve acetaminophen in alcohol in separate vessel and mix it with above solution, add flavor and make up the volume.

Mouthwashes

Mouthwashes are sometimes used synonymously with gargles because of their intended route of administration and approximately same site of action. Mouthwashes can be used for cosmetic as well as therapeutic purposes in oral cavity and are not intended to be administered to cure the ailments of throat. Their intended use is in buccal cavity and oral mucosa only. The desired antiseptic action of mouthwashes helps to protect gums and buccal mucosa.

Evaluation and stability testing of monophasic formulations

In the case of oral solutions, organoleptic properties are of great importance. Organoleptic evaluation is usually done subjectively, i.e., a tester (operator, technician) will judge the product and score it, either numerically or descriptively or both. In the case of appearance of solutions, there should always be a subjective statement (quantitative or subjective description) even if more quantitative instrumental parameters are recorded.

Polyvinyl pyrrolidone-iodine mouthwash	
Ingredients	**Quantity**
Polyvinyl pyrrolidone-iodine	100 g
Sodium saccharin	5 g
Menthol	2 g
Aniseed oil	0.5 g
Eucalyptus oil	0.5 g
Polyethylene glycol 400	160 g
Ethanol	300 g
Purified water	440 mL

Procedure: Dissolve PVP-iodine powder and sodium saccharin in specified quantity of water to obtain a clear solution. In a separate container add alcohol and mix and dissolve aniseed oil, eucalyptus oil, menthol, and polyethylene glycol 400 to obtain a clear solution. Mix both the solutions with stirring.

For organoleptic testing it is important to establish a test panel early in the stability program. First of all, the depth of organoleptic capacity should be tested. This can be by asking the tester to taste serial dilutions of a bitter substance (e.g., quinine) i.e. a sensitivity level can be established. A control of water or high dilutions should always be part of the protocol. It should be noted that the technicians are not taste testers in the ordinary sense. That is, it is not necessary to match their "likings" to that of the general public. Rather, it is important that they can (a) duplicate their results, and (b) remember them, since they will be asked to taste a preparation that they originally tested 3 or 6 months earlier. In so doing, they would have to score the degree of flavoring, i.e., whether the flavor being lost or its intensity is lesser than initial. For example, if the chemical is slightly anesthetizing, the duration of the anesthesia would be important. Finally, it is important to screen several testers to ascertain

that they give the "same result." In describing the flavor, several categories can be used (degree of sourness, degree of saltiness, level of flavor, type of flavor). Each of these may be assigned to a level of, for example, 1-5. A flavor profile may hence be established, and this can then be reestablished at several time points in the room-temperature storage. It is not recommended to evaluate results from higher temperature.

When it is not possible to establish either the source of the color or the level of the substance causing it, a good practice would be to use a color standard to describe the "intensity" of the discoloration. For instance the so-called Roche Color Standard (RCS) can be utilized, that can be reliably reproduced and has exceptional color stability. The main types of changes in appearance of oral solutions (syrup, elixirs etc.) are loss of dye, precipitation, and bacterial growth. Scott et al. [1960] showed the loss of dye in a vitamin syrup, as it could be treated exactly like a substance.

Stability Guidelines also states that high oxygen atmosphere should be evaluated in stability studies on solutions or suspensions of the bulk drug substances. Oxidation reactions are relatively rare in pharmaceutical dosage forms as a main reaction but some oxidation probably takes place in many cases and results in small amounts of unidentified degradation products e.g. vitamin preparations [Chakrabarti et al., 1993]. So, the stability of liquid dosage forms against oxidation is to be checked in open as well as closed systems as described by Carstensen, [2001].

The powder for reconstitution should be evaluated for flowability (using angle of repose method) to ensure uniform filling of material in the final containers and the reconstituted formulation should be evaluated for sedimentation volume and ease of redispersion. Drugs degraded by hydrolysis, oxidation or photolysis in solution should be evaluated in container of the same material and size in which the product is marketed.

Biphasic systems

Suspensions

Oral suspensions are oral liquids containing one or more active ingredients suspended in a suitable vehicle. Suspended solids may slowly separate on standing but are easily resuspended [British Pharmacopoeia, 2007]. Suspension is a mode of supplying insoluble and often distasteful substances in a form that is pleasant to the taste. It provides a suitable form for the application of dermatological materials to the skin and sometimes to the mucous membranes and parenteral administration of insoluble drugs. Therefore, the suspensions may be classified into three groups: (i) oral mixtures; (ii) topical lotions; and (iii) parenteral suspensions. The major problem is uniformity and accuracy of dose, which is not as comparable to tablets, capsules or solutions. Sedimentation and compaction of the sediment cause problem that is by no means always easy to solve. Additionally, the product is liquid and relatively bulky; these properties are disadvantageous to both pharmacist and patient. Formulation of an effective and pharmaceutically elegant suspension is usually much harder to achieve than that of tablet or capsule of same drug.

An acceptable suspension possesses certain desirable qualities. The suspended material should not settle rapidly, the particles that do settle to the bottom of the container must not form a hard cake but should be rapidly redispersed into a uniform mixture when the container is shaken, and suspension must not be too viscous to pour freely from the orifice of the bottle or to flow through the syringe needle. Suspension must have an acceptable color and odor.

Product development of suspensions

A generalized consideration of the selection of ingredients and equipments for manufacturing of suspensions is not possible. If the suspension is to be prepared by dispersion technique, it is better to pulverize the solids first. The particles are subjected to a stream of turbulent air, which makes them to colloid with each other and fracture. Particles below 5 μm sizes are easily obtained. In case of controlled crystallization technique, the supersaturated solution is quickly cooled with rapid stirring. The later action ensures the formation of large number of crystals and avoids crystal growth. Homogenization, if required at any stage, can be accomplished by colloid mills. Although ultrasonic techniques can also be used yet they are of less commercial value.

A few general guidelines are stated below:

Wetting of the particles is better achieved by keeping them in contact with a small portion of vehicle containing an appropriate quantity of wetting agents without agitation. Suspending agent should be dissolved or dispersed in main portion of the vehicle and sufficient time and dispersion equipment should be employed. This helps in attainment of proper viscosity. The slurry of wetted particles should be added at low shear to main portion of suspending agent, and not the other way round. Electrolyte addition should be properly controlled to prevent variations in the particle charge. All the finished suspensions must be carefully preserved against bacterial growth.

- **Aggregated (open network system):** A controlled aggregate system can be made by using an electrolyte. Schulze – Hardy rule can be used to determine the amount of electrolyte needed. Electrolytes promote aggregation by reducing zeta potential, which acts as an electrical barrier between the particles. In some cases in which incompatibility factors are absent, very small amount of aluminium chloride or potassium biphosphate may act as aggregating agent. Surfactants, both ionic and nonionic, can also be used for the purpose. One must be careful in case of non-ionic surfactants because above critical micelle concentration they tend to get adsorbed on the particle surface, forming a continuous film, leading to coagule formation. Long chain high molecular weight polymers act as aggregating agents because part of their chain gets adsorbed on the particle surface, with the remaining part projecting out into dispersion medium. Bridging between these latter portions leads to the formation of flocs.

Oral suspensions, due to high solid contents, exhibit poor drainage from bottles. This may be improved by the use of protective colloids. Protective colloids differ from surfactants in that they do not reduce interfacial tension. They not only increase the zeta potential but also form mechanical barrier around the particles. Example of this approach is the use of silica gel, aluminium hydroxide gel etc.

- **Dispersed system:** Individual particles in disperse system are generally dispersed with the aid of an agent that lowers the interfacial tension. To maintain this state, however, a viscosity imparting suspending agent is usually required as an adjunct [Wen-Yen & Trong-Ming, 1989]. These agents retard settling and agglomeration of particles by functioning as an energy barrier, which minimizes inter-particle interaction and ultimate aggregation. The general choice of suspending agents includes protective colloids, viscosity inducing agents, surfactants and dispersing agents. Combination of different types of suspending agent may also be used to achieve desired rheologic properties. Formula for Sulfamethoxazole and Trimethoprim Suspension is given below.

Stabilizing suspensions

Various pharmaceutical excipients with different functions can be used for stabilizing suspensions. The following groups of products can be offered for stabilizing oral and topical suspensions. Soluble Kollidon products can be used at low concentrations; for example, Kollidon 90 F (2–5%) suffices to stabilize aqueous suspensions. A combination consisting of Kollidon 90 F (2%) and Kollidon CL-M (5 to 9%) has proved to be an effective system for stabilizing suspensions.

Sulfamethoxazole and trimethoprim suspension	
Ingredients	**Quantity**
Sulfamethoxazole	80 g
Trimethoprim	16 g
Kollidon CL-M	30 g
Sucrose	100 g
Purified water, q.s.	1000 mL
Vanillin	2 g
Chocolate flavor	2 g

Procedure: Dissolve sucrose in water with aid of heat and then allow cooling to 40°C. Pass sulfamethoxazole, trimethoprim and kollidon CL-M through 200-mesh sieve and mix to dissolve. Add flavors, mix and fill.

Kollidon 30 is also used for this purpose. It can be combined with all conventional suspension stabilizers (thickeners, surfactants etc.). The use of Kollidon CL-M as a suspension stabilizer has nothing whatever to do with the principle of increasing the viscosity. The addition of 5 to 9% Kollidon CL-M has practically no effect in changing the viscosity, but it strongly reduces the rate of sedimentation and facilitates the redispersibility, in particular - an effect that is consistent with the low viscosity. One of the reasons for this Kollidon CL-M effect is its low (bulk) density, which is only half of that of conventional crospovidone (e.g., Kollidon CL).

The poloxamers, Lutrol F-68 and Lutrol F-127, in concentrations of 2–5% of final weight of suspension, offer a further opportunity of stabilizing suspensions. They also do not increase viscosity when used in these amounts and can be combined with all other conventional suspension stabilizers.

Evaluation of stability

A. *Sedimentation volume:* Sedimentation volume is the ratio of the ultimate height (H_u) of the sediment to the initial height (H_o) of the total suspension as it settles in a cylinder under standard conditions. The larger this ratio better is the suspendibility. For better formulations a plot of sedimentation volume versus time yields more horizontal, less steep line. In case of highly concentrated suspensions, supernatant available is very little to determine the H_u and hence a modified experimental method is used. The concentrated suspensions are diluted with additional vehicle; H_u values for diluted suspensions are determined, H_o value equals to the original volume of sample before dilution. Sedimentation volumes, thus obtained, are plotted against the time and compared for different formulations.

B. *Rheologic method:* A practical rheologic method utilizes a Brookfield viscometer mounted on a helipath stand. The T-bar spindle is made to descend slowly into suspension, the resistance that spindle meets at various levels in sediment is measured. This resistance is direct measure of structure formation due to agglomeration at different levels. Data can be obtained for variously aged and stored samples. A plot of resistance versus the number of turns a spindle takes may also be useful. Better suspensions show a lesser rate of increase of resistance with spindle turns, that is, curve is horizontal for a longer period.

C. *Particle size analysis:* The suspensions under evaluation study are subjected to freeze–thaw cycle, which causes particle growth and may indicate the probable future particle behavior on long storage at room temperature. The changes in particle size, particle size distribution, and crystal habit are noted. Particle size can be determined by microscopic means and photomicrographs can serve as permanent records.

Certain adjuvants have a profound effect on physical performance of the suspension under freeze–thaw conditions. When a low solid content steroid injectable preparation containing sodium CMC and benzoyl alcohol and other containing CMC, methyl paraben, and propyl paraben were subjected to freezing and thawing, the former suspension caked badly while the later remained unaffected. Protective colloids thus may be adversely affected by freezing thawing or elevated temperatures i.e. gelatin is sensitive to low temperatures whereas methylcellulose is adversely affected by higher temperatures. Although, freeze thaw cycle studies are useful guides, the best stability information is still obtained from studies conducted at room temperature.

D. *Electrokinetic techniques:* Zeta potential has a considerable influence on the physical stability of the suspension. Zeta potential can be measured by microelectrophoresis, in which a sample of suspension is mounted on a special microscopic slide across which a known potential is applied. The speed of movement of the particles across the field is a function of zeta potential and is determined visually. The apparatus is standardized by use of particles of known zeta potential. Rabbit erythrocytes are commonly used for this purpose. Alternatively, more elaborate semi-automated and fully-automated equipments are available. The zeta potential then can be correlated to stability.

E. *Preservation stability:* The various ingredients present in the formulation may interact with the preservatives and thus may lead to either certain chemical incompatibilities or loss of preservative efficacy. Hence to retain preservation capacity of formulation certain analytical procedures should be developed. One such assay developed by Schieffer et al. [1984] describes the rationale for using methyl, ethyl, propyl, and butyl esters of 4-hydroxybenzoic acid in combination with antacids and other pharmaceutical products. The antacids have high pH values, and hence hydrolysis of the esters occurs, but the decomposition of the parent compound can be prevented by properly controlling the concentration.

Emulsions

Oral emulsions are almost exclusively of the oil-in-water type. They provide a degree of taste masking as the aqueous external phase effectively isolates the oil from the tongue. Mineral and castor oils have been emulsified in water and administered orally for the local treatment of constipation for many years, as have various nutritional oils from fish liver (halibut or cod) or vegetable origin to produce oral liquid food supplements. It has long been established that the use of o/w emulsions as carriers for lipophilic drugs may improve oral bioavailability and efficacy [Block, 1996; Rosoff, 1997]. For example, Griseofulvin formulated as an o/w emulsion has enhanced gastrointestinal absorption when compared with suspensions, tablets, or capsule dosage forms.

An emulsion is a thermodynamically unstable system consisting of at least two immiscible liquid phases, one of which is dispersed as globules (dispersed phase) throughout the other (dispersion medium), stabilized by the presence of an emulsifying agent. In an oil-in-water (o/w) emulsion, oil globules are dispersed in aqueous phase. The reverse is true for water-in-oil (w/o) emulsion. The diameter of the dispersed phase globules is generally in the range of about 0.1–10 μm, though some as small as 0.01 μm and as large as 100 μm are not uncommon.

Ordinarily, but not always, emulsions for internal use is of o/w type and emulsion for external use is of either type. Water-in-oil emulsions are insoluble in water, not water-washable, will absorb water, are occlusive, and may be 'greasy' and are meant for external purpose exclusively. Oil-in-water emulsions are miscible with water, are water washable, will absorb water, are non-occlusive, and are non-greasy.

Heterogeneous systems comprising emulsions offer greater difficulties in manufacturing, where not only a careful calculation of formulation additives such as surfactants is required but also the manufacturing techniques

such as mixing times, intensity of mixing, and temperature become critical [Becher,1965]. Microemulsion manufacturing requires special equipment, and recently the use of nanoparticles has created a need for highly specialized handling systems. Homogenizers are used to emulsify liquids along with ultrasonifiers and colloid mills. In some instances, spontaneous emulsification is obtained by a careful order of mixing. The choice of emulsifying agent depends on the type of emulsion desired and determined by the use of hydrophilic–lipophilic balance evaluation. The temperature at which an emulsion is formed can often affect the particle size and, thus, later, the tendency to coalesce or break. Auxiliary emulsification aids include use of fine solids. Hydrophilic colloids are commonly used to impart proper viscosity that enhances stability of emulsions. However, there is a tendency to build-up viscosity with time in freshly prepared emulsions. The flow characteristics of emulsions are important and are determined by the emulsion's yield value. Consistency in the density character of emulsion is therefore important. Clear emulsions have a lower proportion of internal phase and require solubilization techniques more frequently than do opaque emulsions.

The antimicrobial preservatives used in emulsions are selected on the basis of the type of emulsion manufactured (o/w or w/o). Because water is one of the phases often encountered in emulsions, these must be properly preserved. Classical preservatives are used, but care must be exercised in not selecting preservatives that might interact with surfactants; get adsorbed onto the packaging material such as plastic bottles, caps, or cap liners; and be lost to a point at which they are rendered inactive. Parabens remain a good choice. The presence of oil phase also requires inclusion of antioxidants where necessary, and these may include such examples as gallic acid, propyl gallate, butylated hydroxyanisole (BHA), butylated hydroxytoluene (BHT), ascorbic acid, sulfites, l-tocopherol, butyl phenol, and so forth. Scaling-up of emulsion formulations from laboratory scale to manufacturing scale often presents significant problems related to temperature distribution studies; often the two phases are mixed at a specific temperature that may change during the mixing process and thus require a certain mixing rate. Stability testing of emulsions is subject to protocols different from those used for other liquid products; for example, higher-temperature studies may cause an emulsion to break but may not be reflective of the log-linear effect of temperature but, rather, of phase change or inversion. Centrifugation is a common technique to study emulsion stability, and so is the agitation test, which may cause suspended phases to coalesce. Of prime importance in the stability evaluation of emulsions are the phase separation, changes in light reflection, viscosity, particle size, electrical conductivity and chemical composition.

Stability of the emulsions

A. *Creaming:* Movement of individual droplets of dispersed phase or aggregation of the droplets of the dispersed phase to top or bottom of emulsion is called as creaming. The creamed portion can, however, be uniformly redistributed by mechanical shearing. This is possible because the interfacial film of the emulsifying agent is still intact and functioning as mechanical barrier. Though creaming is a less serious problem, it is not esthetically acceptable and also increases the risk of coalescence. Stokes' equation relates the rate of separation to factors such as globule size of the dispersed phase, difference in the densities between the two phases, and the viscosity of the dispersion medium. The possibility of creaming is reduced by reducing the globule size to as minimum as practically possible, minimizing the difference in the density, and with a relatively high viscosity of the dispersion medium. Thickeners like tragacanth, microcrystalline cellulose are used to increase the viscosity of the dispersion medium. Upward creaming (movement of dispersed phase globules to the top) is observed if dispersed phase is lighter than dispersion medium and downward creaming (movement of dispersed phase globules to the bottom) results under opposite conditions.

B. *Coalescence:* A more serious problem is coalescence. This irreversible separation of the dispersed phase arises due to collapse of the interfacial film of the emulsifying agent. Additional emulsifying agent and reprocessing are usually necessary to reproduce the emulsion. For most emulsions, the stability evaluation tests are performed at 5°C and 40°C for 3 months. Shorter exposure periods at 50°C may be used alternatively. Formula for Chloramphenicol Palmitate Emulsion is given below.

Chloramphenicol palmitate emulsion	
Ingredients	**Quantity**
Chloramphenicol palmitate	25 g
Lutrol E 400	40 g
Cremophor RH 40	40 g
Sucrose	400 g
Purified water, q.s.	1000 mL

Procedure: Charge chloramphenicol palmitate, lutrol E 400 and cremophor RH 40 in a suitable stainless steel vessel. Heat to 70°C to obtain a clear solution and then cool to 40°C. In a separate vessel, dissolve sugar in purified water and then add this solution to preformed mixture. Bring to volume with purified water and mix.

Evaluation of emulsion

A. *Emulsion shelf-life:* There are no quick and sensitive methods available to the formulators for the determination of potential instability in an emulsion. It takes a long time for the development of signs of instability at ambient conditions. To accelerate the stability programme the emulsion is subjected to various stress conditions like temperature, centrifugation.

B. *Temperature stress:* Many emulsions may be perfectly stable at 40–45°C, but cannot tolerate temperatures in excess of 55–60°C even for a few hours. Thus, it becomes unrealistic to submit the emulsions to temperatures higher than 50°C even for shorter periods of time. A more useful method is to cycle the emulsion between two temperatures. There is no general consensus on the temperature conditions. Some tests cycle the product for 24 hrs. between –5 to 40°C for 24 cycles while other tests use 12 hrs. cycle between 5 and 35°C for 10 cycles.

C. *Centrifugation stress:* Creaming or coalescence on centrifugation in an emulsion can be used to predict its stability at normal shelf-life storage conditions. Becher [1965] claimed that centrifugation at 3750 rpm in 10-cm radius centrifuge for a period of 5 hrs. is equivalent to the effect of gravity on separation for about one year. The moderate speed suggested by Becher is probably reasonable. There is, however, no general agreement on centrifugation test conditions as well. Test conditions may involve a 5 min test using high-speed centrifuge, however, a 20 min test using a low speed centrifuge may also be used.

D. *Chemical parameters:* Chemical composition of the emulsion components needs to be established e.g. polyethylene glycol or its derivatives are prone to auto-oxidation, which may lead to undesirable odors, formation of acidic components and other oxidative byproducts. Hydrolytic degradation of non-ionic esters leads to changes in dielectric constants of the emulsion.

E. *Physical parameters:* Commonly evaluated physical parameters include:

(a) *Particle size and size distribution:* Size and size distribution of dispersed phase globules can be used as parameters of emulsion stability. A simple visual inspection can give an idea of change in globule size. Emulsion appearance as a function of globule size is given in Table 2.10. Increase in the globule size changes emulsion appearance and can be taken as measure of emulsion instability.

Table 2.10. Globule size and appearance of emulsion

Globule size (μm)	Appearance
> 1	White
0.1–1.0	Blue-white
0.05–0.1	Opalescent, semi-transparent
< 0.5	Transparent

(b) *Phase separation and coalescence:* The rate and extent of phase separation on aging of an emulsion may be observed visually or by measuring the volume of separated phase. A simple but trivial method for determination of phase separation involves withdrawing small specimens of the emulsion from the top and the bottom of the preparation after some period of storage and comparing the composition of the two samples by appropriate analysis of water content, oil content or any suitable constituent.

Simple techniques like visual observation before and after shaking, and photo microscopy can be useful for testing emulsions for coalescence. Particle size counters like coulter counter or light scattering techniques can be used for emulsion globule size determination and particle size distribution.

Tingstad [1964] proposed a very simple test to evaluate coalescence. An oil phase containing all the hydrophobic components of emulsion is very carefully poured over the aqueous phase, which contains all the water-soluble substances. A drop of oil is transferred by means of a syringe into the aqueous phase and released at a specific distance below the phase boundary. The time required for the droplet to coalesce with the bulk of oil phase is recorded. The longer the coalescence time, more is the stability of the emulsion.

(c) *Viscosity:* Change in the viscosity of an emulsion on aging can be determined using viscometer. Cone and plate viscometers are particularly suitable for emulsions but instruments using coaxial cylinders are easy to use. Penetrometers can be used when the preparation is too viscous. A Brookfield viscometer with helipath attachment can be used to determine creaming or sedimentation. The Brookfield viscometer determines the resistance encountered by a rotating spindle or cylinder immersed in a viscous material. The degree of resistance is correlated to degree of separation in an emulsion. The helipath attachment slowly lowers the rotating spindle into the medium so that the resistance encountered is always that of previously undisturbed sample. Almost all emulsions show change in consistency on aging; an emulsion with least changes should be considered most stable.

(d) *Electrophoretic properties:* Zeta potential of emulsion can be measured with the aid of moving boundary method, or more quickly and directly, by observing the movement of particles under the influence of electric current. The zeta potential is essentially useful for assessing flocculation since electrical changes on particles influence the rate of flocculation.

Electrical conductivity measurement also serves as a means to evaluate emulsion stability. It is determined using platinum electrodes (diameters 0.4 nm, distance 4 mm) micro-amperometrically to produce a current of 15 to 50 mA. Measurements are made on emulsions stored at room temperature or 37°C for short time. Stable o/w emulsions offer less resistance, but droplet aggregation increases the resistance. A stable w/o emulsion doesn't conduct electricity, but conductivity increases with droplet coagulation.

Microemulsion

The concept of microemulsion was introduced as early as in 1940s by Schulman and Cockbain. Hoar & Schulman [1943], generated a clear single phase by titrating a milky emulsion of hexanol. Schulman and co-workers, subsequently, coined the term microemulsion [Schulman et al., 1959].

Different scientists have defined micro-emulsions in different ways. Danielsson & Lindman [1981] defined microemulsions as a system of water, oil and amphiphile, which is a single optically isotropic and thermodynamically stable liquid solution. Microemulsions differ from emulsions on parameters more than the size. Microemulsions have globule size in the range of 10–100 nm as compared to 100 nm–100 mm in case of conventional emulsions. Emulsions exhibit excellent kinetic stability, but are fundamentally thermodynamically unstable. Microemulsions, on the contrary, are stable thermodynamic systems. Emulsions have milky or cloudy appearance whereas the micro-emulsions are transparent or translucent. For emulsion preparation large energy is required while this is not a requisition for microemulsions. It's obvious implication is relatively higher production cost in case of emulsion than micro-emulsion. Yet another important difference is the quantity of surfactant used; while in emulsions it is 2–3%, in microemulsions it is higher 6–8%.

o/w microemulsions are formed when the volume of oil is low whereas w/o systems are likely when the volume fraction of water is low. A third type, bicontinuous microemulsion, results when amounts of both water and oil are similar [Keipert & Schulz, 1994]. In this system, both water and oil exist as continuous phases in the presence of continuously fluctuating surfactant film. For further knowledge, the readers are advised to consult the book "Progress in Controlled and Novel Drug Delivery Systems" by N.K. Jain, published by CBS Publishers, New Delhi.

Microemulsion preparation: o/w microemulsion can be prepared starting with w/o emulsion containing lipophilic surfactant. In this process, hydrophilic surfactant is added by stirring, which initially forms cubic structure, but on further addition of hydrophilic surfactant forms o/w microemulsion. An exactly opposite procedure can be adopted for the preparation of w/o microemulsions [Li et al., 1995]. Formula for a multivitamin microemulsion is given below.

Multivitamin microemulsion	
Ingredients	**Quantity**
Vitamin A palmitate	7.35 g
Vitamin D	0.021 g
Polysorbate 80	75.0 g
Lemon oil	0.5 g
Vitamin E	0.88 g
Disodium edetate	0.5 g
Ascorbic acid	108.33 g
Saccharin sodium	1.0 g
Thiamine hydrochloride	3.75 g
Nicotinamide	17.5 g
Pyridoxine hydrochloride	0.88 g
Riboflavin sodium phosphate	2.16 g
Glycerin	700.0 g
Water, purified	250.0 g

Procedure: To prepare this formulation about 80% of purified water is to be taken in a container and disodium edetate, ascorbic acid, thiamine hydrochloride, nicotinamide, pyridoxine and saccharin sodium are added with continuous stirring, until dissolved completely. Required amount of glycerin is added to the above mixture, stirred for 5 minutes and kept aside. In another container specified amount of polysorbate 80 is taken and vitamins A, D, E and lemon oil are added with continuous stirring for 1 hr. Two portions are mixed by pouring oily phase at a rate of 4 mL/min into aqueous one with continuous stirring. The oil phase container is washed with purified water and added into aqueous phase. Adjust the volume and mix for 15 minutes, filter through 0.2 mm membrane filter and bubble with nitrogen for 15 minutes. It being a thermolabile preparation, the temperature of solution must not exceed 25°C.

Multiple emulsions

Multiple emulsions are also called as double emulsions as the internal phase itself contains dispersed phase globules, which are miscible with external medium. In both, w/o/w and o/w/o emulsions the central phase acts as a membrane that allows interphase transfer of solute. In most w/o/w emulsions the aqueous phases are identical giving rise to second order two component system. $o_1/w/o_2$, however, is a three-component system where the oil phases used are not identical [Lin et al., 1992]. For advanced knowledge about multiple emulsion and its processing, the readers are advised to consult the book "Advances in Controlled and Novel Drug Delivery Systems" by N.K. Jain, published by CBS Publishers, New Delhi.

- *Preparation:* A multiple emulsion can be prepared by double emulsification and phase inversion techniques.

  A. *Double emulsification:* In this method primary emulsion is emulsified in an external phase to produce a multiple emulsion. A w/o primary emulsion is emulsified in an aqueous vehicle containing hydrophilic surfactant to produce w/o/w system. Emulsification of w/o primary emulsion in an oily medium containing hydrophobic emulsifier produces w/o/w multiple emulsion.

  B. *Phase inversion:* Multiple emulsion can be readily formed by phase inversion of a primary emulsion. Phase inversion of o/w emulsion forms o/w/o emulsion and that of w/o emulsion will form w/o/w emulsion. Formula for a Multiple Emulsion is given below.

Nanoemulsions

Nanoemulsions can be defined as extremely small droplet emulsions, so small that the interaction of matter with light is negligible and they appear transparent, or translucent with bluish coloration. Nanoemulsion is actually a misnomer because the drop size is far larger than a nano-

Multiple emulsion	
Ingredients	**Quantity**
Primary emulsion	
Triglycerides	15 g
Flumethrin	15 g
Xanthan gum	5 g
Purified water	65 g
Multiple emulsion	
Primary emulsion	20 g
Triglycerides	76 g
Polyether–polysiloxane copolymer	4 g

Procedure: Multiple emulsions of the o/w/o type, where both the inner and the external oil phases were medium chain triglyceride, can be prepared by the two-step emulsification method, in which primary emulsion has been prepared by conventional methods and stabilized by xanthan gum and subsequently utilizing it in preparation of multiple emulsion using Polyether-polysiloxane copolymer in different ratios with xanthan gum.

meter. It is usually around 100 nm and broadly speaking in 50–500 nm range. In fact the globule size of microemulsions is smaller than that of nanoemulsions. Microemulsions are really single phase systems in which fusioned oil balls and fusioned water balls are present with no actually dispersed phase. They are flexible near zero curvature structures whose thermodynamic stability implies an ultra low interfacial tension, so that interfacial deformation is easy. In other words microemulsions are not emulsions with small droplets but some kind of weaved complex fabric with oil and water incorporated domains. Emulsions with small droplets in the range 50 nm–1 μm should be called **miniemulsions**, but the term nanoemulsions has prevailed, probably because it implies an even smaller droplet size and it has become more suitable for commercial issues. Thus, nanoemulsions (miniemulsions) are true emulsions with dispersed phase droplets and continuous phase and a surface area, which is much smaller than microemulsions, thus, requiring much less surfactant.

Preparative techniques: There are at least two techniques both called as phase transition methods. The first technique utilizes destabilizing the microemulsion structure to produce a nanoemulsion. It is a tricky method as the coalescence of droplets may lead to formation of droplets too big for nanoemulsion. The second technique utilizes a phenomenon called catastrophic inversion. In this an emulsion containing drops of oil in water suddenly becomes dispersion of w/o and vice versa. In some cases this transition may take place through an intermediate stage of multiple emulsions. This multiple emulsion breaks to release the extremely fine innermost droplets.

STANDARDS [IP, 2014]

Uniformity of content

For oral liquids (single dose in suspension form or powders or granules presented in single dose containers) containing more than one active ingredient (each active ingredient is less than 10 mg or less than 10% of all active ingredient), each container is to be emptied as completely as possible and the test on individual contents of active ingredients is to be carried out.

The test for uniformity of content should be carried out only after the content of active ingredient(s) in a pooled sample of the preparation has been shown to be within the accepted limits of the stated content. The content of active ingredient(s) of each of 10 containers taken at random using the suitable analytical method should be determined.

The preparation complies with the test if the individual values, thus, obtained are all between 85 to 115% of the average value. The preparation fails to comply with the test if more than one individual value is outside the limits 85–115% of the average value or if any one individual value is outside the limits 75–125% of the average value. If one individual value is outside the limits 85–115% but within the limits 75–125% of the average value, repeat the determination using another 20 containers taken at random. The preparation complies with the test if in the total sample of 30 containers not more than 3 individual values are outside the limits 85–115% and not more than one is outside the limits 75–125% of the average value.

Uniformity of weight/volume

Viscous preparations

Select a sample of 10 filled containers and determine the weight of the contents of each container as directed. A thoroughly clean and dry pycnometer is calibrated by filling it with recently boiled and cooled water at 25°C and weighing the contents. Adjust the temperature of the substance being examined, to about 20°C and fill the pycnometer with it. Adjust the temperature of the filled pycnometer to 25°C, remove any excess of the substance and weigh. Subtract the tare weight of the pycnometer from its fill weight. Determine the weight per mL by dividing the weight in air, in g, of the quantity of liquid, which fills the pycnometer at the specified temperature, by the capacity expressed in mL, of the pycnometer at the same temperature.

Non-viscous and free-flowing liquids

Pour completely the contents of each container into calibrated volume measures of the appropriate size and determine the volume of the contents of the 10 containers. The average net volume of the contents of the 10 containers is not less than the labelled amount, and the net volume of the contents of any single containers is not less than 91% and not more than 109% of the labelled amount where the labelled amount is 50 mL or less; or not less than 95.5% and not more than 104.5% of the labelled amount where the labelled amount is more than 50 mL but not more than 200 mL, or not less than 97% but not more than 103% of the labelled amount where the labelled amount is more than 200 mL but not more than 300 mL.

If this requirement is not met, determine the net volume of the contents of 10 additional containers. The average net volume of the contents of the 20 containers is not less than the labelled amount, and the net volume of the contents of not more than 1 of the 20 containers is less than 91% or more than 109% of the labelled amount where the labelled amount is 50 mL or less, or less than 95.5% or more than 104.5% of the labelled amount where the labelled amount is more than 50 mL but not more than 200 mL, or less than 97% or more than 103% of the labelled amount where the labelled amount is more than 200 mL but not more than 300 mL.

CONCLUSION

Oral liquids are useful in drug delivery for a variety of reasons. Patient compliance is often problematic with oral solid dosage forms, especially with young children and the elderly. Such difficulties can be overcome by administering the active compound in a palatable liquid form. Furthermore, the medication is uniformly distributed throughout the preparation; the dose can be fractionally adjusted by simply diluting it to meet the needs of patients. In addition, some deliquescent and hygroscopic powders are easily dispensed as liquids. The fact that drugs are rendered dispersed in oral liquids is advantageous in enhancing drug absorption.

However, oral delivery of drugs via various liquid dosage forms is not free from limitations. Drug substances are generally less stable in liquid form and masking the taste of inherently bitter drugs can also be difficult. Also, improvements in the palatability or pourability of liquid formulations may require the addition of viscosity imparting agents, which may themselves form complexes with drug molecules and hence result in undesired mitigations in drug activity. Extremely potent drugs with low-therapeutic indexes may be problematic when dosed in oral liquid preparations as the patients could easily err in dosage measurement. Therefore, processing and development of oral liquids necessitates the use of various tactics and techniques along with skilled operation.

While oral liquids may always be a smaller niche than solid dosage forms, increased patient demands are making this drug type more viable to pursue. Pharmaceutical companies who respond to market demands for new medicines and appropriate delivery systems such as oral liquids stand to reap the economic benefits.

REFERENCES

- Abdalla, A. Klein, S. Mäder, K. (2008). A new self-emulsifying drug delivery system (SEDDS) for poorly soluble drugs: Characterization, dissolution, *in vitro* digestion and incorporation into solid pellets, *Eur. J. Pharm. Sci.*, 35: 457–464.
- Agharkar, S., Lindenbaum, S., Higuchi, T. (1976). Enhancement of solubility of drug salts by hydrophilic counterions: properties of organic salts of an antimalarial drug, *Am. Pharm. Sci.*, 65: 747–749.
- Barr, M., Tice, L.F. (1957). The preservation of aqueous preparation containing non-ionic surfactants, *J. Am. Pharm. Ass.* (Sci. Edn.) 46: 445–451.
- Becher, P. (1965). **Emulsion: Theory and Practice**, Reinhold, New York.
- Block, L.H. (1996). Pharmaceutical emulsions and microemulsions, *In:* **Pharmaceutical Dosage Forms: Disperse Systems**, Lieberman, H.A., Rieger, M.M., Banker, G.S., Eds., Marcel Dekker, Inc., New York, 2: 47–109.
- Boylan, J.C. (1996). Liquids, *In:* **The Theory and Practice of Industrial Pharmacy**, 3rd ed., Lachman, L., Lieberman, H.A., Kanig, J.L., Eds., Lea & Febiger, Philadelphia, 457–458.
- Breitkreutz, J., Boos, J. (2007). Pediatric and geriatric drug delivery, *Exp. Opin. Drug Deliv.*, 4: 37–45.
- **British Pharmacopeia** (2007). Published by Her Majesty's Stationary Office for the Department of Health, London.
- Brown, D., Ford, J.L., Nunn, A.J., Rowe, P.H. (2004). An assessment of dose-uniformity of samples delivered from paediatric oral droppers, *J. Clin. Pharm. Ther.*, 29: 521–529.
- Carstensen, J.T. (2001). **Drug Stability Practices and Principles**, Marcel Dekker, Inc., New York.
- Carstensen, J.T. (1989). **Advanced Pharmaceutical Solids**, Marcel Dekker, Inc., New York.
- Carstensen, J.T. (2000). Solution kinetics, *In:* **Drug Stability: Principles and Practices**, Marcel Dekker, Inc., New York, 19–56.
- Chakrabarti, P.K., Harindran, J., Saraf, P.G., Wamburkar, M.N. (1993). Role of new anti-oxidants in the stabilization of ophthalmic and ear dosage form preparation of hamycin, *Drug Dev. Ind. Pharm.*, 19: 2595.
- Dainelsson, I., Lindman, B. (1981). The definition of microemulsion, *Colloids Surfaces B*, 3: 391–392.
- **Furia E. Fenaroli's Handbook of Flavor Ingredients**, Bellanca, N., Ed., CRC Press, Cleveland, OH, 1971.
- Gennaro, A.R., Ed., **Remington's Pharmaceutical Sciences**, 16th ed., Mack: Easton, PA, 1980; Ch. 69.
- Goncalves, E., Almeida, L.M., Dinis, T.C.P. (1998). Antioxidant activity of 5-aminosalicylic acid against lipid peroxidation in the presence of vitamins C and E, *Int. J. Pharm.*, 172: 219–228.
- Griessmann, K., Breitkreutz, J., Schubert-Zsilavecz, M., Abdel-Tawab, M. (2007). Dosing accuracy of measuring devices provided with antibiotic oral suspensions, *Paediatr. Perinat. Drug Ther.*, 8: 61–70.
- Heyd, A., Dhabhar, D. (1979). Particle shape effect on caking of coarse granulated antacid suspension, *Drug. Cosmet. Ind.*, 125: 42–45.
- Hiestand, E.N. (1964). Theory of coarse suspension formulation, *J. Pharm. Sci.*, 53: 1.
- Higuchi, T. (1958). Some physical chemical aspects of a suspension formulation, *J. Pharm. Sci.*, 59: 776–782.
- Hoar, T.P., Schulman, J.H. (1943). Transparent oil in water dispersions, *Nature*, 152: 102–103.
- Huang, L.F., Tong, W.Q. (2004). Impact of solid state properties on developability assessment of drug candidates, *Adv. Drug Deliv. Rev.*, 56: 321–334.
- **Indian Pharmacopoeia** (2014). Published by The Controller of Publications, Ministry of Health and Family Welfare, Government of India, New Delhi.
- International Conference on harmonisation of technical requirements for registration of

pharmaceuticals for human use (ICH), *Q1A & B stability guidelines*.

- Jain, N.K. (2007). **A Text Book of Forensic Pharmacy**, Vallabh Prakashan, Delhi.
- Kearns, G.L., Abdel-Rahman, S.M., Alander, S.W., Blowey, D.L., Leeder, J.S., Kauffman, R.E. (2003). Developmental pharmacology – drug disposition, action, and therapy in infants and children. *N. Engl. J. Med.*, 349: 1157–1167.
- Keipert, S., Schulz, G. (1994). Microemulsions with sucrose fatty acid surfactants, Part I: *In vitro* characterization, *Pharmazie*, 49: 195–197.
- Ková, J., Fortelný, I. (1984). Effect of poly-dispersity on the viscosity of a suspension of hard spheres, *Rheologica Acta*, 23: 454–456.
- Kruyt, H.R. (1953). **Colloid Science: Irreversible Systems**, Elsevier, Amsterdam.
- Li, M.J., Lee, H., Shim, C.K. (1995). Inverse targeting of drugs to reticuloendothelial system-rich organs by lipid microemulsions emulsified with by polaxamer 338, *Int. J. Pharm.*, 113: 175–187.
- Li, P., Zhao, L., Yalkowsky, S.H. (1999). Combined effect of cosolvent and cyclodextrin on solubilization of non-polar drugs, *J. Pharm. Sci.*, 88: 1107–1111.
- Lin, S.L., Kawashima, Y. (1985). The influence of three poly(oxyethylene) poly (oxypropylene), surface-active block copolymers on the solubility behavior of indomethacin, *Pharm. Acta Helv.*, 60: 339–344.
- Lin, S.Y., Wu, W.H., Lui, W.Y. (1992). *In vitro* release, pharmacokinetics and tissue distribution studies of doxorubicin hydrochloride encapsulated in lipidiolized w/o emulsion and w/o/w multiple emulsion, *Pharmazie*, 47: 439-443.
- Loftsson, T., Brewster, M.E. (1996). Pharma-ceutical applications of cyclodextrins: Solubili-zation and stabilization, *J. Pharm. Sci.*, 85: 1017–1025.
- Magnuson, B.A., Burdock, G.A., Doull, J. (2007). Aspartame: A safety evaluation based on current use levels, regulations, and toxicological and epidemiological studies, *Crit. Rev. Toxicol.*, 37: 629–727.
- Martin, A. (2005). **Physical Pharmacy**, Lippincott Willams & Wilkins, Maryland, USA.
- Mortensen, A. (2006). Sweeteners permitted in the European Union: Safety aspects, *Scan. J. Food Nutri.*, 50: 104-116.

- Pinco, R.G. (1991). Hurdling international barriers to existing and new excipients, *World Pharm. Stand. Rev.*, 2: 14–19.
- Rajewski, R.A., Stella, A.J. (1996). Pharmaceutical applications of cyclodextrins: *In vivo* drug delivery, *J. Pharm. Sci.*, 85: 1142–1168.
- Rasool, A.A., Hussain, A.A., Dittert, L.W. (1991). Solubility enhancement of some water-insoluble drugs in the presence of nicotinamide and related compounds, *J. Pharm. Sci.*, 80: 387–393.
- Rosoff, M. (1997). Specialised pharmaceutical emulsions. *In:* **Pharmaceutical Dosage Forms: Disperse Systems**, Lieberman, H.A., Rieger, M.M., Banker, G.S., Eds., Marcel Dekker, Inc., New York, 3: 1–22.
- Rowe, R.C., Sheskey, P.J., Weller, P.J. (2003). **Handbook of Pharmaceutical Excipients**, American Pharmaceutical Association, Pharma-ceutical Press, London.
- Roy, G.M. (1994). Taste masking in oral pharmaceuticals. *Pharm. Technol.*, 18: 84–90.
- Saiki, J.H., Thompson, S., Smith, F., Atkinson, R. (1972). Paraplegia following intrathecal chemotherapy, *Cancer*, 29: 370–374.
- Schieffer, G.W., Palermo, P.J., Pollard-Walker, S. (1984). Simultaneous determination of methyl, ethyl, propyl, and butyl 4-hydroxybenzoates and 4-hydroxybenzoic acid in liquid antacid formu-lations by gas chromatography, *J. Pharm. Sci.*, 73: 128–131.
- Schulman, J.H., Stoeckenius, W., Prince, L.M. (1959). Mechanism of formation and structure of microemulsions by electron microscopy, *J. Phys. Chem.*, 63: 1677–1680.
- Schulman, J.H., Cockbain, E.G. (1940). Molecular interactions at oil water interface. I. Molecular complex formation and the stability of oil in water emulsion, *Trans. Faraday Soc.*, 36: 651.
- Scott, M.W., Goudie, A.J., Huetteman, A.J. (1960). The stability of oral liquids, *J. Am. Pharm. Assoc. Sci.*, 49: 467.
- Seedher, N., Bhatia, S. (2003). Solubility enhance-ment of cox-2 inhibitors using various solvent systems, *AAPS Pharm. Sci. Technol.*, 4: 33–39.
- Shami, E.G., Bernardo, P.D., Rattie, E.S., Ravin, L.J. (1972). Kinetics of polymorphic trans-formation of sulfathiazole form I. *J. Pharm. Sci.*, 61: 1318–1321.

- Smith, J.M., Dodd, T.R.P. (1982). Adverse reactions to pharmaceutical excipients, *Adv. Drug React. Pois. Rev.*, 1: 93–142.
- Standing, J.F., Tuleu, C. (2005). Paediatric formulations – getting to the heart of the problem, *Int. J. Pharm.*, 300: 56–66.
- Stegemann, S., Ecker, F., Maio, M., Kraahs, P., Wohlfart, R., Breitkreutz, J., Zimmer, A., Bar-Shalom, D., Hettrich, P., Broegmann, B. (2010). Geriatric drug therapy – neglecting the inevitable majority, *Ageing Res. Rev.*, 9: 384–398.
- Streng, W.H. (1985). The stability of oral liquids, *Drug Dev. Ind. Pharm.*, 11: 1869–1888.
- Sznitowska, M., Janicki, S., Dabrowska, E.A., Gajewska, M. (2002). Physicochemical screening of antimicrobial agents as potential preservatives for submicron emulsions, *Eur. J. Pharm. Sci.*, 15: 489–495.
- Tingstad, J.E. (1964). Physical stability testing of pharmaceuticals, *J. Pharm. Sci.*, 53: 955–961.
- Tinwalla, A.Y., Hoesterey, B.L., Xang, T., Lim, K., Anderson, B. (1993). Solubilization of thiazolo-benzimidazole using a combination of pH adjustment and complexation with 2-hydroxypropyl-beta-cyclodextrin, *Pharm. Res.*, 10: 1136–1143.
- Varagunapandiyan, N., Gandhi, N.N. (2008). Enhancement of solubility and mass transfer coefficient through hydrotropy, *Int. J. Appl. Sci. Eng.*, 6: 97–110.
- Wen-Yen, C., Trong-Ming, D. (1989). A study on viscosity of suspensions, *J. App. Polymer Sci.*, 37: 2973–2986.
- Zhang, Y.G., Wright, W.J., Tam, W.K. (1990). Effect of inhaled preservatives on asthmatic subjects. II. Benzalkonium chloride, *Am. Rev. Respir. Dis.*, 141: 1405–1408.

3

Tablets

Ambikanandan Misra and Naazneen Surti

INTRODUCTION

Historical background

Oral drug delivery remains the preferred route of drug administration. For systemic effects, about 90 percent of drugs are administered via oral route. Most common solid oral dosage forms are tablets and capsules that account for more than half the total number and cost of all prescriptions issued. In Dec. 1843, a patent was granted to the Englishman, William Brockedon, for a machine to compress powders to form compacts. This machine consisted of a hole (or die) bored through a piece of metal within which the powder was compressed between two cylindrical punches; one was inserted into the base of the die and at a fixed depth, the other was inserted at the top of the die and struck with a hammer. The invention was first used to produce compacts of potassium bicarbonate and later on was adopted by a number of pharmaceutical companies. Wellcome, in Britain, was the first company to use the term tablet to describe this compressed dosage form. Novel technologies with improved performance, patient compliance, and enhanced quality have emerged in the recent past. Oral administration is the most popular route due to natural route for food ingestion, versatility to accommodate various types of drug candidates, no medical intervention in administration and, most importantly, patient compliance. A tablet is usually administered orally, but can be administered sublingually, rectally or intravaginally. The tablet is just one of the many forms that an oral drug can take such as syrups, elixirs, suspensions, and emulsions. It consists of an active pharmaceutical ingredient (A.P.I.) with biologically inert excipients in a compressed, solid form. Tablets are manufactured in non-sterile area with high manufacturing efficiency and hence are least expensive to manufacture. They have been in widespread use since the latter part of the 19th century, and their popularity continues.

The British Pharmacopoeia defines tablets as circular in shape with either flat or convex faces and prepared by compressing the medicament or mixture of medicaments usually with the added excipients. Tablets are now the most popular dosage form, accounting for some 70% of all ethical pharmaceutical preparations produced. British Pharmacopoeia in 1932 included only one tablet monograph (glyceryl trinitrate), which rapidly increased to 82 in 1953

BP. By 1963, the BP had 183 tablet preparations and in 1973, this figure had risen to 310 and 384 in the 1980 edition. The term compressed tablet is believed to have been used first by John Wyeth and Brother of Philadelphia. During this same period, molded tablets were introduced for use as hypodermic tablets for the extemporaneous preparation of solutions for injection.

Tablets remain popular as a dosage form because of the advantages afforded both to the manufacturer (e.g., simplicity, economy of preparation, stability, convenience in packaging, shipping, and dispensing, etc.) as well as patient (e.g., accuracy of dosage, compactness, portability, blandness of taste, and ease of administration, etc.).

Although, tablets frequently are discoid in shape, they may also be in round, oval, oblong, cylindrical, or triangular shapes. They may differ greatly in size and weight depending on the amount of drug substance present and intended method of administration.

Advantages of tablet medication

Tablets are unit dosage forms, which offer the highest dose precision and least content variability. They are lightest and most compact dosage forms, hence easiest and cheapest to package and ship. Product identification requires no additional processing steps when employing an embossed or monogrammed punch face. Tablets provide greatest ease of swallowing with the least tendency for hang-up above the stomach. They lend themselves to certain special release profile products e.g. enteric coated or delayed release profiles. It is easier to scale-up production than other oral dosage forms. They have the best combined properties of chemical, mechanical and microbiological stability among all the oral dosage forms. The patient can conveniently carry the emergency supply of the drug(s) as tablets.

Disadvantages of tablet medication

All the drugs cannot be formulated into tablets because some drugs are resistant to compression into dense compacts, owing to their amorphous nature or flocculent, low density properties. Drugs with bitter taste, objectionable odor, sensitivity towards oxygen or hygroscopic nature may require encapsulation/entrapment prior to compression, or coating of tablets is required. Elderly, ill and children could have problem in swallowing the tablets.

TYPES OF TABLETS

Tablets are divided into classes based on their route of administration and functions (Aulton., 2000; Gennaro., 2000'; Liberman et al., 1989).

Tablets administered orally

Compressed tablets

The tablets are prepared using compression and do not require special coatings. They are composed of powdered, crystalline, or granular material, alone or in combination with diluents such as binders, disintegrants, controlled-release polymers, lubricants, diluents, and colorants etc.

Sugar-coated tablets

These are compressed tablets are subjected to sugar coating.

Film-coated tablets

These are compressed tablets covered with a thin layer or film of a water soluble coating material.

Enteric-coated tablets

These are compressed tablets coated with substances that resist solution in gastric fluid but disintegrate in the intestine. Enteric coating of tablets is done for drugs, which are inactivated or degraded at stomach pH, irritant to gastric mucosa, or for delayed release of the medication.

Chewable tablets

These tablets are intended to be chewed by the patient. Patients who have difficulty in swallowing whole tablets or for children especially prefer it. Mannitol is normally used as a chewable base diluent, since it has a pleasant, cooling sensation in the mouth and can mask the taste of some objectionable medicaments. Chewable tablets are prepared by wet granulation. A disintegrating agent is not required, since the teeth perform this function. Antacid tablets are invariably presented as chewable tablets to obtain quick relief from indigestion.

Controlled release tablets

Compressed tablets can be formulated to release the drug slowly over a prolonged period of time. Hence, these dosage forms have been referred to as prolonged-release or sustained-release dosage forms as well. These tablets can be categorized into three types:

1. Those that respond to some physiological condition to release the drug, such as in enteric coating.
2. Those that release the drug in a relatively steady, controlled manner.
3. Those that combine combinations of mechanisms to release pulses of drug, such as repeat action tablets.

Multiple compressed tablets

These are compressed tablets manufactured by application of more than one cycle of compression.

Layered tablets

Layered tablets are prepared by compressing additional tablet granulation on a previously compressed granulation. The operation may be repeated to produce multilayered tablets of two or more layers. Special tablet presses are required to make layered tablets such as the Versa press (Stokes/Pennwalt).

Press coated tablets

Press coated tablets also referred as dry-coated tablets are prepared by feeding previously compressed tablets into a special tableting machine and compressing another granulation layer around the preformed tablets. An example of a press-coated tablet press is the Manesty Drycota. Press-coated tablets also can be used to separate incompatible drug substances; in addition, they provide a means of giving an enteric coating to the core tablets.

Tablets administered in oral cavity

Buccal and sublingual tablets

These are small, flat, oval shaped tablets. Tablets placed under tongue (sublingual) or in the side of the cheek (buccal) can produce an immediate systemic effect by enabling the drug to be directly absorbed through the mucosa in the systemic circulation, e.g. Isoprenaline sulphate (bronchodilator) and Glyceryl trinitrate tablets (vasodilator). These tablets are usually small in size and flat; they do not contain a disintegrant and are compressed at low pressure to produce a fairly soft tablet.

Lozenges and troches

Lozenges

Lozenges are compressed tablets, usually at least 18 mm in diameter, which do not contain a disintegrant and which are sucked to dissolve in the mouth. Generally, there are two types, depending on the required action. The first type produces a local effect in mouth or throat. Usually, these types of lozenges contain an antiseptic (e.g. benzalkonium) or antibiotic. The second type of lozenge produces a systemic effect. An example is a lozenge containing vitamin supplements, which is required to be sucked and is a palatable way of administering vitamins.

Troches

Troches are small square shaped tablets that dissolve in the mouth. They are now being used for natural hormone replacement therapy (NHR), anesthetics, antibiotics, and other combinations of medicines.

Dental cores

Dental cores are tablets to be placed in the empty socket following tooth extraction to prevent multiplication of bacteria by use of antibacterial compounds and reduce bleeding by using astringent/coagulant. The tablet should be formulated to dissolve or erode slowly in 30–40 minutes period and should not contain any component that might provide media for bacterial proliferation.

Tablets administered via other routes

Implants

Implants are very small pellets (2–3 mm dia) composed only of drug substance and prepared aseptically. Implants are inserted into body tissues by surgical procedures, where they are very slowly absorbed over a period of months. Implant pellets are used largely for the administration of hormones such as stilbestrol, testosterone etc. The particle size of the drug is usually kept large to produce a slow rate of absorption. In addition, implants are made very hard to achieve a gradual release.

Compressed suppositories or inserts

Occasionally, vaginal suppositories, such as metronidazole tablets are prepared by compression.

Tablets administered in solution form

Effervescent tablets

In addition to drug substances, these contain sodium bicarbonate and an organic acid such as tartaric or citric acid. In the presence of water, these additives react, liberating carbon dioxide that acts as a disintegrant and produces effervescence. Except for small quantities of lubricants present, effervescent tablets are soluble.

Dispensing tablets

These provide a convenient quantity of potent drug that can be incorporated readily into powders and liquids, thus circumventing the necessity to weigh small quantities.

Hypodermic tablets

Hypodermic tablets are soft, readily soluble tablets and originally were used for the preparation of solutions to be injected. The resulting solutions are not sterile. No hypodermic tablets ever have been recognized by the official compendia

Tablet triturates

Tablet triturates are usually made from moist material, using a triturate mold that gives them the shape of cut sections of a cylinder. The problem arising from compression of these tablets is the failure to find a lubricant that is completely water-soluble.

COMPONENTS OF TABLET

Active ingredients

The physicochemical properties of active ingredient provides rational basis for a particular tablet design. Preformulation investigations are designed to identify those physicochemical properties of drug substances and excipients that may influence the formulation design, method of manufacture, and pharmacokinetic-bio-pharmaceutical properties of the resulting product. Following is a generalized **preformulation protocol** appropriate for tablet dosage forms.

Identity and purity

These tests are necessary to identify degradation products and contaminants and may include organoleptic tests for color, odor, and taste. Alternative methods can be employed only if they are validated against the USP procedure. Tests other than potency, which can help to identify or determine the purity of compounds, are melting point, specific rotation, pH, heavy metals, residue on ignition, etc. An ordinary impurity test estimates impurities by thin-layer chromatography (TLC).

Crystal properties and polymorphism

Many drug substances appear in more than one polymorphic form. Even though they are chemically identical, the different polymorphic forms of a compound have different physical properties that can significantly influence the product performance. Polymorphic transformation can take place during pharmaceutical processing, such as particle size reduction, wet granulation, drying, and even during the compaction process. Tests employed to determine crystal properties include differential thermal analysis (DTA), differential scanning calorimetry (DSC), and X-ray diffraction.

Particle size, shape, and surface area

Particle characteristics are the most important characteristics in determining the performance of a drug substance in a formulation. This is particularly true in those cases where the drug is a poorly soluble non-electrolyte or a free acid form with poor solubility at low pH values. Such drugs are likely to exhibit dissolution-rate-limited absorption, the peak plasma concentration may be significantly delayed, or much of the drug may bypass that region of the gastrointestinal (GI) tract where absorption is best.

Particle size reduction (e.g., micronization) is often utilized to enhance dissolution rate. Particle size and shape also play an extremely important role in the homogeneity of powder blends and the unblending of powders in a mixer. Segregation in handling or during the compaction process has a significant effect on the content uniformity of the finished products. Surface area is critical for interaction with excipients in tablet dosage forms and can greatly affect stability. Methods to determine particle size and shape include light microscopy, scanning electron microscopy, sieve analysis, and various electronic sensing-zone particle counters. Methods available for surface area measurement include air permeability and various gas adsorption techniques.

Bulk powder properties

Knowledge of the true and bulk densities of the drug substance as well as of the excipients is extremely useful in providing perspective as to the size of the final tablet and the size and type of processing equipment needed, in anticipating problems in the physical mixing of powders and the homogeneity of intermediate and final products (significant differences in true densities can result in segregation), in anticipating problems in flow properties, and in identifying differences in different lots and raw materials from different suppliers because different polymorphic forms can be expected to exhibit different true densities.

A comparison of true particle density, apparent particle density, and bulk density can provide information on total, interparticle, and intraparticle porosity. Methods include true particle density measurements via helium pycnometry, mercury intrusion porosimetry, and poured and tapped bulk density.

The compactibility of relatively large-dose drug substances and formulations is another important property. Measures of compact mechanical strength include hardness (or crushing force), tensile strength, and friability.

For the evaluation of flow properties, angle of repose, minimum orifice diameter, Carr index, flow rate and weight variation during tableting runs are studied. The ultimate goal of flow analysis is to identify the powder or powder blend that provides the least weight variation in the finished tablet.

Solubility and permeability

In many cases, the rate of dissolution in gastrointestinal fluids is the rate-limiting step in absorption. The bioequivalence requirements established by the FDA define low solubility as < 5 mg/mL in water, and slow dissolution rate to be < 50% in 30 minutes. However, the solubility of a drug should be considered together with its dose; that is, even a very poorly soluble drug having a sufficiently small therapeutic dose may completely dissolve under physiological conditions. Thus, Amidon et al. (1995) defined a **high solubility** drug as one which at the highest human dose is soluble in 250 ml (or less) water throughout the physiological pH range (1–8) at 37°C. A **low solubility** drug is, thus, one which requires more than 250 ml of water to dissolve the largest human dose at any pH within the physiological range.

The intrinsic dissolution rate (IDR) of drugs is frequently measured by the rotating disk method or Wood's apparatus. The IDR may be used to detect different polymorphs as well as to judge the risk of a drug exhibiting dissolution-rate-limited absorption.

Excipients

Excipients are inactive, non-medicinal ingredients that are critical to the design of the delivery system and play a major role in determining its quality and performance. They may be selected to enhance stability (anti-oxidants, UV absorbers), optimize or modify drug release (disintegrants, hydrophilic polymers, wetting agents, biodegradable polymers), provide essential manufacturing technology functions (binders, glidants, lubricants), enhance patient acceptance (flavors), or aid in product identification (colorants). The excipients should be kept to a minimum in number and quantity and multifunctional excipients may be given preference over unifunctional excipients (Stephen et al., 2006).

Excipients may be classified as follows according to their general function.

Diluents/Fillers

Diluents are also referred to as bulking agents. These are inert substances, which are added to the active ingredient in sufficient quantity to make a reasonably sized tablet. This agent may not be necessary if the dose of the drug per tablet is high. Generally, a tablet should weigh at least 50 mg and therefore very low dose drugs will invariably require a diluent to bring the overall tablet weight to at least 50 mg.

The selection of a diluent will depend on the type of processing and plasticity of materials to be used. A direct-compression formulation will require a diluent with good flow and compaction properties. If the material is extremely plastic, it is appropriate to add a diluent that compacts by brittle fracture; similarly, a brittle drug substance should be combined with plastic filler.

A soluble drug is normally formulated with an insoluble filler to optimize the disintegration and dissolution. Drugs with low water solubility should never be formulated solely with insoluble fillers, including calcium salts (calcium sulfate, calcium phosphate, etc.)

Examples of commonly used diluents include lactose, calcium carbonate, dibasic calcium phosphate, microcrystalline cellulose, starches, mannitol, sorbitol etc.

Binders (Granulating agents)

Before tableting the powder mixture by compression, generally powders are granulated to form bridges followed by drying process. This granulation process can make powders of larger particle size and more free flowing for tablet production. The most common method of adding binders is as a solution in the granulating fluid. It is also possible to add synthetic polymers such as PVP and HPMC as powders and use water as the granulation agent. Inclusion of granulating agents or binders to increase granule strength is necessary. Granulating agents are usually hydrophilic polymers that have cohesive properties that both aid the granulation process and impart strength to the dried granulate. They form hydrophilic films on the surface of granules, which can aid in the wetting of hydrophobic drugs. However, if added at too great concentrations, the films can form viscous gels on the granule surface and will retard dissolution. Some commonly used binders are:

Starch

Corn starch is used widely as a binder in concentration ranging from 10 to 20%. It is not only useful as a binder, but also as a method to incorporate some disintegrant inside the granules.

Pre-gelatinized starch

It is soluble in cold water so easier to prepare than starch paste. It is used in the concentration of 0.1–0.5 %.

Gelatin solution

Gelatin generally is used as a 2–10% solution. Gelatin solutions are freshly prepared and used when warm or they will solidify.

Cellulosic solutions

Various celluloses have been used as binders in solution form. Most commonly used cellulose is HPMC. Others are HEC and HPC. All cellulosics are not soluble in water. EC solutions in alcohol have been effectively used as binders.

Polyvinylpyrrolidone

It can be used either as alcoholic/hydro alcoholic or aqueous solutions in a concentration range up to 20%.

Disintegrants

The drug solubility mainly depends on physical–chemical characteristics of the drug. However, the rate of drug dissolution is greatly influenced by disintegration of the tablet. The drug will dissolve at a slower rate from a non-disintegrating tablet due to exposure of limited surface area to the fluid. Disintegrants, an important excipient of the tablet formulation, are always added to tablet to induce breakup of tablet when it comes in contact with aqueous fluid and this process of desegregation of constituent particles before the drug dissolution occurs is known as **disintegration process**. This is especially important for immediate release products where rapid release of drug substance is required. The objectives behind addition of disintegrants are to increase surface area of the tablet fragments and to overcome cohesive forces that keep particles together in a tablet.

Mechanism of action of tablet disintegrants

The tablet breaks to primary particles by one or more of the mechanisms listed below:

By capillary action

When a tablet is put into suitable aqueous medium, the medium penetrates into the tablet and replaces the air adsorbed on the particles, which weakens the intermolecular bond and breaks the tablet into fine particles. Water uptake by tablet depends upon hydrophilicity of the drug/excipient and on tableting conditions.

By swelling

Tablets with high porosity show poor disintegration due to lack of adequate swelling force. On the other hand, sufficient swelling force is exerted in the tablet with low porosity.

Heat of wetting

When disintegrant with exothermic properties gets wetted, localized stress is generated due to capillary air expansion, which helps in disintegration of tablet.

Due to disintegrating particle/particle repulsive forces

The electric repulsive forces between particles are the mechanism of disintegration and water is required for it. Repulsion is believed to be secondary to wicking.

Due to deformation

During tablet compression, disintegrant particles get deformed and these deformed particles get into their normal structure when they come in contact with aqueous media or water. This increase in size of the deformed particles produces a break-up of the tablet.

Due to release of gases

Carbon dioxide is released within tablets on wetting due to interaction between bicarbonate and carbonate with citric acid or tartaric acid. The tablet disintegrates due to generation of pressure within the tablet.

Methods of addition of disintegrants

Disintegrating agent can be added either prior to granulation (intragranular) or prior to compression (after granulation i.e. extragranular) or at the both processing steps. Extragranular fraction of disintegrant (usually, 50% of total disintegrant) facilitates break-up of tablets to granules and the intragranular addition of disintegrants produces further erosion of the granules to fine particles. The greater the level of disintegrant, the faster the tablet will disintegrate. However, the compaction properties of many disintegrants, including starch, are not satisfactory and use of high concentration could also reduce tablet strength. Disintegrant activity can be affected by mixing with hydrophobic excipients.

The oldest and most popular disintegrant is corn and potato starch which has been powdered and well dried. Starch has a great affinity for water and swells when moistened, thus, facilitating the rupture of the tablet matrix. In addition to starches, a large variety of materials have been used and reported to have dis-integrating properties. These include MCC, CMC, MC, agar, bentonite, Veegum, etc.

Incorporation of super-disintegrants (crospovidone, croscarmellose sodium, sodium starch glycolate) has improved dissolution from both direct-compression and wet-granulation formulations. **Superdisintegrants** are effective at low concentrations, have greater disintegrating efficiency and are more effective intragranularly. They act by swelling and due to swelling pressure exerted in the outer direction or radial direction, they cause tablet to burst or the accelerated absorption of water leads to an enormous increase in the volume of granules to promote disintegration.

Some super-disintegrants are listed below:

Croscarmellose sodium

Cross-linked sodium carboxymethylcellulose has high absorption capacity, contains no sugar or starch, high swelling capacity, and is effective at low concentrations (0.5–2.0% but can be used up to 5.0%).

Crospovidone

A synthetic homopolymer of cross-linked *N*-vinyl-2-pyrrolidone, completely insoluble in water, acids, alkalis, and all organic solvents, hygroscopic, swells rapidly in water, rapidly disperses in water but does not gel even after prolonged exposure. It has greatest rate of swelling compared to other disintegrants as well as, greater surface area to volume ratio than other disintegrants typically used at a level of 1–3%.

L-HPC

A low-substituted hydroxypropyl ether of cellulose swells rapidly in water whereas types with a larger average particle size and higher hydroxypropyl content show higher degree of swelling. Recommended concentration is 1–5%.

Sodium starch glycolate

It is a sodium salt of carboxymethyl ether of starch, practically insoluble in organic solvents. It absorbs water rapidly, resulting in swelling that leads to rapid disintegration of tablets and granules. Recommended concentration is 1.0–4.0% but may need to use up to 6.0%.

Lubricants

Lubricants are required during manufacture to ensure that the tableting powder (i.e. the raw

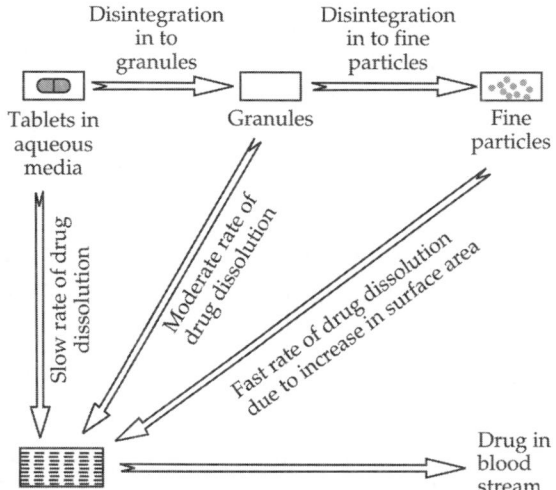

Fig. 3.1. Diagrammatic representation of disintegration and dissolution steps.

ingredient blend) does not stick to the pressing equipment. Lubricants improve the flow of powder mixtures through the presses and help finished tablets release from the equipment with a minimum of friction and breakage.

Based on their action, lubricants are classified into **antiadherent** excipients, which reduce the friction between the tablet faces and tablet punches, and **die wall lubricant** excipients, which reduce the friction between tablet surface and the die wall during and after compaction to enable easy ejection of the tablet. Most die wall lubricants also have anti-adherent actions.

Some commonly used lubricants are:

Magnesium stearate

It is a widely used and extremely effective lubricant, works in concentrations from 0.5–5%, although, it is best to use this lubricant in the lowest effective concentration. Magnesium stearate is not only hydrophobic but also has a laminar crystal structure. When blended with other ingredients, it tends to make them hydrophobic by delaminating to coat their surfaces. The problems with magnesium stearate are thus highly process dependent. For example, blending time differences of as little as 2 min can significantly alter the dissolution pattern of finished tablets.

Stearic acid

Stearic acid is frequently used in combination with magnesium stearate, to get a synergistic lubricant effect on punch faces and die walls. It does not have the over blending problems observed with magnesium stearate.

Other lubricants used are sodium stearyl fumarate and glyceryl behanate.

Glidants

Glidants are substances that improve the flow characteristics of a powder mixture. These materials are always added as dry powders just prior to compression. Colloidal silicon dioxide is the most commonly used glidant in concentrations up to 5%. Talc is also used and may serve the dual purpose of lubricant as well as glidant.

Coating agents

Coating agents are used to impart a finished look and a smooth surface to tablets, and to mask any unpleasant flavors that the tablet ingredients may have. Coating agents are applied after tablet pressing in a separate operation. Some examples of coating agents are beeswax, cellulosic derivatives, titanium dioxide etc.

Preservatives

Antimicrobials and antioxidants are added to pharmaceutical products to prolong shelf life and maintain sterility. Common **antimicrobial agents** include chlorbutol, benzyl alcohol, sodium benzoate, sorbic acid, phenol, thimerosal, parabens, and benzalkonium chloride. **Antioxidants** used in pharmaceutical products include butylated hydroxyl toluene and hydroxyanisole, as well as propyl gallate and sulfites.

Sweetening and flavoring agents

Sweetening and flavoring agents are commonly added to chewable tablet formulations to improve taste, texture and overall palatability. Mannitol, sucrose, lactose, dextrose etc. are natural sweeteners as well as saccharin, cyclamate and aspartame are examples of artificial sweeteners. Saccharin is 500 times sweeter than sucrose. Its major disadvantages are that it has a bitter aftertaste and is carcinogenic. Aspartame is about 180 times sweeter than sucrose. The primary disadvantage of aspartame is its lack of stability in the presence of moisture.

Flavors are commonly used to improve the taste of chewable tablets as well as mouth dissolved tablets. Flavors are incorporated either as solids (spray dried flavors) or oils or aqueous (water soluble) flavors. The maximum amount of oil that can be added to granulation without affecting tableting characteristics is 0.5–0.75%

w/w. Aqueous flavors are less used because of their instability on aging.

Dyes and coloring agents

Dyes and coloring agents are used to provide a unique product identity, to overcome color change on aging, disguising of off-color drugs, for brand image in the market and to enhance the aesthetic appearance of the product to have better patient acceptance.

There are currently more than 100 dyes and lakes approved by the Food and Drug Administration for use in pharmaceutical preparations. One of the important advantages in using lakes is reduced risk of interaction between the drug and other ingredients, color development is rapid; which reduces processing time.

Miscellaneous excipients

Wetting agents

In tablet formulation these aid water uptake and thereby enhance disintegration and assist in drug dissolution. Wetting agents are mainly added when hydrophobic drug is to be formulated into tablet. SLS, Sodium diisobutyl sulfosuccinate are used as wetting agent in tablet formulation.

Dissolution retardants

These are incorporated into tablet formulation only when controlled release of drug is required. Waxy materials like stearic acid and their esters can be used as dissolution retardants.

Adsorbents

These are the agents that can retain large quantities of liquids. Most commonly used adsorbents in pharmaceuticals are anhydrous calcium phosphate, starch, magnesium carbonate, bentonite, kaolin, magnesium silicate, magnesium oxide and silicon dioxide.

Modified excipients

Introduction of novel drug delivery systems and new drug moieties lead to the need for new excipients with varied characteristics. Development of new excipient entities and their evaluation is a costly procedure; modification of existing excipients is very easy, more economical and less time consuming. The development of excipients that are capable of fulfilling multifunctional roles such as enhancing drug bioavailability and drug stability as well as controlling the release of the drug according to the therapeutic needs is one of the most important prerequisites for further progress in the design of novel drug delivery systems (Joshi et al., 2004).

Moreover, direct-compression process and high-speed machines have increased the demands on the functionality of excipients in terms of flow and compression properties. Particle engineering of individual excipients and excipient combinations using co-processing, by virtue of subparticle modifications, has provided an attractive tool for developing high-functionality excipients that are suited to modern tablet manufacturing processes. Excipients with improved functionality can be obtained by developing new chemical excipients, new grades of existing materials, and new combinations of existing materials. Developing new grades of existing excipients (varying physicochemical properties) has been the most successful strategy for the development of new excipients in past three decades, a process that has been supported by the introduction of better performance grades of excipients such as pre-gelatinized starch, croscarmellose, and crospovidone. However, functionality can be improved only to a certain extent because of the limited range of possible modifications.

A new combination of existing excipients is an interesting option for improving excipient functionality because all formulations contain multiple excipients. Many possible combinations of existing excipients can be used to achieve the desired set of performance characteristics. However, the development of such combinations is a complex process because one excipient may interfere with the existing functionality of another excipient. Over the years, the development of single-bodied excipient combinations at a subparticle level, called co-processed excipients, has gained importance.

Co-processed excipients

A co-processed excipient is a combination of two or more compendial or non-compendial excipients designed to physically modify their properties in manner not achievable by simple physical mixing, and without significant chemical change. Co-processed excipients are used mainly in solid dosage forms such as tablets, capsules, powder and in liquid dosage forms such as emulsions, suspensions, injections and in semisolid dosage forms such as creams, ointments and pastes (Chaudhary et al., 2012).

Co-processed excipients (Table 3.2) are prepared by incorporating one excipient into the particle structure of another excipient using processes such as co-drying. Thus, they are simple physical mixtures of two or more existing excipients mixed at the particle level. Particle engineering is a broad-based concept that involves the manipulation of particle parameters such as shape, size, size distribution, and simultaneous minor changes that occur at the molecular level such as polytypic and poly-morphic changes (Nagacheri et al., 2004). All these parameters are translated into bulk-level changes such as flow properties, compressibility, moisture sensitivity, and machine ability. The success of any pharmaceutical excipient depends on quality, safety, and functionality. Although, the first two parameters have remained constant, significant improvements in functionality open the door for the increased use of co-processed excipients. The advantages of these excipients are numerous, but further scientific exploration is required to understand the mechanisms underlying their performance. The main obstacle to the growth of this area of excipients is the non-inclusion of their monographs in pharma-copoeias, which discourages pharmaceutical manufacturers to use them. With recommen-

dations from International Pharmaceutical Excipients Council (IPEC), these products could find their way into official monographs either as mixtures or as single bodied excipients. Once the obstacles are overcome, the use of co-processed excipients can be expected to increase dramatically.

Multifunctional excipients

Multifunctional excipients are a class of excipients that includes preprocessed and co-processed excipients that provide added functionalities to the formulation (for example, Silicified Micro-Crystalline Cellulose, which is a processed combination of MCC and colloidal silicon dioxide). These functionalities include flowability, compressibility, particle size distribution, shape, porosity, etc. The term multifunctional excipient is also extended to products that serve multiple roles in the formulation e.g. Ludipress, which is co-processed product containing lactose, Kollidon and Kollidon-CL, serves the role of directly compressible diluent with binder and disintegrant properties

Some examples of Innovative Multi-functional excipients are galenIQTM-The smart excipient, MCC SANAQ®burst, NEUSILIN, SYLOID® FP, UNI-PURE™ WG, Pharmaburst™ "Quick Dissolve".

High functionality excipients

High Functionality Excipients (HFE) are inactive ingredients that meet four unique criteria. Firstly, they are multifunctional; they combine two or more functions through a single ingredient. Secondly, they have high inherent functional performance allowing for increased batch sizes and higher drug-loading, even at low usage levels. Thirdly, HFE require no complex processing, making them ideal for direct compression processes. Lastly, they impart their high inherent performance characteristics to the overall formulation. This last criterion is critical and separates HFE from other multi-functional

Table 3.1. Commonly used tablet excipients

DILUENTS

LACTOSE ANHYDROUS

Applications	Commercially available	Suppliers/manufacturers
Wet granulation filler/binder	Pharmatose® DCL 21	CHR Hansen
Direct compression filler/binder	Sheffield DT, Sheffield 60M	Sheffield (Quest)

LACTOSE MONOHYDRATE

Product category	Typical examples
Crystalline, sieved	Pharmatose 50M, 80M, 90M, 100M, 110M & 125M, PrismaLac® 40 & 50, Capsulac® 60, Sachelac® 80 and Spherolac® 100
Crystalline, milled	Granulac® 70,140 & 200, Pharmatose® 150M, 200M, 325M, 350M & 450M and Sorbolac® 40
Agglomerated	Tablettose® 70 and Tablettose® 80.
Spray-dried	FlowLac® 100 and Pharmatose® DCL 11.

Applications

Wet granulation	Crystalline, milled products like GranuLac® 70, 140, 200, 230; and Pharmatose® 150M, 200M, 350M, 450M
Powder blends, capsule/sachets	Crystalline products like PrismaLac® 40, Capsulac® 60, Sachelose® 80, Pharmatose®150M, 200M, 350M, and 450M; Spray-dried products like FlowLac® 100 provide excellent flow properties, and Pharmatose DCL-11
Direct compression	Agglomerated products like Tablettose® 70/80, combine the flowability of coarse lactose crystals with the good flow properties of milled lactose. Highly stable and non-hygroscopic. High surface area provides easy water intrusion for fast tablet dissolution. White appearance leads to absolutely white tablets. Spray-dried products like FlowLac® 100 provide superior flowability with exceptional hardness yield. Useful for low-dose formulations. Good water solubility leads to fast tablet disintegration. Porous surface provides an adhesion of actives leading to high content uniformity. Crystalline products like Pharmatose 50M, 80M, 90M, 100M, 110M and 125M. Spray-dried products like Pharmatose DCL-11
Effervescent tablets	Tablettose® 70/80, FlowLac®100
Spheronization	Crystalline, sieved products like Spherolac® 100
Chewable tablets	Spray dried products like FlowLac® 100 provide pleasant taste and mouth feel. Good water solubility leads to fast tablet disintegration. Porous surface of the particles provides an adhesion of actives leading to high content uniformity
Dry powder inhalers and blend premixes	Crystalline, milled products with superior surface area like Pharmatose® 325M and Sorbolac® 400
Sweetener	Tablettose® 70/80, Highly stable and non-hygroscopic. Ideal for table-top sweeteners due to its particle-structure, whiteness, and sugar like appearance

Suppliers

CHR Hansen/DMV International	Lactose monohydrate, NF
	Crystalline, sieved Pharmatose® 50M, 80M, 90M, 100M, 110M, 125M, & 325M
	Crystalline, milled Pharmatose® 150M, 200M, 350M, and 450M
	Spray-dried Pharmatose® DCL 11

(Contd.)

Meggle	Lactose monohydrate, JP, Ph.Eur., NF
	Crystalline, Sieved Prismalac® 40, Capsulac® 60, Sachelac® 80, SpheroLac® 100, and Inhalac®
	Crystalline, milled Granulac® 70, 140, 200 and 230, and Sorbolac® 400
	Spray-dried FlowLac® 100
	Agglomerated Tablettose® 70/80 and 100
Sheffield	Lactose monohydrate, NF
Wyndale, New Zealand	80 mesh sifted
	300 mesh milled
Lactose, New Zealand	Lactose monohydrate, NF Super Tab®

MICROCRYSTALLINE CELLULOSE

Product, Original	Product, Small particle size	Product, Large particle size	Product, Low moisture	Product, High density
Avicel® PH 101, PH 102	Avicel® PH 105	Avicel® PH 200	Avicel® PH 113, 112, 103	Avicel® PH 301, 302
Vivapur® 101, 102	Vivapur® 99, 105	Vivapur® 12, 200	Vivapur® 103, 112	Vivapur® 301, 302
Tabulose® 101, 102	—	Tabulose® 250, 500	Tabulose® 103, 112	Tabulose® 301, 302

Applications	Grades used
Direct compression	12, 102, 200, 302 or 112
Wet granulation	101 or 301
Slugging or roller compaction	102, 302 or 112
Encapsulation	102, 302 or 112
Spheronization	101 or 301

Suppliers	
Blanver	Tabulose, microcrystalline cellulose, BP, DAB, NF, Ph. Eur.
	Grades:
	Original: 101, 102
	Low Moisture: 103, 112
	Large particle size: 250, 500
	High density: 301, 302
FMC	Avicel , microcrystalline cellulose, BP, JP, NF, Ph. Eur.
	Grades:
	Small particle size: PH 105
	Original: PH 101, PH 102
	Low moisture: PH 103, PH 112, PH 113
	Large particle size: PH 200
	High density: PH 301, PH 302
JRS	Vivapur, microcrystalline cellulose, DAB, JP NF, Ph. Eur.
	Grades:
	Small particle size: 99, 105
	Original: 101, 102

(Contd.)

Low moisture: 103, 112
Large particle size: 12, 200
High density: 301, 302

OTHER DILUENTS

	Trade names	Manufacturers/suppliers
Mannitol	Mannogem®	SPI Pharma
	Mannitol Powder	
	GetecMannitol, Pyrogen Free	
	Mannitol Granular	
	Mannitol Granular 2080	
	Mannitol Granular 3215	
	Pearlitol®	Roquette
	Partech M®	EM Industries
Calcium carbonate		
Calcium carbonate USP		
Oyster shell powder	Pharma-carb® LL	
Calcium carbonate and maltodextrin	Oyster Shell Powder 4402	CHR Hansen
Calcium carbonate and pregelatinized starch	Cal-Carb® 4450 PG	
Precipitated calcium carbonate and pregelatinized starch	Carb® 4457 Cal-Carb® 4462	
Compressible sucrose	Compressuc®	Beghin-Say (France)
	NU-TAB® Compressible Sugar NF, also available in different colors	CHR Hansen
	SugarTab® Compressible Sugar, NF	Penwest
	Di-Pac® Compressible Sugar NF	Tate and Lyle
Dextrose (D-glucose)	C*Pharm Dextrose Monohydrate	Cerestar
Maltodextrin	Maltrin®	Grain Processing Corporation
	C*Pharm Maltodextrins	Cerestar
Maltose	Advantose® 100	SPI Pharma
Xylitol, DC	Xylitab®	Danisco
Sorbitol, Crystalline	C Sorbidex P®	Cerestar
	C Sorbidex S®	
Directly compressible starch	C*Pharm® DC 93000	Cerestar
	Sta-Rx 1500	
Hydrolyzed starch	Emdex	—
	Celutab	
Modified starches (Carboxymethyl starch)	—	—
Dibasic calcium phosphate	A-Tab	—
Tribasic calcium phosphate	Tri-Cafos	—
Calcium sulfate dihydrate	Destab	—

(Contd.)

BINDERS

Binder	Usual concentration
Polyvinylpyrollidone (various grades)	5–20% (Dry/aqueous, alcoholic or hydro alcoholic solution)
Methylcellulose (various viscosity grades)	2–10% (Aqueous solution)
Ethylcellulose (various viscosity grades)	2–15% (Alcoholic solution)
Starch	5–10% (Aqueous paste)
Starch 1500	5–10% (Dry/aqueous paste)
Pregeltinized starch	5–10% (Dry/aqueous solution)
Gelatin (various types)	2–10% (Aqueous solution)
Sucrose	10–85% (Aqueous solution)
Acacia	5–20% (Dry/aqueous solution)
Sodium carboxymethylcellulose (low viscosity grade)	2–10% (Aqueous solution)
Polyvinyl alcohol (various viscosity grades)	2–10% (Aqueous or hydro alcoholic solution)
Polyethylene glycol 6000	10–30% (Aqueous, alcoholic or hydro alcoholic solution)

DISINTEGRANTS

Disintegrant	Usual concentration in granulation (% w/w)
Starch	5–20
Starch 1500	5–15
Avicel PH 101, PH 102 (microcrystalline cellulose)	5–15
Alginic acid	5–10
Methycellulose, sodium carboxymethylcellulose, hydroxypropylmethylcellulose	5–10
Guar gum	2–8
Amberlite IPR 88 (Ion exchange resin)	0.5–5
Sodium starch glycolate (Explotab, Vivastar, Primojel)	2–8
Croscarmellose sodium (Ac-diSol, Vivasol, Solutab)	0.5–5
Crosslinked polyvinylpyrrolidone (Polyplasdone XL-10, INF 10)	1–3

GLIDANTS

Glidant	% w/w
Silica aerogels (Cab-o-Sil M-5, Aerosil 200 M, QUSO F-22)	0.1–5.0
Calcium stearate	0.5–2.0
Magnesium stearate	0.2–2.0
Zinc stearate	0.2–1.0
Calcium silicate	0.5–2.0
Starch, dry flow	1.0–10.0
Starch 1500	1.0–10.0
Magnesium lauryl sulfate	0.2–1.0
Magnesium carbonate, heavy	1.0–3.0
Magnesium oxide, heavy	1.0–3.0
Purified Talc	1.0–5.0

(Contd.)

LUBRICANTS

Lubricant	% w/w
Hydrophobic	
Metal stearate, calcium, magnesium, zinc	0.5–2.0
Stearowet C (Water wettable mixture of calcium stearate and sodium lauryl sulfate)	0.5–2.0
Stearic acid, fine powder	1.0–3.0
Hydrogenated vegetable oils (Sterotex, Duratex, TriStar)	1.0–3.0
Glycerylbehenate (Compritol 888 ATO)	0.5–3.0
Purified Talc	5.0–10.0
Starch	5.0–10.0
Light mineral oil	1.0–3.0
Hydrophilic	
Sodium benzoate	2.0–5.0
Sodium chloride	5.0–20.0
Sodium and magnesium lauryl sulfate	1.0–3.0
Sodium stearylfumarate	0.5–3.0
Polyethylene glycol 4000 and 6000 (Carbowax 4000 and 6000), fine powder	2.0–5.0

COLORS, FLAVORS AND SWEETENERS

FD & C and D & C dyes and lakes
Spray dried and other flavors
Natural sweeteners
Artificial sweeteners

Table 3.2. Co-processed excipients

Co-processed excipients	Trade name	Manufacturer	Added advantage
Lactose, 3.2% Kollidon 30, Kollidon CL	Ludipress	BASF, AG, Ludwigshafen, Germany	Low degree of hygroscopicity, good flowability, tablet hardness independent of machine speed
Lactose, 25% cellulose	Cellactose	Meggle GmbH & Co. KG, Germany	Highly compressible, good mouthfeel, better tableting at low cost
Sucrose, 3% dextrin	DiPac		Directly compressible
MCC, silicon dioxide	Prosolv	Penwest Pharmaceuticals Company	Better flow, reduced sensitivity to wet granulation, better harness of tablet, reduced friability
MCC, guar gum	Avicel CE-15	FMC Corporation	Less grittiness, reduced tooth packing, minimal chalkiness, creamier mouthfeel, improved overall palatability
Calcium carbonate sorbitol	ForMaxx	Merck	Controlled particle size distribution
MCC, lactose	Microcelac	Meggle	Capable of formulating high dose, small tablets with poorly flowable active
95% [beta]-lactose + 5% lactitol	Pharmatose	DMV Veghel	High compressibility, low lubricant sensitivity
85% α lactose MH + 15% native corn starch	StarLac	Roquette	Good flow

excipients or conventional specialty excipients, e.g. PROSOLV SMCC (Silicified microcrystalline cellulose) and Captisol (Modified beta cyclodextrin)

Patents on novel excipients

Joan CucalaEscoi published a patent (US20050031862 A1 10, Feb, 2005) on modified calcium phosphate excipient. The invention is based on the discovery that calcium phosphate can be modified with a fatty acid wax and further such a modified calcium phosphate can provide advantageous properties. Accordingly, a first aspect of the invention relates to an excipient composition comprising calcium phosphate modified with a fatty acid wax, wherein a weight ratio of calcium phosphate to wax is within the range of 50:50 to 95:5, respectively. The excipient composition is generally provided in a free flowing particulate form and the fatty acid wax is generally selected from palmitic acid, behenic acid, stearic acid, glyceryl behenate, glyceryl palmitostearate, hydrogenated castor oil, and mixtures thereof. The particles generally have an average size in the range of 20 to 1000 microns, typically 50 to 500 microns, and in some embodiments from 125 to 250 microns. The calcium phosphate is normally an anhydrous dibasic calcium phosphate (Joan CucalaEscoi et al., 2005).

Gorgegoan published a patent (EP1697050A2, Sep 6, 2006) on Fiber rich fraction (FRF) of trigonellafoenum-graceum seeds and its use as a pharmaceutical excipient. The invention relates to a novel solvent free process of obtaining an insoluble fiber rich fraction from TrigonellaFoenum-graceum seeds. The invention further relates to the fraction obtained from TrigonellaFoenum-graceum seeds, having at least 50% of dietary fiber with a ratio of insoluble dietary fiber to soluble dietary fiber greater than 0.8 and a protein content not more than 10 weight % with a viscosity greater than 10000 cps at 2% w/v concentration. The invention also relates to the process of purifying the fiber rich fraction to obtain a highly purified fiber rich fraction. The invention further discloses use of FRF or highly purified FRF as a pharmaceutical excipient in various pharmaceutical dosage forms (Gorgegoan et al., 2006).

Vincent Green published a patent (US 2006/0008521 A1, Jan, 2006) entitled Tablet excipient. This invention relates to a composition comprising physically modified, partially pregelatinized starch, which is useful as a multifunctional excipient for solid dosage forms, a method of making such composition, and solid dosage forms prepared using the composition. The starch composition according to this invention is a multi-functional excipient, which possesses excellent binding, disintegrating, and flow properties. It is also capable of accelerating drug dissolution from a solid dosage form (Vincent Green et al., 2006).

Romain Callaird published a patent (US20110076326, March 31, 2011) entitled 'modified protein excipient for delayed-release tablet'. The invention relates to the delayed release of molecules when formulated in a compressed tablet that is protein-based of which the protein's isoelectric point has been modified in order to reduce solubility and swelling. Particularly, the invention relates to tablets that comprise an excipient comprising chemically modified food proteins such as soy proteins or β-lactoglobulin useful for delaying release of an active ingredient, namely a pharmaceutical drug or a probiotic (Romain Callaird et al, 2011)

Gordon Bardley published a patent (US8226967 B2, July 24, 2012) entitled 'Surface-active proteins as excipients in solid pharmaceutical formulations'. The invention provides a method for utilizing surface-active proteins as excipients in pharmaceutical technology, particularly in galenics. The hydrophobins may be used either by admixture to pharmaceutically utilized polymers and compounds, by incorporation into/formation of a matrix or by coating of galenic forms to achieve a modulation of release kinetics. The pharmaceutical form to be treated with the method according to the present invention can be designated for oral application or other routes of administration (e.g. rectal application). Examples for galenic forms according to the present invention are capsules, pills, tablets, matrix tablets, microgranules and suppositories, but not limited to these (Gordon Bardley et al., 2012).

In summary, the use of pharmaceutical excipients is necessary to produce the wide variety of medications available to patients. While most patients tolerate these inert ingredients without problems, it should be remembered that these compounds are capable of inducing adverse effects. The trend towards more prudent use of these chemicals by pharmaceutical manufacturers and the increasing availability of labelling information will help clinicians to select appropriate products for their patients.

Drug-excipient compatibility

Knowledge of the interaction of drugs and excipients is essential in the initial formulation of a product. It may also be necessary later on during processing scale-up, when problems arise, to determine if incompatibilities exist which affect manufacturing or stability. Drug-excipient interactions are often directly related to the moisture present in one or another of the components or to the humidity to which the formulation is exposed during processing or storage. Hence these studies are always carried out at accelerated temperature and humidity conditions. Tests for excipient drug interactions are usually conducted on blends of the pure drug and excipient in ratios similar to those in the final dosage form. Powders are physically mixed and may be granulated or compacted to accelerate any possible interaction. Samples can be exposed in open pans or sealed in bottles or vials to mimic product packaging. Evaluation of samples includes visual inspection for changes in color or texture. Both HPLC and

TLC are commonly employed with unstressed samples being used as controls. Other tests employed are differential thermal analysis, isothermal microcalorimetry as well as a thermal activity monitor (TAM) technique.

MANUFACTURING

The manufacturing of tablets involves a number of unit processes such as (i) dispensing, (ii) particle size reduction (milling) and sizing, (iii) blending, (iv) granulation, (v) drying, and (vi) compaction/compression (Shayne et al., 2006).

Dispensing

Dispensing may be done by purely manual scooping from primary containers and weighing each ingredient by hand on a weigh scale, manual weighing with material lifting assistance like vacuum transfer and bag lifters, manual or assisted transfer with automated weighing on weigh table, manual or assisted filling of loss-in weight dispensing system, automated dispensaries with mechanical devices such as vacuum loading system and screw feed system. Issues like weighing accuracy, dust control (laminar air flow booths, glove boxes), during manual handling, lot control of each ingredient, material movement into and out of dispensary should be considered during dispensing.

Particle size reduction and sizing

Mixing or blending of several solid ingredients of pharmaceuticals is easier and more uniform if the ingredients are approximately of same size. This provides a greater uniformity of dose. **Size reduction** increases surface area, improves the tablet-to-tablet content uniformity by virtue of the increased number of particles per unit weight, improves flow properties of raw materials, improves colour and/or active ingredient dispersion in tablet excipients and promotes uniform drying of sized granules.

Equipment employed for size reduction include Fluid energy mill, Colloidal mill, Ball mill, Hammer mill, Cutting mill, Roller mill, Conical mill, etc.

Blending

The powder/granules blending is involved at stage of pre-granulation and/or post-granulation stage of tablet manufacturing. The various blenders used include "V" blender, Oblicone blender, Container blender, Tumbling blender, Agitated powder blender, etc.

Granulation

Granulation is the process in which primary powder particles are made to adhere to form larger, multi-particle entities called granules. Granulation, normally, commences after initial dry mixing of the necessary powdered ingredients so that a uniform distribution of each ingredient through the mix is achieved. After granulation the granules may be mixed with other excipients prior to tablet compaction.

Reasons for granulation

The reasons why granulation is often necessary are as follows:

To prevent segregation of the constituents of the powder mix

Segregation is due to differences in the size or density of the components of the mix, the smaller and/or denser particles concentrating at the base of a container with the larger and/or less dense ones above them. An ideal granulation will contain all the constituents of the mix in the correct proportion in each granule, and segregation of the ingredients will not occur. It is also important to control the particle size distribution of the granules because although the individual components may not segregate, if there is a wide size distribution the granules themselves may segregate. If this occurs in the hoppers of tablet machines, products with large weight variations will result. This is because these machines fill by volume rather than weight, and if different regions in the hopper contain granules of different sizes (and hence bulk density), a given volume in each region will contain a different weight of granules. This will lead to an unacceptable distribution of the drug content within the batch of finished product, even though the drug is evenly distributed through out the granules.

To improve the flow properties of the mix

Many powders, because of their small size, irregular shape or surface characteristics, are cohesive and do not flow well. Granules produced from such a cohesive system will be larger and more iso-diametric, both factors contributing to improved flow properties.

To improve the compaction characteristics of the mix

Some powders are difficult to compact even if a readily compactable adhesive is included in the mix but granules of the same formulation are often more easily compacted and produce stronger tablets. This is associated with the distribution of the adhesive within the granule and is a function of the method employed to produce the granules. Often solute migration occurring during the post-granulation drying stage results in a binder-rich outer layer to the granules. This, in turn, leads to direct binder–binder bonding, which assists the consolidation of weakly bonding materials.

Granulation methods

Granulation methods can be divided into two types:

Dry granulation

In the dry methods of granulation the primary powder particles are aggregated under high pressure. There are two main processes. Either a large tablet (known as a **slug**) is produced in a heavy-duty tabletting press (a process known as **slugging**) or the powder is squeezed between two rollers to produce a sheet of material (**roller compaction**). In both cases these intermediate products are broken using a suitable milling technique to produce granular material, which is usually sieved to separate the desired size fraction. The unused fine material may be reworked to avoid waste. This dry method may be used for drugs that do not compress well after wet granulation, or those which are sensitive to moisture.

Wet granulation

Wet granulation involves the massing of a mix of dry **primary powder particles** using a **granulating fluid**. The fluid contains a solvent, which must be volatile, so that it can be removed by drying, and be non-toxic. Typical liquids include water, ethanol and isopropanol, either alone or in combination. The granulation liquid may be used alone, or more usually, as a solvent containing a dissolved **adhesive** (also referred to as a **binder** or **binding agent**), which is used to ensure particle adhesion once the granule is dry. Water is commonly used for economical and ecological reasons. Its disadvantages as a solvent are that it may adversely affect drug stability, causing hydrolysis of susceptible products, and it needs a longer drying time than do organic solvents. This increases the length of the process again may affect stability because of the extended exposure to heat. The primary advantage of water is that it is non-flammable, which means that expensive safety precautions such as the use of flame-proof equipment need not be taken. Organic solvents are used when water-sensitive drugs are processed, as an alternative to dry granulation, or when a rapid drying time is required. In the traditional wet granulation method the wet mass is forced through a sieve to produce wet granules, which are then dried. A subsequent screening stage breaks agglo-merates of granules and removes the fine material, which can than be recycled. Variations of this traditional method depend on the equip-ment used but the general principle of initial particle aggregation using a liquid remains in all of the processes.

Effect of granulation method on granule structure

The method and conditions of granulation affect inter-granular and intra-granular pore structure by changing the degree of packing within the granules. It has been shown that pre-compressed granules, consisting of compressed drug and binder particles, are held together by simple bonding during compaction. Granules prepared by wet massing consist of intact drug particles held together in a sponge-like matrix of binder. Fluidized-bed granules are similar to those prepared by the wet massing process, but possess greater porosity and the granule surface is covered by a film of binding agent. With spray-dried systems the granules consist of spherical particles composed of an outer shell and an inner core of particles. Thus, the properties of the granules are influenced by the manufacturing process.

ADVANCES IN GRANULATIONS TECHNOLOGY

Advancements in technology and a need to improve commercial output has lead to development of newer granulation technologies such as :

Fluidized hot melt granulation (FHMG)

This is an emerging technique combining the advantages of both dry and wet granulation methods. It is a process conducted at elevated temperatures and involves meltable binders to agglomerate fluidized dry powders. Use of solvents is avoided negating the problems associated with in-process hydrolysis and solvent removal. It is a simple and rapid technique that does not require powder blends to possess high levels of fluidity and compressibility, and reflects the simplicity of dry techniques in that it may be performed in one step. This is in contrast to conventional wet techniques whereby transfer from the granulator to the drying equipment is usually necessary – commonly involving losses in transfer, contamination of manufacturing equipment, increased processing and operator time, and increased dust levels: issues that are particularly pertinent when manufacturing dosage forms containing potent drugs.

Steam granulation

It is a modification of wet granulation where steam is used as a binder instead of water. Its advantages include higher distribution uniformity, higher diffusion rate into powders and more favorable thermal balance during drying step. Steam granules are more spherical, have large surface area hence increased dissolution rate of the drug from granules, processing time is shorter, therefore, more number of tablets are produced per batch, compared to the use of organic solvent water vapour is environmentally friendly, no health hazards to operators, no restriction by ICH on traces left in the granules, freshly distilled steam is sterile and, therefore, the total count can be kept under control. However, this method is unsuitable for thermolabile drugs. Moreover, special equipments are required and are unsuitable for binders that cannot be later activated by contact with water vapour.

Melt granulation/Thermoplastic granulation

Here granulation is achieved by the addition of a binder that is solid at room temperature but melts in the temperature range of 50–80°C. Melted binder then acts like a binding liquid. The process of granulation consists of a combination of three phases: wetting and nucleation, coalescence and attrition and breakage. During the nucleation step the binder comes into contact with the powder bed and some liquid bridges are formed, leading to the formation of small agglomerates i.e. nuclei. Coalescence involves successful fusion of nuclei. Attrition and breakage refer to the phenomenon of granulation fragmentation that are solidified by cooling to ambient temperature without the need for drying by a tumbling process. 10–30% w/w of meltable binder, with respect to that of fine solid particles, is generally used. Hydrophilic meltable binders

(e.g. polyethylene glycol (PEG)) are used to prepare immediate-release dosage forms while the hydrophobic meltable binders (stearic acid, cetyl or stearyl alcohol) are preferred for prolonged-release formulations. The melting point of fine solid particles should be at least 20°C higher than that of the maximum processing temperature. Melt granulation is useful for granulating water sensitive materials but not suitable for thermolabile substances. When water soluble binders are needed, polyethylene glycol (PEG) is used as melting binders. When water insoluble binders are needed, stearic acid, cetyl or stearyl alcohol, various waxes and mono-, di-, & triglycerides are used as melting binders.

Moisture activated dry granulation (MADG)

In this method moisture is used to activate the granules formation but the granules drying step is eliminated by moisture absorbing materials. The process consists of two steps, wet agglomeration of the powder mixture followed by moisture absorption stages. A small amount of water (1–4%) is added first to agglomerate the mixture of the API, a binder, and excipients. Moisture absorbing material is then added to absorb any excessive moisture. After mixing with a lubricant, the resulting mixture can then be compressed directly into tablets. Hence, this process offers the advantage of wet granulation without the need for a drying step.

The binders used in the agglomeration stage should be easily wettable and become tacky with the addition of a small amount of water. Examples of binders commonly used are low-viscosity polyvinylpyrrolidones (PVPs). If PVP is not an acceptable choice because of formulation concerns then hydroxypropyl cellulose (HPC), copovidone, maltodextrins, sodium carboxymethylcellulose (Na CMC), or hydroxypropyl methylcellulose (HPMC) can be used instead. The binders can be used singly or in multiple combinations to achieve the desired effects.

Microcrystalline cellulose (e.g., Avicel PH101, PH102, and PH200), silicone dioxide, and crospovidone can be used as moisture absorbing excipients.

Moist granulation technique (MGT)

MGT works on the same principle as Moisture Activated Dry Granulation (MADG) described earlier. It involves binder activation by adding a minimum amount of liquid. Then, excess of moisture present in the blend is removed by adding moisture-absorbing material like microcrystallinecellulose (MCC), which eliminates the drying step. It is applicable for developing a controlled release formulation.

Thermal adhesion granulation process (TAGP)

TAGP is performed under low moisture content or low content of pharmaceutically acceptable solvent by subjecting a mixture containing excipients to heating at a temperature in the range from about 30ºC to about 130ºC in a closed system under mixing by tumble rotation until the formation of granules. This method utilizes less water or solvent than traditional wet granulation method. It provides granules with good flow properties and binding capacity to form tablets of low friability, adequate hardness and have a high uptake capacity for active substances whose tableting is poor.

Foam granulation

Here liquid binders are added as aqueous foam. Foam granulation takes advantage of the tremendous increase in the liquid surface area and volume of polymeric binder foams to improve the distribution of the water/binder system throughout the powder bed of a solid dose pharmaceutical formulation. A simple foam generation apparatus is used to incorporate air into a conventional water-soluble polymeric excipient binder such as hydroxypropyl methylcellulose. Hypromellose polymers are ideal candidates for this technology because they are excellent film formers and create exceptionally stable foams. The key to the effectiveness of foam binder performance is rapid and extremely efficient particle coverage. Compared to sprayed liquid binders, foamed binders offer much higher surface area, and they spread very rapidly and evenly over powder surfaces. The foamed binders and the powder particles show excellent mutual flow through one another. Compared to conventional spray processing, foamed binder technology can shorten processing times by reducing water requirements. It can improve reproducibility through more uniform binder distribution. Moreover, it eliminates spray nozzles and their many variables in granulation processing equipment. Foam processing also offers better end point determinations and reduced equipment clean-up time. While foamed binder processing offers many advantages, this technology doesn't demand new equipment or radical changes in processing techniques. Overall, foam binder processing is easier, faster, and allows safer handling of potent drug compounds.

Freeze granulation technology

Swedish Ceramic Institute (SCI) has adopted and developed an alternative technique that is freeze granulation, which enables preservation of the homogeneity from suspension to dry granules by spraying a powder suspension into liquid nitrogen, the drops (granules) are instantaneously frozen. In a subsequent freeze-drying the granules are dried by sublimation of the ice without any segregation effects as in the case of conventional drying in air. The result will be spherical, free flowing granules, with optimal homogeneity. Freeze granulation provides optimized condition for the subsequent processing of the granules, for example easy crushing to homogeneous and dense powder compacts in a pressing operation. The granule size distribution can be controlled by the suspension rheology (flow properties) and the process parameters (pump speed and air pressure). [www.powderpro.se/uploads/media/ Freeze_Granulation_of_Nano_Materials_ London_ June_ 2010.pdf]

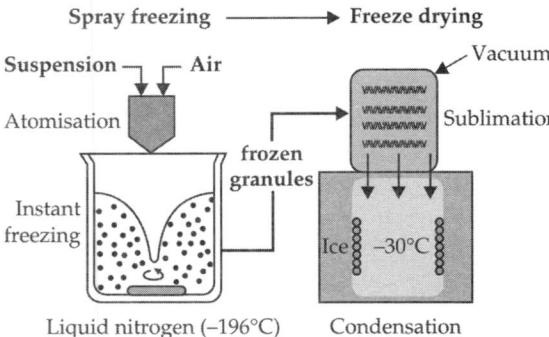

Fig. 3.2. Freeze granulation.

Pnuematic dry granulation

Dry granulation techniques and more specifically roller compaction can provide many advantages over the more established wet granulation techniques. There are still problems with roller compaction such as high amount of fines and poor flow of granulate. Pneumatic dry granulation (PDG^{TM}) has a potential to improve and extend the use of dry granulation processes, which can result in substantial contribution to drug delivery system development and drug product manufacture.

Granulation mechanisms

To form granules, bonds must be formed between powder particles, so that they adhere and these bonds must be sufficiently strong to prevent breakdown of the granule to powder in subsequent handling operations. The primary bonding mechanisms between particles are as follows:

Adhesion and cohesion forces in immobile films

If sufficient liquid is present in a powder to form a very thin, immobile layer, there will be an effective decrease in interparticulate distance and an increase in contact area between the particles. The bond strength between the particles will be increased because of this, as the Van der Waals forces of attraction are proportional to the particle diameter and inversely proportional to the square of the distance of separation. Although, such

films may be present as residual liquid after granules prepared by wet granulation have been dried, it is unlikely that they contribute significantly to the final granule strength. In dry granulation, however, the pressures used will increase the contact area between the adsorption layers and decrease the inter-particulate distance, and this will contribute to the final granule strength. Thin, immobile layers may also be formed by highly viscous solutions of adhesives, and so the bond strength will be greater than that produced by the mobile films. The use of starch mucilage in pharmaceutical granulations may produce this type of film.

Interfacial forces in mobile liquid films

During wet granulation liquid is added to the powder mix and will be distributed as films around and between the particles. Sufficient liquid is usually added to exceed that necessary for an immobile layer and to produce a mobile film. There are three states of water distribution between particles. At low moisture levels, termed the pendular state, the particles are held together by lens shaped rings of liquid. These cause adhesion because of the surface tension forces of the liquid/air interface and the hydrostatic suction pressure in the liquid bridge. When all the air has been displaced from between the particles the capillary state is reached, and the particles are held by capillary suction at the liquid/air interface, which is now only at the granule surface. The funicular state represents an intermediate stage between the pendular and capillary states. Moist granule tensile strength increases about three times between the pendular and the capillary state. It may appear that the state of the powder bed is dependent upon the total moisture content of the wetted powders, but the capillary state may also be reached by decreasing the separation of the particles. In the massing process during wet granulation, continued kneading/mixing of material originally in the pendular state will densify the wet mass, decreasing the pore volume occupied by air and eventually producing the funicular or capillary state without further liquid addition. In addition to these three states, a further state, the droplet, is reached. This will be important in the process of granulation by spray drying of a suspension. In this state, the strength of the droplet is dependent upon the surface tension of the liquid used. These wet bridges are only temporary structures in wet granulation because the moist granules will be dried. They are, however, a prerequisite for the formation of solid bridges formed by adhesives present in the liquid, or by materials that dissolve in the granulating liquid.

Solid bridges

It can be formed by partial melting, hardening binders and crystallization of dissolved substances.

Partial melting

It is possible that the pressures used in dry granulation methods may cause melting of low melting-point materials where the particles touch and high pressures are developed. When the pressure is relieved, crystallization will take place and bind the particles together.

Hardening binders

This is the common mechanism in pharmaceutical wet granulations when an adhesive is included in the granulating solvent. The liquid will form liquid bridges, as discussed above, and the adhesive will harden or crystallize on drying to form solid bridges to bind the particles. Adhesives such as PVP, the cellulose derivatives (such as CMC) and pregelatinized starch function in this way.

Crystallization of dissolved substances

The solvent used to mass the powder during wet granulation may partially dissolve one of the powdered ingredients. When the granules are dried, crystallization of this material will take place and the dissolved substance then acts as a hardening binder. Any material soluble in the granulating liquid will function in this manner, e.g. lactose incorporated into dry powders

granulated with water. The size of the crystals produced in the bridge will be influenced by the rate of drying of the granules; the slower the drying time, the larger the particle size. It is therefore important that the drug does not dissolve in the granulating liquid and re-crystallize as it may adversely affect the dissolution rate of the drug if crystals larger than that of the starting material are produced.

Attractive forces between solid particles

In the absence of liquids and solid bridges formed by binding agents, there are two types of attractive force that can operate between particles in pharmaceutical systems. **Electrostatic forces** may be important in causing powder cohesion and the initial formation of agglomerates, e.g. during mixing. In general, they do not contribute significantly to the final strength of the granule. **van der Waals forces**, however, are about four orders of magnitude greater than electrostatic forces and contribute significantly to the strength of granules produced by dry granulation. The magnitude of these forces will increase as the distance between adjacent surfaces decreases, and in dry granulation this is achieved by using pressure to force the particles together.

Drying

After the process of granulation, the product exists as a wet mass from which the liquid must be removed, since the presence of water leads to the impairment of flow properties and chemical instability. The traditional means of drying is tray drying but the most commonly used device for drying tablet granules is fluidized bed drying.

Microwaves (incident microwave radiation frequencies of 2450 and 960 MHz) are being increasingly employed in the pharmaceutical industry for drying purposes. The water vapor is removed under vacuum, and hence the product dries rapidly at a relatively low temperature. As the bed of solid is stationary, particle attrition does not occur, and dust formation is minimized.

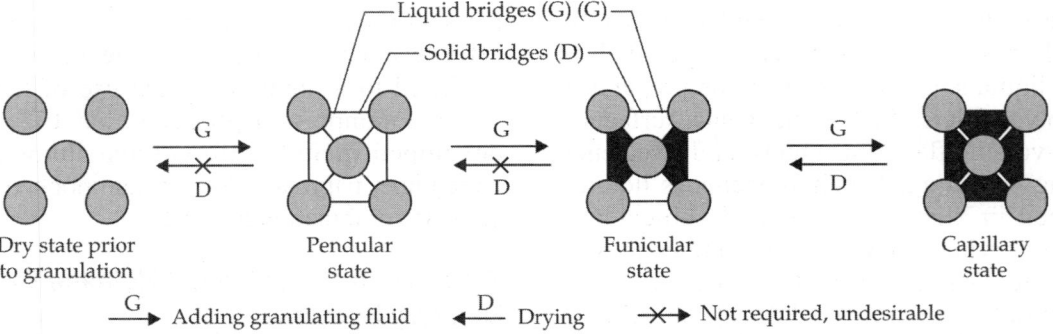

Fig. 3.3. Water distribution between particles of a granule during formation and drying.

When the drying process is complete, it is likely that the product will have cohered into relatively large masses, especially if tray drying has been used. The dried material is, therefore, passed through a sieve (usually 250–700 µm) to break-up aggregates and to give a relatively uniformly sized granule. A second mixing stage now follows in which several important ingredients like glidants, lubricants and disintegrants are added.

Compaction/Compression

After the preparation of granules (in case of wet granulation) or sized slugs (in case of dry granulation) or mixing of ingredients (in case of

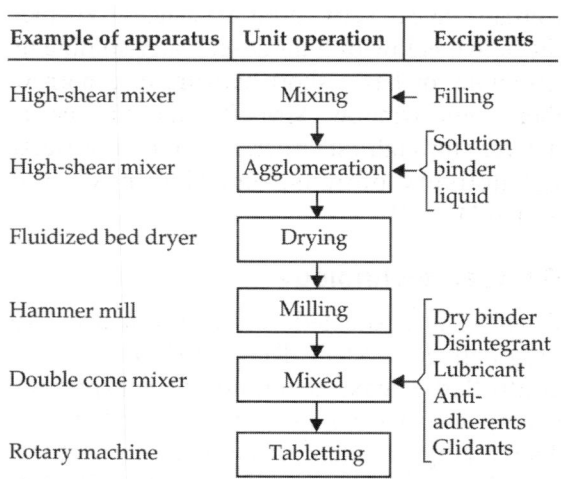

Fig. 3.4. Overview of sequence of operations used in production of tablets by wet granulation.

direct compression), they are compressed to get final product. Granules are contained in a die and a compressing force of several tons is applied to it by means of punches. The shape of the die governs the cross-sectional shape of the tablet, and the distance between the punch tips at the point of maximum compression governs its thickness. The conformation of the tablet faces, usually flat or convex, is a reflection of those of the punches. The compression is done either by single punch machine (stamping press) or by multi-station machine (rotary press).

Direct compression

Both wet and dry granulation methods of tablet manufacture are complex multistage processes, but are necessary to convert the components of the formulation into a state that can be readily compressed into acceptable tablets. If, however, a major component of the formulation already possesses the necessary degree of fluidity and compressibility, granulation would be unnecessary. This is the basis of the direct compression method of tablet manufacture. The key component here is the diluent that must not only possess those properties, which are necessary for satisfactory tablet formulation, but also retain those properties when mixed with the other constituents of the formulation such as the active ingredient. The process of direct compression is shown in Fig. 3.5. The ingredients are mixed together and then compressed. Almost invariably a lubricant must

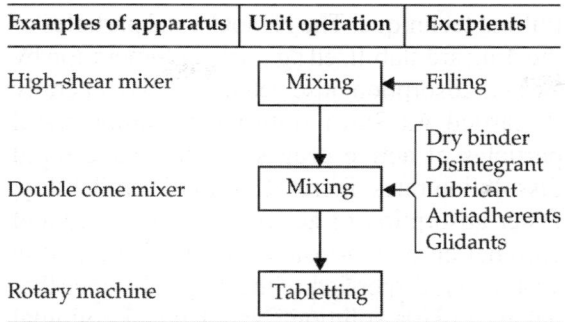

Examples of apparatus	Unit operation	Excipients
High-shear mixer	Mixing ← Filling	
Double cone mixer	Mixing ←	⎧ Dry binder ⎪ Disintegrant ⎨ Lubricant ⎪ Antiadherents ⎩ Glidants
Rotary machine	Tabletting	

Fig. 3.5. Sequence of operations used in production of tablets with direct compression.

be added, and a glidant and a disintegrating agent included when necessary. The process does not involve the use of a liquid, and hence a drying stage with its attendant energy costs is avoided.

Problems encountered during tablet manufacture

Tabletting problems, their causes and solutions are summarized in Table 3.3.

EQUIPMENTS

Granulation equipment

Wet granulators

There are three main types of granulators used in the pharmaceutical industry for wet granulation.

Shear granulators

In the traditional granulation process a planetary mixer is often used for wet massing of the powders. The mixed powders are fed into the bowl of the planetary mixer and granulating liquid is added as the paddle of the mixer agitates the powders. The planetary action of the blade during mixing is similar to that of a household mixer. The moist mass has then to be transferred to a granulator, such as an oscillating granulator. The rotor bars of the granulator oscillate and force the moist mass through the sieve screen, the size of which determines the granule size. The mass should be sufficiently moist to form discrete granules when sieved. If excess liquid

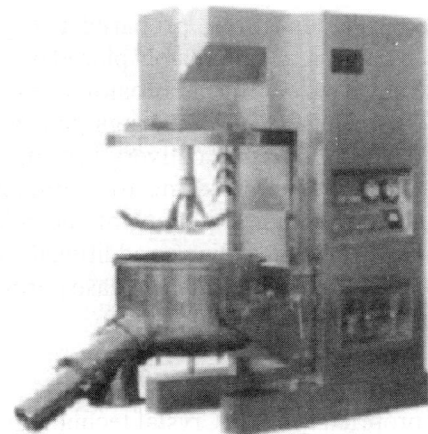

Fig. 3.6. Mixer granulator.

is added, strings of material will be formed and if the mix is too dry the mass will be sieved to powder and granules will not be formed. The granules can be collected and subjected to drying.

High-speed mixer/Granulators

This type of granulator (e.g. Diosna, Fielder) is used extensively in pharmaceutics. The machines have a stainless steel mixing bowl containing a three-bladed main impeller, which revolves in the horizontal plane, and a three-bladed auxiliary chopper (breaker blade) which revolves either in the vertical or the horizontal plane. The unmixed dry powders are placed in the bowl and mixed by the rotating impeller for a few minutes. Granulating liquid is then added via a port in the lid of the granulator while the impeller is turning. The granulating fluid is mixed into the powders by the impeller. The chopper is usually switched on when the moist mass is formed, as its function is to break up the wet mass to produce a bed of granular material. Once a satisfactory granule has been produced, the granular product is discharged, passing through a wire mesh which breaks up any large aggregates, into the bowl of a fluidized-bed drier.

The advantage of the process is that mixing, massing and granulation are all performed within a few minutes in the same piece of equipment.

Table 3.3. Problems encountered during tablet manufacture

Problem	Identification	Causes	Solutions
Capping	Partial or complete separation of the top or bottom crown	• Can be the result of dirty or worn out punches. • Result from air entrapment during processing. • Large amount of fines. • Improperly dried granules.	• Polish dies and use flat punches. • Remove fines. • Check and adjust moisture content of granules.
Lamination	Separation of a tablet into two or more layers	• Results from air entrapment during processing. • Too much of hydrophobic lubricant.	• Reduce turret speed and reduce the final compression pressure. • Use a less amount of lubricant or change the type of lubricant. • Add fines.
Picking	Removal of a tablet's surface material by a punch	• Due to excessive moisture, low melting point substances, insufficient lubricants. • When punch tips have engraving or embossing letters.	• Check moisture and add lubricants. • Design lettering as large as possible.
Sticking	Adhesion of the tablet material to the die wall	• Due to excessive moisture, low melting point substances, insufficient lubricants. • Too little pressure or high compression speed.	• Check moisture and add lubricants. • Increase pressure and reduce speed.
Chipping	Breaking of tablet edges while the tablet leaves the press or during subsequent handling	• Too dry granules. • Incorrect machine settings, specially mis-set ejection take-off.	• Check moisture. • Polish dies and punches.
Mottling	Unequal distribution of color	• Due to drug and excipients of different colors or formation of degradation products. • A dye migrates to the surface of granulation while drying.	• Uniform color distribution and protection of active ingredient. • Change the solvent system, reduce drying temperature and use a smaller particle size.
Weight/ Hardness variation	Variation in individual weight/ hardness of tablets	• Any alteration in the die filling process, e.g., granule size and size distribution, poor flow, poor mixing, punch variation, etc.	• Improve the flow properties and size distribution of granules.
Double impression	Seen with punches that have a monogram or engraving	• If a punch rotates during its free fall, it makes a lighter impression on the bottom of the tablet.	• Installation of antiturning devices.

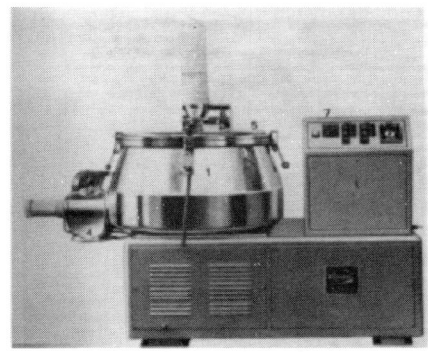

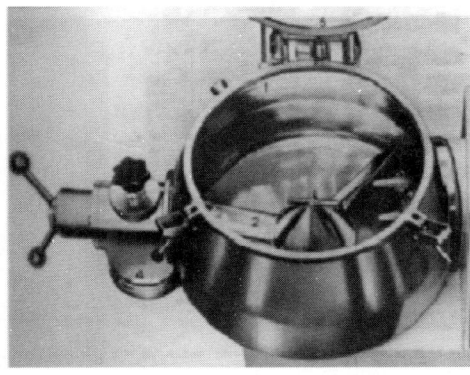

Fig 3.7. Diosna mixer-granulator. (A) Side view, (B) Top view.

The process needs to be controlled with care as the granulation progresses so rapidly that a usable granule can be transformed very quickly into an unusable, over-massed system. Thus, it is often necessary to use a suitable monitoring system to indicate the end of the granulation process, i.e. when a granule of the desired properties has been attained. The process is also sensitive to variations in raw materials, but this may be minimized by using a suitable end-point monitor.

A variation of the Diosna/Fielder type of design is the Collette–Gral mixer. This is based on the bowl and overhead drive of the planetary mixer, but the single paddle is replaced by two mixing shafts. One of these carries three blades, which rotate in the horizontal plane at the base of the bowl, and the second, carries smaller blades, which act as the chopper and rotate in

the horizontal plane in the upper regions of the granulating mass. Thus, the operating principle is similar.

Fluidized-bed granulators

Fluidized-bed granulators (e.g. Aeromatic, Glatt) have a similar design and operation to fluidized bed driers, i.e. the powder particles are fluidized in a stream of air, but in addition granulation fluid is sprayed from a nozzle on to the bed of powders. Heated and filtered air is blown or sucked through the bed of unmixed powders to fluidize the particles and mix the powders; fluidization is actually a very efficient mixing process. Granulating fluid is pumped from a reservoir through a spray nozzle positioned over the bed of particles. The fluid causes the primary powder particles to adhere when the droplets and powders collide. Escape of material from the granulation chamber is prevented by exhaust filters, which are periodically agitated to reintroduce the collected material into the fluidized bed. Sufficient liquid is sprayed to produce granules of the required size, at which point the spray is turned off but the fluidizing air continued. The wet granules are then dried in the heated fluidizing air stream.

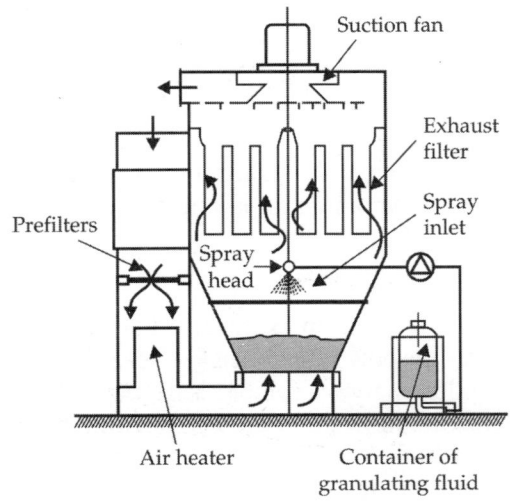

Fig. 3.8. Schematic cross-section of fluid bed spray granulator.

Fluidized bed granulation has many advantages over conventional wet massing. All the granulation processes, which require separate equipment in the conventional method, are performed in one unit, saving labour costs, transfer losses and time. Another advantage is that the process can be automated once the conditions affecting the granulation have been optimized. On the downside, the equipment is initially expensive and optimization of process (and product) parameters affecting granulation needs extensive development work, not only during initial formulation work but also during scale-up from development to production.

Dry granulators

Dry granulation converts primary powder particles into granules using the application of pressure without the intermediate use of a liquid. It, therefore, avoids heat–temperature combinations that might cause degradation of the product. Two pieces of equipment are necessary for dry granulation: first, a machine for compressing the dry powders into compacts or flakes, and secondly, a mill for breaking up these intermediate products into granules.

Sluggers

The dry powders can be compressed using a conventional tablet machine or, more usually, a large heavy duty rotary press can be used. This process is often known as 'slugging', the compact made in the process (typically 25 mm diameter by about 10–15 mm thick) being termed a 'slug'. A hammer mill is suitable for breaking the compacts.

Roller compactors

Roller compaction is an alternative gentler method, the powder mix being squeezed between two rollers to form a compressed sheet. The sheet normally is weak and brittle and breaks immediately into flakes. These flakes need gentler treatment to break them into granules, and this can usually be achieved by screening alone. Since no liquid is used, no granulation

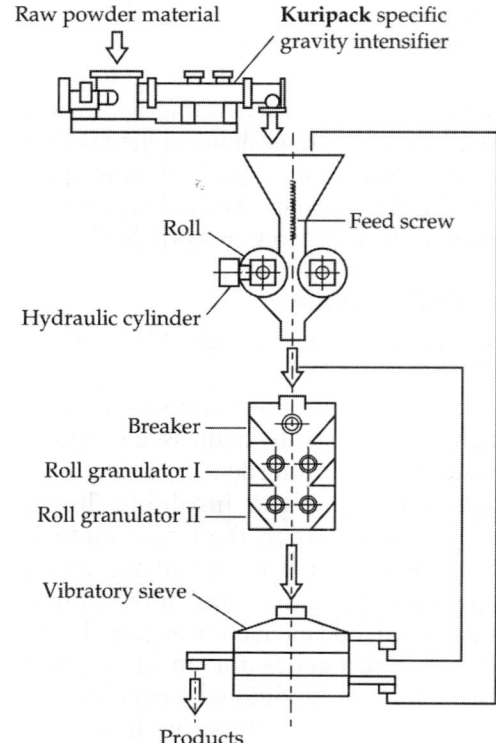

Fig. 3.9. Roller compactor.

liquid has to be prepared beforehand. Also, no additional drying step is required and investments in drying capacity (time, expenses, and space) are unnecessary. This is the cause for a high throughput of the small dry granulation equipment (expressed in kg per hour or kg per m^3 of overall equipment). Furthermore, dry granulation is a continuous process that can be run in continuous mode, while the other granulation methods usually run in batch mode and do not allow a continuous process. Except for electrical connections (e.g. typical power requirements for production machines are less than 10 kW), no additional supplies such as hot air or pressurized air are needed to start roll compaction. Due to absence of water, no capillary forces exist to contribute to binding forces within the granule particles. Granule formation has to take place only by means of the powder particle's own compressibility.

Therefore, excipients will have to be used that assure good compactibility during dry granulation and subsequent tabletting. The missing of capillary forces also contributes to the comparably higher number of fines usually found in granules produced by dry granulations in comparison to wet granulation.

Tablet machines

The basic mechanical unit in tablet compression involves the operation of two steel punches within a steel die cavity. The tablet is formed by the pressure exerted on the granulation by the punches within the dye cavity. The tablet assumes the size and shape of the punches and dies used.

Single-punch machine

This is the simplest of all tabletting machines. Most of these are motor driven models. A feed shoe filled with the granulation is positioned on the die cavity that it fills. The feed shoe retracts

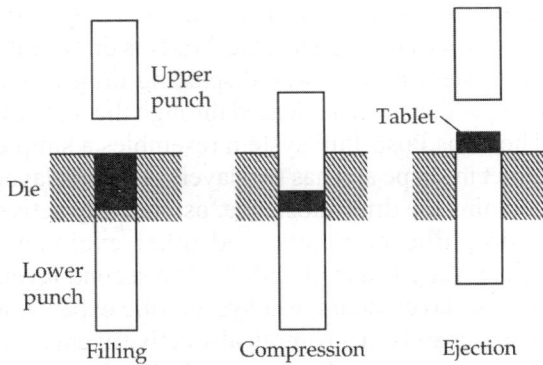

Fig. 3.10. Cycles of operations on an eccentric tablet press.

and scrapes all excess granulation away from the die cavity. The upper punch retracts, and the lower punch rises to eject the tablet. As the feed shoe returns to fill the die cavity, it pushes the compressed tablet from the die platform. The weight of the tablet is determined by the volume of the die cavity; the lower punch is adjustable to increase or decrease the volume of

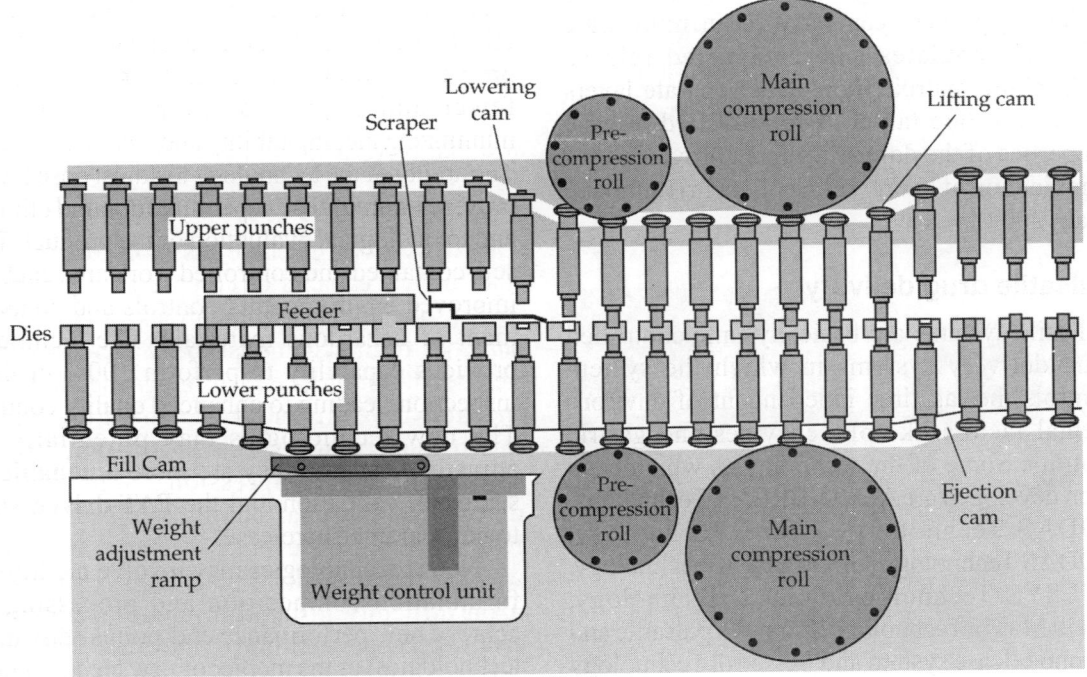

Fig. 3.11. Schematic of multistation tablet press.

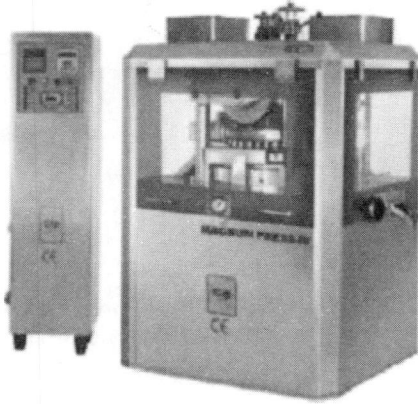

Fig. 3.12. High speed rotary tablet press.

granulation, thus increasing or decreasing the weight of the tablet. As tablets are ejected from the machine after compression, they are usually accompanied by powder and uncompressed granulation. To remove this loose dust, the tablets are passed over a screen, which may be vibrating, and cleaned with a vacuum line.

Rotary tablet machines

For increased production, rotary machines offer great advantages. A head carrying a number of

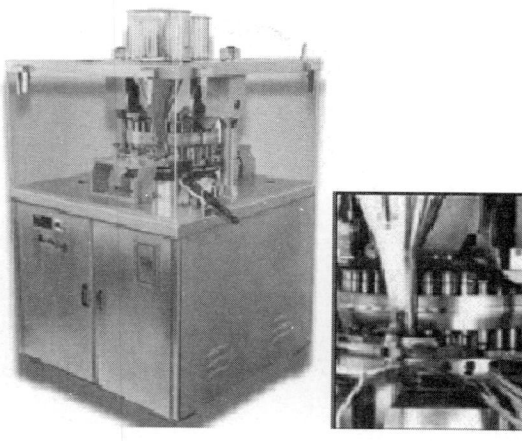

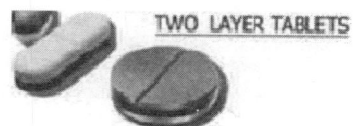

Fig. 3.13. Double side rotary tablet press.

sets of punches and dies revolves continuously while the tablet granulation runs from hopper, through a feed frame and into the dies placed in a large, steel plate revolving under it. This method promotes a uniform fill of the die and therefore an accurate weight for the tablet. Compression takes place as the upper and lower punches pass between a pair of rollers. This action produces a slow squeezing effect on the material in the die cavity from the top and bottom and so gives a chance for the entrapped air to escape. The lower punch lifts up and ejects the tablet. Adjustments for tablet weight and hardness can be made without the use of tools while the machine is in operation. One of the factors that contribute to the variation in tablet weight and hardness during compression is the internal flow of the granulation within the feed hopper. On most rotary machine models there is an excess pressure release that cushions each compression and relieves the machine of all shocks and undue strain. The punches and dies can be removed readily for inspection, cleaning, and inserting different sets to produce a great variety of sizes and shapes. It is possible to equip the machine with as few punches and dies, as the job requires, and thus economize on installation costs.

High speed rotary tablet machines

The rotary tablet machine has evolved gradually into models capable of compressing tablets at high production rates (Swarbick et al., 2007). This has been accomplished by increasing the number of stations, i.e., sets of punches and dies, in each revolution of the machine head, improving feeding devices, and on some models installing dual compression points. Rotary machines with dual compression points are referred to as double rotary machines, and those with one compression point, single rotary. The main difficulty in rapid machine operation is ensuring adequate filling of the dies. With rapid filling, dwell time of the die cavity beneath the feed frame is insufficient to ensure the

Table 3.4. High speed rotary tablet presses and their characteristics

Manufacturer	Number of stations available		Output, tables per minute (TPM)	
	Min	Max	Min	Max
Colton/Vector	12	90	480	16,000
Manesty Machines Ltd., Liverpool, England	16	69	600/1500	3330/10,000
Stokes-Merill	33	65	1200/3300	3500/10,000
Sejong, Korea	12	65	600/1800	1300/5200
Killan & Co., GmbH, Köln, Germany	14	67	140/383	1083/10,000
Hata Iron Works, Hori Engineering Co., Osaka, Japan	28	71	420/1420	1960/7100
Karnavati Engineerig, Ahmedabad, India	37	81	888/4440	12,960

requirements of uniform flow and packing of the dies. Presses with triple compression points permit the partial compaction of material before final compaction. This provides for partial de-aeration and particle orientation of material before final compaction. This helps in the direct compacting of materials and reduces laminating and capping due to entrapped air.

Multilayer rotary tablet machines

The rotary tablet machines also have been developed into models capable of producing multiple-layer tablets; the machines are able to make 1-, 2- or 3-layer tablets e.g. Versa Press, Stokes/Pennwalt. Originally, the tablets were prepared by a single-compression method. The dies were filled with different granulations in successive layers, and the tablets were formed by a single compression stroke. The separation lines of the tablets prepared by this method tended to be irregular. In the machines available now for multilayer production the granulation receives a pre-compression stroke after the first and second fill, which lightly compacts the granulation and maintains a well-defined surface of separation between each layer with the machine running at any desired speed for periodic weight and analysis check. Other multiple-compression pressed can receive previously compressed tablets and compress another granulation around the preformed tablet.

An example of a press with this capability is the Manesty Drycota.

QUALITY CONTROL

Quality control during the manufacture of the tablets becomes essential for the assurance that the tablets do not vary from one production batch to another. The specifications of tablets include the following:

Physical appearance

Generally, tablets are discoid in shape, although they may be oval, oblong, round, cylindrical, concave, or convex. The concave punches are referred to as shallow, standard, and deep, depending on the concavity. The size and shape of the tablet are governed by the choice of tabletting machine, on the die and the punches selected for the compression of the tablet, the best particle size for granulation, production lot sizes, and the best type of tablet process, packaging operation, and cost to produce the tablet.

Identification

The first and foremost important test in tablet testing is to establish that the tablets contain the labelled active ingredient. For this purpose, usually, a fixed number of tablets (10–20) are ground and extracted with appropriate solvent extraction. The extract, with or without a concentration step, is usually chromatographed along with an authentic standard solution. The identity of drug is confirmed based on similarity of ultraviolet (UV) spectrum and/or retention times using chromatographic analysis. This test is generally qualitative in nature. More sophisticated techniques such as chromato-graphic techniques with or without coupling with mass-spectrometry may be used. However, for routine quality control purposes, the simpler techniques such as thin layer chromatography (TLC) or high-performance liquid chromato-graphy (HPLC) with UV detection are mostly employed.

Assay

For assay, 10–20 tablets are ground and the active ingredient is dissolved or extracted in a suitable solvent using the described procedure. The concentration of the extracted solution is determined using a specific and validated spectroscopic or chromatographic method against a solution of reference standard. These results are reported as percent of expected/labelled value. Although, the specifications for assay results differ from product-to-product, generally, the expected range for individual active ingredient is to be within 90–110% of the labelled amount.

Uniformity of dosage units

This test is conducted to establish consistency in the content of active ingredient from tablet to tablet. There are generally two approaches taken in establishing uniformity of dosage units: weight variation or content uniformity.

Weight variation

If the active ingredient represents not less than 50% weight of the tablet and greater than 50 mg, then one may establish uniformity of dosage units using the weight variation method. The USP and BP provide tolerances for the average weight of uncoated compressed tablets. Twenty tablets are weighed individually and the average weight is calculated. The variation from the average weight in the weights of not more than two of the tablets must not differ by more than the specified percentage, no tablet differs by more than double that percentage. Coated tablets are exempt from these requirements but must conform to the test for content uniformity, if applicable.

Content uniformity

Tablet monographs with a content uniformity requirement do not have a weight variation requirement. This test is done to ensure that every tablet contains the amount of drug substance intended, with little variation within a batch. A sample of 10 tablets is individually analyzed using the analytical method described under the assay procedure. It is mandatory to use content uniformity for tablets with less than 50 mg of active ingredient and/or representing less than 50% total mass of the tablets. The content uniformity approach is preferred over the weight variation approach as it more precisely reflects the variation of the active ingredient from tablet to tablet. The required specification for this test is that uniformity of dosage unit should be within a range of 85%–115% with a relative standard deviation of less than or equal to 6%.

Friability

The tablets may be subjected to a tumbling motion, mechanical shock or attrition, e.g. during coating, packaging or transport, which may cause small particles to abrade from the surface of the tablet. To examine this, test to measure the friability or resistance to abrasion is done. Commercially available apparatuses, known as friabilators, are used for the test. A friabilator consists of a drum with diameter between 283 mm and 291 mm and having width of 36–40 mm, made of transparent plastic material. The drum is attached to the horizontal axis of a device that rotates at 25 rpm. The tablets are tumbled at each turn of the drum by a curve projection with an inside radius of 75.5–85.5 mm that extends from middle of the drum to outer wall. Thus, at each turn, the tablets roll or slide and fall from a height of about 6 inches onto the drum wall or onto each other. Usually, a sample of 10 tablets are tested at a time, unless tablet weight is 0.65 g or less, where 20 tablets are tested. After 100 turns, the tablet samples are evaluated by weighing. If the reduction in the total mass of the tablets is more than 1%, the tablets fail the friability test. Generally, the test is done once. If cracked, cleaved, or broken tablets are obvious, then the sample also fails the test. The Roche Friabilator is the most frequently used friability tester.

Hardness

The need for testing hardness or crushing strength, in addition to friability, may be explained with an analogy that friability determines how fragile a tablet is. If a tablet is more fragile than expected, then the friability test will detect its substandard quality. However, on the other hand, if the tablets are more robust than desired, a friability test would not detect this deficiency. It is the tablet hardness test that will detect the deficiency. This test normally consists of breaking or crushing the tablet by application of a compressive load. A number of devices have been designed to measure crushing strength. The simplest are hand-operated, the tablet being held between a fixed and a movable jaw. Typical examples of this type are the Monsanto tablet hardness tester, in which the force is applied via a screw-driven spring; and the Pfizer tester, in which a gripping action transfers force to the tablet. In experienced hands, these can give fairly reproducible results, but it has been found that the crushing strength so obtained is in part governed by the rate at which the force is applied. Even if the load is applied at a uniform rate, the variation in strength within a batch of tablets can be considerable. Also since crushing strength is dependent on tablet dimensions, comparing the strengths of tablets of different sizes is difficult. In an attempt to overcome these problems, the parameter **tensile strength** is frequently used. This is given by the formula:

$$St = 2p/\pi.d.t\,(1-e)$$

where, S is the tensile strength, p is the crushing strength, d is the tablet diameter, t is the tablet thickness, and e is the tablet porosity.

This definition also compensates for the fact that porous tablets, having proportionally less inter-particulate contact, will be expected to be weaker. A further development is to determine tablet toughness in which the flexing of the tablet as a load is applied is also measured, analogous to force-displacement data obtained during tablet compression.

Thickness

The thickness of a tablet from batch-to-batch needs to be controlled. Thickness may vary with no change in weight because of difference in the density of granulation and the pressure applied to the tablets, as well as the speed of tablet compression. Not only is the tablet thickness important in reproducing tablets identical in appearance but also to ensure that every batch will be usable with selected packaging components.

Disintegration test

Although, this test is in use for some products in pharmacopeias, its use is generally diminishing in favor of drug dissolution testing. When required, the test is conducted using a specially designed instrument known as disintegration apparatus. The apparatus employs a basket of six tubes with a base of metal sieve. A tablet is placed in each tube and is held in place by a plastic weight. The six-tube assembly, containing six tablets, is suspended using a hanger with a mechanism of vertical motion at a frequency of between 29 to 32 cycles per minute. While hanging the six-tube assembly on the hanger, the assembly is moved in vertical motion in water or a buffer solution. The time for disintegration of each tablet is recorded and should meet the required time specification. For compressed, uncoated tablets the testing fluid is usually water at 37°C.

Dissolution test

The best standard to establish drug release characteristics of a product is based on an *in vivo* study, i.e., testing bioavailability of the drugs in humans. However, conducting such studies is often one of the most expensive and time-consuming processes in the manufacturing of a product. In addition to the cost and time considerations, ethical concerns also limit the conduct of these studies in humans. For this purpose, an *in vitro* dissolution test for tablet products has been developed and has become a tool for both product development and quality assurance.

As a dissolution test is conducted to simulate drug release in the human GI tract, the generally recommended media are based on aqueous buffers in the pH range of 1–8. Commonly used media are hydrochloric acid (0.01–0.1 N) to simulate gastric fluid and phosphate or acetate buffer in the range of pH 4.0–6.8 to represent intestinal fluids. Volumes are usually in the range of 250–1000 ml. In the case of low solubility drugs, solubilizing agents, such as sodium lauryl sulfate, are added to enhance the solubility. A low concentration of alcohol may be used to facilitate dissolution for low solubility drugs. The dissolution tests are conducted in media kept at a temperature of 37°C.

Apart from the dissolution media, the second major determinant for drug dissolution testing concerns the device for stirring or mixing of the product with the dissolution medium. Four different types of apparatuses based on different types of mixing approaches are available commercially and have compendial recognition. These apparatuses are known as: (1) paddle; (2) basket; (3) flow-through; and (4) reciprocating cylinder apparatus.

Generally, dissolution results are reported as cumulated percent drug release vs. time. Presently, most of the tolerances are based on a single time point, such as not less than 85% dissolved or released in 30 min. However, more reports are appearing with percent drug release values at multiple time points, resulting in a drug release pattern, commonly known as a "profile." Most commercially available apparatuses can run a test in a set of six units (tablets), thus resulting in saving of time and resources and leading to better reproducibility.

TABLET COATING

Tablets are coated for a number of reasons: to protect the drug from its surrounding environment (air, moisture, light) with a view to improving stability, to mask unpleasant taste and odor, to improve product identity, to facilitate handling (coating minimizes cross-contamination due to dust elimination), to reduce the risk of interaction between incompatible components, to improving product mechanical integrity because coated products are more resistant to mishandling and to modify drug release, as in enteric-coated, repeat action and sustained-release products.

Following types of tablet coatings are in common use:

Sugar coating

Sugar coating is the oldest method of tablet coating and involves the deposition of aqueous solution of coatings based predominantly on sucrose as a raw-material, because, sucrose is one of the few materials that enables smooth, high quality coatings to be produced that are essentially dry and tack-free at the end of the process. Since sugar coating is a multi-step process, where esthetics of the final product is an important goal, still in many companies, it is highly dependent on the use of highly skilled manpower. However, in the last few decades, adoption of modern techniques and by the introduction of automation, processing times have been reduced.

Film coating

It involves the deposition of a thin polymeric film onto the dosage form from organic-solvent based solutions. Organic solvent is being replaced with water because of the obvious advantages. This is a popular alternative to sugar coating.

Compression coating

This involves the use of modified tabletting machine that allows the compaction of a dry coating around the tablet core produced on the same machine. The main advantage of this type of coating is that it eliminates the use of any solvent. However, the process is mechanically complex.

Electrostatic coating

Electrostatic coating is employed for applying films of electro-conductive materials. In this, an ionic charge is imparted to the core and an opposite charge to the coating material. This technology ensures thin, continuous and electronically perfected film to the surface.

Laminate coating

Laminated coating provides multiple layers for incorporation of medicament; for example (1) Repeat-action tablet, here a portion of the drug is kept in outer lamella or coating; (2) Enteric tablet, here one drug could be made available for gastric absorption while another for release in intestine; and (3) Buccal-swallow tablet, this could first be administered sublingually, and upon a signal, such as release of flavour from the inner core, the same may be swallowed as a normal peroral tablet.

Vacuum film coating

This employs a specially designed baffled pan, which is water-jacketed and could be sealed to achieve vacuum. Tablets are placed in the sealed pan, the vacuum is applied and the coating material is introduced through airless hydraulic spray system. Since the pan is completely sealed,

organic solvents could be effectively used with minimal environmental or safety concern.

Solvent-free coatings

Solvent less coating technologies can overcome many of the disadvantages associated with the use of solvents (e.g., solvent exposure, solvent disposal, and residual solvent in product) in pharmaceutical coating. Solvent less processing reduces the overall cost by eliminating the tedious and expensive processes of solvent disposal/treatment. In addition, it can significantly reduce the processing time due to reduction of step of drying/evaporation. The conventional pan coater, fluidized bed coater and spray dryer can be used with slight modification for most of the solvent less coating methods. These processes are performed without any heat in most cases and thus can provide an alternative technology to coat temperature-sensitive drugs.

1. Compression coating

This involves the use of modified tabletting machine that allows the compaction of a dry coating around the tablet core produced on the same machine. The main advantage of this type of coating is that it eliminates the use of any solvent. However, this process is mechanically complex.

2. Electrostatic coating

Electrostatic coating is employed for applying films of electro-conductive materials. In this, an ionic charge is imparted to the core and an opposite charge to the coating material. This technology ensures thin, continuous and electronically perfected film to the surface (Chrai et al., 1998). Qtrol^{TM} is the core technology platform of PhoqusPharmaceuticals, which is derived from electrostatic deposition. Qtrol^{TM} enables solid oral dosage forms such as tablets to be coated in a controlled and precise manner that can then be used to modify the way that a drug is released into the body. Chronocort® is specially formulated dosage form invented by

Phoqus Pharmaceuticals to enable sustained release of Hydrocortisone based on Qtrol™ core technology.

3. Magnetically assisted impaction coating (MAIC)

Many food and pharmaceutical ingredients, being organic and relatively soft, are very sensitive to heat and can quite easily be deformed by severe mechanical forces. Soft coating methods that can attach the guest (coating material) particles onto the host (material to be coated) particles with a minimum degradation of particle size, shape and composition caused by the build-up of heat are the better candidates for such applications. The rise in temperature is negligible; this is an added advantage when dealing with temperature-sensitive powders such as pharmaceuticals. Apparatus for MAIC consists of processing vessel surrounded by the series of electromagnets connected to the alternating current. The host and guest materials are placed in the vessel along with the measured mass of the magnetic particles. When a magnetic field is present, the magnetic particles are agitated and move furiously inside the vessel, resembling a fluidized bed system. These agitated magnetic particles then impart energy to the host and guest particles, causing collisions and allowing coating to be achieved by means of impaction of the guest particles onto the host particles. The magnetic particle motion studies suggests that the primary motion due to the magnetic field is the spinning of the magnetic particles, promoting de-agglomeration of the guest particles as well as the spreading and shearing of the guest particles onto the surface of the host particles. Various steps in MAIC process are excitation of magnetic particle, de-agglomeration of guest particles, shearing and spreading of guest particles on the surface of the host particles, magnetic-host-host particle interaction, magnetic–host–wall interaction and formation of coated products (Singh P. et al., 2001; Ramlakhan M. et al., 2000).

4. Supercritical fluid coating

The supercritical fluid spray coating process consists of dissolving the coating material or drug in supercritical carbon dioxide, and gradually reducing the solvent power of carbon dioxide to enable the coating material to precipitate onto drug particles dispersed in the medium. Although, this process is technically a solvent-based coating process, the use of carbon dioxide as the supercritical fluid avoids some of the challenges associated with traditional solvent-based processes. In the absence of co-solvents, the coating materials used in supercritical fluid coating are limited mainly to lipids (fats and waxes). Carbon dioxide is the most widely used supercritical fluid because of its relatively low critical temperature (31°C) and pressure (74 bar). (Ribeiro Dos Santos et al., 2002; Thies et al, 2003)

5. Photocurable coating

Photocuring can be defined as a process of rapid conversion of specially formulated (usually liquid) solvent less compositions into solid films by irradiation with ultraviolet or visible light. It is a chemical approach proposed to rapidly coat tablets at or below room temperature with an extremely rapid rate. Photocuring systems generally consist of 4 major components: a) Specially functionalized liquid pre-polymers or monomers, an initiator, and b) UV/visible light source and pore forming agents. (Luo et al., 2008)

6. Hot melt coating

In hot melt coating method, the coating material is applied in its molten state on the substrate and then solidified by cooling. Hence, the necessity of the application of any solvent is fully eliminated in coating of pharmaceutical formulation like tablets and pellets. Lipid, waxes, fatty bases and hydrogenated vegetable oils are the most suitable coating material in hot melt coating. As the lipid based coatings are less expensive, less weight gain and processing time is short, hot melt coating is also cost effective (Padsalgi et al., 2008). Examples of some marketed hot melt coating excipients are Gelucires, Precirol, Stearines, Myvaplex, Compritol 888ATO.

Supercell technology

Supercell coating technology is an invention of NiroPharma, which uses a small modular design where tablets are coated in batches ranging from 30 to 40 grams, and which is amenable to linearly scale up to the production capacities.

In this, typically tablets are coated with coating spray in the same direction as the drying gas, hence, resulting in a more efficient process. This technology provides unique air distribution and the tablets moves quickly and predictably through the spray zone, receiving only a small amount of coating per pass, and therefore, achieving higher coating accuracy. The process time is short, seconds or minutes are required as opposed to hours required in other techniques, and therefore, it is gentler on the tablets. It allows for coating of friable tablets, as well as, flat or highly oblong tablet shapes and even extremely hygroscopic cores. The accuracy of deposition is high, therefore, if required the active ingredients could be layered onto tablets, and uniform layers of taste masking or modified release coatings could also be applied.

Soflet technology

This is an invention of Banner Pharmacaps and it employs application of gelatin layers over the table cores. Specially designed machines form two ribbons in which tablets are sandwiched and then cut-sealed by thermal compression. The tablets may have two different colours at two different sides. This technology is claimed to providing better swallowability in addition to other features like oxygen barrier capabilities of the gelatin. BioProgress, a new entrant in coating technology, has come out with a similar technology where gelatin is replaced by HPMC film.

One step dry coating method (OSDrC)

The manufacturing method for OSDrC is different from conventional methods in that dry-coated tablets can be made with only one process. The schematic sequence of the OSDrC manufacturing method is shown in Fig. 3.14. This OSDrC manufacturing method is developed by a rotary type tabletting machine using a single set of punches and die. Every upper and lower punch in the OSDrC system has a double structure as shown in Fig. 3.14. Each punch consists of a center punch (diameter: 6 mm) and an outer punch (diameter: 7, 8 and 10 mm). The OSDrC-system employs three compression processes. The first compression forms lower outer layer (indicated as the first-outer layer), the second compression to builds up the first-

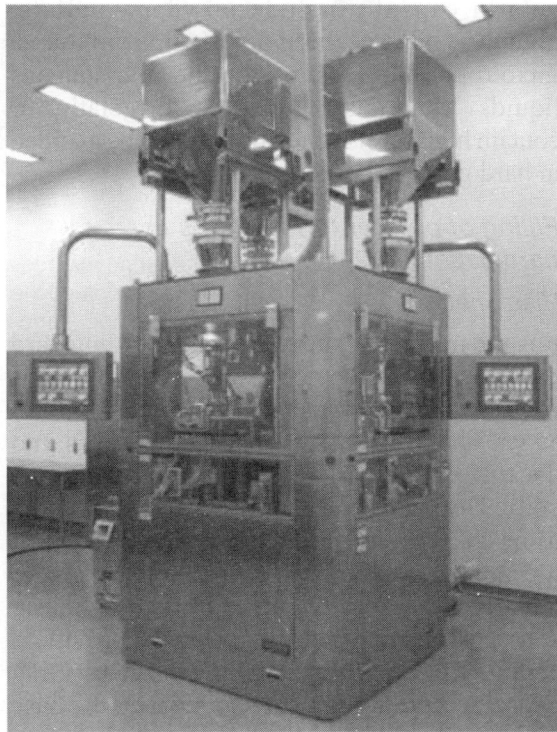

Fig. 3.14A. OSDrC® tablet press.

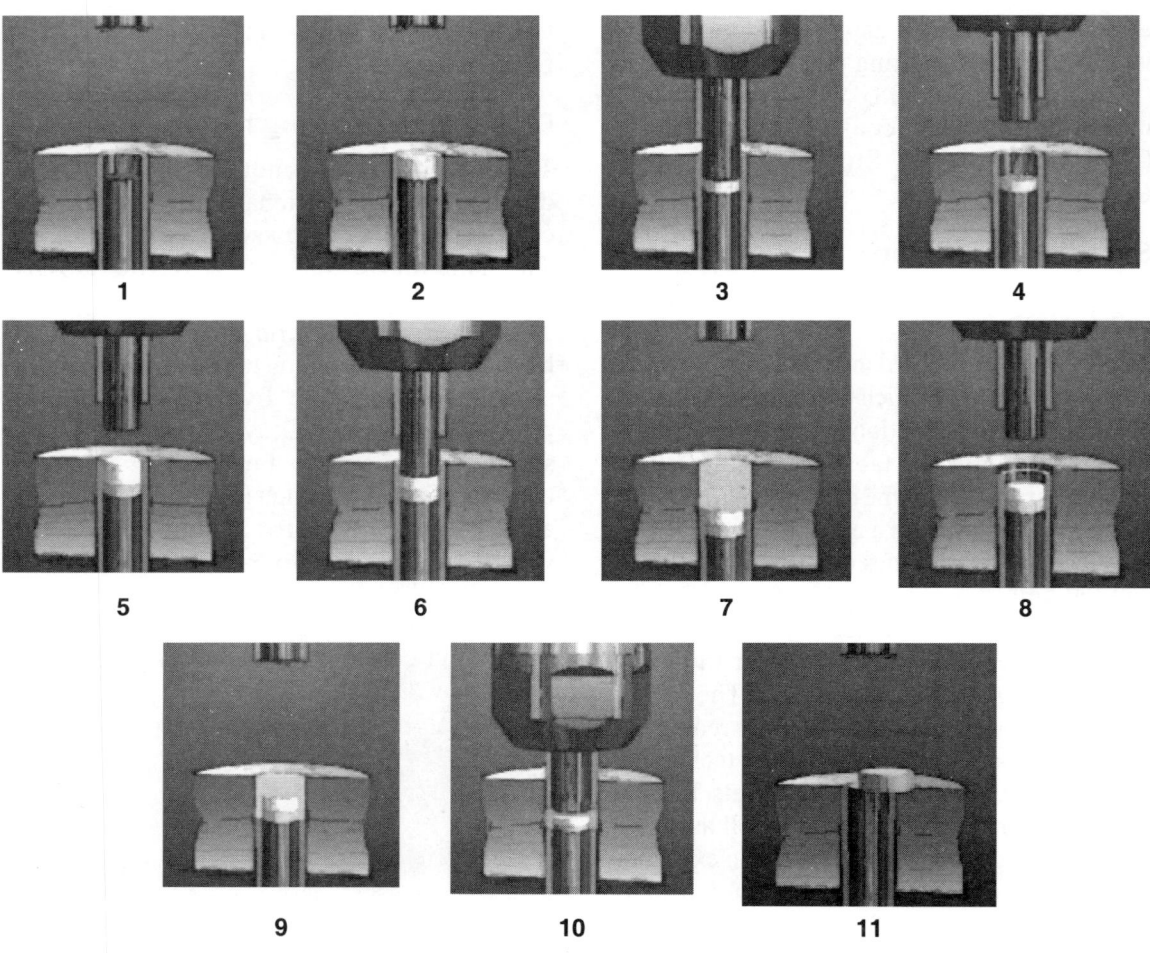

Fig. 3.14B. Steps of OSDrC manufacturing method. (1) Only the lower center punch slides down. (2) Space is filled with powder for the coating, which becomes the base layer of the tablet; at this time, the lower outer punch acts as a die. (3) Pre-compression by the upper and lower center punches. (4) Upper punch retracts. (5) Space is filled with powder for the API layer. (6) Pre-compression by the upper and lower center punches. (7) Upper punch retracts. (8) Die is filled with remaining powder for the coating. (9) Pre-shaped API layer is pushed up inside the die; the API layer is now completely surrounded by the coating. (10) Compression is completed by the upper and lower punches in flush alignment. (11) Finished tablet is released.

outer layer/core complex and the third compression shapes the whole tablet, including both the upper-outer and side-outer layers (indicated as the second-outer layer). In the first step to form the first-outer layer, the lower-center punch is slid down to fill up the space made by the lower-center punch with the powder for the first-outer layer (polymer). Then, the powder is pre-compressed by the upper-center punch.

While the upper-center punch is pushing down the pre-compressed first-outer layer to downward, the lower-center punch slid down at the same time. After pre-compression, the upper-center punch is pull up to create a space, which was to be filled up with the drug powder for the core. Drug powder is then subjected to pre-compression by the upper-center punch, this form complex of first outer layer with core powder. While the upper-center punch is pre-compressing, the lower-outer punch is sliding down, that creates the space over the pre-compressed complex of the first-outer/core, which is filled up with the remaining powder (polymer) to build up the second-outer layer. At the last compression, the remaining powder is compress by the upper and lower punches with the pre-compressed complex. The final compression employs simultaneous movement of the center and outer punches at a fixed speed of 1mm/min under constant pressures. The tips of the center and outer punches were adjusted to create a flat face like a normal punch. The quantity of powder for the second-outer layer was adjusted to create the same thickness as that of the 1st-outer layer.

Soflet technology

This is an invention of Banner Pharmacaps and it employs application of gelatin layers over the table cores. Specially designed machines form two ribbons in which tablets are sandwiched and then cut-sealed by thermal compression. The tablets may have two different colours at two different sides. This technology is claimed to providing better swallowability in addition to other features like oxygen barrier capabilities of the gelatin.

BioProgress, a new entrant in coating technology, has come out with a similar technology where gelatin is replaced by HPMC film.

Sugar coating

The sugar coating process cān be divided into different steps:

Sealing

Sugar coating is an aqueous process during which the tablet cores are thoroughly wetted by syrup applications. A tablet sealant is, therefore, applied to protect the tablet. The seal coat provides a moisture barrier and hardens the surface of the tablet in order to minimize attritional effects. In addition, core tablets having very rapid disintegration rates conceivably could start the disintegration process during the initial phase sugar coating. Depending on the hygroscopicity of the core, four sealing applications may be required. Dusting powder is added in between applications to prevent tablets from sticking together and to the pan.

Tablet sealants are generally water-insoluble polymers or film formers applied from an organic solvent solution. Examples of tablet sealants are: (a) shellac – very commonly used and is best in combination with PVP, which prevents hardening of the polymer on ageing; (b) cellulose acetate phthalate; (c) polyvinyl acetate phthalate; and (d) acrylate polymers. The sealing stage must be conducted with some caution as over- application of tablet sealants can lead to disintegration problems. Because shellac, CAP, PVAP, and zein also have enteric properties, care must be taken not to apply more coating than is required for sealing purposes. This amount will vary with the porosity, hardness, and hygroscopicity of the core tablet and must be determined experimentally.

Sub-coating

Sub-coating is the actual start of the sugar-coating process and provides the rapid build-up necessary to round the tablet edge. It also functions as the foundation for the smoothing and color coats. Sub-coating can be accomplished by two methods, either (1) the application of a gum/sucrose solution followed by dusting with powder and then drying; this routine is repeated many times until the desired shape is achieved; or (2) the application of a suspension of dry powder in the gum/sucrose solution followed by drying. The above procedure is repeatedly performed until the correct shape is evident. The solution used is sucrose based and contains a gum such as gelatin, acacia or a starch derivative, which aid in the adhesion of the powder fillers such as calcium carbonate or talc. If a coating suspension is used then the solids content is made as high as possible in order to reduce each application. The solution is normally used at a temperature between 60 and 70°C, because of the reduced viscosity at the elevated temperature.

Smoothing/Grossing

The grossing process is for the specific purpose of smoothing and filling the irregular surface generated during the sub-coating layer. If the sub-coated tablets are relatively smooth with hardly any depressions and the difference between the finished size and the sub-coat is small, simple 70% w/w sugar syrup is enough. If the sub-coating is rough with much irregularity, the use of grossing syrup containing suspended solids will provide more rapid build-up and better filling qualities. These syrups generally contain pigments, starch, and gelatin or acacia.

Color-coating

The colors used in sugar coating are those permitted in national legislation of the countries where the product will be sold. There are two groups of coloring substances generally used in colored tablet coatings: water-soluble dyes and water-insoluble pigments. The use of water-soluble dyes is part of the traditional method of sugar coating tablets. However, their use demands a great deal of skill and patience and the process is prone to coating faults such as poor and uneven coverage and variation in color from batch to batch. Most modern sugar coating procedures utilize pigments such as the aluminum lakes or iron oxides. They are easier to use and permit comparatively fast color coating times compared with soluble dye coating.

Polishing

After color coating, the tablets will require a separate polishing step for them to achieve an attractive appearance. This step is carried out in a clean pan but sometimes a wax or canvas lined pan is used. The tablets receive one or two applications of a wax dissolved in an organic solvent. The waxes may be applied directly to the tablets as finely divided powders. Usually, beeswax or carnauba wax is used. In order to achieve good finish due consideration must be given to optimum temperature and humidity condition.

Printing

The use of indented monograms on sugar coated tablet cores is not feasible because the considerable thickness of coating obliterates any core markings. Instead, if identification is required then this can be accomplished by printing. The printing process used is an offset rotogravure and this is used in conjunction with special edible printing inks.

Application procedure

The basic application process consists of three steps: application of appropriate volume of coating liquid to a cascading bed of tablets, distribution of the coating liquid uniformly across the surface of each tablet in the batch, and drying of the coating liquid once uniform distribution is achieved. The coating pan should exhibit good mixing characteristics so that dead spots are avoided.

Sugar coating defects

These are usually associated with processing.

Chipping of coatings

Addition of small quantities of polymers (such as cellulosics, polyvinyl pyrrolidone, acacia or gelatin) to the coating formulation helps to improve structural integrity, and thus reduces chipping problems.

Cracking of the coating

Tablet cores may expand during or after coating due to moisture absorption or due to stress relaxation of the core after compaction. This expansion leads to cracking of the core. Cracking can be avoided by minimizing moisture absorption by using seal coat and allowing sufficient time between compaction and coating for relaxation of post-compaction stress.

Non-drying coatings

When sugar coating solutions containing aluminium lakes are kept hot for too long, or constantly reheated to redissolve sugar, inversion of sucrose takes place. Such sugar coatings show inability to get dried.

Twinning (or build-up or multiples)

Sugar coating solutions are very sticky, particularly when they begin to dry. This results in sticking of the adjacent tablets. This problem usually occurs when the tablets being coated have a flat surface or high dose, capsule shaped tablets that have high edge walls.

Uneven color

This is more apparent with darker colors and it occurs due to poor distribution of coating liquids during application, color migration of water-soluble dyes while the coating is drying, unevenness of the surface of sub-coat, washing back or pigment-colored color coatings and excessive drying between color applications.

Blooming and sweating

Residual moisture in the finished tablet diffuses out and causes the polish of the tablet to take on fogged appearance (blooming). If the residual moisture content is high, it may appear like beads of perspiration on the tablet surface (sweating).

Prior to the application of further coating suspension, it should be assured that the earlier coat has thoroughly dried.

Marbling

This problem occurs as the result of the collection of wax in the small surface depressions of rough coating and is particularly evident with darker colors.

Film coating

Film coating has proved successful as a result of many advantages. There is minimal weight increase (2–3% of the tablet core weight). There is significant reduction in processing times. Only thin film is applied, so there is decrease in the amount of coating material and solvent, which must be applied, and organic solvents evaporate fast. There is increased process efficiency and output as it lends itself easily to automation. Unlike sugar coating, the flexibility afforded in film coating allows additional substrates, other than just compressed tablets to be considered e.g. powders, granules, capsules etc. as compared to sugar coating, film coating is resistant to chipping. The major process advantages result from the greater volatility of the organic solvents used. The use of organic solvents has created many potential problems including flammability hazards, toxicity hazards, and concerns over environmental pollution and cost.

Raw material used in film coating

Raw materials commonly used in the preparation of coating suspension are film forming resin, solvent system, plasticizers, colorants, opaquants etc. Numerous ready-to-use coating materials with variety of functional properties are available commercially.

Film formers

Materials used to coat pharmaceutical products are primarily based on acrylic and cellulosic polymers. Water-soluble films are produced using polymers like hydroxypropyl cellulose, hydroxypropyl methylcellulose, sodium carboxymethylcellulose, and polyvinyl pyrrolidone, are often used for rapidly disintegrating film-coated tablets. Examples of sustained release polymers are ethyl cellulose and commercially available water-insoluble polymethacrylates.

Common commercially available enteric polymers are cellulose acetate phthalate, hydroxypropyl methylcellulose phthalate, hydroxypropyl methylcellulose acetate succinate, polyvinyl acetate phthalate, and several methacrylic acid copolymers.

Solvents

The primary criteria for the selection of a solvent for a particular polymer system include solvency, volatility, toxicity, and pollution control. The most superior films, showing the greatest combined strength of cohesiveness, have been reported when the coating solution solvation and polymer chain extension are at a maximum.

Film coating technology, however, has shifted toward aqueous-based systems for environmental and economic reasons and the majority of polymeric materials used today are applied as aqueous-based solutions and dispersions.

With aqueous-based systems, the risk of explosion is diminished, costs of disposing of the solvents are reduced, and concerns of potential toxicities due to residual solvents within the film are eliminated.

Plasticizers

Many pharmaceutical polymers exhibit brittle properties and require the addition of a plasticizing agent to obtain an effective coating, free of cracks, edging, or splitting. Plasticizers function by weakening the intermolecular attractions between the polymer chains and generally cause a decrease in the tensile strength and the glass transition temperature and an increase in the flexibility of the films. Plasticizers used in a polymeric system should be miscible with the polymer and exhibit little tendency for migration, exudation, evaporation, or volatilization. Many compounds can be used to plasticize polymers, including water. Phthalate esters such as diethyl phthalate, sebacate esters such as dibutylsebacate, and citrate esters such as triethyl citrate and tributyl citrate are commonly used as plasticizing agents. Various glycol derivatives including propylene glycol and polyethylene glycol have also been used to plasticize polymeric films. In addition, surfactants, preservatives, and other compounds have been shown to function as plasticizing agents in cellulosic and acrylic polymers.

For aqueous-based dispersed systems, water-insoluble plasticizers should be emulsified first and then added to the polymer. Sufficient time must be allowed for plasticizer uptake into the polymer phase prior to the initiation of coating.

The effectiveness of a plasticizing agent is dependent, to a large extent, on the amount of plasticizer added to the film coating formulation and the extent of polymer–plasticizer interaction. Forces involved in polymer–plasticizer mixtures include hydrogen bonding, dipole–dipole, and dipole-induced dipole interactions, as well as dispersion forces.

Other additives

In addition to the polymer, plasticizer, and solvent, other water-soluble and water-insoluble compounds such as pigments, anti-adherents, surfactants, and antifoaming agents may be added to coating formulations to improve the appearance of the final dosage form, to facilitate processing, and to reduce the tackiness of the films.

Conventional film coatings

Conventionally film coating has been applied to improve product appearance, improve stability and ease of ingestion without altering drug-release characteristics from the dosage form. The selection of raw materials is often based on factors that affect the mechanical properties of the coating, allow smooth, glossy coats to be obtained and produce coating that readily dissolve in GI tract. Conventional coating is the area where aqueous technology has gained the highest acceptance.

Modified-release film coatings

Film coating techniques can be effectively used either to sustain the release (extended release) or delay the release (enteric coating) of drug.

Sustained release film coatings

The film coating acts as a membrane that allows infusion of GI fluids and the outward diffusion of drugs or the release process may be augmented

Table 3.5. Commercially available coating materials with various functional properties

METHACRYLATE-BASED COATINGS

Polymer	Trade name
Cellulose Acetate Phthalate (CAP)	Aquacoat® CPD, Aqueous Dispersion (30% solids)
	C-A-P NF Eastman
Hydroxypropylmethylcellulose (HPMC)	Sepifilm™ LP
Hydroxypropylcellulose (HPC)	Klucel®
Hydroxypropylethylcellulose (HPEC)	
Ethylcellulose	Aquacoat® ECD, Aqueous Dispersion (30% solids)
	Aqualon®
	Surelease® Aqueous Dispersion (25% solids)
Methylcellulose	Metolose® SM-4, extremely low viscosity methylcellulose for film coating
Microcrystalline Cellulose and Carrageenan	LustreClear™, All-in-one coating system

Applications

Enteric Coatings	Aquacoat® CPD, Cellulose acetate phthalate aqueous dispersion
	C-A-P NF Eastman is used in solvent-based coatings
Polymer Extenders	Klucel® EF and LF enhance the utility of HPMC. Eliminates bridging, improves adherence to problem tablet substrate, reduces the incidence on film cracking on the tablet edge
Immediate Release Coatings	*Moisture barrier/sealant:* Use Aquacoat® ECD, Opadry® AMB, Sepifilm™ LP, Surelease®
	Taste masking: Use Aquacoat® ECD, LustreClear™, Metolose® SM-4, Surelease®
	LustreClear™ is used as an aqueous clear film coating. It allows for short hydration time prior to coating and fast drying. Its smooth satin-like finish eliminates edge wear and logo bridging.
	Sepifilm™ LP is a ready-to-use, gastrosoluble composition for the film-coating of moisture-sensitive solid particles. Plasticized with stearic acid. Shows significantly lower moisture permeability compared to PVA and other HPMC-based coating formulations.
Sustained Release Coatings	Ethylcellulose-based coatings
	Aquacoat® ECD
	Aqualon®
	Surelease®, a complete, optimally plasticized system for modified release.
Subcoat	Klucel® EF is a highly flexible film former, and is an excellent subcoat for tablets that are difficult to coat.
Pellet Coating	Metolose® SM-4, low viscosity (4mPas), less tacky, and therefore better than HPMC for fine pellet coating

Suppliers

Supplier	Trade Name	Regulatory Status
Colorcon	Opadry®	
	Opadry®	
	Surelease®	

(Contd.)

Eastman	C-A-P	NF
FMC	Aquacoat® CPD Aqueous Dispersion	NF
	Aquacoat® ECD Aqueous Dispersion	NF
	LustreClear™	NF
Hercules	Aqualon®	NF
	Klucel®	NF
	Klucel® EF	Pharm grade for NF, EP, JP
SEPPIC	Sepifilm™ LP	Pharm grade for NF, EP, JP
Shin-Etsu	Metolose® SM-4	EP, JP, USP/NF

METHACRYLATE-BASED COATINGS

Functionality	Trade Name
Anionic polymer of methacrylic acid and methacrylates with a –COOH group	Eudragit® L 100-55 – powder, spray dried L 30 D-55 which can be reconstituted for targeted delivery in the duodenum
	Eudragit® L 30 D-55 – aqueous dispersion, pH dependent polymer soluble above pH 5.5 for targeted delivery in the duodenum
	Eudragit® L 100 – powder, pH dependent polymer soluble above pH 6.0 for targeted delivery in the jejunum
	Eudragit® S 100 – powder, pH dependent polymer soluble above pH 7.0 for targeted delivery in the ileum
	Eudragit® FS 30 D – aqueous dispersion, pH dependent polymer soluble above pH 7.0, requires no plasticizer
Cationic polymer with a dimethylamino-ethyl ammonium group	Eudragit® E 100 – granules, pH dependent, soluble in gastric fluid up to 5.0, swellable and permeable above pH 5.0
	Eudragit® E PO – powder form of E-100
Copolymers of acrylate and methacrylates with quaternary ammonium group	Insoluble, high permeability
	Eudragit® RL 30D – aqueous dispersion, pH independent polymer for sustained release formulations
	Eudragit® RL PO – powder, pH independent polymer for matrix formulations
	Eudragit® RL 100 – granules, pH independent
	Insoluble, low permeability
	Eudragit® RS 30D – aqueous dispersion, pH independent polymer for sustained release formulations
	Eudragit® RS PO – powder, pH independent polymer for matrix formulations
	Eudragit® RS 100 – granules, pH independent
Copolymers of acrylate and methacrylates with quaternary ammonium group in combination with sodium carboxymethylcellulose	Eudragit® RD 100 – powder, pH independent for fast disintegrating films

Applications

Enteric Coatings	Eudragit® L 100-55 or L 30 D-55 – delivery to the duodenum (pH > 5.0). Exact pH controlled drug release can be adjusted by a combination of polymers and coating thickness

(Contd.)

	Eudragit® L 100 – delivery to the jejunum (pH > 6.0)	
	Eudragit® S 100 – delivery to the intestine (pH 6.0 to 7.5), site specific delivery can be achieved by combining with Eudragit® L types	
	Eudragit® FS 30 D – delivery to the colon (pH > 7.0)	
	Acryl-eze® – one step dry enteric coating system, soluble at pH 5.5	
Sustained Release Coatings	Eudragit® RL and RS – release profile determined by the ratio of RL to RS polymers, and the film thickness applied	
Taste Masking	Eudragit® RD 100 – pH independent, fast disintegrating film	
	Eudragit® E 100 and EPO – pH dependent cationic polymer, soluble in gastric fluid up to pH 5.0, swellable and permeable above pH 5.0	
Rapidly Disintegrating Films	Eudragit® RD 100	

Suppliers

Supplier	Trade Name	Regulatory Status
Degussa	Eudragit® L 100-55 – powder	Ph. Eur., USP/NF
	Eudragit® L 30 D-55 – aqueous dispersion	Ph. Eur., JPE, USP/NF
	Eudragit® L 100 – powder	Ph. Eur., JPE, USP/NF
	Eudragit® S 100 – powder	Ph. Eur., JPE, USP/NF
	Eudragit® FS 30 D – aqueous dispersion	
	Eudragit® E 100 – granules	DAB, JPE
	Eudragit® E PO – powder	DAB, JPE
	Eudragit® RL 30 D – aqueous dispersion	
	Eudragit® RL PO – powder	JPE
	Eudragit® RL 100 – granules	JPE, USP/NF
	Eudragit® RS 30 D – aqueous dispersion	
	Eudragit® RS PO – powder	JPE
	Eudragit® RS 100 – granules	JPE, USP/NF
	Eudragit® RD 100 – powder	
Colorcon	Acryl-eze®	
Eastman	Eastacryl®	

by a coating that slowly dissolves/subjected to digestion by enzymes. Currently, the two most popular types of coatings are ethylcellulose-based Aquacoat® (FMC) and Surelease® (Colorcon) or the acrylic based Eudragit® NE and RS lines (Rohm Tech) and Kollicoat® SR 30D (BASF).

When used as an external coating, ethylcellulose coatings allow a gradual zero-order release of the drug substance where as acrylic-based systems produce a more sigmoidal dissolution profile, delaying drug release based on the thickness of the coating, with a relatively rapid release thereafter. Sustained-release coating permeability can be enhanced with water-soluble excipients such as HPMC for the ethylcellulose systems or water-insoluble, but freely permeable, Eudragit® RL 30D (Rohm Tech) in the acrylic systems. The most common application of sustained-release coatings is on microparticles that are subsequently encapsulated or tabletted.

Enteric film coatings

Enteric coatings allow the drug delivery system to pass through the stomach intact and dissolve upon reaching the intestine. Aqueous-based suspensions such as Eudragit® L30D-55 (Rohm

Tech) and Kollicoat® MAE 30 DP (BASF) or coating materials supplied as powders like Eudragit® L100 or AQOAT® AS (Shin-Etsu) are used to protect the tablet or microparticles from the low pH of the stomach. Upon reaching the near-neutral pH of the small intestine, these coatings dissolve rapidly and allow for immediate availability. Two fully formulated, aqueous enteric coating systems are commercially available in dry dispersible powders form and these use one-step process and are simple to apply. The first 'Sureteric System' is based on polyvinyl acetate phthalate (PVAP), and the second 'Acryl-Eze System' is based on methacrylic acid copolymer type C (Eudragit L100-55).

Application procedure

Film coatings can be applied by either manual ladling techniques or by means of spray atomization, the latter being more popular. Spray atomization allows coating liquids to be applied in a much more controlled and reproducible manner. Three basic types of spray-atomization techniques are airless spray techniques, air spray techniques and ultrasonic spray techniques.

Problems associated with film coating process, reasons and solutions

Problems, along with the causes and solutions are enlisted in Table 3.6.

Table 3.6. Problems associated with film coating process, reasons and solutions

Problem	Reason	Solution
Sticking and picking	• Over-wetting. • Excessive film tackiness.	• Decrease spray rate. • Increase drying temperature and air volume.
Peeling (extension of picking)	• Tablet bed becomes too wet.	• Decrease spray rate. • Increase drying temperature and air volume.
Bridging and filling	• Adhesion related problem.	• Use more dilute coating solutions. • Increase/change plasticizer. • Include wetting agents.
Orange peel effects	• Inadequate spreading of the coating solution before drying.	• Decrease viscosity of the coating solution.
Color variation/mottling	• Use of soluble dyes.	• Use pigments.
Cracking	• Higher molecular weight polymers or polymer blends.	• Adjust the plasticizer and pigment type and concentration.
Blistering	• Too rapid evaporation of the solvent from the core. • High drying temperature.	• Use milder drying conditions.
Roughness	• Faulty spray technique.	• Move the nozzle close to the tablet bed. • Increase spray rate. • Milder drying conditions.
Hazing/dull film	• High processing temperature for formulations consisting of cellulose polymers in aqueous media. • High humidity conditions on storage.	• Reduce drying temperature.

Methods of evaluating film coats

Free films

Evaluation of free films has proved a popular means of assessing the properties of polymer films and to optimize the coating formulation. Free films samples should be prepared by a spray technique rather than by the film casting technique (cast films can be prepared by spreading the coating composition on a teflon, glass or aluminium foil surface using a spreading bar to get a uniform film thickness. Sprayed films can be obtained by mounting a plastic-coated surface in a spray hood or coating pan, spraying should be such that a uniform film representative of the type achieved in tablet technology.

Free films are studied mainly for permeability and tensile properties. The assessment of the permeability properties of the polymer provides useful information regarding the potential effect of the film on the stability of the product. Tensile properties are measured to determine the mechanical properties of the films. These are useful for determining the qualitative and quantitative effects of additives such as plasticizers and pigments. Strips of the film are tested on tensile strength tester by applying a known force at a constant rate.

In-situ films

Even under the best conditions, it is difficult for free films to mimic exactly those, which have been applied to tablets. So, applied film is examined. **Diametric crushing strength** of a coated tablet gives the information on the relative increase in the crushing strength provided by the film and contribution made by change in film composition. It shows the ability of the film to absorb some of the applied stress or significantly modify the stress distribution within the sample. Surface hardness measurements, determined by a **micro-indentation technique,** provide a useful means of predicting how well the coated tablets will resist attrition during coating process and in automatic handling and filling equipment. A practical qualitative measure of the resistance of a coated tablet to abrasion can be obtained by merely rubbing the coated tablet on a white sheet of paper. Resistant films remain intact and no color is transferred to the paper. Very soft coatings are readily erased from the tablet surface to the paper. **Film adhesion test** is performed using tensile strength testers to measure the force required to peel the film from the tablet surface. This is done to ensure that the films do not bridge across break lines etc. Unless the coating is intended to control drug release, the coating should have a minimal effect on tablet DT and dissolution.

Coating equipment

There are three types of coating equipment used to apply polymeric materials: conventional coating pans, perforated coating pans, and fluidized beds. The **conventional coating pan** system consists of a round coating pan that rotates on an inclined axis. Tablets in the coating pan tumble due to pan rotation. Heat is blown across the surface of the tumbling tablets and exhaust air is withdrawn. Aqueous polymeric film coating, however, requires more rapid solvent evaporation and the drying efficiency of conventional coating pans is improved by adding perforations. These perforations allow air to be forced through the tablet bed. A schematic of a perforated coating pan is shown in Fig. 3.15. Baffles in the perforated coating pans contribute to the tumbling action of the tablets and facilitate uniform film coverage. In contrast to the coating

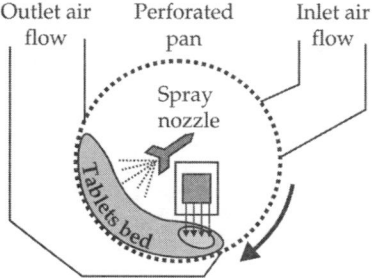

Fig. 3.15. Schematic of a perforated coating pan apparatus.

pans, the **fluidized bed** or **air suspension** method, utilizes a carrier gas to keep the tablet cores in motion. The high air current makes this technique more efficient at water removal. The bottom spray technique is one of the most common fluidized bed application methods and a schematic of this process is shown in Fig. 3.16. The bottom spray method provides ideal conditions for complete film coalescence.

The **top spray method** (Fig. 3.16), also known as the granulator mode, sprays the polymeric material counter currently into the fluidizing tablets. The rotary or tangential spray technique, shown in Fig. 3.16, uses a rotating disk to add a centrifugal force to fluidization and gravity. Irrespective of the type of coating equipment used, polymeric solutions and dispersions are generally applied using a spray-atomization technique and two types of spray nozzles namely pneumatic nozzles and hydraulic nozzles are employed.

Standards for coated tablets

There are differences in the requirements for coated and uncoated tablets in the general tablet monograph in the B.P. For coated tablets, the requirement for uniformity of weight and diameter has been deleted. Also, the disinteg-

ration test for coated tablets specifies a maximum disintegration time of 60 min. in water but permits the test to be repeated in 0.1 M HCl should the tablets fail. As with uncoated tablets, if the individual tablet monograph requires a dissolution test, then the disintegration test may be justifiably omitted. However, the uncoated tablets have to be tested prior to coating, including in the test schedule parameters appropriate for an uncoated tablet. The BP treats press coated tablets as for uncoated tablets for the purposes of compendial control. The BP disintegration test for enteric coated tablets directs that six tablets should withstand 2 hours in 0.1 M HCl without disintegrating, but on replacing the fluid with pH 6.8 phosphate buffer, all six should disintegrate within 1 hour.

AUTOMATION IN TABLET MANUFACTURING SYSTEM

In a tablet manufacturing system, some of the unit operations may include particle size reduction, sieving or classification, mixing, particle size enlargement, drying, compression, sorting and packaging. The traditional systems to control critical process parameters affecting product characteristics involve establishment of

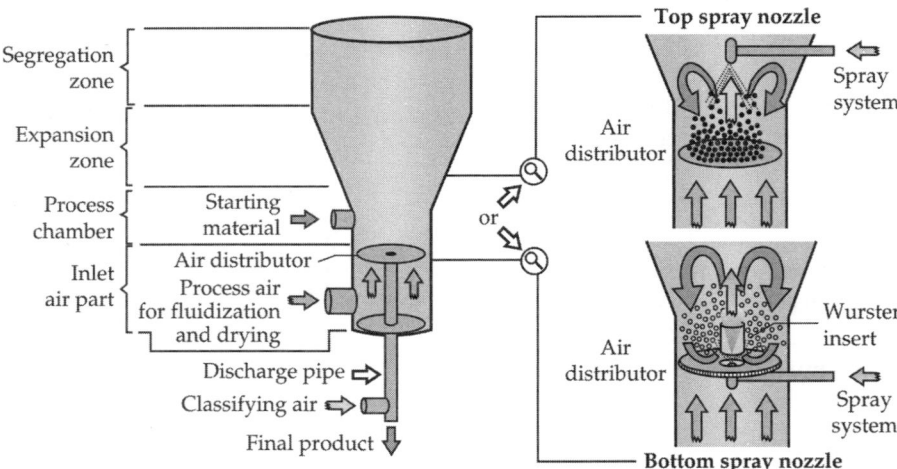

Fig. 3.16. Schematic of a fluidized bed coating apparatus.

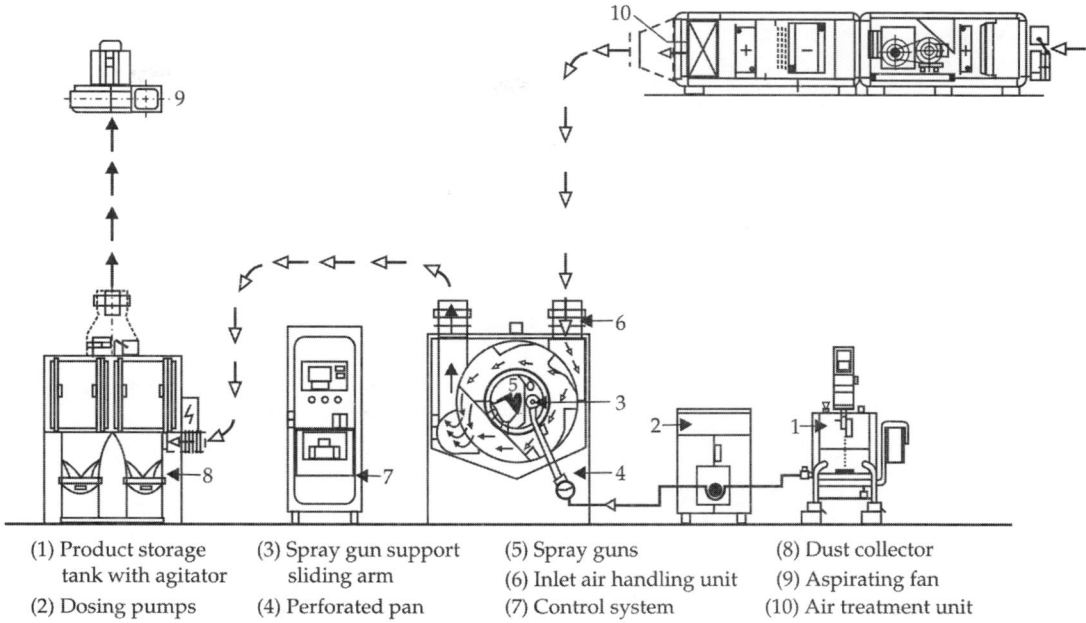

(1) Product storage tank with agitator
(2) Dosing pumps
(3) Spray gun support sliding arm
(4) Perforated pan
(5) Spray guns
(6) Inlet air handling unit
(7) Control system
(8) Dust collector
(9) Aspirating fan
(10) Air treatment unit

Fig. 3.17. Diagram showing high efficiency film coating machine system.

specific operating limits for unit operations to ensure production system is under control for production of safe, effective and reliable tablets.

Most tablet manufacturing systems are batch operations, whereby a series of manufacturing steps are used to prepare a single batch or lot of particular product. A relatively few products are manufactured by true continuous-processing procedures whereby raw materials continuously fed into and through the production sequence and the finished product is continuously discharged from the final processing step(s). Development of continuous-processing procedures requires specially designed and interfaced equipment, special plant layouts and dedicated plant space. In the tablet manufacturing system automation of granulation system eliminates the conventional/manually controlled steps of dry grinding, dry mixing, granulating, wet grinding, fluid-bed drying, post-dry-grinding, and lubrication (all done heretofore in separate piece of equipment). The automated granulating system consists of a dumping station, a mixer with vacuum drying and forced air

drying capabilities, a comminutor, a lubricant-addition station, a blender and pneumatic conveyer system for transporting the bulk material for compression. The automated system is enclosed and uses one field operator to load raw materials into loading hopper and to unload lubricated product into portable totes. In addition the process shares the services of two computer operators with another automated process. The computer operator works at a central control panel in the room that houses the computer and its peripheral equipment. In an automated production facility fork trucks or pallets never enter the facility. Instead, drums enter on roller conveyers and are discharged through a trash chute (at the bottom of which is positioned a drum crusher and compactor). The wheeled totes always remain within the facility's walled boundaries; washing the totes always done entirely within the facility. Such a total segregation of product eliminates any possibilities of cross-contamination and may be especially useful for toxic and other dangerous products.

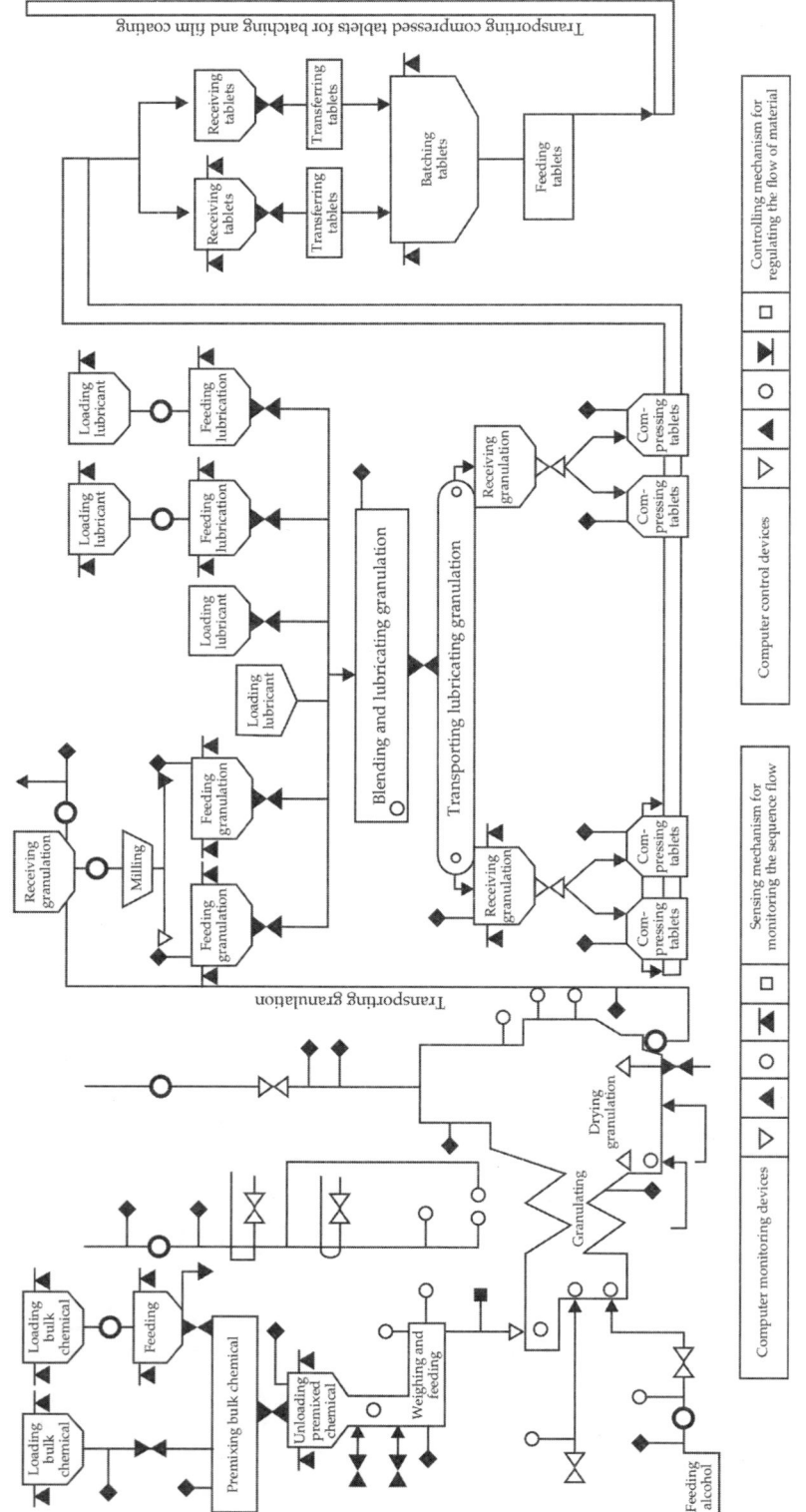

Fig. 3.18. Schematic flow diagram of automated tablet manufacturing system.

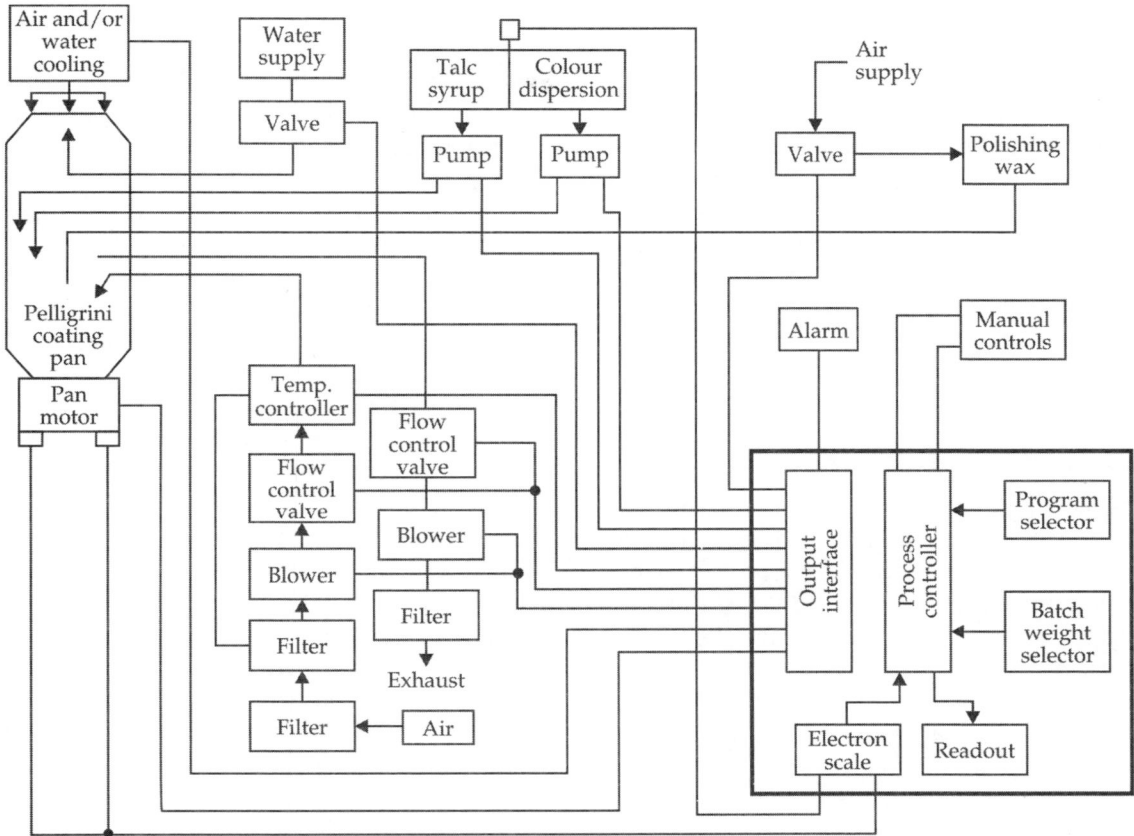

Fig. 3.19. Schematic diagram of microprocessor-based automated sugar-coating system.

Automatic control of modern, tablet rotary presses is essential because of the high speed and high output of such presses (Fraade et al., 2002). Manual tablet checks cannot suffice, because by nature they tend to vitiate the advantages of high speed and high output. The use of microprocessor technology differs from conventional two point control systems in both function and structure, and the system can be used to produce tablets within tolerances heretofore unavailable to the industry. The system corrects automatically for weight variation, monitors mean and individual tabletting values (hardness, thickness), controls sorting shifts that discard faulty tablets, and can include an optional quick-stop control that operates when tolerances are exceeded. The printer displays optimum speeds for the centrifugal filling shoe, helps optimize tool use, evaluates tabletting data, records errors, and offers opportunity to conduct statistical evaluations. In short, the system will allow rotary presses to operate to maximum capacity without sacrificing either high speed or high output levels.

The process of tablet coating usually includes many time-consuming steps, especially in sugar coating the entire process takes at least two or three eight-hour shifts and a worker must be at each pan at all times during the coating operation. If, however, this process is automated and totally controlled by microprocessor or mini-computer, it can be completed in about one eight hour shift. A **microprocessor-based automated sugar-coating system** monitors weight as the output of load cells mounted both on the pan and on the tank containing the coating suspensions and syrups. The system executes entire cycle – subcoating, coloring and polishing the tablets – in one pan, uninterrupted and unattended. The system gives accurate and reproducible uniformity of size, shape, weight distribution and color from batch to batch. This system can coat a pan load of tablets through the polishing stage, automatically in approximately one eight-hour shift.

FUTURE TRENDS

Advances in tablet formulation

The stellar growth of the pharmaceutical industry in the 1980s and 1990s has slowed during the last few years. In 1998, FDA approved 41 new molecular entities, but in 2002, the agency approved only 17, the fewest since 1983. These kinds of numbers have worried pharmaceutical companies that are now scrambling to maintain or enhance their product offerings by turning to advances in tablet technology. Significant advances have been made in the development of elegant systems to modify the oral drug delivery, but the basic approaches have remained greatly unchanged with the major systems being insoluble, slowly eroding, or swelling matrices, effervescent tablets, polymer-coated tablets, pellets, or granules, osmotically driven systems, systems controlled by ion exchange mechanisms, and various combinations of these approaches.

A summary of patented technologies is given below.

Mouth dissolving tablets

OraSolv and DuraSolv:
Efficient technologies for orally disintegrating tablets

Mouth-dissolving tablets, also known as fast melt/ fast dissolving or oro-disperse tablets (ODT) are one of the novel drug delivery systems (Mcgee et al., 2004). ODT is a unit dosage form that disintegrates in the oral cavity, usually in few seconds, to enhance compliance and overcome difficulty in swallowing by pediatric and geriatric patients (Danckwerts et al., 2003). A key attribute of the OraSolv technology is the fact that saliva causes the relatively soft tablet to rapidly disintegrate in the mouth (Habib et al., 2000). An essential feature is the presence of an effervescent couple that acts as a disintegrating agent while also assisting with taste masking and providing a pleasant sensation in the mouth (Weyhling et al., 1993). Orasolv tablets comprise of taste masking active(s), fillers, sweeteners, disintegrating agents, lubricants, glidants, flavors, and coloring agent. Tablets are manufactured by direct compression technique using conventional blending techniques and high speed tablet presses (Amborn et al., 2001a;, Amborn et al., 2001b; Katzner et al., 2000). The specially designed package and processing system, referred to as Pak-AolvTM for Orasolv tablets is also available. **DuraSolv** is second-generation fast-dissolving/ disintegrating tablet formulation. Produced in a fashion similar to OraSolv, DuraSolv has much higher mechanical strength than its predecessor due to the use of higher compaction pressures during tabletting. DuraSolv utilizes indirectly compressible fillers in fine form (Khankari et al., 2000, 2001). Product is packed in a blister or pouches (Myers et al., 1999).

Zydis oral fast-dissolving dosage form

The Zydis fast-dissolving dosage form is a unique freeze-dried medicinal tablet, made from well-known and acceptable materials (Seager, 1998; Danckwerts et al., 2003). Zydis tablet can be swallowed without water, because it dissolves instantly on the tongue in less than 3 seconds (Grother et al., 1998). The manufacturing process requires the active ingredients to be dissolved or suspended in an aqueous solution of water-soluble structure formers. The resultant mixture is poured in blister pockets of laminate film and freeze dried (Iles et al., 1993; Yarwood et al., 1998; Green et al., 1999).

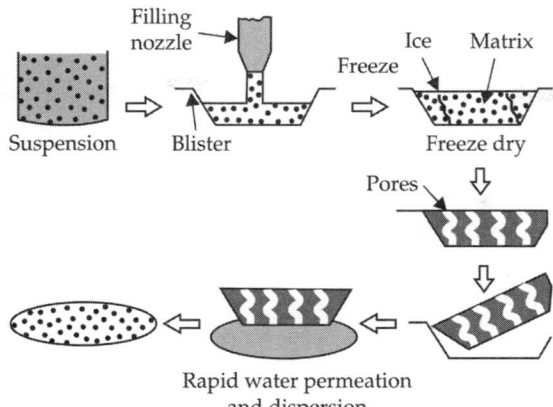

Fig. 3.20. Zydis manufacturing process.

Flash dose technology

Two platform technologies called Sheaform and Ceform are currently being utilized in the preparation of a wide range of oral fast disintegrating products. The Sheaform technology is based on preparation of floss that is known as 'Sheaform matrix' which is produced by subjecting a feedshock containing a sugar carrier to flash heat processing. In this procedure, the sugar is simultaneously subjected to centrifugal force and to a temperature gradient, which raises the temperature of the mass to create an internal flow condition, which permits part of it to move with respect of the mass. The flowing mass exits through the spinning head that flings the floss. The floss so produced is amorphous in nature so it is further chopped and recrystallised by various techniques to provide uniform flow properties and thus facilitate blending. The recrystallised matrix is then blended with other tablet excipients and an active ingredient. The resulting mixture is compressed into tablet.

In Ceform technology microspheres containing active ingredient are prepared. The essence of Ceform microsphere manufacturing process involves placing dry powder, containing either substantially pure drug material or a special blend of drug material plus other pharmaceutical compounds, and excipients into a precision engineered rapidly spinning machine. The centrifugal force of the rotating head of ceform machine throws the dry drug blend at high speed through small, heated openings; the carefully controlled temperature of the resultant microburst of liquefied the drug blend to form a sphere without adversely affecting drug stability. The microsphere are then blended and/or compressed into the pre-selected oral delivery dosage form.

Wowtab technology

Yamanauchi pharmaceutical company patented this technology. 'wow' means 'without water'. The active ingredients may constitute up to 50% w/w of the tablet. In this technique, saccharides of both low and high mouldability are used to prepare the granules. Active ingredients are mixed with low mouldability saccharides and then granulated with high mouldability saccharides and then compressed into tablet. The Wowtab product dissolves quickly in 15 seconds or less. Wowtab product can be packed in both conventional bottle and blister packs.

Flashtab technology

Prographarm Laboratories have a patent over this technology wherein microgranules of the taste-masked active drug are used. These may be prepared by using conventional techniques like coacervation, microencapsulation, and extrusion-spheronisation. All these processes utilize conventional tabletting technology. These taste-masked microcrystals of active drug, disintegrating agent, a swelling agent and other excipients like soluble diluents etc. are compressed to form a multiparticulate tablet that disintegrates rapidly.

Oraquick

This technology is patented by K.V. Pharmaceuticals. It utilizes taste masking microsphere technology called as micro mask, which provides superior mouth feel, significant mechanical strength, and quick disintegration/

dissolution of product. This process involves preparation of micro particles in the form of matrix that protects drug, which can be compressed with sufficient mechanical strength. Low heat of production accommodates high doses of drug and offers improved mechanical strength.

Pharmaburst technology

SPI Pharma, New Castle, patented this technology. The Pharmaburst ODT uses a proprietary disintegrant (Pharmaburst) that is based on mannitol blended with conventional tabletting aids. It utilizes the co-processed excipients to develop ODT, which dissolves within 30-40 s. This technology involves dry blending of drug, flavor, and lubricant followed by compression into tablets.

Frosta technology

Akina patented this technology. The Frosta technology is based on the compression of highly plastic granules at low pressure to prepare fast melting tablets. The highly plastic granules are composed of three components: a plastic material, (Maltrin QD M580 and MaltrinM180 are maltodextrin and corn syrup solids), a water penetration enhancer (Mannogem EZ Spray), and a wet binder (sucrose, poly vinyl pyrolidone and hydroxyl propyl methylcellulose). Each of the three components plays an essential role in obtaining tablets with higher strengthened faster disintegration time.

Advantol™ 200

Advantol™ 200 is a directly compressible excipient system offering "Soft-Melt" functionality and specially formulated for nutraceutical applications. SPI Pharma's Advantol platform uses proprietary co-processing technology. Advanto requires no special manufacturing equipment or tooling. Advantol formulations utilize a standard rotary tablet press with standard tooling under normal tabletting temperature and humidity conditions to make robust "soft-melt" tablets.

AdvaTab 53

AdvaTab tablets disintegrate rapidly in less than 30 seconds. These tablets are prepared using polymer-coated drug particles that are uniformly dispersed in an ultra-fine, low water content, rapidly disintegrating matrix with superior organoleptic properties. AdvaTab tablets are compressed using a proprietary, patented, external lubrication system in which the lubricant is applied only to the tablet surface, resulting in robust tablets that are hard and less friable and can be packaged in bottles or blister.

Quicksolv technology

This technology is patented by Janssen Pharmaceuticals. It uses two solvents in formulating a matrix, which disintegrates instantaneously. Methodology includes dissolving medium components in water and the solution or suspension is frozen. Then dry the matrix by removing water using an excess of alcohol (solvent extraction). Thus, the product formed has uniform porosity and adequate strength for handling.

Ziplet technology

In Ziplet technology water-insoluble drugs or drugs as coated micro particles are used. The addition of a suitable amount of water-insoluble inorganic excipients combined with disintegrants imparted an excellent physical conflict to the oral dissolving tablet (ODT) and the simultaneously maintained optimal disintegration. The use of water-insoluble inorganic excipients offers better enhancement of disintegration in comparison with the most commonly used water-soluble sugars or salts. Tablets primarily of water-soluble components often tend to dissolve rather than disintegrate and concentrated viscous solution is formed, which reduces the rate of water diffusion into the tablet core.

Lyoc technology

Lyoc technique was owned by Cephalon Corporation. Lyoc utilizes a freeze-drying process but differs from Zydis in that the product is frozen on the freeze dryer shelves. The liquid solution or suspension preparation involves fillers, thickening agents, surfactant, non-volatile flavoring agents, and sweeteners along with drug. This homogeneous liquid is placed in blister cavities and subjected to freeze-drying. To prevent in-homogeneity by sedimentation during this process, these formulations require a large proportion of undissolved inert filler (mannitol), to increase the viscosity of the in-process suspension. The high proportion of filler reduces the potential porosity of the dried dosage form and results in denser tablets with disintegration rates that are comparable to loosely compressed fast melt formulations.

AdvaTab technology (Eurand)

In this technology, microencapsulation process is used for coating the drug particles with gastro soluble polymer to mask the taste along with restriction of drug dissolution in mouth cavity. AdvaTab tablets disintegrate rapidly in the mouth, typically in less than 30 seconds. These tablets are especially suited to those patients that have trouble in swallowing capsules and tablets. AdvaTab is distinct from other orally disintegrating tablet technologies as it can be combined with Eurand's complimentary particle technologies like its world leading Microcaps® (taste-masking technology) and its Diffucaps® (controlled-release technology)

EFVDAS technology (Elan Corporation)

EFVDAS or Effervescent Drug Absorption System is a drug delivery technology that has been used in the development of a number of both OTC and prescription medications. This is particularly advantageous for conditions such as colds and flu, for which Elan has modified its EFVDAS technology to develop hot drink sachet products that combine medicines and vitamins for OTC use. The granular contents of the sachets can be added to boiling water to produce

pleasant-flavored solutions. In these cases the effervescence of the granulate mixture is modified to accommodate the use of heated water. Examples of products that Elan has developed include effervescent ibuprofen, cimetidine, naproxen, and acetaminophen and codeine combination product.

Time Rx Oral Controlled-Release Drug Delivery Systems

The novel oral controlled release drug delivery system TIMERx is a pre-granulated blend composed of synergistic heterodisperse polysaccharides (usually xanthan gum and locust bean gum) together with a saccharide component such as dextrose (Staniforth et al., 1993; Baichwal et al., 1991). The synergism between the homo- and hetero-polysaccharide components of the system enables formulation manipulation of different rate-controlling mechanisms and rate of drug release is controlled by the rate of water penetration into the matrix. TIMERx tablet formulations consist of drug, bulk TIMERx and lubricant, and are processed using conventional tabletting equipment (Staniforth et al., 1993; Baichwal et al., 1991). The TIMERx delivery system is compatible with a broad range of active drug substances. Whether the active is low or high dose, water-soluble or insoluble, or has a short half-life or a narrow therapeutic window, TIMERx can enhance its delivery through 1st Order, Zero Order or Burst CR delivery options, e.g. Geminex® and SyncroDose™.

RingCap technology

RingCap is a patented, oral controlled-release drug delivery system. RingCap™, a new oral controlled-release technology, incorporates several insoluble polymeric rings around a tablet. These rings control erosion of the tablet, modulating the release of drug in the GI tract. RingCap systems can deliver the total dose evenly over an extended period. Compounds suitable for are traditional small molecule therapeutics, including calcium channel blockers, ACE inhibitors, NSAIDS and vitamins. The dosage form is a capsule-shaped matrix tablet to which bands of insoluble material are applied circumferentially to the surface of the tablet. These bands modify the release of drug from RingCap through the control of surface area (Wong et al., 1996, 1997). Release of drug from RingCap is proportional to the surface area exposed to the dissolution media. The exposed surface area is controlled by the number, width, and placement of bands of insoluble material applied to the tablets (Dickason et al., 2000a, 2000b; Dalton et al., 2001). The matrix core tablet can be prepared by multiple techniques such as low- or high-shear wet granulation, fluid bed granulation, or dry blending. Capsule shaped tablets are compressed using high-speed tabletting equipment. A film coat is applied to the matrix tablets to prepare the surface for the application of bands. The banding material for RingCap tablets is selected from a group of polymers that are insoluble and impermeable. The banding formulation may contain plasticizers, colorants, or other additives depending on the specific application. Conventional capsule banding equipment is employed to apply the bands around the circumference of the matrix tablets.

TheriForm technology

TheriForm technology originated at the Massachusetts Institute of Technology (MIT), is distinguished by its ability to spatially control, with extreme precision, the placement of multiple materials into complex three-dimensional constructs (Wu et al., 1996; Cima et al., 1993). The process provides a high degree of flexibility in the design of macro- and micro-architecture, material composition, and internal and external surface textures. TheriForm is capable of high accuracy placement of liquid droplets, high accuracy metering of active dosage and the ability to construct oral dosage forms

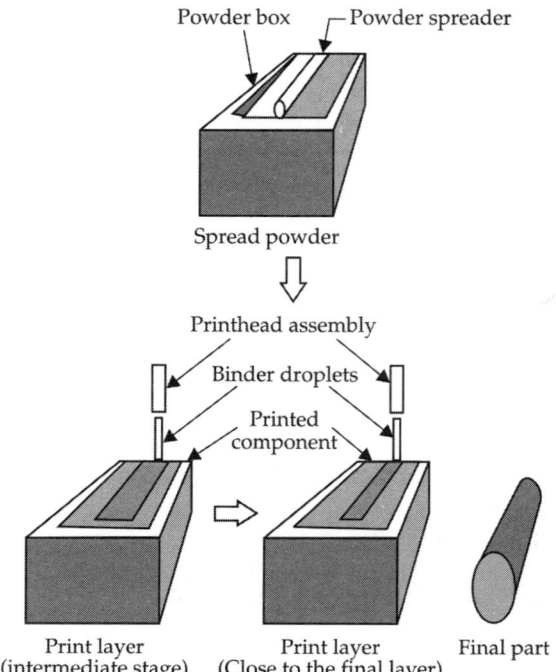

Fig. 3.21. TheriForm technology process.

with complex release profiles. TheriForm manufacture of drug delivery devices is a novel method of fabrication based on Three Dimensional Printing (3DP), a solid free form fabrication technology (Katstra et al., 2000; Rowe et al., 2000). Dosage forms are fabricated in a layer-by-layer fashion using ink-jet printing technology to allow fine spatial placement of specific substances within the body of the dosage form, thus providing control over the release of active drug from the assembled structure. TheriForm process consists of a motion-controlled print head that dispenses liquid into a thin powder layer. Each layer printed is a two-dimensional slice of the dosage form being manufactured. The powder bed is lowered after each printing pass, additional powder is spread, and the printing process is repeated with a new two-dimensional slice until the dosage form is completely built. The process allows placement of one or more active substances within selected locations inside the dosage form, along with other pharmaceutical materials that controls the release properties of these actives. These complex release profiles are generally achieved by placing the active substance within various matrices to control the release of the active (Yoo et al., 1997). TheriForm technology is applicable to Microdose, Pulsatile release, and Zero-order or release kinetics following specific pharmacokinetic/pharmacodynamic models, delivery of protein molecules such as proteins and peptides, Implantable delivery systems, Tissue repair scaffold products, Plasma rich platelet solution, Bone chips, Bone marrow, Blood and Human demineralized bone matrix (DBM) etc.

Procise™

Procise™ was originally developed in the early 90s by GlaxoSmithKline (GSK) Canada, Inc, 1991. Procise™ is a complex technology that combines the geometry of a pill with the formulation of its ingredients (DePrince, 1987), that combination will dictate the drug release profile. Various design models can be programmed into Procise™ so that the drug can be released at different times and at different rates, depending on the need. By varying the geometry of the core, the profile of drug release can be adjusted to follow zero-order, first order, or a combination of these orders, also allows delivery of two different release profiles drugs simultaneously. Procise™ system consists of a core that contains uniformly dispersed drug and has a hole in the middle. A slowly permeable inactive coat surrounds the entire surface of the core except the surface of the cylindrical face. Drug release mechanism is based on diffusion and dissolution mechanism (Theeeuwes et al., 1983). The drug release profile can be easily modulated in predicted manners simply by changing the geometric configuration of core and dose dumping is avoided (Fahie et al., 1998). Manufacturing technique includes granulation of core using conventional, dry or wet granulation technique, followed by core

compression and pre-compressed core are compression coated using a core coater

Accudep technology (Dry powder deposition)

Electrostatic powder deposition is being used to develop novel dosage forms and drug delivery systems. In this process (call Accudep), drug powder is charged and deposited onto thin, water-soluble films. The depositions are covered, sealed, and cut into Accudep Cores. These Cores are further processed into tablets, capsules, controlled release systems, or novel formulations such as Overwraps. Accudep technology is a controlled release system under development by Delsys. The system design avoids the conventional pharmaceutical processes such as mixing, blending, granulation, drying, sizing and compression. Proposed system utilizes active drug moieties as pure active ingredient, and achieves controlled release through the use of polymeric films of various release characteristics. In the Accudep process, pharmaceutical powders acting as toner are charged, and then transported to a chamber wherein dispersion and deposition take place (Chrai et al., 1998). For the purpose of controlled

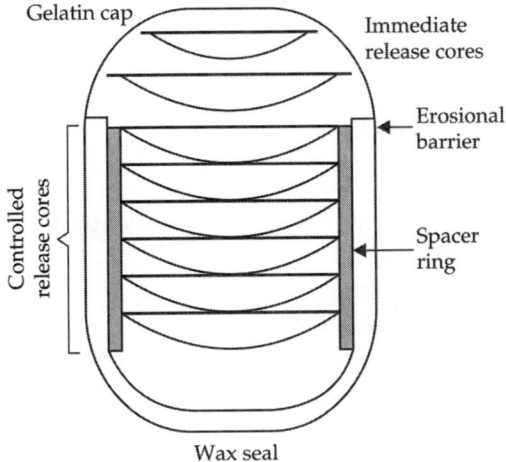

Fig. 3.22. Capsule with cores and CR discs is placed in a two-piece hard shell gelatin capsule.

release, Accudep cores, prepared using the Accudep process, are alternately placed between polymeric films acting as erosional barriers (Friend et al., 2002). Two drugs can be co-delivered from the same delivery system. This design variable permits one to engineer an immediate release component of the release profiles as well as providing an additional means for modulating the controlled-release portion of the drug (Kupperblatt et al., 2000).

NanoCrystal™ technology

Elan's proprietary NanoCrystal technology can enable formulation and improve compound activity and final product characteristics of poorly water-soluble compounds. The NanoCrystal technology can be incorporated into all dosage forms both parenteral and oral, including solid, liquid, fast-melt, pulsed release and controlled release dosage forms. NanoCrystal particles are small particles of drug substance, typically less than 1000 nanometers (nm) in diameter, which are produced by milling the drug substance using a proprietary wet milling technique. The NanoCrystal particles of the drug are stabilized against agglomeration by surface adsorption of selected GRAS (Generally Regarded As Safe) stabilizers. NanoCrystal particles of active drug substance have rapid dissolution rates, increased oral bioavailability, faster absorption of active drug substance and elimination of fed-fasted effects. The result is an aqueous dispersion of the drug substance that behaves like a solution (NanoCrystal colloidal dispersion), which can be processed into finished dosage forms for all routes of administration.

NanoCrystal technology can be incorporated in a variety of oral dosage presentations includes tablets – Immediate-release film coated, modified-release, Orally Disintegrating tablets, Capsules – Immediate-release, modified-release, Liquid dispersions and Powders.

Parenteral Administration: NanoCrystal dispersions of poorly water-soluble drugs can also provide improved performance characteristics for intravenous, subcutaneous or intramuscular dosage forms with higher dose loading, no organic solvents or pH extremes,

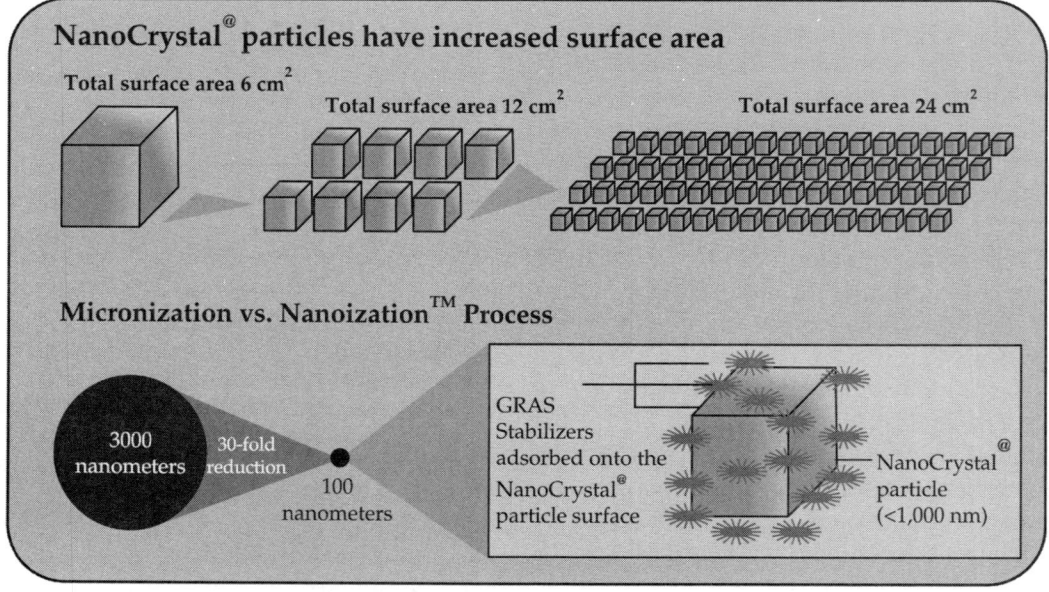

Fig. 3.23. NanoCrystal technology process.

capability for sterile filtering, Longer dose retention in blood and tumors.

Current marketed products are Rapamune® (Sirolimus) received marketing approval from the U.S. Food & Drug Administration (FDA) and Emend® (Aprepitant, MK 869) was approved by the FDA in March 2003 and launched in the United States by Merck in April 2003.

IDD formulations

A novel approach, Insoluble Drug Delivery (IDDTM) technology, is a phospholipids-based drug delivery system for water-insoluble drugs, which has successfully addressed the problems of water-insoluble drug delivery to improve drug bioavailability. Water insoluble drug pose intricate problems in their formulation and delivery with respect to poor GI absorption and bioavailability, inter- and intra-individual variation and food interaction in their absorption. Delivery approaches for an insoluble drug delivery includes traditionally micronization by air-jet milling, anew approaches includes nano-particles, microparticles, nanospheres, and hydrophobic drug carrier systems etc. However, these systems have characteristic limitations narrowing its suitability to only certain types of the drugs. The principal excipients used in IDD® formulations are biocompatible and have been previously-accepted by the US FDA.

The IDD involves formulation of micro-particles of water-insoluble drugs modified by surface modifying agents such as phospholipids with or without other surface modifiers. Size reduction of drugs particles dispersed in aqueous medium in the presence of phospholipids results in association of the latter with the newly cleaved plan of the freshly generated drug surface, which includes hydrophobic, van der Waals, dipolar, or combinations thereof. IDD particle core results in very high drug pay loads, e.g. 200mg/ml in IDD-P suspension. IDD® formulated water insoluble drugs can be used for injectable, oral, inhalation, and topical routes of administration and offer benefits namely Lower toxicity formulations; Sustained-release depot

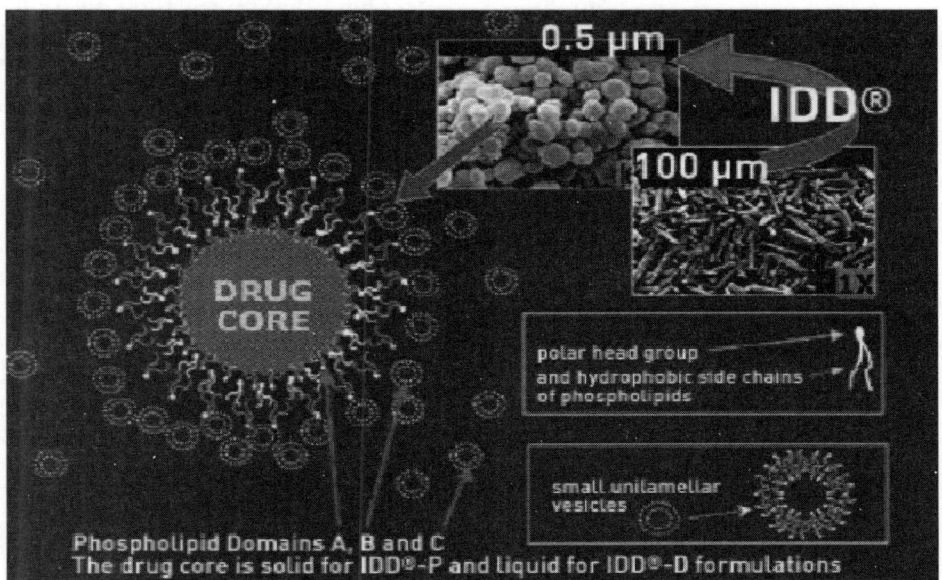

Surface modified micrometer to submicrometer sized particles form the basis of IDD® Solubilization Technologies

Fig. 3.24. IDD solubilization technology.

formulations; Improved oral bioavailability; Oral, intravenous or ophthalmic formulations of drugs that currently are available only in other dosage forms; High drug payloads and, Broad patent coverage providing extension of market exclusivity (Haynes, 1992).

IDD manufacturing technology includes (a) particle fracture processes and (b) particle nucleation processes. The particle size reduction has been achieved using M-210B Microfluidizer (Microfluidics, Newton, MA). The homogenized formulation is converted into solid form using spray drying or lyophilization technique. IDD formulations display excellent physical and chemical stability. Clinical trials of IDD CTM650 (free-flowing powder placed in hard gelatin capsule) results in two fold improvement in bioavailability as compared to micronized drug in fasting state.

Self-repairing tablets

BASF (The Chemical Company, Germany) has developed a new raw material that helps protect tablets from mechanical stress. The sustained-release film coating is called Kollicoat SR 30 D. (SR stands for "sustained release" and 30 D means it is polyvinyl acetate at 30% dispersal). Tablets coated with Kollicoat SR 30 D, if subjected to strong mechanical stresses, including a friability test (500 revolutions, 15.5 cm drop height) and 20 drops from a height of 1.5 m., did not give any noticeable effect on the release characteristics. Tests on isolated films show that Kollicoat SR 30 D has far greater elasticity than ethyl cellulose or ammonium methacrylate copolymer. In addition, the release rate can be adjusted by using water-soluble polymers and by varying the coating thickness. E.g. Kollicoat® contains Polyvinyl acetate stabilized with polyvinylpyrrolidone and sodium lauryl sulfate by BASF AG Chemical Company.

Effervescent tablets

Effervescents are not new, having been used in OTC products for years. A majority of effervescents today are used in neutraceuticals but that could change in the coming years. Effervescent tablet's major advantage is that the drug product is already in solution at the time that it is consumed. This way absorption is a lot faster and more complete than with a conventional tablet (Wehling et al., 1993). Effervescent tablets offer an alternative to standard tablets that some patients may find difficult to swallow and can have a buffering effect against pH changes in the GI tract, improve tolerance after ingestion and improve palatability. But effervescents have been ignored because they do not always dissolve into a clear solution, a factor that has made them less popular with consumers. A combination of glycine carbonate and glycine citrate, and a combination of L-lysine carbonate and glycine citrate can be used in sodium-restricted formulations. Glycine plays an important role in dissolution and absorption; because it is neutral and amphoteric, it is an efficient buffer in both acidic and basic pH ranges. E.g. Redoxon Double Action Vitamin C + Zinc Effervescent 1000 mg Tablets, Roche Consumer Health UK.ACC™ 200 effervescent tablets, HexalPharma (SA) (PTY) Ltd., Westmead.

DissoCubes

DissoCubes is a novel formulation for poorly soluble and poorly bioavailable drugs (Muller et al., 1999, Rasenack et al., 2002).DissoCubes combine the advantages of using a size reduction technique with the advantages of a precipitation technique opening the opportunity to induce structural changes, which means increasing the amorphous fraction. DissoCubes technology basically means production of a suspension of drug nanoparticles (nano-suspension) by high-pressure homogenization. The powdered drug is dispersed in a aqueous surfactant or polymer solution to yield a traditional macro-suspension. The dispersion is performed by high-speed stirring. This pre-suspension is then high-pressure-homogenized using pressures between 500-1500 bars. The increase in the dissolution velocity due to increased surface area, and increased adhesiveness of fine particles help improve the bioavailability of drugs. The structural changes depend very much on the means of production (e.g. the introduction of high energy to increase the amorphous fraction as performed by high-pressure homogenization).

Bilayer tablets

Interest in developing a combination of two or more active pharmaceutical ingredients in a single dosage form has increased in pharmaceutical industry. Bilayer tablet is suitable for sequential release of two drugs in combination,

separate two incompatible substances and also for sustained release dosage form, wherein one layer is immediate release as initial dose and second layer is maintenance dose. So, use of bilayer tablets is important in delivery of anti-hypertensive, diabetic, anti-inflammatory and analgesic drugs where combination therapy is often used.

A. OROS push-pull technology

ALZA Corporation pioneered the solid tablet osmotic dosage form (Oros system) in the 1970s (Theeuwes et al., 1975; Wong et al., 1986). The basic Oros system is the elementary osmotic pump (EOP), which consists of a drug-containing core, a semi-permeable membrane

Technology	Marketed product	Patented by	References
OraSolv/DuraSolv	Tempra* Firs, Tabs, RemeronSoltab, NuLev, Zomig ZMT	Habib et al.	Habib et al., 2000
Zydis	Temesta, Seresta, Imodium, Motilium	Danckwerts et al.	Danckwerts et al., 2003
TIMERx	Geminex®, SyncroDose™	Staniforth et al.	Staniforth et al., 1993 Baichwal et al., 1991
RingCap Technology	Acetaminophen RingCap tablets	Wong et al.	Wong et al., 1996
TheriForm Technology	TheriFil EXT, TheriLink	Cima et al.	Cima et al., 1993
Procise™	PROCISE™	GlaxoSmithKline (GSK), Canada Inc.	GlaxoSmithKline (GSK), Canada Inc., 1991
Accudep Technology	Accudep technology	—	—
Osmotically controlled tablets	Alpress LP, Cardura Xl, Covera–HS, Glucotrol	ALZA Corporation	ALZA Corporation
NanoCrystal™ Technology	—	Elan's proprietary	http://www.elan.com/DrugDelivery
IDD Formulations	IDD-PTM, IDD-TM, IDD-TM, Glucotrol	Pace et al.	Pace et al., 1999
Self-Repairing Tablets	Kollicoat®	BASF A Chemical Company	www.pharmasolutions.basf.com
Effervescent Tablets	Redoxon Double Action Vitamin C + Zinc Effervescent 1000 mg Tablets, ACC™ 200 effervescent tablets	Roche Consumer Health, UK HexalPharma (SA) (PTY) Ltd., Westmead	Roche Consumer Health, UK HexalPharma (SA) (PTY) Ltd., Westmead
DissoCubes	DissoCubes	Muller et al.	Muller et al., 1999

made of water-permeable cellulose polymers, and orifices for drug release. Water is drawn into the system by osmosis, displacing drug in the core, which is then released through the orifices. The Oros Push-Pull system resembles a simple tablet in shape and has two layers. The first layer contains the drug substance, osmotically active hydrophilic polymers, and other excipients (Shan-Yang Lin et al., 2002). The second layer, or push layer, contains a hydrophilic expansion polymer and other osmotically active agents and tablet excipients (Rani et al., 2003). The basic Oros EOP and push-pull designs, which allow zero-order delivery of drugs, can be modified to provide patterned release (e.g. pulsed, ascending, delayed release).

B. DUREDAS™ Technology

This system was developed by Elan drug technologies. DUREDAS™ Technology is a bilayer tablet, which can provide immediate or sustained release of two drugs or different release rates of the same drug in one dosage form. The tabletting process can provide an immediate release granulates and a modified release hydrophilic matrix complex as separate layers within the one tablet. The modified-release properties of the dosage form are provided by a combination of hydrophilic polymers (Rathbone et al., 2002).

Pulsatile drug delivery

Pulsatile systems are basically time controlled drug delivery systems in which the system controls the lag time independent of environmental factors like pH, enzymes and gastric motility. Some of the technologies which have been developed are ACCU-BREAK Technology, SODAS Technology, IPDAS Technology, CODAS Technology, GEOCLOCK Technology, PULSYS Technology, OSDrC Technology, Intelli Matrix Technology, Eurand's pulsatile and chrono release system and Versetrol Technology (Anantha Nayaki Ravula et. al., 2011).

PROCESS ANALYTICAL TECHNOLOGY

Improving excipients and other ingredients can make drug delivery much more effective at lower costs, but those benefits can be mitigated when quality control problems arise during manufacturing. That's where process analytical technology (PAT) plays a role. With PAT, state-of-the-art technology using laser and infrared sensors provide real-time information on active ingredients, inactive ingredients and the distribution of moisture in a product. A desired goal of the PAT framework is to design and develop processes that can consistently ensure a predefined quality at the end of the manufacturing process. Such procedures would be consistent with the basic tenet of 'quality by design' and could reduce risks to quality and regulatory concerns while improving efficiency.

Technologies demonstrate how recent advances in formulation development and processing tablet technologies are evolving to meet efforts to achieve more therapeutically effective as a dosage form. An enhanced stability profile is expected to result in the presence of fewer and improved excipients, thereby minimizing incompatibility and analytical issues. The ability of the technology to adjust dose levels provides a multidose capability for rapid clinical and toxicological evaluation of the product. The self-contained and controlled work area enables improved environmental controls and containment of hazardous materials. The technique provides capability to perform 100% on-line inspection, leading to enhanced quality control. The new technologies may potentially be attractive, because they are more **amenable** to **scale-up**, validation and the **PAT-driven** shift to non-parametric release.

Newer technologies may involve modifying formulation composition and processing to achieve new performance end-points (fast-melt technologies) or the merger of new technological advances (three-dimensional printing and electrostatic powder deposition) with traditional pharmaceutical processing techniques for the production of new and novel tablets. The future of drug delivery might well see, for example, microchips in tablets of medicines lodged in specific parts of the body programmed to release treatments at various times. It is reasonable to expect that future trends in drug delivery system innovation will continue to bring together different technological disciplines to create novel technologies.

REFERENCES

- Amborn, J., Tiger, V. (2001). Apparatus for handling and packaging friable tablets. **US Patent 6,269,615**.
- Amborn, J., Tiger, V. (2001). Apparatus for handling and packaging friable tablets. **US Patent 6,311,462**.
- Amidon, G.L., Lennernas, H., Shah, V.P., Crison, J.R. (1995). A theoretical basis for a bio-pharmaceutic drug classification: The correlation of *in vitro* drug product dissolution and *in vivo* bioavailability. *Pharm. Res.*, 12, 413–420.
- Anantha Nayaki Ravula, Bairi Agaiah Goud (2011). A review on recent advances in oral pulsatile drug delivery. *J. Adv. Pharm. Sci.*, 1(1), 132–145.
- Aulton, M.E. (2000). **Pharmaceutics: The Science of Dosage Form Design**. Churchill Livingstone, UK, 304–321; 616–677.
- Baichwal, A.R., Staniforth, J.N. (1991). Directly compressible sustained release excipient. **US Patent 4,994,276**.
- Chaudhary, P.D., Pathak, A.A., Desai, U. (2012). A review: Co-processed excipients – An alternative to novel chemical entities. *Int. J. Pharm. Chem. Sci.*, 1(4), 1480–1498.
- Chrai, S.S., Singh, B., Kopcha, M., Murari, R., Sun, S., Kumar, N., Desai, N., Levine, A., Rivenburg, H., Kaganowick, G. (1998). Electrostatic dry deposition technology. *Pharm. Tech.*, 4, 17–20.
- Cima, M.J., Haggerty, J.S., Sachs, E.M., Williams P.A. (1993). Three-dimensional printing techniques. **US Patent 5,204,205**.
- Dalton, J.T., Straughn, A.B., Dickason, D.A., Grandolfi, G.P. (2001). Predictive ability of level A *in vitro–in vivo* correlation for RingCap controlled-release acetaminophen tablets. *Pharma. Res.*, 18(12), 1729–1734.
- Danckwerts, M.P. (2003). Intraoral drug delivery: A comparative review. *Am. J. Drug Del.*, 1(3), 171–186.
- DePrince, R.B. (1987). Disc like sustained release formulation. **US Patent 4,663,147**.
- Dickason, D., Grandolfi, G., Leenellett, M. (2000). An *in vitro* study of the effect of band configuration on the release profile of RingCap tablets. *Int. Symp. Control. Rel. Bioact. Mater.*, 2000; 27: 435–436.
- Dickason, D., Grandolfi, G., Rotty, E., Leenellett, M., Dalton, J. (2000). An *in vitro– in vivo* correlation from a RingCap human pharmaco-kinetic study. *Int. Symp. Control. Rel. Bioact. Mater.*, 27, 439–440.
- Fahie, B.J., Nangia, A., Chopra, S.K., Fyfe, C.A., Grondey, H., Blazek, A. (1998). Use of NMR imaging in the optimization of a compression coated regulated release system. *J. Contr. Rel.*, 51, 179–184.
- Fraade, D.J. (2002). **Automation of Pharmaceutical Operations**. Pharmaceutical Technology Publications, Springfield, Oregon.
- Friend, D.R. (2002). Oral drug delivery: A new approach to dosage forms. *Pharma. News*, 9, 375–380.
- Gennaro, A.R. (2000). **Remington: The Science and Practice of Pharmacy**, 20th ed., Lippincott Williams and Wilkins: Baltimore, 858–902.
- Gordon Bardley (2012). Surface active proteins as excipients in solid pharmaceutical formulations. **US Patent US8226967 B2**.
- Gorgegoan (2006). Fiber rich fraction of trigonella-foenum-graceum seeds and its use as a pharma-ceutical excipient. **US Patent EP1697050A2**.
- Habib, W., Khankari, R., Hontz, J. (2000). Fast dissolving drug delivery systems. *Crit. Rev. Ther. Drug Carr. Syst.* 17, 61–72.
- Haynes, D.H. (1992). Phospholipid coated microcrystal injectable formulations of water insoluble drugs. **US Patents 5,091,187 and 5,091,188**.
- http://www.cardinal.com/pts/content/delivery/dd-oral-zydis.asp (downloaded: 9/1/04)
- http://www.elan.com/DrugDelivery/drug_delivery/nanocrystal_technology.asp (down-loaded: 22/7/04)

- http://www.emea.eu.int/Inspections/PAThome.html (downloaded: 25/4/04)
- Iles, M.C., Atherton, A.D., Copping, N.M. (1993). Freeze-dried dosage forms and methods for preparing the same. **US Patent 5,188,825**.
- Joan CucalaEscoi (2005). Modified calcium phosphate excipient. **US Patent 20050031862 A1**.
- Joshi, A., Duriez X. (2004). Added functionality excipients: An answer to challenging formulations. Pharmaceutical Technology. *Excipients and Solid Dosage Forms*, Jan 1, 12–19.
- Katstra, W.E., Palazolo, R.D., Rowe, C.W., Giritlioglu, B., Teung, P., Cima, M.J. (2000). Oral dosage form fabricated by three dimensional printing. *J. Contr. Rel.*, 66, 1–9.
- Katzner, L.D., Jones, B., Khattar, J., Kosewick J. (2000). Blister package and packaging tablets. **US Patent 6,155,423**.
- Khankari, R.K., Hontz, J., Chastain, S.J., Katzner, L. (2000). Rapidly dissolving robust dosage form. **US Patent 6,024,981**.
- Khankari, R.K., Hontz, J., Chastain, S.J., Katzner, L. (2000). Rapidly dissolving robust dosage form. **US Patent 6,221,392**.
- Kupperblatt, G., Katdare, A., Slack, G., Chen, J.C., Karetny, M., Chrai, S. (2000). Oral delivery using a novel controlled release technology: System design and material selection. *Proc. Int. Symp. Control. Rel. Bioact. Mater.*, 27, 1226–1227.
- Lieberman, H., Lachman, L. (1982). **Pharmaceutical Dosage Forms: Tablets**. Marcel Dekker, New York, 3, 1–69.
- Luo Y, Zhu J, Ma Y, Zhang H. (2008). Dry coating, a novel coating technology for solid pharmaceutical dosage forms. *Int. J. Pharm.* 358(1–2), 16–22.
- McGee, P. (2004). Tablet technology: Sophisticated excipients, fast-dissolve technology and self-repairing coatings are new developments transforming tablet technology. *Pharmaceutical Formulation and Quality*.
- Muller, R.H., Grau, M.J. Increase of dissolution rate and solubility of poorly water soluble drugs as nanosuspension. Proceedings. (1998). *World Meeting APGI/APV*, Paris; 2: 62–624.
- Myers, G.L., Battist, G.E., Fuisz, R.C. (1999). Process and apparatus for making rapidly dissolving dosage units and products therefrom. **US Patent 5,866,163**.
- Nachaegari, S.K., Bansal, A.K. (2004). Co-processed excipients for solid dosage forms. *Pharma. Tech.*, 28(1), 52–64.
- Padsalgi, A., Bidkar, S., Jadhav, V., Sheladity, D. (2008). Sustained release tablet of theophylline by hot melt wax coating technology. *Asian J. Pharm.*, 2(3), 26–29.
- Ramlakhan, M., Wu, C.Y., Watano, S., Dave, R.N., Pfeffer, R. (2000). Dry particle coating using magnetically assisted impaction coating: Modification of surface properties and optimization of system and operating parameters. *Powder Tech.*, 112(1), 137–148.
- Rani, M., Surana, R., Mishra, C.B. (2003). Development and biopharmaceutical evaluation of osmotic pump tablets for controlled delivery of diclofenac sodium. *Acta Pharm.*, 53, 263–273.
- Rasenack, N., Müller, B.W. (2002). Dissolution rate enhancement by *in situ* micronization of poorly water-soluble drugs. *Pharm. Res.*, 19(12), 1894–1900.
- Rathbone, M.J., Hadgraft, J., Roberts, M.S. (2002). **Modified-Release Drug Delivery Technology**. Marcel Dekker, New York, 11–215.
- Ribeiro Dos Santos I., et al. (2002). Micro-encapsulation of protein particles within lipids using a novel supercritical fluid process. *Int. J. Pharm.*, 242, 69–78.
- Romain Callaird (2011). Modified protein excipient for delayed-release tablet. **US Patent 0076326**.
- Rowe, C.W., Katstra, W.E., Palazolo, R.D., Giritlioglu, B., Teung, P., Cima, M.J. (2000). Multimechanism oral dosage forms fabricated by three dimensional painting. *J. Contr. Rel.*, 66, 11–17.
- Seager, H. (1998). Drug-delivery products and the Zydis fast-dissolving dosage form. *J. Pharm. Pharmacol.*, 50(4), 375–82.
- Self-repairing tablet: http://www.pharmaquality.com/Feature5.htm (downloaded: 30/3/04)
- Singh P., Solanky T., Mudryy R., Pfeffer R., Dave, R. (2001). Estimation of coating time in the magnetically assisted impaction coating process. *Powder Technology*, 121(2), 159–167.
- Shan-Yang, L., Kung-Hsu, L., Mei-Jane, L. (2002). Influence of excipients, drugs, and osmotic agent in the inner core on the time-controlled disintegration of compression coated ethyl cellulose tablets. *J. Pharm. Sci.*, 91(9), 2040–2046.

- Shayne, C.G. (2008). **Pharmaceutical Manufacturing Handbook: Production and Processes**. Wiley-Interscience Publication, USA.
- Staniforth, J.N., Baichwal, A.R. (1993). Synergistically interacting heterodisperse polysaccharides: Function in achieving controlled drug delivery. *In:* M.A. El-Nokaly, D.M. Piatt, B.A. Charpententier (1993) eds. **Polymeric Drug Delivery System: Properties and Applications**. ACS, 327–350.
- Staniforth, J.N., Baichwal, A.R. (1993). Synergistically Interacting Heterodisperse Polysaccharides: Function in Achieving Controllable Drug Delivery. **Polymer Delivery Systems**, ACS Symposium Series, USA, American Chemical Society, 327–350.
- Staniforth, J.N., Baichwal, A.R. (1993). Synergistically Interacting Heterodisperse Polysaccharides: Function in Achieving Controlled Drug Delivery. American Chemical Society, 327–350.
- Stephen, M., Borowitz, A. (1996). Guide to Pharmaceutical Excipients. *Pharmacotherapy*, 2(9), 1–5.
- Swarbrick, J. (2007). **Encyclopedia of Pharmaceutical Technology**, 3rd ed, Informa Healthcare Inc., USA.
- Theeuwes, F., Swanson, D., Wong, P., Bonson, P., Place, V., Hiemlich, K., Kwan, K.C. (1983). Elementary Osmotic Pump for Indomethacin. *J. Pharm. Sci.*, 72, 253.
- Thies C, Ribeiro I, et al. (2003). A supercritical fluid-based coating technology 1: Process considerations. *J. Microencapsul.*, 20(1), 87–96.
- Vincent Green (2006). Tablet Excipient. **US Patent 0008521 A1**.
- Wehling, F., Schuele, S., Madamala, N. (1993). Effervescent Dosage Form with Microparticles. **US Patent 5,178,878**.
- Wong, P.S.L., Edgren, D.E., Dong, L.C., Ferrari, V.J. (1996). Active Agent Dosage Form Comprising a Matrix and at least Two Insoluble Bands. **US Patent 5,534,263**.
- Wong, P.S.L., Edgren, D.E., Dong, L.C., Ferrari, V.J. (1997). Banded Prolonged Release Active Agent Dosage Form. **US Patent 5,667,804**.
- Wu, B.M., Borland, S.W., Giordano, R.A., Cima, L.G., Sachs, E.M., Cima, M.J. (1996). Solid freeform fabrication of drug delivery devices. *J. Control. Rel.*, 40, 77–87.
- www.gsk.ca/en/careers/student/q104_ innovation_ excellence.php (downloaded: 21/3/04)
- Yarwood, R.J., Kearney, P., Thompson, A.R. (1998). Process for Preparing Solid Pharmaceuticals Dosage Form. **US Patent 5,837,287**.
- Yoo, J., Bornancini, E., Yang, A., Shanahan, G., Monkhouse, D. (1997). Content uniformity study of microdose tablets fabricated by the Theriform process. *Annual Meeting of the American Association of Pharmaceutical Scientist*, Boston.

4

Capsules

Sonia Trehan

Rapidly budding nutraceutical and pharma-ceutical companies, rising demand of alternative capsules like hydroxypropyl methylcellulose/non-gelatin or non-animal origin and increase in therapeutic applications of capsules are driving the global empty capsule market. The word 'capsule' is derived from the Latin word 'capsula', which means a small box or container. In pharmacy, capsule is used to describe an edible package made from gelatin or other suitable material, which is filled with medicines to produce a unit dosage, mainly for oral use. There are many forms of capsules and they can be divided into main two categories which in current usage are described as 'hard' and 'soft'; better adjectives would be 'two-piece' instead of hard, and 'one-piece' instead of soft. The hard capsule consists of two pieces, each a semi-closed cylinder in shape, one part being called the 'cap' (shorter piece), fits over the open end of the longer piece, called the 'body'. The soft gelatin capsule is a one-piece container, which has a variable shape, may be seamed or seamless.

HISTORY OF GELATIN CAPSULE

In nineteenth century the gelatin capsule was invented. The first recorded patent for a gelatin capsule was French Patent 5648, granted in Paris on 25th March 1834 to Dublanc and Mothes, which covered a method for producing single-piece, olive-shaped, gelatin capsules, which were closed after filling by a drop of concentrated warm gelatin solution. The actual inventor of the gelatin capsule was Mothes. It was stated that Mothes was a pharmacy student, and so was under the legal age to obtain his pharmacy diploma; in order to present the patent he became associated with Dublanc, who was already an established pharmacist [Ridgway, 1987].

In USA, the first mention of capsules in the pharmaceutical literature was in 1835 in the American Journal of Pharmacy, which published an abstract of the paper by Cottereau [Anon, 1835-6]. The first American capsule business was started in New York in 1836 by H. Planten, a Dutchman who had emigrated there in 1835 [Alpers, 1896]. He was described as using French manufacturing methods, selling his capsules as 'Mothes' capsules. In German-speaking states the invention appears to have been first reported by Buchner [Schlenz, C., 1897]. He described Mothes' capsules as copaiba balsam covered in a bubble of glue.

One successful way of overcoming Mothes' patent resulted in the production of a new type of capsule, the hard two-piece, invented by Parisian pharmacist, J.C. Lehuby, who was granted a patent on 20th October 1846 [French patent 4435]. Although, Lehuby was the undoubted inventor of the two-piece capsule, many have credited it to J. Murdoch, who was granted British Patent 11937 in London on May 2nd 1848. The first recorded large scale manufacture of hard two-piece capsule was by an American company, H. Planten of New York, but were discontinued due to their poor fit.

The first successful manufacturer of hard gelatin capsules on a commercial scale was a Detroit pharmacist, F.A. Hubel [Wilkie, 1913]. The capsule quickly achieved popularity, particularly after 1875, when the whole of Hubel's output was sold for him by another Detroit company, Parke Davis [Stadler, 1959]. In 1910, the estimated world production was over one thousand million capsules per year, of which 90% were made in U.S.A. The two factors, which have contributed most to the vast increase in capsule output are air-conditioning and machinery design.

In 1913, the first fully automatic machine for making hard gelatin capsules, designed by B.W. Scott, of the Arthur Colton Co. of Detroit, for Eli Lilly & Co eliminated the manual procedure. The design on which nearly all modern large-scale machines are based was patented by Arthur Colton and assigned to Parke Davis Co. [U.S. Patent 1787777 and British Patent 360427]. Augmented demand for innovative drug delivery formulations and increased daily intake of dietary supplements have a positive impact on capsule market. Current market of $1300 billion in 2014 has been expected to grow at CAGR of 7% by 2019 [*http://www.marketsandmarkets. com/Market-Reports/empty-capsules-market-218018190.html*]. After the introduction of first non-animal HPMC capsule, more than a decade ago, vegetarian capsules are achieving big share in the hard capsule market. Unique features of these capsules offer lots of benefits in global marketing and certification as well as in novel drug delivery.

HARD GELATIN CAPSULES

Capsules are made principally of gelatin and may contain small amounts of certified dyes, opaquing agents, plasticizers, preservatives and water. Denatured gelatins have been used to produce a shell with low moisture content [Ogura, 1998].

Advantages

Manufacturing advantages

1. Simpler manufacturing process
2. Fewer production steps as compared to tablets
3. Fewer analytical tests
4. Less manufacturing equipment
5. Fewer validation requirements
6. Reduced risk of mix-up.

(http://www.capsugel.com/pdf/brochure_conisnap.pdf)

Formulation advantages

1. Granules, powders, semi-solids, and minitablets can be easily filled alone or in combination.
2. Ideal for controlled release in particular pellets
3. Requires fewer excipients
4. Reduces stability problems with sensitive drugs
5. Easy to differentiate
6. Ideal container for traditional medicines

Consumer advantages

1. Unique color and shape configurations enhance product identity
2. Easy to swallow
3. Masks tastes and odors
4. Improves patient compliance
5. Promotes image of efficacy

Gelatin

Gelatin is a major component of capsule, which is a heterogeneous product derived by irreversible hydrolytic extraction of treated animal collagen. Gelatin has all the properties required to meet the needs of capsule, which include non-toxicity, solubility, and viscosity enabling it to produce strong flexible film, thermally reversible gelation properties in water. The origin of gelatin manufacture can be traced back as far as 4000 B.C.

There are two main types of gelatin: Type A, which is produced by acid hydrolysis, and Type B, which is produced by basic hydrolysis. The acid process takes about 7–10 days and is used mainly for animal skins and basic process takes about 10 times as long and is used mainly for bovine bones. The bones must be washed with acid for few days to give soft sponge like material, called ossein, which is then soaked in lime pits for few weeks, lime is removed, pH adjustment is done and gelatin is extracted from treated material using hot water. Gelatin solution is concentrated and chilled to form gel, air dried and milled to desired size. The properties of the gelatin that are most important to the capsule manufacturers are bloom strength and the viscosity. Bloom strength is a measure of gel rigidity and is determined by preparing a standard gel (6.66% w/v) and maturing it at 10°C. It is defined as the load in grams required for pushing a standard plunger 4mm into gel. The gelatin used in hard capsule manufacturing is of higher bloom strength (200–250 g) [Jones, 2007].

Gelatin additives

The materials which are used in gelatin shell can be classified into main four categories: colouring agents, plasticizers, process and performance aids, and preservatives.

Colouring agents

Colouring agents are added in products for aesthetic effects, ease of identification, psychological effect on patient and light protection. The colouring agents mainly used for colouring capsules are synthetic water-soluble dyes (azo, indigoid, quinophthalone, triphenylmethane and xanthene), pigments (especially titanium dioxide) and certain dyes of natural origin (carotenoids and flavones) [FAO/WHO, 1984].

Plasticizers

Hard capsules have been defined as having less than 5% by weight of plasticizer present. The function of the plasticizer in the capsule wall is to reduce the rigidity of the gelatin and make it pliable. Examples include glycerol, sorbitol, propylene glycol, sucrose and acacia. Materials, which enhance the effect of main plasticizer when added in concentrations of 2–6% include mannitol, glycine, acetamide, formamide and lactamide.

Process and performance aids

Types of process aids are: surfactants, which enable the gelatin solution to take up the shape of the moulds better, and substances which enable the capsules to be further processed, e.g. a silicone fluid which allows formaldehyde treatment to produce an enteric product more readily. Performance aids are materials to improve the patient acceptability of the product, such as flavoring agents.

Preservatives

The simplest way to control the microbial content of capsules is to use a preservative, which is usually added during the processing of the gelatin solution. Sulphur dioxide has been most widely used. Several esters of *p*-hydroxybenzoic acid have been used as preservatives. The most commonly used combination is methyl paraben and propyl paraben. Most preservatives are used at concentrations upto 1% w/w.

Manufacture of hard gelatin capsules

The process for the manufacture of hard gelatin capsules in use today is essentially the same as that proposed by Lehuby in his original patent in 1846, but it has been refined and automated by successive generations. Two companies, which have done most of the pioneering work in this field, have been making capsules for 100 years: Shionogi (formerly Eli Lilly) and Warner Lambert's Capsugel (formerly Parke Davis).

Gelatin solution

A concentrated solution of gelatin 35–40% is prepared by dissolving gelatin in hot demineralized water in jacketed stainless steel tanks and the solution is stirred until the gelatin is dissolved and then vacuum is applied to remove any entrapped air bubbles. Other additives are added and viscosity is adjusted to target value. The viscosity adjustment is important as it governs the thickness of the capsule shells.

Capsule formation

The manufacturing machines consist of two parts, which are mirror images of each other; on one half the capsule cap is made and on the other capsule body. The moulds on which capsules are formed are called pins mounted in sets on metal strips, called pin bars. The gelatin solution is placed in the machine in a jacketed stirred container, which is called a dip pan or dip pot, and its level is kept constant automatically by a feed from the holding hopper. Capsules are formed by dipping set of moulds, which are at room temperature, into this solution. A film is formed on the surface of each mould by gelling. To spread the gelatin evenly over the surface of the mould pins, the pin bars are rotated about a horizontal axis as they are transferred from the lower level to the higher level of the machine.

Drying

Groups of 'pin bars' are passed through a series of drying kilns, in which large volumes of controlled humidity air are blown over the pins to dry the film. A balance has to be struck between drying the film until it is strong enough to handle, and over drying with consequent brittleness.

Capsule removal and sorting

Dried films are removed from the moulds, cut to the correct length, the two parts joined together and the complete capsule delivered from the machine. The mould pins are then cleaned and lubricated for the start of the next cycle.

Capsules are now made to pass through a series of sorting and checking processes, which can be manual, mechanical or electronic to remove as many defective ones as possible. The faults, which are generally looked upon are defects caused by poor initial formation of the capsule film, poorly cut edges, splits or holes caused by the stripper jaws.

Capsule printing

Capsules are printed with variety of information such as product name, product strength, company name, logo or symbol. This allows rapid identification of the contents of the capsule. The process, which is used most often is an "offset" method using an edible pharmaceutical grade ink.

Capsule filling

Hard gelatin capsules are available in a variety of sizes and are designated by numbers from 000 to 5. Numbers 0 or 00 to 5 are normally used for human medicines (Table 4.1 shows different fill volumes in different capsule sizes). The simplest way to estimate the fill weight for powder is to multiply the body volume by its tapped bulk density. For liquids, the fill weight is calculated by multiplying the specific gravity of the liquid by the capsule body volume $\times$ 0.8 [Jones, 1998]. Alternately, it is important to determine the size of the capsule to be used for particular formulation. We need to know the tapped density for powder formulations and bulk density value for pellets and granules and then look for the right capsule size in the capacity chart from capsule supplier. Table 4.1 shows the information compiled from the capsule capacity chart from Capsugel®.

To accommodate special needs some intermediate sizes are produced, termed as 'elongated' (e.g. 0el, 1el, 2el) that are typically having 10% extra of fill volume over standard sizes.

Capsule size	Capsule volume (mL)	Capsule capacity (mg)			
		Powder tapped density (g/mL)			
		0.6	0.8	1.0	1.2
000	1.37	822	1096	1370	1644
00el	1.02	612	816	1020	1224
00	0.91	546	728	910	1092
0el	0.78	468	624	780	936
0	0.68	408	544	680	816
1el	0.54	324	432	540	648
1	0.50	300	400	500	600
2el	0.41	246	308	410	492
2	0.37	222	296	370	444
3	0.30	180	240	300	360
4	0.21	126	168	210	252
5	0.13	78	104	130	156

Table 4.1. Capsule size and fill capacity

Types of material that can be filled in hard gelatin capsule include powders, pellets, granules, tablets, thermo-softening mixtures, thixotropic mixtures, pastes and non-aqueous liquids. Materials that react with gelatin, or contain high level of moisture should be avoided in hard gelatin capsule.

Filling of powder formulations in hard capsules

Plate method

It is the traditional method used for filling hard capsules. A development of the plate method is the use of a hopper fitted with an agitator and an auger. The agitator is used to feed material into the auger, which, in turn, feeds into the capsule body. Hofliger and Karg produced a machine using this type of feed system, which filled at the rate of 3000 capsules per hour. Powder initially flows into the holes in a dosage disk, which is machined to thickness to provide a certain fill-weight in the capsule. A tamping punch compresses the powder against the base plate and then rises. Filling and retamping takes place in five successive stages. After the fifth stage the dosage hole moves off the base plate and the plug of powder is ejected into the capsule body.

Intermittent compression filling

It was used by Zanasi and later introduced by mG2. Powder is fed into the dosage hopper and its level adjusted to about twice the depth of the compressed plug. The dosage tube enters the powder bed and the powder inside it is pressed by the dosage punch just sufficiently to form a coherent plug that can be lifted by the dosator, carried to the capsule body, and ejected into it by the piston.

Continuous compression filling

This was first developed by the mG2 company. The dosage trough here is annular, rotates and is fed from a bulk hopper. The dosators dip into it whilst it is in motion. As the speed of filling increases, the dwell time becomes shorter.

Vacuum filling

Perry Industries developed this concept of using vacuum to dose vials with volumetric quantities of powders. Powder is drawn into the dosator by suction, applied through a filter pad. The machine is continuous in operation and similar in action to the mG2 models. The material is held in place by the vacuum until the dosage tube is in position over the capsule body, when the powder is ejected by releasing the vacuum and applying the positive pressure [Ridgway, 1987].

Filling of pellet formulations in hard capsules

Pellets are filled using modified machinery having a dosing system based on chamber with a volume that can be easily changed. Pellets are not compressed in the process and may have to be held inside the measuring devices by mechanical means i.e. either by inverting the dosator or by applying suction to the dosing tube. In general, when evaluating a pellet-filling device the most important points to consider are dosage accuracy, the extent to which pellets are damaged at various filling rates, the degree of segregation if a mixture is used, the effect of batch variations in pellets on attainable filling speeds, the type of flow from the storage hopper, the effect of ambient conditions on the filling characteristics, and the filling speeds at which partial fills start to occur.

Filling of tablets in hard capsules

The reasons for the use of pellets also apply to the use of tablets. Tablets for capsule filling are normally film coated to prevent dust, and are sized so that they can fall freely into the capsule body. Tablets are placed in hoppers and allowed to fall down tubes, at the bottom of which is a gate device that will allow a set number of tablets to pass. Mechanical probe detects the exact number of tablets inserted in capsule.

Filling of semisolids and liquids

Dosing of liquids is done by volumetric pumps. Leakage needs to be stopped from filled capsule. For non-aqueous liquids it is done by sealing by applying gelatin band around the centre of capsule, which forms a hermetic seal. There are many formulations, which exhibit thixotropic behavior, i.e. while filling they are heated to form a liquid and later on, on cooling they solidify to form a solid plug.

Capsule filling machinery

Capsule filling machinery can be categorized into hand-operated, semi-automatic and automated. Some of the most widely used machines were manufactured by Whitfield [US Patent 210589, 1878], Davenport [US Patent 221534, 1879], Reymond [US Patent 244308, 1881], Schmidt [US Patent 255680, 1882] and Ihrig [US Patent 596813, 1898]. The machine invented by Walsh in 1886 was subsequently marketed by Parke Davis.

Hand-operated machines

Hand-operated machines at the end of nineteenth century include Davenport capsule filler, which filled only one capsule at a time; Reymond capsule filler and Walsh capsule filler, which filled 12 capsules at a time; and Ihrig capsule filler which filled 48 or 56 capsules at a time. The advanced versions of hand operated machines include Feton machine (Fig. 4.1) which can fill up to 100 capsules at a time, ChemiPharm capsule fillers which has an output of 1000 capsules per hour, and Tevopharm machine having an output of 3000 capsules per hour.

Semiautomatic machines

Semiautomatic machines include Pedini Model having an output of 2000 capsules per hour, LAF multifill machine claiming an output of 5000 capsules per hour, Colton machine having an output up to 20000 capsules per hour.

STI model 10 ver 4.2 capsule filling machine

The STI model 10 ver 4.2 by Schaefer Technologies, Inc. is a semi-automatic capsule filling machine for powder and pellets with capacity of 18000 to 25000 capsules per hour for sizes 000 through 5. It has horizontal,

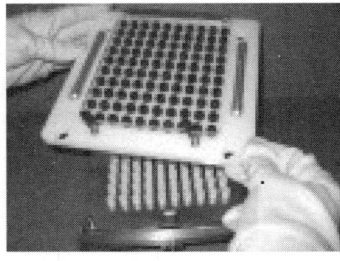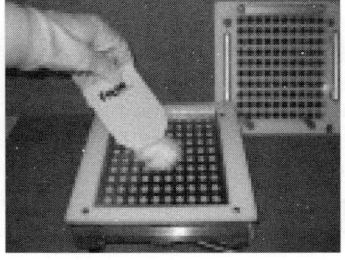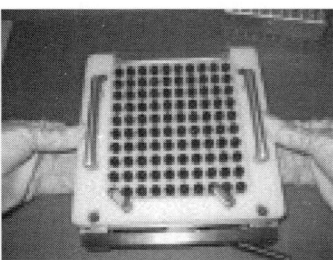

Fig. 4.1. Feton hand operated capsule filler. (http://www.feton.com/products-capsule-fillers.php)

pneumatic closing station with variable speed drive motors (Fig. 4.2), HMI touch screen control and quick changeover from size-to-size. It has a feature of temper-evident capsule banding.

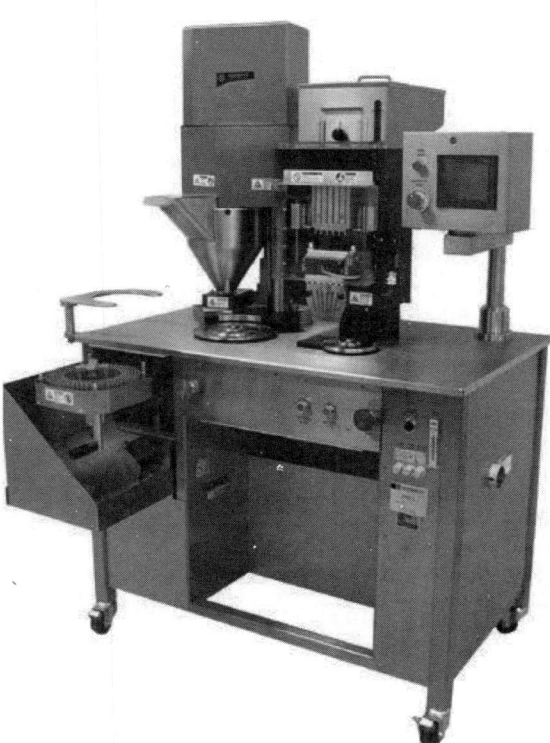

Fig. 4.2. STI capsule filling machine. (http://www. schaefer-technologies.net/capsule_filling_machines/model_10/default.htm)

Automatic machines

They can be categorized as intermittent motion machines or continuous motion machines:

Intermittent motion machines

Zanasi

Five machines ranging in capacity from 60 to 1000 filled capsules per minute are now available by this machine maker. They are LZ-64 at 60, RM-63 at 160, the RV-59 at 250, the AZ-30 at 500, AZ-40 at 700 (Fig. 4.3) and the AZ-60 at 1000 capsules per minute. It works on dosator principle.

The dosator principle has been previously described [Small & Augsburger, 1977; Stoyle,

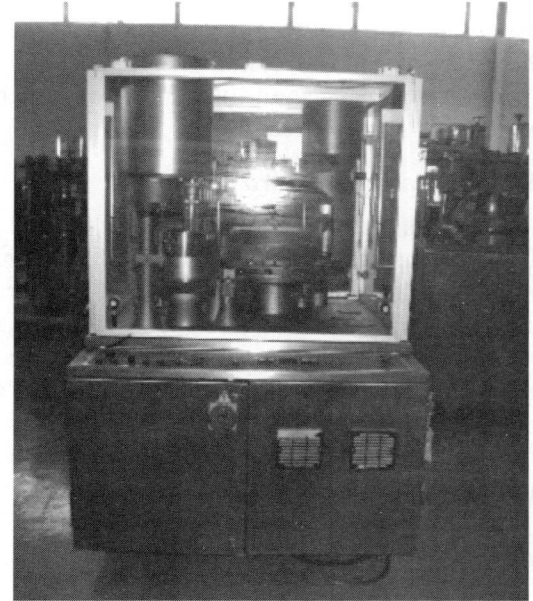

Fig. 4.3. Zanasi AZ-40 capsule filling machine. (http://pharmasurplusequipment.com/inventory.php?p_ID=89)

1966]. The dosator consists of a cylindrical dosing tube fitted with a moveable piston. The end of the tube is open, and the position of the piston is preset to a particular height to define a volume (again, comparable with a tablet press die cavity) that would contain the desired dose of powder. In operation, the dosator is plunged down into a powder bed maintained at a constant preset level by agitators and scrapers. The powder bed height is generally greater than the piston height. Powder enters the open end and is slightly compressed against the piston (termed as precompression [Small & Augsburger, 1977]. The piston then gives a tamping blow, thus forming the powder into a plug. The dosator, bearing the plug, is withdrawn from the powder hopper and is moved over to the empty capsule body where the piston is pushed downward to eject the plug. In certain machines, such as the Macofar machines, the body bushing is rotated into position under the dosator to receive the ejected plug. The primary control over fill weight (for a given set of tooling) is the initial piston height in the dosing tube. A secondary control of weight is the height of the powder bed into which the dosator dips.

In one of the earliest reports evaluating the Zanasi machine, Stoyle [Stoyle, 1966] suggests that formulations should have the following characteristics for successful filling:

1. Fluidity is important for powder feed from the reservoir to the dipping bed and also to permit efficient closing of the hole left by the dosator.
2. A degree of compatibility is important to prevent loss of material from the end of the plug during transport to the capsule shell.
3. Lubricity is needed to permit easy and efficient ejection of the plug.
4. It was suggested that formulations have a moderate bulk density. Low-bulk density materials or those that contain entrapped air will not consolidate well, and capping similar to what occurs in tabletting may result.

The quantitative retention of powder within the dosator during transfer from the powder bed to the capsule shell is essential to a successful filling operation. Jolliffe et al., [1979] have studied this theoretically by the application of hopper design theory. The retention of powder during transfer requires the formation of a stable powder arch at the dosator outlet, and this depends on the angle of wall friction. Generally, theory predicts that cohesive materials will be retained with minimal compressive stress on rough dosator walls and that smoother walls provide the best conditions for retaining more freely flowing powders.

Hofliger and Karg

Hofliger–Karg models include GKF-70 at 70, GKF 330 at 330, GKF 602 at 635, GKF 1200 at 1270 and GKF 2400 at 2540 capsules per minute. All are based on tamp filling as well as dosing disk filling principle.

The dosing-disk-filling principle has been described [Shah, 1983] and the dosing-disk, which forms the base of the dosing or filling chamber, has a number of holes bored through it. A solid brass "stop" plate slides along the bottom of the dosing disk to close off these holes, thereby forming openings similar to the die cavities of a tablet press. The powder is maintained at a relatively constant level over the dosing disk. Five sets of pistons (Hofliger-Karg machines) compress the powder into the cavities to form plugs. The cavities are indexed under each of the five sets of pistons so that each plug is compressed five times per cycle. After the five tamps, any excess powder is scraped off as the dosing disk indexes to position the plugs over empty capsule bodies where they are ejected by transfer pistons. The dose is controlled by the thickness of the dosing disk (i.e., cavity depth), the powder depth, and the tamping pressure. The flow of powder from the hopper to the disk is auger-assisted. A capacitance probe senses the powder level and activates an auger feed if the level falls to below the preset level. The powder is distributed over the dosing disk by the centrifugal action of the indexing rotation of the disk. Baffles are provided to help maintain a uniform powder level. However, while working with a Hofliger–Karg model 330, Shah et al., [1983] noted that a uniform powder bed height was not maintained at the first tamping station because of its nearness to the scrape-off device. Kurihara & Ichikawa, 1978 reported that variation in fill weight was closely related to the angle of repose of the formulation; however, a minimum point appeared in the plots of the angle of repose versus coefficient of variation of filling weight. In fact, at higher angles of repose, the powders did not have sufficient mobility to distribute well under the acceleration of the intermittent-indexing motion. The powder was apparently too fluid to maintain a uniform bed when the angle of repose was low. However, the investigators did not appear to make use of powder compression through tamping, and this complicates the interpretation of their results. These machines, generally, require that formulations be adequately lubricated for efficient plug ejection, to prevent filming on pistons, and to reduce friction between any sliding components that may come into contact with powder. A degree of compatibility is important, as coherent plugs appear to be desirable for clean, efficient transfer at ejection. However, there may be less dependence on formulation cohesiveness than exists for dosator machines.

The Harro-Hofliger machine is similar to Hofliger-Karg machines, except that it employs only three tamping stations. However, at each station, the powder in the dosing cavities is tamped twice before rotating a quarter turn to the next station. One other difference is that the powder in the filling chamber is constantly agitated to help in the maintenance of a uniform powder bed depth.

Continuous motion machines

mG2

It is first commercially available continuous motion capsule filler. mG2 range of models include G36/4 at 150, G36/2 at 300, G36 at 600, G37 at 1600 and G140 at 2300 capsules per minute (Fig. 4.4). The following identifications apply to mG2 models; empty capsule holder and rectifier; cap holder removal station; bulk powder hopper; powder dosing head; cap holder replacing station; capsule closing and ejection station; cleaning station.

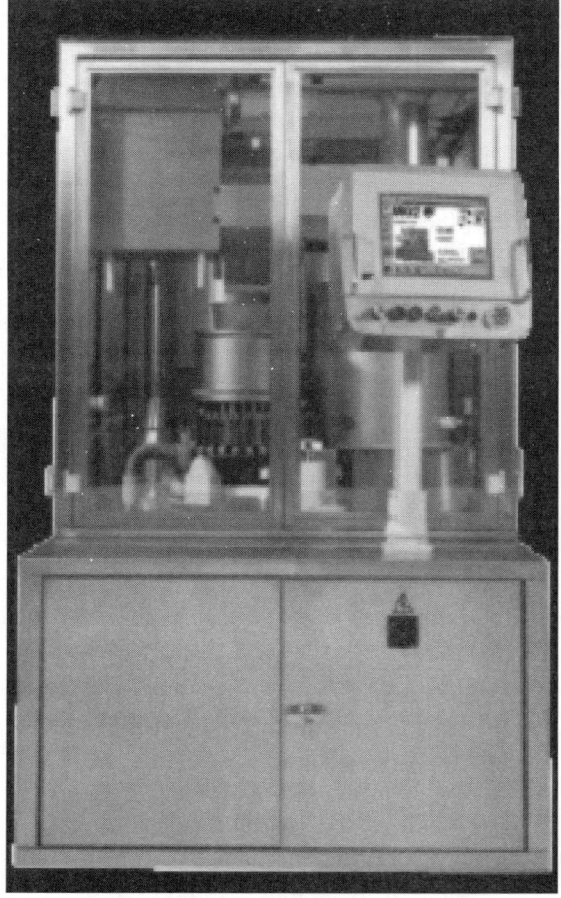

Fig. 4.4. mG2 G140 capsule filling machine. (http:// mpiaust.com.au/products/mgcaps.htm)

Perry Accofil Model CF

It has an output of 36000, 48000, 60000 capsules per hour. The machine has four rotating assemblies; rectification, filling, closing turrets and rotary powder hopper. The three turrets are linked together by a unique swing like capsule conveying system. The filling turret, closing turret and powder pan are synchronously driven by a sprocket and timing chain system located in the machine base. The rectifier has no moving parts but rotates because it is driven by the capsule-conveying system.

Zanasi BZ-72, 150 and Z 5000 Range

BZ-72 fills capsules from 00 to 5 and has an output of 72000 capsules per hour. BZ-150 has an output up to 150,000 capsules per hour. Zanasi Z 5000 series include Z 5000 R1, Z5000 R2 and Z 5000 R3 with maximum outputs in capsules per hour of 70000, 110000 and 150,000 respectively. The dimensions of the machine in 5000 R series have been reduced, and the control console has been attached to the main frame of the machine. Zanasi's high production machines include Adapta series at 100,000 capsules per hour and Imatic series, which include Imatic 100 at 100,000, Imatic 150 at 150,000 and Imatic 200 at 200,000 capsules per hour (Fig. 4.5).

Farmatic machines

It consists of 2000/15, 2000/30 and 2000/60 with maximum outputs of 40,000, 80,000 and 160,000 capsules per hour, respectively. These machines have a single operating tower with a separate turret to hold the powder. A central hopper holds the empty capsules, which are fed into special scoops for intercepting and rejecting damaged and distorted capsules. In a lower part of this central turret, the capsules are rectified, separated, filled and reunited. In addition to these few other popular, well accepted industrial capsule filling machines with digital controls are also available.

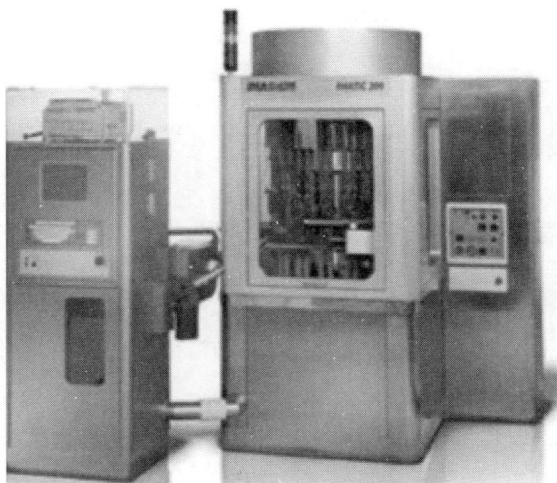

Fig. 4.5. Zanasi Imatic capsule filler. (http://www.ima.it/Imatic-Continuous-Motion-Capsule-Fillers_1l1c50f82m.asp)

Fully Automatic Model YX-CF800

The model is the latest equipment that completely meets the GMP, ISO, and USFDA requirements and the safety of the operator. It automatically processes capsule feeding, detaching, filling, ejecting defective capsule, closing capsule, discharging finished capsule. PLC program control panel with LCD touch screen operation and highly automation machine of water, electricity and pneumatic with 99% capsule upload due to capsule vacuum positioned mechanism (Fig. 4.6). Many attractive features like Auto-trouble shooting of lack of material, lack of capsule, block in material channel and other mechanical trouble, make alarm and stop automatically, closed capsule length adjustment, fully enclosed dosing stations and easy to remove rotating table, quick and accurate change part set-up and ring carrier assembly makes it suitable for integration of whole capsule filling plants.

Qualicaps® unequalled LIQFIL automated filling equipment

Qualicaps® is a market leader in hard shell filling equipment manufacturing for customized liquid

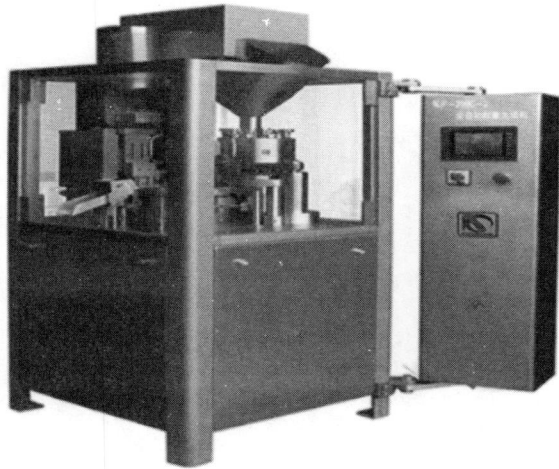

Fig. 4.6. Fully automatic model YX-CF800. (http://www.penglaichina.com/capsule-filling-machine-GMP-pharma.html)

fill technology (http://qualicaps.com/pharmaceutical-equipment/capsule-filling-machine/). This machine has a capacity of 500 to 150,000 capsules per hour for drugs in early stage development, pilot study and full scale commercialization. It has a patented three drum rectification system for gentle capsule transport and other industry leading features like capsule filling solutions, removable filling unit, automatic removal of defective capsules from feed drum and rectifier rollers. F-Labo: LIQFIL super Labo Capsule Filling Machine has been developed for filling of every drug dosage form and multilayer filling for lab study of drug formulation and manufacturing investigational new drugs. F-40/80: LIQFIL super 40/80 Capsule Filling Machine features a compact size with easy conversion, highly accurate filling and the ability to handle a variety of dosage forms. These machines have output ranges from 40,000-80,000/hour and temper-evident capsule banding feature.

Formulation

Formulations for filling into capsules must be capable of being filled uniformly to give a stable product, must release their active contents in a form that is available for absorption by the patient, must be compatible with excipients and must comply with pharmacopoeial and regulatory requirements. Powder formulations for encapsulation should be developed in consideration of the particular filling principle involved. The requirements on the formulation imposed by the filling process, such as lubricity, compatibility, and fluidity are not only essential to a successful filling operation, but also may be expected to influence drug release from the capsules. Indeed, the various filling principles themselves may be expected to influence drug release. This seems particularly evident for those machines that form compressed plugs.

Various factors, which influence filling of powder formulations in capsule include active ingredient, dose of active, solubility of active, particle size of active and excipients, shape of active and size of capsule to be used. Excipients that can be used in powder filled capsules include diluents, lubricants, glidants, wetting agents, and disintegrants.

Diluents

These are often needed to increase the bulk of the formulation and to give plug forming properties. The most common capsule diluents are starch, lactose, and dicalcium phosphate. Modifications of these materials for direct-compression tabletting, such as pre-gelatinized starch or spray-processed lactose or unmilled dicalcium phosphate, can also be used. These substances improve flow and compatibility while maintaining the basic properties of the original materials. Australian physicians noted an increase in the number of patients exhibiting phenytoin toxicity while using a particular sodium phenytoin capsule product. This occurrence coincided with the manufacturer changing the filler from calcium sulfate to lactose and was the result of increased bioavailability when lactose was the filler. Here, the effect may not be solely due to the greater solubility of lactose. Bastami & Groves [1978] have reported that the *in vitro* dissolution of phenytoin may not be complete in the presence of calcium sulfate and suggested the formation of an insoluble calcium salt of the drug. It has also been reported that lactose, at a concentration of 50%, enhanced the dissolution of phenobarbital from capsules, but had no effect on the dissolution of the water-soluble sodium salt [York, 1980].

Glidants

These are used to improve the fluidity of powders. They are fine particles that appear to coat the particles of the bulk powder and enhance fluidity by one or more of several possible mechanisms [York, 1975]: (a) reducing roughness by filling surface irregularities; (b) reducing attractive forces by physically separating the host particles; (c) modifying electrostatic charges; (d) acting as moisture scavengers; and (e) serving as ball bearings between host particles. Usually, there is an optimum concentration for flow; generally, less than 1% w/w and typically 0.25–0.50% w/w. Glidants include colloidal silica, corn starch, talc, and magnesium stearate.

Lubricants

They ease the ejection of plugs, reduce filming on pistons and adhesion of powder to metal surfaces, and reduce friction between sliding surfaces in contact with powder. Metallic stearates, talc, stearic acid are the commonly used ones. Increasing the concentration of hydrophobic lubricants, such as magnesium stearate, is generally understood to retard drug release by making formulations more hydrophobic [Newton et al., 1971, 1971a; Samyn & Jung, 1970; Murthy & Samyn, 1977]. However, exceptions to that rule are possible. Stewart et al. [1979] reported that the effect of magnesium stearate concentration on the dissolution of a model low-dose drug, riboflavin, from capsules was dependent in some manner on the type of filler. Soluble fillers exhibited the anticipated prolonged times with increasing lubricant levels. However, the trends with insoluble fillers were less predictable.

Disintegrants

These produce disruption of the powder mass. Commonly used ones include starch, croscarmellose sodium, sodium starch glycolate and crospovidone. Botzolakis et al. [1982] compared various levels of these newer disintegrants against 10% starch and 0% disintegrant as controls in dicalcium phosphate-based capsules filled on an instrumented Zanasi LZ-64 at a uniform compression force. In most cases, the dissolution rate of hydrochlorothiazide was dramatically enhanced. Disintegrant efficiency was concentration-dependent. Although, the typical use levels of these disintegrants in tablets are 2–4%, the most effective disintegrants required 4–6% for fast dissolution.

Surfactants

These may be included in capsule formulations to increase the wetting of the powder mass and enhance drug dissolution. The "water-proofing" effect of hydrophobic lubricants may be offset by the use of surfactants. The most common surfactants employed in capsule formulations are sodium lauryl sulfate and sodium docusate. Levels of 0.1–0.5% w/w are usually sufficient to overcome wetting problems.

Capsule finishing

Capsules after filling require some sort of dusting or polishing operation before the operations of inspection, bottling, and labelling are completed. The methods used are:

Salt polishing

In this procedure some materials, which stick to capsule surface, are removed by rotating filled capsules in pan along with sodium chloride. Following rotation capsules are separated from the salt by a screening operation. Salt polishing may have a deleterious effect on imprinted capsules.

Pan polishing

A polyurethane cloth liner in coating pan is used to trap the removed dust from capsules as well as to impart a gloss to the capsules.

Cloth dusting

For removing dust and for imparting shine to capsules, filled capsules are rubbed with cloth by hand.

Brushing

In this procedure, dust is removed by placing capsules under rotating soft brushes. This procedure must be accompanied by a vacuuming for dust removal.

Modified release capsules

Modified-release capsules are hard or soft capsules in which the contents or the shell or both contain excipients or are prepared by special procedures such as microencapsulation which, separately or together, are designed to modify the rate, place or time of release of the active ingredient(s) in the GI tract. It can be sustained release (extended- or prolonged-release) capsules that are designed to slow the rate of release of the active ingredient(s) in the GI. Capsules are usually required to dissolve in the stomach as rapidly as possible, releasing their contents, but for certain purposes they are designed to pass through the stomach and into the intestine before dissolving. Such products are defined by terms such as **gastro-resistant**, **entero-soluble** or **enteric coated** capsule. Their production was first suggested in the 1880s as means of administering medicines, which were very irritating to the gastric mucosa or which degrade in stomach.

Initially, in 1895, Dr. Weyland suggested use of formaldehyde solution to harden the capsules, which was patented in Germany by Hausmann (employer of Weyland) in 1895. Hausmann obtained a second patent in same year for another aldehyde, acrolein. Later on, cocoa butter, paraffin wax, or other suitable vegetable, animal or mineral fats were used for enteric coating the capsule. Further, during the first half of this century, shellac, tolu, mastic, resin, carnauba wax and salol were also tried. But all such coatings lead to poor *in vivo* results. It was not until the development of modified cellulose derivatives such as phthalates, which had the correct solubility properties i.e. insoluble in strong acid solution but soluble at slightly acid pH values, the satisfactory products were produced [John, 1960].

Capsules for dry powder inhalation devices

Dry Powder Inhalation (DPI) is an important drug delivery technology for the treatment of respiratory diseases, and progressively for systemic drug delivery. It is not an easy job to optimize a DPI capsule. It involves the key understanding of the relationship between the device, formulation and capsule to improve drug performances like good powder aerosolization and delivery of the active ingredient deep into the lungs [Edwards, 2010]. Many industries like Capsulgel, Qualicaps etc. have developed capsules to match the specific requirements of DPI device and formulation. It includes strict microbial limits, moisture content, lubrication level, weight tolerances, minimum powder adhesion for consistent dose delivery and capsules with optimum cutting and puncturing performance [Richardson, 2011]. Besides, storage condition of the DPI capsules also affect the formulation efficiency and device performance [Borgstrom, 2005]. Aerodynamic particle size distribution is an important factor for any dry powder for inhalation formulation. Such formulations can be either conventional carrier (lactose, mannitol and other sugar alcohols) based API formulation or non-carrier based multimodal particle size distribution of one or more APIs, which can be formulated using spray drying or other particle engineering techniques. Such formulations should be subsequently tested for particle size distribution, emitted dose and fine powder fraction (FPF) using gravimetric determination and cascade impaction, amorphous content and dose content uniformity using dose uniformity sampling apparatus (DUSA).

Packing and storage

Finished capsules normally contain an equilibrium moisture content of 13–16%. This moisture is critical to the physical properties of the shells, since at lower moisture contents (< 12%), shells become too brittle; at higher moisture contents (> 18%) they become too soft [Scott, et al., 1992; Murthy & Ghebre-Sellassie, 1993]. It is beneficial to avoid extremes of temperature and to maintain a relative humidity between 40–60% and temperature between 10–30 degrees when handling and storing capsules.

The bulk of the moisture in capsule shells is physically bound, and it can readily transfer between the shell and its contents, depending on their relative hygroscopicity [Ito, et al.,1969; Strickland & Moss, 1962]. The removal of moisture from the shell could be sufficient to cause splitting or cracking, as has been reported for the deliquescent material, potassium acetate. Sodium cromoglycate has been reported to act as a "sink" for moisture, in that moisture was continuously removed from hard gelatin shells, especially at higher temperatures [Bell, et al., 1973]. Conditions that favor the transfer of moisture to powder contents may lead to caking and retarded disintegration or other stability problems. It may be useful to pre-equilibrate the shell and its contents to the same relative humidity within the acceptable range [Kontny & Mulska, 1989; Zographi et al., 1988].

One issue that is receiving current attention is the loss of water solubility of shells, apparently as a result of sufficient exposure to high humidity and temperature or to exposure to trace aldehydes [Schweir et al., 1993]. Such capsules develop a "skin" or pellicle during dissolution testing, exhibit retarded dissolution, and may fail to meet the U.S. Pharmacopeia (USP) drug dissolution specifications. This insolubilization of gelatin capsules has been attributed to "gelatin cross-linking." In one example, photo-instability compounded by humidity has been suggested as the explanation for the retarded dissolution of model compounds from hard gelatin capsules containing certified dyes, particularly when FD & C Red No. 3 was incorporated in both the cap and the shell [Murthy et al., 1989]. The problem also has been attributed to the presence of trace aldehydes in excipients [Mohmad, 1986], as well as to the liberation of furfural from the rayon stuffing in bottles. These results point to the need for appropriate storage conditions and moisture-tight (air-tight) packaging, as well as to the need to exclude aldehydes.

Pharmacopoeial capsule standards

Weight variation

In this test, 20 intact capsules are individually weighed and the average weight determined. The test requirements are met if none of the individual weights differ by 10% of the average. If the original 20 do not meet these criteria, the individual net weights are determined. These are averaged, and differences between each individual net content and the average. The test requirements are met if (i) not more than two of the individual differences are greater than 10% of the average, or (ii) in no case is any difference greater than 25%.

If more than two, but less than 6, net weights determined above deviate by more than 10%, but less than 25%, the net contents are determined for an additional 40 capsules, and the average calculated for the entire 60 capsules. Sixty deviations from the new average are calculated. The requirements are met if (i) the difference does not exceed 10% of the average in more than 6 of the 60 capsules, and (ii) in no case does any difference exceed 25%.

Uniformity of content

In this case, 30 capsules are selected, 10 of which are assayed by the specified procedure. The requirements are met if 9 of the 10 capsules are within the specified potency range of 85 to 115%, and the tenth is not outside 75 to 125%.

If more than 1, but less than 3, of the first 10 capsules fall outside the 85 to 115% limits, the remaining 20 are assayed. The requirements are met if all 30 capsules are within 75 to 125% of the specified potency range, and not less than 27 of the 30 are within the 85 to 115% range.

Disintegration test

This test is conducted to simulate movement within the stomach by the use of an oscillating tube apparatus, which consists of a vertically-mounted tube made of glass or Perspex, with a wire mesh base. The capsule is placed in the tube, which is then raised and lowered in the test solution at a frequency of approximately 30 strokes per minute through a specified distance. The end point is given as 'no residue remains, it consists of fragments of shell or is a soft mass with no palpable core.' The time allowed for disintegration varies but is usually in the range of 15 to 30 minutes as per different pharmacopoeial standards. For enteric capsules, two different media are used i.e. acidic and basic. Normally, the enteric capsule is required to be resistant to the first acidic solution for 2 hours, but they must disintegrate in the second basic solution within 1 hour. For capsules in which the contents, rather than the shell, resist the action of gastric fluid, a suitable dissolution test should be carried out to demonstrate the appropriate release of the active substance(s) [http://www. who.int/medicines/publications/pharmacopoeia/en/].

ALTERNATIVE TO HARD GELATIN CAPSULES

For the past few years, hard capsules have been manufactured from some alternative materials like HPMC, polyvinyl alcohols and pullulan etc.

to meet the dietary and cultural needs of vegetarian patients. Besides vegetarian customer demand, non-animal capsules can meet various other manufacturing, marketing and regulatory mandate. Although, gelatin had been used as the sole material for manufacturing capsules traditionally, yet it has many disadvantages of cost and stability issues like crosslinking of unmodified gelatin, solubilty with certain fill formulations, difficulty to produce transparent capsules, moisture and temperature sensitivity and, thus, requirement of special packaging and storage conditions. Gelatin is not suitable for readily hydrolyzable drugs due to its high water content of 13–15%. Further, due to its bovine origin, there is a potential risk posed by bovine spongiform encephalopathy (BSE). Many patents describe the use of alternative synthetic polymers and/or plant derived hydrocolloids, however, only few have gained commercial interest.

WO 0103677 (Draper et al., 1999] described the use of a combination of iota carrageenan (12–24% w/w of dry shell) and modified starch, namely hydroxypropyl starch (30–60% w/w of dry shell), as a gelatin substitute. WO 0137817 [Menard et al., 1999] described the formulation of soft capsules from potato starch (45–80% w/w), with a specific molecular weight distribution and amylopectin content, together with a conventional plasticizer such as glycerol (> 12% w/w), a glidant and a disintegrant. WO 9735537 [Brown, et al., 1996] described the preferable use of polyvinyl alcohol (PVA) and optional use of some other materials, all-being film forming polymers that lack the gelling properties that are necessary for soft capsule production using the conventional rotary die press.

Hypermellose (HPMC) is the most successful gelatin alternative due to its good machinability, better stability under extreme storage conditions without the risk of capsule cross-linking and amenability to modified release coatings. First such capsules were produced as Quali V® by Shionogi Qualicaps for eventual use. HPMC capsules are suitable even for moisture sensitive, hygroscopic formulation as well as under low humid conditions as it does not become brittle or act as plasticizer. G.S. Technologies Inc.(now R.P. Scherer Technologies) developed the first vegan capsules Vegicaps from HPMC in 1989. Other popular HPMC capsules are Vcaps® and Vcaps Plus®(Capsulgel, A division of Pfizer). The production technology is same as that of gelatin based hard capsules with a little modifications like dipping of rather heated pins in the HPMC solution. These capsules have been patented pertaining to without or with the use of gelling agents and its types. These capsules have become very popular for its pharmaceutical application in dispensing various DPI (dry powder for inhalation) formulations as it remains resistant to breakage even under low humid conditions as well as to the application of desiccant and hence exhibit good DPI device compatibility [Borgstrom, 2005]

PVA copolymer (PVA, acrylic acid (AA) and methyl methacrylate (MMA) is another gelatin substitute under development to formulate less moisture sensitive, non-cross linking and more soluble soft gelatin capsules with low electric propensity and no Maillard reaction. Capsules prepared with PVA copolymer are compatible with hydrophilic materials like PEG 400, Tween 80 and LABRASOL contrary to those prepared with HPMC and gelatin.

Another vegetable derived highly stable, well characterized water soluble polysaccharide,

Pullulan has been approved by regulatory agencies to successfully manufacture non-animal capsules that are marketed as NPcaps®. It can produce crystal clear transparent capsules with very low oxygen permeability [Rabadia, 2013]. Overall there is changeover from gelatin to vegan capsules due to comparable (Table 4.2) benefits of plant based products.

For the past few years, due to socio-cultural and health-related concerns, the ultimatum of capsules is towards organic, vegan, herbal, all natural, non-allergenic, soy or gluten free landscapes.

SOFT GELATIN CAPSULES

Soft gelatin capsules (referred to as soft elastic gelatin capsules, liquid gels or softgels) are a unique drug delivery system that can provide distinct advantages over traditional dosage forms such as tablets, hard gelatin capsules and liquids. However, due to economic, technical and patent constraints, there are relatively a few manufacturers of softgels in the world. Softgel is a hermetically sealed, one-piece capsule with a liquid or semisolid fill. Soft gelatin capsules may be oblong, elliptical, spherical, or tube shape.

The softgel consists of two major components, the gelatin shell and the fill. In the finished product gelatin shell is primarily composed of gelatin, plasticizer and water. Soft gelatin capsules, generally, contain the drug in a non-aqueous solution or suspension. The vehicle

Table 4.2. Comparison of gelatin-based and plant-based capsules

Type of capsule	Source	Stability	Moisture content (%)	Allergy/Disease	Suitability
Gelatin capsule	Bovine or cow skin	Cross-linking with aldehyde	13–15	BSE (mad cow disease) and TSE (transmissible spongiform encephalopathy) to humans	Not suitable for kidney and liver disease patient
Vegetarian capsule	Plant line pine tree bark gum	No cross-linking with aldehyde	2–7 (suitable for moisture sensitive and hygroscopic ingredient)	Non-GMO (Genetically Modified Organisms)	Suitable

may be water immiscible liquid, such as PEG, and non-ionic surface-active agent, such as Polysorbate 80. Soft gelatin capsules are especially important to contain liquid drugs or drug solutions. Also, volatile drug substances or drug materials susceptible to deterioration in the presence of air may be better suited to a soft gelatin capsule than to hard gelatin capsule. Softgels can be formulated as chewable, suckable or twist-off softgels having pharmaceutical applications through various routes as an oral dosage form, as suppository for rectal or vaginal use and as a single dose application for topical, ophthalmic and optic use [Reddy, et al., 2013].

Advantages

1. Improved rate and extent of absorption mainly for poorly soluble drugs.
2. Patient compliance and consumer preference as easy to swallow with possibility of small to large size.
3. Safe for potent and cytotoxic drugs.
4. Overcomes manufacturing problems with tablets or hard gelatin capsules.
5. Dose uniformity for low-dose drugs as drug solutions provide homogeneity over powder or granule mixtures.
6. Product stability as drugs are protected against degradation by lipid vehicles and soft gel shells.
7. Uniquely suited for liquids and volatile drugs as soft gels are hermetically sealed [Hutchinson & Ferdinando, 2007].
8. Elegant and portable with odor and taste masking capability.

Disadvantages

1. Soft gelatin products must be contracted out to a limited number of firms having the necessary filling equipment and expertise.
2. Interaction possibility is increased as there is more intimate contact between the shell and its liquid contents than hard gelatin capsules.
3. Drug migration can occur from an oily vehicle into the shell.

Manufacture of soft gelatin capsule

Soft gelatin capsules have been available since the middle of nineteenth century. The capsules were filled by medicine dropper and sealed by hand with a glob of molten gelatin [Stanley, 1976].

Plate process

It is an oldest process that involved (a) placing the upper half of a plasticized gelatin sheet over a die plate containing numerous die pockets; (b) application of vacuum to draw the sheet into die pockets; (c) filling the pockets with liquid or paste; (d) folding the lower half of the gelatin sheet back over the filled pockets; and (e) inserting the "sandwich" under a die press where the capsules are formed and cut out.

Rotary die process

Scherer invented this process that reduced manufacturing losses to a negligible figure and content variation to an excellent ± 1 to 3%. In this process, die pockets are machined into the outer surfaces of two die-rollers. The die pockets on the two rollers match as the rollers rotate. Two gelatin ribbons are continuously and simultaneously fed with liquid or semi-solid fill between the rollers. Forceful injection of feed material between two ribbons causes the gelatin to swell into the left and right hand die-pockets as they converge. As the die rolls rotate, the convergence of the matching die pockets seals and cuts out the filled capsules. The early success of the rotary die process led others to develop continuous methods of soft gelatin capsule manufacture. One such method was developed by Norton, known as reciprocating die process and is now owned by Banner Gelatin Products. It involves careful control of three parameters viz; temperature, timing and pressure. Temperature controls the heat available for capsule seal formation. Timing of dosing of unit quantities of fill matrix into softgel during its formation is critical. The pressure exerted between the two rotary dies controls the soft gels shape and the final cut-out from the gel ribbon. Pharmagel's machine for soft gel preparation based on rotary die process is shown in Fig. 4.7.

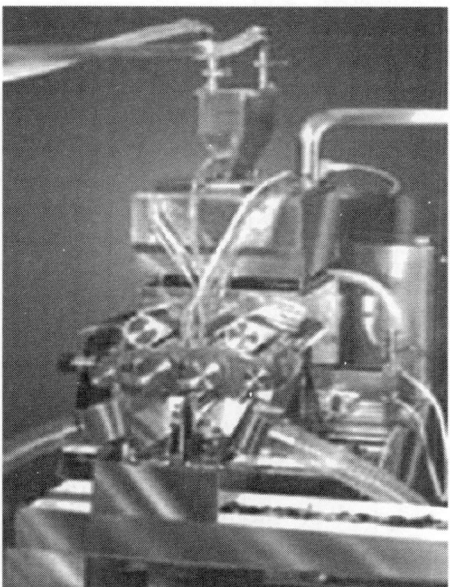

Fig. 4.7. Pharmagel's rotary die process machine for soft gel preparation. (http://www.pharmaceutical-technology.com/contractors/process automation/pharmagel/) US 6805818

Accogel process

This continuous process was developed by Lederle Labs. It is unique in that it is the only equipment that can fill powdered dry solids, with accuracy into soft gels. Machine may be adapted for liquid/granule filling also. This process also involves measuring roll, a die roll and a sealing roll. The measuring roll rotates directly over the die-roll, and the pockets in the two rolls are aligned with each other. The powder or granular fill material is held in the pockets of the measuring roll under vacuum. A gelatin sheet is drawn into the die-pockets of the die-roll under the vacuum. As the measuring roll and die rolls rotate, the measured doses are transferred to the gelatin-lined pockets of the die-roll. Pressure developed between the die-roll and sealing roll seals and cuts the capsules.

Formulation of soft gelatin capsules

Gelatin shell

The capsule shell is composed of gelatin, plasticizer, water and additives like preservatives, colorants, chelating agents and opacifiers. The same has already been described in detail under hard gelatin capsules.

Nature of capsule content

The maximum capsule size and shape convenient for oral use in humans is the 20 minim oblong, the 16 minim oval or the 9 minim round. Different types of soft gel fill materials include lipophilic liquids or oils, hydrophilic liquids, self-emulsifying oils, microemulsions, nanoemulsions, semi-solids or pastes, and suspensions. The choice of components is made based on capacity to dissolve the drug, rate of dispersion in GI tract after softgel shell ruptures and releases the fill matrix, capacity to retain the drug in solution in GI tract, compatibility with soft gel shell, ability to optimize the rate, extent and consistency of drug absorbed.

Quality controls

Due to the nature of materials contained in the capsule shell and comprising capsule shell, unprotected soft gelatin capsules rapidly reach equilibrium with the atmospheric conditions under which they are stored. For the unprotected capsule, low humidities i.e. less than 20%, low temperatures i.e. less than 35°F and high temperatures i.e. greater than 100°F or combinations of these will have only transient effects, which include brittleness, and greater susceptibility to shock. High humidities (more than 60%) produce more lasting effects on the capsule shell since as moisture is absorbed, the capsules become softer, tackier and bloated. Presence of impurities i.e. aldehydes and peroxides which may be present in polyethylene glycol should be controlled as high levels of such impurities lead to cross-linking of the gelatin polymer leading to slow dissolution of capsule shell and subsequent release of drug. Capsules often show "soft spot" at the site at which they lie next to the tray or against another capsule. This spot is due to slower drying and is of no consequence, since such areas will firm up and are not flaws in the capsule shell. If such areas do not firm up, then physical stability problems are anticipated. In process quality controls include gel ribbon thickness, soft gel seal thickness, fill matrix weight, capsule shell weight and soft gel moisture level and hardness at the end of drying stage. Finished product is subjected to number of pharmacopoeial or non-pharmacopoeial tests, which include assay, fill weight, content uniformity, microbiological testing etc.

A new technological advancement in this area is development of solid state capsule, which will allow the encapsulation of 30 to 50% aqueous solutions and suspensions of active coupled with macromolecular gel-lattice matrix.

MICROENCAPSULATION

Microcapsules and microspheres have found extensive use in the field of drug delivery. Microencapsulation is an interdisciplinary field that requires knowledge of polymer science, emulsion technology (in most cases) and an understanding of drug and protein stabilization. Encapsulation is a very standard practice in the food, consumer products and cosmetics industries. Flavors have been encapsulated since the 1930s, vitamins since the 1940s and ink for carbonless paper since 1956. The concept of using semi-permeable microcapsules for the delivery of therapeutic biological reagents was pioneered by T.M.S. Chang almost 40 years ago and over the years a wide range of drugs such as steroids, vitamins and antibiotics has been encapsulated [Li & Vert, 1999].

Microcapsules offer several advantages in their use as drug delivery systems, the most important being that the kinetics of drug release can be altered by changing the properties of the microcapsule. The delivery of drugs can be varied from several days to several months. Also,

the surface of the microcapsules can be modified by attaching ligands such as antibodies, which would enable them to target specific organs and sites in the body.

Microspheres of biodegradable and non-biodegradable polymers have been investigated for sustained release depending on their final application. Non-biodegradable polymers pose problems of toxicity; difficulty in removal and also a constant rate of drug release can't be achieved from CR devices using these polymers [Hermann & Bodmeier, 1995]. To overcome these problems, concept of biodegradable polymers for sustained release drug delivery systems was developed. Thus, interest in biodegradable polymers developed for two reasons; firstly, surgical removal of drug depleted delivery system of non-biodegradable polymers is difficult and non-removal may pose toxicological problems; secondly, diffusion controlled delivery systems though are excellent means of achieving predetermined rates of drug delivery, it is limited by polymer permeability and characteristics of the drug. Basic mechanisms in non-degradable devices being diffusion and drugs, which have either high molecular weight or poor solubility in polymer, are not amenable to diffusion controlled release. Various drugs have been encapsulated in these polymeric systems like recombinant interferon alpha [Diwan & Park, 2003], curcumin [Kumar, et al., 2002], hepatocyte growth factor [Oe, et al., 2003], bromocriptine mesylate [Arica, et al., 2002], cisplatin [Chandy et al., 2002], calcitonin polypeptide [Prabhu, et al., 2002], etc.

A key factor in the design of delivery systems is the choice of an appropriate biodegradable polymer. The usefulness of polymers in drug delivery system is well established. Continued improvement and accelerating research and development in polymeric materials has played a vital role in progress of most controlled release technologies. In the past 25 years, there has been a considerable increase in interest in this technology, as shown by the increasing number of publications and patents in the area of controlled drug release system using synthetic as well as naturally occurring polymeric materials.

Microspheres of biodegradable and non-biodegradable polymers have been investigated for sustained release depending on their final application. For more than two decades, fabricating drugs in polymeric device has attracted the attention of investigators throughout the scientific community. Polymer chemists, chemical engineer and pharmaceutical scientists are engaged in bringing out predictable and controlled delivery of agents ranging from small molecules to proteins and peptides. Examples of early polymeric devices for parenteral administration were prepared from silicon rubber [Folkman & Long, 1964] and polyethylene [Desai, et al., 1965]. A serious drawback to using these inert polymers as parenteral depots is their non-biodegradability and toxicological problems. To overcome these problems, the concept of biodegradable polymers delivery began to develop in the early 1970's.

Biodegradable polymers

Biodegradable polymers may be defined as synthetic or natural polymers, which degrade *in vivo* either enzymatically/non-enzymatically to produce biocompatible or non-toxic by products along with the progressive release of dissolved/dispersed drug. These can be further metabolised/excreted via normal physiologic pathways.

Biodegradable polymers are preferred because surgical removal of drug depleted delivery system is not required, so no possibility of toxicological problems, and they have the properties of degrading in biological fluids to produce bio-compatible or non-toxic products, which can be removed from body by normal physiological pathways. These polymers, as carriers are being used in controlled release technology to achieve many of its objectives [Murthy, 1997]. In addition to biocompatibility

[Visscher, et al., 1985, Kulkarni et al., 1966] and other properties [Miller, et al., 1997, Ellis & Tipton, 1994, English, et al., 1985] of these polymers that make them uniquely suited for these and other applications include; thermo-plasticity, high tensile strength, controlled crystallinity, controlled degradation rates, controlled hydrophilicity and proven non-toxicity.

Classification of biodegradable polymers

A variety of synthetic and naturally occurring polymers have been intensively studied over past 30 years [Murthy, 1997], which include the natural and synthetic ones (Table 4.3). Degradation times of various polymers are shown in Table 4.4 and Fig. 4.8. Polyesters have attracted the most because of the following reasons:

- Outstanding biocompatibility.
- Versatility regarding physical, chemical and biological properties [Li & Vert, 1999].
- Available toxicological and clinical data.
- Easy preparation in a wide range of molecular weights.
- Forming naturally occurring non-toxic metabolites by undergoing simple hydrolysis.
- Relatively strong and long-standing safe use, and regulatory approval.

Preparation techniques

A variety of microencapsulation techniques have been developed till date [Deasy, 1979]. The selection of a particular technique is dependent on the nature of the polymer and core and also the intended use. The method of preparation has much influence on the properties of micro-particles and therefore the desired properties should be kept in mind during the selection of particular method of preparation. For the formulation of particles from the biodegradable polymer matrix it is essential to select an encapsulation process, which fulfills the requirements of the ideal controlled release

Table 4.3. Classification of biodegradable microspheres

Class	General structure
Synthetic	
(a) Polyorthoesters	$(OO-P)_n$ with central ring structure
(b) Polyanhydrides	$\{\!\!-\overset{O}{\overset{\|}{C}}-R-O-(CH_2)_x-\overset{O}{\overset{\|}{C}}-O-\!\!\}_n$
(c) Polyamides	$\{\!\!-R-\overset{O}{\overset{\|}{C}}-NH-\!\!\}_n$
(d) Polyalkylcyanoacrylates	$\{\!\!-CH_2-\overset{CN}{\underset{COOR}{C}}-\!\!\}_n$
(e) Polyesters (i) Lactides/Glycolides	$\{\!\!-R-\overset{O}{\overset{\|}{C}}-O-\!\!\}_n$
(ii) Polycaprolactones	seven-membered lactone ring
(f) Polyphosphazenes	$\cdots\{\!\!-N-\overset{R}{\underset{R}{P}}-\!\!\}_n\cdots$
(g) Pseudopolyamino acids	$\overset{R}{\underset{H_2NCOOH}{\wedge}}$
Natural	
(i) Proteins – albumin, globulin, gelatin, collagen, casein, etc.	
(ii) Polysaccharides – starch, cellulose, chitosan, dextran, alginic acid	

system. The following requirements of the encapsulated polymer particles should be met while choosing a particular method of encapsulation:

1. *Optimal drug loading:* The encapsulation efficiency of the drug should be high. The ratio of the drug to the polymer should be such that the highest amount of drug is encapsulated in the minimal amount of polymer. This reduces the mass of the material to be administered.

2. *High yield of particles:* The process of encapsulation should generate high yield of particles of the targeted size.

Table 4.4. Degradation times of various polymers

Polymer	Degradation time (months)
Poly (l-lactide)	18–24
Poly (dl-lactide)	12–16
Poly (glycolide)	2–4
dl-lactide-co-glycolide) (50:50)	2
dl-lactide-co-glycolide (65:35)	3–4
dl-lactide-co-glycolide (85:15)	5

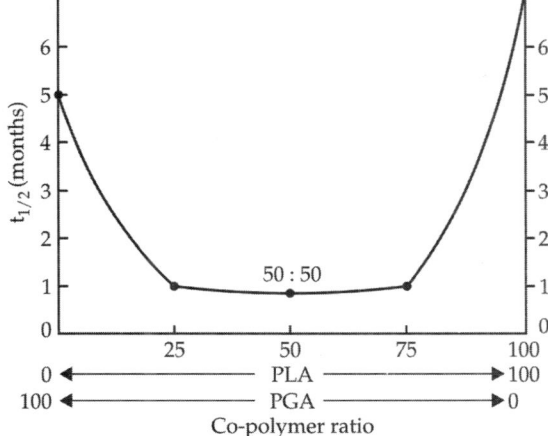

Fig. 4.8. Degradation chart of various polymers.

3. *Stability of the encapsulated drug:* The biological activity of the encapsulated drug should be maintained during the process of particle formulation. It is desirable to use a process where the exposure of the labile drug into strong denaturing solvent is low.

4. *Batch uniformity and inter-batch reproducibility:* The process should be simple and scaleable so that batches of particles having same properties and desired release characteristics can be produced.

5. *Adjustable release profiles:* The method of encapsulation should be such that by manipulating the formulation conditions, different types of release profiles of the encapsulated material can be produced.

6. *Low burst effect:* The particles should be formulated in such a way that minimum of the encapsulated drug is released during the burst phase. This will help in extending the release of the drug for a longer period of time.

7. *Free flowing particles:* The encapsulation method used should always produce free flowing particles, which do not aggregate. This will help in producing uniformly syringeable suspension of the particles.

8. *Syringeability:* Apart from the adjuvanticity considerations, a major requirement of the microsphere system is syringeability through hypodermic needles.

9. *Residual solvent:* In order to gain US FDA approval for any microsphere formulation, it is necessary to consider regulatory requirements of residual solvents content in microspheres. Virtually all microsphere fabrication processes require the use of an organic solvent such as dichloromethane, ethyl acetate for polymer dissolution. FDA limit of dichloromethane (class II) based on recommendations of ICH and USP is 600 ppm.

Many procedures have been used for the preparation of lactide-glycolide microparticles for parenteral delivery. Some of the techniques are discussed below:

Phase separation by emulsification – Solvent evaporation/solvent extraction

O/W emulsion technique

In o/w emulsion technique, polymer is dissolved in dichloromethane or chloroform (Fig. 4.9). The core is either solubilised or suspended in this solution, which is then emulsified with water phase containing a suitable emulsifier as polyvinyl alcohol, methylcellulose, sodium alginate, sodium oleate gelatin, tweens, etc. alone or in combination.

Subsequent removal of organic solvent by heat, vacuum or both results in phase separation of the polymer and core to produce microspheres. This technique was originally developed by

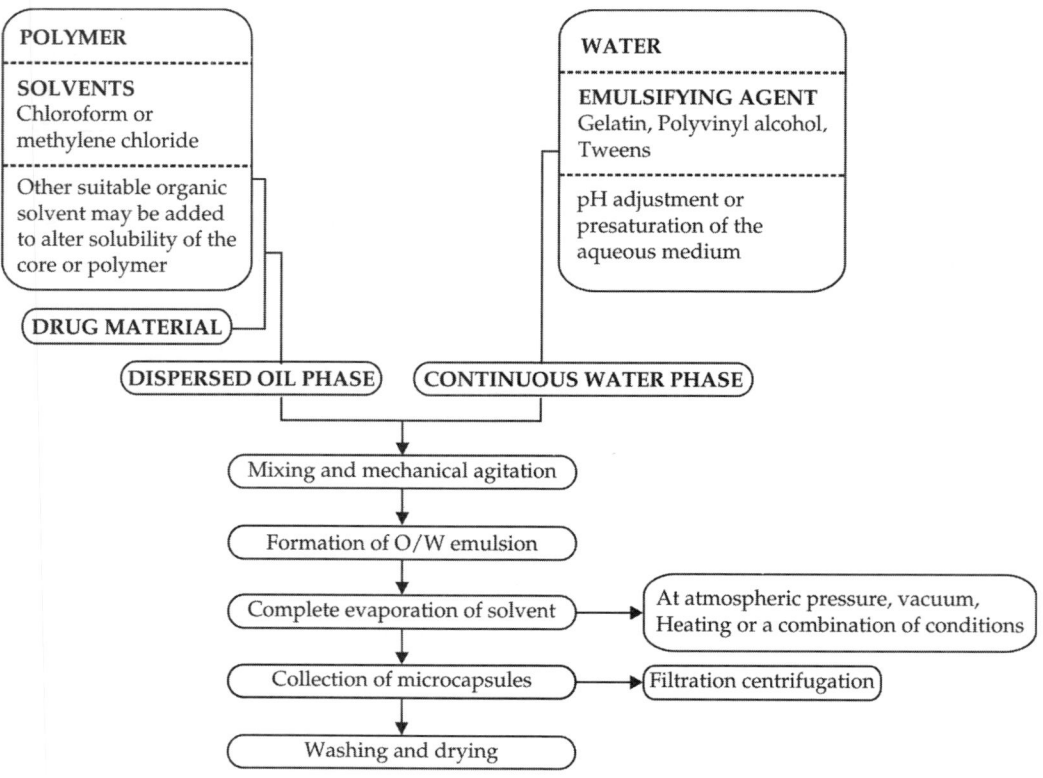

Fig. 4.9. Preparation of microspheres by o/w emulsion technique.

Beck, et al. [1979; 1979a] to encapsulate progesterone with PLA and subsequently by several workers to encapsulate hydrocortisone (Cavalier, et al., 1986), chlorpromazine [Suzuki & Price, 1985], quinidine and quinidine sulphate [Bodmeier & McGinity, 1987], local anaesthetics [Juni, et al., 1985], prednisolone [Smith & Hunneyball, 1986] and narcotic antagonists [Mason, et al., 1976]. A major problem with this technique is the poor encapsulation efficiency of moderately water-soluble and water-soluble compounds, which partitioned out from the organic dispersed phase into the aqueous continuous phase. Adjusting pH of the aqueous phase to suppress ionization could minimize diffusion into aqueous phase, which led to loss of water-soluble drugs. Drug partitioning between the organic dispersed phase and the aqueous continuous phase can also be reduced by prior saturation of the continuous phase with the same drug.

W/O emulsion technique

In w/o emulsion technique, polymer is dissolved in acetonitrile or small amounts of other organic solvent may be added. Core material is either dissolved or suspended in this solution (dispersed aqueous phase), which is then emulsified with liquid paraffin (continuous oil phase) or any other suitable vegetable oil containing emulsifying agents like spans etc.

Subsequent removal of the acetonitrile, at 55°C, results in precipitation of both the polymer and the drug and their incorporation into the microspheres. In order to improve the loading of water-soluble compounds within polyester microspheres, Tsai, et al. [1986] used w/o emulsion system, dissolving polymer such as

PLA and mitomycin C in acetonitrile (dispersed aqueous phase) and emulsifying with liquid paraffin (continuous oil phase) containing Span 65 as an emulsifier. Subsequent removal of acetonitrile, at 55°C, led to formation of drug-loaded microspheres.

W/O/W multiple emulsion

This is another approach for efficient encapsulation of water-soluble active principles by solvent evaporation in aqueous continuous phase. In this method, the organic phase acts as a barrier for diffusion of drug towards external aqueous phase. In this technique, drug is dissolved in aqueous solution (internal phase), which is then emulsified in a polymer solution of methylene chloride (external phase) to form w/o emulsion. This emulsion is further emulsified with aqueous solution of polyvinyl alcohol (PVA) to form w/o/w multiple emulsion. Evaporation of organic solvent by continuous stirring of the multiple emulsion results in hardening of microspheres. This technique is widely used for encapsulation of proteins and peptides. This was first proposed by Ogawa, et al., [1988] for encapsulation of peptide analogue of LHRH (Fig. 4.10). Other agents encapsulated by this technique include Influenza-A vaccine [Hilbert, et al., 1999], BSA and chicken egg-white lysozyme [Fu, et al., 1999], etc.

Instead of solvent evaporation, solvent extraction can be undertaken in which the organic solvent of dispersed phase is eliminated by diffusion of the solvent in the dispersing phase. This is achieved by using large volumes of dispersing phase with respect to dispersed phase or by choosing a dispersed phase consisting of cosolvents of which at least one has a great affinity for dispersing phase. Also, one may formulate a dispersing phase with 2 solvents, in which one acts as a solvent extractor of dispersed phase.

O/O emulsion

Here the dispersed phase needs to be totally immiscible with continuous phase. Dispersing

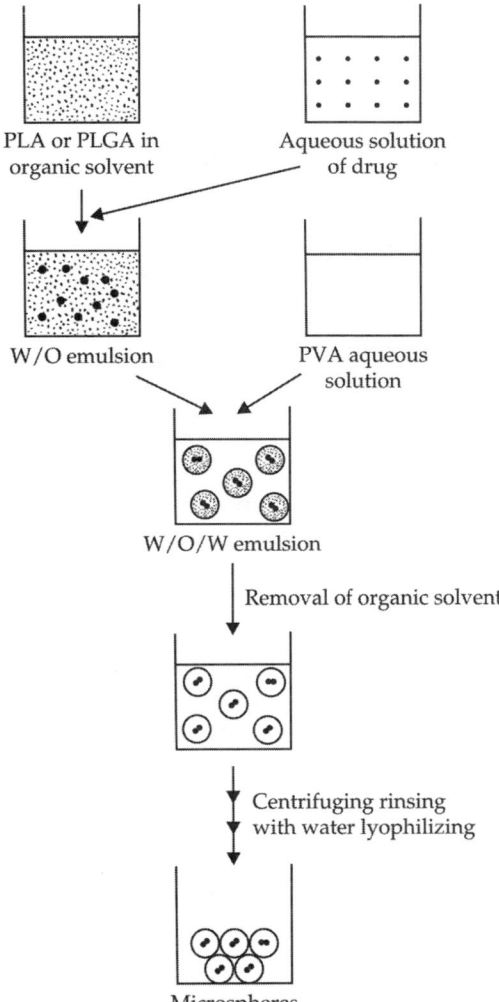

Fig. 4.10. Preparation of microspheres by w/o emulsion technique.

medium is a mineral/vegetable oil/non-volatile organic solvent. In this technique, polymer is dissolved in organic solvent like dichloromethane or acetone. The core is either solubilised or suspended in this solution, which is then emulsified with oily phase that may be liquid paraffin, silicone oil or any other suitable oil containing a suitable emulsifier alone or in combination. Subsequent removal of organic solvent results in phase separation of the polymer and core to produce microspheres. This process permits one to avoid the loss of water soluble active principles, e.g. near zero order release over 60 days from gentamycin sulfate loaded PLGA microspheres was obtained which were prepared by this method [Leel, et al., 1990].

Phase separation by non-solvent addition

Polymer phase separation in non-aqueous media by non-solvents or polymer addition also called coacervation is an excellent technique for entrapment of water-soluble drugs. This technique involves suspending the drug (either solid crystals or aqueous solution) in an organic solution of polymer and subsequent phase separation by addition of a second miscible organic solvent in which polymer is miscible. Luteinizing hormone releasing hormone (LHRH) analogues have been entrapped using this technique. Various drugs that have been encapsulated using this technique include; nafarelin acetate [Sanders et al., 1984], oxytetracycline hydrochloride [Vidmar et al., 1984], sulphamethazole [Nakano et al., 1980], pilocarpine hydrochloride [Vidmar et al., 1985] etc.

Spray drying

In principle, the biodegradable polyester is dissolved in a volatile organic solvent, such as dichloromethane or acetone, the drug in solid form is dispersed in polymer solution by high-speed homogenization, and this dispersion is atomized in stream of heated air. From the droplets formed, the solvent evaporates instantaneously yielding microspheres in typical size ranges from 1 to 100 microns depending upon atomizing conditions. The microspheres are collected from air stream by a cyclone separator. Residual solvents are removed by vacuum drying. The process can be operated under aseptic conditions, and in closed loop configurations. Spray drying in a nitrogen atmosphere is technically feasible. Important advantages of this technique over other encapsulation techniques are proven reproducibility, well defined control of particle size, control of drug release properties of resulting microspheres and process is quite tolerant to small changes of polymer specifications. The disadvantages include high capital investment; encapsulation of proteins using this technique requires lyophilization of protein before dispersion and homogenization in organic polymer solution. These processing conditions are likely to induce aggregation and denaturation to sensitive proteins and antigens, so, stability of microencapsulated proteins during processing, release and storage becomes a major concern. Examples of drug encapsulated using this technique include Tetracycline HCl [Bittner, et al., 1999], and Diazepam [Guinchedi, et al., 1998].

Interfacial deposition

This technique was reported by Uno et al. 1984 in preparing ethyl cellulose and polystyrene microspheres containing water. Makino, et al., 1985 also prepared drug free microspheres of L-PLA and DL-PLA to study the degradation of these polymers. They emulsified *n*-heptane in aqueous Pluronic F68 solution (emulsifier) to yield an o/w emulsion. On addition of polymer solution in dichloromethane, the polymer precipitated at the surface of *n*-heptane droplets and concomitant removal of organic solvent resulted in microspheres. It is difficult to encapsulate water-soluble compounds by this method as partitioning of core with the aqueous continuum occurs. However, water insoluble compounds may be encapsulated using this method.

In situ polymerization

Speiser & Hinjsbroek [1992] patented this process for the preparation of PLA microspheres. A mixture of lactide and estrone was added to dried and degreased silicone oil and heated at 130°C to melt the lactide, and estrone was allowed to dissolve in the melted lactide. After dispersion diethyl tin was added as a catalyst, to induce polymerization. Reaction was allowed to proceed for 5 minutes. Estrone, embedded in PLA matrix was separated by centrifugation. Their technique produced microspheres from 100 to 1000 μm size. In this technique, degree of polymerization is difficult to control in the presence of the drug.

Chemical and thermal cross-linking

A cross-linking process prepares microspheres made from natural polymers. Polymers include chitosan, gelatin, albumin, starch and dextran. A w/o emulsion is prepared, where the water phase is a solution of polymer containing drug. Oil phase is suitable vegetable oil or oil-organic solvent mixture containing an oil-soluble emulsifier. Once w/o emulsion is formed, water-soluble polymer is solidified by thermal/ chemical cross-linking e.g. glutaraldehyde forms stable chemical cross-links as in albumin. If a chemical or heat process is used to cross-link the protein, the amount of chemical and the period and intensity of heating are critical in determining the release rates and swelling properties of the microspheres. If glutaraldehyde is the cross-linking agent, residual amounts can have toxic effects.

Hot melt microencapsulation

This process was developed in 1970's for photographic applications. In this process the melted polymer is mixed with drug, which can be encapsulated as solid or liquid particles. The mixture is then suspended in a immiscible solvent that is heated 5°C above the melting point of the polymer and stirred continuously. Once the emulsion is stabilized, it is cooled until the core material has solidified. The solvents used in this process could be silicon oil and olive oil. The low solubility of various drugs in these organic solvents makes them effective. In general, the drug particle size should be less than 50 μm. Using drugs with small particle sizes was found to improve the drug distribution within microspheres. After cooling, the microspheres

are washed by decantation with petroleum ether to give a free flowing powder. This micro-encapsulation procedure is reproducible with respect to yield and size distribution, but the disadvantage of this approach is the moderate temperatures to which the drug must be exposed. Synthesising polymers with lower melting points can overcome this problem. This can be achieved by changes in the backbone of the polymer. Polyanhydride microspheres have been prepared using this method.

Characterization of microspheres

Microspheres are very delicate systems. They have a distinct microstructure that depends strongly on the manufacturing conditions [Schugens, et al., 1994]. The microstructure, in return, affects the stability of drugs and drug release. The careful microstructural characterization of microspheres, therefore, enables us to solve problems in which drug release and drug stability issues are involved. The various physico-chemical methods by which microspheres might be characterized are as follows:

Particle size analysis

Particle size is an important variable affecting parameters like rates of dissolution and drug release, injectability and dose delivery. The most widely used methods include microscopy, coulter analysis and laser light scattering methods. In some cases, where particle size is very less, photon correlation spectroscopy is also used.

Examination of particles by optical micro-scopy is time-consuming method for measuring particles. Optical microscopy is most often used for particles between 3 and 150 μ. Three major statistically acceptable measures of size in optical microscopy are Martin's diameter, Feret's diameter and Projected area diameter. Another limitation of optical microscopy is the small depth of focus, i.e. for wide size distributions, only some particles in a particular view will be visible at any one time.

The electrical sensing zone method, also known as the Coulter technique, was presented in 1956 as an automatic method for counting and sizing blood cells and was soon applied to many kinds of particulate materials [Miller, et al., 2005]. A coulter counter can count and size thousands of particles in a few seconds. The large number of particles analysed, often may be thousands, greatly improves the accuracy of a number-based distribution, and also improves the accuracy when data are converted to a volume distribution. Care must be taken to control the concentration of suspended particles, as passage of two particles through the orifice at roughly the same time, leads to oversizing and it becomes significant at higher concentrations.

Instruments that use light scattering principles for particle size analysis have become popular because they allow quick and absolute determination of particle size, i.e. without the need for calibration. Although, all of these approaches use a laser to measure particle size, there are really three major light scattering methods, each based on different principles. These are Static Light Scattering (SLS), Laser Diffraction and Dynamic Light Scattering (DLS) [Bodner, et al., 2005]. The first two are sometimes referred to as total intensity light scattering (TILS) methods [Aboofazeli, et al., 2000] and use time averaged measurements of scattered light flux, whereas DLS measure fluctuations in the intensity of scattered light and relate them to size-dependent parameters such as diffusion coefficients. Broad particle size distributions of 0.1–1000 µm can easily be measured with instruments based on laser diffraction principles. All these methods require dilute concentrations where interactions between particles and secondary scattering are minimized, although, this must be balanced against the requirement for enough sample to obtain a sufficient signal to noise ratio.

Surface analysis

Surface characterization of microspheres provides important information about microstructure, topography, texture, porosity, physical state, nature of diffusion barriers, biocompatibility, erosion, etc.

Scanning Electron Microscopy (SEM) is one of the standard techniques for microsphere surface characterization with a much higher resolution. SEM allows investigation of microsphere surfaces, texture and morphology of fractured or sectioned surfaces. The modern SEM has a resolution of 3 nm and provides magnifications ranging from less than 30-fold to 300,000-fold. Tremendous versatility of this method is its biggest advantage over other techniques.

Electron Spectroscopy for Chemical Analysis (ESCA) is another technique, which allows investigation of the surface chemistry of microspheres. It is possible to determine atomic composition, within a few nanometers of a material surface. This can be used effectively for the investigation of degradable polymer surfaces.

The degradation of polymers can be investigated using Fourier-transformed infrared (FTIR) spectroscopy by following the changing IR signals that are obtained from degrading polymers. ATR (Attenuated total reflectance)-FTIR spectroscopy yields valuable information on the surface composition of microspheres depending on the manufacturing procedure as well as on the degradation processes.

Surface charge analysis is determined by microelectrophoresis. Surface charge provides important information regarding microsphere aggregation [Labhasetwar & Dorle, 1991]. Surface charge is an important parameter with respect to the interaction of microspheres within the body. Following intravenous injection, microspheres can be taken up by the macrophage or monocyte cells present in the plasma; surface charge is one of the parameters that determine whether this takes place [Tabata & Ikada, 1988].

Thermal analysis

A large number of techniques, which are available for collecting information necessary for preformulation and formulation of microspheres, are: differential thermal analysis (DTA), differential scanning calorimetry (DSC), modulated differential scanning calorimetry (MDSC), thermogravimetric analysis (TGA), isoperibol calorimetry and heat conduction calorimetry. Out of all these DSC has been one of the most widely used calorimetric techniques for the determination of various thermal parameters, which allow a better understanding of drug-polymer interactions, drug excipient interactions and thermal denaturation of polymers. DSC measures the heat capacity of the system as a function of temperature. Following the change in heat capacity of the sample as a function of temperature, allows for the detection of phase transitions of various orders.

Release studies

The release from the microspheres is dependent both on diffusion through the polymer matrix and on polymer degradation. If during the desired release time, polymer degradation is considerable, then the release rate may be unpredictable and erratic due to breakdown of microspheres. However, the release of core material from such systems is dependent on diffusivity through the polymer barrier, solubility of core in bulk phase, size of drug molecule and distribution of core throughout the matrix etc. Nature of polymer plays a major role in release process. Route of administration of injectable microspheres may also alter the duration of release. Release from PLA (polylactic acid) and PLGA (polylactic-glycolic acid) is dependent both on diffusion and polymer degradation [Johnson et al., 1996]. Theoretically, release from biodegradable microspheres has been classified into 4 different categories.

Degradation controlled monolithic system

Here the drug is strongly attached to the polymer matrix and is released only on degradation of the matrix. Diffusion is slow as compared to degradation, which can be homogeneous/ heterogeneous. In case of heterogeneous degradation, release from sphere is governed by the equation:

$$\frac{M_t}{M_\infty} = 1 - \left[\left(1 - \left[\frac{t}{t_\infty}\right]\right)\right]^3$$

where M_t is amount of agent released at time t, M_∞ is the amount of agent released at infinite time, and t and t_∞ are times for erosion.

Release from PLA and PLGA is dependent both on diffusion and polymer degradation. The possible mechanisms of release are: initial release from microsphere surface, release through the pores, diffusion through the intact polymer barrier, diffusion through a water swollen barrier and polymer erosion, and bulk degradation. All these mechanisms together play a part in release process. Nature of core also influences release kinetics either by increasing polymer degradation or by physically binding with the polymer chain. Drug polymer interaction leads to decreased release. Additives such as plasticizers decrease Tg, which leads to increased diffusion rates.

Diffusion controlled monolithic system

Diffusion of drug is prominent as compared to degradation of the polymer matrix. Degradation of the polymer matrix affects the rate of release. Rate of release also depends on whether the polymer degrades by homogeneous or heterogeneous mechanisms.

Diffusion controlled reservoir system

In this case, the drug diffuses through the rate controlling membrane and the membrane erodes only after complete delivery. Drug release is unaffected by degradation of matrix.

Erodible polyagent system

Here the active agent is chemically attached to the matrix and rate of biodegradation of matrix is slow as compared to rate of hydrolysis of drug polymer bond.

Applications of microencapsulation

Although, most of the current applications that have been realized using encapsulation are undoubtedly useful, they do not directly address the field of human health insofar as life-threatening conditions are concerned. Encapsulation has been used for decades for vitamins and other drugs, but nowadays encapsulation is used for efficient and prolonged delivery of many drugs. Various microencapsulated depot based products currently in market (Rxlist.com) include:

Decapeptyl® (Ipsen-Beaufour/Ferring)

It is a triptorelin sustained-release preparation based on lactide/glycolide microspheres for monthly intramuscular administration developed by Debio R.P. (Valais, Switzerland). After injection, an initial plasma peak is observed during 3 hours, and then triptorelin plasma levels decrease and remain stable at a plateau for 28 days. This preparation developed by Debio R.P. was the first sustained-release formulation of LHRH agonist allowing continuous release of the drug over 30 days. This was the first injectable, long-acting microparticle product on the market.

Lupron Depot® (TAP)

Lupron Depot belongs to a class of drugs called gonadotropin-releasing hormone (GnRH) agonists. It contains luprorelin in injectable microsphere form. It is used to decrease the body's production of specific hormones, natural chemicals that influence the behavior of certain cells. Because Lupron Depot can reduce the production of both male and female hormones, it is used to treat specific conditions in men,

women, and children. Lupron Depot is indicated for treatment of advanced prostate cancer. Doses are available as 1-, 3-, and 4-month products. Lupron Depot (-4 month 30 mg, -3 month 22.5 mg, and -1 month 7.5 mg) is indicated for the palliative treatment of advanced prostate cancer.

Suprecur®MP (Aventis)

It is a controlled release microsphere formulation of buserelin (GnRH analogue), which enables a long lasting suppression of pituitary and gonad function with one monthly subcutaneous injection. Suprecur® MP launched in February 1999, improves endometriosis, shrinkage of uterine leiomyoma and alleviation of symptoms linked with uterine leiomyoma: hypermenorrhea, lower abdominal pain, back pain, anemia.

Sandostatin LAR® Depot (Novartis)

Sandostatin LAR® Depot (octreotide acetate for injectable suspension) is a long acting dosage form consisting of microspheres of bio-degradable glucose star polymer, D,L-lactic and glycolic acids copolymer, containing octreotide. It is a long-acting octapeptide with pharma-cological properties mimicking those of the natural hormone somatostatin.

Nutropin Depot® (Genentech)

Nutropin Depot consists of thousands of micro-spheres made of a substance commonly found in medical products such as the "thread" used for dissolvable stitches. Each of these microspheres contains molecules of GH. Once Nutropin Depot suspension is injected under the skin (sub-cutaneously), its microspheres degrade, releasing the GH into the body in 2 phases—this is known as biphasic release. Nutropin Depot is the only GH available for patients who prefer the convenience of once- or twice-a-month dosing.

Trelstar™ Depot (Pfizer)

Trelstar™ Depot is a sterile, lyophilized bio-degradable microsphere formulation supplied as a single-dose vial containing triptorelin pamoate as the peptide base, poly-d,l-lactide-co-glycolide, mannitol, carboxymethylcellulose and sodium polysorbate 80. The recommended dose of Trelstar™ Depot is 3.75 mg incorporated in a depot formulation and is administered monthly as a single intramuscular injection.

Somatuline® LA (Ipsen-Beaufour)

Somatuline LA is a prolonged release microsphere based formulation of lanreotide. Lanreotide is an octapeptide, an analogue of a naturally occurring hormone, somatostatin. Lanreotide lowers the levels of hormones in the body such as GH (growth hormone) and IGF-1 (insulin-like growth factor-1) and inhibits some digestive hormones and intestinal secretions. Somatuline LA, a long acting formulation controls plasma GH levels for up to 14 days and improves acromegaly symptoms, and hence improves patient compliance and quality of life.

Boniva® (Ibandronate sodium)

Boniva® (Roche) is a nitrogen-containing bisphosphonate that inhibits osteoclast-mediated bone resorption [DeLuca et al., 2010], used for the treatment of osteoporosis in postmenopausal women. It is available as ready-to-use solution in a prefilled syringe that delivers 3.375 mg of Ibandronate monosodium salt monohydrate in 3 mL of solution, equivalent to a dose of 3 mg Ibandronate free acid. The recommended dose is 3 mg every 3 months administered intravenously only, over a period of 15 to 30 seconds.

Vitrasert® (Bausch and Lomb)

The Vitrasert Implant contains the antiviral drug ganciclovir [DeLuca, et al., 2010]. Each Vitrasert Implant contains a ganciclovir tablet which contains the inactive ingredient, magnesium stearate (0.25%). Each tablet is coated with polyvinyl alcohol and ethylene vinyl acetate polymers. It is indicated for the treatment of cytomegalovirus (CMV) retinitis in patients with acquired immunodeficiency syndrome (AIDS). This implant contains a minimum of 4.5 mg of ganciclovir, and is designed to release the drug over a 5 to 8 month period of time.

Ozurdex® (Allergan)

Ozurdex® is an intravitreal implant containing 0.7 mg (700 mcg) dexamethasone in the Novadur® solid polymer sustained-release drug delivery system. Ozurdex® is preloaded into a single-use, DDS® applicator to facilitate injection of the rod-shaped implant directly into the vitreous. The Novadur® system contains poly (D,L-lactide-co-glycolide) PLGA intravitreal polymer matrix without a preservative. It is indicated for the treatment of macular edema.

Risperdal® Consta™ (Johnson & Johnson)

Risperdal® Consta™ is the most recently approved depot formulation. It was approved in the US on October 29, 2003. Risperidone is micro-encapsulated in 75:25 polylactide-co-glycolide (PLG) at a concentration of 381 mg risperidone per gram of microspheres. This is an injectable, microparticle formulation that provides a 2-week release of the antipsychotic risperidone. It is indicated for the treatment of schizophrenia.

Zoladex® (AstraZeneca)

Zoladex® (goserelin acetate implant) is a GnRH agonist. It is indicated in the palliative treatment of advanced carcinoma of the prostate and for the management of endometriosis (DeLuca, et al, 2010). Goserelin acetate is dispersed in a matrix of D,L-lactic and glycolic acids copolymer (13.3–14.3 mg/dose) containing less than 2.5% acetic acid and up to 12% goserelin-related substances and presented as a sterile, white to cream colored 1-mm diameter cylinder, preloaded in a special single use syringe with a 16-gauge × 36 +/− 0.5 mm siliconized needle with protective needle sleeve (SafeSystem™ Syringe) in a sealed, light- and moisture-proof, aluminum foil laminate pouch containing a desiccant capsule. Zoladex, at a dose of 3.6 mg, should be administered subcutaneously every 28 days into the anterior abdominal wall.

REFERENCES

- Aboofazeli, R., Barlow, D., Lawrence, M.J. (2000). Particle size analysis of concentrated phospholipid microemulsions II. Photon correlation spectroscopy. *AAPS Pharm. Sci.*, 2, E19.
- Alpers, W.C. (1896). Gelatine capsules. *Am. J. Pharm.*, 68, 481–494.
- Anon (1835–36). Gelatine capsules. In report on article by Cottereau, Traite de pharmacologie, *Am. J. Pharm.*, 1, 351–352.
- Arica, B., Kas, H.S., Orman, M.N., Hincal, A.A. (2002). Biodegradable bromocriptine mesylate microspheres prepared by a solvent evaporation technique. I: Evaluation of formulation variables on microspheres characteristics for brain delivery. *J. Microencapsul.*, 19, 473–484.
- Augsburger, L.L. (1995). Hard and Soft Gelatin Capsules. *In:* **Modern Pharmaceutics**. Banker G., Rhodes C.T. (editors). Marcel Dekker Inc., New York, 3rd ed.
- Bastami, S.M., Groves, M.J. (1978). Some factors influencing the *in vitro* release of phenytoin from formulations. *Int. J. Pharm.*, 1, 151.
- Beck, L.R., Cowsar, D.R., Lewis, D.H., Gibson, J.W., Flowers, C.E. (1979a). New long-acting injectable microcapsule contraceptive system. *Am. J. Obst. Gyne.*, 135, 419–426.
- Beck, L.R., Cowsar, D.R., Lewis, D.H., Cosknowe, R.J., Riddel, C.T., Lowry, S.L., Epperly, T. (1979). A new long-acting microcapsule system for administration of progesterone. *Fertilisation and Sterility*, 31, 545–551.
- Bell, J.H., Stevenson, N.A., Taylor, J.E. (1973). A moisture transfer effect in hard gelatin capsules of sodium cromoglycate. *J. Pharm. Pharmacol.*, 25 (Suppl.), 96P.
- Bittner, B., Mader, K., Kroll, C., Borchert, H., Kissel, T. (1999). Tetracycline-HCl loaded poly (Dl-lactide-co-glycolide) microspheres prepared by a spray drying technique: Influence of gamma irradiation on radical formation and polymer degradation. *J. Control. Rel.*, 59, 23–32.
- Bodmeier, R., McGinity, J.W. (1987). Poly(lactic acid) microspheres containing quinidine base and quinidine sulphate prepared by solvent evaporation technique. II. Some process parameters influencing the preparation and properties of microspheres. *J. Microencap.*, 4, 289–297.
- Bodnar, M., Hartmann, J.F., Borbely, J. (2005). Preparation and characterization of chitosan-based nanoparticles. *Biomacromolecules*, 6, 2521–2527.
- Borgstrom, L. (2005). An *in vivo* and *in vitro* comparison of two powder inhalers following storage at hot/humid conditions. *J. Aerosol. Med.*, 18(3), 304–310.
- Botzolakis, J.E., Small, L.E., Augsburger, L.L. (1982). Effect of disintegrants on drug dissolution from capsules filled on a dosator-type automatic capsule-filling machine. *Int. J. Pharm.*, 12, 341.
- Catlapalli, R., Rohera, B.D. (1998). Physical characteristics of HPMC and HEC and investigation of their use as pelletization aids. *Int. J. of Pharm.*, 179–193.
- Cavalier, M., Benoit, J.P., Thies, C. (1986). The formation and characterization of hydrocortisone loaded poly(D,L-lactide) microspheres. *J. Pharm. Pharmacol.*, 38, 249–253.
- Chandy, T., Wilson, R.F., Rao, G. H., Das, G.S. (2002). Changes in cisplatin delivery due to surface-coated poly(lactic acid)-poly(epsilon-caprolactone) microspheres. *J. Biomater. Appl.*, 16, 275–291.
- Coles, G.C. (1987). The Mechanical Operations of Filling Hard Capsules. *In:* **Hard Capsules**. Ridgway, K. (editor). Development and Technology, London: Pharmaceutical Press, 92–103.
- Deasy, P.B. (1979). Microencapsulation Processing and Technology. *In:* Ade Van Valkenburg, J. (editor). Marcel Dekker Inc., New York, 361.
- DeLuca, P.P., Mansour, H., Rhee, Y.S., Park, C.W. (2010). Sustained-release injectable drug delivery. *Pharm. Tech.*, 11, 16–22.
- Desai, S.J., Simonelli, A.P. and Higuchi, W.I. (1965). Investigation of factors influencing release of solid drug dispersed in inert matrices. *J. Pharm. Sci.*, 54, 1459–1464.
- Diwan, M., Park, T.G. (2003). Stabilization of recombinant interferon alpha by pegylation for encapsulation in PLGA microspheres. *Int. J. Pharm.*, 252, 111–122.
- Edwards, D. (2010). Applications of capsule dosing techniques for use in dry powder inhalers. *Ther. Del.*, 1, 195–201.
- Ellis, D.N., Tipton, A.J. (1994). Influence of injection rate on tensile strength and molecular weight of moulded poly(L-lactide) test pieces.

Transactions of 20th Annual Meeting of the Society for Biomaterials (Boston, Massachusetts). Abst. 17.

- English, J.P., Lawler, T.E., Tipton, A.J., Dunn, R.L. (1985). Properties of lactide/caprolactone copolymers and polyblends. *Transactions of the 11th Annual Meeting of the Society of Bio-materials: San Diego, California,* Abst. 8.
- FAO/WHO (1984). Specifications for Identity and Purity of Food Colors. *Joint Expert Committee on Food Additives, FAO Food and Nutrition Paper.* 31 (1), 200.
- Folkman, J., Long, D.M. (1964). The use of silicone rubber as a carrier for prolonged drug therapy. *J. Surg. Res.,* 4, 139–142.
- Fu, K., Griebenow, K., Hsieh, L., Klibanov, A.M., Langer, R. (1999). FTIR characterization of the secondary structure of proteins encapsulated within PLGA microspheres. *J. Control. Rel.,* 58, 357–66.
- Giunchedi, P., Conti, B., Scalia, S., Conte, U. (1998). *In vitro* degradation study of polyester microspheres by a new HPLC method for monomer release determination. *J. Control. Rel.,* 56, 53–62.
- Reddy, G., Muthukumaran, R., Krishnamoorthy, B. (2013). Soft gelatin capsules – Present and future prospective as a pharmaceutical dosage forms – A Review. *Int. J. Adv. Pharm. Gen. Res.,* 1(1), 20–29.
- Hermann, J., Bodmeier, R. (1995). The effect of particle microstructure on the somatostatin release from poly(lactide) microspheres prepared by a W/O/W solvent evaporation method. *J. Control. Rel.,* 36, 63–71.
- Hilbert, A.K., Fritzsche, U., Kissel, T. (1999). Biodegradable microspheres containing influenza-A vaccine: Immune response in mice. *Vaccine,* 17, 1065–73.
- http://qualicaps.com/pharmaceutical-equipment/capsule-filling-machine/
- http://www.capsugel.com/ihc/dry-powder-inhaler-capsules
- http://www.capsugel.com/media/library/ConiSnap_brochure_full.pdf
- http://www.marketsandmarkets.com/Market-Reports/empty-capsules-market-218018190. html. (2014) 'Empty Capsules Market by Product (Hard gelatin, Non-gelatin capsules), Raw Material (Pig meat, Bovine, HPMC), Therapeutic Application (Antibiotics, Vitamins) & by End User (Pharmaceutical, Health Supplements) - Global Forecast to 2019.' marketsandmarkets.com. Report Code: PH 2935.
- http://www.penglaichina.com/capsule-filling-machine-GMP-pharma.html
- http://www.schaefer-technologies.net/capsule_filling_machines/model_10/default. htm
- Hutchison, K.G., Ferdinando, J. Soft Gelatin Capsules. *In:* Aulton, M.E. (editor) **Aulton's Pharmaceutics: The Design and Manufacture of Medicines**, 3rd edition., Elsevier. 527–538.
- Incompatibilities in prescriptions IV. (1940) The use of inert powders in capsules to prevent liquefaction due to deliquescence. *J. Am. Pharm. Assoc.* (Sci. Ed.), 29, 136.
- Ito, K.S., Kaga, I., Takeya, Y. (1969). Studies on hard gelatin capsules I. Water vapor transfer between capsules and powders. *Chem. Pharm. Bull.,* 17, 1134.
- John, G.W., Stuart, L. (1960). Enteric coatings III. An improved enteric coating and its *in vitro* evaluation. *J. Am. Pharm. Assoc.,* 49(3), 121–127.
- Johnson, O.L., Cleland, J.L., Lee, H.J., Charnis, M., Duenas, E., Jaworowicz, W., Shepard, D., Shahzamani, A., Jones, A.J., Putney, S.D. (1996). A month long effect from a single injection of microencapsulated human growth hormone. *Nat. Med.,* 2, 795–799.
- Jolliffe, I.G., Newton, J.M., Walters, J.K. (1979). A theoretical approach to optimizing capsule filling by a dosator nozzle. *J. Pharm. Pharmacol.,* 31(Suppl), 70.
- Jones, B.E (2007). Hard Gelatin Capsules. *In:* Aulton, M.E. (editor) **Aulton's Pharmaceutics: The Design and Manufacture of Medicines**, 3rd edition, Elsevier, 515–527.
- Jones, B.E. (1987). The History of the Gelatin Capsules. *In:* **Hard Capsules**, Ridgway K. (editor). Development and Technology, London: Pharmaceutical Press, 1–13.
- Jones, B.E. (1998). New thoughts on capsule filling. *S.T.P. Pharma Sci.,* 8, 277–283.
- Juni, K., Ogata, J., Nakano, M., Ichihara, T., Mori, K., Akagi, M. (1985). Preparation and evaluation *in vitro* and *in vivo* of poly(lactic acid) micro-spheres containing doxorubicin. *Chem. Pharm. Bull.,* 33, 313–318.

- Kontny, M.J. and Mulski, C.A. (1989). Gelatin capsule brittleness as a function of relative humidity at room temperature. *Int. J. Pharm.*, 54, 79.
- Kulkarni, R.K., Pani, K.C., Mewman, C., Leonard, F. (1966). Polylactic acid for surgical implants. *Arch. Surg.*, 93, 839–43.
- Kumar, V., Lewis, S.A., Mutalik, S., Shenoy, D.B., Udupa, N. (2002). Biodegradable microspheres of curcumin for treatment of inflammation. *Ind. J. Physiol. Pharmacol.*, 46, 209–217.
- Kurihara, K., Ichikawa, I. (1978). Effect of powder flowability on capsule filling weight variation. *Chem. Pharm. Bull.*, 26, 1250.
- Labhasetwar, V.D., Dorle, A.K. (1991). A study on the zeta potential of microcapsules during ageing. *J. Microencapsul.*, 8, 83–85.
- Leel, H.B., Khang, G., Cho, J.C., Rhee, J.M., Lee, J.S. (1990). Near zero order release over 60 days from gentamycin sulfate-loaded PLGA microspheres for osteomyelitis treatment. *Proc. Int. Symp. Control. Rel. Bioact. Mater. Control. Rel. Soc. Inc.* Abst. 1088–90.
- Li, S., Vert, M. (1999). Biodegradable Polymers: Polyesters. *In:* Mathiowitz, E. (editor). **Encyclopedia of Controlled Drug Delivery**, John Wiley and Sons, Inc., New York. (1) 71–93.
- Makino, K., Arakawa, M., Kondo, T. (1985). Preparation and *in vitro* degradation properties of poly(lactide) microcapsules. *Chem. Pharm. Bull.*, 33, 1195–1201.
- Mason, N.S., Thies, C., Cicero, T.J. (1976). *In vitro* and *in vivo* evaluation of a microencapsulated narcotic antagonist. *J. Pharm. Sci.*, 65, 847–850.
- Miller, C.R., Vogel, R., Surawski, P.P., Jack, K.S., Corrie, S.R., Trau, M. (2005). Functionalized organosilica microspheres via a novel emulsion-based route. *Langmuir.*, 21, 9733–9740.
- Miller, R.A., Brady, J.M., Cutright, D.E. (1997). Degradation rates of oral resorbable implants (polylactates and polyglycolates): Rate modification with changes in PLA/PGA copolymers ratio. *J. Biomed. Mat. Res.*, 11, 711–719.
- Mohamad, H., Aiche, J.M., Renoux, R., Mougin, P., Kantelip, J.P. (1986). Etude De La Stabilite Biopharmaceutique Des Medicaments Application A Des Gelules De Chlorohydrate De Tetracycline IV. Etude Complimentaire *in vivo*. *STP Pharm. Sci.*, 3, 407.
- Mohamad, H., Renoux, R., Aiache, S., Aiache, J.M. (1986). Etude de La Stabilite Biopharmaceutique Des Medicaments Application A Des Gelules de Chlorohydrate de Tetracycline I. Etude *In Vitro*. *STP Pharma.*, 2, 531.
- Mohan, P., Ansari, A., Patel, S., Khinchi, M.P. (2013). A review on recent advancement in capsule formulation. *Am. J. PharmTech Res.*, 3 Suppl 1.
- Mony, C., Sambeat, C., Cousin, G. (1977). The measurement of compression during the formulation and filling of capsules. In: *Proceedings of the 1st International Conference on Pharmaceutical Technology, Paris.* 98–108.
- Murthy, K.S., Ghebre-Sellassie, I. (1993). Current perspectives on the dissolution stability of solid oral dosage forms. *J. Pharm. Sci.*, 82, 113.
- Murthy, K.S., Samyn, J.C. (1977). Effect of shear mixing on *in vitro* drug release of capsule formulations containing lubricants. *J. Pharm. Sci.*, 66, 1215.
- Murthy, K.S., Enders, N.A., Fawzi, M.B. (1989). Dissolution stability of hard-shell capsule products. Part I: The effect of exaggerated storage conditions. *Pharm. Technol.* 13(3), 72.
- Murthy, K.S.; Reisch, R.G. Jr., Fawzi, M.B. (1989). Dissolution stability of hard-shell capsule products. Part II: The effect of dissolution test conditions on *in vitro* drug release. *Pharm. Technol.*, 13(6), 53.
- Murthy, R.S.R. (1997). Biodegradable Polymers. *In:* Jain, N.K. (editor). **Controlled and Novel Drug Delivery**, CBS Publishers & Distributors, New Delhi, 27–51.
- Nakano, M., Itoh, M., Juni, K., Sekikawa, H., Arita, T. (1980). Sustained urinary excretion of sulphamethazole following oral administration of enteric coated microcapsules in humans. *Int. J. Pharm.*, 4, 291–298.
- Newton, J.M., Rowley, G., Torablom, J.F.V. (1971). The effect of additives on the release of drug from hard gelatin capsules. *J. Pharm. Pharmacol.*, 23, 452.
- Newton, J.M., Rowley, G., Tornblom, J.F.V. (1971a). Further studies on the effect of additives on the release of drug from hard gelatin capsules. *J. Pharm. Pharmacol.*, 23, 156S.
- Oe, S., Fukunaka, Y., Hirose, T., Yamaoka, Y., Tabata, Y. (2003). A trial on regeneration therapy of rat liver cirrhosis by controlled release of hepatocyte growth factor. *J. Control. Rel.*, 88, 193–200.

- Ogawa, Y., Yamamoto, M., Takada, S., Shimamoto, T. (1988). Controlled release of leuprolide acetate from polylactic acid or co-polymer ratio of polymer. *Chem. Pharm. Bull.*, 36, 1502–1507.
- Ogura, T., Furuya, Y., Matsuura, S. (1998). HPMC capsules: An alternative to gelatin. *Pharm. Tech. Eur.*, 11, 32–42.
- Prabhu, S., Sullivan, J.L., Betageri, G.V. (2002). Comparative assessment of *in vitro* release kinetics of calcitonin polypeptide from biodegradable microspheres. *Drug Deliv.*, 9, 195–198.
- Rabadiya, B. (2013). A review: Capsule shell material from gelatin to non-animal origin. *Int. J. Pham. Res. Bio. Sci.*, 2(3), 42–71.
- Richardson, M. (2011). Impact of capsule selection on formulation stability in dry powder inhalers (DPIs). *Inhalation*.
- Rxlist.com. http://www.rxlist.com/script/main/hp.asp (Last searched on Jan 2015).
- Samyn, J.C., Jung, W.Y. (1970). *In vitro* dissolution from several experimental capsules. *J. Pharm. Sci.*, 59, 169.
- Sanders, L.M., Kent, J.S., McRae, G.I., Vickery, B.H., Tice, T.R., Lewis, D.H. (1984). Controlled release of leutinizing hormone-releasing hormone analogue from poly(D,L-lactide-co-glycolide) microspheres. *J. Pharm Sci.*, 73, 1294–1297.
- Schlenz, C. (1897). Zur Geschichte der Gelatine Kapseln. *Apotheker-Zeitung*, Berlin. 34, 275–276.
- Schugens, C., Laruelle, N., Nihant, N., Grandfils, C., Jerome, R., Teyssie, P. Effect of emulsion stability on the morphology and porosity of semi-crystalline poly(l-lactide) microparticles prepared by W/O/W double emulsion-solvent evaporation. *J. Control. Rel.*, 32, 161–176.
- Schwier, J.R., Cooke, G.G., Hartauer, K.J., Rayon, L. Yu. (1993). A source of furfural—A reactive aldehyde capable of insolubilizing gelatin capsules. *Pharm. Technol.*, 17(5), 78.
- Scott, D., Shah, R., Augsburger, L.L. (1992). A comparative evaluation of the mechanical strength of sealed and unsealed hard gelatin capsules. *Int. J. Pharm.*, 84, 49.
- Shah, K.B., Augsburger, L.L., Small, L.E., Polli, G.P. (1983). Instrumentation of a dosing disc automatic capsule filling machine. *Pharm. Technol.*, 7(4), 42.
- Small, L.E., Augsburger, L.L. (1977). Instrumentation of an automatic capsule filling machine. *J. Pharm. Sci.*, 66, 504.
- Smith, A., Hunneyball, I.M. (1986). Evaluation of poly(lactic acid) as a biodegradable drug delivery system for parenteral administration. *Int. J. Pharm.*, 30, 215–220.
- Spieser, P., Hijnsbroek, R. Micropellets in bio-degradable carrier. **German Patent 2,824,112**.
- Stadler, L.B. (1959). The gelatin capsule. *J. Am. Pharm. Assoc. Pract. Pharm. Edn.* 20, 723–724.
- Stanley, J.P. (1986). Capsules II. Soft gelatin capsules. *In:* Lachman, L., Lieberman, H.A., Kanig, J.L. (Editors). **The Theory and Practice of Industrial Pharmacy**, 3rd ed. Lea and Febiger: Philadelphia. 404–420.
- Stewart, A.G., Grant, D.J.W., Newton, J.M. (1979). The release of a model low-dose drug (riboflavine) from hard gelatin capsule formulations. *J. Pharm. Pharmacol.*, 31, 1.
- Stoyle, L.E. (1966). Evaluation of the Zanasi automatic capsule machine. *Paper presented to the Industrial Pharmacy Section, A.Ph.A. 113th Annual Meeting*, Dallas, TX.
- Strickland, W.A. Jr., Moss, M. (1962). Water vapor sorption and diffusion through hard gelatin capsules. *J. Pharm. Sci.*, 51, 1002.
- Suzuki, K., Price, J.C. (1985). Microencapsulation and dissolution properties of neuroleptic in a biodegradable polymer, poly(d,l-lactide). *J. Pharm. Sci.*, 74, 21–24.
- Tabata, Y., Ikada, Y. (1988). Effect of the size and surface charge of polymer microspheres on their phagocytosis by macrophage. *Biomaterials*, 9, 356–362.
- **The International Pharmacopoeia**, 4th ed. (2013) – Capsules in General Monograph (http://www.who.int/medicines/publications/pharmacopoeia/en/).
- Vidmar, V., Pepeljnjak, S., Jalsenjak, I. (1985). The *in vivo* evaluation of poly(lactic acid) microcapsules of pilocarpine hydrochloride. *J. Microencapsul.*, 2, 289–292.
- Vidmar, V., Smolcic-Bubalo, A., Jalsenjak, I. (1984). Poly(lactic acid) microencapsulated oxytetracycline: *In vitro* and *in vivo* evaluation. *J. Microencapsul.*, 1, 131–136.
- Visscher, G.E., Robinson, R.L., Maulding, H.V., Fong, J.W., Pearson, J.E., Argentieri, G.J. (1985). Biodegradation of and tissue reaction to 50:50 poly(D,L-lactide-co-glycolide) microcapsules. *J. Biomed. Mat. Res.*, 19, 349–65.

- Wilkie, W. (1913). The manufacture of gelatin capsules. *Bull. Pharm.*, Detroit, 27, 382–384.
- York, P. (1975). Application of powder failure testing equipment in assessing effect of glidants on flowability of cohesive pharmaceutical powders. *J. Pharm. Sci.*, 64, 1216.
- York, P. (1980). Studies of the effect of powder moisture content on drug release from hard gelatin capsules. *Drug Dev. Ind. Pharm.*, 6, 605.
- Zographi, G., Grandolfi, G.P., Kontny, M.J., Mendenhall, D.W. (1988). Prediction of moisture transfer in mixtures of solids: Transfer via the vapor phase. *Int. J. Pharm.*, 42, 77.

5

Parenteral Formulations

K.C. Jindal, S.P. Boldhane and N.K. Jain

INTRODUCTION

Parenteral preparations are sterile products intended for administration by injection, infusion or implantation into the body. They may be preparations intended for direct parenteral administration or to be administered after constituting or diluting.

The term parenteral is derived from Greek word '*para*' meaning beside and '*enteron*' meaning the intestine. Thus, parenteral administration should include the administration of drugs by any route other than intestine. In pharmaceutical practice, however, parenteral preparations are considered to be those sterile drugs, solutions, suspensions or emulsions that are administered by hypodermic injection either directly or after constituting or diluting prior to administration.

Historically, Sir Christopher Wren in about 1657 injected drugs into the veins of living animals. In 1855 Dr. Alexander Wood of Edinburgh described the first subcutaneous injection of drugs for therapeutic purposes using a true hypodermic syringe. The importance of sterilizing both the syringe and the solution was realized by the 1890s. Injections were not official upto 1926 when for the first time 6 injections were included in NF V under the name 'Ampoules'. Subsequently, injections became official in many pharmacopoeias. IP 2014 includes more than 100 monographs on injections.

PARENTERAL ADMINISTRATION OF DRUGS – NECESSITY

Oral route is the most preferred route for drug administration, however, certain situations demand delivery of drugs through parenteral route like:

(a) For quick restoration of fluid and electrolyte imbalances in patients suffering from severe dehydration or electrolyte depletion for a variety of reasons (such as severe diarrhoea) and vomiting, electrolyte solutions are administered intravenously.

(b) Intravenous feeding of essential nutrients like necessary amino acids, glucose, minerals and vitamins for short and prolonged periods of time to patients who cannot eat e.g. during unconscious or coma states or who have undergone surgery of gastrointestinal tract.

(c) Administration of drugs to the uncooperative or uncontrollable patients, like the ones suffering from epileptic seizures, delirium or psychosis.

(d) To elicit desired local effect like local anesthetics for minor surgeries.

(e) In emergency conditions to get quick response, for example, the intravenous or direct.

(f) Cardiointraventricular routes may be desirable to achieve immediate effects in emergencies such as life-threatening hypotension, arrhythmias or bronchospasm.

(g) To ensure patient compliance, when the patient cannot be relied upon to self-medicate e.g. the use of long acting (monthly) intramuscular penicillins may be used to manage children prophylactically for rheumatic heart disease.

(h) To achieve adequate concentrations of the drug into diseased tissues e.g. intraventricular injection of aminoglycoside antibiotics in certain patients suffering from acute bacterial or fungal meningitis or ventriculitis.

(i) Administration of drugs which are poorly absorbed from the alimentary canal or degraded by gastric contents e.g. many peptides and proteins such as erythropoietin, insulin, human growth hormone etc.

ROUTES OF ADMINISTRATION FOR PARENTERALS

Intravenous

This route is most common. It has the advantages of quick response, absolute bioavailability, convenience of administering large volumes (up to 1 L) and convenience of dose titration against a physiological response. This route, however, is not suitable for suspensions, water-in-oil emulsions and oil-in-water emulsions having large droplet size.

Injection is administered directly into a prominent vein, normally in the forearm. These are usually aqueous solutions but may also be oil-in-water emulsions in which the droplet size is small and carefully controlled. Intravenous administration, however, bypasses protective mechanisms of the body, and the onset of adverse reactions, which may come about from many causes, can be as rapid as the beneficial effects.

Intramuscular

This route is convenient and common for small volumes. Absorption is relatively faster than subcutaneous but slower than intravenous route. Injection is administered into a muscle mass. A common site is the deltoid muscle of the upper arm into which as much as 2 mL volume may be injected. Larger volumes, up to 5 mL, may be administered into the gluteal medial muscle of each buttoc. Absorption of drug can be prolonged by administration of the drug as a suspension in an aqueous or oily vehicle.

Subcutaneous

This route is frequently used for local action e.g. the administration of local anaesthetics and it has the advantage that a relatively low dose of drug can be used to elicit a significant local response without large quantities of drug reaching the blood stream, thus avoiding the systemic adverse cardiac effects of some local anaesthetics. Injection volumes do not normally exceed 1 mL.

Injection is administered into the loose tissue immediately below the dermis layer of the skin. The most popular sites for subcutaneous injections are the arm and thigh. Absorption after subcutaneous administration is slower than that following intramuscular administration. Injections are normally aqueous solutions or suspensions.

Intradermal

This route is used for diagnostic test injections for allergy or immunity. A limited number of vaccines is also administered by this route.

Injection is injected into the skin between the epidermis and the dermis. This route is also referred to as the intracutaneous route. Injection volumes should not exceed 0.2 mL and 0.1 mL is the most common volume. Absorption from intradermal injections is prolonged with slow onset of drug action. Consequently, allergens used in diagnostic tests are taken into the blood very slowly in very small quantities, which are less likely to elicit a major allergenic response in the body. Thus, allergenic response is contained around the site of administration.

Intra-arterial

This route is sometimes used to target a particular organ, which the artery serves, for example, the heart.

Because of the large flow of blood through the arteries, the drug is rapidly diluted. This is an advantage in the administration of radio-opaque materials for diagnostic purposes, such as arteriograms.

Injection is administered directly into an artery. This route can be used to administer some cytotoxic drugs such as methotrexate. However, administration via the intra-arterial route can be hazardous and arterial spasm and subsequent gangrene can result. Intra-arterial injections must not contain bactericide.

Intra-cardiac

This route is used in emergencies only. Injections are administered directly into either the cardiac muscle or a ventricle. However, due to the growing success of intensive care for patients with coronary heart disease or cardiac arrest, the use of this route of administration is increasing. These injections are aqueous solution and must not contain a bactericide.

Intra-spinal

Injections are also aqueous solutions injected into particular areas of the spinal column. Volumes should not exceed 20 mL and solutions should not contain bactericides or antioxidants. They should be presented as single dose containers. In many instances there is a preference for ampoules that are sterilized in a transparent outer wrap that maintains the sterility of the external ampoule surfaces so as to ensure administration of contamination-free solution, since the spinal fluid contains no natural body defence mechanism. Intraspinal injections are further subdivided according to the area of the spinal cord into which the injections are administered, like intracisternal, epidural or peri-dural injections.

Local anaesthetics like Lidocaine, Bupivacaine, etc. for spinal injection are formulated at different specific gravities in order to target the portion of the spinal column where nerve block is required. The position at which the anaesthetic acts will depend on both the specific gravity of the solution and the positioning of the patient. Hypobaric solutions have a specific gravity lower than that of the cerebrospinal fluid and, thus, move upwards after administration. Isobaric solutions have approximately the same specific gravity as the cerebrospinal fluid and exert their effect at about the same level as the injection site. Hyperbaric solutions have a greater specific gravity than the cerebrospinal fluid and exert their effects at sites lower than the injection site.

Intra-articular

Injections are aqueous solutions or suspensions that are injected into the synovial fluid in a joint cavity.

Intrathecal

Injection into the subarachnoid space surrounding spinal cord, which contains cerebrospinal fluid.

Injections for ophthalmic use

This route is commonly used for the administration of local anaesthetics used in eye surgery. The injections are aqueous solutions or suspensions and the volume injected is generally small (not exceeding 1 mL). The most common ophthalmic injections are subconjunctival injections, which are administered beneath Tenon's capsule, close to the eye but not into it. Intracameral injections are administered into the anterior chamber, intravitreous injections into the vitreous humour, and retrobulbar injections into the posterior segment of the globe.

The use of antimicrobial preservatives is permissible in subconjunctival injections but not in intracameral or intravitreous injections. The inclusion of antioxidants should be avoided because of their irritant effects on the eye.

Other routes

These include intraperitoneal (into the peritoneum), intra-amniotic (into the amniotic fluid) intralymphatic (into the lymph), intraureteral (into the uretra) and intrapleural (into the pleural cavity) intracisternal (the cistern containing cerebrospinal fluid, peridural (between the duramater and inner aspects of the vertebrae, intrasynovial (into a joint fluid area) etc.

Intramammary

This route is used in mammal animals. The drug solution or suspension is administered into the mammary gland through the teat canal.

CATEGORIES OF PARENTERAL PRODUCTS BASED ON VOLUME

Sterile preparations are classified into two major categories:

A. Small volume parenterals

The term small volume parenteral (SVP) has been officially defined by the United States Pharmacopeia (USP, 2004) as "… an injection that is packaged in containers labelled as containing 100 mL or less."

The USP categorizes sterile preparations for parenteral use according to the physical state of the product as follows:

(a) [Drug] Injection: Liquid preparations that are drug substances or solutions thereof

(b) [Drug] for Injection: Dry solids that, upon addition of suitable vehicles, yield solutions conforming in all respects to requirements for injections

(c) [Drug] Injectable Emulsion: Liquid preparations of the drug substances dissolved or dispersed in a suitable emulsion medium.

(d) [Drug] Injectable Suspension: Liquid preparations of solids suspended in suitable liquid medium.

(e) [Drug] Injectable Suspension: Dry solids that, upon the addition of suitable vehicles, yield preparations conforming in all respects to the requirements for injectable suspensions.

B. Large volume parenterals

The USP defines the large volume parenterals (LVPs) as "single dose injection that is intended for intravenous use and is packaged in containers labelled as containing 100 mL or more." (USP, 2004). The FDA has adopted broader definition to include:

"A terminally sterilized aqueous drug product packaged in a single-dose container with a capacity of 100 mL or more and intended to be administered or used in man. It includes intravenous infusions, irrigating solutions, peritoneal dialysates and blood collecting units with anticoagulant.

Large volume parenterals are used for following purposes:

(a) Supply the water, electrolytes, and simple carbohydrates needed by the body.

(b) Act as the vehicle for infusion of drugs that are compatible in the solution.

(c) Supply nutritional requirements when the nutrients cannot be taken orally e.g. fat emulsions and amino acid preparations.

(d) Provide solutions to correct acid-base balance in the body.

(e) Act as plasma expanders.

(f) Promote diuresis when the body is retaining fluids.

(g) Act as dialyzing agents in patients with impaired kidney function.

(h) Act as x-ray contrast agents to improve diagnostic abilities.

(i) Specialized solutions for renal support, hepatic support, and the newborn.

When a patient is admitted to a hospital, generally, large volume parenteral, often dextrose and electrolytes, are infused shortly after admission to the hospital. Besides providing fluids and electrolytes to achieve an optimum balance for further treatment, this is to provide a readily accessible link to the venous systems if additional medications are required.

FORMULATION ADDITIVES

Excipients used in the parenteral preparations must be non-pyrogenic, non-toxic, non-haemolytic and non-irritating, should be physically and chemically compatible with active ingredient(s), must not interfere with the therapeutic effect of the active ingredient(s), must maintain stability during sterilization and during the shelf-life of the product, should be effective at low concentration and should be acceptable from a regulatory point of view. Every additive to a formulation must be justified by a clear purpose and function. International regulatory requirements should be considered for products intended for international marketing. Such stringent requirements limit the actual number of parenterally acceptable formulation additives used in parenteral suspensions, and most formulations contain relatively few ingredients. Any additive to a formulation must be justified by a clear purpose and function.

Added substances such as antioxidants, buffers, bulking agents, chelating agents, anti-microbial agents, solubilizing agents, surfactants, and tonicity adjusting agents are incorporated into parenteral formulae in order to provide safe, efficacious, and elegant parenteral dosage forms.

Pharmacopeias often specify the type and amount of additive substances that may be included in injectable products. These requirements often vary from compendia to compendia, so, it is important to refer to the specific pharmacopeia that applies to the product in question. Two examples are sulfites and chelating agents. The USP allows the use of up to 3.2 mg of sodium bisulfite per mL of solution, whereas the French Pharmacopeia allows only 1.6 mg per mL.

Vehicles for parenterals

Solvent systems used in parenteral formulation are classified as either aqueous or nonaqueous vehicles. Choice of a typical solvent system depends on solubility, stability, and the desired release characteristics of the drug. Nonaqueous vehicles include both water miscible and water-immiscible vehicles.

Aqueous vehicles

The most frequently used solvent in the large-scale manufacture of injections is Water for Injection (WFI). This water is purified by distillation or by reverse osmosis and may not contain added substances. Although, water for injection is not required to be sterile, it must be pyrogen free. Water for injection should be stored in tight containers at temperatures below or above the range in which microbial growth occurs. Water for injection should be used within 24 hours following its collection. The water should be collected in sterile and pyrogen-free containers and frequently tested to assure that it is of quality as specified in official compendia.

Sterile Water for Injection (SWFI)

It is Water for Injection, which has been sterilized and packaged in single dose containers of not greater than 1.0 L, it must be pyrogen free and may not contain an antimicrobial agent or other added substance. This water should be used as a solvent, vehicle or diluent for already sterilized and packaged injectable medications.

Bacteriostatic Water for Injection (BWFI)

It is Sterile Water for Injection containing one or more suitable antimicrobial agents. It is packaged in prefilled syringes or in vials containing not more than 30 mL of the water. The container label must state the name and proportion of the antimicrobial agent(s) present. The presence of the bacteriostatic agent gives the flexibility for multiple-dose vials. If the first person to withdraw medication inadvertently contaminates the vial contents, the preservative will destroy the microorganism. Because of the presence of antimicrobial agents the bacteriostatic water must only be used in parenterals that are administered in small volumes. Its use in parenterals administered in large volume is restricted due to the excessive and perhaps toxic amounts of the antimicrobial agents, which would be injected along with the medication. Generally, if volumes of greater than 5 mL of solvent are required, sterile water for injection rather than bacteriostatic water for injection is preferred. While using bacteriostatic water for injection the chemical compatibility of the bacteriostatic agent(s) present with the drug product being dissolved or suspended should be duly considered.

Sodium chloride injection

It is a sterile isotonic solution of sodium chloride in Water for Injection. It contains no anti-microbial agents. The sodium and chloride ion contents of the injection are approximately 154 mEq of each per litre. The solution may be used as a sterile vehicle in preparing solutions or suspensions of drugs for parenteral adminis-tration.

Bacteriostatic sodium chloride injection

It is a sterile isotonic solution of sodium chloride in Water for Injection, containing one or more suitable antimicrobial agents. When this solution is used as a vehicle, care must be exercised to assure the compatibility of the added medicinal agent with the preservative(s) present as well as with the sodium chloride. The relative tonicity of preservative should be considered. Further, USP specifies that the label state, "Not for Use in Newborns." This labelling statement was the result of problems encountered with neonates and the toxicity of the bacteriostat, i.e., benzyl alcohol. This toxicity may result from the high cumulative amounts (mg/kg) of benzyl alcohol and the limited detoxification capacity of the neonate liver. This solution has not been reported to cause problems in older infants, children, or adults.

Ringer's injection

It is a sterile solution of sodium chloride, potassium chloride, and calcium chloride in Water for Injection. The three agents are present in concentrations similar to that found in physiologic fluids. The solution is employed as an electrolyte replenisher and fluid extender or as a vehicle for other drugs. Lactated Ringer's injection has different quantities of the same three salts in Ringer's injection and contains sodium lactate. This injection is a fluid and electrolyte replenisher and a systemic alkalizer.

Nonaqueous water – Miscible vehicles

The nonaqueous water-miscible agents such as ethanol, glycerin and propylene glycol are used as cosolvents with Water for Injection to promote the solubility and stability in parenteral preparations. Water-miscible cosolvents could have undesirable side effects. The intramuscular injections of products containing propylene glycol, ethyl alcohol or polyethylene glycol 400 are reported to cause muscle damage in animal experimentation. Too rapid intravenous administration of such products could result in the precipitation of the drug in blood stream.

Nonaqueous water – Immiscible vehicles

The fixed oils as well as ethyl oleate, isopropyl myristate, and benzyl benzoate are some of the water immiscible vehicles used in parenterals. Fixed oils must be fluid at room temperature, and vegetable in origin, and should have good thermal stability at both high and low temperatures. An antioxidant is, generally, required to ensure the stability of fixed oils over the shelf-life of the drug product.

Regardless of the type of oil selected, purity is critical for any oil employed in parenteral products. Extensive purification must be performed to remove undesirable components such as peroxides, pigments, thermal and oxidative decomposition products, and certain unsaponifiable matter, for example sterols and polymers (Chang, 1978). Natural oils must also be free of aflatoxins, herbicides and pesticides, which might be present as a result of inadvertent contamination.

In addition to the distribution of related substances, the lecithins undergo hydrolysis to form the corresponding lysoderivatives: lyso-phosphatidylcholine and lysophosphatidyl-ethanolamine. Levels of these lyso derivatives must be controlled to reduce their hemolytic potential. Although, purified lecithins reduce the incidence of side effects, they are not optimal emulsifiers (Herman & Groves, 1992). It is believed that the formation of a complex inter-facial film among these substances might improve the overall stability of an emulsion (Davis, 1974; Benita & Levy, 1993).

The fixed oils, like olive oil, corn oil, sesame oil, arachis oil, almond oil, peanut oil, poppyseed oil, soya oil, cottonseed oil and castor oil are being used in parenterals. Of these, sesame oil is the preferred oil as it is the most stable due to its content of natural antioxidants, except in light. The fixed oils are normally well tolerated, however, some patients may have allergic reactions to some vegetable oils, and specific oils should always be listed on the product label. Excessive unsaturation of oils can produce tissue irritation. Isopropyl myristate, ethyl oleate, benzyl benzoate, polyoxyethylene oleic triglycerides (Labrafils™), thin vegetable oil (fractionated coconut oil) and the liquid poly-ethylene glycols are some of the synthetic

alternative vehicles available. Ethyl oleate is sometimes preferred over fixed oils due to its lower viscosity, and consequently, better syringeability and injectability. Spiegel and Nosesworthy (1963) reviewed the use of non-aqueous solvents in parenteral products and listed some lesser-used vehicles, e.g., ethyl lactate and glycerin.

Ideally, the water-immiscible parenteral vehicle should have following attributes:

(a) Ability to dissolve or disperse adequate quantities of the drug, such that sufficient drug can be administered in minimum volumes.

(b) The vehicle should also remain fluid over a fairly wide range of temperature.

(c) Low viscosity for good syringeability and injectability

(d) Stable and non-reactive.

(e) Free from rancidity.

(f) Free from mineral oil or solid paraffins, which are not metabolized by the body and might eventually cause tissue reaction and even tumours.

(g) Biologically inert, non-toxic, non-antigenic, non-irritant, biocompatible and pyrogen free.

(h) Ability to be absorbed from tissues after administration, leaving no residues.

(i) The breakdown products should also be non-toxic and be absorbed from the injection site.

(j) Free from any inherent pharmacological action.

(k) Should not potentiate the activity of the medicament.

The selection of vehicle is based on characte-ristics of drug to be dissolved or suspended and the desired release profile.

Cottonseed, soybean, safflower, sesame, cod liver, linseed, coconut, corn, peanut, olive, cocoa butter and butter oil have been studied for preparations of nutritional parenteral emulsions (Graves, 1973). The long chain triglycerides (LCTs) from vegetable sources (soybean or safflower oil) that contain a significant percent of linoleic acid, an essential fatty acid are commonly used. Medium chain triglycerides (MCTs) are being used more frequently in combination with LCTs because they provide a more readily available source of energy. MCTs are reported to be 100 times more soluble in water than are LCTs. Thus, they may have an increased ability to solubilize liposoluble drugs.

Because of water solubility the triacetin (1 part triacetin in 14 parts water) has been used to solubilize taxol. It is expected to dissolve rapidly in the body, thus, preventing phagocytosis and accumulation in the RES.

The rubber plunger tips of plastic syringes may absorb oil and swell, with a consequent increase in the force needed to expel the syringe contents (Halsall, 1985; Dexter and Shott, 1979). Such oil absorption by the rubber plunger tip may alter the formulation through loss of oil. The use of glass syringes for the injection of oil-based formulations is therefore strongly recommended.

Antimicrobials

Agents with antimicrobial activity must be added to preparations packaged in multiple-dose containers unless prohibited by the monograph or unless the drug itself is bacteriostatic (an example being methohexital sodium for injection). In the case of multiple-dose preparations the antimicrobial agent is required as a bacteriostat to inhibit any microbes accidentally introduced while withdrawing doses. Similarly, preservatives should be added to formulations aseptically packaged and not terminally sterilized in single-dose vials, if the active ingredient(s) does not have bactericidal or bacteriostatic properties or is growth-promoting. A growth-promoting study should be conducted to determine the microbiological properties of the preservative-free formulation.

The antimicrobial agents should also be present as adjunct in intermittent heat sterilization methods (tyndallization) in which the product is subjected to two or more heat treatments at temperatures below that normally used for sterilization. The use of antimicrobial agents, however, is not a substitute for good manufacturing practices.

The antimicrobial agents fall into five basic classes of chemicals: the quaternary ammonium compounds, alcohols, esters, mercurials, and acids. The quaternary ammonium compounds are incompatible with negatively charged ions and proteins. They are most often used in ophthalmic products. The alcohols and esters are generally employed in parenteral products.

Antimicrobial agents are specifically excluded in the large volume injections that are used to provide fluids, nutrients, or electrolytes, such as Dextrose and Sodium Chloride Injection, Dextrose Injection, Ringer's Injection, Lactated Ringer's Injection, and Sodium Chloride Injection.

Where the inclusion of an antimicrobial preservative is deemed to be necessary in a formulation the stability and effectiveness of the preservative in combination with the active ingredient and other added substances must be considered. There are many reports describing the incompatibilities or binding of preservatives with surfactants, medicaments, and rubber closures. Selection of an appropriate rubber formulation will minimize the absorption of preservative from solution and will, thus, prevent a loss of preservative efficacy during the shelf-life of the product.

The effectiveness of antibacterial agents can be tested by challenging the product with selected organisms to evaluate the bacteriostatic or bactericidal activity in a formulation; as described in Pharmacopoeias.

Preservative challenge tests should be performed throughout the projected shelf-life of the product and near the expiry date of the product to ensure that adequate levels of preservative are still available. Consequently, preservative efficacy tests are routinely included in stability testing protocols for formulations containing preservatives. The BP requires a 10^3

reduction in the surviving bacterial cells within 24 hours following inoculation of each mL or gram of the product with at least 10^6 bacterial cells. The USP requires the same 10^3 reduction in bacterial cells within 14 days.

However, with the availability of accurate and selective analytical methods for measuring low preservative concentrations in the presence of high concentrations of medicaments, it is more convenient and more economical to perform chemical assays for preservatives provided that such assays can be related to preservative efficacy.

The pH of the formulation can sometimes affect the efficacy of the preservative and the chemical stability of the preservative itself. Some preservatives are active in the unionised form, for example, phenolics and benzoic acid, which are inactivated at high pH. Others are preferentially active as the anion or cation. Cationic antibacterials such as quaternary ammonium compounds are more active at alkaline pH. Chlorbutol is less active above pH 5.0 and unstable above pH 6.0. The best preservative is one which is active at the pH of the formulation and is not affected by small changes in pH.

Some of the commonly used preservatives and the concentrations in which they are normally used to provide effective bacteriostasis are listed in Table 5.1.

Antioxidants

Many drugs in aqueous solution are subject to oxidative degradation. Antioxidants are added in the formulation to minimize this degradation by preferentially undergoing oxidation as the result of their lower oxidation potential or by terminating the propagation step in the free radical oxidation mechanism. Therefore, parenteral products that contain such drugs will frequently require the addition of an antioxidant. An antioxidant is an agent that has a lower oxidation potential than the drug and can be preferentially oxidized, until all of the oxygen present in the system has been taken up, thus

Table 5.1. Commonly used antimicrobial preservatives

Antimicrobial preservative	Concentration range (% w/v)
Benzyl alcohol	0.5–10.0
Benzethonium chloride	0.01
Butylparaben	0.015
Chlorobutanol	0.25–0.5
Metacresol	0.1–0.25
Methylparaben	0.01–0.18
Myristylgamma picolinium chloride	0.17
Phenol	0.065–0.5
2-Phenoxyethanol	0.5
Phenylmercuric nitrate	0.001
Propylparaben	0.005–0.035
Thiomersal	0.001–0.002

providing protection from oxidation for the drug molecule. An antioxidant must have a lower oxidation potential than the medicament itself; otherwise oxygen will preferentially attack the medicament.

As pH increases, the oxidation potential of the system increases. For example, at pH 4.58, ascorbic acid has an EO of –0.136 V and at pH 5.20 this increases to –0.115 V. Therefore, many oxygen sensitive compounds, provided they are still soluble, are formulated at lower pH values to increase their resistance to oxidation. However, the salts of sulphur dioxide are most effective at varying pH values. Metabisulphite is used as antioxidant at low pH, bisulphite at intermediate pH, and sulphite at higher pH values.

The other factor that influences the choice of antioxidant is toxicity. The number of antioxidants that are universally acceptable is limited. Regulatory authorities publish guidelines on the compounds that are regarded as acceptable for use as excipients. A loss of antioxidant, during processing and during the first few weeks of storage of the product, is normally seen. The extent and the rate of this loss will be dependent upon the amount of oxygen present in the container and the redox potential of the antioxidant. The process of oxidation in parenterals involves a reaction between oxygen and the medicament. The process is spontaneous and is often referred to as autoxidation. Autoxidation is a chain reaction involving free radicals formed by the loss of a hydrogen atom. It may be catalysed by variations in temperature or hydrogen ion concentration, the presence of trace metals or peroxides, or exposure to light (Alkers, 1982). While the solubility of oxygen is less at higher temperatures, the rate of oxidation will increase as temperature is increased.

The use of antioxidants can sometimes be avoided by reducing the amount of oxygen dissolved in solution and the amount present in the container headspace. This is achieved by sparging solutions with an inert gas, such as nitrogen, to displace the oxygen in solution before filling and by purging the container with inert gas both before and after filling. The amount of oxygen present will depend upon the efficiency of sparging and purging and on the speed with which the container is sealed after purging. The manufacturing process can be closely monitored by specialized equipment for monitoring dissolved and headspace oxygen.

The oil-based formulations such as emulsions may contain antioxidants such as alpha-tocopherol, deferoxamine mesylate, or ascorbic acid to prevent peroxidation of unsaturated fatty acids. Preservatives such as methylparaben and butylparaben can be dissolved in the aqueous phase prior to emulsification.

Metals can react directly with oxygen and with hydroperoxides to form free radical, which could initiate the chain reaction of autoxidation. Copper and iron are the most active catalysts. Chelating agents such as ethylenediaminetetraacetic acid (EDTA) derivatives and salts are used to complex the trace amounts of heavy metals, which otherwise would catalyze oxidative reactions.

In addition to chelating agents, there are other additives that are used in parenteral solutions as antioxidant synergists. Citric, phosphoric, and tartaric acids are used to reduce the pH of the solution and povidone, lecithin, glycerol, and propylene glycol are used to increase viscosity and, thus, reduce the rate of diffusion of oxygen. Surfactants, such as polysorbates, and certain amino acids such as glycine, cysteine, and tryptophan have also been used as antioxidant synergists.

Exposure to light will also catalyse autoxidation reactions. Low wavelength (high energy) light has the greatest effect and oxygen-sensitive products are least stable in ultraviolet light. The product should be protected from light adequately.

Buffers

The solubility and stability of the medicament in water can be greatly affected by the pH of the solution. Many drugs that are administered parenterally are the salts of organic acids or bases. These salts are selected because of their water solubility. However, in these cases it is essential that extensive pH-solubility and pH-stability profiles be undertaken in order to determine the optimum pH for the formulation. Many organic salts (for example, acetate, mesylate, or sodium salts) have a considerable buffering capacity at higher concentrations. Nevertheless, many compounds are particularly susceptible to pH changes, which can be brought about by heat sterilisation, contact with containers and closures, degradation of the medicament, or dissolution of carbon dioxide from the headspace of the container. In these cases it is necessary to introduce a buffer.

The ideal pH of a parenteral product is 7.4 i.e. the pH of blood. Extreme deviation from this pH can cause complications (Deluca & Rapp, 1982). Above pH 9, tissue necrosis often occurs, whereas below pH 3 extreme pain is experienced at the site of injection. The acceptable pH range (3.0 to 10.5) for intravenous preparations is wider than the acceptable range for other routes (pH 4 to 9). This is because blood itself is an excellent buffer and it can dilute and distribute the solution throughout the circulatory system very rapidly.

Determination of the desired pH for a particular product will normally determine the choice of the buffer. For optimum solubility the pH of the buffer will be at least 2 pH units away from the pKa of the salt being considered. However, this may not be the optimum pH for stability or for biological activity. The desired pH is normally a compromise between the optimum for solubility, the optimum for stability, and the ideal pH 7.4.

The most common buffers used in parenterals are acetate buffers (pH range 4 to 6), phosphate buffers (pH range 6 to 8), glutamate buffers (pH range 2 to 5 and 8.5 to 10.5), and citrate buffers (pH range 2 to 6). Buffers exert their greatest buffering capacity when the pH is equal to the pKa of the buffer. Buffers are normally selected with a pKa within 1 pH unit of the desired pH. Glutamate and citrate buffers have more than one pKa, hence may be used over the wide pH range.

The Henderson-Hasselbalch equation is used to calculate the quantities of buffer species required to provide the desired pH:

$$pH = pKa + \log C_{salt} / C_{acid}$$

where, C_{salt} and C_{acid} are the molar concentrations of the salt form and acid form, respectively. The commonly used buffering agents for parenterals are listed in Table 5.2.

Tonicity contributors

Isotonic solutions exert the same osmotic pressure as blood plasma. Solutions may also exert less (hypotonic) or more (hypertonic) osmotic pressure than plasma. Red blood cells (erythrocytes) when introduced into hypotonic solutions will swell and often burst because of diffusion of water into the cell (hemolysis), and when placed in hypertonic solutions, they may lose water and shrink (crenation). In isotonic solutions (e.g., 0.9% sodium chloride) the cells

Table 5.2. Commonly used buffering agents

Buffering agent	Concentration (% w/v)
Acetic acid	0.22
Adipic acid	1.0
Benzoic acid and sodium benzoate	5.0
Citric acid	0.5
Lactic acid	0.1
Maleic acid	1.6
Potassium phosphate	0.1
Sodium phosphate monobasic	1.7
Sodium phosphate dibasic	0.71
Sodium acetate	0.8
Sodium bicarbonate	0.005
Sodium carbonate	0.06
Sodium citrate	4.0
Sodium tartrate	1.2
Tartaric acid	0.65

maintain their "tone" and the solution is isotonic with human erythrocytes.

To minimize tissue damage and irritation, reduce hemolysis of blood cells and prevent electrolyte imbalance upon administration, the parenteral products should be isotonic, or nearly so, for small volume injectables. This is not always feasible, because of the high concentration of drug used and the low volumes required for some injections, the wide variety of dose regimens, methods of administration, or product stability considerations. Historically, there has been concern over the osmolarity or tonicity of intravenous infusion fluids because of the large amounts of solution administered to hospitalized patients, but in the last few years there has also been interest in the osmolarity of other parenteral dosage forms. Aqueous solutions for subcutaneous, intradermal, or intramuscular injection should be made isotonic, if possible. As mentioned previously, sodium or potassium chloride and dextrose are commonly added to adjust solution tonicity.

If a solution is hypertonic either it can be diluted with water prior to administration or administered slowly to permit dilution by the blood. There are several methods available to calculate tonicity (Martin, et.al., 1991). The sodium chloride equivalent method is the most convenient.

The cell membrane, which does not always behave as a truly semipermeable membrane, results in variable diffusibility of different medicinal substances across the cell membrane, solutions that are theoretically isoosmotic with the cells may cause hemolysis because solutes diffuse through the cell membrane. For example, 1.8% solution of urea has the same osmotic pressure as 0.9% sodium chloride, but the urea solution produces hemolysis, because urea permeates the cell membrane.

The effect of isotonicity on reducing the pain on injection is somewhat vague; although it may atleast reduce tissue irritation. Pain on injection may occur during and immediately following the injection or it may be a delayed or prolonged type of pain, which increases in severity after subsequent injections. In some cases, pain is more inherent to the drug and the problem is more difficult or impossible to resolve. Pain, soreness, and tissue inflammation are often encountered in parenteral suspensions, especially those containing a high amount of solids. In some cases, where injection of such solutions produces pain, as in an intramuscular injection, a local anesthetic such as Benzyl alcohol or Lidocaine hydrochloride may be added.

Suspending agents

The parenteral suspensions must be of a regular small particle size and must not cake during storage. These should also be easy to resuspend and inject through an 18 to 20-gauge hypodermic needle. In order to achieve these parameters it is necessary to control the degree of crystallization, the particle size range, and the method of sterilization of the drug substance. Micronization may be necessary. The processes involved in wetting the drug, aseptic dispersion and milling, and filling into final containers must all be carefully controlled. Uniform distribution of the drug is required to ensure that a controlled and adequate dose is administered to the patient. Suspending agents play a vital role in controlling these processes. Carmellose sodium, povidone, and gelatin are all commonly used as suspending agents in parenterals. Gelatin and carmellose sodium are derived from natural sources and consequently must be carefully monitored for microbial contamination during routine production. Some of the commonly used suspending agents in parenterals are listed in Table 5.3.

Table 5.3. Commonly used suspending agents

Suspending agent	Concentration range (% w/v)
Gelatin	2.0
Methylcellulose	0.03–1.05
Pectin	0.2
Polyethylene glycol 4000	2.7–3.0
Sodium carboxymethylcellulose	0.05–0.75
Sorbitol solution	50.0

Flocculating agents

The flocculated suspensions are easy to dispense compared to structured suspensions.

Typical flocculating agents used in injectable suspensions include:

Surfactants

Lecithin, Polysorbate 20, Polysorbate 40, Polysorbate 80, Pluronic F-68, Sorbitan trioleate.

Hydrophilic colloids

Sodium carboxymethylcellulose, Acacia, Gelatin, Methylcellulose, Polyvinylpyrrolidone.

Electrolytes

Potassium/Sodium chloride, Potassium/Sodium citrate, Potassium/Sodium acetate.

Wetting agents

There are a number of drugs, which are hydrophobic. For preparation of aqueous suspensions, the wetting agents are added to facilitate their dispersion.

The wetting agents reduce the contact angle between the surface of the particle and the wetting liquid. The surfactants with hydrophilic-lipophilic balance (HLB) value in the range of 7 to 9 show maximum wetting efficiency. The usual concentration of surfactant varies from 0.05% to 0.5% depending on the solid content of the suspension. Only optimum amount of wetting agents should be used, since the excessive amounts may cause foaming or caking or provide an undesirable taste/odor to the product.

Emulsifiers

The oils have hydrophobic surface. For their dispersion in aqueous system, suitable emulsifying agents are essential. Natural lecithin is obtained from both animal (egg yolk) and vegetable (soybean) sources. An advantage of using natural lecithin is that it is metabolized in the same way as fat and is not excreted via the kidneys, as are many synthetic agents. Another advantage is that some phosphatide emulsions are very stable, resisting hydrolysis and oxidation if processed under inert atmosphere.

Various antioxidants can be added to prevent peroxidation of unsaturated fatty acids in the oxidation of the drug substance (Levy & Benita, 1991). α-Tocopherol is most commonly selected, probably because of its successful incorporation into two commercial lipid emulsions (Lipofundin® and Trive 1000®).

Poloxamers are also promising emulsifiers for parenteral emulsions. Cholesterol is sometimes added to increase stability of emulsions.

Miscellaneous additives

Sugars such as sorbitol, sucrose, or fructose have been used in Procaine benzylpenicillin and Sodium benzylpenicillin parenteral suspensions to enhance stability. Injectable suspensions of tetracycline in Miglyol are stabilized by the addition of maleic acid or its salts. Aluminum monostearate is used mostly in long-acting parenteral suspensions to reduce the interfacial tension and enhance the suspension stability.

DEVELOPMENT OF PARENTERAL PRODUCTS

The successful formulation of an injectable preparation requires a broad knowledge of physical, chemical, and biological principles as well as expertise in the application of these principles. Such knowledge and expertise are required to effect rational decisions regarding the selection of:

(i) A suitable vehicle (aqueous, non-aqueous or cosolvent)
(ii) Added substances such as antimicrobial agents, antioxidants, buffers, chelating agents, and tonicity contributors
(iii) The appropriate container and container components

Inherent in the above decisions is the obligatory concern for product safety, effectiveness, stability and reliability. The study of physical-chemical aspects of preparing a stable product in a suitable container is required, recognizing that safety must be established through evaluation of toxicity, tissue tolerance, pyrogenicity, sterility, and tonicity. The efficacy must be demonstrated through controlled clinical investigations.

The majority of parenteral products are aqueous solutions, preferred because of their physiologic compatibility and versatility with regard to route of administration. Chemically, the high dielectric constant of water makes it possible to dissolve ionizable electrolytes and its hydrogen-bonding potential facilitates the solution of alcohols, aldehydes, ketones, and amines. However, co-solvents or non-aqueous substances are often required to affect solution or stability. For instance, nonpolar substances such as alkaloidal bases possess limited solubility in water and it is necessary to add a co-solvent such as glycerin, ethanol, propylene glycol or polyethylene glycol. Furthermore, the desired properties are sometimes attained through the use of a suspension or an emulsion. Although, each of these dosage forms have distinctive characteristics and formulation requirements, certain physical-chemical principles are common.

In other cases, to prevent chemical degradation (i.e., hydrolysis, oxidation, decarboxylation, or racemization) water may have to be eliminated partially or totally. Most proteins and peptides require an aqueous environment; and the addition of salt, buffer, or other additives for solubility purposes often leads to conformational changes. Consequently, the formulator should be aware of not only the nature of the solvent and solute in parenterals but also the solvent-solute interactions and the route of administration.

For discussing formulation development the parenteral products are classified below according to their presentation, as they require different formulation approaches.

Solutions

Aqueous solution

The simplest and most convenient form of presentation of an injectable product is an isotonic aqueous solution, which has a pH close to that of blood and body tissues (pH 7.4). The inclusion of buffers in the formulation may be necessary to stabilise the injection at a suitable pH. Such a presentation is suitable for all routes of administration provided that the active ingredients are sufficiently soluble to ensure that the required dose is dissolved in an injection volume appropriate to the desired route. This consideration is of particular importance for medicaments intended for administration by the intradermal, subcutaneous, or subconjunctival routes where the injection volume must be small. However, medicaments administered by these routes are generally intended to mediate a local effect and therefore doses are usually small.

If the medicament is susceptible to oxidation, antioxidants may be added to stabilize the product. The use of antioxidants in injection formulations is not permissible for a number of parenteral routes of administration because of their toxic or irritant properties. If injected into the spinal column they interact with the nerve endings causing traumatic effects, including paralysis. Many antioxidants are also irritating to mucous membranes and to the eye.

Injectable solutions can be presented in either single-dose or multidose containers. Multidose containers are normally glass vials with rubber stoppers suitable for multiple withdrawals. The major pharmacopoeias require multidose injections to contain an antimicrobial preservative. However, because of the toxicity of most antimicrobial preservatives and the potential for contamination of multidose containers, the multidose injection formulations are developed for only those products for which the normal indication of the product requires such presentations. Such products might be required for multiple self-administrations by the patient, for example, insulin preparations; or for multiple administrations in a specific clinical situation, such as the injection of vaccines. In the UK and in a number of other EC countries, the use of multidose injections is increasingly regarded as poor pharmaceutical practice. Consequently, the majority of newly developed parenteral products are single-dose preparations, which should not contain an antimicrobial preservative.

Large volume parenterals

Infusion fluids are aqueous solutions that are presented in larger volumes than those normally administered by intravenous injection. Injection volumes range from 50 mL to 1 L and are normally presented in polyvinyl chloride infusion bags. Products presented as infusions include preparations used for:

(a) Basic nutrition, for example, glucose injection
(b) Restoration of electrolyte balance, for example, compound sodium chloride injection, which contains sodium, potassium, and calcium ions

(c) Fluid replacement, for example, a combination such as glucose and sodium chloride injection

(d) A number of special uses, such as parenteral hyperalimentation.

Since the dose of LVP administered at any one time is usually large, any additives added in the product could have a significant effect on the patient. Hence only those additives should be incorporated in the formulation, which are essential for product stability and effectiveness and must not be harmful to the patient. The chelating agents, antioxidants, buffering agents, preservatives etc., which are commonly added to SVP's are rarely, added to LVP's. These ingredients, if essential, must be in bare minimum concentrations. The LVPs should be isotonic and isoosmotic to body fluids as far as possible. Hypertonic and hypotonic solutions if used should be administered slowly.

Solubility of solutes is rarely a consideration during formulation and since most of the solutes are readily soluble. Once in solution, the ingredients remain dissolved under normal storage and handling conditions. Highly concentrated solutions, such as 15% mannitol may show signs of crystallization at low temperature; however, crystals go back into solution readily when the bottle is warmed. Freeze thaw studies i.e. exposure of product to alternating cycles of low and high temperatures provide information about behaviour of solution and container under adverse storage conditions.

The pH of blood serum is normally between 7.35 and 7.45. The solution is rapidly diluted in the bloodstream, and the body's buffering system can maintain the proper pH level when high or low-pH LVPs are administered. Besides this, the pH of a formulation is important for its effect on product stability and stability of drugs that are added.

The sensitivity of a solution when exposed to light and changes that might occur during exposure should be determined during the preformulation developmental phase of a formulation. Sensitive products like vitamin solutions require protection from light by use of amber bottle pack or an opaque unit carton. A light protective cover must be put over containers of solutions to which photodegradable drug has been added during use. Light sensitivity can be determined by exposing samples in a light cabinet to a specified number of luxes and comparing the results of tests for color and degradation with the results from samples that have been shielded from light.

The drug sensitive to oxidation should be protected by flushing solution head space with an inert gas such as nitrogen or use of a safe antioxidant. LVPs are terminally sterilized by steam sterilization process or hot water immersion, or hydrostatic pressure.

The USP requires that LVP must contain not more than 25 particles per mL that are equal to or larger than 10 μm and no more than 3 particles per mL that are equal to or larger than 25 μm in effective linear measurement.

Colloidal solutions

The colloidal solutions for injection preparations are sterilized by heating in an autoclave since they may be retained on bacterial filters. Iron Dextran Injection BP and Iron Sorbitol Injection BP are two such preparations. Iron Dextran Injection BP contains dextrans complexed with ferric ions while Iron Sorbitol Injection BP contains sorbitol, dextrins, and citric acid complexed with ferric ions. Both are given by deep intramuscular injection.

Mixed solvent systems

Poorly water-soluble drugs are difficult to formulate as aqueous solutions. To formulate such drugs as a true solution, which is readily and completely miscible with serum for intravenous administration, it may be necessary to formulate the product in a mixed solvent system. A co-solvent is used to reduce the polarity of the vehicle and render the medicament more soluble. Ethanol, propylene glycol, and glycerol have all been used as co-solvents either singly or in combination. The choice of co-solvent is restricted due to the danger of toxicity and the concentrations of such co-solvents must be restricted to ensure that there is a safe quantity of co-solvent being administered in the maximum recommended injection volume. In many cases the formulator must strike a fine balance between the concentration of co-solvent and the injection volume required. Some formulations contain a number of co-solvents, thus, avoiding the use of a toxic quantity of a single co-solvent.

The products containing these solvents may exhibit incompatibility with intravenous fluids, bags infusion, sets, or plastic syringes. They should be used with care in patients with compromised liver function since clearance of the co-solvent may be impaired. The use of mixed solvent systems is, therefore, normally restricted to a small number of products that are required to be administered intravenously in critical clinical circumstances. However, these solvents when used in SVPs in low concentrations may not have significant problem.

The most common examples of injections formulated in mixed solvent systems are Digoxin Injection BP, which has a mixture of ethanol, propylene glycol, and water as vehicle, and Ergotamine Injection BP, which has a vehicle that comprises ethanol and glycerol.

Oily solutions

The use of oils is necessitated by very low water solubility of certain drugs. Oily solutions are intended primarily for intramuscular administration and, under normal circumstances, should not be administered by other routes. The vehicle used varies widely from vegetable oils such as arachis oil (used with benzyl benzoate in Dimercaprol Injection BP) and sesame oil (used in the depot injections: Fluphenazine Decanoate Injection BP and Fluphenazine Enanthate Injection BP) to simple esters such as ethyl oleate (used as the vehicle in a range of pharmacopoeial

products such as Nandrolone Decanoate Injection BP), which is relatively non-toxic and therefore very popular.

SUSPENSIONS

Suspensions are thermodynamically unstable heterogeneous systems consisting of a solid phase dispersed in a liquid phase that may be either aqueous or non-aqueous. Injectable suspension should be sterile, pyrogen free, stable, resuspendable, syringeable, injectable, isotonic, and non-irritating. Because of these requirements injectable suspensions are one of the most difficult dosage forms to develop in terms of their stability, manufacture and usage. Another disadvantage of injectable suspension lies in difficulty to administer accurate and uniform dose. These suspensions may be formulated as a ready-to-use injection or require a reconstitution step prior to use. Injectable suspensions usually contain 0.5% to 5.0% solids and should have a particle size less than 5 μm for IM or SC administration. Certain antibiotic preparations, for example, Procaine Penicillin G may contain up to 30% solids.

The physicochemical properties of drugs that profoundly influence the formulation and stability of suspensions include particle size distribution, dissolution and recrystallization, pKa, solvates and polymorphs, solubility, pH stability and pH solubility profiles.

The problems that are specific to suspension dosage forms include viscosity, rheological behavior, suspendibility, cake formation, crystal formation, syringeability and particle size distribution. These parameters should be monitored as a part of stability program.

Typical excipients used in formation of parenteral suspensions include antioxidants, wetting agents, solvent systems, preservatives, flocculating/suspending agents, chelating agents, buffering agents, and tonicity agents

Following approaches are used to formulate a suspension:

(a) Controlled flocculation
(b) Structured vehicle
(c) A combination of (a) and (b)

The choice depends on whether the particles in a suspension are to remain flocculated or deflocculated.

The controlled flocculation approach uses flocculating agent(s) to form loosely bound aggregate or flocs in a controlled manner that settles rapidly but redisperses easily upon agitation. The flocculating agent is added in optimized concentration to maximise sedimentation volume and prevents cake formation. Electrolytes (like potassium/sodium chloride), surfactants (like lecithin, polysorbates), and hydrophilic colloids (like PVP, Sodium CMC) are typically used as flocculating agents.

For structured vehicles approach the suspending or thickening agents are used to keep the dispersed particles in the suspension in a deflocculated state. These agents impart viscosity and reduce the rate of sedimentation of the dispersed particles.

The particle size distribution of solids in suspension is controlled to ensure that the particles pass readily through a hypodermic needle during administration. Particle size must not increase and caking must not occur during storage.

Gel-forming agents such as carmellose sodium, methylcellulose, and gelatin may also be included to increase viscosity and hence aid the stability of the suspension. Ideally, the vehicle should provide a stable dispersion during storage and be sufficiently fluid to allow administration via a syringe. A thixotropic vehicle may, therefore, be desirable.

Aqueous suspensions

Insoluble drugs can be formulated as aqueous suspension. Some examples of injectable aqueous suspensions include Methylprednisolone Acetate Injection BP, Medroxyprogesterone Acetate Suspension USP and Chloramphenicol Injection BP (Vet). Sterile Chloramphenicol USP is a sterile (micronised) powder, which can be reconstituted to an injectable suspension.

Suspensions are generally administered by IM or SC route and should never be administered by the intravenous, intra-arterial, intra-spinal, intra-cardiac, or ophthalmic routes. Development of novel delivery systems for suspensions containing drug in the microparticulate forms have made it feasible to inject parenteral suspensions by the intravenous or intra-arterial route.

The factors affecting the release of drug from the suspension and absorption from the intra-muscular or subcutaneous injection site should be considered while developing suspension formulations. The rate of drug release from a suspension can be affected by dissolution of drug particles, perfusion of the area by blood, oil-water partition coefficient, and diffusion through the highly viscous adipose layer to the vascular system. In addition, the injection depth and constitution of muscle and adipose tissue at injection site are important variables because the mean absorption times are considerably longer when the drug is shallowly injected in the adipose layer.

The properties of the active medicament that are important for formulation of a suspension include particle size and size distribution, pKa, solubility in water and in biological fluids (at injection site), lipid solubility, partition coefficient, crystallinity or amorphous nature.

The possibility of product-package interactions should also be considered during the development of parenteral suspensions. Because the surface free energy of fine particles is greater than that of coarse particles, fine particles will be more soluble. For such systems, fluctuations in temperature will result in crystal growth as the fine particles dissolve with increase in temperature and the coarse crystals will grow at the expense of the fine particles. Certain agents like Tweens and TritonX-100 at very low concentrations (0.005%), gelatin and polyvinyl-pyrrolidone at concentrations < 0.1 %, adsorb on crystal surface and retard the crystal growth. Freeze-thaw and elevated temperature tests can be useful in evaluating the crystal growth and crystal growth inhibitors.

Oily suspensions

Injectable suspensions can also be presented in an oily vehicle, although such preparations are far less common than aqueous suspensions. They can provide an effective slow release or depot mechanism by the deep intramuscular route. Aluminium monostearate is sometimes included in oily vehicles to produce thixotropic gels, for example, in Sterile Procaine Penicillin G with Aluminum Stearate Suspension USP.

Manufacturing considerations

Unlike solutions the suspensions are difficult to terminally sterilize by conventional methods like autoclaving or aseptic filtration. This makes the manufacturing of suspensions little complicated. The process involves sterilization of the vehicle system, aseptic wetting and dispersion of the sterile active and inactive ingredient(s), aseptic milling of the bulk suspension, and aseptic filling of the bulk suspension into suitable sterile containers.

The solid active ingredient may be sterilized prior to compounding into the suspension in a number of ways, such as sterile precipitation and/or crystallization, spray drying, lyophilization, dry heat, ethylene oxide, and radiation. The vehicle system may be sterilized by steam (for aqueous solutions) or heat (for oily vehicles) or by sterile filtration. The second process, which is relatively uncommon, involves in-situ crystallization. In this method active ingredient(s) are solubilized in a suitable solvent system, a sterile vehicle system or counter solvent is added that causes the active ingredient to crystallize, the organic solvent is aseptically removed, the resulting suspension is aseptically milled as necessary, and then filled into suitable containers. Testosterone and Insulin parenteral suspensions are prepared by this process.

Gamma irradiation can be used to sterilize bulk drug and/or finished product. Relatively low temperatures are required, no residual matter is deposited in the product, and maximum sterility assurance is achieved. Gamma irradiation can cause physical and/or chemical degradation of the product and/or the packaging component; therefore, preliminary experiments should be conducted to determine if stability is affected. The primary source used for gamma irradiation is cobalt-60.

Suspension characteristics and evaluation

Due to their thermodynamically unstable nature, the physical stability of suspensions becomes as important as the chemical and biological stability. Parenteral suspensions are frequently administered through 19 to 22 gauge needles. Besides common requirements for parenterals, these suspensions are evaluated for following parameters initially and on storage stability.

(a) Viscosity: An ideal suspension should exhibit a high viscosity at low shear (storage) with significant yield value and a low viscosity at high shear (agitation and syringeability).

(b) Resuspendibility describes the ability of the suspension to uniformly disperse with minimal shaking after it has stayed undisturbed for any length of time during shelf-life.

(c) Sedimentation volume describes the amount of settling in a suspension on standing. Sedimentation volume is used to evaluate the changes in suspension characteristics over shelf-life and also to compare different suspension formulations.

(d) Crystal growth in suspensions is affected by the particle size distribution, changes in pH, temperature, crystal form, and solvate formation and by dissolution and recrystallization of the particles. Crystal growth should be monitored by examining changes in particle size over time and comparing that with the initial particle size distribution.

Susceptibility of suspension to crystal growth could be determined by subjecting the suspension to freeze thaw cycles.

(e) Syringeability determines suspension characteristics such as the ease of withdrawal, clogging and foaming tendencies, and accuracy of dose measurements. Increase in the viscosity, density, particle size, and concentration of solids in suspension hinders the syringeability of suspension. The entire suspension should pass through a 25-gauge needle of internal diameter 0.3 mm.

(f) Injectability measures the performance of suspension during injection. It reflects the pressure or force required for injection, evenness of flow, aspiration qualities, and freedom from clogging. Clogging could result from aggregates or suspension inhomogeneity.

(g) Drainage refers to the ability of the suspension to break cleanly away from the inner walls of the primary container-closure system. It is an important characteristic of a well-formulated suspension and could be improved by siliconisation of containers and closures.

(h) Particle size distribution: Particle size distribution in suspensions on storage could result from the changes in pH (caused by drug decomposition) and temperature.

(i) Zeta potential is important if the controlled flocculation approach is used to formulate the suspension. The electrokinetic method measures the migration velocity of the suspended particles with respect to the net effective charges on the surface.

During development the product should be evaluated for the following tests. Formulation could be optimized based on results as required.

Parenteral suspensions may require dilution or mixing with other products prior to use. Dilution with water or normal saline will often causes the system to defloculate; it may not be necessarily detrimental in the light of the time frame of suspension administration, because of slow settling of deflocculated particles. Agglomeration or coagulation of suspension on mixing with other parenterals may cause serious incompatibilities.

During transportation the suspension undergoes stress due to vibration, impaction, and shaking which may seriously affect its physical characteristics. Common laboratory test methods (like vibrators, shakers, and impact devices) can be used to evaluate effects.

Antimicrobial preservatives and antioxidants present in the suspension formulation may adsorb on to the stopper resulting in the less stable suspension or agglomeration of fine particles on the surface of glass. The probability of particle agglomeration can be reduced by uniform siliconization of the vial, which also promotes efficient drainage of the suspension.

The freeze-thaw cycle promotes particle growth and may predict the results of long-term storage at room temperature. A total of three complete cycles with each cycle consisting of 24 hours at 40°C followed by 24 hours at 0°C is suggested, although various cycles are suitable.

EMULSIONS

Parenteral emulsions are best known as a source of calories and essential fatty acids for non-ambulatory patients (Davis, 1974; Jeffrey et.al., 1977), but significantly their physical properties and low toxicity make them excellent vehicles for the formulation and delivery of drugs with a broad range of applications. These applications extend from enhanced solubilization or stabilization of the contained drug to sustained release and site-specific delivery.

Advantages of parenteral emulsions

(a) For many drugs, insufficient aqueous solubility and/or water hydrolysis are the major formulation challenges. The use of an oil-in-water (o/w) emulsion can reduce or overcome these problems by incorporating the drug into the interior oil phase.

(b) An emulsion formulation can avoid the use of conventional co-solvent systems and the associated undesirable effects caused by precipitation of the drug at the injection site, as seen in the case of the anti-cancer drug Taxol of Bristol-Myers Squibb (Lundberg, 1997).

(c) Protein binding and hydrolytic degradation of drugs such as barbiturates (Jeppsson, 1972) do not occur as long as the drug remains in the oil phase, thus, further contributing to an improved therapeutic index for emulsion formulations compared with aqueous solutions.

(d) The potential to provide for sustained release (Prankard et al., 1988; Khopade et al., 1996). Delayed absorption of the total dose form the emulsion can be achieved for drug with a large partition coefficient.

An emulsion is a heterogeneous dispersion of one immiscible liquid in another. This inherently unstable system is made possible through the use of emulsifying agents, which prevent coalescence of the dispersed droplets. Parenteral emulsions are rare because it is necessary (and difficult) to achieve stable droplet of less than 1 mm to prevent emboli in the blood vessels. Formulation options are severely restricted through a very limited selection of stabilizers and emulsifiers primarily due to the dual constraints of autoclave sterilization and parenteral injection.

The lipophilic drugs can also be presented as oil-in-water emulsions. The oily solution of drug is then emulsified to a very small droplet size. The oil droplet size must be carefully controlled. Intravenous infusions formulated as emulsions normally contain up to 15% of emulsified vegetable oil and glucose. They are used for parenteral nutrition in patients who may rely entirely on intravenous feeding for long periods of time. Emulsifiers and stabilizers for intravenous emulsions must be non-toxic. Such materials include lecithin, polysorbate 80, gelatin, methylcellulose, and serum albumin.

Formulation of a stable emulsion

Unique to parenteral emulsions are strict requirements for globule size and surface charge. These two aspects are important in the manufacture and control of emulsions beside pH and will be discussed in more detail.

Globule size

The main feature common to all injectable emulsions is their strict globule size requirement, as this has a direct effect on both toxicity and stability. Emulsions containing globules ranging in size from 0.5 to 1.0 µm are utilized more rapidly by the body than emulsion with 3–5 µm globules (Laval-Jeantet, et al., 1982).

Small particle size promotes good physical stability because creaming is prevented by Brownian movement. In addition, large oil droplets (greater than 4 to 6 µm) can cause emboli.

Surface charge

The surface potential of lecithin-stabilized emulsions plays important role in stabilizing drug-containing emulsions through electrostatic repulsion (Washington, 1996). Ionized lipids are thought to have a favourable effect on emulsion globule size, stability and plasma clearance through an increase in the surface charge and bilayer thickness of phospholipids films (Rubino, 1990). A reduction in the electrical charge is known to increase the rate of flocculation and coalescence, and, thus, the measurement of surface charge is useful in stability assessments (Yalabik-Kas, et al., 1985). Selection of lecithins with varying amounts of negatively charged phosphatides could optimize surface charge and, thus, enhance stability (Hansrani et al., 1983).

Zeta potential measurement is typically performed using a Doppler electrophoresis apparatus such as the Zetasizer (Malvern Instruments, Malvern, UK).

Emulsions with globules size from 0.5 to 1.0 µm are utilized more rapidly by the body than emulsions with 3 to 5 µm particles. Globules greater than 4 to 6 µm are known to increase the incidence of emboli and blood pressure changes.

Microemulsions in the size range of 1 to 100 nm can be formulated by the use of a primary surfactant (which will be adsorbed at the oil/water interface and determine whether the emulsion is O/W or W/O) and a secondary surfactant, known as a cosurfactant, besides oil and aqueous phases. The cosurfactant interacts with high specificity at the interface and forms a mixed duplex film. These microemulsions are more stable than emulsions of bigger globule size.

pH

The pH is important for maintenance of the desired particle size because of its effect on the surface charge of the particle. A breakpoint in the profile occurs at the isoelectric point for lecithin at pH 6.7 ± 0.2. A low pH (< 5) can reduce the electrostatic repulsion between emulsified oil particles, thus resulting in coalescence and generation of large particles.

The fat emulsions have been found to have pH dependent stability, with an optimum in the range of 6.6 to 6.8 or, more generally, 6 to 7. The final pH of intravenous lipid emulsion varies from approximately 4.5 up to 7.2 due to liberation of free fatty acids.

The pH of the emulsion is usually adjusted little higher to approximately 8.0 prior to sterilization. The pH of the emulsion usually falls on autoclaving, and on storage, as the result of glyceride and phosphatide hydrolysis liberating free fatty acids (FFA). The rate of FFA production is minimal if the pH of the emulsion is between 6 and 7 after sterilization.

The surface potential plays an important role in the stability of emulsions through electrostatic repulsions.

However, emulsions of equal zeta potential were found to have different flocculation behaviours in the presence of added electrolyte, thus, indicating factors other than zeta potential can also influence the physical stability.

Various substances have been added to the aqueous phase to adjust or control osmolarity, pH, oxidation, and microbial growth. Because emulsified oil exerts no osmotic effect, additives are required to produce isotonic conditions in large-volume parenterals such as the injectable fat emulsions. Commonly used tonicity modifying agents i.e. both ionic agents (sodium chloride) and reducing sugars (glucose, dextrose) are unsatisfactory because of interaction with the lecithin emulsifying agent, resulting in brown discoloration and/or phase separation of the emulsion. Glycerol, sorbitol and xylitol have, however, been used successfully.

Emulsion manufacture

A sterile emulsion has important requirements such as very small droplet size (below 2.0 µm), terminal heat sterilization, low bioburden and sensitivity of lipid components to microbial growth.

Formulation preparation

The emulsifier, an osmotic agent, preservatives or any other water soluble ingredient are usually dissolved or dispersed in the aqueous phase. The phospholipids, antioxidants, and any lipophilic drugs are usually dissolved or dispersed in the oil phase. Filtration of every component of the emulsion is required to ensure low foreign particulate levels and bioburden before further processing. Hydrophilic membrane filtration is suitable for the aqueous phase. Hydrophobic filters are suitable for the oil and ethanol solution of the phosphatides, if used. Both phases are then heated to 70 to 85°C with agitation, preferably under inert atmosphere, to minimize oxidation.

The final pH adjustment takes place after the emulsion is prepared before the batch is brought to final volume and homogenized to reduce the particle size even further by homogenization or microfluidization.

Colloid mills are effective only at reducing the average oil droplet size to approximately 5 µm and are thus not suitable for the preparation of injectable emulsions.

Microfluidization, a relatively new proprietary technology (Cook & Lagace, 1985), has been used very successfully to produce parenteral emulsions. A combination of shear, turbulence, and gravitation forces results in the energy-efficient production of consistently fine droplets with a narrow size distribution. Greater emulsion stability may be achieved with micro-fluidization because of its superior ability to decrease the mean particle size and provide a narrower size distribution. The homogenized emulsion is then filtered to remove large particles.

Injectable fat emulsions are generally sterilized by autoclaving. Sterilization conditions must be selected carefully to ensure a sterile product but minimize degradation of the thermolabile product. Sterilization causes some hydrolysis of lipids and lecithins resulting in the liberation of free fatty acids (FFA), which are known to lower the pH of the emulsion. The alternate approaches to terminal sterilization include:

(a) Preparation of emulsion using individually sterilized components aseptically

(b) Sterile filtration through a 0.22µm cartridge filter for a parenteral emulsion is described for a microfluidized emulsion. This approach minimizes or eliminates the heat input into the emulsion but does not provide the degree of sterility assurance provided by terminal sterilization

Packaging

The LVP emulsions are packaged in USP type I or type II glass bottles [Hansrani, et al., 1983]. Some manufacturers siliconize their bottles to provide a hydrophobic surface in contact with the emulsion. Plastic containers are, generally, unsuitable because they are permeable to oxygen and contain oil-soluble plasticizers, which may be extracted by the emulsion.

The stoppers used to package injectable emulsions must not be permeable to oxygen or become softened by contact with the oil phase of the emulsion. Coated stoppers provide an inert barrier between the rubber compound and the product. The headspace of the final container may be flushed with nitrogen or evacuated prior to sealing to minimize oxidation of the emulsion.

The stability of emulsions is influenced by electrolytes, additives, or any change in the continuous phase composition. Processing conditions, autoclaving, storage conditions and excessive shaking also influence stability of emulsions.

Powders for injection

For convenience the injectable products should be in ready-to-use solution or suspension or emulsion forms. However, some drugs, which are not sufficiently stable in these forms are presented as powders for injection. These can be dry-filled powders in vials or in situ lyophilized (freeze-dried) products. Dry-filled powders must be sterilized as powders, before filling, either by dry heat or by gamma irradiation. The medicaments that are sensitive to heat or irradiation may be sterilized in solution by filtration and subsequently lyophilized.

A large number of products are available as lyophilized powder dosage form, such as penicillins, cephalosporins, penams, large molecular weight peptides and some vaccines. Many diagnostic agents, blood products, immunological products, and vaccines are presented as lyophilized products.

In-vial lyophilization results in a very light, fluffy porous cake in the vial, which gets readily reconstituted, using an aqueous diluent, than a dry-filled powder. The resultant product is very elegant and particle-free preparation. Lyophilization process, however, is very expensive.

PARENTERAL PRODUCTS OF PEPTIDES AND PROTEINS

Peptides and proteins play a key role in physiological activities (e.g. reproduction, growth, etc.)

and have been used for the treatment of various pathologic conditions such as diabetes mellitus, endocrine disorders, autoimmune disorders and specific metabolic abnormalities. Recent developments in the field of biotechnology, recombinant DNA technology and analytical methods for peptides and proteins are resulting in a greater availability of peptides and proteins for therapeutic use e.g., vasopressin, insulin, growth hormone, interferons and calcitonin etc.

Proteins and peptides are made of aminoacids in specific sequence, which determines the protein's structure. With the advances in biotechnology, the proteins can be produced by over expression through use of recombinant DNA technology. The gene responsible for producing a protein having a particular sequence can be isolated, modified, and recombined with a plasmid DNA. The modified plasmid is then implanted into a host cell which then replicates and transcribes the recombinant DNA to produce the specific protein in large quantities e.g. the yeast can be modified to produce hepatitis B vaccine and mammalian cells to produce erythropoietin. The advantages of such production are practically unlimited supplies of protein of high purity and consistent quality in lot-to-lot production.

Protein pharmaceuticals are (and will be) the most rapidly growing sector in the pharmaceutical repertoire. The scientific community has reached a new stage in the understanding of the properties of peptides and proteins and in the manufacturing of these therapeutic agents. Therapeutic peptides and proteins will give the solution for most "cures" for difficult diseases such as Alzheimer's, cancer, autoimmune diseases, etc., however, proteins are difficult to work with and most protein delivery is via injection only. Newer methods of protein delivery are being reported and are promising.

The peroral route is considered to be the most convenient way of drug application for the patient. The application of peptides through the intestine, however, faces several severe obstacles. These are the deterioration of the peptide structure by gastric pH and intestinal enzymes, as well as the poor absorption of intact peptide structures through the gut wall. The absorption barrier in the intestine is represented by epithelial cell membranes, interconnected by proteinaceous tight junctions.

The pulmonary route provides a large surface area, good vascularization, and immense capacity for drug exchange and ultra-thinness of the alveolar epithelium are unique features of the lung that can facilitate systemic delivery via pulmonary administration of protein and peptides. Recent progress has been made in the development of inhaled insulin as an alternative to insulin injections. Oral mucosa offers excellent accessibility, is not easily traumatized and avoids degradation of proteins and peptides. Peptide absorption occurs across oral mucosa by passive diffusion and the principal pathway is probably via the intercellular route. The transdermal route provides generally poor delivery of proteins and peptides because of highest efficient skin barrier. The major disadvantage with the nasal route has been the low bioavailability for macromolecules due to low intranasal absorption.

Regardless of the route of administration, the aims of a formulator are to maintain the stability of peptides and proteins prior to their absorption and localization at or near the target site, decrease their antigenicity properties, prolong their half-life and increase their absorption through biological membranes.

In systemic delivery of proteins the biodegradable parenteral depot formulations (e.g. microspheres, nanospheres, etc.) occupy an important place because of several aspects like protection of sensitive proteins from degradation, prolonged or modified release, and pulsatile release patterns. Specialized hydrogel implants are being under research for developing self-regulated protein and peptide delivery system in which a reversible gel-sol transformation controls the delivery of protein and peptide as a function of biochemical agent or pH or temperature in its surroundings. The controlled release protein depot injectables avoid regular invasive doses, which, in turn, provide patient compliance, comfort as well as control over blood levels.

The protein molecules are too large and too heavy to be absorbed into the body other than by injection. And once in, they do not remain in the blood stream long enough to maintain a therapeutic effect thereby needing frequent or high dosing. Two of the most successful protein drugs are Insulin and Erythropoietin. Insulin is injected up to five times a day and Erythropoietin on a biweekly basis. Attempts are on to develop alternate delivery systems for insulin such as pulmonary or buccal delivery (Jackylaw, 2001)

The parenteral formulations of proteins and peptides are mostly in aqueous solution or in freeze-dried form. Leuprolide and bovine somatotropin have been developed as erodable microspheres for depot injection.

The protein formulations utilize multiple ingredients in parenteral products. To formulate a stable protein formulation the environment in the product should be similar to that present in a cell. The essential features of the environment in a cell are: (1) a concentrated soup of protein, at least 100 mg/mL, and other carbohydrates, salts, etc., (2) low oxygen tension, with a variety of reducing compounds such as glutathione, used to maintain a high reducing potential, (3) immobilized water. Thus, the stable protein formulation would demand multiple ingredients to create such an environment.

Protein and peptide drugs are of great therapeutic interest because of their high potency and generally low toxicity. As these therapeutic proteins and peptides are made available, it will be essential to formulate these drugs into safe and effective delivery systems. The most important challenge to the formulation of peptides and proteins into effective dosage forms is to ensure their stability over their shelf-lives. Physical instability (including denaturation,

aggregation, precipitation and adsorption onto surfaces) and chemical instability (including oxidation, hydrolysis, deamidation, beta-elimination, racemization and disulfide exchange) may occur for a given peptide or protein, due to the presence of multiple susceptible sites. It should be noted that in most cases, more than one pathway of physical and/or chemical instability may be responsible for the degradation of peptides and proteins. Therefore, compared to the formulation of traditional dosage forms, formulation of peptide and protein drugs is very difficult and, regardless of the route of administration, product development should start with preformulation studies including physico-chemical characterization, solubility determination, stability determination under various conditions, isoelectric point determination, optimal pH determination and characterization of impurities. Also, choice of buffer system, pH of the vehicle, selection of an appropriate solvent system and preservation of the formulation, as well as selection of appropriate pharmaceutical excipients, are among the factors that should be considered in the formulation development of peptides and proteins, in order to prevent or minimize the various physical and chemical degradation pathways.

The degradation of proteins and peptides can be divided into two main categories: those that involve a covalent bond and those involving a conformational change. The latter process is often referred to as denaturation.

PARENTERAL DRUG DELIVERY SYSTEMS

Injection is invasive and painful route of dug delivery, definitely not enjoyed by patients. Hence it is clearly desirable for such products to be administered as infrequently as possible. Sustained release systems are attractive because they add value to patient, the physician and pharmaceutical company (Guy Furness, 2004). For the patient it is convenient to take less injection, maintenance of constant blood levels above therapeutic concentrations (hence better therapy) and compliance. Where compliance is an issue, for example, for schizophrenia patients, the Johnson & Johnson's Risperdal consta, a two weekly formulation of Risperidone has proved to be very useful. For physician, the patient's compliance to therapy is better assured and for companies, it is the product life extension and better product acceptance by patients and clinicians.

There are considerable challenges in developing long acting injectable technologies (Guy Furness, 2004) like:

(a) Problem of drug loading: For intramuscular use the volume should not be more than about 2.5 mL. As the duration of action of a single dose increases, so must the amount of active substance contained within it. Moreover, sustained release formulations require more excipients, increasing the volume further.

(b) Long acting formulations contain relatively larger particles, thus, blocking the hypodermic needle during administration.

(c) Internal burst: 10–30% of dose is released immediately, which may cause adverse effects.

(d) Once the injections are administered, the effects including adverse effects of long-acting product cannot be stopped.

Parenteral drug delivery systems are, generally, used to improve the therapeutic response by providing appropriate dosing strategies (which may be constant or pulsatile release). Such systems can be considered safer than conventional parenteral dosage forms because less drug is required, as the drug may be targeted to the *in vivo* site and avoiding high systemic levels. Due to the lower dosing frequency and simpler dosage regimes, patient compliance can be improved with these dosage forms. For example, microspheres and larger implantable devices can be used to modify release over periods of months to years.

Liposomes may achieve targeted delivery, both by passive and active means, following intravenous administration and are utilized to target toxic drugs, such as anti-cancer agents, to avoid systemic side effects.

Controlled release (CR) drug delivery systems are used to improve the therapeutic response by providing blood levels that are more consistent and stable compared to immediate release dosage forms. With targeting and more sustained, predictable levels, efficacy may also be enhanced. CR parenteral drug delivery systems include: suspensions, liposomes, microspheres, gels, implants and others. Tiny microspheres and larger implantable devices can be used to modify release over periods of months to years. Suspensions, liposomes and gels may not achieve quite as long durations of action, however, they can be localized at the site of action *in vivo* and liposomes may achieve targeted delivery both by passive and active means following intravenous administration.

Not all drugs are candidates for controlled delivery via the parenteral route. The candidate drug should be potent with known toxicity and pharmacokinetic profiles. A CR parenteral dosage form is usually selected when there are problems associated with oral delivery (e.g. gastric irritation, first pass effects or poor absorption) and a need for extended release or targeted delivery (e.g. rapid clearance). Both systemic and localized delivery can be achieved using CR parenterals. In addition, the drug must be compatible with the manufacturing process, which may be fairly harsh for some of these products. Examples of disease applications for CR parenteral delivery include: fertility, hormone therapy, protein therapy, infections (antibiotics and antifungals), cancer therapy, orthopedic surgery and post-operative pain, chronic pain, vaccination/immunization, CNS disorders, and immunosuppression. Approved CR parenteral products are listed in Table 5.4.

Although, CR parenteral products are relatively low volume in sales compared to oral

Table 5.4. Some USFDA approved CR parenteral products

Trade name	Active ingredient	Date of approval by USFDA
Suspension products		
Depo-Medrol	Methylprednisolone	Pre-1982
Depo-Provera	Medroxyprogesterone	Pre-1982
Celestone Soluspan	Betamethasone	Pre-1982
Insulin	Lente/Ultralente/NPH	Pre-1962
Plenaxis	Abarelix	2003
Microsphere products		
Lupron Depot	Leuprolide	1989
Sandostatin LAR	Octreotide	1998
Nutropin Depot	Somatropin	1999
Trelstar Depot	Triptorelin	2000
Liposome products		
Doxil	Doxorubicin	1995
Daunoxome	Daunorubicin	1996
AmBisome	Amphotericin B	1997
DepoCyt	Cytarabine	1999
Lipid complex products		
Abelcet	Amphotericin B	1995
Amphotec	Amphotericin B	1997
Implant products		
Norplant	Levonorgestrel	1990
Gliadel	Carmustine	1996
Zoladex	Goserelin	1989
Viadur	Leuprolide	2000

products. They offer significant and distinct therapeutic advantages for certain types of drugs and, consequently, their use is becoming more prevalent. CR parenterals are complex formulations and thereby present significant challenges in regulation and the development of standards. In addition, they are considered high-risk products since they are complex, are designed for prolonged and targeted release and, in the case of dispersed system CR parenterals, are almost impossible to remove from the body, once administered.

Controlled and novel drug delivery systems for parenteral administration fall outside the scope of this book. Interested readers are, however, suggested to refer any standard text including: **Controlled & Novel Drug Delivery** by N.K. Jain (Editor) 1st Ed., 1997; **Advances in Controlled and Novel Drug Delivery** by N.K. Jain (Editor), 2001; **Progress in Controlled and Novel Drug Delivery** by N.K. Jain (Editor), 2004; **Introduction to Controlled & Novel Drug Delivery Systems** by N.K. Jain, 2010.

STABILITY TESTING

The finished products are subjected to stability testing to establish an expiration period.

The vials should be studied in both the upright and either inverted or on the side positions to increase contact of stopper components with product constituents. The comparison between upright and inverted or on-the-side position is important to determine whether contact of drug product with the closure results in extraction of closure components or absorption and desorption of product components into container/closure.

Stability samples of all parenteral products should be evaluated for appearance, colour, assay, degradation products, preservative content (if present), pH, sterility, pyrogenicity, preservative effectiveness, particulate matter (where feasible) or foreign matter.

The sterility testing is recommended initially and at yearly time intervals till the proposed expiry date. Pyrogen testing is recommended only initially and at the proposed expiry date. The stability protocol can be designed based on the type of dosage form.

Besides above common test the products should be evaluated for following dosage form specific tests.

Solutions products

Clarity of solution.

Dry Powder for injection

Moisture content and reconstitution time. After reconstitution the product is subjected to other tests for solution or suspension, as the case may be. Most of these solids have optimism moisture range for stability. Besides stability the moisture can affect polymorphic form of drug.

Suspensions

Particle size and size distribution, redispersibility, rheological properties phase separation. Low-temperature storage data is needed for suspension formulations to evaluate crystal-growth potential and thermal sensitivity.

Emulsion

Creaming, coalescence, phase separation, viscosity, mean size and size distribution of dispersed phase globules. Besides degradation substances of drug, the degradants of oils like FFA should be monitored.

Large Volume Parenterals (LVPs)

Volume (there could be volume loss from plastic containers), clarity of solution.

CONTAINER AND CLOSURES

Containers for parenterals preparations must be made from materials that are sufficiently transparent to permit visual inspection of the contents, do not adversely affect the quality of the contents and do not permit diffusion of foreign substances into the product.

Glass

Glass has excellent clarity, thermal resistance, barrier properties, and is chemically inert. Glass is inorganic product having silicon dioxide (silica) as the major constituent. The fusion temperature of silica is very high, over 1700°C, making it impractical to form containers from it. Inorganic oxides are added to silica to lower fusion temperatures, and confer desired physical and chemical properties to the final product.

Example: Sodium oxide (Na_2O), calcium oxide (CaO), potassium oxide (K_2O), boron oxide (B_2O_3) and aluminium oxide, (Al_2O_3). Glass produced from these oxides is essentially colourless. Other materials can be added to confer a desired colour to glass. For example, small amounts of iron oxide and sulphur produce amber, iron and chromium oxides produce green and cobalt oxide produces blue. The amber glass is used for light sensitive products. However, these metal oxides are reported to get extracted from glass and degrade several drugs like L-ascorbic acid.

As per USP-NF, four types of glass are used for pharmaceutical containers.

Type I Glass (Borosilicate)

It is highly resistant borosilicate glass, relatively low in Na_2O. It has a superior resistance to alkaline products particularly because of the high Al_2O_3 content. B_2O_3 acts as non-alkaline flux to facilitate the melting of the low Na_2O glass.

It is used for buffered and unbuffered aqueous solutions, SVPs of all kinds regardless of pH and LVPs that are mildly alkaline or when high thermal shock resistance is required. It is the best all-purpose glass for injectables and should be the only glass used for alkaline products.

Type II Glass (Treated Soda Lime)

It is soda lime glass where contact surfaces are dealkalized to enhance chemical resistance. Dealkalization can be accomplished by using sulphur-containing gas such as SO_2, SO_3 or by fluorine containing gas such as 1,1-difluoro-ethane. It is less expensive than type I glass.

It is mainly used for LVPs, intravenous solutions, irrigating solutions, blood components and diagnostic preparations. It is more suitable for acidic and neutral products.

Thermal shock tests, internal pressure tests, and impact resistance tests are measures of how well a glass container will withstand the rigors of sterilization and subsequent handling. The tests are conducted by the glass suppliers on a scheduled basis, the LVP manufacturer may not have the equipment needed and will have to work with the supplier in order to get test results.

Type III Glass (Soda-Lime Glass)

It is untreated soda-lime glass container. These are generally used for solutions, suspensions in vegetable oil or for dry powders that are sub-sequently dissolved to make a buffered solution added at the time of use and liquid formulations that prove to be insensitive to alkali. It is normally used for small volume parenterals for which containers are pre-sterilized and filled under aseptic conditions with sterile product. It is not normally used for terminally sterilised products.

Type NP Glass (General Purpose Soda-Lime Glass)

This is also soda-lime glass but does not comply with type III. It is generally not recommended for parenterals. It is mainly used for cough syrups, elixirs, tinctures, extracts, creams, tablets, capsules and other dry products.

Siliconisation of glass containers is usually necessary to facilitate the draining of solid products (dry powders, suspension) from the walls of the container. This also helps in improving the appearance of product and also helps dose uniformity by maximizing drainage of product from vial. Siliconisation is carried out by spraying dilute aqueous silicone emulsion inside the vials via a standard vial washing machine followed by baking in dryer oven at 250°C for 5 hours. This way silicone gets baken on vial surface. Dry heat also dehydrogenates the vials.

Design of glass parenterals containers

Two methods are used for formation of glass containers for all types of glass i.e. blowing or tubing.

Blowing

Blow-moulded containers are mainly made-up of soda-lime glass. The greater strength blown vials and bottles may be essential for handling by mechanical processing equipment. Large vials and bottles are manufactured by blow molding process.

Tubing

Most tubing made containers are of borosilicate glass. Tubing is made in a wide variety of diameters and wall thicknesses, with excellent dimensional control and uniformity. Containers made from tubing are lighter in weight than blown containers because they have thinner walls and bottoms with resultant improved heat transfer characteristics. It is used for making ampoules, vials and cartridges.

Limit test used for glass (USP2004a)

Powdered glass test

Containers are crushed and exposed to the action of high purity water at 121°C for 30 minutes in autoclave. The resulting extract solution is titrated with acid to measure the alkaline ingredients of the glass that have been extracted during the test. This test is an indicator of the extrinsic chemical durability of glass as material. Glass types and test limits as per USP are summarized in Table 5.5.

Water attack at 121°C

Glass containers are rinsed and filled to 90% of overflow capacity with water, suitably covered and autoclaved at 121°C for 60 minutes. The resulting extract solution is titrated with acid. This test is used to check chemical durability to an internal surface treatment carried out at the time of manufacture to reduce leaching.

Plastics (USP 2004b)

Because of weight and susceptibility to breakage, glass containers have been largely replaced by plastic. Glass is essential only for those products basically incompatible with plastic e.g. lipid emulsions which may extract plasticizers from plastic, or bicarbonate solutions requiring carbon dioxide barrier not offered by the existing plastic containers. Flexible containers fabricated from polyethylene or polyvinylchloride are commonly used. Recently, modified polyethylenes and laminated structures made from polyethylene, modified polyethylene and/or plasticized PVC have been developed.

Plastics are polymers both synthetic and natural, which can be shaped when softened and then hardened to produce the desired structure. Plastics are relatively unbreakable and extremely light compared with glass. They are readily fabricated into a variety of complex shapes thereby providing ease of handling and packaging. Lastly, the cost for plastic products is generally less than glass.

For parenterals packaging the thermoplastic materials are preferred over the thermoset polymers due to their availability, reusability and processability. Additives such as antioxidants, heat stabilizers, lubricants, plasticizers, fillers, and colourants are frequently used to modify the physical and chemical properties of the plastic. These additives are combined with the polymers during its manufacture, or compounded in as a post-operation. During the storage of these parenterals, the additives could extract or leach into a drug solution in intimate contact with plastic container. Therefore, it is important to evaluate the physical and chemical compatibility of the drug formulation in a packaging system under various storage conditions to ensure safety and stability of the drug product.

Plastic containers do not require the rubber closure typical of glass bottles. Plastics are permeable to water and air to differing extents hence packaged products could loose water and are susceptible to oxidation. Polyolefins are less permeable to water hence could be used for over pouches for PVC containers. For light and oxygen protection, aluminum foil or combination thereof could be used.

The formulator of LVPs would look with interest at polyvinyl chloride resins that do not

Type	General description	Type of test	Limits	
			Size mL (Overflow capacity in mL)	mL of 0.020 N Sulphuric acid
I	Highly resistant, borosilicate glass	Powdered glass	All	1.0
II	Treated soda-lime glass	Water attack	100 or less	0.7
III	Soda-lime glass	Powdered glass	Over 100	0.2
NP	General purpose	Powdered glass	All	8.5

Table 5.5. Glass types and test limits (USP 2004a)

contain DEHP (diethyl hexyl phthalate) as a plasticizer. The fat-containing fluids, such as fat emulsions extract DEHP from the plastic. Examples of plastics used for parenterals drug container are given in Table 5.6.

Table 5.6. Examples of plastics used for parenterals drug container

Sterile plastic device	Plastic material
Containers for blood products	Polyvinyl chloride
Disposable syringe	Polycarbonate, Polyethylene, Polypropylene
Irrigating solution container	Polyethylene, Polyolefins, Polypropylene
I.V. infusion fluid container	Polyvinyl chloride, Polyester, Polyolefins
Administration sets	Acrylonitrile butadiene styrene, Nylon, Polyvinylchloride (tube), Polymethylmethacrylate (needle adaptor), Polypropylene
Catheter	Teflon, Polypropylene

The USP has provided test procedures for evaluating the toxicity of the plastic materials. Essentially the tests consist of three phases.

(i) Implanting small precise piece of the plastic material intramuscularly in rabbits.

(ii) Injecting eluates using Sodium Chloride Injection, with and without alcohol, intravenously in mice, and

(iii) Injecting eluates using polyethylene glycols and sesame oil intraperitoneally in rabbit. The reaction from the test samples must not be significantly greater than non-reactive control samples.

Elastomeric closures for parenterals (USP 2004c)

Elastomers, sometimes known as "rubbers", are moldable into almost limitless varieties of permanent shapes and forms to meet specific package design requirements. Examples of desirable properties of elastomers are compressibility and resealability. Elastomers are easily penetrated by a hypodermic syringe needle and reseal rapidly after needle withdrawal.

Typical physical and chemical properties of elastomers

(a) A rubber rated excellent for moisture vapour or gas transmission resistance will be impermeable to water vapor or gases such as O_2, N_2 and CO_2. Butyl rubber has excellent gas resistance.

(b) Bromobutyl rubber closures of new formulations or improved coatings that have the potential for reducing particle levels or extractables.

(c) Coring resistance is the ability to resist fragmentation during puncture. A multidose vial, requiring many seal punctures during its use, would be better sealed with natural rubber stopper than with silicone.

(d) Compression recovery is a measure of the resiliency of the rubber. It is the ability to recover to its original dimensions after being compressed for a given time at a given temperature. A natural rubber would be a better choice than a butyl for a syringe piston, which must remain resilient and not leak during storage or use.

(e) Shelf-life is related to the chemical properties of rubber compound. It is the ability to maintain its properties after exposure to oxygen, ozone, heat, light and moisture.

(f) Resistance to solvent is an important property for pharmaceutical rubber items since they are frequently in contact with liquids. The ability of a rubber to resist solvent transmission, swelling, extraction, and degradation is an important packaging parameter. Butyl rubber is compatible with vegetable oil but not mineral oil.

(g) Abrasion resistance: The ability to resist surface disruption and the generation of particles is important in all parenteral applications.

(h) Radiation resistance: The ability to resist a change in properties after exposure to gamma rays or an electron beam is more important now since radiation sterilization of many pharmaceutical items is common.

(i) The most common compatibility problems, which occur with stoppers are leaching of ingredients from the stopper and reaction of these stoppers with the product leading to turbidity, discolouration, precipitation or drug degradation. The solution ingredients could get sorbed into stoppers like preservative or active resulting in inadequate preservation or sub-potency.

Vial closures

Elastomer vial stoppers, used as primary closures for parenteral vials, are one of the most commonly used forms of pharmaceutical closures. A flange stopper consists of a hollow plug and disk designed as one unit. Both the cylindrical surface on the inside of the vial neck and the circular surface at the top of the neck finish are sealed with a properly placed flange stopper. The flange stopper is held in place by a metal seal applied over it and crimped around the bottom edge of the glass finish.

A special design of flange stopper, a lyophilizing stopper, permits evacuation of the liquid vial contents prior to final stopping. The closures are used for freeze-drying of products in vials.

Manufacture of elastomers

Rubber manufacturers combine the elastomers with other ingredients to produce a vulcanized product having specific physical and chemical properties that meet defined packaging needs. Elastomers are classified by chemical functionality into saturated and unsaturated types. Elastomers may also be classified by the source of origin as either natural rubber or synthetic. Pharmaceutical rubber manufacturers use a grade of natural rubber that is virtually free of mold, specks of foreign matter, resinous

matter, sand, bark, and blemishes. Synthetic elastomers are those produced chiefly from petroleum products in a well-controlled, highly automated continuous process.

Rubber closures are designed to possess a slight "interference fit" with their mating parts. An interference fit is one, in which the closure diameter is slightly larger than the diameter of the hole into which it fits. The amount of interference ranges from 2 to 10%, varying with the hardness of the rubber and the performance requirements of the closure system.

Following factors should be considered during selection of rubber closures:

(a) Buffer system
(b) Colour
(c) Configuration of closure
(d) Drug/medicament
(e) Metallic sensitivities
(f) Method of sterilization
(g) Moisture vapor/gas protection required
(h) pH of packaged product
(i) Preservative
(j) Solvent vehicle

The closure manufacturer occasionally performs several auxiliary finishing operations for special purposes. Surface chlorination (oxiglazing) is a process in which the surface of the rubber is oxidized in a controlled manner, causing a marked decrease in the coefficient of friction, to aid in the movement of rubber components during high-speed automatic assembly during the drug-packaging operation.

Another auxiliary operation required by pharmaceutical packagers is siliconization of the rubber closures. The silicon film acts as a lubricant, aiding in stopper transport during high speed filling operations. The siliconization process is achieved by tumbling a quantity of closures with a measured amount of silicone fluid followed by heat treatment. Silicon fluid may have deleterious effects on some parenterals like removal of silicon from closures leading to high particulate levels. The pharmaceutical manufacturer performs auxiliary extraction procedure by extending autoclaving cycle or cycling with vacuum to reduce the residual extractable substances. Testing of elastomers can be performed as per United States Pharmacopoeia (USP 2004c).

MANUFACTURING OF PARENTERALS

The use of superior quality materials alone in the preparation of parenteral products is not sufficient because parenteral products are subject to a variety of stringent requirements. If the processing is done in an environment, which is contaminated, or the manufacturing process is not carried out properly, then the purpose of selecting best quality components is automatically defeated.

Parenteral preparations should be prepared by methods that ensure their sterility and avoid the introduction of foreign contaminants, pyrogens, bacterial endotoxins and micro-organisms.

The general requirements for the manufacture of parenteral products have been laid down under Schedule M (Good Manufacturing Practices) and Schedule L1 (Good Laboratory Practices) of the Drugs and Cosmetics Act and Rules. The specific requirements for the manufacture of sterile products are prescribed in Schedule M (1A) of the Drugs and Cosmetics Act and Rules.

Recently introduced concepts in parenteral manufacturing include **Clean In Place** (CIP) and **Sterilise In Place** (SIP) so as to minimize contamination and attain preparations of highest quality.

Use of ready for use i.e. prefilled syringes is yet another improvement in maintaining the absolute sterility of the parenteral preparations. Modern parenteral manufacturing plants are fully automatic, which produce the preparations with zero defect.

Manufacturing facility

All sterile products must be manufactured under controlled and monitored conditions. A sole reliance can not be placed on terminal processing or on the tests for assurance of sterility or microbial or particulate quality in the final product; hence special precautions are taken in the manufacturing of sterile products especially for products which are aseptically filled.

Construction

The main consideration in the design and construction of sterile manufacturing facility is the elimination of microbial and particulate contaminants, which is achieved by clear separation of different areas of operation and an exceptionally high standard of environmental cleanliness in all areas where sterile products are manufactured.

The basic design comprises a complex of rooms arranged in a way that men, materials and components move from the relatively less clean areas to the more critical areas like filling and sealing only after all the materials and equipments have been processed and sterilized and the personnel have been adequately covered with sterilized garments. The surrounding area should provide a buffer area in which standards of cleanliness are only slightly lower than those for aseptic rooms. The prevention of contamination must be primary objective in design of these facilities. The product in the sealed containers is then transferred to less critical areas for final finishing. The facility should have compact layout to minimize movement of materials. Materials and men movement should be unidirectional.

Construction standards for sterile processing areas should be higher than that for other areas because frequent repairing of premises is not advisable. Walls, ceilings and floors in the aseptic areas must have a smooth, cleanable finish. It should be continuous and non-shedding and resistant to detergents, disinfectants used in the area. Epoxy or vinyl flooring is recommended as cleaning is very easy. Ceilings should be solid and continuous, light fittings and air grills should be flushed and not hanging from the ceilings. There should be no drains in the aseptic areas. Painting in the sterile area should be antifungal, polyurethane foam (PUF) is generally preferred. Door interlocking system should be provided to prevent the opening of more than one door at a time. The facility must be internally finished in a manner, which facilitates cleaning and disinfection and minimizes growth of contaminants.

Manufacturing area of sterile products is classified into aseptic areas, clean areas and change rooms. This classification is based on the positive pressure, temperature and humidity conditions, criterion for cleaning and quality of air that is supplied to the area.

Aseptic area

It is important area in which the sterilized product, containers and closures are exposed to the environment. This area includes gowning rooms, air locks, sterile corridors, hold area for equipments, containers and closures, filling rooms and container sealing room.

Clean area

The second area is called as support area where it is equally important to control the environment. In this area the unsterilized product, in-process materials, containers and closures are prepared and cleaned for further use.

Change room

It should be air locked and effectively flushed with filtered air at a positive pressure lower than that in the aseptic and support areas. Change rooms should be strictly used for entry and exit of personnel only. All personnel entering aseptic areas must pass through change rooms. There should be three change rooms in series to enter the aseptic area. In first change room, factory uniform and footwear are removed, in second change room, hand disinfection and sterile gowning are done and in third change room sterilized hand gloves are put and checked in the full length mirror so that no part of body is being exposed to the environment, and then entry is made to aseptic area. At the time of exit this order is reversed.

Basic design requirements

Sterile processing area should be isolated from the general factory environment and should be viewable from the outside, from observation corridors only. It should be designed taking account of operator safety and comfort of temperature and humidity conditions. Proper provision should be provided for verbal and visual communication to ensure good contact between aseptic and support areas. Hands free telephone set should be provided. Double door dry heat sterilizers and steam heat sterilizers should be installed between the aseptic and support area.

Air quality

An important aspect of environmental quality is the particulate content of air. Particulates may enter a product and contaminate it physically or, by acting as a vehicle for microorganisms. It is, therefore, necessary to minimize the particle content of air.

All air that is supplied to the sterile products manufacturing area has therefore to be filtered. The various processing rooms should be supplied and effectively flushed with air under positive pressure, which is passed through filters of appropriate efficiency and which will maintain a positive pressure differential relative to adjacent areas under all operational conditions. Terminal air filtration should be at point of input to a room. A warning system should indicate failure in the air supply, and an indicator of pressure differentials should be fitted between areas where this differential is critical. Air supplied to the aseptic areas must be passed through terminal HEPA (High Efficiency

Particulate Air) filters and may be considered to be of acceptable particulate quality when it has a per cubic metre particulate count of not more than 3000 in a size range of 0.5 microns and larger (class 100) when measured at the time of filling and sealing operation. The air may be supplied at the point of use as HEPA filtered laminar flow air having a velocity of about 0.07 metre per second, although, higher velocities may be needed where the operations generate high levels of particulates. The sterile area should have positive pressure differential areas of 1.25 mm.

Air handling facility

Air handling system is the core part of the sterile manufacturing facility. The minimum air changes in critical aseptic areas should not be less than 20 per hour, in a room with good air flow pattern and appropriate HEPA filters. Temperature and relative humidity in the aseptic areas should be 25°C and 55%, respectively unless there are product-specific requirements. Air handling systems should be validated at periodic intervals for air velocity, HEPA filter integrity, airflow pattern, direction study, non-viable particle count, and finally, calculation of air changes. Air classification for sterile products manufacturing area is given in Table 5.7.

Compressed gases

Nitrogen, carbon dioxide and air may be used during the processing of parenterals. The gases must be of assured quality and free from microbes, moisture, oil droplets and other contaminants.

Nitrogen is frequently used to protect a product from oxygen in bulk stage and in the final container. Carbon dioxide may be employed to displace air or for pH adjustments. Compressed air is used to drive equipment or to clean and air dry parts.

Fumigation

Fumigation is a process of gaseous sterilization, which is used for killing of microorganisms and prevention of microbial growth in air, on surface of wall or floor. It is commonly used in pharmaceuticals. Generally, for fumigation, chemicals like formaldehyde and potassium permanganate are used. Its mechanism of action is intermolecular cross-linking between proteins together with interaction with RNA and DNA.

In order to be effective, the gas has to dissolve in the film of moisture surrounding the bacteria and for this reason relative humidities in the order of 75% are required. Steam can be used to increase humidity and temperature in room upto a required limit. Following are the two different concentrations for fumigation

(a) 500 mL formaldehyde and 1 L distilled water for 28 cubic metre of area for 4 hours or overnight.
(b) 170 g potassium permanganate and 500 mL formaldehyde for 28 cubic metres of area for 4 hours or overnight.

Table 5.7. Air classification for sterile products manufacturing area			
Grade (Class)	Maximum no. of permitted particles per cubic metre of air equal to or above		Maximum no. of viable micro-organisms permitted per cubic metre of air
	0.5–5.0 µm	> 5 µm	
A (Class 100) Laminar air flow	100 – at rest; 3500 – in operation	None	Less than 1
B (Class 100)	3,500	None	5
C (Class 10,000)	3,50,000	2,000	100
D (Class 1,00,000)	35,00,000	20,000	500

Water systems

Water is used as the main solvent in sterile preparations. Water for injection for the manufacturing of liquid injectables should be freshly collected from distillation plant or from storage tanks through re-circulation loop system, where the water for Injection is stored at 80°C to prevent the growth of microorganisms. The purified water and water for injection should be stored in S.S. jacketed tanks, which should have hydrophobic bacteria retentive 0.2 μm vent filters. All parts coming in contact with Water for Injection and Purified Water should be constructed with S.S. 316 grade. Diaphragm valves should be used in the water system to avoid the dead legs formation. There should be a periodic sanitization of recirculating loops.

To keep the bacterial endotoxins under control and to assure final sterility, the bioburden of water should be controlled and limits of microbial count should be imposed. The source water entering the plant (municipal supply or private well) should have less than 50 CFU/mL (colony forming units per mL) with no coliforms, water for cleaning less than 50 CFU per 100 mL, and water for final rinsing of equipment less than 10 CFU per 100 mL.

Cleaning of equipments and area

Principles of cleaning of equipment used in the manufacturing of sterile products are similar to those applied for other equipments except that all the equipments coming in contact with end product must be free from microbiological contaminants. Final rinse of all the equipments whether subjected to sterilization or not must be carried out with Water for Injection. Filling lines, being of silicone tubes, can easily be autoclaved.

There should be written procedures for sanitization of sterile processing facilities. Employees engaged in the sanitization activities should be trained. All equipment and surrounding work area must be cleaned thoroughly at the end of the working day, leaving no contaminating residue from the concluded process. Different sanitizing agents should be used in rotation and the concentrations of the same should be as per recommendations of the manufacturer and records of all should be maintained. All disinfectants should be aseptically filtered prior to use. Some of the commonly used cleaning agents are listed in Table 5.8.

The equipments, which are to be cleaned, should be transferred to the cleaning areas for cleaning, disinfection or sterilization as required. Where this is not possible, equipment must be so located that it is accessible to a complete cleaning system. Nowadays Clean-in-place (CIP) and Steam-in-place (SIP) systems are most commonly used for this purpose. Items of equipment, those are difficult or impossible to sterilize, should be kept out of aseptic area. They should remain there and be continuously exposed to disinfecting processes. Whenever possible, operating machinery should be enclosed in stainless steel housing.

High bacterial counts can be brought under control by treatment with alkaline sanitizing chemicals (sodium hypochlorite or organic chloro compounds) followed by mild detergents.

Anionic detergents like sodium alkyl sulfonates are preferred because they do not leave residuals. Before any sterilization process is adopted, its suitability for the product and its efficacy in achieving the desired sterilizing conditions in all parts of load pattern should be confirmed and demonstrated by physical measurements and by biological indicators.

Cleaning of rubber and plastic components

Closures are subjected to gentle agitation with air bubbles, basket rotation accompanied by spray rinsing followed by autoclaving as a part of cleaning process. Rubber closures are then washed by mechanical agitation in a tank of hot detergent solution (such as 0.5% sodium pyrophosphate) followed by series of thorough water rinse, the final rinse being WFI. This treatment is required to remove surface debris and leachable constituents at or near the surface.

Table 5.8. Commonly used cleaning agents			
Disinfectant	**Active ingredient**	**Concentration (v/v)**	**Use**
Teepol	Sodium benzene sulphonate	0.1%	A multipurpose cleaning agent useful for most equipments, floors and glasswares
Liquid soap	Soap	As is	For washing hands, gloves and machine parts
Savlon	Chlorhexidinegluconate and cetrimide	2.5%	Treatment of all surfaces within the aseptic area; useful for floors, hands and equipments entering aseptic areas
Lysol	Chlorocresol in soap	1%	For treatment of all surfaces within the aseptic areas
Dettol	Chloroxylenol and terpineol	2.5%	Antiseptic for hand as a spray
Cidex	Glutaraldehyde	2%	Used without dilutions as an anti-microbial agent in aseptic area
Benzalkonium chloride	Benzalkonium chloride	0.1%	Fungicidal, bactericidal
Isopropyl alcohol	Isopropyl alcohol	70%	Treatment of equipments and work surfaces, hand disinfectant
Formalin	Formaldehyde	–	As a gas for disinfection of aseptic areas
Hypochlorite solution	Sodium hypochlorite	0.1% to 1.0%	Treatment for all clean surfaces

Filling procedures

Liquids

(a) For SVPs, syringe-based system is used. LVPs are filled by gravity, pressure or vacuum filling devices.
(b) The delivery tube must freely enter the constricted neck of container and deliver the liquid deep enough to permit air to escape without sweeping the entering liquid into the neck or out of the container.
(c) Retention device is designed to avoid wetting of ampoule neck.

Solids

Solids should be preferably free flowing, uniform particle size, no electrostatic charge within mass of dry solid particles, free from clumping of particles and no formation of air pockets. One of the methods employs an auger in the stem of funnel-shaped hopper. The size and rotation of the auger can be adjusted to deliver a regulated volume or weight of material from funnel stem into the container.

Sealing

Containers should be sealed in the aseptic area immediately adjacent to the filling machine. Sterile container, once opened, can no longer be considered to be sterile. Therefore, tamper-proof sealing is essential.

Sealing of ampoules

(a) Before and after filling of solution into ampoules, purging of inert gas such as nitrogen or carbon dioxide may be performed to displace the air in the headspace to prevent oxidative degradation of sensitive drugs.
(b) Ampoules are closed by melting a portion of the glass of the neck to form either bead seals (tip-seals) or pull seals.
(c) Wet glass at the neck increases the frequency of bubble formation and unsightly appearance and contaminating deposits of carbon as a result of the effect of heat of sealing on the droplets of product.
(d) Excessive heating of air and gases in the neck causes expansion against the soft glass with

the formation of fragile bubbles at the end point of seal.

(e) When ampoules are used for lyophilization, they must be filled and loaded into lyophilization chamber unsealed. When lyophilization is complete, they must be removed from the chamber and transported back to the filling line for sealing.

Sealing of vials, bottles and cartridges

(a) Rubber closures must fit the opening of the container snugly enough to produce a seal. It may be inserted by hand, using forceps. When closures are to be inserted by machines, the surface of closure is usually halogenated or coated with silicone to reduce friction.

(b) Aluminum caps are used to hold rubber closures in place. Single caps may have a permanent center hole or a center that is torn away at the time of use to expose the rubber closure.

Visual inspection

Filled containers of sterile products should be inspected individually for extraneous contamination and other defects. Generally, black particles, fibers or glass particles are observed as defects. Visual inspection is done under suitable and controlled conditions of illumination and background. Generally, container should be checked against white and black background.

Operators doing the inspection should pass regular eyesight checks and should be allowed frequent rest from inspection. Where other methods of inspection are used, the process should be validated and performance of equipment should be checked at regular intervals and recorded.

Sterilization

Before any sterilization process is adopted, its suitability for the product and its efficacy in achieving the desired sterilizing conditions in all parts of load pattern should be assessed and demonstrated by physical measurements and by biological indicators.

All the sterilization processes should be properly validated and verified at regular intervals. Sterilization records of each load should be maintained with thermograph and sterilization monitoring strip. The process used for sterilization by dry heat should include air circulation pattern within the sterilizing chamber and positive pressure should be maintained to prevent the entry of non-sterile air. Air inlets and outlets should be provided with microorganism-retaining filters. Challenge tests using endotoxins should be performed as a part of validation. Sterilization methods are summarized in Table 5.9.

Bacterial endotoxin is not lost with loss of viability. Of the sterilization processes commonly used in pharmaceutical manufacturing, only dry heat at above 250°C is capable of destroying bacterial endotoxins within reasonable time frame. The water used in preparation of parenteral products should contain no more than 0.25 EU/ml.

The endotoxins can be removed from product contact packaging components and equipment by washing and rinsing with water of WFI quality for at least the final rinse.

QUALITY CONTROL REQUIREMENTS FOR PARENTERALS

Most important quality parameters required to be assured specific to parenteral products are discussed below.

Freedom from particulate matter

As per USP definition the particulate matter consists of mobile, randomly sourced, extraneous substances, other than the gas bubbles, that cannot be quantitated by chemical analysis due to the small amount of material that it represents and to its heterogeneous composition. Freedom from visible evidence of

Table 5.9. Sterilization methods

Sterilization method	Conditions	Principle	Usage	Biological indicators
Moist heat (autoclave)	121°C/15 min, 115°C/30 min, 126°C/10 min	Irreversible coagulation of proteins	To sterilize filling vessels, machine parts, garments, membrane assembly, rubber stoppers and hand gloves	*Bacillus stearothermophilus* (*Clostridium sporogenes*)
Dry heat	160°C/120 min, 170°C/60 min, 180°C/30 min	Thermal inactivation destroys by oxidation	To sterilize ampoules, vials, pressure vessels	*Bacillus subtilis* var. *niger*
Ethylene oxide	Gas concentration 800–1200 mg/L at 45-63°C/30–70% RH for 1–4 h	Alkylation, sulphydryl, hydroxyl, carboxyl and amino group on proteins	Medical devices, dressings, catheters and tubing, IV infusion set, intraocular lens	*Bacillus subtilis* var. *niger*
Irradiation	25 kgy (2.5 mrad dose) Gamma rays or accelerated electrons	Disorganization of enzymes and DNA, cell death	Medical devices, plastic disposable equipments	*Bacillus pumilus*
Filtration	< 0.22 µ pore size sterile membrane filter	Physical separation of microorganisms	Filtration of bulk solution	*B. diminuta*

particulate matter is basic and essential requirement of injectable products. Parenteral products should be essentially, free from particles that can be observed with an unaided eye in visual inspection. The term essentially free is debatable and subjective. A single discrete particulate entity with a diameter of 50–100 µm is just about at the edge of visual. Good pharmaceutical practice requires that each final container of injection be subjected individually to a physical inspection, whenever the nature of the container permits, and that every container whose contents show presence of contamination with visible foreign material, be rejected.

The smallest capillary blood vessels are considered to have a diameter of approximately 7 µm. Thus, all the particles having a size equal to or greater than 7 µm can conceivably become entrapped in and occlude a blood capillary resulting in multiple infractions. Particles greater than 7 µm in diameter are viewed to be more threatening than particles of smaller size.

Although, ideally the injectable solutions should be completely free from particulate matter, it is, however, impossible to remove every particle and there is no objective evidence about the hazard to the patient at levels currently accepted as being realistic without significant increase in production costs. Particulate matter found in injectable could be:

Intrinsic materials

Contributed by components of fill material or glass container e.g. formation of insoluble sodium or magnesium acid phosphates from phosphate buffer solutions or reaction of citrates with glass components.

Extrinsic materials

Contributed by environment, contact surfaces, machines, personnel etc. during processing or leachings from elastomer closure such as silicon oil, antioxidants, lubricants, etc.

Visual inspection

Manual method

Visual inspection of products is done against nonreflecting black and white surface lightened with non-glaring light. Normally, fluorescent light source is used with 15-watt capacity. Containers are held 10 inches from the light source. The white background aids in the detection of dark colored particles. Light or retractile particles will appear against the black background.

Automation methods

- **By using imaging optics:** Particles suspended in the solution are illuminated by a fiber optic light system and imaged on video display.
- **Light scattering:** Light scattering from particulate matter, which is then received by a detection system and projected onto a television camera system e.g. Autoskan, Eisai AIM System, Seideneider and Schering PDS/A-V System.

The quantitative analysis of particulate matter is best carried by instruments to get generally accurate and precise counts at faster rate.

IP 2014 has prescribed the **Limit Test for Particulate Matter**. Particulate matter is defined as extraneous, mobile, undissolved substances, other than gas bubbles, unintentionally present in injections. All injectable solutions including solutions constituted from sterile solids must be essentially free from particles of approximately 50 μm or more that can be observed by inspection with the unaided eye. The test applies to single dose large volume injections for IV infusion in containers containing 100 ml or more. The detailed procedure is specified in IP 2014.

The permitted limits of particulate matter are given below:

Particle size in μm (equal to or larger than)	Maximum No. of particles per ml
10	50
25	5
50	Nil

Limits as per USP (USP 2004d) for particulate matter in injections are given in Table 5.10.

Sterility

Parenteral products must be sterile because their route of administration overrides the body's external barriers in infection. Sterility is defined as total absence of viable life forms. Exponential inactivation is the basis of the concept of sterility assurance. With an exponential order of microbial death, the form of the survival curve is linear. The logarithmic axis of survival curve has no zero point. There can, therefore, be neither time of exposure nor dose of radiation that can guarantee inactivation of 100% of any microbial population. These can only be greater and greater confidence of sterility. The major compendia now define sterility for pharmaceuticals in terms of there being assurance of less than one chance in one million that viable contaminants survive in any one unit. The probability microbial survival is called Sterility Assurance Level (SAL). The acceptable standard is an SAL of 10-6. In process contamination of aseptically filled products is generally demonstrated through filling placebos (media fill test). The contamination of aseptically filled products may occur in not more than 1 in 1000 units. However, this does not mean that SALs of 10^{-3} are acceptable. The SALs better than 10^{-3} are difficult to demonstrate because of the very large and probably uneconomical number of placebo units required to be filled.

A sterility testing is very exacting procedure, where the asepsis of the procedure must be ensured for the correct interpretation of results. It is important that personnel be properly trained and qualified. The test for sterility is carried out under aseptic conditions. It is performed by either membrane filtration or direct inoculation of the culture medium. Detailed procedure, sample preparation, method and interpretation shall be done as per USP (USP, 2004e)

Pyrogens and bacterial endotoxins

Pyrogens or bacterial endotoxins are substances that when injected into the human body in

Table 5.10. USP limits (USP 2004 d) for particulate matter in injections				
	Particle count			
	Light obscuration test		**Microscopic method**	
	≥ 10 μm	**≥ 25 μm**	**≥ 10 μm**	**≥ 25 μm**
Small-volume parenterals (per container)	6000	600	3000	300
Large-volume parenterals (per ml)	25	3	12	2

sufficient amounts, give rise to a variety of symptoms of which the most recognizable is an increase in body temperature. Endotoxin levels of about 50 pg/mL may induce clinical pyrogenic response in humans. In extreme cases pyrogens can be fatal because of endotoxic shocks. All microbes appear to be capable of producing pyrogens but Gram (–)ve bacteria produce the most potent ones.

The pyrogen test is designed to limit an acceptable level, the risk of febrile reaction in the patient to injection of the product concerned. The test involves measuring the rise in temperature of rabbits following the intravenous injection of a test solution and is designed for the products that can be tolerated by the test rabbit in a dose not to exceed 10 mL per kg injected intravenously within a period of not more than 10 minutes (USP, 2004f)

The rabbit pyrogen test suffers from several limitations, which established the opportunity for the Limulus Amebocyte Lysate test (LAL test) as a possible alternative for the rabbit test, as an official pyrogen test procedure. LAL test is used to detect or quantify bacterial endotoxins that may be present in or on the sample of the articles to which the test is applied. It uses Limulus Amebocyte Lysate (LAL) obtained from the aqueous extract of circulating amebocytes of horseshoe crab (Limulus-polyphemus or Tachypleus-tridentatus) which can be prepared and characterized for use as LAL reagent.

The advantages of LAL test over rabbit pyrogen test are greater sensitivity, less variation, quantitative test, less time-consuming, less expensive and an easier test.

There are two types of techniques for this test: the gel-clot techniques and turbidimetric method.

Gel-Clot techniques

It is based on gel formation, and the photometric techniques. End point is determined from dilutions of the material under test in direct comparison with parallel dilutions of a reference endotoxin and quantities of endotoxin are expressed in USP endotoxin units. It detects or quantifies endotoxins based on clotting of the LAL reagent in the presence of endotoxin.

Turbidimetric method

It includes a turbidimetric method, which is based on the development of turbidity after cleavage of an endogenous substrate, and a chromogenic method, which is based on the development of color after cleavage of a synthetic peptide chromogen complex.

Package integrity testing

Package integrity is a measure of a package's ability to keep the product in and to keep potential contaminants out. Leakage occurs when a discontinuity exits in the wall of the package that can allow the passage of gas under the action of a pressure or concentration differential existing across the wall.

Following are the commonly used leak tests:

(a) Visual inspection
(b) Bubble test
(c) Pressure/vacuum decay
(d) Dye tests
(e) Chemical tracer test

Leaker test is intended to detect incompletely sealed ampoules, so that they may be discarded. Tip sealed ampoules are more likely to be incompletely sealed than pull sealed. Leakers are usually detected by producing negative pressure within an incompletely sealed ampoule, usually in vacuum chamber, while the ampoule is entirely submerged in a deeply colored dye solution (usually 0.5 to 1.0 % methylene blue). Subsequent atmospheric pressure then causes the dye to penetrate an opening, being visible after the ampoule has been washed externally to clear the dye. The vacuum (27 inches Hg or more) should be sharply released after 30 minutes. Vials and bottles are not subjected to such a leaker test because rubber closure is not rigid.

REFERENCES

- Alkers, M.J. (1982). Antioxidants in pharmaceutical products. *J. Parenter. Sci. Technol.*, 36 (5), 222–28.
- Benita, S., Levy, M.L. (1993). Submicron emulsions as colloidal carriers for intravenous administration: Comprehensive physicochemical characterization. *J. Pharm. Sci.*, 82 (11), 1069–79.
- Bennett, W.F., Builder, S.E., Gatlin, L.A. (1988). Stabilized Human Tissue Plasminogen Activator Composition. **U.S. Patent No. 4,908,205**.
- Bringer, J., Heldt, A., Grodsky, G.M. (1981). Prevention of insulin aggregation by dicarboxylic amino acids during prolonged infusion. *Diabetes*, 30(1), 83–5.
- Chang, S.S. (1978). Silicic acid or silica gel adsorbent. **US Patent No. 75,598,568**.
- Coval, M.L. (1979). Injectable gamma globulin. **U.S. Patent No. 4,165,370**.
- Crowe, J.H., Crowe, L.M., Carpenter, J.F., Aurell-Wistrom, C. (1987). Stabilization of dry phospholipid bilayers and proteins by sugars. *Biochem. J.*, 242, 1.
- Davis, S.S. (1974). Pharmaceutical aspects of i.v. fat emulsion. *J. Hosp. Pharm.*, 32, 149–70.
- Deluca, P.P., Rapp, R.P. (1982). Parenteral Drug Delivery Systems. *In:* Banker G.S., Chalmers R.K. (editors). **Pharmaceutical and Pharmacy Practice**, Philadelphia: Lippincott, 238–278.
- Dexter, M.B., Shott, M.J. (1979). The evaluation of force needed to expel oily injection vehicles from syringes. *J. Pharm. Pharmacol.*, 31, 497–500.
- Fukushima, T., Matsunaga, T., Funakoshi, S. (1981). Process for Heat Treatment of Aqueous Solution Containing Human Blood Coagulation Factor XIII. **European Patent No. 37078**.
- Graves, M.J. (1973). **Parenteral Products**. William Heirmann Medical Books Ltd., London. 30.
- Guy, F. (2004). A renaissance for injectables. *Scrip Magazine*, 135(5), 7–9.
- Halsall, K.G. (1985). Calcitrol injection and plastic syringes. *Pharm. J.*, 235, 99.
- Hansrani, P.K., Davis, S.S., Groves, M.J. (1983). The preparation and properties of sterile intravenous emulsions. *J. Parenter. Sci. Technol.*, 37(4), 145–50
- Hellman, K., Miller, D.S., Cammack, K.A. (1983). The effect of freeze-drying on the quaternary structure of asparaginase. *Biochim. Biophys. Acta*, 749, 133.
- Herman, C.J., Groves, M.J. (1992). Hydrolysis kinetics of phospholipids in thermally stressed intravenous lipid emulsion formulations. *J. Pharm. Pharmacol.*, 44, 539–42.
- Jackylaw (2001). Cashing on proteins. *Scrip Magazine*, 5, 17–19.
- Jansen, V. (1976). Process of stabilizing therapeutically useful plasmin solutions. **U.S. Patent No. 3,950,513**.
- Jeffrey, L.P., Johnson, P.N., Stonka, D.J., Randall, H.T. (1977). Intravenous fat emulsion. *Hosp. Formul.*, 12(11), 772–73.
- Jeppsson, R. (1972). Effects of barbituric acids using an emulsion form intravenously. *Acta Pharm. Suec.*, 9, 81–90.
- Johnson, D.M., Pritchard, R.A., Taylor, W.F., Conley, D., Zyniga, G., McGreevy, K.G. (1986). Degradation of the LHRH analog nafarelin acetate in aqueous solution. *Int. J. Pharm.* 31, 125.
- Laval-Jeantet, A.M., Laval-Jeantet, M., Bergot, C. (1982). Effect of particle size on the tissue distribution of iodized emulsified fat following intravenous administration. *Invest. Radiol.*, 17(6), 617–20.
- Levy, M.Y., Benita, S. (1991). Short and long-term stability assessment of new injectable diazepam submicron emulsion. *J. Parenter. Sci. Technol.*, 45(2), 101–7.

- Lundberg, B.B. (1997). A submicron lipid emulsion coated with aliphatic polyethylene glycol for parenteral administration of paclitaxel (Taxol). *J. Pharm. Pharmacol.*, 49(1), 16–21.
- Manning, M.C., Patel, K., Borchardt, R. (1989). Stability of protein pharmaceuticals. *Pharm. Res.*, 6, 903.
- Martin, A.N., Swarbrick, J., Cammarata, A. (1991). **Physical Pharmacy**, 3rd ed. Lea & Febiger, Philadelphia.
- Pearlman, R., Nguyen, T. (1989). Formulation strategies for recombinant proteins: hGH and tPA. *In:* D. Marshak, D. Liu (eds). **Therapeutic Peptides and Proteins: Formulation Delivery and Targeting**, Cold Spring Harbor Lab.
- Peters, T. Jr. (1985). Serum albumin. *Adv. Protein Chem.*, 37,161–245.
- Quinn, R., Andrade, J.D. (1983). Minimizing the aggregation of neutral insulin solutions. *J. Pharm. Sci.*, 72, 1472.
- Rubino, J.T. (1990). The influence of charged lipids on the flocculation and coalescence of oil-in-water emulsions. I: Kinetic assessment of emulsion stability. *J. Parenter. Sci. Technol.*, 44(4), 210–15.
- **United States Pharmacopoeia, National Formulary (2004)**, 27th Ed., 22nd Ed., United States Pharmacopoieal Convention, Inc., Rockville, MD, 20852, 2108.
- **United States Pharmacopoeia, National Formulary**, 27th Ed., 22nd Ed (2004a) Containers (661) United States Pharmacopoieal Convention, Inc., Rockville, MD, 20852: 2289–90.
- **United States Pharmacopoeia, National Formulary**, 27th Ed., 22nd Ed (2004b) Biological tests – Plastics and other polymers. United States Pharmacopoieal Convention, Inc., Rockville, MD, 20852, 2290–2292.
- **United States Pharmacopoeia, National Formulary**, 27th Ed., 22nd Ed., Elastomeric closures for injection (381) (2004c), United States Pharmacopoieal Convention, Inc., Rockville, MD, 20852, p 2214.
- **United States Pharmacopoeia, National Formulary**, 27th Ed., 22nd Ed. (2004d) Particulate matters in Injections (788), United States Pharmacopoieal Convention, Inc., Rockville, MD, 20852, 2338–2344.
- **United States Pharmacopoeia, National Formulary**, 27th Ed., 22nd Ed. (2004e) Sterility tests (71) United States Pharmacopoieal Convention, Inc., Rockville, MD, 20852, 2157–2162.
- **United States Pharmacopoeia, National Formulary**, 27th Ed., 22nd Ed. (2004f) Pyrogen test (851) United States Pharmacopoieal Convention, Inc., Rockville, MD, 20852, 2194–2195.
- **United States Pharmacopoeia, National Formulary**, 27th Ed., 22nd Ed. (2004g) Bacterial Endotoxin Tests (85). United States Pharmacopoieal Convention, Inc., Rockville, MD, 20852, 2169–2171.
- Wang, Y.J., Hanson, M.A. (1988). Technical Report No. 10. Parenteral formulations of proteins and peptides: Stability and stabilizers. *J. Parent. Sci. Tech.*, 42: S3–S26.
- Washington, C. (1996). Stability of lipid emulsions for drug delivery. *Adv. Drug Del. Rev.*, 20, 131–45.
- Wolfert, R.R., Cox, R.M. (1975). Room temperature stability of drug products labeled for refrigerated storage. *Am. J. Hosp. Pharm.*, 32, 585.
- Yalabik-Kas, H.S., Eylimaz, S., Hincal A.A. (1985). *STP Pharma. Sci.*, 1978–1984.

6

Ophthalmic Products

Virendra Gajbhiye and N.K. Jain

INTRODUCTION

Ophthalmic preparations are sterile products essentially free from foreign particles, suitably compounded and packaged for instillation into the eye. They are intended to be applied to the eyelids or employed in the space between the eyelids and the eyeball. Generally, solutions, suspension, ointments and inserts are commonly used as ophthalmic products. Preparations intended for eye disorders can be traced back to antiquity. Egyptian papyri writings describe eye medications. The Greeks and Romans expanded such uses and invented the term *collyria*. Ophthalmic products are administered to the eye for local effects, for example, miosis, mydriasis, and anesthesia, or to diminish intraocular pressure in glaucoma patients. Drug penetration into the eye (i.e., transcorneal transport) is not a very effective route. It is assessed that only one-tenth of a dose penetrates into the eye. Most of the ophthalmic products are no longer prepared in the hospital pharmacy. Ophthalmic drug delivery, in turn, had become interesting and challenging endeavors for the pharmaceutical product development scientists. However, it is necessary for the formulation scientist to be familiar with the significant characteristics of these important products. The specific aim of designing ophthalmic product is to achieve an optimal concentration of a drug at the active site for the appropriate durations. A significant challenge to the formulator is to circumvent the protective barriers of the eye without causing permanent tissue damage. Ocular disposition and elimination of a therapeutic agent is dependent upon its physicochemical properties and relevant ocular anatomy and physiology. It is possible to get systemic effects after ophthalmic administration. Drug reaches the systemic circulation either by entering into lacrimal canalicula followed by emptying into the GI tract or by absorption through the conjunctiva. Drugs such as antibiotics and corticosteroids can be administered systemically to treat certain eye conditions, but this route of administration is not often favored because of the poor drug penetration into the eye from the systemic circulation. Subsequently, high doses of drugs have to be administered, leading to systemic side effects and toxicity. Periocular injections are also used to administer anti-infective drugs, mydriatics or corticosteroids. However, injections tend to be reserved for serious conditions affecting the anterior portion of the eye where the topical therapy is ineffective. By far, the most popular route of administration for drug treatment in the ocular diseases and diagnostics is the topical route and this route is, therefore, the main focus of this chapter. There are many diseases affecting the eye that are treated with various types of drugs and drug delivery systems. Table 6.1 lists some of the main therapeutic classes of drugs currently used to treat eye diseases and types of dosage forms available commercially.

In the recent years there have been increasing efforts to find safer and effective drugs to treat various ocular conditions and diseases that are poorly controlled now, as well as to develop novel dosage forms and delivery systems to improve the topical delivery of existing drugs. There is an unmet demand for new products in some markets, such as antiglaucoma products for patients that do not respond to currently available marketed products. Carbonic anhydrase inhibitors, which were formally avail-

Table 6.1. Examples of therapeutic classes of drugs currently used to treat ocular diseases

Drugs	Class	Clinical use	Dosage form
Acyclovir	Antiviral	Against viral infection	Eye ointment
Idoxuridine			Eye ointment
			Eye drop solution
Trifluridine			Eye drop solution
Oxybuprocaine	Local anesthetic	Tonometry and prior to minor surgery	Eye drop solution
Procaine		Contact lens fitting	Eye drop solution
Dexamethasone	Anti-inflammatory	Inflammation	Eye drop solution
Hydrocortisone			Eye drop solution
Chloramphenicol	Antibacterial	Eye infection	Eye drop solution
			Eye ointment
Sulfacetamide			Eye drop solution
			Eye ointment
Tetracycline			Eye drop solution
			Eye ointment
Tropicamide	Mydriatics	Examination	Eye drop solution
			Eye ointment
Ephedrine			Eye drop solution
			Eye ointment
Cyclopentolate	Cycloplegics	Examination	Eye drop solution
			Eye ointment
Atropine		Temporarily paralyze the accommodation reflex	Eye drop solution
Betaxolol	β-Adrenergic blocker	Treatment of glaucoma	Eye drop solution
			Eye suspension
			Eye ointment
Timolol			Eye drop solution
Pilocarpine	Miotic	Treatment of glaucoma	Ocular insert
			Eye drop solution
Carbachol			Eye drop solution

able as oral products only, are being developed as topical products for glaucoma treatment. The majority of research so far was aimed at delivery to the anterior segment tissues, but recently it had been aimed for delivery to posterior globe (Fig. 6.1).

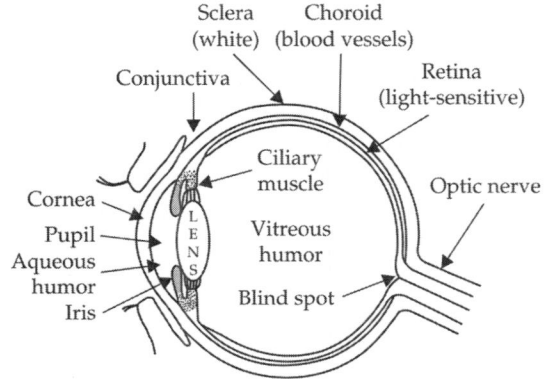

Fig. 6.1. Anatomy of the eye.

ISSUES AND CHALLENGES IN OCULAR DRUG DELIVERY

Ocular topical drug delivery is particularly challenging because of inherent difficulties associated with absorption of topically applied drugs into the eye. Ophthalmic dosage forms are administered via the topical route to treat both surface and intraocular conditions. Consideration of the anatomical and physiological features of the eye as well as the physicochemical properties of the drug, are all important when developing a topical ophthalmic delivery system. A good overview of the structure of the outside of the eye and a cross-section of the anterior segment of the eye can be seen in Fig. 6.1. The front part of the globe of the eye is clear and colorless and is called the *cornea*. It contains no blood vessels, but is rich in nerve endings. The cornea consists of three major layers: the *outer epithelium*, *middle stroma* and *inner endothelium*. When topical products are administered to the eye, they first encounter the cornea and conjunctiva, representing the primary barriers to drug penetration. The epithelium and endothelium of

the cornea are rich in lipid content, making them barriers to drug penetration of polar, water soluble compounds. The stroma, on the other hand, is a hydrophilic layer containing 70 to 80 percent water, presenting a barrier to the permeation of non-polar, lipid soluble compounds. The other part of the boundary layer to the front of the eye is the *sclera*. This is white in color and opaque, and contains most of the blood vessels supplying the anterior tissues of the eye. The outer surface of the sclera is loosely covered by the conjunctival membrane, which is continuous with the inner surface of the eyelids, and also presents a significant permeability barrier to most drugs. For drugs that permeate the vascular systems of the sclera and conjunctiva, transport tends to be away from the eye into the general circulation.

Other major physiological barrier mechanisms are due to tear production and the blink reflex. The conjunctival and corneal surfaces of the eye are continuously lubricated by a film of fluid secreted by the conjunctival and lacrimal glands. The lacrimal glands secrete watery fluid called tears, and the sebaceous glands on the margin of eyelids secrete an oily fluid that spreads over the tear film. The latter reduces the rate of evaporation of the tear film from the exposed surface of the eyes. Blinking assists to evenly spread the tear film over the surface of the eye and to drain the tears via the nasolacrimal duct into the nose, and ultimately down the back of the throat into gastrointestinal (GI) tract. Upon administration of topically applied eye drops, removal from the eye is rapid due to tear production and the blinking processes occurring simultaneously. The precorneal volume is very less, about 7 to 8 µL, but volumes up to 25 to 30 µL can be held in this area before spillage occurs. The volume over this simply spill out or lost rapidly with tears. The eye drops causing irritation are likely to stimulate tear production rate and increase the rate of drug removal from the eye. The removal of the drug by dilution is also aided by the blink reflex.

Other physiological factors affecting ocular delivery of topical drugs are protein binding and drug metabolism. Protein accounts for up to 2 percent of the total content of the normal tears and can be higher under certain pathological conditions such as uveitis. The increased size of the protein-drug complex will render the bound drug molecules unavailable for absorption, and lacrimal drainage will rapidly remove them from the eye. Tears are also known to contain a range of enzymes, such as esterases, monoamino oxidases and aminopeptidases, which can metabolize many ocularly applied drugs. Most of the ophthalmic solutions and suspensions are packaged in eye dropper bottles. Patients should be demonstrated how to properly instill the drops in their eyes, and every effort should be made to emphasize the need for instilling only one drop per administration, not two or three.

ABSORPTION OF DRUGS IN THE EYE

The drug given by ocular route must be:

(a) potent,
(b) non-toxic,
(c) sufficiently stable such that neither significant loss in potency from diminished availability nor little increase in toxicity from byproducts of degradation arises,
(d) targetable either to tissues and location of primary disease-state etiology or to sites responsible for symptomatic response, and
(e) sufficiently compatible with the dosage form, and with the tissues exposed to it, to achieve an effective pharmacokinetic tissue profile.

The major routes of administration for ocular therapeutics comprise of topical, periocular, intraocular and systemic. Furthermore, ionic drugs can be delivered to the intraocular tissues through the cornea by corneal iontophoresis technique. This method has the advantage of attaining drug penetration even with the presence of corneal epithelium, an anatomical barrier to transcorneal drug permeation. Constant irrigation through the use of catheters or miniature infusion pumps, though not in common practice, are the other routes of administration.

The various factors affecting drug availability are:

1. Loss of drug from the palpebral fissure and spillage of drug from the eye and its removal by the nasolacrimal drainage.
2. Drainage from an administered drop through the nasolacrimal system into the GI tract begins immediately on instillation. The clinical significance of drainage is so well recognized that manual nasolacrimal occlusion has been recommended as a means of improving the therapeutic index of anti-glaucoma medications.
3. Superficial absorption of drug into the palpebral and bulbar conjunctiva, with generally concomitant rapid removal from ocular tissues by the peripheral blood flow due to the extensive vascularity of the uvea that lies under the bulbar conjunctiva (a mucous membrane), the sclera (white part of eye) and a tough covering, to which it is attached anteriorly.
4. Binding of drug to either external sites (e.g., by mucins) or internal tissues (e.g., sclera) can be detrimental to efficacy.
5. Removal from the palpebral fissure, instilled volume drainage, drug protein interactions, non-productive conjunctival uptake, productive corneal absorption, tear production and evaporation are also major factors affecting the concentration of topically applied drug in the precorneal space.

Transcorneal transport

Although, transport of hydrophilic and macro-molecular drugs has been reported to occur by limbal or scleral routes, often this is at rates significantly reduced from those expected for transcorneal transport of conventional, modestly lipophilic agents of low molecular weight

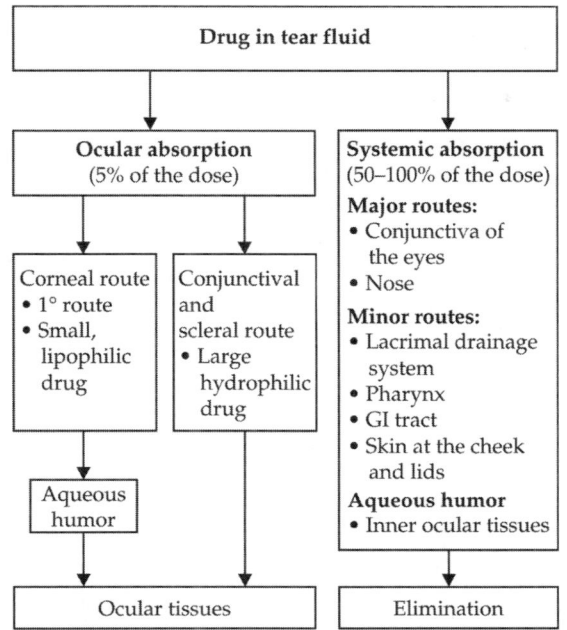

Fig. 6.2. Schematic diagram of ocular distribution.

(Fig. 6.2). Even here, transmembrane transport is a significant requirement for availability.

Simple hydrodynamic analysis of the *in vitro* mechanism indicates that the elution concentration, in the absence of absorption, is a linear kinetic process, with a release profile that scales as the ratio of the tear production to tear volume, V/V_R specifically, as per Eq. 1.

$$N_{T(t)} = N_1(1 - \exp(-V/V_R)) \qquad ...(1)$$

where
V_R = volume of the reservoir;
V = flow rate through reservoir;
N_1 = amount of drug in reservoir at time zero;
$N_{T(t)}$ = time dependent total amount eluted from reservoir volume

and where, the complementary amount contained in reservoir $N_{C(t)}$, the amount of drug in the reservoir, is defined as

$$N_{C(t)} = N_1 - N_{T(t)} \qquad ...(2)$$

This amount contained in reservoir is the characteristic of the stirred-tank chemical reactor models. Combining these containment profiles,

$N_{C(t)}$, with diffusional transmembrane transport, yields expected tissue profiles the rates of which are dictated by both containment profile and tissue affinities, and the magnitude of which is often dominated by trans-membrane flux.

Ex vivo studies of trans-corneal transport can be used to establish the characteristics of passive diffusional motion, the conventional means by which drugs reach internal ocular tissues (Fig. 6.3). Although such analysis neglects the complications of tear flow, tear drainage, non-productive membrane absorption, elimination from the aqueous humor, and so forth, the corneal transport results are crucial and can be grafted into the primarily hydrodynamic effects subsequently (Figs. 6.2 and 6.3).

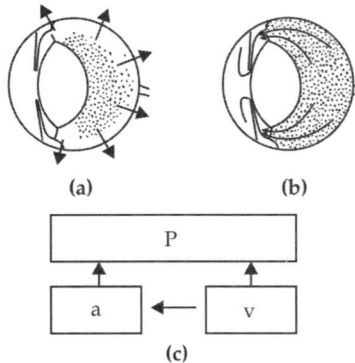

Fig. 6.3. Schematic representation of exit pathways from the vitreous humor: (a) transretinal; (b) by drainage out of aqueous humor; (c) compartmental model showing kinetic relationships between a, anterior chamber, p, plasma, and v, vitreous.

One of the key parameters for correlating molecular structure and chemical properties with bioavailability has been transcorneal flux, or alternatively, the corneal permeability coefficient. The epithelium is modelled as a lipid barrier (possibly, with a limited number of aqueous "pores" that, for this physical model, serve as the equivalent of the extracellular space in a more physiological description) and the stroma as an aqueous barrier. The endothelium is very thin and porous compared with the epithelium and can be ignored in the analysis, although, mathematically it can be included as part of the lipid barrier. Diffusion through bilayer membranes of various structures has been modelled for some time and adapted to ophthalmic applications more recently. For a series of molecules of similar size, it was shown that the permeability increases with the partition coefficient until a plateau is reached. Modelling of this type of data has led to the conclusion that drugs need to be both oil- and water-soluble. If pores are not included in the analysis, the steady-state corneal flux, J_s, can be written as:

$$J_s = PC_w / [(Pl_s/D_s) + (l_e/D_e)] \qquad ...(3)$$

where

C_w = concentration of drug in donor phase;
l_s, l_e = stromal and epithelial thickness, respectively;
D_s, D_e = corresponding diffusion coefficients; and
P = oil-to-water distribution coefficient.

The permeability coefficient is just the flux divided by C_w. It is apparent that the permeability coefficient is linear with P for small distribution coefficients and constant for large P. Thus, for small P the epithelium is the barrier, and for large P the stroma is the barrier.

A simple estimate of the diffusion coefficients can be approximated from examining the effects of molecular size on transport through a continuum for which there is an energy loss for displacing solvent. Since the molecular weight dependence of the diffusion coefficients for polymers obeys a power law equation, a similar form has been chosen for the corneal barriers. That is, the molecular weight (M) dependence of the diffusion coefficients can be expressed as:

$$D_e = D_e^{(0)} M_a$$
$$D_s = D_s^{(0)} M_g$$

One observes a rapid reduction in permeability coefficient with decreasing P and increasing M. The addition of pores to the model, a mathematical construct, is necessary to account for permeability of polar molecules, such as mannitol and cromolyn. These would also be required for correlating effects of compounds, such as benzalkonium chloride, which may compromise the epithelial barrier by increasing the volume of the extracellular space. Another perspective provided by this model is the effect of three physicochemical parameters; solubility, distribution coefficient, and molecular mass on transcorneal flux. In case of agents with low molecular mass, flux depends significantly on the mass.

Since direct determination of ophthalmic bioavailability in humans is not possible without endangering the eye, investigators have used fluorescein to study factors affecting bio-availability in the eye, because its penetration can be quantitated in humans through the use of a slit-lamp fluorophotometer. The use of fluorescein data to extrapolate vehicle effects to ophthalmic drugs in general would be questionable owing to the large differences in chemical structure, properties, and permeability existing between fluorescein and most ophthalmic drugs. For ocular pharmacokinetic studies target tissue drug concentration measurements can be made using non-invasive approaches such as nuclear imaging using SPECT (single-photon emission computed tomography) and PET (photon emission tomography), magnetic resonance imaging, magnetic resonance spectroscopy, and laser scanning fluorophotometry. Non-invasive approaches are particularly feasible with the eye, an external organ that has a transparent surface. The transparency of cornea, aqueous humor, lens, and vitreous humor, which facilitate the access of light signal to the retina, can be utilized to access these compartments for the assessment of drug contents using spectrophotometry. With laser scanning fluorimetry, estimation of drug levels at various depths and individual layers of tissues is now possible for fluorophores. Also, non-invasive PET and NMR studies can be used to assess the disposition of some drugs.

BIOAVAILABILITY IN OCULAR REGION

Absolute bioavailability of topically administered ophthalmic products in the eye can be sub-categorized into, pre-absorption bioavailability, biophasic availability and systemic bioavailability. Absolute bioavailability of the drug is characterized by the patterns of the rates and extents at which the drug molecules enter into the body or released at the pre-absorption sites to subsequently enter the body. Biophasic availability and systemic bioavailability refer to the drug's entry to its site of action and into systemic circulation, respectively. Drug remains in equilibrium between the two compartments, if the distribution between systemic circulation and biophase is sufficiently rapid. Therefore, systemic and biophasic availabilities are identical. The bioavailability of topically applied ocular drugs is, generally very poor. It is estimated that less than 10%, and typically 1% or less, of the topically instilled dose into the eye actually permeates the cornea and is distributed within the various compartments of the eye. This poor availability is attributed to physiological protective mechanisms comprising nasolacrimal drainage, permeability and metabolic obstacles imposed by the corneal epithelia, and the inherent physicochemical insufficiencies of the drug molecules. Currently, the major focus is on the mechanistic understanding of corneal and conjunctival transport pathways. The dynamic properties of the epithelial barriers and their reversible modulation under physiological conditions offer great promise in improving the ocular bioavailability of topically administered drugs through either the corneal or non-corneal pathway. In recent years, research in ophthalmic drug delivery has been directed towards the design of novel drugs and drug delivery systems with improved corneal permeability and, in turn, improved ocular bioavailability.

PRODUCT DEVELOPMENT

Products designed for the ophthalmic use undergo a process of design optimization owing to characteristic problems associated with absorption proficiencies of topically applied drugs. It has been realized that the process of ocular product design and development necessitates a thorough understanding of the numerous anatomical, physiological and metabolic considerations of the eye, in addition to the physicochemical properties of the drug. Because the official compendia require all topically administered ophthalmic medication to be sterile, the manufacturer of such medication must consider all the current concepts in the manufacture of sterile pharmaceuticals in designing a manufacturing procedure for sterile ophthalmic pharmaceutical products. It is quite rare that the composition or the packaging of the ophthalmic pharmaceutical will lend itself to terminal sterilization, the simplest form of manufacture of sterile products. Only a few of those drugs formulated in simple aqueous vehicles are stable to normal autoclaving temperatures and times (121°C for 20-30 min). Such drug products must be packaged in glass or other heat-deformation-resistant packaging and, thus, can be sterilized in this manner.

To sustain longer contact between the drug and the surrounding eye environment, suspensions, ointments, and inserts have been developed. In case of aqueous suspensions, the particle size is retained to a minimum to avoid irritation of the eye. It is likely to find particles that stick to the conjunctiva after administration of this dosage form. Ointments tend to retain the drug in contact with the eye longer than suspensions. Most ophthalmic ointment bases are a mixture of mineral oil and white petrolatum and have a melting point close to body temperature. But ointments tend to blur patient vision as they remain viscous and are not removed easily by the tear fluid. Therefore, ointments are generally used at night as adjunctive therapy to eye drops, which are used during the day. Ophthalmic ointment tubes are typically small and fitted with narrow gauge tips which permit the extrusion of narrow bands of ointment.

Most ophthalmic products, however, do not fall into the foregoing category. In general, the active principle is particularly physically or chemically unstable at higher temperature. Moreover, to impart viscosity, aqueous products are generally formulated with the inclusion of high molecular weight polymers, which may, similarly, be adversely affected by heat. Finally, the convenience of plastic dispensing bottles has led to the use of modern polyolefins that resist heat deformation and, with a proper sterilization cycle, are now being used for some ophthalmic pharmaceutical products.

Because of these product sensitivities, most ophthalmic pharmaceutical products are aseptically manufactured and filled into previously sterilized containers in aseptic environments using aseptic filling and capping techniques. This is the case for ophthalmic solutions, suspensions, and ointments, and rather specialized technology is involved in their manufacture. In general, however, the manufacture of sterile ophthalmic pharmaceutical products requires special attention to environment, manufacturing techniques, raw materials (including packaging components), and equipments. In addition to the design selection criteria, there are some other design specification criteria and critical quality parameters that should be emphasized. Ophthalmic products should comply with compendial requirements specified for the territory in which the product is to be registered. Reference to the major pharmacopoeias should highlight the majority of requirements. The British and European Pharmacopoeias offer the most detailed guidance for the different types of preparations, eye drops, eye lotions, semi-solid preparations or ophthalmic inserts. There are also pharmacopoeial requirements relating to the

container to be used, which have been discussed in pack design consideration. One very important design requirement worth stressing is that the container/delivery system be easy to use. Glaucoma is a common eye condition affecting many elderly patients who may have poor eyesight and manual dexterity, and thus are not capable of administering a complex delivery system. Design of a new delivery system should include consumer trials and customer feedback to ensure the new device is acceptable.

Ophthalmic products are required to be sterile up to the point of use and must comply with the pharmacopoeial tests for sterility. Terminal sterilization method is preferred method from a regulatory point of view, as opposed to aseptic manufacture. If terminal sterilization is not used, for example, because the drug substance cannot withstand the processing conditions, good supporting documentation will be required to gain regulatory approval.

The advantage of using established excipients in a topical formulation is to improve the chance of patient tolerability and patient compliance. An essential product design requirement is to minimize ocular side effects such as irritation, burning, stinging and blurring of vision, any of which may provide a reason for patient to stop their medication. Typical finished products specification and control tests for an ophthalmic multi-dose solution product, required to demonstrate that the product is of a quality suitable for intended use, may include the following:

- Appearance, description, e.g. clear, colored, absence of foreign particles
- Identification tests for the drug
- Quantitative drug assay/impurities and degradation products; limits based on analytical capability and stability data
- Quantitative preservative assay; limits based on analytical capability and levels required for antimicrobial preservative efficacy
- pH; limits based on stability, solubility and physiological acceptability

- Osmolarity; limits based on physiological acceptability
- Volume/weight of contents; to ensure that labelled or claimed number of doses can be dispensed, but not more than 10 µL unless otherwise justified
- Sterility

A. Environment

Ophthalmic products must be prepared in a precise environment that is designed to ensure their sterility. Aside from drug safety, stability, and efficacy, the major design criteria of an ophthalmic pharmaceutical product are the additional safety criteria of sterility, preservative efficacy, and freedom from extraneous foreign particulate matter. Monitoring of air and water system is critical in confirming that they are being controlled and that the levels of particulates, microbial matter, and other contaminants are within pre-established limits. Current U.S. standards for Good Manufacturing Practices (GMP) provide for the use of specially designed, environmentally controlled areas for the manufacture of sterile large and small volume injections for terminal sterilization. These environmentally controlled areas must meet the requirements of Class 100,000 space in all areas where open containers and closures are not exposed, or where product filling-and capping operations are not taking place. The latter areas must meet the requirements of Class 100 space.

As defined in Federal Standard 209, Class 100,000 and 100 space contain not more than 100,000 or 100 particles (either viable or non-viable), respectively, per cubic foot of air of a diameter of 0.5 mm or larger. Often these design criteria are coupled with laminar airflow concepts. Class 100,000 conditions can be achieved in the conventionally designed clean room where proper filtration of air supply and adequate turnover rates are provided. Class 100 conditions over open containers can be achieved with properly sized HEPA (high-efficiency particulate air) filtered laminar airflow sources. Depending on the product need and funds available, some aseptic pharmaceutical manufacturing environments have been designed totally to class 100 laminar-flow specifications, although, during actual product manufacture, the generation of particulate matter by equipment, product, and people, may cause these environments to demonstrate particulate matter levels two or more times greater than that designed. It is for this reason that specialists in the design of pharmaceutical manufacturing and hospital operating room environments are beginning to view these environments not from the standpoint of total particles per cubic foot of space alone, but also from the standpoint of the ratio of viable to non-viable particles.

When dealing with the environment in which a sterile product is manufactured, the materials used for construction of the facility, as well as personnel attire, training, conduct in the space; the entrance and egress of personnel, equipment, and packaging, and the product; all bear heavily on the assurance of product sterility and minimization of extraneous particulate matter. Walls, ceilings, and floors should be constructed of materials that are hard, non-chipping/non-flaking, smooth, and unaffected by surface-cleaning agents and disinfectants. All lights and windows should be flush-mounted in walls and ceilings for ease of cleaning and disinfection. Ultraviolet lamps may be provided in recessed, flush-mounted fixtures to maintain surface disinfection. Separate entrances for personnel and equipment should be provided through specially designed air locks that are maintained at a negative pressure relative to the aseptic manufacturing area and at a positive pressure relative to non-environmentally controlled area. Equipment should be designed for simplicity of operation and should be constructed for ease of disassembly, cleaning, and sterilization or sanitization.

The importance of personnel training and behavior cannot be overemphasized in the maintenance of an acceptable environment for the manufacture of sterile ophthalmic products or sterile pharmaceutical agents. The staff working on the process and for the filling of the product must be suitably trained and certified to work within cleanrooms. Training of personnel is a critical issue. Any activities conducted by human personnel represent a high risk of contamination. Personnel training, retraining, and ongoing monitoring of performance must be a continuing consideration in manufacturing of sterile products. Personnel must be trained in the proper mode of gowning with sterile, non-shedding garments, and also in the proper techniques and conduct for aseptic manufacturing. For the maximum in personnel comfort and to minimize sloughing of epidermal cells and hair, a cool working environment should be maintained, with relative humidity controlled between 40 and 60%.

B. Manufacturing techniques

The manufacturing techniques should meet the requirements of GMP and GLP, specifically with regard to cross-contamination. During manufacturing, all procedures should be validated and supervised by doing suitable in-process controls. These should be considered to guarantee the efficiency of each stage of production. In-process controls during production of ophthalmic products should comprise monitoring environmental conditions (especially regarding particulate and microbial contamination), pyrogens (use of a limulus amoebocyte lysate (LAL) test), pH and clarity of solution and integrity of the container (absence of leakage). Appropriate limits should be set for the particle size of the active ingredients. It is mandatory that ophthalmic preparations are sterile. Therefore, aseptic manufacturing process is usually employed when the dosage form precludes routine sterilization methods.

Aqueous ophthalmic solutions are generally manufactured by dissolving the active ingredient and all or a portion of the excipients into all or a portion of the water, and then sterilizing this solution by heat or by filtration through sterile membrane filter media into a sterile receptacle. If incomplete at this point, this sterile solution is then mixed with the additional required sterile components, such as previously sterilized solutions of viscosity-imparting agents, preservatives, and so on, and the batch is brought to final volume with additional sterile water. Aqueous suspensions are handled in almost similar manner, except that before bringing the batch to final volume with additional sterile water, the solid that is to be suspended is previously rendered sterile by heat, or by exposure to ethylene oxide, or ionizing radiation (gamma or electrons), or by dissolution in an appropriate solvent, sterile filtration, and aseptic crystallization. The sterile solid is then added to the batch, either directly or by first dispersing the solid in a small portion of the batch. After adequate dispersion, the batch is brought to final volume with sterile water. Because the eye is sensitive to particles not much larger than 25 mm in diameter, proper raw material specifications for particle size of the solid to be dispersed must be established and verified on each lot of raw material and final product.

When an ophthalmic ointment is manufactured, all raw material components must be rendered sterile before compounding, unless the ointment contains an aqueous fraction that can be sterilized by heat, filtration, or ionizing radiation. The ointment base is sterilized by heat, and appropriately filtered while molten to remove extraneous foreign particulate matter. It is then placed into a sterile steam jacketed kettle to maintain the ointment in a molten state under aseptic conditions, and the previously sterilized active ingredients(s) and excipients are added aseptically. While still molten, the entire ointment may be passed through a previously sterilized colloid mill for adequate dispersion of the insoluble components.

After the product is compounded in an aseptic manner, it is filled into previously sterilized containers. Commonly employed methods of sterilization of packaging components include exposure to heat, ethylene oxide gas, and ^{60}Co (gamma) irradiation. When a product is to be used in conjunction with ophthalmic surgical procedures and must enter the aseptic operating area, the exterior of the primary container must be rendered sterile by the manufacturer and maintained sterile with appropriate packaging. This may be accomplished by aseptic packaging or by exposure of the completely packaged product to ethylene oxide gas, ionizing radiation, or heat.

C. Raw materials

All raw materials used in the compounding of ophthalmic pharmaceutical products must be of the highest quality available. Complete raw material specifications for each component must be established and verified for each lot purchased. When raw materials are rendered sterile before compounding, the reactivity of the raw material with the sterilizing medium must be completely evaluated, and the sterilization must be validated to demonstrate its capability of sterilizing raw materials contaminated with large numbers (10^5–10^7) of microorganisms that have been demonstrated to be most resistant to the mode of sterilization appropriate for that raw material. The manufacturing of ophthalmic products requires careful consideration of numerous physicochemical parameters. These comprise the necessity for isotonicity, required pH, addition of antioxidants and antimicrobial agents, a certain buffering capacity, usage of viscosity enhancers, and the choice of suitable packaging. Ophthalmic products can be considered isotonic when the tonicity is equal to that of a 0.9% sodium chloride solution. The eye typically tolerates solutions equivalent to 0.5–1.8% of sodium chloride. The pH of ophthalmic drops must correspond to that of tear fluid (pH 7.4). To accomplish this, buffer may need to be added to the ophthalmic preparation. The requirement to add a buffering agent is based on stability considerations. Selected pH must be the optimum for both physiological tolerance and stability of the active pharmaceutical ingredient. Buffer system must not cause deterioration or precipitation of the API. The effect on the lacrimal flow should also be considered. The various commonly used excipients are:

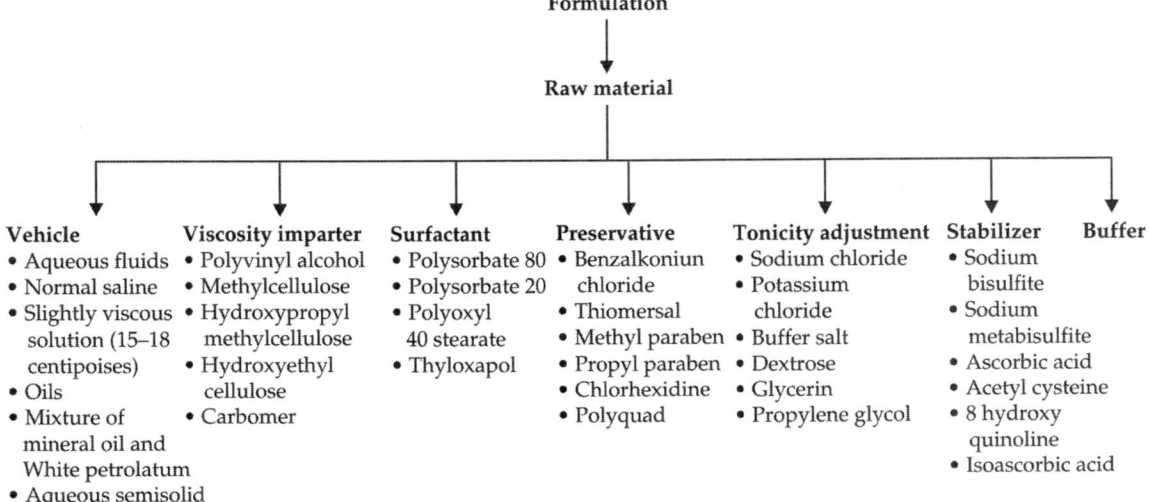

Fig. 6.4. Ophthalmic product excipients.

1. Vehicles

Vehicles used in ophthalmic preparation must have excellent wetting capability to penetrate cornea and other tissues. Ophthalmic drops are, with few exceptions, aqueous fluids using any official Purified Water, as the solvent. Purified Water meeting pharmacopeial standards may be obtained by distillation, de-ionization, or reverse osmosis. Water For Injection (WFI) is the most extensively used solvent/vehicle for ophthalmic products. WFI can be acquired by distillation of de-ionized water or a reverse osmosis procedure. Inorganic traces from the vehicle can be separated by reverse osmosis, distillation, de-ionization, or by combination of these processes. Membrane filters are also employed to eliminate particulate impurities, and charcoal beds may be used to remove organic materials. Sodium chloride solution (0.9% w/v), also known as normal saline is also a common and an acceptable vehicle for ophthalmic drugs, slightly viscous solutions are generally recognized as more satisfying to use by the patients. Increasing the viscosity is also exploited as a means to increase the bioavailability of drugs, due to an increased time of residence of the medication in the eye. However, there appears to be only a narrow band of acceptable viscosity (15–18 centipoises), since the products must have negligible visual effects, should not obstruct the puncti and canaliculi and should be filterable and sterilisable. Recently, much research has been dedicated to mucoadhesive polymers, i.e. macromolecules capable of retaining the medication in the precorneal area not only by viscosity effects, but also by establishing physicochemical interactions with the mucin layer covering the corneal epithelium.

Oils have been used as vehicles for several topical eye drop products that are extremely sensitive to moisture. White petrolatum and its combination with liquid petrolatum to obtain a proper consistency is routinely used as the vehicle for ophthalmic ointments. When oils are used as vehicles in ophthalmic fluids they must be of the highest purity. Vegetable oils such as olive oil, castor oil, and sesame oil have been used for extemporaneous compounding. These oils are subject to rancidity and, therefore, must be used carefully. Some commercial oils, such as peanut oil, contain stabilizers that could be irritating. The purest grade of oil, such as that used for parenteral products would be advisable for ophthalmics.

The ointment vehicle is usually a mixture of mineral oil and white petrolatum. The mineral oil is added to reduce the melting point and modify the consistency. The principal advantages of the petrolatum-based ointments are their blandness and their anhydrous and inert nature, which make them suitable vehicles for moisture-sensitive drugs.

The anhydrous petrolatum base may be made more miscible with water through the use of an anhydrous liquid lanolin derivative. Drugs can be incorporated into such a base in aqueous solution if desired. Polyoxyl 40 stearate and Polyethylene glycol 300 are used in an anti-infective ointment to solubilize the active principle in the base, so that the ointment can be sterilized by aseptic filtration. The cosmetic-type bases, such as the o/w emulsion bases popular in dermatology, should not be used in the eye, nor should liquid emulsions, owing to the ocular irritation produced by the soaps and surfactants, used to form the emulsion. The non-aqueous portions of the base were either glycerin or polyethylene glycols in high concentrations. The matrix used to form the phases included silica, Gantez AN-139, and Carbopol 940. The bases may be quite irritating in rabbit eyes. The irritation is believed to be primarily due to the high concentration of the polyols used as vehicles.

An aqueous semisolid gel base has been developed that provides significantly longer residence time in the cul-de-sac and increases drug bioavailability and, thereby, may prolong the therapeutic level in the eye. The gel contains a high molecular weight, cross-linked polymer to provide the high viscosity and optimum rheological properties for prolonged ocular retention. Only a relatively low concentration of polymer is required, so that the gel base comprises of more than 95% water. The use of other polymers, such as cellulosic gums, polyvinyl alcohol, and polyacrylamides at comparable apparent viscosities, did not provide a significant prolonged effect. The prolonged effect of pilocarpine has also been demonstrated in human clinical trials, in which a single application of 4% pilocarpinc HCl-containing carbomer gel at bedtime, provided a 24 hr duration of reduced intraocular pressure (IOP), compared with the usually required q.i.d. dosing for pilocarpine solution. As a result, some glaucoma patients can now use pilocarpine in this aqueous gel base (Pilopine HS Gel), dosing only once a day at bedtime to control their IOP without the significant vision disturbance experienced during the day for the use of conventional pilocarpine eyedrops.

2. Tonicity adjusting agents

Generally used tonicity-adjusting ingredients include NaCl, KCl, buffer salts, dextrose, glycerin, and propylene glycol. A range of 0.5–2.0% NaCl equivalency does not cause a marked pain response, and a range of about 0.7–1.5% should be acceptable to most persons. In certain instances, the therapeutic concentration of the drug will necessitate using what might otherwise be considered an unacceptable tonicity, e.g. sodium sulfacetamide, for which the isotonic concentration is about 3.5%, but the drug is used in 10–30% concentrations. Fortunately, the eye seems to tolerate hypertonic solutions better than hypotonic ones. Ophthalmic products instilled into the eye may be tolerated over a fairly wide range of tonicity (0.5–1.5 percent NaCl equivalent). However, to minimize irritation and discomfort, ophthalmic solutions should ideally be isotonic with the tears, equivalent to 0.9 percent w/v solution of sodium chloride. Hypotonic ophthalmic solutions or suspensions

can be rendered isotonic by the addition of tonicity agents such as sodium chloride, potassium chloride, dextrose, glycerol and buffering salts. As with other adjuvants; the formulator should give due consideration to possible interaction between the tonicity agent and other components of the formulation, including the drug itself.

3. Buffers

The stability of most commonly used ophthalmic drugs is largely controlled by the pH of their environment and hence manufacturers place particular emphasis on this aspect. In addition to stability effects, pH adjustment can influence the comfort, safety, and activity of the product. Comfort can be described as the subjective response of the patient after instillation of the product in the cul-de-sac (i.e., whether it causes a pain response such as stinging or burning). Eye irritation is normally accompanied by an increase in tear fluid secretion (a defense mechanism) to aid in the restoration of normal physiological conditions. Accordingly, in addition to the discomfort encountered, products that produce irritation will tend to be flushed from the eye and, hence, a more rapid loss of medication may occur, with a probable reduction in the therapeutic response.

Owing to the small buffer capacity of tear fluids, acidic or basic pH solutions may result in excessive secretion of tears and may cause damage to the corneal epithelial cells. Therefore, pH adjustments are made close to the pH of tears. Likewise, pH adjustments are done to retain drug compounds in un-ionized form, which permits fast penetration across the corneal epithelial barrier. The pH values of ophthalmic solutions are adjusted to a range in which an acceptable shelf-life of at least 2 years can be achieved. Ideally, every product would be buffered to a pH of 7.4 (the normal physiological pH of tear fluid) so that it would be comfortable and possibly have optimum therapeutic activity. Various experiments, primarily in rabbits, have shown an enhanced effect when the pH was increased, owing to the solution containing higher concentration of the non-ionized lipid–soluble drug base, which is the species that can more rapidly penetrate the corneal epithelial barrier. This would not be true if the drug were an acidic moiety. The tears have some buffer capacity of their own, and hence they can neutralize the pH of an instilled solution if the quantity of solution is not excessive and if the solution does not have a strong resistance to neutralization. Pilocarpine activity is apparently the same whether applied from vehicles with nearly physiological pH values or from more acidic vehicles, provided the latter are not strongly buffered. A pH difference of 6.6 versus 4.2 produced a statistically insignificant difference in pilocarpine miosis. The pH values of ophthalmic solutions are adjusted to a range at which an acceptable shelf-life stability of at least 2 years can be achieved, and if necessary, they are buffered to remain within this range. If buffers are required, their capacity is controlled to be as low as possible, thus, enabling the tears to bring the pH of the eye back to the physiological range. Since the buffer capacity is determined by buffer concentration, the effect of buffers on tonicity must also be taken into account and is another reason that ophthalmic products are usually only lightly buffered.

The pH value is not the sole contributing factor to discomfort of some ophthalmic solutions. It is possible to have a product with a low pH and little buffer capacity that is more comfortable than a similar product with a higher pH and a strong buffer capacity. Epinephrine hydrochloride and Dipivefrin hydrochloride solutions, used for treatment of glaucoma, have a pH of about 3, yet they have acceptable comfort such that they can be used daily for many years. The same pH solution of epinephrine bitartrate has an intrinsically higher buffer capacity and will produce much more discomfort. A variety of regulatory approved buffers are available covering the useful pH range. For acidic pH

adjustment acetic acid/sodium acetate or citric acid/sodium citrate are often employed. For alkaline buffered solutions phosphate or borate buffers are frequently used. Buffering agent may also affect the activity of other components. For example, the anti-microbial preservative parabens (esters of para-hydroxybenzoic acid) is inactive at alkaline pH and more active as pH becomes more acidic. Another example is the viscosity of aqueous ophthalmic gels formulated with acrylic acid polymers (Carbomer), Carbopol resins, which are particularly sensitive to pH changes. To maintain a low viscosity in the dosing solutions, the pH is typically in the 4 to 5 range. When placed in the eye, the immediate increase in pH causes a rapid gelation, which results in an increase residence time and bioavailability.

If pH manipulation fails to increase the drug solubility sufficiently, the next logical step is to try adding the solubility enhancing materials to the formulation. The choice of approved material for use in ophthalmic products is somewhat limited because of irritation potential of many adjuvants. Co-solvents, for example, are not generally acceptable. Materials approved and typically used include polyethylene glycol, propylene glycol, polyvinyl alcohol, Poloxamers, glycerin, cellulose derivatives and surfactants.

4. Surfactants

Surfactants are mainly employed to solubilize or disperse drugs in solutions and dispersions. The use of surfactants is greatly restricted in formulating ophthalmic solutions due to irritation and toxicity issues. The order of surfactant toxicity is anionic > cationic >> nonionic. Several nonionic surfactants are used in lowest possible concentrations to aid in dispensing steroids in suspensions and to achieve or to improve solution clarity. Those principally used are Polysorbate 20 and 80, tyloxapol, and polyoxyl 40 stearate. Their effect on preservative efficacy, ocular irritation and their possible binding by macromolecules must be taken into account. Furthermore, surfactants are being used to prevent drug loss due to adsorption on the container walls. For example, polyoxyl hydrogenated castor oil has been used for stabilization of ophthalmic preparation, which is indicated for lessening of raised intraocular pressure in patients with glaucoma or ocular hypertension.

5. Stabilizers

Stabilizers are ingredients added to a formula to decrease the decomposition of the active ingredients. Antioxidants are the principal stabilizers added to some ophthalmic solutions, primarily those containing epinephrine and other oxidizable drugs. Sodium bisulfite or meta-bisulfite are used in concentration up to 0.3% in epinephrine hydrochloride and bitartrate solutions. Epinephrine borate solutions have a pH in the range 5.5–7.5 and offer a more difficult challenge to formulators who seek to prevent oxidation. Several patented antioxidant systems have been developed specifically for this compound. These consist of ascorbic acid and acetyl cysteine, and sodium bisulfite and 8–hydroxyquinoline. Isoascorbic acid is also an effective antioxidant for this drug. Sodium thiosulfate is used with sodium sulfacetamide solutions. For drugs that are susceptible to oxidative degradation, stabilizers such as anti-oxidants and/or chelating agents can be included in the formulation to improve the product shelf-life. The use of plastic bottles, which allow gases to permeate through the container, will be particularly susceptible to oxidative degradation. There are a variety of regulatory approved anti-oxidants commonly used in liquid ophthalmic products, such as sodium metabisulphite, sodium sulphite, ascorbic acid acetylcysteine, 8-hydroxyquinoline and antipyrine. Trace metal sources in drug materials, solvents, excipients, containers and closures are a continuous source of oxidation. Oxidation reactions are frequently catalyzed in the existence of heavy metals ions.

These trace metals can be removed in free-form from ophthalmic products through chelation (complexation). Chelating agents are supplemented to complex and inactivate metals like copper, iron and zinc which catalyze oxidation of drug substances. Common chelating agents comprise disodium edetate, tartaric acid and citric acid. In some instances, chelating agents and antioxidants are added together to stabilize ophthalmic products.

6. Antimicrobial preservatives

In certain cases, ophthalmic formulations need to be chronically administered in order to assure their efficacy e.g. dry eye and glaucoma. Nevertheless, although preservatives have been frequently used in eye drops, its frequent use has been associated with alterations in the precorneal film, while in patients suffering from dry eye they tend to aggravate the already existing problem. Alternatively, in glaucoma patients the prolonged use of eye drops with preservatives has been associated with changes in the ocular surface accompanied by inflammation. In fact, conjunctival biopsies in patients suffering from glaucoma have revealed an increased number of immune cells. However, the use of preservatives is mandatory in the case of multi-dose containers, since bacterial contamination takes place when handling containers twice a day.

Preservatives are included as a major component of multiple dose eye solutions for the primary purpose of maintaining sterility of the product after opening and during use unless prepared sterile in a unit dose package. U.S. Food and Drug Administration (FDA) regulations permit unpreserved ophthalmic solutions to be packaged in multi-dose containers too, as long as they are packaged and labelled in a way that have acceptable protection and diminishes microbial contamination. This can be achieved by using a re-closable container with a lowest number of doses that is to be discarded 12 hours after initial opening. Unit dose ophthalmic preparations, generally, do not contain preservative. Stricter microbiological guidelines have recently been imposed in the area of flexible hydrophilic contact lens accessory products. Specific guidelines have been devised by the FDA for this area of ophthalmic products and differ primarily in the necessary kill rate, depending on whether or not the solution is to be used as a cleaning or rinsing product or as a flexible hydrophilic lens disinfectant. However, the use of preservatives is prohibited in products that are used at the time of eye surgery on account of the risk of the solution contacting the internal eye tissues causing toxicity. If sufficient concentration of the preservative is in contact with the cornea endothelium for a sufficient time period; the cells can become damaged to the point of causing clouding of the cornea and possible loss of vision. These products should be packaged in sterile, unit-of-use containers without preservatives.

The mechanism of action of preservatives may be divided into two main categories: surfactants and oxidants. Surfactants act upon microorganisms altering the cellular membrane and resulting in the lysis of the cytoplasm content. Cells in mammals cannot neutralize chemical preservatives, and, thus, preservatives become part of the cell and results in toxic effects. The classical example for this type of agents is benzalkonium chloride. Oxidizing preservatives are usually smaller molecules interfering with cell functions. They may destabilize membranes, although to a lesser extent than chemical agents. They are less toxic for mammal cells.

The choice of preservative is limited to only a few chemicals that have been found, over the years, to be safe and effective for this purpose. These are benzalkonium chloride, Polyquad, thimerosal, methyl and propylparaben, phenylethanol, chlorhexidine, and polyaminopropylbiguanide. The chelating agent, disodium edetate (EDTA), is sometimes used to increase the activity against certain *Pseudomonas* strains, particularly with benzalkonium chloride.

Refrigeration of the product should also be required as a precautionary measure. To reduce the potentially largest source of microbial contamination, only sterile Purified Water should be used in compounding ophthalmic solutions. Sterile Water For Injection, USP, from unopened IV bottles or vials is the highest quality water available. Prepackaged sterile water with bacteriostatic agents should not be used. The commonly used preservatives and their properties are enlisted in Table 6.2.

Ophthalmic products have to be manufactured sterile and free from microorganisms. Once opened, the sterility of the multi-dose product must be maintained during its period of the use. This is usually required for at least 4 weeks, after which the product is discarded. If the drug itself does not possess antimicrobial properties, then an antimicrobial preservative must be included in the formulation to ensure that any microorganism accidentally introduced during use are destroyed. There are limited number of regulatory approved antimicrobial preservatives which can be used in ophthalmic products, and some of these are becoming less favored because of increasing awareness of ocular toxicity concerns. Therefore, it can be a challenging exercise for the formulator to find a preservative to use with the following attributes:

- Effective at the optimal formulation pH
- Stable to processing, possibly heat sterilization
- Stable over the product shelf-life
- Does not physically interact with other components in the formulation
- Does not interact with the package components.

A list of regulatory approved antimicrobial preservatives used in ophthalmic formulations with recommended concentration ranges is shown in Table 6.3. The use of methyl- and propylparabens, thimerosal and other mercurial preservatives has decreased in recent years due to adverse reactions inherently associated with their use.

Table 6.2. Profile of some commonly used preservatives in ophthalmic formulations

Types	Typical structure	Concentration range	Incompatibility	Properties
Quaternary ammonium compounds	$\begin{bmatrix} R_2 \\ R_1-N-R_4 \\ R_2 \end{bmatrix} Y^-$	0.004–0.02%; 0.01% (mostly)	Soaps, anionic materials, salicylates, nitrates	Good antimicrobial; excellent chemical stability (benzalkonium chloride, benzethonium chloride)
Organic mercurials (phenyl-mercuric acetate and nitrate, thimerosal)	$SHgC_2H_5$ ... COONa	0.001–0.01%	Certain halides with phenylmercuric acetate	Slow in action to kill especially *P. aeruginosa*; sensitization; iatrogenic mercury deposits; yellowing of lens in long use
Parahydroxy benzoate	HO— —COOCH₃	Maximum 0.1%	Adsorption by macro-molecules with marginal activity	Good antimicrobial; excellent chemical stability
Chlorobutanol	$\begin{matrix} CH_3 \\ H_3C-N-CCl_3 \\ OH \end{matrix}$	0.5%	Stability is pH-dependent; activity concentration is maximum near solubility; heating releases hydro-chloric acid and can lower pH	Slow, ineffective; not considered suitable
Aromatic alcohols	—CH₂OH	0.5–0.9%	Lower solubility in water; marginal activity	Good antimicrobial against *P. aeruginosa*, *S. aureus*, *P. vulgaris*

Table 6.3. Regulatory approved ophthalmic antimicrobial preservatives

Antimicrobial preservatives	Concentration range (%)
Phenylmercuric acetate	0.001–0.002
Thimerosal	0.001–0.15
Phenylmercuric borate	0.002–0.004
Phenylmercuric nitrate	0.002–0.004
Chlorhexidine	0.002–0.01
Propylparaben	0.005–0.01
Benzalkonium chloride	0.01–0.02
Benzethonium chloride	0.01–0.02
Methylparaben	0.015–0.05
Chlorobutanol	Upto 0.5
Phenylethyl alcohol	Upto 0.5

By far, the most widely used antimicrobial preservative used in ophthalmic is BKC (70 percent of all commercial products). It is often used in combination with disodium edetate because of the synergistic effects, allowing lower concentrations of BKC to be used. Even the use of BKC has been questioned because of some evidence of eye toxicity in rabbits, and some people have developed hypersensitivity to this preservative. However, BKC does possess good pharmaceutical properties, being stable in solution, stable to autoclaving, and at the usual concentration of 0.01 percent, is an effective preservative over the range of pH values typically used in ophthalmic formulations.

The effectiveness of any antimicrobial preservative in a formulation must be demonstrated by using specified test procedures described in relevant Pharmacopoeias. Unfortunately, the preservative challenge test procedures and acceptance criteria are different in major Pharmacopoeias in the world. All the tests involve mixing the preserved formulation with standard cultures of Gram (+)ve and Gram (–)ve bacteria, yeast and moulds, and counting the number of viable microorganism remaining at different time points after inoculation. The preservative is effective in the formulation if the concentration of each test microorganism remains at or below the stipulated levels during the test periods.

7. Viscosity imparter

Polyvinyl alcohol, methylcellulose, hydroxypropyl methylcellulose, hydroxyethylcellulose, and carbomers, are commonly used to increase the viscosity of ophthalmic solutions and suspensions. Although, they reduce surface tension significantly, their primary benefit is to increase the ocular contact time, thereby decreasing the drainage rate and increasing drug bioavailability. A secondary benefit of the polymer solutions is a lubricating effect that is largely subjective, but noticeable to many patients. One disadvantage to the use of the polymers is their tendency to dry to a film on the eyelids and eyelashes; however, this can be easily removed by wiping with a damp tissue. Increasing the viscosity of ophthalmic products increases contact time and pharmacological effect, but there is a plateau reached after which further increases in viscosity produce only slight or no increases in effect.

Methylcellulose solutions increase contact time in rabbits up to 25 cP (centipoise) and an optimum at 55 cP. This decrease in drainage rate increased the concentration of drug in the precorneal tear film at zero time and subsequent time periods, which resulted in a higher aqueous humor drug concentration. The magnitude of aqueous humor drug concentration increase was smaller than the increase in viscosity, about 1.7

times, for the range 1.0–12.5 cP, and only a further 1.2-fold increase at 100 cP. The major commercial viscous vehicles are hydroxypropyl methylcellulose (Isopto) and polyvinyl alcohol (Liquifilm). Isotonic products most often use 0.5% of the cellulosic and range from 10 to 30 cP in viscosity, such products have viscosities of about 4–6 cP and use 1.4% polymer. It is, generally, agreed that an increase in vehicle viscosity increases the residence time in the eye, although, there are conflicting reports in the literature to support the optimal viscosity for ocular bioavailability. Products formulated with a high viscosity are not well tolerated in the eye, causing lacrimation and blinking until the original viscosity of the tears is regained. Drug diffusion out of the formulation into the eye may also be inhibited due to high product viscosity. Finally, administration of high viscosity liquid product tends to be more difficult. Therefore, most commercial liquid eye drop products are adjusted to within the range of 10 to 25 cP, using an appropriate viscosity-enhancing agent.

Ophthalmic ointments are designed to be of very high viscosity to prolong the residence time in the eye, compared to solutions and suspensions. However, ointments are the least tolerated and so tend to be restricted to application at night when the patient is asleep.

Table 6.4. FDA approved ophthalmic viscosity-enhancing agents

Viscosity enhancer	Concentration range (%)
Methylcellulose Hydroxypropyl cellulose Hydroxypropyl methylcellulose Hydroxyethylcellulose	0.2–2.5
Polyvinyl alcohol	0.1–5.0
Povidone	0.1–2.0
Polyethylene glycol	0.2–1.0
Carbomer 940/934P	0.05–2.0
Poloxamer 407	0.2–5.0

D. Equipment

The design of equipment for use in controlled environment areas follows similar principles, whether for general injectable manufacturing or for the manufacture of sterile ophthalmic pharmaceuticals. All tanks, valves, pumps, and piping must be of the best available grade of corrosion-resistant stainless steel. In general, stainless steel type 304 or 316 is preferable. All product contact surfaces should be finished either mechanically or by electropolishing to provide a surface as free as possible from scratches or defects that could serve as a nidus for the commencement of corrosion. Care should be taken in the design of such equipment to provide adequate means of cleaning and sanitization.

For equipment that will be placed in aseptic filling areas, such as filling-and-capping machines, care should be taken in their design to yield equipment as free as possible from particle-generating mechanisms. Wherever possible, belt or chain-drive concepts should be avoided in favor of sealed gear or hydraulic mechanisms. Additionally, equipment bulk should be held to an absolute minimum directly over open containers during filling-and-capping operations to minimize introduction of equipment-generated particulate matter and to minimize creation of air turbulence, particularly when laminar flow is used to control the immediate environment around the filling-capping operation. In the design of equipment for the manufacture of sterile ophthalmic (and non-ophthalmic) pharmaceuticals, manufacturers and equipment suppliers are turning to the relatively advanced technology as (clean in place) (CIP), clean out of place (COP), automatic heliarc welding, and electropolishing have been in use for several years.

GENERAL SAFETY CONSIDERATIONS

The single dominant factor characteristic of all ophthalmic products is the special specifications of general safety considerations. Any product intended for eyes regardless of form, substances, or intent must be sterile.

A. Sterility

Every ophthalmic product must be manufactured under conditions validated to render it sterile in its final container. Sterility testing is conducted on each lot of ophthalmic product by suitable procedures, as set forth in the Pharmacopeia, and validated in each manufacturer's laboratory. The USP recognizes six methods of achieving a sterile product:

(a) steam sterilization,
(b) dry heat sterilization,
(c) gas sterilization,
(d) sterilization by ionizing radiation,
(e) sterilization by filtration, and
(f) aseptic processing.

The British Pharmacopoeia suggests similar five methods of sterilization:

(a) sterilization by autoclaving,
(b) dry heat sterilization, usually to $> 60°C$,
(c) sterilization by filtration,
(d) ionizing radiation (electron accelerator or gamma radiation), and
(e) ethylene oxide, which IP also recommends.

For ophthalmic products packaged in plastic containers, a combination of two or more of these six methods is routinely used in manufacturing of ophthalmic formulations. For example, for a sterile ophthalmic suspension, bottles, dropper tips, and caps may be sterilized by ethylene oxide or gamma radiation; the suspended solid may be sterilized by dry heat, gamma radiation, or ethylene oxide; and the aqueous portion of the composition may be sterilized by filtration. The compounding is completed under aseptic conditions, and the product is filled into the previously sterilized containers, again under aseptic conditions. The sterile manufacturing procedure must then be validated to prove that no more than 3 containers in a lot of 3000

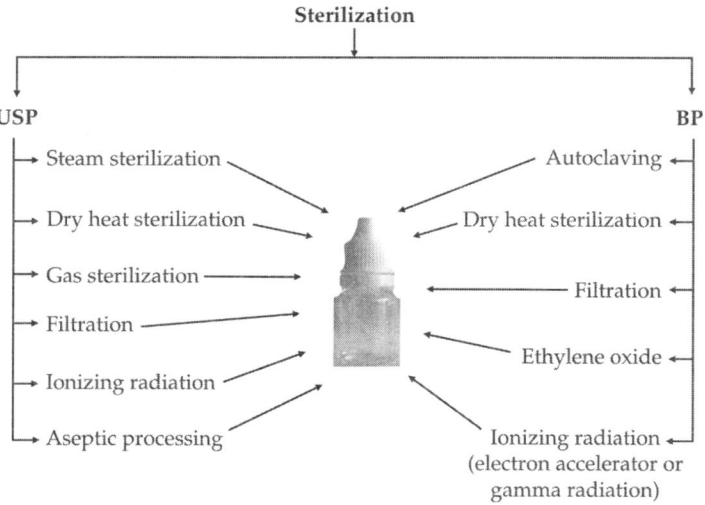

Fig. 6.5. USP & BP sterilization techniques for ophthalmic products.

containers (0.1%) are non-sterile. For ophthalmic products sterilized by terminal sterilization (e.g. steam under pressure), the sterilization cycle must be validated to ensure sterility at a probability of 10^6 or greater. It is the responsibility of manufacturer to ensure the safety and efficacy of the manufacturing process, such as the possible formation of substances toxic to the eye, an ever-present possibility with gas sterilization when using ionizing radiation.

During the manufacture of ophthalmic products, sterility may be checked while the finished product is in its bulk form before filling. It is then also tested on a random sampling basis in the finished package. The number of samples suggested in guidelines is dependent on whether or not sterilization has taken place in the sealed final container. Class A products are those sterilized in bulk form and filled aseptically into sterile final containers without further sterilization. Class B products are those sterilized in sealed final containers. Class B is further subdivided according to method of sterilization: type I comprises those products sterilized by steam under pressure while type II comprises those products sterilized by any other means. Class A products require a minimum random

sample number of no fewer than 30 items from each filling operation. Class B products require varying sample sizes, depending on whether the sterilization occurs in a chamber or by a continuous process. This generally ranges from 5 to 30 units per lot, depending on conditions of sterilization.

B. Ocular toxicity and irritation

Assessment of ocular irritation potential of ophthalmic solutions is an extremely important step in the development of both, over the counter (OTC) and prescription pharmaceuticals. Albino rabbits are currently used to test the ocular toxicity and irritation of ophthalmic formulations. The rabbit has obvious advantages associated with its use. It is readily available, docile, easily handled, relatively inexpensive, easy to maintain, has a large eye, both the corneal surface and the bulbar conjunctival areas are large and easily observable, and the iris is unpigmented, allowing ready observation of the iridal vessels. The primary differences of rabbit and human eye in ophthalmic studies are the low tear in rabbits, lower blinking rate, loosely attached eyelids, presence of a nictating membrane, differences in the structure of

Bowman's membrane, and a slower re-epithelialization of cornea. Currently, the primate has also gained popularity as an ocular model for the evaluation of drugs and chemicals.

It is the manufacturer's responsibility to determine those specific studies appropriate to test the safety of the ophthalmic formulation. The USP presents guidelines for a 72 hr ocular irritation test in rabbits using saline and cottonseed oil extracts of plastic containers used for packaging ophthalmic products. Containers are cleaned and sterilized as in the final packaged product and extracted following submersion in saline and cottonseed oil. Topical ocular instillation of the extracts and blanks in rabbits is completed and ocular changes examined. If ocular changes between extracts and blanks are similar, the plastic passes the test.

A modified **Draize test** has been adopted as the official method for eye irritancy evaluation as a part of the Federal Hazardous Substances Act (FHSA). The best way to determine the degree of irritation or differences between may not be the FHSA or Draize methods, as these are pass/fail procedures. A better judgment for irritancy is based on degree, frequency, and duration of ocular changes. These changes are graded by examination, and a provision allows slit-lamp (biomicroscope) examination or fluorescein staining of the cornea, or both.

Current guidelines for toxicity evaluation of ophthalmic formulations involve both single and multiple applications except for contact lens solutions. The multiple applications extend over a 21 day period and involve both irritation and systemic toxicological studies. Contact lens products have specific guidelines for testing accessory solutions used with contact lens materials (other than polymethyl methacrylate). These solutions are viewed as new drug devices and require testing with the contact lenses with which they are to be used. These testing guidelines are in addition to the guidelines necessary for ophthalmic solutions. The tests include a 21 day ocular study in rabbits,

employing various types (group I, II, III, or IV) of the lenses as they are to be used clinically, including solutions that may be used with the lens (Table 6.5).

Table 6.5. Types of tests and requirements for ophthalmic product development

I. Chemistry/manufacturing
  A. Solution/container descriptions
  B. Solution stability testing
  C. Lens group selection for solution testing
II. Toxicology
  A. Solution testing
    1. Acute oral toxicity assessment
    2. Acute systemic toxicity assessment
    3. Acute ocular irritation and cytotoxicity assessment
    4. Sensitization/allergic response assessment
      a. Preservative uptake and release test
      b. Guinea pig maximization testing
  B. Container/accessory testing
    1. *In vitro* testing
    2. Systemic toxicity testing
    3. Primary ocular irritation testing
III. Microbiology
  A. Sterilization of the solution by the manufacturer
    1. Validation of the sterilization cycle
    2. USP sterility tests
    3. USP type preservative effectiveness test
    4. USP microbial limits test
  B. Shelf-life testing requirements
    1. Shelf-life sterility
    2. Shelf-life preservative effectiveness
    3. Extension of shelf-life protocol
  C. Disinfection of the lens
    1. Chemical disinfection systems
      a. Contribution of elements test
      b. D-value determinations
      c. Multi-item microbial challenge test
    2. Thermal (heat) disinfection system
      Same as for chemical disinfection system
IV. Clinical
  A. Patient characteristics
  B. Number of eyes duration and number of investigators
  C. Initial patient visit parameters

During the application of the various guidelines for both ophthalmic and contact lens products, ocular and biomicroscopic examination on rabbit eyes are completed with reproducible grading for conjunctival congestion, conjunctival swelling, conjunctival discharge, aqueous (humor) flare, iris involvement, corneal cloudiness, severity, area of corneal opacity or cloudiness, pannus, and intensity of fluorescein staining. In addition to *in vivo* testing of ophthalmic preparations, primarily in rabbit eyes and; secondarily, in primate eye; numerous *in vitro* methods have been developed over the past few years as alternatives to *in vivo* ocular testing. *In vivo* methods that incorporate new technology and reduced numbers of animals have also been developed. Particular attention has recently been given to evaluation of preservative effect on corneal penetration, cytotoxicity, and effects on wound healing. Several manufacturers are currently using *in vitro* toxicity tests in the development of ophthalmic solutions.

C. Preservation

The popular plastic eye drop "suck back" an unreleased drop when pressure on the bottle is released, thereby introducing contamination, if the tip is allowed to touch a non-sterile surface. The contamination hazard is magnified in the busy clinical practice of the eye care professional where numerous diagnostic solutions of cycloplegics, mydriatics, and dyes are used in many patients from the same container. The single use packages still contain (as a large scale manufacturing necessity) an amount in excess of the several drops (0.05–0.20 ml) to be used and there is the tendency to use the entire contents and, thereby, reintroduce the contamination hazards and defeat the purpose of this special packaging.

Considerable emphasis in the ophthalmic literature is placed on the effectiveness of preservatives against *Pseudomonas* spp. because of the reports of the loss of eyes through corneal ulcerations from eye solutions contaminated with *P. aeruginosa*. This organism is not the most prevalent cause of bacterial eye infections, even

though it is a common inhabitant of human skin, but it is the most opportunistic and virulent. *Staphylococcus aureus* is responsible for most bacterial infections of the eye. The eye seems to be remarkably resistant to infection when the corneal epithelium is intact. When there is a corneal epithelial abrasion, organisms can enter freely and *P. aeruginosa* can grow readily in the cornea and rapidly produce an ulceration and loss of vision.

The test procedure for antimicrobial effectiveness is not a mandatory requirement of the USP or the FDA, but it is used by the manufacturers to guide them in developing adequately preserved products. This testing of formulas is carried out as a part of the formulation development sequence. A standardized inoculum with organism counts of 10^5–10^6 million/ml for microorganism (*Candida albicans/Apergillus niger/Escherichia coli/Pseudomonas aeruginosa*, or *Staphylococcus aureus*) is prepared and tested against the preserved formula. The inoculated samples are incubated at 20° or 25°C for 28 days and examined at days 7, 14, 21, and 28. The preservative is effective in the product if:

(a) the concentrations of viable bacteria are reduced to no more than 0.1% of the initial concentrations by day 14,

(b) the concentrations of viable yeasts and molds remain at or below the initial concentrations during the first 14 days, and

(c) the concentration of each test microorganism remains at or below these designated levels during the remainder of the 28-day test period.

An additional test procedure employed by one manufacturer in the evaluation of the preservative is "cidal" test. A formulation is tested against 5–14 microorganisms, including Gram (+)ve and Gram (–)ve bacteria, fungi, and yeasts in a standardized inoculum. Cidal times (no growth) are measured for each organism within 24, 48, and 72 hr of contact.

D. Drug and excipient interaction

The consequences of having several components in an ophthalmic formulation are the increased possibility of physical or chemical incompatibilities occurring, resulting in an unstable product, or one component not functioning in the presence of another. The presence of interaction between the drug, excipients or pack does not necessarily mean that they cannot be used together. However, the formulator will be required to determine the extent and nature of such an interaction, and conduct sufficient testing to develop an effective formulation. A systematic approach to formulation development of an ophthalmic product is, therefore, recommended. The product design requirements should be evaluated systematically to try and achieve the targets and limits for specification tests, such as appearance, drug solubility, pH, viscosity, osmolarity and preservative effectiveness. By experimentation and iteration, the selection and quantity of each type of component can be established, until the acceptance criteria are met for each product design requirements. For example, in the first stage of experimentation, the requirement might be to achieve the target drug solubility. If the solubility in an aqueous vehicle is insufficient, pH manipulation or the addition of various solubility enhancers can be evaluated over a range of concentrations, to establish the optimum combination which meets the design criteria. In the next stage of experimentation, viscosity enhancers and tonicity agents can be evaluated to meet the specification test limits for viscosity and osmolarity. Finally, a variety of antimicrobial preservatives are evaluated, but at the same time, the formulator checks to ensure that drug solubility, viscosity, osmolarity are not significantly affected. Further experimentation and testing is continued until all of the various components have been added in this iterative manner, and the product design requirements have been met. Alternatively, an experimental design approach could be attempted to reduce the number of excipients, but this can be very complex if a large number of components are involved.

Accelerated stress stability testing of the final product, with all the components added, should establish whether there are any compatibility problems between the drug, excipients and packaging. Stability data from accelerated studies can be used to predict shelf-lives at ambient conditions. It is worthwhile including temperature cycling from low (4°C) to high (40°C) temperatures in the stability program, particularly if solubility enhancers have been used.

E. Administration and use

As part of optimization program, it is important to evaluate the ocular irritation potential of formulation prototypes. The Draize test, established in 1940s, is the most widely used method for identification of primary irritants. There have been modifications to the original test, but they all involve instilling a drop of the formulation into the conjunctival sac of one eye of an albino rabbit, the other eye acting as a control. The condition of both eyes is then evaluated after stipulated time periods and scored relative to the control eye. A high score indicates that the formulation is likely to be an irritant and would not be recommended for progression.

CONVENTIONAL OPHTHALMIC DOSAGE FORMS

A. Topical eyedrops

Although, many methods of instilling drugs to the eye have been experimented with, the use of eyedrops remains the major mode of administration for the topical ocular route. Eye drops are one of the few dosage forms that are not administered by exact volume or weight dosage, yet this seemingly imprecise method of dosing is quite well established and accepted by ophthalmologists. The volume of a drop is dependent on the physicochemical properties of the formulation, particularly surface tension; the design and geometry of the dispensing orifice; and the angle at which the dispenser is held in relation to the receiving surface. The manufacturer of ophthalmic products controls the tolerances necessary for the dosage form and dispensing container to provide a uniform drop size.

Solutions

Solutions are undoubtedly the most commonly used and accepted forms. They are relatively simple to make, filter and sterilize. Nearly all the major ophthalmic therapeutic agents are water-soluble or can be formulated as water-soluble salts. A homogeneous solution offers greater assurance of uniformity of dosage and bioavailability and simplifies large-scale manufacture. The selection of the appropriate salt form depends on its solubility; the therapeutic concentrations required; the ocular toxicity; the effect of pH, tonicity, and buffer capacity; its compatibility with the total formulation; and the intensity of any possible stinging or burning sensations produced (i.e., discomfort reactions).

For compounds having a low aqueous solubility, there are numerous methods that can be employed to increase the concentration of drug in the solution. Various drugs remain weak bases or acids which can be formulated as water-soluble, pharmaceutically suitable salts. Ideally, salt assortment must be fixed while selecting preclinical candidate. It is not advised to alter the salt form during clinical development since it could result to significant deviations in the drug absorption and bioavailability studies. The most common salt forms used are the hydrochloride, sulfate, nitrate, and phosphate, however, salicylate, hydrobromide, and bitartrate salts are also used. For acidic drugs like the sulfonamides, sodium and diethanolamine salts are used. The effect that choice of salt form can have on resulting product properties is exemplified by the epinephrine. The bitartrate form is a 1:1 salt, and the free carboxyl group acts as a strong buffer resisting neutralization by the tears,

causing considerable stinging. The borate form results in a solution with lower buffer capacity, a more nearly physiological pH, and better patient tolerance; however, it is less stable than the other two salts. The hydrochloride salt combines better stability than the borate with acceptable patient tolerance.

Suspensions

Suspensions, while not as common as solutions, are widely used for formulations involving anti-inflammatory steroids (e.g. prednisolone alcohol and acetate). A proper particle size and a narrow size range, ensuring low irritation and adequate bioavailability, should be sought for every suspended drug. Other formulation factors, i.e. the use of correct wetting, suspending and buffering agents, protective colloids, preservatives, etc., should also be considered attentively. If the drug is not sufficiently soluble, it can be formulated as suspension. A suspension may also be desired to improve stability, bioavailability, or efficacy.

The major topical ophthalmic suspensions are the steroidal anti-inflammatory agents; water-soluble salts of prednisolone phosphate and dexamethasone phosphate are available. However, they have lower steroid potency and are poorly absorbed. An ophthalmic suspension should use the drug in a microfine form, usually 95% or more of the particles have a diameter of 10 μm or less. This is necessary so that the particles do not cause irritation of the sensitive ocular tissues and ensure that a uniform dosage is delivered to the eye. Since a suspension is made up of solid particles, it is at least theoretically possible that they may provide a short-lived reservoir in the cul-de-sac for slightly prolonged activity. However, it appears that this is not so, since the drug particles are extremely small, and with the rapid tear volume turnover rate, they are washed out of the eye relatively quickly. Formulation scientists are developing improved suspension dosage forms to overcome hurdles of poor solubility. A significant development facet of ophthalmic suspension is the capability to re-suspend effortlessly any settled particles earlier to instillation in the eye and confirm that an even dose is delivered.

Powders for reconstitution

Several ophthalmic drugs are prepared as sterile powders for reconstitution by the pharmacist before dispensing to the patient. These include α-chymotrypsin and echothiophate iodide. The sterile powder is usually manufactured by lyophilization and is packaged separately from the diluent, and a sterile dropper assembly is provided. In powder form these drugs have a much longer shelf-life than that of their solution forms. The pharmacist should use only the diluent provided with the products, since it has been developed to maintain the optimum potency and preservation of the reconstituted solution.

B. Semisolid dosage forms: Ophthalmic ointments and gels

Semisolid, petrolatum-based ointments presented problems for years because they could not be filtered to eliminate particulate matter, could not be made truly sterile and no adequate tests had been devised to indicate the suitability of added preservatives. In time, most of these problems have been solved, and sterile, filtered ophthalmic ointments are currently available on the market. These preparations, however, occupy a position of minor importance since they are ill-accepted on account of their greasiness, vision-blurring effects, etc., and are generally used as night-time medications.

Formulation

The principle semisolid dosage form used in ophthalmology is an anhydrous ointment with a petrolatum base. Ophthalmic ointments containing antibiotics are used quite frequently following operative procedures. After applying the ointment to the eye, it decomposes into small drops, which stay for a longer time period in conjunctival sac, thus increasing drug's bio-availability. The chief disadvantages of the use of ophthalmic ointments are their greasy nature and the blurring of vision they produce and sometimes have irritating effects, because of which they are mainly applied night-time. They are most often used as adjunctive nighttime therapy, with eye drops administered during the day. The nighttime use obviates the difficulties produced by blurring of vision and is stated to prolong ocular retention when compared with drops. Ointments are used almost exclusively as vehicles for antibiotics, sulfonamides, anti-fungals, and anti-inflammatories. The petrolatum vehicle is also used as an ocular lubricant following surgery or to treat various dry eye syndromes. Anesthesiologists may prescribe the ointment vehicle for the non-ophthalmic surgical patients to prevent severe and painful dry eye conditions that could develop during prolonged surgeries.

In situ gels are another type of semisolid ophthalmic dosage form, which are viscous liquids, showing the ability to undergo sol-to-gel transitions when influenced by external factors, like appropriate pH, temperature, and the presence of electrolytes. This property causes slowing of drug drainage from the eyeball surface and increase of the active ingredient bio-availability. Polymers employed in developing these drug forms include gellan gum, poloxamer, and cellulose acetate phthalate, whereas examples of active ingredients used in the course of research on in situ gels include ciprofloxacin hydrochloride, timolol maleate, fluconazole, ganciclovir, and pilocarpine. The gel is applied in a small strip in the lower conjunctival sac from an ophthalmic ointment tube. The Carbomer polymeric gel base itself has been used success-fully to treat moderate to severe cases of dry eye (keratoconjunctivitis sicca). The dry eye syndrome is usually characterized by a deficiency of tear production and, therefore, requires frequent instillation of aqueous artificial tear eye drops to keep the corneal epithelium moist. The gel base applied in a small amount provides a prolonged lubrication to the external ocular tissues, and some patients reduce the frequency of dosing to control their symptoms to three times a day or fewer.

Sterility and preservation

Since October 1973, FDA regulations require that all U.S. ophthalmic ointments be sterile. The time lag in imposition of a legal requirement for sterility of ointments compared with solutions and suspensions was due to the absence of a reliable sterility test for the petrolatum-based ointments until isopropyl myristate was employed to dissolve these ointments and allow improved recovery of viable microorganisms by membrane filtration. A suitable substance or mixture of substances to prevent the growth of microorganisms must be added to ophthalmic ointments that are packaged in multiple-use containers, regardless of the method of sterilization employed, unless otherwise directed in the individual monograph, or unless the formula itself is bacteriostatic.

Sterile ointment cannot become excessively contaminated by ordinary use because of its consistency and the fact that in non-aqueous medium microorganisms merely survive, but do not multiply. An official test for effectiveness of a preservative in a non-aqueous medium has not been devised, thus, making rational selection by the formulator an even more difficult task. Chlorobutanol and methyl- and propylparaben are the most often used when an ophthalmic ointment contains a preservative, and they are used in the same concentration as in aqueous systems.

Processing considerations

For ophthalmic products, like parenterals, process development can be quite challenging because the formulation must be manufactured sterile. Quite often, it is discovered that some formulations cannot withstand a stressful sterile process such as autoclaving. Chemical degradation or changes to the formulation

properties of multi-phase system, such as suspensions and gels, can occur. In all cases, the compendial sterility test requirements described in the various Pharmacopoeias must be complied with. There are certain expectations and requirements for acceptable sterile products from the regulatory agencies, advising that for products intended to be sterile (including ophthalmic products), an appropriate method of sterilization should be chosen and the choice justified. Whenever possible, all such products should be terminally sterilized in their final container, using a fully validated terminal sterilization method using steam, dry heat or ionizing radiation. The guidance emphasizes that heat lability of a packaging material should not itself be considered adequate justification for not utilizing terminal sterilization, for otherwise heat stable products. Alternative packaging material should be thoroughly investigated before making any decision to use a non-terminal sterilization process. However, it could be that the drug candidate, or one or more of the formulation excipient, are not stable to heat.

For ophthalmic products, there is a dilemma because recent market trends show that flexible LDPE plastic dropper bottles are popular with users because they offer several advantages, including ease of administration, better control of drop delivery and lower risk of contamination during patient use; plastic dropper bottles are lightweight, yet more robust than glass. However, the disadvantage of LDPE containers is that they cannot withstand terminal heat sterilization using Pharmacopoeial recommended heat cycles.

According to the decision trees, where it is not possible to carry out terminal sterilization by heating due to formulation instability, a decision should be made to utilize an alternative method of terminal sterilization, filtration and/or aseptic processing. If this alternative route is taken, then a clear scientific justification for not using terminal heat sterilization will be required. Commercial reasons will not be acceptable because terminal sterilization offers the highest

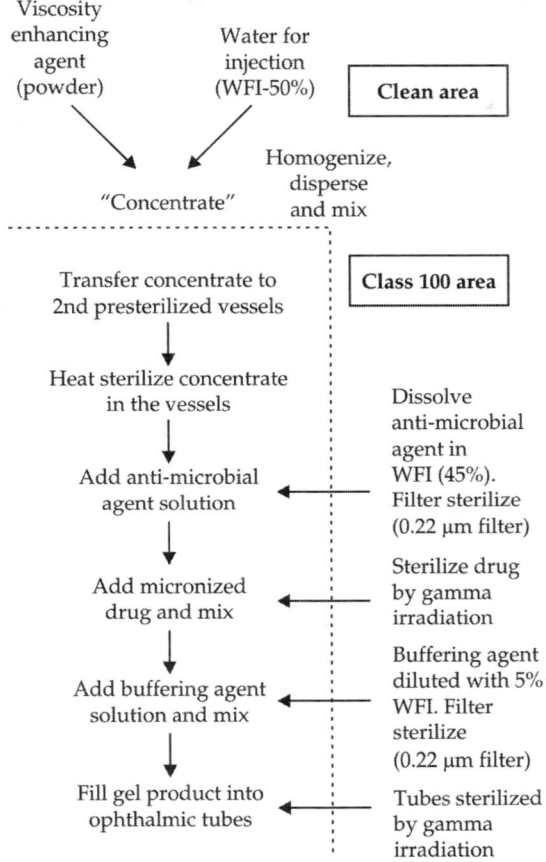

Fig. 6.6. Steps in manufacture of a semi-solid ophthalmic gel suspension.

possible level of sterility assurance. If using non-terminal sterilization methods, it is important to ensure that a low level of pre-sterilization bio-burden is achieved prior and during manufacture. The FDA guidance on sterile drug products produced by aseptic processing and the recently revised Annex 1 of the EC GMP guide manu-facture of sterile medicinal products should be referred for further guidance. It will be necessary to conduct preliminary feasibility studies to establish an acceptable and effective method for sterilization of the product. There is a clear responsibility with the manufacturer to provide evidence to the regulatory agencies that the product can or cannot be terminally sterilized.

Preformulation studies will indicate whether the candidate drug and proposed formulation can withstand the sterilization process using small samples of the product. Careful selection of the processing equipment and design features are important for successful manufacture. Stainless steel vessels fitted with a paddle stirrer for general mixing, and a homogenizer head for high speed mixing of the drug and excipient can be used.

PACKAGING AND STORAGE

The choice of packaging for ophthalmic products will depend on type of dosage form, such as whether it is a liquid solution/suspension or semisolid gel or ointment. Also, choice will depend on how the product is to be used by the patient, such as whether it is intended to be a unit-dose or multi-dose application. For any formulation type, the packaging design acceptance criteria must ensure that the:

(a) materials are compatible with the formulation and ensure product stability;
(b) sterility of the product can be achieved and assured for the entire shelf life;
(c) materials meet pharmacoepoeial and regulatory standard requirements;
(d) container should be temper-evident; and
(e) pack design offers ease of administration to the patient.

Eye drops have been packaged almost entirely in plastic dropper bottles since the introduction of the Drop–Tainer plastic dispenser in the 1950s. A few products still remain in glass dropper bottles because of special stability constraints. The main advantages of the Drop–Tainer and similarly designed plastic dropper bottles are convenience of use by the patient, decreased contamination potential, lower weight, and lower cost. The plastic bottle has the dispensing tip as an integral part of the package. The patient simply removes the cap and turns the bottle upside down and squeezes gently to form a single drop that falls into the eye. The dispensing tip can be designed to deliver only

1 drop or a stream of fluid for irrigation, depending on the pressure applied. When used properly, the solution remaining in the bottle is only minimally exposed to airborne contaminants during administration; thus, it will maintain very low to non-existent microbial content as compared with the old-style glass bottle with separate dropper assembly.

The plastic bottle and dispensing tip is made of low-density polyethylene (LDPE) resin, which provides the necessary flexibility and inertness. Because these components are in contact with the product during its shelf-life, they must be carefully chosen and tested for their suitability for ophthalmic use. In addition to stability studies on the product in the container over a range of normal and accelerated temperatures, the plastic resins must pass the USP Biological and Chemical Tests for Suitability. The LDPE resins used are compatible with a very wide range of drugs and formulation components. Their one disadvantage is their sorption and permeability characteristics. Volatile ingredients such as the preservatives chlorobutanol and phenylethyl alcohol can migrate into the plastic and eventually permeate through the walls of the container. The sorption and permeation can be detected by stability studies if it is detectable. If the permeating component is a preservative, a repeat test of the preservative effectiveness with time will determine if the loss is significant. If necessary, a safe and reasonable excess of the permeable component may be added to balance the loss over the shelf-life. Another means of overcoming permeation effects is to employ a secondary package, such as a peel-apart blister or pouch composed of non-permeable materials (e.g., aluminum foil or vinyl). The plastic dropper bottles are also permeable to water, and weight loss by water vapor transmission becomes less significant as the size of the bottle increases. The consequences of water vapor transmission (WVT) must be taken into consideration when assessing the stability of a product, and appropriate corrections for loss of water on the analysis of components must be applied.

The LDPE resins are translucent, and if the drug is light-sensitive, additional package protection may be required. This can be achieved by using a resin containing an opacifying agent such as titanium dioxide, by placing an opaque sleeve over the exterior of the container, or by placing the bottle in a cardboard carton. Extremely light-sensitive drugs, such as epinephrine and proparacaine, may require a combination of these protective measures. Colorants, other than titanium dioxide, are rarely used in plastic ophthalmic containers; however, the use of colorants is common for the cap for a very important purpose. Red is used to denote a mydriatic drug, such as atropine, and green a miotic drug, like pilocarpine. This is an aid to the physician and the dispensing pharmacist to prevent potentially serious mistakes. Table 6.6 provides some examples of color codes used for few important class of pharmaceuticals. The LDPE resin used for the bottle and the dispensing tip cannot be autoclaved, and they are sterilized either by ^{60}Co gamma irradiation or ethylene oxide. The cap is designed such that when it is screwed tightly onto the bottle, it mates with the dispensing tip and forms a seal. The cap is usually made of a harder resin than the bottle, such as polystyrene or polypropylene, and is also sterilized by gamma radiation or ethylene oxide gas exposure.

Table 6.6. Ophthalmic cap color coding for important class of pharmaceuticals

Color	Class of pharmaceuticals
Red	Mydriatics
Orange	Carbonic anhydrase inhibitors
Green	Miotics
Yellow	Beta blockers
Pink	Steroids
Grey	Non-steroids
Brown	Anti-infectives
Turquoise	Prostaglandins

A special plastic ophthalmic package has been introduced that uses a special grade of polypropylene that is resistant to deformation at autoclave temperatures. With this specialized packaging, the bottle can be filled, the dispensing tip and cap applied, and the entire product sterilized by steam under pressure at 121°C. The glass dropper bottle is still used for products that are extremely sensitive to oxygen or contain permeable components that are not sufficiently stable in plastic. Powders for reconstitution also use glass containers, owing to their heat-transfer characteristics that are necessary during the freeze-drying process. The glass used should be USP type I for maximum compatibility with the sterilization process and the product. The glass container is made sterile by dry-heat or steam autoclave sterilization. Amber glass is used for light–resistance and is superior to green glass. A sterile dropper assembly is usually supplied separately. It is usually gas sterilized in a blister composed of vinyl and Tyvek, a fused, porous polypropylene material. The dropper assembly is made of a glass or LDPE plastic pipette and a rubber, dropper bulb. The manufacturer carefully tests the appropriate plastic and rubber materials suitable for use with the product; therefore, they should be dispensed with the product. The pharmacist should aseptically place the dropper assembly in the product before dispensing it and advice the patient on precautions to be used to prevent contamination.

The pure tin tube is compatible with a wide range of drugs in petrolatum-based ointments. Aluminum tubes have been considered and may eventually be used because of their lower cost and ease of availability. Until internal coating technology for these tubes advances, the aluminum tube will be a secondary packaging choice. Plastic tubes made from flexible LDPE resins have also been considered as an alternative material, but do not collapse and tend to suck–back the ointment. Plastic tubes recently introduced as containers for toothpaste have been investigated and may offer the best alternative

to tin. These tubes are laminates of plastic and various materials, such as paper, foil, and so on. A tube can be designed by selection of the laminate materials and their arrangement and thickness to provide the necessary compatibility, stability, and barrier properties. The various types of metal tubes are scaled using an adhesive coating covering only the inner edges of the bottom of the open tube to form the crimp, which does not contact the product. Laminated tubes are usually heat-sealed. The crimp usually contains the lot code and expiration date.

Filled tubes may be tested for **leakers** by storing them in a horizontal position in an oven at 60°C for at least 8 hr. No leakage should be evidenced except for a minute quantity that could come only from within the crimp of the tube or the end of the cap. The screw cap is made of polyethylene or polypropylene. Polypropylene must be used for autoclave sterilization, but either material may be used when the tubes are gas sterilized. A **tamper-evident** feature is required for sterile ophthalmic ointments, and may be accomplished by sealing the tube or the carton holding the tube such that the contents cannot be used without providing visible evidence of destruction of the seal. The Teledyne Wirz tube used by most manufacturers has a flange oil cap that is visible only after the tube has been opened the first time. The tube can be a source of metal particles and must be cleaned carefully before sterilization. The test procedure limits the level of metal particles in ophthalmic ointments. The total number of metal particles detected under 30 times magnification that are 50 mm or larger in any dimension is counted. The requirements are met if the total number of such particles counted in ten tubes is not more than 50, and if not more than one tube is found to contain more than 8 such particles (USP).

Freezing of ophthalmic products, particularly suspensions should be avoided. A freeze-thaw cycle can induce particle growth or crystallization of a suspension and increase the chances of causing ocular irritation and loss of dosage uniformity. Glass-packaged liquid products may break owing to the volume expansion of the solution when it freezes. It is especially important that the pharmacist fully advise the patient on proper storage and use of ophthalmic products to ensure their integrity and their safe and efficacious use.

Traditionally, ophthalmic products were packed in glass containers fitted with rubber teats for the eye dropper. Glass containers find limited use today when there are product stability or compatibility issues that exclude the use of flexible plastic containers made of polyethylene or polypropylene. Most liquid eye products in the market are plastic container fitted with nozzles from which, the contents may be expressed as drops by gentle squeezing. Plastic containers have several advantages over the glass-dropper combination such as minimizing the risk of the contents being contaminated with microorganisms by the replacement of a pipette that may have become contaminated by touching the infected eye. Also, plastic containers are cheap, light in weight, more robust to handle and easier to use than glass dropper type container. Multi-dose plastic bottle can comprise of conventional dropper bottles or a form-fill-seal (FFS) bottle, where the dropper tip is an integral part of the bottle.

However, there are some disadvantages of plastic eye drop containers. Some plastic material such as polyethylene can absorb some anti-microbial preservatives [e.g., benzalkonium chloride (BKC)], or some drugs. They may also leach plasticizers into the product or printing inks from the label through the plastic into the products. It is necessary to conduct compatibility and stability studies to ascertain whether this is likely to be a problem. For ophthalmic solutions, that require the addition of a preservative because the drug product itself has no adequate anti-microbial properties, it may be necessary to use glass. Alternatively, a preservative free product could be considered. The challenge is to develop a packaging system for preservative free products, which maintains the stability of the product throughout its shelf-life and during use.

Unit dose system offers a easiest technical solution to this problem, but has the disadvantages of higher cost of manufacture and of not being as compact as a multiple-dose product containing equivalent doses. Unit dose products are usually made of low density polyethylene (LDPE), with the formulated sterile solution being without a preservative, and sealed using the FFS process. An alternative approach is to develop a multiple dose preservative free system. The container is required to be collapsible, and the suck-back of air, which could contain bacteria, has to be avoided. Containers are being developed that contain a valve mechanism to achieve this. Due to the safety and regulatory concerns raised by preservatives used in ophthalmic products, there have been efforts to develop new eye drop packaging systems which can remove the preservative from the formulation during administration. BKC is the most common preservative used in commercial eye drops, and yet there are reports of side effects such as allergic reactions, irritation, decreased lacrimation and damage to the corneal endothelium caused by its multiple uses in eye products. Also, BKC can accumulate in soft contact lenses and is therefore not recommended for the patients. A French pharmaceutical research company, Transphyto, have patented a multi-dose preserved ophthalmic product with an adsorbent membrane in the neck of the bottle to remove the preservative during administration. It also contains 0.2 μm bacteriological membrane to prevent the ingress of bacteria into the bottle during use (ABAK device).

Plastic containers can also be permeable to water vapor and oxygen over prolonged period of storage. This can lead to gradual loss of liquid or oxidation of an unstable drug over time. Polyethylene containers are not able to withstand autoclaving and are usually sterilized by ethylene oxide or by irradiation before being filled aseptically with pre-sterilized product.

Polypropylene containers can be autoclaved, but are not flexible as polyethylene for eye-dropper use. Guidance recently available on the manufacture of sterile medicinal products from a number of regulatory sources suggests that there is a changing attitude to the use of manufacturing processes other than terminal sterilization. The implication is that the type of container is not the satisfactory reason for not autoclaving the product, and manufacturer should use a package, which is currently available as a heat stable alternative (such as polypropylene), and use standard terminal sterilization by heat as recommended in the Pharmacopoeias. If a non-heat stable container is processed, and terminal sterilization is not possible, a full justification will be required for this approach.

A variety of novel ophthalmic liquid pack design features are in development recently. For example, the 'Optidyne system' being developed by Scherer DDS is an atomized spray which delivers a tiny volume (about 5 μL) directly to the front of the eye ball so fast that it beats the blink reflex. The volume is similar to the capacity of the precorneal volume in the eye. Unlike the traditional eye drops, the spray product can be directed more easily and should reduce the wastage associated with conventional eye drops, which have a typical volume of 40 μL.

Another device to aid administration is an eyecup fitted to a metered dose pump to help the patient position the product correctly over the eye during administration. Novel devises have been developed to accommodate moisture and/or oxygen sensitive drugs, such as a dual chamber container that can hold drug, or freeze dried drug, and diluent separately in a single package. The drug, or lyophilized drug, is contained in a glass bottle, and the reconstitution liquid is contained in a plastic bottle. Prior to use the liquid contents are transferred into the glass bottle by rupturing a membrane, and a drug solution is produced by mixing ready for administration.

Semi-solid products have been traditionally packed in collapsible tin tubes. Metal tubes are a potential source of metal particles in ophthalmic products, and so the tubes have to be cleaned carefully prior to sterilization. Also, the final product must meet limits for the number of metal particles found. Plastic tubes are not suitable because of their non-collapsible nature, which causes air to enter the tube after withdrawal of each dose. However, collapsible tubes made from laminates of plastic, aluminium foil and paper are a good alternative to tin tubes. Laminated tubes fitted with polypropylene cap can be sterilized by autoclaving, whereas tubes fitted with polyethylene caps are sterilized by gamma irradiation. The tubes are usually filled aseptically, sealed with an adhesive and then crimped.

APPROACHES FOR EFFICIENT DRUG DELIVERY

In recent years, extensive efforts has been dedicated to prolonging the retention time of medications on the eye surface and to the improvement of transcorneal penetration of traditional and of novel therapeutic agents such as protein and peptide drugs. For anterior-segment drug delivery, common routes of administration are topical instillation and sub-conjunctival injection; whereas for posterior segment drug delivery common routes include systemic dosing, periocular and intravitreal injections. Some recently developed systems aim at prolonging the preocular retention and therefore reducing the frequency of administration. Other delivery systems are designed to provide controlled, continuous drug delivery with the dual goal of avoiding or minimising the initial drug concentration peak in the aqueous humour (with its associated side effects) and of avoiding the periods of under dosing that may occur between eye-drop instillations.

Two particular physical factors in ocular formulations that, among others, have been

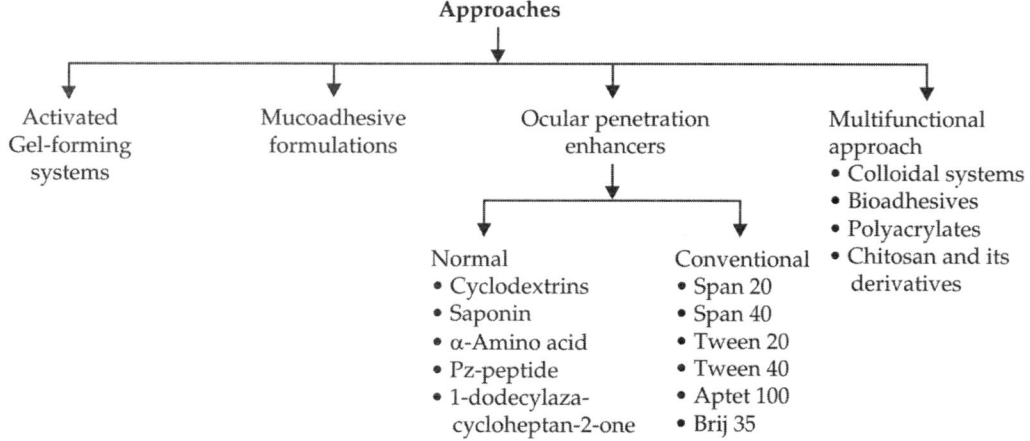

Fig. 6.7. Approaches for efficient ocular drug delivery.

investigated attentively are the drug solubility and physical form and the vehicle viscosity. In the case of poorly soluble drugs, as in steroids, two aspects of the solubility parameter are relevant to ocular absorption; the presence in the cul-de-sac of the eye of a reservoir of insoluble particles could lead to a sustaining effect, and different esters of the drug could show different transcorneal permeation characteristics.

A. In-situ activated gel-forming systems

These (liquid) vehicles undergo a viscosity increase upon instillation in the eye, thus, favouring precorneal retention. Such a change in viscosity can be initiated by a change in temperature, pH or electrolyte composition. Poloxamer 407 (a polyoxyethylene polyoxypropylene block copolymer) is a polymer with a solution viscosity that increases when its temperature is raised to the eye temperature. Cellulose acetophthalate (CAP) is a polymer undergoing coagulation when the original pH of the solution (4.5) is raised to 7.4 by the tear fluid. Both systems, however, are characterised by a high polymer concentration (25% for Poloxamer 407 and 30% for CAP). By contrast, Gelrite® is a polysaccharide (low acyl gellan gum) that forms clear gels at a much lower concentration

in the presence of mono or divalent cations typically found in tear fluids. It is marketed as a once-a-day dosing vehicle for timolol maleate (Timoptic XE, Merck & Co., Inc.). The in situ gel-forming devices can be described as viscous liquids, which undergo a transition to the gel phase upon exposure to certain changes in physiological conditions *in vivo*. The system utilizes polymers that demonstrate transition from a sol to a gel phase, when applied to the corneal surface. The phase transition occurs either due to change in the pH (from 4.5 to 7.4) or due to a change in temperature (from a lower temperature to the temperature of the corneal surface). Another factor is the change in electrolyte composition when polymers like Carbopol, methylcellulose, Pluronics, Tetronics, and cellulose acetate phthalate (CAP) undergo phase transition and gel.

B. Mucoadhesive formulations

This approach relies on vehicles containing polymers that adhere via non-covalent bonds to conjunctival mucin, thus, ensuring contact of the medication with the precorneal tissues until mucin turnover causes elimination of the polymer. Mucoadhesive polymers are usually hydrocolloids with numerous hydrophilic functional groups such as carboxyl, hydroxyl, amide and sulphate. These groups can establish electrostatic interactions, hydrophobic interactions, van der Waals intermolecular interactions and hydrogen bonding with mucus substrates. For many polymers, hydrogen bonding appears to play a significant role in mucoadhesion, thus the presence of water seems to be a prerequisite for a majority of mucoadhesive phenomena.

Some synthetic, semi-synthetic and naturally occurring polymers like hydroxypropylcellulose, polyacrylic acid, high-molecular-weight (> 200,000) polyethylene glycols, dextrans, hyaluronic acid, polygalacturonic acid, xyloglucan, etc. may be used for mucoadhesion for the development of more efficient ocular delivery systems.

Current status of mucoadhesives in ocular drug delivery

The successful development of newer mucoadhesive dosage forms for ocular delivery still poses numerous challenges, particularly important among these are the determination of exact nature of the interactions occurring at the tissue mucoadhesive interface and the development of an ideal, non-toxic, non-immunogenic mucoadhesive for clinical applications. Some of the potential candidates used for ocular drug delivery and retarding the removal of formulations from the corneal sites are:

1. Erodible inserts of polyvinyl alcohol film or silicone rubber for the ocular delivery of pilocarpine and oxytetracycline, respectively.
2. Poly(vinyl methyl ether-maleic anhydride) matrices containing timolol.
3. Polycyanoacrylate nanoparticles to improve the corneal penetration of hydrophilic drugs.
4. An aqueous dispersion with limited water solubility.
5. In-situ forming gel preparations.
6. Sustained-release liposomes coated with a mucoadhesive polymers.
7. Microspheres preparations.
8. Mucoadhesive polysaccharides etc.

C. Ocular penetration enhancers

The use of substances facilitating drug penetration through the corneal tissues is a potentially interesting, yet little-explored approach to improve ophthalmic bioavailability. The effect of these substances (mainly surface-active agents) on the cornea is to enhance the permeability of superficial cells by destroying the cell membranes and causing cell lysis in a dose-dependent manner. The following substances have shown positive results: benzalkonium, chloride, polyoxyethylene glycol lauryl ether (Brij® 35), polyoxyethylene glycol stearyl ether (Brij® 78), polyoxyethylene glycol oleyl ether (Brij® 98), ethylenediaminetetraacetic acid (EDTA), sodium salt, digitonin, sodium taurocholate, saponins, Cremophor EL, etc. Unfortunately, some agents, while effective, cause transient irritation or produce irreversible damage to corneal tissues.

Ideally ocular penetration enhancers should have following characteristics:

1. The enhancing action should be immediate and unidirectional, and the duration should be specific and predictable.
2. There should be immediate recovery of the tissue after removal of the enhancers.
3. The enhancers should be safe i.e. there are no systemic or local effects associated with the enhancers.
4. The enhancers should be physically and chemically compatible with a wide range of drugs and excipients.

However, the currently available enhancers do not so much satisfy the required conditions. None were yet approved by FDA because of safety concerns. The penetration enhancers work by one or more of the following mechanisms.

1. Altering membrane structure and enhancing transcellular transport by extracting membrane components and/or increasing the fluidity.
2. Enhancing paracellular transport by chelating calcium ions leading to opening of tight junctions. They can induce high osmotic

pressure that transiently opens up the tight junctions, which, in turn, can disrupt the structure of the tight junctions.

3. Altering mucus structure and rheology, so that the diffusion barrier is weakened.
4. Modifying the physical properties of the drug enhancer entity, and
5. Inhibiting enzyme activity.

The various penetration enhancers, in turn, can be classified as:

1. Conventional

Surfactants and the surface active agents like Span (20, 40 and 85), Tween (20, 40, and 81), Aptet 100, G1045, Brij (35, 48, 58, 98), bile acids, Myrj (52, 53), taurocholic acid, taurodeoxycholic acids, urodeoxycholic acids etc., can be used in various concentration ranges for a range of drugs. Enhanced aqueous humour concentrations and higher HLB values of 16–17 make them most effective and dose dependent. Fatty acids like capric acid in concentration range of 0.5%; preservatives like benzalkonium chloride (0.005–0.025%), chlorhexidine digluconate (0.01%), benzyl alcohol (0.5%), chlorbutanol (0.5%), 2, phenylethanol (0.5%), paraben (0.04%), propyl paraben (0.02%), chelating agents like EDTA (0.1–0.5%) etc. can be considered for enhancement of drug permeation.

2. Newer and novel penetration enhancers

(a) Cyclodextrins

Poorly soluble ophthalmic drugs can be solubilised by the use of cyclodextrins (CDs), a group of cyclic oligosaccharides capable of forming inclusion complexes with many drugs. In ophthalmic preparations, co-administration of CDs has been reported to increase corneal penetration, ocular absorption and the efficacy of poorly water-soluble drugs such as dexamethasone, cyclosporin, acetazolamide, etc. These positive results are attributed to the ability of CDs to increase the aqueous solubility of lipophilic drugs without affecting their intrinsic ability to permeate biological membranes. It is thought that CDs act as true carriers by keeping the hydrophobic drug molecules in solution and delivering them to the surface of the corneal epithelium where they partition. The recent study had shown that β-cyclodextrin can directly interact with corneal epithelium leading to subsequent destabilization of the cell membrane for enhancing penetration of pilocarpine. However, damage to cornea was minimal at 8% concentration.

(b) 1-dodecylazacycloheptan-2-one (Azone)

It is a highly lipophilic component, which can be incorporated into lipoidal cell membrane and exert penetration enhancing activity. It can enhance corneal penetration of hydrophilic components by at least 20 folds but can inhibit penetration of lipophilic components e.g. flurbiprofen. It was speculated that incorporation of azone in corneal epithelium changed the structure and fluidity of cell membrane. Loosening of tight junctions and subsequent water and drug influx also might be a possible mechanism. Azone can be used in a concentration upto 0.1% since higher concentration causes ocular discomfort, conjunctival hyperemia and epithelial thinning as a result of erosion and/or atrophy.

(c) Saponin

Saponin is an amphiphile isolated from the bark of Quillaja saponaria tree that has surface activity. The activity relies solely on its detergent action. Saponin was used in concentration range of 0.5% to increase penetration of atenolol but can only slightly improve the delivery of lipophilic compounds timolol and befunolol. It was also extensively studied as a penetration enhancer for systemic delivery of macromolecules like insulin and glucagon via the eye. Concentrations higher than 0.5% are irritating to the eyes.

(d) Amino acid

Emisphere Technologies (New Jersey, USA) synthesized a series of small molecular weight α-amino acids which can be used to promote oral delivery. It was clear that these carriers do not damage cell membranes or tight junctions and thus are unlike classical penetration enhancers. They form drug-carrier complex and are not absorbed by an active transport process but promote transport by shielding those hydrophilic groups on the molecule that restrain absorption. Works had shown that these can increase the permeability of human growth hormone by ten folds.

(e) Pz-Peptide

Also called as 4-phenylazobenzoxycarbonyl-Pro-Leu-Gly-Pro-D-Arg, Pz-Peptide is a hydrophilic collagenase-labile pentapeptide with a molecular weight of 777 D. It is capable of triggering opening of tight junctions in a transient reversible manner, facilitating paracellular transport of the drugs as well as its own. Pz-peptide increases penetration across the cornea and conjunctiva for a wide range of compounds such as atenolol, propranolol, mannitol, fluorescein, FITC-Dextran 4000 etc. The exact mechanism of enhancement of permeation is yet to be established. However, the enhancement activity is more pronounced *in vitro* than *in vivo*. This may be due to the dilution effects of resident tears on Pz-peptide and the applied dose or binding of peptide with mucin in tear proteins.

3. Multifunctional approach (Polymeric penetration enhancers)

(a) Colloidal systems

These systems were extensively used for enhancement of ocular drug delivery. The mechanism of enhancement is generally believed to be related to prolonged residence time in the cul-de-sac. Poly-ε-caprolactone nanoparticles, nanocapsules and sub-micron emulsions improved ocular bioavailability when compared with aqueous solutions and with the suspensions of microparticles. It was believed that the colloidal nature rather than the inner structure or the specific compositions of the colloidal carriers plays a key role in the enhancement of penetration since all the three carriers can equally cause an improvement of drug release to the same extent. Confocal microscopy reveals that the colloidal carriers can penetrate into the epithelium layers and cells of the cornea without causing any damage to the cell membrane. This suggests that these carriers enter the epithelium via endocytosis and hence act as a penetration enhancer or an endocytotic stimulator.

(b) Bioadhesives

Various means were employed to enhance the residence time in cul-de-sac, which can, in turn, increase the amounts of drug penetration. Obviously it is desirable to have a delivery system that can stay in the precorneal area for an extended period of time but at the same time enhance corneal penetration. A number of bio-adhesive polymers have such properties. Typically these are the macromolecules that have already been approved by FDA for other purposes. Therefore, safety is not a problematic issue.

(c) Polyacrylates

Poly(acrylic acid) derivatives such as carbomer and polycarbol are used extensively as bio-adhesives. They donot have membrane penetration enhancing activity but exact mechanism of action is still not well understood. It was demonstrated that the solvent drug is responsible for enhanced absorption of low molecular weight compounds. The gels cannot increase penetration solely by surface activity as these inhibit hemolysis caused most commonly by most of the surfactants. Another proposed mechanism can be calcium chelating activities, which is an essential component for normal activity of tight junctions and metabolizing enzymes.

(d) Chitosan and its derivatives

The positively charged chitosan, a hydrophilic, biodegradable and biocompatible polymer of lower toxicity is chemically poly[(β-(1-4)-2-

amino-2-deoxy-D-glucopyranose)] that can reduce elimination rate by increasing viscosity and by its interactions with negatively charged mucus (mucoadhesive). This, in addition to increasing residence time of the drug in precorneal area, can be used as potential penetration enhancer to improve delivery across the cornea. The exact mechanism of action is still not known but could be due to partial alteration of cytoskeleton.

D. Intraocular dosage forms

A special class of ophthalmic drugs and irrigating solutions requiring the application of parenteral dosage form technology in their design and manufacture comprises those that are introduced into the interior structure of the eye during surgery. Presurgical therapy to maintain pupil dilation and enhance the surgeon's ability to remove the cataract and insert a plastic intraocular lens replacement (IOL) is widely practiced.

Most ophthalmic surgeons also use a viscous solution of sodium hyaluronate alone or in combination with chondroitin sulfate as an aid to help maintain anterior chamber depth and visibility and to minimize interaction between tissues or surgical trauma to them during the procedure. It is also used to provide a hydrophilic coating for the plastic intraocular lens before and during insertion. These polymers are naturally occurring high molecular weight linear polysaccharides. They form viscoelastic solutions in water, which give them unique properties for use in ocular surgery. For this use, they must be specially purified to remove pyrogenic, inflammatory, and antigenic components. The molecular weight fraction must be selected and carefully controlled to provide the desired degree of viscoelasticity, without excessive viscosity, which can detract from their handling characteristics and could result in prolonged retention in the anterior chamber, where the polymers can block aqueous outflow and cause a dangerous increase in intraocular pressure.

These solutions must be refrigerated until just before use.

The plastic IOL, that the surgeon implants as an artificial lens, is primarily made of polymethyl methacrylate (PMMA), silicone and the hydroxyethyl methacrylic acid (HEMA). However, systemic toxicity is seldom encountered in the use of intraocularly administered drug products, but the prime concern in the design of such products is that of tissue compatibility. For such drug products, it is mandatory to design specific *ex vivo* testing protocols that amount to continuous infusion of the specific product composition, both freshly made and aged, into the anterior chamber of excised rabbit eyes for prolonged periods. Judgments for product-tissue compatibility can then be made by observing the corneal endothelium by specular microscopy and histopathology.

In vitro these materials can also be evaluated against specific cell lines in tissue culture. As tissue culture technology progresses, cell lines for the other tissues in the anterior segment of the eye will be established and will become useful in tissue compatibility testing as well. In considering the design of a drug for intraocular use, simplicity of composition is the key. In general, the fewer the ingredients, the lesser is the likelihood of tissue incompatibility.

Packaging system for drug products of this type need to use more specialized packaging designed to circumvent some of the recognized difficulties in use of ampoules and single- or multiple dose vials. Glass fragments and elastomer particles generated during ampoule fracture and stopper penetration may be there, so very specialized stopper design, cleaning procedures, and lubrication should be considered when this type of packaging is used. Also packaging sterility must be considered.

E. Viscoelastics and hydrogels in ophthalmic formulations

Viscoelastic polymer solutions are widely used to separate and protect fragile tissues, and maintain the shape of the eye during cataract surgery and intraocular lens implantation. Anionic polysaccharides similar to HA (hyaluronic acid) but having much lower cost and greater stability (e.g. carboxymethyl-cellulose – CMC), are of particular interest. Animal studies suggest that CMC compositions with properties like those of HA products can be autoclave sterilized and exhibit good shelf-life. Concepts have been developed for bene-ficially incorporating drugs into these bio-materials to produce 'medicated devices'. Gamma-polymerized N-vinylpyrrolidone produced unique gel-like PVP polymers of interest for artificial vitreous replacements for the eye and for retinal tamponades.

With the change in ocular implant technology to rigid lenses to flexible-foldable polymers, studies have been devoted to improved hydro-gels, silicones, and low Tg-acrylics with greater strength and toughness and with refractive indexes of > 1.48. More efficient vinyl-functional UV absorbers for covalent binding to ocular lens polymers have also been developed. Hydrophilic radiation surface modification of hydrogels has yielded "super-hydrophilic" hydrogels and an unusual method was developed to prepare "hydrophobic hydrogels."

F. Other modes of administration

1. Packs

These sometimes are used to prolong contact of the solutions with the eye. A cotton pledget is saturated with an ophthalmic solution, and this pledget is inserted into the superior or inferior fornix e.g., packs saturated with phenylephrine solutions may be used to produce maximal mydriasis.

2. Intracameral injections

Injections may be added directly into the anterior chamber (e.g. acetylcholine chloride, certain antibiotics, steroids) or directly into the vitreous chamber (amphotericin B, gentamicin sulfate

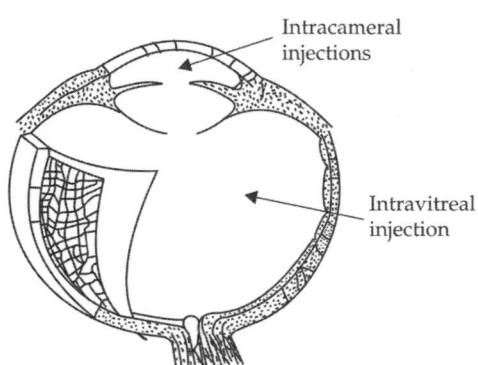

Fig. 6.8. Mode of administration.

and steroids). Injections are not made into posterior chamber (Fig. 6.8).

3. Iontophoresis

This procedure keeps the solution in contact with the cornea by means of an eyecup bearing an electrode. Diffusion of the drug (e.g. fluorescein sodium, an antibiotic) is effected by the difference in electrical potential.

4. Subconjunctival injections

These are used frequently to introduce medications that if applied topically either do not penetrate into the anterior segment or penetrate too slowly to attain the concentration required. The drug is injected underneath the conjunctiva and probably passes through the sclera and into the eye by simple diffusion. The most common use of subconjunctival injections is for the administration of antibiotics in infections of the anterior segment of the eye. Subconjunctival injections of mydriatics and cycloplegics also are used to achieve maximal pupillary dilatation or relaxation of the ciliary muscle.

5. Retrobulbar injections

Drugs administered by retrobulbar injection may enter the globe in essentially the same manner as the medications given subconjunctivally. The orbit is not well vascularized and the possibility of significant effects from these injections is very remote. In general, such injections are given for the purpose of getting medications (e.g., antibiotics, local anesthetics, enzymes with local anesthetics, steroids, vasodilators) into the posterior segment of the globe and to affect the nerves and other structures in that space.

6. Artificial tears

Solutions intended to rewet hard lenses in situ are referred to as rewetting solutions or artificial tears. Such preparations are intended to reinforce the wetting capacity of the normal tear film. Early products of this type tended to be somewhat viscous wetting solutions acceptable for direct instillations into the eye. More recent preparations mimic tears more accurately, and their viscosity is rather low, thus user acceptability is improved.

G. Non-corneal routes in drug delivery

The non-corneal penetration routes create a framework for rational design of drug delivery systems for therapeutic agents that are poorly absorbed across the cornea or require delivery to the posterior segment of the eye.

The non-corneal route of delivery is best suited for the large polar drug components, which have poor permeability across the cornea and are less likely to be cleared by systemic losses via absorption into the ocular blood vessels. The effective non-corneal routes of drug delivery require special consideration in dosage form design and methods of administration that can minimize precorneal exposures and retain higher concentrations of drug at the absorptive surfaces or the conjunctiva and sclera. Delivery system options include bioadhesive polymeric vehicles, controlled release inserts, prodrugs, microparticulate and scleral implants. The method of administration most likely to enhance such delivery opportunities is via subconjunctival or subtenon's injection or implantation as these methods are best suited to administer the drugs in close proximity of the absorbing surfaces as a depot form.

The non-corneal penetration pathways, thus, involve the permeation of drug across the conjunctiva and sclera and may contribute significantly to drug penetration into intraocular tissues for some drugs. Recent advances in drug delivery systems that minimize precorneal losses and can retain higher concentrations of drug at the absorptive surfaces of sclera and conjunctiva may be particularly suited for non-cornea delivery. The non-corneal approach, thus, appears to be a potential area for intraocular delivery of molecules.

H. Microemulsion as newer emerging carriers

The microemulsions are different from emulsions in having an extra cosurfactant phase, which makes the systems thermodynamically very stable and very transparent as compared to the emulsions. The stability of such microemulsions were described in terms of droplet model for lower concentrations of internal oil phase (~10%), where stabilization is achieved by interfacial film of surfactant and cosurfactant; and bicontinuous models, where the water and oil phases were separated by regular or irregular interfacial layer. The microemulsions are liquid and behave as a Newtonian liquid and are not very viscous, their formation is spontaneous and does not require much energy, and are thermodynamically stable. The physicochemical parameters and other factors deciding designing and formulations of microemulsions relating its use in ophthalmic delivery can be summarized as follows:

(a) Improvement in drug solubilization

The main advantage of the microemulsions is the solubilization of drugs. In the aqueous solutions each constituents of the microemulsions viz. oil phase, surfactant and cosurfactant should have intrinsic solubility for the drug or at least synergistically increase the solubility of the drug for the formulation of stable microemulsions for ophthalmic delivery.

(b) Formulation variables

1. Surfactants

The preferential adsorption of surfactant enables modification of the physicochemical properties of the interface due to its amphiphilic nature. Higher amounts of surfactants are generally required in microemulsions as compared to its lower concentrations in emulsions, which may lead to its ocular toxicity. Non-ionic surfactants are the most preferred ones. The most commonly used surfactants are Poloxamers, polysorbates, Tyloxapol and other polyethylene glycol (PEG) or polyoxyethylene terminated derivatives, etc. Amphoteric surfactants like lecithin are also interesting due to their lower toxicity, but are mostly dependent on their source of origin.

2. Cosurfactants

The cosurfactants provide very low interfacial tensions required for the formation of microemulsions and are thermodyanamically stable. They can also modify the curvature of the interface based on the relative importance of their apolar groups other than providing fluidity to the interfacial film. If the film is too rigid, it can prevent the formation of microemulsion and results in a more viscous and birefringent phase. The cosurfactant provides additional fluidity and is equivalent to a branched surfactant. The cosurfactants used are generally small molecules, which are alcohols and glycols of low molecular weights and chain length ranging from C2 to C10. Amongst these PEGs, PEG 200 is preferred due to its lower viscosity as cosurfactants other than propylene glycols. Some alcohols like pentanol and hexanol are not used in pharmaceuticals especially ophthalmics because of irritating nature. Benzyl alcohol and ethanol can be used in rare circumstances. Amine with short chains can also be used as co-surfactants.

3. Oily phase

The oil phase is responsible for the formation of microemulsion and solubilization of drug within it. The same type of oil does not satisfy both the conditions in most cases. Therefore, it is necessary to find an appropriate combination. Oils with excessively long hydrocarbon chains do not result in microemulsions. The shorter the chains the deeper the penetration of the organic phase into the interfacial film and more important is the existence of the range of the microemulsion. On the contrary, the capacity of solubilization by the organic phase increases with the length of the chain. Therefore, the choice is based on solubility of the drug.

The most often used external phase consists of vegetable oils like soya oils, castor oils, triglycerides for which 90% of fatty acids are made of 8–10 carbon chains. Myglyol 812 (triesters of glycerol, capric acids, and caprylic acids), isopropyl myristate, fatty acids such as oleic acids, and esters of sacchrose, such as mono-, di- or tri-palmitates of sacchrose. As these excipients are well tolerated by the eye, their degree of purity must be high to prevent any contamination by irritating substances.

4. Aqueous phase

The aqueous phase must contain several additives, such as buffers, antibacterial and isotonic agents. They can affect the area of existence of the microemulsions, and, therefore, they must be studied in the presence of other ingredients of the microemulsions. Salinity can affect the phase diagram when ionic surfactants are added and can reduce the phase inversion temperatures of non-ionic surfactants. The preparation of microemulsions is very sensitive to the temperature, if the PIT is close to the operating temperature. Adjustment of pH to 7–8 is needed as to minimize the hydrolysis of phospholipids and triglycerides to fatty acids, which can reduce the pH of the microemulsion.

The preservatives which are usually used in eye drops formulations are not suitable for microemulsions. The preservatives in most cases should neither interact with the surfactant (result in complex formation) nor get adsorbed in nanodroplets, which can considerably decrease the bacterial activity and preservative efficacy of the microemulsions. Thiomersal and chlorbutanol with concentrations of 0.01–0.2% can be used; that combination increases their preservative efficacy.

5. Preparation techniques

There are generally two techniques in preparation of microemulsions, which can be the exact processes by autoemulsification and process based on supply of energy. Due to the spontaneous formation of microemulsions they can be prepared by one step by mixing the constituents with reduced roughness. The order of addition of surfactants is not considered as a critical factor for the formulation of microemulsion but can determine the time required to attain the equilibrium. The time required will increase if the cosurfactant is added because of its greater solubility in this phase that will prevent the diffusion in the aqueous phase. In the other case, where the microemulsions are not obtained freely, the high pressure homogenizers can be used to obtain the desired size of droplets that constitute the internal phase. In this the first step produces a coarse emulsion (100 micron) and then followed by high speed mixer and the second step consists of using high pressure homogenization. The dispersion can also be done by heating the phases before mixing depending on the sensitivity of the drug to heat followed by cooling and homogenization. A blue opalescent microemulsion is formed of 0.65 μm diameter of droplets.

(c) Zeta potential

The charge of the internal droplet phase could increase the residence time of droplets at the site by binding to the sites. The charge can be imparted by various lipophilic solutes that can get incorporated into the droplets. The pair of ions in the internal phase can provide a delayed release by a reservoir effect. The concentration of drug in the internal phase can be modified by the concentration of counter ions and the partition coefficient of the drug. Also the pair of ions located in the external phase could easily penetrate the lipophilic epithelium and thus can increase the corneal bioavailability of the drug.

(d) Future challanges

The production and sterilization of microemulsions being easier, they are considered as simple and inexpensive alternative for solubilization and ophthalmic delivery system for lipophilic drugs and that could at the same time increase the systemic bioavailability of the drugs from ocular route. The appropriate delivery is dependent on choice of oil phase, surfactants, cosurfactants and their relative and additive undue toxicity. It is, thus, preferable to keep the level of surfactants below 5% and may require dispersion and homogenization. The choice of oily phase for the emulsions is also to be taken into consideration in existence range of microemulsions. The future challenge is, thus, development of microemulsion-based carriers of drugs that could deliver the drug in zero order rate kinetics. Also, using charged microemulsions one can increase the affinity between the cornea and microemulsions and can increase the corneal residence time.

OPHTHALMIC IMPLANTS AND SHUNTS

A. Inserts

In earlier times, it has been reported that lamellae or disks of glycerinated gelatin were used to supply drugs to the eye by insertion beneath the eyelid. The aqueous tear fluids dissolved the lamella and released the drug for absorption. The medical literature also describes a sterile paper strip impregnated with drug for insertion in the eye. These appear to have been the first attempts at designing sustained-release dosage form. Ophthalmic inserts are solid devices intended to be placed in the conjunctival sac and to deliver the drug at a relatively slow rate. These devices might present valuable advantages, such as:

(a) increased ocular contact time with respect to standard vehicles, hence prolonged drug activity and a higher drug bioavailability;

(b) accurate dosing as all of the drug is retained at the absorption site;

(c) capacity to provide, in some cases, a constant rate of drug release;

(d) possible reduction of systemic absorption, as in case of standard eye drops through nasal mucosa;

(e) better patient compliance, resulting from a reduced frequency of medication and a lower incidence of visual and systemic side effects;

(f) possibility of targeting internal ocular tissues through non-corneal conjunctival-scleral penetration routes; and

(g) increased shelf-life with respect to eye drops due to the absence of water.

An interesting device developed by Alza Corp. is the Ocusert®, a diffusion unit consisting of a drug reservoir e.g. pilocarpine HCl in alginate gel enclosed by two release-controlling membranes made of ethylene-vinyl acetate co-polymer and enclosed by a white ring, allowing positioning of the system in the eye. Clinical studies with the pilocarpine Ocusert® demonstrated that slow release of the drug can effectively control the increased intraocular pressure in glaucoma, with a minor incidence of side effects such as miosis, myopia, browache, etc. Other inserts, both erodible and non-erodible e.g. medicated contact lenses, collagen shields, the Minidisc®, etc. have also been shown capable of diminishing the systemic absorption of ocularly applied drugs as a result of a decreased drainage into the nasal cavity, which is one of the major systemic absorption sites of topical ocular medications.

Another potential advantage of insert therapy is the possibility of promoting non-corneal drug penetration, thus increasing the efficacy of some hydrophilic drugs that are poorly absorbed through the cornea. But, in spite of the advantages demonstrated by extensive investigations and clinical tests, inserts have not gained acceptance. The prolonged, constant-rate release pattern achievable by inserts, resulting in increased therapeutic efficacy and reduction of ocular and systemic side effects, can be considered as the most desirable condition for long-term therapy. Various types of ophthalmic inserts are given in Table 6.7.

Table 6.7. Types and examples of ophthalmic inserts

Type	Examples
Nonerodible ocular inserts	• Ocusert Pilo-20 and Pilo-40 • Ocusert (Diffusion or Osmotic) • Bioadhesive eye insets • Contact lenses
Erodible ocular inserts	• Lacrisert • Ocular therapeutic system (OTS) or minidisc • Soluble ocular drug insert (SODI) • Collagen shields • Ocufit SR

Nonerodible ocular inserts

In 1975, the first controlled-release topical dosage form was marketed in the United States by the Alza Corporation. The Alza therapeutic system is described as a drug-containing device or dosage form that administers a drug or drugs at programmed rates, at a specific body site, for a prescribed time period to provide continuous control of drug therapy and to maintain this control over extended periods, e.g. therapeutic systems for uterine delivery of progesterone, transdermal delivery of scopolamine, and oral delivery of systemic drugs have also been developed.

The Ocusert **Pilo-20** and **Pilo-40** system is an elliptical membrane that is soft and flexible and designed to be placed in the inferior cul-de-sac between the sclera and the eyelid and to release pilocarpine continuously at a steady rate

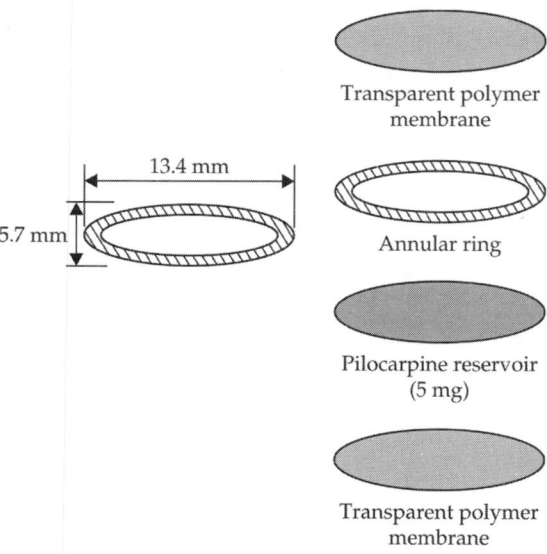

13.4 mm

5.7 mm

Transparent polymer membrane

Annular ring

Pilocarpine reservoir (5 mg)

Transparent polymer membrane

Fig. 6.9. Formulation and design of ocular inserts.

for 7 days. The design of the dosage form is described by Alza in terms of an open-looped therapeutic system, having three major components: (a) the drug, (b) a drug delivery module, and (c) a platform. In the Ocusert Pilo-20 and Pilo-40 systems, the drug delivery module consists of (a) a drug reservoir, pilocarpine (free base), and a carrier material, alginic acid; (b) a rate controller, ethylene vinyl acetate (EVA) copolymer membrane; (c) an energy source, the concentration of pilocarpine in the reservoir; and (d) a delivery portal, the copolymer membrane.

The platform component for the Ocusert consists of the EVA copolymer membranes, which serve as the housing, and an annular ring of the membrane impregnated with titanium dioxide that forms a white border for visibility. The free-base form of pilocarpine is used, since it exhibits both hydrophilic and lipophilic characteristics. Use of extremely water-soluble salts of pilocarpine would have necessitated the use of a hydrophilic membrane which, if it osmotically imbibed an excessive amount of water, would cause a significant decline in the release rate with time. Use of the free base allowed a choice of more hydrophobic

membranes that are relatively impermeable to water; accordingly the release rate is independent of the environment in which it is placed. EVA, the hydrophobic copolymer chosen, was found to be very compatible with the sensitive ocular tissues.

The pilocarpine Ocusert is claimed to offer a number of theoretical advantages over drop therapy for the glaucoma patient. The Ocusert exposes a patient to only one-fourth to one-eighth the amount of pilocarpine, compared with drop therapy. This could lead to reduced local side effects and toxicity. It provides continuous round-the-clock control of intraocular pressure (IOP), whereas drops used four times a day can permit periods where the IOP might rise. Additionally, the Ocusert provides for more patient convenience and improved compliance, as the dose needs to be administered only once a week. However, the clinical experience seems to indicate that the Ocusert has a compliance problem of its own (i.e., retention in the eye for the full 7 days).

Erodible ocular inserts

Since polymers have been added to solutions to increase their conjunctival retention time, it is not surprising that similar solutions have been dried to form films of the polymer drug system. These films have been inserted in the cul-de-sac and have been reported to increase retention time, increase the penetration of the drug, and prolong its effect. Polymers used in soluble ophthalmic film inserts are polyacrylamide, ethylacrylate, and vinylpyrrolidone. A solid disk of pilocarpine alginate provides a greater degree of miosis and prolonged activity compared with aqueous solutions of the hydrochloride and alginate salts.

These solid inserts absorb the aqueous tear fluid and gradually erode or disintegrate. The drug is slowly leached from the matrix, but a constant zero-order delivery is not achieved. They quickly lose their solid integrity and are squeezed out of the eye with eye movement and blinking. If they are made more hydrophobic, they become irritating when placed in the eye. These erodible inserts possess an advantage over the nonerodible inserts as they do not have to be removed at the end of their useful dosing cycle.

Lacrisert is a sterile ophthalmic insert that is used in the treatment of moderate to severe dry eye syndrome and is generally used in patients when an adequate trial of artificial tear solutions failed to provide symptomatic relief. The insert is composed of 5 mg of hydroxypropyl cellulose in a rod-shaped form of about 1.27 mm diameter by about 3.5 mm long. No preservative is used, since it is essentially anhydrous. The cellulose rod is placed in the lower conjunctival sac and first imbibes water from the tears and forms a gel-like mass after several hours, which gradually erodes as the polymer dissolves. This action thickens the tear film and provides increased lubrication, which can provide symptomatic relief for dry eye states. It is usually used once or twice daily.

B. Contact lens

Contact lenses are optical devices that are either fabricated from preformed polymers or polymerized during lens manufacture. The main purpose of contact lenses is to correct defective vision. For this application, they are called cosmetic lenses. Contact lenses used medically for the treatment of certain corneal diseases are called bandage lenses.

Evolution of contact lenses

In 1508, Leonardo da Vinci conceived the concept of the contact lens. It was not until 1887 that scleral contact lenses were fabricated by Dr. A.E. Fick, a physician in Zurich; F.A. Mueller, a maker of prosthetic eyes in Germany; and Dr. E. Kalt, a physician in France. Muller, Obrig, and Gyorry fabricated contact lenses made from polymethyl methacrylate (PMMA) in the late 1930s. K. Tuohy filed the patent for contact lens design in 1948, which were made of PMMA material. Although they were safe and effective, these lenses were uniformly uncomfortable, thus suppressing their potential growth for contact lens wear. Lenses made from polyhydroxyethyl methacrylate (HEMA), the so called soft lenses or hydrophilic lenses were introduced in 1970. Since then, significant technological advances have been made in the lens materials, lens fabrication, and lens designs. Today, rigid lenses made from materials polymerized with PMMA and in combination with various siloxanes and fluorocarbons are available to meet the broadest needs of lens wearers.

Composition of contact lenses

Contact lenses are broadly classified as rigid gas-permeable (made of PMMA), and soft hydrogel (HEMA) lenses. Dyes may be added during polymerization or after fabrication to improve lens handling or to change the color of the lens wearer's eyes. Lenses made from numerous polymers are available today. In soft hydrogel lenses, HEMA is a commonly used monomer. However, to avoid infringement of existing patents, many co-monomers, e.g., methyl methacrylic acid or a blend of co-monomers, are used. Co-monomers produce changes in the water content or ionic nature of lenses that is significantly different from HEMA lenses. For example, addition of acrylic acid in HEMA increases the water content and ionic nature of lenses. Some lenses are made from N-vinyl-pyrrolidone and have high water content. Such lenses have pore sizes that are much larger than low water content lenses. Desired properties of these lenses include flexibility, wettability, and gas transmissibility.

Cross-linkers, such as ethyleneglycol dimethacrylate, and initiators like benzyl peroxide, in appropriate amounts, are added for polymerization and to achieve desirable physical and chemical properties. Table 6.8 gives a list of monomers, co-monomers and cross-linkers along with their effects on polymer properties. In 1985, FDA published a classification for soft hydrophilic lenses based on their water content and ionic nature. Adequate levels of oxygen are

Table 6.8. Commonly used monomers, co-monomers, and cross-linkers in contact lens polymers

Name	Abbreviation	Lens properties
Acrylic acid	AA	Flexibility, hydrophilicity, pH sensitivity, acidic, reactivity, ionically interacts with positively charged tear components, wettability
Butyl methacrylate	BMA	Softness, flexibility, hydrophobicity, attracts lipids, wettability, gas transmisssibility
Cellulose acetate butyrate	CAB	Clarity, wettability, gas transmissibility
Dimethyl siloxane	DMS	Hydrophobicity, wettability, gas transmissibility, physical stability
Diphenyl siloxane	DPS	Hydrophobicity, wettability, gas transmissibility, physical stability
Ethonyethyl methacrylate	EOEMA	Flexibility, softness, hydrophobicity, wettability, gas transmissibility
Ethylene glycol dimethacrylate	EGDME	Hydrophilicity, wettability
Glyceryl methacrylate	GMA	Wettability, gas transmissibility, hydrophilicity, machinability
Hydroxyethyl methacrylate	HEMA	Flexibility, wettability, gas transmissibility, softness, machinability
Methacrylic acid	MA	Hardness, hydrophilicity
Methyl methacrylate	MMA	Hardness, machinability, wettability, gas transmissibility, hydrophobicity
Methylphenyl siloxane	MPS	Hydrophobicity, gas transmissibility
Methyl vinyl siloxane	MVS	Hydrophobicity, gas transmissibility
N-Vinylpyrrolidone	NVP	Hydrophilicity, wettability, machinability, color, clarity
Siloxanyl methacrylate	SMA	Hardness, wettability, gas transmissibility

necessary to maintain normal corneal metabolism. Lenses that are poorly designed and worn overnight deprive the cornea of oxygen, causing edema. Contact lenses made from PMMA materials are virtually impermeable to gases. The PMMA lenses are also inflexible, causing discomfort in a large percentage of individuals while the lens is worn. During the 1980s, lenses that were somewhat flexible and permeable to oxygen were introduced. These lenses were made from either cellulose acetate butyrate (CAB), or silicone elastomer. Although comfortable and flexible, such lenses accumulated lipids, were non-wettable, and adhered to the cornea. Lenses made from fluorocarbons, and in various combinations of fluorocarbon, silicone, methyl methacrylate, and acrylic acid are currently available.

Complications of contact lens wear and the need for care products

Lens design, user compliance with manufacturers' instructions, hygiene, environmental conditions, poor fit, lens materials, and tear chemistry are the major causes of lens wear complications. Knowledge of tear chemistry is important in understanding the complex chemical processes between tear components and contact lenses. The tear film can be broadly divided into three distinct layers: lipids, aqueous, and mucin. Each layer of the tear film performs a specific function. The mucin layer spreads and coats the hydrophobic corneal cells and extends into the aqueous layer. The aqueous layer contains 98% water and 2% solids. Solids in this layer are predominantly the electrolytes (Na^+, K^+, Ca^{++}, Mg^{++}, Cl^-, and HCO^-), nonelectrolytes (urea and glucose), and proteins. The lipid layer, which consists of cholesterol esters, phospholipids, and triglycertides, prevents and regulates aqueous evaporation from the tear film.

Components of the tear attach to contact lenses by electrostatic and van der Waals forces, and build up to form deposits. Deposits on the surface and in the lens matrix may result in reduced visual acuity, irritation, and in some instances, serious ocular complications. The composition of deposits vary because of the complexity of an individual's ocular physiology. Lysozyme is a major component of soft lens deposits, especially found on high water content ionic lenses. Calcium and lipids are infrequent components of deposits, occurring as inorganic salts, organic salts, or as an element of mixed deposits, or as combination thereof.

Lenses are exposed to a broad spectrum of microbes during normal wear and handling and become contaminated relatively quickly. Failure of effective removal of microorganisms from lenses can cause ocular infections. Ocular infections, particularly those caused by pathogenic microbes, such as *P. aeruginosa*, can lead to loss of the infected eye if left untreated.

Types of lens care products

Contact lens care products can be divided into three categories: cleaners, disinfectants, and lubricants. Improperly cleaned lenses can cause discomfort, irritation, decrease in visual acuity, and giant papillary conjunctivitis (GPC). This latter condition often requires discontinuation of lens wear, at least until the symptoms clear. Deposits can also accumulate preservatives from lens care products and produce toxicity, and can act as a matrix for microbial attachment to the lens. Thus, cleaning is one of the most important steps in successful lens wear. It helps in removal of surface debris, tear components, and contaminating microorganisms, resulting in safety and efficacy of lens-wearing.

Daily cleaners and weekly cleaners are employed to clean deposits that accumulate on lenses during normal wear. Single cleaning agents or combinations of cleaning agents may be used in a cleaner. Surfactant(s), solvent(s), and complexing agent(s) chosen for cleaner formulations must be capable of solubilizing lens deposits and must have low irritation potential. They must be easily rinsed, leaving very low or nondetectable residue levels on the lens. Nonionic and amphoteric surfactants are commonly used in daily cleaner products. Because of their toxicity to the cornea and binding to the lenses, anionic and cationic surfactants are avoided. Solvents capable of solubilizing lens deposits, without altering the lens's polymer properties, should be carefully selected. Complexing agents, such as citrates, are included in daily cleaner formulations. They counter the binding of positively charged proteins to the lenses and render the proteins more soluble in the media by ion-pair or salt formation.

Mechanical force is a key aspect in the cleaning process. For daily cleaning, mechanical force is generally provided through tile rubbing action of the fingers over the lens during the actual cleaning process. Cleaning lenses by rubbing typically removes 1.7 ± 0.5 logs of microorganisms, rinsing the lens removes 1.9 ± 0.5 logs of microorganisms, and cleaning plus rinsing the lens removes 3.7 ± 0.5 logs of microorganisms of a typical 10^6 colony forming units (CFU)/ml challenge. Abrasive particles are included in products to enhance the mechanical force applied to the lens during the cleaning process. The abrasive properties are evaluated by testing the hardness of the included abrasive particles. Particles that have Rockwell hardness lower than the hardness of the lens polymers are typically used. If the hardness of abrasive particles is higher than the hardness of the lens polymer, it is possible that the lens would be damaged. Some contact lenses are reported to require special treatment. Abrasive particles may alter surface treatment effects even when their hardness is lower than that of the lens polymer.

Enzymatic cleaners contain enzymes derived from animals, plants, or microorganisms. Plant and microorganism-derived enzymes cause sensitization problems in many lens wearers. Commonly used enzymes are of either animal origin like proteases, lipases and amylases or papain of plant origin or of microbial origin like Subtilisin A and B, etc. All of these enzymes are effective in removing deposits from the contact lens surface. They are biochemical catalysts that are specific for catalyzing certain chemical reactions. Those that aid in removing contact lens debris are protease (protein-specific enzyme), lipase (lipid-specific enzyme), and amylase (polysaccharide-specific enzyme). Such enzymes act by attacking substrate molecules, such as protein, lipid, and mucin, on the lens and catalyzing their breakdown into smaller molecular units. This process yields fragments that are readily removed by mechanical force and rinsing. The newer products are either in a tablet or a solution product form. They require soaking lenses in solutions for a period of 15 min to more than 2 hr before disinfecting the lenses.

Other than the preservatives as discussed earlier, thimerosal and sorbic acid are also commonly used as preservatives in these products; however, concerns over the sensitization potential and discoloration of lenses has led to the introduction of new and safer molecules like Polyquad (a polymerically bound quaternary ammonium compound) and Dymed. Specifically, Polyquad is resistant to absorption into the lenses; thus, it may not diffuse out of the lens into the eye, leading to corneal toxicity, an inherent problem associated with nonpolymerically bound quaternary ammonium compounds. The FDA and the USP have specific Preservative Effectiveness Standards that these products must meet. The FDA standards detailing the method were published in 1985. Oxidizing agents and nonoxidizing chemical disinfectants that are non-toxic at product concentrations are used to chemically disinfect lenses. Mostly, hydrogen peroxide is used as an oxidizing agent. It is used in concentrations of 0.6–3.0%. Peroxides are very toxic to the cornea of the eye. After the disinfection cycle, and before placing the lens in the eye, hydrogen peroxide must be completely neutralized by reducing agents, catalase or transition metals, such as platinum.

Recent developments in contact lenses

1. Bandage lenses

Even with technological and material advances over time, the use of bandage lenses remains somewhat controversial. When used judiciously, they can be an effective way to manage many pathological conditions and provide relief to the patient, although there is risk of complications. There are two principal reasons for using hydrophilic bandage contact lenses (HBLs): pain relief and corneal re-epithelialization, specifically for keratorefractive surgery. Studies have shown that HBLs, compared with pressure patching, expedite the rate of epithelial repair and greatly enhance comfort. Specifically, a HBL provides the traumatized cornea with a mechanical barrier against the shearing forces of the lids. It amplifies drug delivery to the anterior segment. It also possibly heightens lubrication therapy, since the lens acts as a reservoir for continuous sustained hydration. Bandage lenses provide splinting effect and may temporarily treat a corneal laceration when used as a thick/stiff lens. Often a wound leak or perforation can be managed in this fashion, allowing the anterior chamber to reform and restoring near normal intraocular tension. This delays the urgency and, in some cases, eliminates the need for surgical intervention. The major conditions where they are indicated are:

Keratitis sicca (dry eyes)

For keratitis sicca (dry eyes) bandage lens are chosen dependent upon patient's condition. High-water materials are selected for patients with tear deficiency. These deliver additional moisture to the corneal surface (Fig. 6.10). The patient needs to use tear supplements, but the HBL allows water to collect within the lens matrix and ultimately be released to the eye.

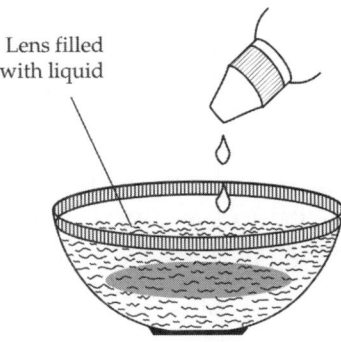

Lens filled with liquid

Fig. 6.10. Lens filled with liquid.

Table 6.9 lists some FDA approved contact lenses used as bandage lenses. Patients with an evaporative problem will benefit from more "stable" materials that are more likely to stay fully hydrated. For these individuals, low-water content lenses are selected. Additionally, Bausch & Lomb's alphafilcon material (Soflens 66) had been shown to be effectively binding water to its polymer matrix, maximizing its retention. Also, Biocompatibles (UK) claims that its omafilcon material (Proclear) offers minimal eye dehydration because the lens contains synthetic phosphorylcholine. But a compromised pre-corneal tear film may develop on long use of such lenses that can dispose individuals to infectious keratitis. Therefore, prophylactic topical antibiotic therapy is needed.

Epithelial disorders

These are the most common applications for bandage lenses. HBL therapy is often beneficial in treating persistent epithelial defects that may occur in neurotrophic cases or diabetic patients with impaired corneal healing. The lens helps to guide epithelial cells in their migration. It also protects them from the disruptive action of the eyelids. This theoretical model led to replacing pressure patching with HBL therapy following keratorefractive surgery.

Two specific applications:

1. Corneal erosions
2. Surface irregularity.

Bullous keratopathy

Bullae are essentially 'water blisters' that develop at the epithelial layer. They are caused by excessive edema from the stromal side. Several conditions may contribute to the development of corneal bullae. Among them: corneal guttata, Fuchs' endothelial dystrophy, uncontrolled glaucoma, surgical trauma and intraocular lens implants. Endothelial compromise is the common denominator. Physiological breakdown of this layer results in stromal edema, which contributes to bullous keratopathy. In milder cases, desiccation therapy with hyperosmotic agents may provide some improvement. If IOP is elevated, treatment of IOP reduction is required firstly before initiating more sophisticated measures, such as bandage lens therapy or surgical alternatives.

Bandage lens therapy can be extremely effective in these cases, offering multifaceted

Lens	Manufacturer	Material, % water
Fre-Flex Custom Bandage Lens	Optech	Focofilcon A, 5%
O4 (plano power)	Bausch & Lomb	Polymacon, 38%
Permalens for Therapeutic E.W.	Coopervision, Inc.	Perfilcon A, 71%
Plano T	Bausch & Lomb	Polymacon, 38%
PROTEK	Ciba Vision	Vifilcon A, 55%
U3 (plano power)	Bausch & Lomb	Polymacon, 38%

Table 6.9. FDA-approved bandage lenses

relief. Thick, high water content lenses are suggested for their ability to 'wick' moisture from the cornea and allow it to evaporate. HBLs also provide a protective barrier to tamponade the bullae and minimize lid interaction. At the same time, they mask irregularity and improve acuity. However, watch for lens-induced hypoxia with a commensurate increase in edema and reduction in acuity.

Complications in use of such lenses

While relatively uncommon with judicious use of bandage lenses, complications may occur. These mirror complications which may present with extended-wear lenses on non-diseased eyes. They include:

- Corneal edema and hypoxia.
- Neovascularization.
- Papillary conjunctivitis.
- Sterile infiltrates.

2. Therapeutic contact lenses in drug delivery

There is overwhelming evidence that HBLs improve the results of concomitant topical medications. Various studies have shown HBLs enhanced the effects of anti-virals (idoxuridine) on rabbit corneas infected with herpes virus; helped keep the agent in contact with the ocular surface for longer periods of time; and resulted in more significant efficacy of a topical aminoglycoside when applied over a high water content HBL.

Bactericidal concentrations of antibiotics have been recovered in the precorneal tear film for up to three days following application of HBLs soaked in the drug. Also, greater anterior chamber concentrations have been measured in the presence of an HBL than by simple topical application without a lens in place. Apparently, the lens can absorb the agent, prolong the contact time with the ocular surface and provide time-released action. Some rules are to be remembered when combining topical medications and bandage lenses such as avoid ointments; not to

alter the prescribed dosage and alternate antimicrobial agents every four to five weeks. Various types of such contact lenses that are available and marketed with other particulars are listed in Table 6.10.

3. Silicone hydrogel-based lenses

Silicone hydrogel lenses have been developed to address the major issues of overnight wear. High levels of oxygen transmission, along with excellent surface wetting, contribute to significant wearer benefits. When considering therapeutic uses, the need for overnight wear without further compromise to an already unhealthy cornea, suggests silicone hydrogel lenses as a significant step forward.

In addition to the routine uses of these lenses for bandage applications, there may be some indications for piggy-back/silicone hydrogel/RGP combinations in keratoconus and other corneal irregularities to limit the hypoxic complications evident when conventional hydrogels are used in this configuration. In addition, the unique characteristics of silicone hydrogel lenses may provide additional benefits for those patients who have marginal dry eye or poor tear film quality. The high oxygen transmissibility of these lenses also permits the management of previous hypoxic stress, even during a continuous wear modality.

For example both CIBA Vision Focus® NIGHT & DAY™ and Bausch & Lomb PureVision® silicone hydrogel contact lenses are designed to permit up to 30 days' continuous wear through their unique properties. For PureVision contact lenses, it is claimed that they are specifically designed to provide a balance of properties (Table 6.9) which, together, help ensure maximised success with overnight wear. In particular, the main obstacle to successful continuous wear has been the inability of conventional hydrogels to prevent significant overnight corneal swelling because of low oxygen transmission. While this has not been a problem with silicone elastomer lenses, the

Table 6.10. Approved and marketed therapeutic contact lenses

Manufacturer	Series	Material	Water content	Dia (mm)
Hydrogel types				
Bausch & Lomb	O4	HEMA	38.6%	14.00
Bausch & Lomb	Plano	Polymacon	38.6%	13.50/14.50
Lunelle ES70	Plano	MMA/PV	70%	15.00
Troy	Plano		62/70/74/85%	15.00–20.00
Igel 67	Igel		67/77 67/77%	14.50
Disposable examples only				
Wessley Jessen Precision UV	Monthly disposables	Vasurfilcon A	74%	14.50
Hydron	Actifresh 400	MMA/VP	55%	14.30
Proclear		Omafilcon A	62%	14.20
B&L Soflens66	Monthly disposables	Alphaphilcon A	66%	14.20
B&L Purevision	Silicone hydrogel	Balafilcon A	36%	14.00
Acuvue, J&J	Vistavue	Genfilcon	48%	14.00
CibaVision	Dailies	Nelfilcon A	69%	13.80
Collagen shields (not currently available in the UK)				
Bio-Cor		Type 1 (porcine)		
Chiron		Type 1 (bovine)		
Silicone rubber				
Wohlk	Silflex	Polysiloxane	0%	11.70–13.70
Scleral lenses				
Innovative Sclerals	Sealed			~22.00
David Thomas	GP Centres	60 Dk		Various

problem of lens adhesion (due to a high modulus of elasticity) and poor wetting (due to the hydrophobic nature of the silicone material) have made this a specialist lens only really indicated for aphakia and, in particular, paediatric aphakia.

C. Collagen shields and implants

Biodegradable collagen shields are now available for use as bandage lenses. These come in a dehydrated state, and are to be reconstituted, often with the appropriate topical medication, before placing them on the eye. The shields dissolve in 12–72 hours, depending upon the cross linking of the material and the patient's tear chemistry. Bandage lens therapy has become a very important tool in treating a variety of clinical problems, including keratitis sicca, epithelial disorders and bullous keratopathy. They could provide pain relief and allow for corneal re-epithelialization.

Collagen shields are made of collagen, a natural protein that can be safely applied to the body for a variety of medical and cosmetic purposes. The creation of the corneal collagen shields has provided a means to promote wound dressing and healing and perhaps more importantly to deliver a variety of medications to the cornea and other ocular tissues (Fig. 6.11). There are many indications that the shields deliver drugs as well as, if not better than, topical drops. The simplicity of use and convenience afforded by shields make them attractive delivery

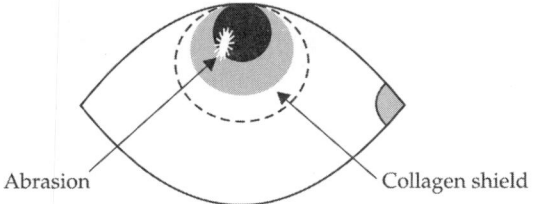

Fig. 6.11. Collagen shield for abrasion.

devices. Although collagen shields produce some discomfort and interfere with the vision, corneal collagen shields could become a commonly employed technological improvement in ophthalmic drug delivery.

In the manufacture of collagen shields, the ability to control the amount of cross-linking in the collagen subunits by exposures to ultraviolet (UV) light is an important physicochemical property, because the amount of cross-linking is related to the dissolution time of the shield on the cornea. The dissolution time of the cross-linked type is more and can prolong the drug delivery times. Cross-linked collagen shields are more useful ocular drug delivery devices because they allow drug concentration to be achieved to higher levels in the cornea and aqueous humor.

The collagen shields were designed to be a disposable, short-term therapeutic bandage lens for the cornea. It conforms to the shape of the eye, protects the corneal surface, and provides lubrication as it dissolves. Unlike the hydrophilic plastic bandage lenses, the collagen shield offers no refractive benefit; but because of not being optically clear, it reduces visual acuity to the 20/80–20/200 range. Also the collagen shield causes some discomfort. Bio-Cor (Bausch & Lomb Surgical Inc., Claremont, CA) was the first commercially available shield that was introduced in 1986. Bausch & Lomb Surgical Inc. is selling only SurgiLens. The shields are derived from bovine collagen and are 14.5 mm in diameter. Dissolution time determined after UV irradiation during the manufacture is about 12 hr. The shields are sterilized by gamma-irradiation, then dehydrated and individually packaged for storage and shipping. Alcon Laboratories Inc. (Fort Worth, TX) is selling ProShield. The rapid dissolution as well as 12, 24, and 72 hr shields are available. The shields have a diameter of 14 mm and compound base curve that is approximately 9 mm when hydrated. The water content is approximately 75%.

The collagen shileds were widely used for the therapy to assist in particularly post-surgical wound healing after penetrating keratoplasty, cataract extraction, epikeratophakia, or non-surgical epithelial healing problems.

A new drug delivery system, collasomes were recently developed. They combine collagen pieces or particles and a viscous vehicle that could be instilled beneath the eyelid, thereby simplifying application and reducing the blurring of vision. The collasomes were well tolerated, and because the collagen particles are suspended in carrier vehicles, they could be instilled safely and effectively by patients in much the same fashion as drops or ointments.

The most obvious use is for ocular surface lubrication. As these shields dissolve, they become gel-like and eventually liquefy. The collagen shield can reduce the necessity for this frequent and inconvenient administration of artificial tears. The Bio-Cor collagen shield is currently available to physicians for use among patients with dry eye syndromes. The collagen shield can serve as a "sponge" to collect medications that are placed in drop form on the surface of the eye and then slowly release them over a period of time as the shield dissolves. Drug released from the collagen shield is high enough to be effectively used for treating a variety of diseases (including infections and inflammation of the ocular surface). This "time release" of topical medications to the eye has obvious benefits for use in several potentially blinding diseases that require frequent administration of drop medications. Collagen shields have not yet been formally approved by the Food and Drug Administration for this use.

Collagen is an essential part of the natural wound healing process. It is conceivable that the collagen in the shield could be incorporated (as the shield dissolves) into a healing wound on the surface of the eye and have beneficial effects. The future for collagen shields is highly promising. The characteristics of providing ocular lubrication, protection, and drug delivery and the potential for better and faster wound healing may eventually make these shields a standard part of ophthalmic practice.

D. Anophthalmos and orbital implants

While it is rare for a person to be born without an eye, it is unfortunately all too frequent occurrence for patients to experience loss of an eye due to trauma, infection or an underlying disease state (Fig. 6.12). The first reported surgical removal of an eye (enucleation) was performed over four centuries ago. It is, however, in the last century that the greatest strides have been made in perfecting this surgical procedure. Once an eye is removed it is important that the loss in orbital soft tissue be replaced with a suitable implant to provide normal cosmesis.

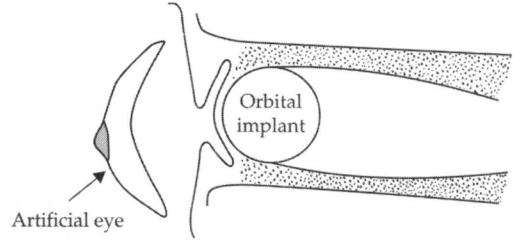

Fig. 6.12. Replacement by suitable implant.

Almost every conceivable material known to man has been used as an orbital implant including magnets, gold, silver, glass, silicone, cartilage, bone, fat, cork, titanium mesh, acrylics, wool, rubber, catgut, peat, agar, asbestos, ivory, cellulose, paraffin, sponge, polyethylene and hydroxyapatite. In addition, a wide variety of implant shapes has been implanted in order to achieve an acceptable cosmetic result including sphere, sphere with a truncated surface, sphere

with a truncated surface and small 'knobs' projecting from the surface, etc.

The most frequent complication associated with the majority of the "older" implants was extrusion of the implant. Other common complications included infection, migration, poor motility, contracted lid fornices and enophthalmos (sunken in appearance). In 1985, hydroxyapatite corraline sphere-shaped implants were introduced. Hydroxyapatite is an inert, biocompatible and nontoxic material that has been in use in the medical field for over 15 years. Hydroxyapatite is a calcium phosphate hydroxide compound made up of multiple interconnecting pores. Because this is an inert porous substance, once implanted into the orbit it becomes vascularized and hence an integral part of the orbit. In recent years, porous polyethylene implants have been utilized in a similar fashion.

E. Glaucoma shunts (Eye valve implant)

Glaucoma is associated with increased intraocular pressure (IOP). The majority (about 90%) of patients with glaucoma have primary open-angle glaucoma (POAG, chronic open-angle glaucoma or chronic simple glaucoma) as a chronic condition in which the IOP is elevated beyond a level compatible with the continued health and function of the eye, with a gonioscopically open angle, and a decreased facility of outflow. Another form of glaucoma is acute angle-closure glaucoma (AACG), which occurs as a dramatic, violent attack with closure of the entire angle. In contrast to POAG, AACG manifests with symptoms of blurred vision with colored halos around lights, pain, redness, and often nausea and vomiting related to the pain. In AACG, the IOP can rise precipitously to more than 50 mm Hg.

The earliest modern implants were developed by Molteno and by Krupin in the early 1970s. Newer implants (Baerveldt, Schocket, Ahmed, Joseph, White, OptiMed) have been introduced with modifications designed to enhance IOP control or limit early post-operative complications. The devices in common use differ primarily on the basis of whether or not the tube contains a pressure-sensitive valve, and the shape and surface area of the scleral explant. The use of glaucoma drainage implants has increased in recent years, especially relative to other surgical glaucoma procedures such as trabeculectomy. The increased utilization of drainage implants is related to a greater experience and appreciation of the efficacy of aqueous shunts, and a growing concern about late complications associated with standard filtering surgery. Only a handful of glaucoma drainage implant types are commercially available and are in common use. Comparisons between the various implant types are, however, difficult because most clinical data are derived from retrospective studies with different study populations, small sample size, limited follow-up, and varied criteria for defining successful outcomes. In addition, the types of glaucoma for which drainage implants are being used has expanded to include eyes with major retinal or corneal surgery and glaucomas associated with pseudophakia, aphakia, uveitis, trauma, epithelial and fibrous downgrowth, anirida, and iridocorneal endothelial syndrome. These refractory glaucoma types can be effectively managed with glaucoma drainage implants, albeit with differing levels of success that affect comparative efficacy results between the varying types of glaucoma drainage implants. When a drainage device with non-valved tube is used, it is necessary to create some restriction to aqueous flow through the tube in the early postoperative period, prior to fibrous encapsulation of the scleral plate.

Currently there are two drainage implants in which the tube has been modified to provide some restriction to aqueous flow – the Ahmed Glaucoma Valve and the Krupin Eye Disk. The need for ligatures or stents at the time of surgery is obviated by a valve mechanism, which is theoretically designed to maintain the IOP within a specific physiologic range (i.e., approx. 8 to 12 mmHg).

Molteno® implants were developed for the treatment of severe and complex cases of glaucoma. The implants consist of a fine bore silicone tube opening onto the upper surface of one or more episcleral plates. The function of the tube is to deliver aqueous from within the eye onto the upper surface of the episcleral plate. The episcleral plate is firmly sutured to the sclera and covered by a thick flap of Tenon's tissue and conjunctiva.

Pharmacia-Baerveldt® glaucoma implants are indicated for use in patients with medically uncontrollable glaucoma and poor surgical prognosis, such as, but not limited to, neovascular glaucoma, aphakic/pseudophakic glaucomas, failed conventional surgery, congenital glaucoma, and secondary glaucoma due to uveitis, epithelial downgrowth, etc. Federal law (USA) restricts this device to sale by a physician. Design features of several available glaucoma drainage implants are given in Table 6.11.

Table 6.11. Design features of available glaucoma drainage implants.

Implant name	Material	Type
Krupin Eye Disk or Krupin Slit Valve	Silastic	Valved
Ahmed Glaucoma Valve	Polypropylene, Silicone	Valved
Baerveldt® Glaucoma Implants	Silicone	Nonvalved
Molteno® Implants	Polypropylene	Nonvalved

F. Particulate-based drug carriers

Controlled and sustained delivery of ophthalmic drug continues to remain a major focus area in the pharmaceutical field. Micro- and nanotechnology involving drug-loaded particles had been proposed as an ophthalmic drug delivery technique that may enhance dosage form acceptability while providing sustained release in the ocular milieu. Particulate drug delivery systems consist of microparticles, nanoparticles, microspheres, nanospheres, microcapsules and nanocapsules, etc. The separate classification and definition of such carriers is out of the scope of the present chapter. These formulations when formulated properly provide controlled drug release and prolonged therapeutic effect. To achieve these characteristics, particles must be retained in cul-de-sac after topical adminis-tration, and the entrapped drug is released from the particles at an appropriate rate. The utility of nanoparticles as an ocular drug delivery system depends on:

(a) Optimizing lipophilic and hydrophilic properties of the polymer-drug system;
(b) Optimizing the rate of biodegradation in the precorneal pocket; and
(c) Increasing retention efficiency in the precorneal pockets.

It is highly desirable to formulate the particles with bioadhesive materials in order to enhance the retention time of the particles in the ocular cul-de-sac. The natural bioadhesive polymers demonstrate promising improvements in ocular bioavailability. Synthetic biodegradable and bioadhesive polyalkylcyanoacrylate systems were also found as the most promising parti-culate drug delivery systems for the future, owing to their lack of toxicity as proven by their safe and successful use for decades in surgery (Table 6.12).

Such carriers can be used as any of the two following systems for ocular drug delivery:

1. Topical systems

Drug-loaded microparticulate systems are suspended in aqueous or non-aqueous medium and instilled in cul-de-sac of the eye wherefrom the drug is slowly released in the lacrimal pool by dissolution and mixing, diffusion, or mechanical disintegration and erosion of the polymer matrix. Microparticles for topical delivery can be of several types including polymer-drug complexes, erodible micro-spheres, responsive particulates, in situ gelling systems, ion exchange systems and nano-particles.

2. Local injectable systems

For diseases like proliferative vitroretinopathy, endophthalmitis and recurrent uveitis require repeated injection of drugs in vitreous cavity to maintain therapeutic levels. Such multiple injection into eye may cause some dangerous clinical and patient-related complications. Development of biodegradable particulate dosage forms of local injections may circum-vent limitations of frequent intravitreal injections by providing a slow release depot of drug in the vitreous cavity and reduce the frequency of injections, thereby increasing patient compliance. The drug like 5-FU was released by simultaneous polymer hydrolysis and drug diffusion from poly(lactide/glycolide) micro-spheres for at least two to seven days as found by *in vitro* and *in vivo* intravitreal kinetic studies without any significant adverse effects on ocular tissues.

Formulation of nanoparticles

A successful nanoparticulate system may be the one that has high loading capacity and reduces the quantity of carrier required for the administration. The drug can either be adsorbed onto the surface of preformed particles or incorporated into the nanospheres during poly-merization process. The loading capacity of nanoparticles has been found to be dependent on the nature and quantities of the monomers used, influencing also the absorption capacity of the carrier. Generally, the longer the chain length, the higher is the affinity of the drug to the polymer, i.e. the capacity of adsorption is related to the hydrophobicity of the polymer and to the specific area of the polymer. Several types of polymeric nanoparticles are used in ophthalmic drug delivery and prepared by the various commonly used methods for the preparation of nanoparticles like emulsion poly-merization in a continuous aqueous phase and

Table 6.12. Summary of various polymers used in ophthalmic particulate drug delivery

Polymer used	Preparation technique	Comments
Polymethylmethacrylate (PMMA)	Emulsion polymerization: 0.1–0.5% in water or phosphate-buffered saline or solution or suspension of drugs or antigens, polymerized by γ-irradiation or chemical initiation using potassium peroxodisulphate and heating to high temperatures.	Drug can be added during polymerization or added to previously produced nanoparticles. Do not degrade biologically or enzymatically, which makes them less attractive for ophthalmic use.
Cellulose acetate phthalate (CAP)	Used for in situ gelling of latex nano-particles. Preparation of these latex particles involves emulsification of polymer in organic solvent followed by solvent evaporation.	Latex suspension upon contact with lacrimal fluid at pH 7.2–7.4 gels in situ, thus averting rapid washout of the instilled solution from the eye leading to vision blurring.
Polyalkyl cyanoacrylate (PACA)	Prepared in the same manner as PMMA. 0.1–3% monomer is added to an aqueous system or to the drug solution. Starts at room temperature and do not require γ-irradiation or addition of special initiators.	Properties of biodegradation and bioadhesion making them suitable as possible drug carriers for controlled ocular drug delivery and drug targeting. Ability to entangle mucin matrix and form noncovalent or ionic bond with mucin layer of the conjunctiva. Merit over acrylic derivatives as these particles do not require high energy input for the polymerization process and there is no effect on stability of adsorbed drug. Demerit is their penetration into the outer layers of cornea causing disruption of the cell membranes.
Poly-ε-caprolactone (PECA)	Starting the polymerization in acidic medium and adjusting the pH providing hydroxyl ions as initiator. The velocity of polymerization and molecular weight of resultant polymer can be controlled by controlling the particle size.	Superior than PACA types for ocular delivery. Yielded highest pharmacological effects, due to agglomeration of the particles in conjunctival sacs.

organic phase, interfacial polymerization, poly-merization by denaturation or desolvation of natural proteins, solvent evaporation method, ionic gelation technique, nanoprecipitation, spray drying methods, etc.

Novel ophthalmic drug delivery systems

Many shortfalls of conventional topical liquid eye drops, like the relatively short precorneal half-life, have resulted in several new ophthalmic drug delivery approaches being investigated in recent years. Promising systems have been evaluated employing small colloidal carrier particles such as liposomes, microspheres, microparticles, nanoparticles or nanocapsules. These systems have the advantage that they may be applied in liquid form, just like eye drop solutions, because of their low viscosity. These novel colloidal carrier systems can be directly applied in liquid form (aqueous suspension) like eye drop solutions. These carrier systems can form a precorneal depot by interaction with the glycoprotein of the cornea and conjunctiva resulting in prolonged release of the bound drug. Nanotechnology-based drug delivery systems are also very effective in crossing anatomical membrane barriers (e.g. the blood-retinal barrier in the eye) and can be employed as excellent systems for chronic ocular diseases requiring frequent drug administration, like chronic cytomegalovirus retinitis (CMV). Thus, they avoid the discomfort often associated with viscous gels and ointments but still provide a reservoir from which the drug can be delivered slowly. Liposomes may increase the ocular bioavailability of certain drugs by increasing the association of the drug with cornea by means of an increased lipophilic liposomal bilayer interaction with the corneal epithelium. They can accommodate both hydrophilic and lipophilic drugs, they are biocompatible and biodegradable, they can protect the encapsulated drug from metabolic degradation and they can act as depot, releasing the drug slowly. Liposomes however have the disadvantages of reduced physical stability and difficulties in sterilizing the product.

Microparticles and nanoparticles are colloidal drug carriers in the micrometer and submicrometer range. Microspheres are monolithic particles possessing a porous or solid polymer matrix, whereas microcapsules consist of a polymeric membrane surrounding a solid or liquid drug reservoir. Nanoparticles, including nanospheres or nanocapsules, have a particle size in the nanometer range from 10 to 1000 nm. Drugs can be incorporated in the core of carrier either dissolved in the polymer matrix in the form of solid solution or suspended in the form of a solid dispersion. Alternatively, the drug may be adsorbed on the particle surface. Release of drug can be attributed to degradation of the polymer, drug desorption from the polymer surface or diffusion through the polymer matrix. Various synthetic and natural biocompatible polymers have been used to prepare microparticles and nanoparticles. These carriers may adhere to inflamed precorneal tissues of the eye. Nanoparticles made up of various biodegradable polymers like polylactide (PLAs), polylactic-co-glycolic acid (PLGA), polycyanoacrylate, poly (D,L-lactides), polyisobutylcyanoacrylate (PIBCA), polyepsiloncaprolactone (PECL), and natural polymers like chitosan, gelatin, sodium alginate and albumin can be used effectively for efficient drug delivery to the ocular tissues. Although there are currently no commercial formulations on the market using novel polymers, these carrier systems show a lot of promise for the future. The challenge will be to demonstrate safety and tolerability and gain acceptance by the regulatory authorities. Recently dendrimers also have been evaluated for ocular drug delivery. Other attempts to improve ocular bioavailability have focused on overcoming poor corneal permeability with penetration enhancers, or by improving the lipophilicity of the drug through ion-pair formation. Delivery of drugs to the posterior site of eye by application of drug solution is very difficult. The possibility of drug-loaded nanoparticles to reach the posterior site of ocular tissues and deliver drugs at targeted sites at effective therapeutic concentration in various disorders like retinitis, diabetic retinopathy, age-related macular degeneration, and corneal/conjunctival squamous cell carcinoma is very high.

Recently, dendrimers (mainly polyamido amine; PAMAM) have gained a lot of attention for ocular drug delivery purpose. Dendrimers are three-dimensional, hyperbranched, macromolecular compounds made up of a series of branches around an inner core. They are attractive systems for drug delivery because of their nanometer size range, huge capacity to encapsulate guest molecules, ease of preparation and functionalization, and presence of a lot of surface groups for biological recognition processes. Because of these properties, they can be used as an effective vehicle for ophthalmic drug delivery.

CONCLUSION

The progress in ophthalmic product development and medical devices in recent past is much thrilling. The abundance of compounds in clinical development, and the recent introduction of new ophthalmic products to the market, indicates the importance of this area. The ophthalmic formulations developed now-a-days have much influence in increasing drug bio-availability, increasing patient compliance, providing greater comfort and ease of application. Continuous studies in general field of ophthalmic pharmaceutics and pharmaco-kinetics lead to advances in ophthalmic drug therapy and delivery. The prosthetics, implants, shunts, lenses, lens care and operative care and products associated is confronted with development of a large range of polymers, viscoelastics and sustained release formulations. Further, many strict requirements for products and the requirements for lens hygiene also have increased utilization of highly suitable and precise means of production and packaging of such formulations, which no doubt helped development and progress of various ophthalmic pharmaceuticals. In future, multiple applications of nanotechnology in ophthalmology should be possible. Nanotechnology may assist in developing nano devices for complex eye surgeries, like glaucoma, retinal vascular surgery and so on. Nanotechnology can also help in the development of new lens materials for the treatment of cataract. Nanotechnology may also benefit in the development of various ophthalmic delivery formats: implantables, injectables, inserts and so on.

REFERENCES

- **Anophthalmos and Orbital Implants** (2003), The American Society of Ophthalmic Plastic and Reconstructive Surgery, ASOPRS, 222 South Westmonte Drive, Suite 101, Altamonte Springs, FL 32714 USA. http://www.asoprs.org/Pages/patients.html

- Banker, G.S., Rhodes, C.T. (Eds.) **Modern Pharmaceutics**, Marcel Dekker, Inc., New York, 4th Revised Edition, Vol. 72, pp. 489–546.
- Buckley, R. In Ed. Efron, N. and Heinemann, B. (2002) **Therapeutic Applications in Contact Lens Practice**, Oxford, 325–331.
- **Clinical Policy Bulletins** (2003), April 18, (CPB0484) http://www.aetna.com/cpb/data/PrtCPBA0484.html, No. 0484, Aqueous Drainage/Shunt Implant for Refractory Primary Open-Angle Glaucoma.
- **Collagen Corneal Shields**. University of Illinois, Eye Center, Ophthalmology and Visual Sciences. http://www.uic.edu/com/eye/LearningAboutVision/EyeFacts/index.shtml.
- Daniele, T., Paolo, C., Giuseppe, R. (2004). *Curr. Opin. Ophthal.* 15(1): 29–32.
- Edwards, K., Atkins, N. (2002). **Silicone Hydrogel Contact Lenses**. Part 2. Therapeutic Applications. www.optometry.co.uk, October 18, OT, 26-30.
- Ehrlich, D. (2001). *Optician*, 222 (5808): 28–32.
- Gennaro, A.R. (Ed.) (2004). **Remington's Pharmaceutical Sciences**. 20th edition, Lippincot Williams & Wilkins, Maryland, USA. 821–835.
- Gibson, M. (Ed) (2009). **Pharmaceutical Preformulation and Formulation**. 2nd edition. CRC Press, USA, 459–487.
- Gaudana, R., Jwala, J., Boddu, S.H.S., Mitra, A.K. (2009). *Pharm. Res.*, 26(5): 1197–1216.
- **Guidance for Industry and for FDA Reviewers/Staff** (1998). Aqueous Shunts – 510(k). Submissions November 16, Intraocular and Corneal Implants, Branch Division of Ophthalmic Devices, Office of Device Evaluation, U.S. Department of Health and Human Services, Food and Drug Administration Center for Devices and Radiological Health.
- Hugkulstone, C.E. (1992). *J. R. Soc. Med.*, 85(6): 322–323.
- Ing, E. (Ed.) (2002). **Neuro-ophthalmic Examination**, http://www.emedicine.com/neuro/topic477.htm.
- Last, R. (2003). Ophthalmic drug delivery through soft hydrogel contact lenses, *Journal of Undergraduate Research*, University of Florida, http://web.clas.ufl.edu/CLAS/jur/0203/lastpaper.html#anchor313189.
- Saettone, M.F. (2002). Progress and Problems in Ophthalmic Drug Delivery, a report in *Business*

Briefing: Pharmatech, Reference Library, 2002, pp. 1–6.

- Mitra, A.K. (Ed.) (2003). **Ophthalmic Drug Delivery Systems**, 2nd Ed., Marcel Dekker, Inc., New York.
- **Molteno Implants® Glaucoma Drainage Devices** (2005) http://www.molteno.com/implants.html#, Molteno Ophthalmic Ltd. also **U.S. Patent Nos. 4,457,757 4,750,901 0600-WWW/A01**.
- Mullin, J.D., Hecht, G. *In:* Gennaro, A.R. (Ed.) (2000). **Remington: The Science and Practice of Pharmacy**, Mack Publishing Company, Philadelphia, 20th Ed. 1581.
- Niazi, S. (Ed.) (2009). **Handbook of Pharmaceutical Manufacturing Formulations: Sterile Products**, CRC Press, USA.
- Perrott, C.M. (Ed.) (1991). Opthalmic Lens Design and Fabrication, *SPIE Proceedings*, Vol. 1529, Pilkington Visioncare, Menlo Park, CA, USA.
- Phakic Intraocular Lenses (2002). Clinical Topics for Ophthalmic Devices Panel, *Discussion*, pp. 1–19.
- **Policy on Recognition and Use of Standards under the Medical Devices Regulations**, (2004). Therapeutic Products Directorate, Medical Devices Bureau, Ottawa, Ontario, Canada.
- Rajasekaran, A., Kumaran, K.S.G.A., Preetha, J.P., Karthika, K. (2010). *Int. J. PharmTech Research*, 2(1): 668–674.
- Rathore, K.S., Nema, R.K. (2009). *Int. J. Pharm. Sci. Drug Research*, 1(1): 1–5.
- Skuta, G.L., Cantor, L.B., Weiss, J.S. (2009). **Fundamentals and Principles of Ophthalmology**, Amer Academy of Ophthalmology, USA.
- Steele, C.F. (2000). **Fitting and Management of Contact Lenses**, Hospital Optometrists Information Series.
- **The Healon: Family of Viscoelastics**, (2004). http://www.healon.com/fivespecs.html, Pfizer, Inc.HE166522.
- Tangri, P., Khurana, S. (2011). *Int. J. Res. Pharm. Biomed. Sci.*, 2(4): 1541–1552.
- Thomas L., Garthwaite, M.D. (2000). **Prescription Optics and Low Vision Devices, VHA Handbook**, 1173.12, Department of Veterans Affairs, Veterans Health Administration, Washington, DC 20420.
- Tsai, J.C., Johnson, C.C., Dietrich, M.S. (2003). *Ophthalmology*, 110(9): 1814–21.
- Veys, J., Davies, I. (1996). *Optician*, 212 (5562): 32–42.

7

Topical Drug Delivery

Subheet Kumar Jain, Lakhvir Kaur,
A.K. Tiwary and N.K. Jain

INTRODUCTION

Skin related issues (dermatological conditions) are becoming prevalent in this hectic world and stats suggest that these dreadful conditions are affecting at least one-third of the US population. These infections have been cited as one of the top 15 medical conditions for which prevalence and healthcare spending increased in the last decade. The pharmaceutical companies due to these reasons have started paying attention towards the dermatological end, the outcome of which is that the topical dermatological drug treatment has been significantly influenced by the choice of vehicle, delivery system, technology of manufacturing these systems and also reformulation of already marketed topical products. The growing market for dermatologicals and the escalating advancements in the life sciences have facilitated the emergence of improved topical formulations and drug delivery systems. The current and emerging break-throughs of optimizing the topical delivery of dermatological agents (small and large molecules) include the use of chemical enhancers, biopolymers (e.g. sodium hyaluronate), liposomes, particulate carriers (micro-spheres and lipid nanoparticles), topical sprays and foams, occlusion (via dressings and patches), topical peels, and temperature (heat). The emphasis is also on the development of electric based technologies such as iontophoresis and ultrasound, which have paved a way for the pronounced development of improved and successful topical drug delivery systems. These delivery approaches (when used solely or in a synergistic manner) are a remarkable improvement over conventional systems (creams, lotions, ointments and pastes) and have the potential to enhance efficacy and tolerability, improve patient compliance (including dermatology life quality) and also fulfill other unmet needs of the topical dermatological market.

Topical dermatological products as sunscreens, keratolytic agents, local anesthetics, antiseptics, anti-inflammatory agents, etc. are intended for localized action on one or more layers of the skin. These topical or dermatological products applied to skin have variable formulation components, which differ in consistency that ranges from liquids to solid powders wherein semisolids among them are considered as the most popular. These components can be categorized as medicated (creams, gels, lotions, etc. intended for one or the other medicinal or therapeutic effect) and as non-medicated (e.g. cosmetics, which are devoid of any therapeutic activity). But these non-medicated systems though devoid of any therapeutic effect give a great hope for the desired outcomes, such as protective, moisturizing, or emollient physical effects on the skin. The effectiveness of both these systems depends upon the extent and rate of percutaneous drug absorption and transportation of these dermatological products across the skin layers, which are further influenced by various factors including skin physiology, physicochemical properties of drugs and excipients, as well as fabrication and design of the delivery systems.

SKIN: THE FINAL FRONTIER

Skin, the heaviest single organ of the body, combines with the mucosal linings of the respiratory, digestive, and urogential tracts to form a capsule, which separates the internal body structures from the external environment. This flexible, self-repairing shell defends the stable internal milieu of living tissues, bathed in the body fluids, from a hostile external world of varying temperature, humidity, radiation and pollution. The integument not only physically protects the internal organs and limits the passage of substance into and out of the body but also stabilizes the temperature and blood pressure with its circulation and evaporation systems. The skin mediates the sensations of touch, pain, heat and cold; it expresses the redness of anger and embarrassment, the seating of anxiety, and the pallor of fear; and the integument identifies individuals through the characteristics of the hair, odor, texture, and color shades, particular to human being.

In the light of many requirements, which the skin must fulfill, it is not surprising that anatomists find that the integument is a very heterogeneous organ. For an average 70 kg human with a skin surface area of 1.8 m^2, a typical square centimeter covers 10 hair follicles, 12 nerves, 15 sebaceous glands, 100 sweat glands, 3 blood vessels with 92 cm total length, 360 cm of nerves and 3×10^6 cells (Schurer, 1991).

Structure and barrier properties of skin

Human skin is, on average, 0.5 mm thick (ranging from 0.05 mm to 2 mm) and is composed of four main layers:

1. Stratum corneum (SC)
2. Viable epidermis
3. Dermis
4. Subcutaneous tissue.

Stratum corneum

The thick (10–20 µm) surface layer, the SC, is highly hydrophobic and contains 10–15 layers of inter-digitated corneocytes, which are constantly shed and renewed. Its organization can be described by the 'brick and mortar' model (Elias, 1983), in which extracellular lipid accounts for ~10% of the dry weight of this layer, and 90% is intracellular protein (mainly keratin) (Schurer, 1991). The SC lacks phospholipids, but is enriched in ceramides and neutral lipids (cholesterol, fatty acids, cholesteryl esters) that are arranged in a bilayer format and form the so called 'lipid channels'. Inter-digitated long-chain ω-hydroxyceramides provide cohesion between corneocytes by forming tight lipid envelopes around the corneocyte protein component (Wertz et al., 1989). The barrier function of the skin is created by lamellar granules, which are synthesized in the granular layer and later become organized into the intercellular lipid bilayer domain of the SC (Landmann, 1986). Barrier lipids are tightly controlled and any impairment to the skin results in active synthetic processes to restore them. The skin's barrier function appears to depend on the specific ratio of various lipids; studies in which non-polar and relatively polar lipids were selectively extracted with petroleum ether and acetone, respectively, indicated that the relatively polar lipids are more crucial to skin barrier integrity (Barry, 1973).

Because of its highly organized structure, the SC is the major permeability barrier to external materials, and is regarded as the rate-limiting factor in the penetration of therapeutic agents through the skin. The ability of various agents to interact with the intercellular lipid, therefore, dictates the degree to which absorption is enhanced.

Viable epidermis

The viable epidermis consists of multiple layers of keratinocytes at various stages of differentiation. The basal layer contains actively dividing cells, which migrate upwards to successively form the spinous, granular and clear layers. As part of this process, the cells gradually lose their nuclei and undergo changes in composition. Several other cells (e.g. melanocytes, Langerhans cells, dendritic T cells, epidermotropic lymphocytes and Merkel cells) are also scattered throughout the viable epidermis, which also contains a variety of active catabolic enzymes (e.g. esterases, phosphatases, proteases, nucleotidases and lipases (Mier & vanden Hurk, 1977). Lipid catabolic enzymes (such as acid lipase, phospholipase, sphingo-myelinase, steroid sulfatase), although mainly concentrated in the SC and granulosum, have been demonstrated throughout the epidermal layers. Although the basal and spinous layers are rich in phospholipids, as the cells differentiate during their migration to the surface, the phospholipid content decreases and the sphingolipid (glucosylceramide and ceramide) and cholesterol content simultaneously increases (Foldvari, 2000).

Dermis and hypodermis

The dermis is largely acellular, but is rich in blood vessels, lymphatic vessels and nerve endings. An extensive network of dermal capillaries connects to the systemic circulation, with considerable horizontal branching from the arterioles and venules in the papillary dermis to form plexuses and to supply capillaries to hair follicles and glands. Dermal lymphatic vessels help to drain excess extracellular fluid and clear antigenic materials (Hadgraft, 2001).

The elasticity of the dermis is attributed to a network of protein fibers, including collagen (types I and III) and elastin, which are embedded in an amorphous glycosaminoglycan ground substance. The dermis also contains scattered fibroblasts, macrophages, mast cells and leukocytes. Hair follicles, sebaceous glands and sweat glands are found in the dermis and subcutis, and might serve as additional specific, albeit fairly limited, pathways for drug absorption. In some cases, for example, hair follicles might act as target sites for drug delivery (Fig. 7.1).

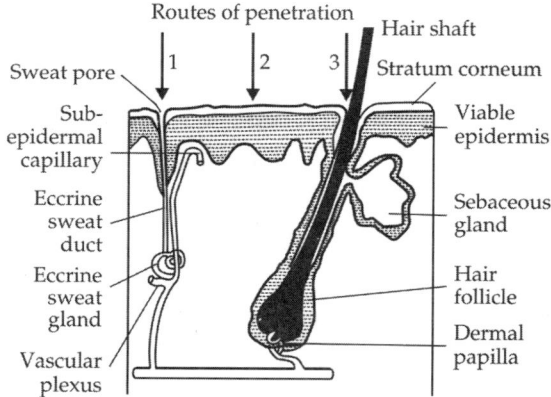

Fig. 7.1. Structure of skin.

MECHANISMS OF SKIN PENETRATION

There are number of routes by which molecules can cross the stratum corneum, i.e. intercellular, transcellular and appendageal (through either the sweat gland or hair follicles) (Fig. 7.2). Under normal conditions, the appendageal route is not thought to be very significant, in part this is due to the low surface area occupied by the appendages. It is more difficult to determine differences between the transcellular and inter-cellular route. Research work, *in vivo*, on the skin absorption of methyl nicotinate was analyzed

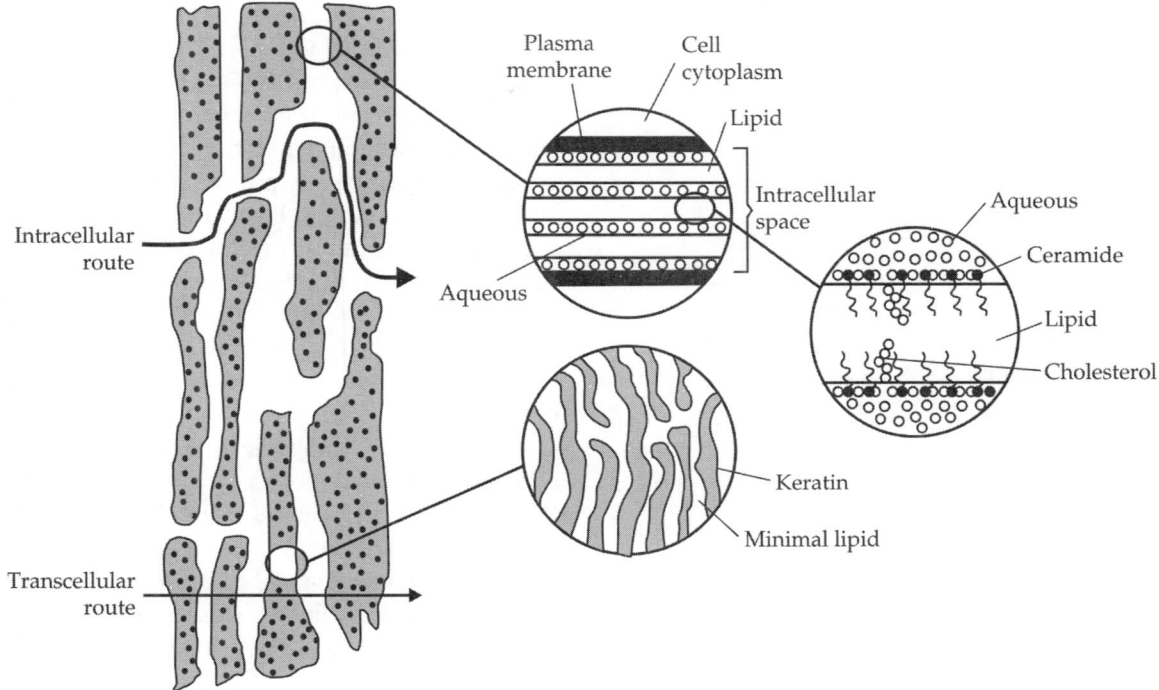

Fig. 7.2. Possible pathways for skin penetration of drug molecules.

using Fick's law of diffusion and the best fit to the data was found for a diffusional path length of 350 μm (Albery & Hadgraft, 1979). Since the thickness of the skin is approximately 1/20 of this, it was postulated that the intercellular route was important. This value was similar to that calculated by 'bricks and mortar' model of the stratum corneum proposed by Michaels, et al., (1975). However, at that time the nature of the intercellular channels was unclear. Later experiments visualized diffusion molecules in the intercellular channels (Bodde, et al., 1989) and work on the diffusion of water suggested that even a small polar molecule transferred along a tortuous pathway. The path length for diffusion of water was quoted as 500 μm (Potts & Francoeur, 1991).

The impermeability is a considerable problem in the delivery of medicines both to and through the skin. It has been estimated that only a few percent of the active material reaches its target site when it is delivered topically. As an example only 1.7% of hydrocortisone alcohol is absorbed (Feldmann & Maibach, 1987). If this could be improved, dermatological formulations could be made much more efficient and effective. For this reason there have been many attempts to identify safe compounds that can be applied to the skin and promote the absorption of the active drug. Now-a-days different carrier systems, e.g. liposomes, niosomes, transfersomes, ethosomes, nanoparticles, solid lipid nanoparticles, nanoemulsions and hydrogels, are extensively studied for the topical delivery of drugs.

Physical chemistry of percutaneous absorption

There has been little evidence to suggest that there are any active processes involved in skin permeation, therefore the underlying transport process is controlled by simple passive diffusion. Fick's laws of diffusion can be used to analyze permeation data and can be used predictively. Fick's first law is used to describe steady state diffusion and can be simplified to:

$$J = DK\Delta C/h \qquad \ldots(1)$$

where

J = flux per unit area,
D = diffusion coefficient in the skin,
K = skin vehicle partition coefficient,
ΔC = concentration difference across the skin, and
h = diffusional path length.

Under normal circumstances the applied concentration (C_{app}) is very much larger than the concentration under the skin and eq. 1 is often simplified to

$$J = K_p \cdot C_{app} \qquad \ldots(2)$$

where K_p is the permeability coefficient ($= KD/h$) and is a heterogeneous rate constant having the units cm/h^{-1}. It is often difficult to separate K and D and their calculated magnitude will depend on h that cannot be accurately estimated because the tortuosity of the intracellular channels is imprecise (Hadgraft, 2001).

PERCUTANEOUS ABSORPTION: CLINICAL SIGNIFICANCE

When the therapeutic target lies beneath the stratum corneum, topical drug delivery becomes more difficult. Regardless of whether the target tissue is local or systemically distant, delivery of sufficient drug is usually a constraining problem. Therefore, there are many potentially useful drugs that do not find a place in topical therapy due to their inability to penetrate the skin adequately. The phenomenon of diffusive penetration by drugs and chemicals into and through the skin is known as percutaneous absorption. There are a number of patho-physiological states that can be treated by concentrating drugs in the skin through percutaneous absorption (Fig. 7.3). For example, most dermatitises result in inflamed skin and

topical steroidal and non-steroidal anti-inflammatory drugs (NSAIDs) are effective in providing symptomatic relief. Corticosteroids are also used in psoriasis, where, in addition to suppressing inflammation, they act on the basal epidermal layer to slow proliferation and return the skin to a normal turnover rate. Pain originating in the skin can be arrested by topically applied local anesthetics, OTC benzocaine and related prescription drugs. Hydroquinone is applied to the skin to lighten excessively pigmented skin by oxidizing melanin.

Another clinical practice that involves percutaneous absorption is the application of 5-fluorouracil (5-FU) for the selective eradication of pre-malignant and some malignant tumors (basal cell carcinomas) of the skin. This cytotoxic drug is topically applied for this purpose without undue toxic complications. In all of the above the key to success is the ability to get therapeutic amount of these drugs through the stratum corneum and into the local tissues.

Systemic actions of a limited number of drugs can also be achieved via percutaneous absorption. The application of warmed, soft masses of bread meal or clay-containing medicinal substances over wounded or aching parts of the body is an ancient practice, probably involving systemic delivery. However, few plasters and poultices (cataplasms) have survived into modern medicine. It was not until the middle of the twentieth century that the means became available to measure the exceedingly low circulating levels of drugs that build up in the body during the course of therapy, an analytical breakthrough foreshadowing breakthroughs in drug delivery. Research soon followed on ways the drug levels could be modulated and extended to drive more benefit from, and lower the risk of toxicity of, each dosage of drug. Novel delivery systems for non-traditional routes of administration were subsequently conceived, constructed, and put to test (Jain & Jain, 2001).

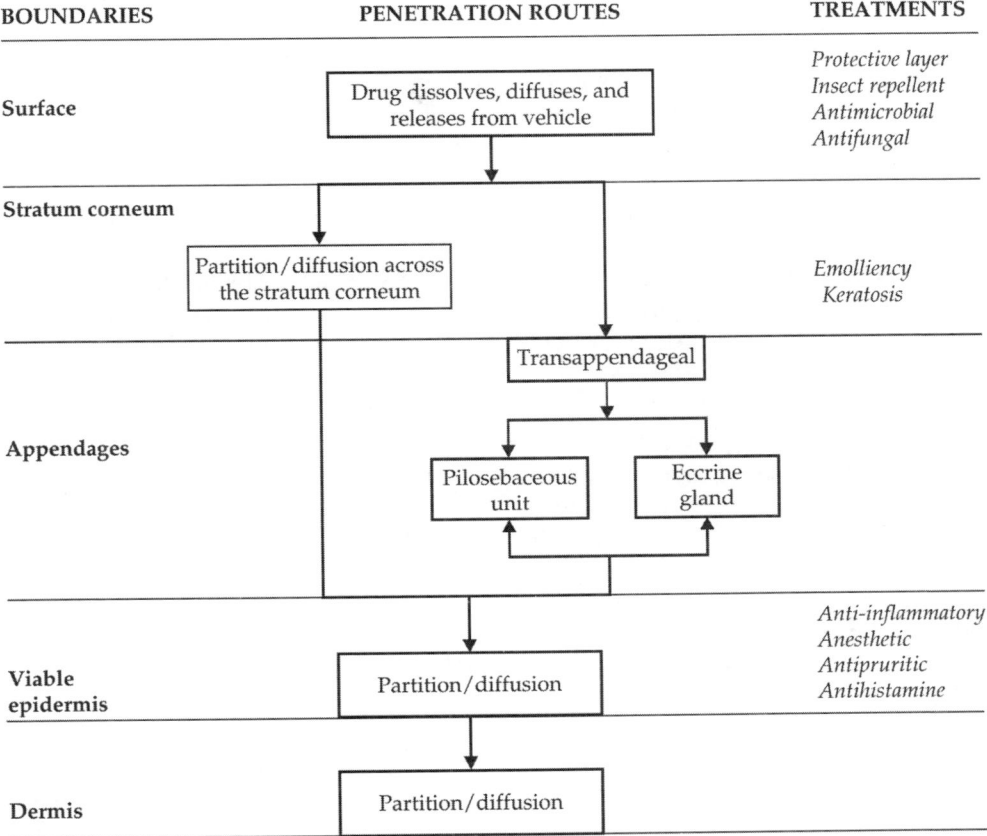

Fig. 7.3. Routes of drug-skin penetration and examples of treatments appropriate to disorders of the various strata.

RATIONALE FOR TOPICAL DRUG DELIVERY

There are two fundamental methods by which we approach the biopharmaceutical problems of formulating a successful topical dosage form. These two methods, as well as a third relatively recent innovation, are described here.

In the first process we assist or manipulate the barrier function of the skin. For example, sunscreening agents increase the power of the horny layer to protect the viable tissues from UV irradiations; topical antibiotics and antibacterials help a damaged barrier to ward off infection; and emollients, ointments, creams, lotions and baths restore the pliability of the skin after low

humidity environments and detergents have desiccated the horny layer.

In the second procedure we attempt to breach the horny layer at the molecular scale so as to direct drugs to the viable epidermal and dermal tissues without using oral, systemic, or other therapies. If we do attempt systemic therapy to treat dermatological conditions, we have the problem that most drugs normally concentrate preferentially in the skin. We therefore usually produce drug levels in highly perfused muscles and organs, which are equal to or greater than the concentration obtained within the skin. In particular, the vascular epidermis is somewhat inaccessible to systemically administered drugs. Using the systemic routes we may therefore invoke side effects because of relatively high dosages required. In contrast, the topical route may allow a drug to diffuse the viable cutaneous tissue in concentrations which are adequate for a therapeutic response and yet, when the medicament finally sweeps into the systemic circulation, the blood volume will so dilute it that undesirable pharmacological effects remain negligible. In addition, of course, there are many traditional valuable dermatological medicaments, which we can apply topically, for example tar, ichthammol or dithranolol (Fig. 7.3).

The third approach is to use the skin deliberately as a portal of entry into the systemic circulation. The transdermal therapeutic systems aim to provide systemic therapy for acute or chronic conditions, which do not involve the skin; the transdermal employs the percutaneous route instead of the more traditional oral, parenteral, pulmonary, or rectal routes.

At the anatomic level, we aim at five main target regions in dermatology:

1. The external objectives of the skin surface
2. The dead stratum corneum or horny layer
3. The viable epidermis and upper dermis
4. The skin glands
5. The target of the systemic circulation

A. Surface treatment

We can minister to the skin surface in three main ways: a simple camouflage or cosmetic application, the formation of a protective film or layer, and an assault on surface bacteria and fungi.

Disfiguring lesions of the exposed skin may psychologically devastate a patient, even to the extent that an abnormality may lead to the person's social ostracism. When physicians and surgeons cannot eradicate such derangements, the patient may cover or disguise them, e.g., portwine nevi (birthmarks) and scars. Di-hydroxyacetone, potassium permanganate, pickled walnut juice, or a mixture of these can disguise depigmented areas of the skin.

An example of a protective film is one which incorporates material to absorb irritating chemicals, e.g., protective pastes which absorb and neutralize the ammonia that bacteria release from infant's urine. For fair-skinned people in sunny climates topically applied agents may protect the skin from actinin rays in two ways: screens absorb light at specific wavelengths, and barriers ('shades'), which are opaque, reflect the radiation. Chemical screens include mexanone, para-aminobenzoic acid, quinine, salicylate esters, cinnamic acid and its compounds, and the coumarins; their protective action continues after the material diffuses into the stratum corneum. Examples of barriers include titanium dioxide or zinc oxide and red veterinary petrolatum.

Another type of protective barrier hinders moisture loss from the skin and averts chapping (e.g. hydrocarbons such as petrolatum), or the application reduces frictions (e.g., powder or silicone oil).

The surface bacteria and fungi are the therapeutic target for topical antibiotics, antiseptics, and deodorants and effective surface bio-availability is important. The formulation must release the medicament so that the antimicrobial may penetrate the surface microcracks and fissures of the skin to attack the microorganisms, which lurk there. The molecules dissolve in the topical preparation (if the agent is in the form of a suspension), diffuse through the formulation matrix, and release onto the dry skin surface (or moist axillae in the case of deodorants). Only then can the bacteria and fungi take up the antimicrobial and be destroyed. Developmental studies should at least confirm that the formulation releases the active medicament and does not bind to the agent (Egbaria, 1991).

B. Stratum corneum treatment

In the main two therapeutic activities aimed at the horny layer we try to improve the emolliency and to stimulate sloughing (keratosis). Water-impermeable film hydrates the stratum corneum and thereby increases its pliability, by inhibiting transepidermal loss. Topical application may also deposit "moisturing agents" within the horny layer.

Salicylic acid, the classic keratolytic, seems to reduce intercellular stickiness within the stratum corneum by directly solubilizing the intercellular cement and causing disintegration and sloughing. In addition to this α-hydroxy acids, propylene glycol, and sulfur are also effective.

C. Skin appendage treatment

We may treat hyperhidrosis of the sweat glands with anti-perspirants such as aluminum salts or other metal salts, for example, aluminium chloride and aluminium hydroxychloride. Anti-perspirants damage the eccrine gland reversibly, but there is little evidence that they have much effect on apocrine glands (Agarwal et al., 2000). Patients may absorb atropine-like drugs in amounts sufficient to produce a beneficial effect without initiating systemic side effects, but the treatment is unreliable.

Acne, a condition that affects the pilo-sebaceous unit, is a malicious disease of adolescence where we can use topical exfoliants in acne, such as salicylic acid, tretionin (retionic acid), and benzoyl peroxide. A recent introduction to the clinic is topical tetracycline in the form of Topicycline, a preparation designed to enhance the skin penetration of the antibiotic. Other topical antibiotics used to treat acne are erythromycin and clindamycin.

Deplitatories, which remove hair at the skin level, usually contain strontium or barium sulfide or thioglycollates. In addition to their cosmetic use, they are valuable in the treatment of hirsutism.

We can treat fungal disease of the nails, together with such infections of other keratin-rich sites (stratum corneum and hair), with topical clotrimazole, miconazole, and thiabendazole.

A particular problem with skin appendage treatment is to ensure that the active ingredient penetrates to the actual site of the disease. For example, it is not easy for the treatment to achieve a high concentration of an antibiotic in a sebaceous gland when, as in acne, a horny accretion blocks the pilosebaceous follicle. Applied percutaneously, the drug may not be hydrophobic to partition from the water-rich viable epidermis and dermis into the sebum-filled gland.

D. Viable epidermis and dermis treatment

The analysis of the possible ways in which a topical drug may reach the viable epidermis and the upper dermis, and in what relative amounts, is quite complicated. In general, a molecule may penetrate to the viable tissue below the horny layer via three potential routes of entry: the medicament may pass through the pilosebacious unit or the sweat duct, or the diffusant may traverse the intact stratum corneum, which lies between these appendages.

We may treat many disease states by topical application, provided that the formulation delivers drug to the site of action in sufficient amounts over a suitable time scale. However, we cannot use many potentially valuable drugs in topical therapy because they cannot cross the impermeable stratum corneum in sufficient quantities. Hence, investigators have a continuing interest in attempting to circumvent the unfavorable physicochemical properties of these drugs by developing "penetration enhancers". Such materials temporarily and reversibly diminish the barrier function of the stratum corneum so that the weakened horny layer allows the percutaneous absorption of drugs (Chowdary & Naidu, 1995; Barry, 1991; Williams & Barry, 1992). Another approach is for scientist to develop pro-drugs that will reach the receptor site readily, there to release the pharmacologically active moiety of the compound (Valia, et al., 1985; Tojo, et. al., 1985).

The common skin diseases that are treated by topical treatment are summarized in Table 7.1

Table 7.1. Common dermatological disorders and their treatment (Barry, 1983)

Skin problems	Examples	Skin problems	Examples
I. GENERAL INVOLVEMENTS		**III. ABNORMALITIES OF THE DERMIS**	
A. Physical damage		**A. Melanocyte abnormalities**	
Blunt instrument	Contusion, bruise	Hyperfunction	Tanning, chloasma
Sharp instrument	Cut, nick, animal bite	Hypofunction	Vitiligo
Scraping, rubbing	Abrasion, blister	Abnormal growth	Mole
Heat	Burns (1°, 2°, 3°), blister	Malignancy	Melanoma
Ultraviolet radiation	Sunburn	**B. Dermal-epidermal interface**	
Insects	Mosquito bite, bee sting, ticks, mites (chiggers), lice	Lifting of the epidermis	Dermatitis herpetiformis
		Overgrowth of papillary layer	Warts
B. Chemical damage		**C. Dermis**	
Contact dermatitis	Poison ivy, poison oak	Vascular reaction	Urticaria, hives
Contact allergy	Cosmetic dermatitis	Abnormal growth of fibrinocyte	Scar, keloid
Solvent extraction	"Dishpan hands"	Abnormal polymerization	Scleroderma
II. ABNORMALITIES OF THE EPIDERMIS		**IV. ABNORMALITIES OF THE GLANDS**	
A. Stratum corneum		**A. Hair follicle**	
Tardigrade sloughing and thickening	Ichthyosis	Hyper-reactivity	Hirsutism
		Hypoactivity	Alopecia, baldness
Hyperdryness	Chapping, windburn	**B. Sebaceous glands**	
Hyperproliferative thickening, abnormal structural organization	Psoriasis	Hyperactivity	Seborrhea
		Occlusion	Acne, pimples
B. Viable epidermis		**C. Eccrine sweat glands**	
Cell damage and inflammation	Eczema, general dermatitis	Hyperactivity	Hyperhidrosis
		Occlusion, inflammation	Miliaria (pricky heat, heat rash)
Fluid correction	Blister		
Abnormal cell growth	Keratosis	**V. INFECTIOUS INFLAMMATION**	
Thickening of granular layer	Lichen planus	Bacterial	Carbuncles (boils)
Hyperproliferation, incomplete keratinization	Psoriasis	Fungal	Athlete's foot, ringworm
		Viral	Chickenpox, herpes simplex (cold sores)
Malignancy	Epithelioma	Protozoal	Topical amebiasis

DESIGN OF TOPICAL DRUG PRODUCTS

Dermatological products applied to skin are diverse in formulation and range in consistency from liquids to solid powders, but the most popular products are semisolid preparations. Some of these may be non-medicated, in the sense that these may be devoid of any thera-peutically active ingredients and are categorized as cosmetics. Nevertheless, these products can provide desired outcomes, such as through their protective, moisturizing, or emollient physical effects on the skin. Topical liquids include aqueous solutions (aluminium subacetate topical solution), hydroalcoholic solutions or tinctures (iodine tincture, Cleocin topical solution), organic solvent-based collodions (salicylic acid collodion), sprays (Benadryl itch relief spray), or the more viscous lotions (Calamine lotion, Selsun shampoo). Lotions are free flowing suspensions, emulsions, or colloidal solutions for external use, and these may be greasy or water-washable. There are only a handful of topical products of solid consistency, and these include powders (Tolnaftate, Desenex), pastes (Zinc oxide), plasters, and soaps. Medicated and non-medicated powders are generally sprinkled over the skin for antisepsis or to absorb skin secretions. Soaps may be medicated or non-medicated, and are used generally for cleansing healthy or infected skin. Use of pastes and plasters is restricted to more specific clinical conditions. Pastes are generally used to protect local skin tissue, and have a higher capacity to absorb skin secretions compared with ointments and creams. On the other hand, plasters are kept on the skin for a longer period and are primarily used to provide mechanical protection to internal tissues beneath the skin. The design and formulation of different types of topical drug products are summarized below (Hadgraft, 1999).

A. Gels (Jellies)

Gel is a two-component system of a semisolid nature, rich in liquid. Although different authors emphasize various properties within their definitions, the one common feature that they identify as characteristic of a gel is the presence of some form of continuous structure, which provides solid-like properties. In a typical polar gel, a natural or synthetic polymer at a relatively low concentration (usually much less than 10%) builds a three-dimensional matrix throughout a hydrophilic liquid. The system may be clear or turbid, because the gelling agent does not fully dissolve or it forms aggregates, which disperse the light. Typical **polymers** include the natural gums tragacanth, carrageenan, pectin, agar, and alginic acid; semisynthetic materials such as methylcellulose, hydroxyethylcellulose, hydroxypropyl methylcellulose, carboxymethylcellulose;

and the synthetic polymer, Carbopol (Kim, et al., 1997).

The cellulose derivatives form colloidal solutions in water, which gel at relatively high concentrations. These celluloses resemble the natural gums in many respects but are not as vulnerable to bacterial or fungal attack. Sodium CMC, an anionic compound, stabilizes and thickens suspensions, lubricating jellies, and topical emulsions.

Sodium alginate, which consists mainly of the sodium salt of alginic acid, produces aqueous solution that gels firmly on the addition of small amounts of soluble calcium salts, e.g., gluconate, tartrate, or citrate. For example, in the presence of calcium citrate a 3% solution yields a stable water-soluble jelly base.

Bentonite, a colloidal hydrated aluminium silicate, is insoluble in water but swells when mixed with 8 to 10 parts of water to generate a slightly alkaline gel resembling petrolatum. Veegum (colloidal magnesium aluminium silicate) and Laponite (a synthetic hectorite) behave somewhat similarly.

Pharmaceutical and cosmetic manufacturers now extensively employ the synthetic polymer Carbopol to formulate gels; for example, the U.S. preparations Topsyn Gel and U.K. preparation Synalar Gel both use this polymer to gel a propylene glycol/water solution of a topical steroid.

The Carbopols (Carbomers), a group of carboxyvinyl polymers crosslinked with allyl sucrose, are hydrophilic colloidal materials, which thicken better than the natural gums. They disperse in water to form cloudy acidic solutions, which are neutralized by strong bases such as sodium hydroxide, amines (e.g. triethanolamine), or weak inorganic bases (e.g. ammonium hydroxide), thereby increasing the consistency and decreasing the turbidity (Yu & Liao, 1996).

B. Liquid preparations

Liquid preparations for external application to the skin include simple baths, application, liniments, lotions, paints, varnishes, tinctures and ear drops. A simple soak or bath provides an active ingredient in an aqueous solution or suspension, which water-miscible solvents may modify. A wide range of gums and gelling agents, either natural and synthetic carbohydrates or clays or synthetic polymers, may vary the consistency from a mobile liquid to a stiff, ringing gel. Bath additives such as Oilatum Emollient (Stiefel) deposit a layer of liquid paraffin on the skin in an attempt to maintain the moisture content of the stratum corneum.

Applications, be they liquid or viscous preparations, often incorporate parasiticides, e.g., dicophane, benzyl benzoate, gamma benzene hexachloride, and malathion.

Patients may apply liniments with or without friction, but they should not treat broken skin with them. Liniments may be alcoholic solutions (Aconite Liniment, BPC), oily solutions (Methyl Salicylate Liniment, BPC), or emulsions (Turpentine Liniment, BP).

Lotions are aqueous solutions or suspensions (shake lotions). After application, the water evaporates to leave a large area of the body covered with a thin uniform coating of powders. Evaporation cools and soothes the skin, so lotions are valuable in treating acutely inflamed areas. Alcohol enhances the cooling effect, and glycerol sticks the powder to the skin. Suspending agents such as bentonite or sodium CMC disperse insoluble powders in shake lotions (Calamine Lotion, BP). Lotions may also be diluted emulsions, usually of the o/w type stabilized by emulsifying wax at a concentration which does not form a continuous matrix in the continuous phase.

Paints, varnishes, and tinctures present solutions of active ingredients in volatile solvents such as water (Crystal Violet Paint, BPC), industrial methylated spirits (Brilliant Green and Crystal Violet Paint, BPC), acetone (Cantharidin Wart Paint), or ether (Flexible Collodion, BP).

Ear drops are often aqueous solutions, although glycerol and alcohol may also be used.

Typical examples include Hydrogen Peroxide Ear drops, BPC, and Phenol Ear drops, BPC.

C. Powders

We may formulate dusting powders for application to skin folds by mixing together several finely divided insoluble powders. Such medicaments function as drying, protective, and lubricating agents. Examples include talc, zinc oxide, starch and kaolin; dusting powders should no longer contain boric acid since abraded skin may absorb it in toxic amounts.

In all systems, which incorporate powders including shake lotions and pastes, the individual powder particles should be compellable i.e., incapable of being perceived as individual particles by touch. The palpability of a powder is a function of its hardness, shape, and size; particles smaller than 20 μm in their longest dimension are impalpable. The coarser powder makes the preparation gritty to the skin.

D. Ointment

A semisolid preparation, intended for external application to the skin or mucous membrane is officially defined as an ointment. These are greasy, semisolid preparations which are often anhydrous and contain the medicament either dissolved or dispersed in the vehicles. We can classify ointment bases into hydrocarbons, fats and fixed oils, silicones, absorption bases, emulsifying bases and water-soluble bases.

1. Hydrocarbon bases

These usually consist of soft paraffin (vaseline, petroleum jelly or petrolatum) or a mixture of soft paraffin with hard paraffin to produce a suitable consistency. Paraffins deposit a greasy film on the skin surface that retards moisture loss. This occlusive property improves the hydration of the horny layer in dry, scaly conditions. Although practitioners usually assume that petrolatum is pharmacologically inert, its wide spectrum of usages in dermatology raises the suspicion that petrolatum may contain traces of compounds, which act at some cell receptors (Woodford & Barry, 1983).

Yellow and white soft paraffin differ only in color, since the latter is bleached. Hard paraffin and microcrystalline waxes are chemically similar to white soft paraffin but contain no fluid components. Petrolatum contains n-paraffins, isoparaffins, and cyclic paraffins; it may also contain saturated and aromatic hydrocarbons. The properties of the various paraffins vary considerably between different batches and grades of petrolatum, and this complexity can lead to difficulties with quality control. The reasons for the variations in the constituents of petrolatum are diverse source of the crude material, different types and extents of refining, and alternative bleaching processes.

As different petrolatums vary so much, pharmacopoeial and other standards are necessarily wide and there is a variety of miscellaneous methods for quality assessment. These techniques assess variables such as melting point, drop point (or congealing point), color, odor, taste, acidity or alkalinity, foreign matter, and sulfated ash. Longworth & French (1990) suggested two additional methods for inclusion in the British Pharmacopoeia – measurement of bleeding tendency and lump forming tendency. Formulators usually subjectively assess ductility i.e., the ability of a material to form filaments on extension, although they can also use instruments.

To alter the consistency of soft paraffins, a manufacturer may incorporate a polymer such as a relatively low-molecular-weight polyisobutylene. If we clap a sample between our hands we may detect the additives as it falls out in the form of fine, fibrous particles.

Hydrocarbon bases may contain ingredients additional to petrolatum, for instance, Paraffin Ointment, BP is a blend of white besswax, hard paraffin, cetostearyl alcohol, and soft paraffin. Ozokerite is a mined wax consisting mainly of C_{35} to C_{55} saturated hydrocarbons, Ceresin is a mixture of ozokerite and paraffin wax (hard paraffin). Ozokerite and ceresin can retain oils within their matrix structures without bleeding or oozing.

Plastibases are soft, smooth, homogeneous, neutral, colorless, odorless, non-irritating, non-sensitizing, extremely stable vehicles. They are compatible with a wide range of medicaments and maintain their consistency even at high concentrations of solids and under extremes of temperature, impart a velvety, non-greasy feel to the skin, and can readily be removed.

The plastibases provide a series of hydrocarbon vehicles in which the manufacturing process incorporates polyethylene into mineral oil at high temperature, followed by rapid cooling. The polyethylene, a large hydrocarbon polymer, forms the structural matrix in a system, which is fluid at the molecular or diffusant scale but is a typical dermatological semisolid at the microscopic level. This feature suggested that drug release should be favored from these vehicles compared to petrolatum systems.

2. Fats and fixed oil bases

Topical vehicles have frequently contained fixed oils of vegetable origin, which consist essentially of the mono-, di- and triglycerides of mixtures of saturated and unsaturated fatty acids. The most common oils include peanut, sesame, olive, cottonseed, almond, arachis, maize and persic oils. Such oils are prone to decompose on exposure to light, air and high temperature, and they may become rancid. Trace metal contamination in the oils catalyze oxidative reactions, which the formulator minimizes with antioxidants such as butylated hydroxytoluene (BHT), butylated hydroxyanisole (BHA), or propyl gallate or with chelating agents such as the salts of ethylene diamine tetra-acetic acid (EDTA). However, antioxidants may themselves introduce problems with respect to drug compatibility or may sensitize some patients.

3. Silicones

Silicones provide formulations with similar

properties to hydrocarbons bases. The silicones are a family of polymers with a structure consisting of alternate atoms of silicone and oxygen, with organic groups such as methyl or phenyl bonded to the silicon atom. The most important are the dimethicones, or dimethyl polysiloxanes. They are fluid polymers with the general formula $CH_3[Si(CH_3)_2O]Si(CH_3)_3$; in each unit two methyl groups and an oxygen atom attach to a silicon atom in the chain. Silicones are water repellent, with a low surface tension; they are used in barrier creams to protect the skin against water-soluble irritants. Creams, lotions, and ointments containing 10 to 30% of dimethicone can prevent diaper rash and bedsores and protect the skin against the trauma associated with colostomy discharge or incontinence.

4. Absorption bases

Absorption bases possess hydrophilic (water-absorbing) properties so that they can soak up water to form w/o emulsions yet retain their semisolid consistencies. In general they are anhydrous vehicles composed of a hydrocarbon base and a substance that is miscible with the hydrocarbon but also carries polar groups and therefore functions as a w/o emulsifier. These polar groups may be hydroxyl, sulfate, sulfonate, carboxyl, or an ether linkage. Typical materials include lanolin, lanolin isolates, cholesterol, lanosterol and other sterols, acetylated sterols, or the partial esters of polyhydric alcohols such as sorbitan monostearate or monooleate.

Anhydrous lanolin (wool fat) is the purified anhydrous fat-like substance derived from the wool of the sheep. It consists mainly of the fatty acid esters of cholesterol, lanosterol, and fatty alcohols and has the remarkable ability of taking up at least twice its own weight of water to form w/o emulsions. It is probable that its emulsifying properties depend on the presence of high-molecular weight diesters of hydroxy acids, although some workers claim that lanolin needs its complex mixture of alcohols to retain its excellent water-absorbing properties.

Several derivatives and modification of wool fat exhibit the fundamental properties of this material together with certain other advantages. Liquid lanolin, a mixture of liquid esters derived from the fractionation of wool fat, is less tacky on the skin. Reaction of wool fat with ethylene oxide yields liquid and solid polyoxyethylene derivatives i.e. the water-soluble lanolin. Hydrogenated wool fat is free from stickiness, and its water-absorbing capacity is 50% greater than that of wool fat. Hydrous wool fat (lanolin) is a mixture of seven parts of wool fat and three parts of water.

The preparations known as **wool alcohols** consist of the alcoholic fraction of the product, obtained by saponifying the wool grease of the sheep. It contains not less than 30% cholesterol, together with 10 to 13% isocholesterol and other steroid and triterpene alcohols; 500 to 1,000 ppm BHA or BHT provide antioxidant protection. Wool alcohol is useful emulsifier since its w/o emulsions do not darken on storage or develop an objectional odor in hot weather. The addition of only 5% of wool alcohol allows soft paraffin to absorb three times more water and weak acids do not crack the resulting emulsion; cetostearyl alcohol further stabilizes the dispersion.

Absorption bases such as Wool Alcohols Ointment and Simple Ointment deposit a greasy film on the skin in a similar manner to that of a hydrocarbon base, but they suppress less transepidermal water loss. However, they may assist the stratum corneum to hydrate by applying a w/o emulsion to the skin and thus prolonging the time during which the horny layer may absorb moisture.

5. Emulsifying bases

These essentially anhydrous bases contain o/w emulsifying agents, which make them miscible with water and so washable or **self-emulsifying**. Often, the preparation incorporates the emulsifying agents in the form of a wax, a granular material which a formulator can more easily handle and weigh, and which can also be used separately to produce a semisolid emulsion (a cream). Depending on the ionic nature of the surface active portion of the water-soluble emulsifying agent, the emulsifying bases can be classified into three main types i.e anionic, cationic, and nonionic.

Emulsifying ointment BP, an anionic base, contains emulsifying wax, white soft paraffin, and liquid paraffin. It is a mixture of sodium lauryl sulfate (an anionic o/w emulsifier); it is incompatible with cationic organic medicaments and the salts of barium and heavy metals.

An example of cationic emulsifying base is Cetrimide Emulsifying Ointment BP. It is blend of cetrimide (a cationic o/w emulsifier) and cetostearyl alcohol, which is compatible with cationic medicaments, and incompatible with anionic.

An official model for a nonionic emulsifying ointment is Cetomacrogol Emulsifying Ointment BPC, a mixture of cetomacrogol emulsifying wax, white soft paraffin, and liquid paraffin. It comprises cetostearyl alcohol and cetomacrogol 1000 (the nonionic o/w emulsifier, a polyethylene glycol ether of cetosterayl alcohol); it is compatible with most ionic medicaments and fairly high concentrations of electrolytes, but the Cetomacrogol is incompatible with phenols.

A recurrent feature of these bases is that they contain a mixture of emulsifiers of the opposite type. The w/o emulsifier is cetostearyl alcohol; it combines with the o/w emulsifier, which may be ionic or nonionic. Formulators employ such or similar blends to stabilize o/w emulsions, particularly dermatological and cosmetic.

Because they contain surfactants, emulsifying bases may help to bring the medicament into more intimate contact with the skin. They mix with aqueous skin secretions and may be readily washed off the skin, hence useful for treating the scalp.

6. Water-soluble bases

Formulators prepare water-soluble bases from mixtures of high- and low-molecular-weight polyethylene glycols (Macrogols, Carbowaxes) with the general formula $CH_2OH (CH_2OCH_2)_n CH_2OH$. These condensation polymers of ethylene oxide and water are liquid when the average molecular weight lies between 200 and 700; those with a molecular weight greater than 1000 increase in consistency with size, changing from soft unctuous material to hard wax-like solids. The number of their name denotes the molecular weight. The liquid and semisolid members of the series are hygroscopic, but this hygroscopicity decreases with increasing molecular weight.

Suitable combinations of Macrogols provide products of an ointment like consistency, which soften or melt on application to the skin. They are non-occlusive, mix readily with skin exudates, and do not stain bed linen or clothing; washing quickly removes any residue from the skin. The Macrogols do not hydrolyze, deteriorate, support mold growth, or irritate the skin.

Macrogol bases are used with local anesthetics such as lignocaine but are incompatible with a wide range of chemicals including phenols, iodine, potassium iodide, sorbitol, tannic acid, and the salts of silver, mercury and bismuth. They reduce the antimicrobial activity of quaternary ammonium compounds and methyl and propyl p-hydroxybenzoates, and rapidly inactivate penicillin and bacitracin.

E. Pastes

Essentially, pastes are ointments that contain a high proportion of powder (as much as 50%) dispersed in a fatty base. Typical powder ingredients include zinc oxide, starch and calcium carbonate. Pastes are stiffer than the parent ointment as the powder contributes its own particle matrix to that of the base. They were originally formulated with the concept that the high solid content would absorb skin exudates, but it is unlikely that a powder coated with a hydrocarbon could take up significant amounts of an aqueous liquid. However, pastes may be more successful in absorbing noxious chemicals such as the ammonia, which bacteria liberate from urine.

Pastes lay down a thick, unbroken, relatively impermeable film on the skin that can be opaque and acts as an efficient sun filter. Skiers use such formulation on the face to minimize windburn (excessive dehydration) and to protect against sun rays.

F. FAPG base

A rather specialized formulation is fatty alcohol/propylene glycol (FAPG) base, which consists mainly of stearyl alcohol and propylene glycol, together with polyethylene glycol and glycerol. The preparation is a smooth, white, soft, non-aqueous hydrophilic semisolid with a slightly pearly sheen. The base is claimed to have significant advantages over traditional ointments and creams. Its main use is as a vehicle for the topical steroid flucinonide, as in the U.K. preparation Metosyn and the U.S. formulation Lidex (Garnier, 1981a, 1981b). The rheological behavior is that of viscoelastic semisolid; continuous shear behavior develops from a mixture of thixotropy and irreversible shear breakdown. The material spreads readily on the skin and adheres there. The combination of rhelogical and sensory properties makes the formulation suitable as a topical vehicle.

G. Aerosols

Aerosols may function as drug delivery systems for solutions, suspensions, powders, semisolids, and emulsions (Sciarra, 1975). Solution aerosols are simple products, consisting of an active ingredient dissolved in a propellant or a mixture of propellant and a miscible solvent. Suitable co-solvents include ethanol, acetone, hexadecyl alcohol, glycol ethers, and polyglycols; and typical dermatological agents are steroids, antibiotics, and astringents.

Powder aerosols (dispersions or suspensions) are similar to solution aerosols but contain solid dispersed throughout the propellant/solvent phase. Such systems encounter problem in respect of particle size growth, agglomeration and caking, and clogging of valves. The formulation may contain oily ingredients such as isopropyl myristate and light liquid paraffin to lubricate the valve and to promote slippage between the particles. Surfactants act as dispersing agents to minimize aggregation and caking. The powder aerosol methodology is useful for poorly soluble compounds such as steroids and antibiotics.

Semisolid preparations, such as ointments and creams, may be dispensed in a flexible bag type of arrangement, which uses compressed nitrogen to expel the contents instead of volatile propellant.

Emulsion systems provide a variety of products, producing foams, which may be aqueous or non-aqueous, and stable or quick breaking. The stable foam, which is similar to a shaving cream preparation but into which the formulator incorporates medicaments, varies in stability depending on the selection of surfactant, solvent and propellant.

The basic quick-breaking aerosol foam contains a foaming agent (i.e., a surfactant), a solvent system, and a propellant. Polawax (an ethoxylated stearyl alcohol and auxillary emulsifying agents) produces a satisfactory product; cetyl/stearyl combinations are less suitable. When the patient actuates the valve, the propellant vaporizes, expelling and cooling the contents. This chilling, together with the loss of volatile co-solvent, crystallizes the foaming agents to form a lattice that initially stabilize the bubbles of foam. The patient breaks the lattice by rubbing it, with his body heat redissolving the surfactant. The concept, then, is of a system which discharges from the container as foam but which readily breaks on the skin. The quick-breaking foams are generally based on ethanol but may incorporate other solvents, such as propylene glycol.

ROLE OF NOVEL DRUG DELIVERY SYSTEM IN TOPICAL DRUG DELIVERY

There has been increased interest during recent years in use of topical vehicle systems that could modify drug penetration into the skin. Optimal vehicles have to exert a high capacity for incorporating both lipophilic and hydrophilic drugs as well as high skin permeability. Many of the dermal vehicles contain chemical enhancers and strong solvents to achieve these goals (Walters & Hadgraft, 1989). This is a major disadvantage, especially in chronic application, where they may usually be irritants. Therefore, it is undoubtedly desirable to develop a topical vehicle system which does not necessitate chemical enhancers or alcohols to facilitate drug penetration into and through the skin. The best way to overcome the limitation of conventional drug delivery system is the use of different carrier systems like liposomes, niosomes, ethosomes, elastic liposomes, microemulsion, solid lipid nanoparticles and nanostructured lipid carrier. For a detailed discussion of various novel drug delivery systems, the readers may refer standard books (Jain & Jain, 2001, 2004).

Different advantages related to use of carrier approach for topical delivery of drug are:

1. Increase the skin permeation and deposition of drug.
2. Increase the drug bioavailability.
3. Minimizes the drug degradation and loss.
4. Sustained or continuous effect of medication.
5. Reduction in skin irritation potential.
6. Increasing the region-specificity at target site.
7. Sustain the release of drug.
8. Reduction in frequency of administration.

Microemulsions

Microemulsions are quaternary systems comprising of an oil phase, a water phase, surfactant and a co-surfactant (Ceglie et al., 1987). These spontaneously formed systems possess specific physicochemical properties such as transparency, optical isotropy, low viscosity and thermodynamic stability. The observed transparency of these systems is due to the fact that the maximum size of the droplets of the dispersed phase is not larger than one-fourth of the wavelength of visible light – approximately 150 nm. Droplet diameter in stable micro-emulsions is usually within the range of 10–100 nm, which means that the term 'microemulsion' is misleading and these systems are actually nano-sized emulsions. Many studies have shown that microemulsion formulations possess improved transdermal and dermal delivery properties, mostly *in vitro* (Osborne, et al., 1991; Trotta, et al., 1996; Delgado-Charro, et al., 1997; Rhee, et al., 2001; Lee, et al., 2003), and several *in vivo* (Kreilgaard, 2001, 2002).

Vesicular approaches for topical drug delivery

The vesicles for effective topical drug delivery can increase drug transport across the skin, e.g liposomes, niosomes, transferosomes, and ethosomes. These vesicles can incorporate both hydrophilic and lipophilic drugs, serve as rate-limiting membrane barrier for systemic absorption of drug, due to its amphiphilic nature may serve as non-toxic penetration enhancer for drugs, and also serve as "organic solvent" for the solublization of poorly soluble drugs.

The vesicular approach in topical drug delivery has been studied for many purposes, and two commercial liposome-based formulations amphotercin B and dithranol (Ambisome, Life Care Innovative Pvt. Ltd., India) evidenced the success of story. Several vesicular carriers like niosomes, proliposomes, proniosomes, pro-transfersomes, elastic liposomes and ethosomes have been developed for topical delivery of drug. The details of these carriers and their uses are summarized below.

The use of **liposomes** is introduced in order to overcome the use of skin penetration enhancers and other chemical methods to increase drug transport across the skin. The first publications on interactions between liposomes and skin appeared in 1980 (Mezei & Gulasekharam, 1980) where liposomes applied to white rabbit's skin *in vivo* favored the deposition of drugs in the epidermis and dermis, while the amount of drug found in various organs was reduced.

Several studies were carried out to evaluate whether liposome composition affects skin penetration of drugs. In the early 1990s, Dowton et al. (1993) compared the effect of liposomal composition on the disposition of encapsulated cyclosporin A in mouse skin when applied non-occlusively *in vitro*. The various liposomes were saturated with cyclosporin A keeping the thermodynamic activity of cyclosporin A equal in all formulations. They observed that application of the drug in non-ionic surfactant vesicles prepared from glyceryl dilaurate/cholesterol/poly-oxyethylene-10 stearyl ether, the amount of cyclosporin A in deeper skin strata and receiver compartment was highest compared to the other formulations Fresta and Puglisi (1997) reported that corticosteroid dermal delivery with skin-lipid liposomes was more effective than delivery with phospholipid vesicles. This concerned the higher drug concentrations in deeper layers of the skin as well as the therapeutic effectiveness. The thermodynamic state of the bilayers of the vesicles plays a crucial role in the effect of vesicles on drug transport rate across skin *in vitro*.

Elastic liposomes are self-optimized aggregates, with the ultraflexible membrane, are able to deliver the drug reproducibly either into or through the skin, depending on the choice of administration or application, with high efficiency. These elastic liposomes are several orders of magnitude, more elastic than the standard liposomes and thus well suited for the skin penetration. Elastic liposomes overcome the skin penetration difficulty by squeezing themselves along the intracellular sealing lipids of the stratum corneum. There is provision for this, because of the high vesicle deformability,

which permits the entry due to the mechanical stress of surrounding, in a self-adapting manner. Flexibility of elastic liposomes membrane is achieved by mixing suitable surface-active components in the proper ratios.. Many reports in the literature supported the better skin penetration ability of elastic liposomes e.g. Honeywell-Nguyen et al. (2002, 2003) reported the enhanced delivery of pergolide using elastic liposomes; El. Maghraby et al. (1999, 2000, 2001a, 2001b) reported better skin permeation ability of elastic liposomes using oestradiol and 5-fluorouracil as a model drug; Essa et al. (2002) reported the combination of iontophoresis and ultradeformable liposomes for delivery of estradiol; Trotta et al. (2003) reported the elastic liposomes for skin delivery of dipotassium glycyrrhizinate; Guo et al. (2000a, 2000b) reported the elastic liposomes for systemic delivery of cyclosporin A; Hofer et al. (2000) reported the elastic liposomes for systemic transdermal delivery of immunomodulatory proteins Interleukin-2 and Interferon-α; vanden Bergh et al. (1999a, 1999b, 2001) in their different studies also proved the better skin permeation ability of these elastic liposomes; Paul et al. (1995a, 1995b, 1998) in their studies reported the transfersomes as a means of transdermal immunization. The use of surfactant as edge activator to provide the flexibility to vesicle membrane in case of elastic liposomes can lead to problem of physical instability.

In 2000, Touitou, et al. developed the new vesicular carrier system "**Ethosomes**" in which liposomes are combined with ethanol. The ethosomes are vesicular carrier comprised of hydroalcoholic or hydro/alcoholic/glycolic phospholipid in which the concentration of alcohols or their combination is relatively high. Such a composition enables delivery of high concentration of active ingredients through skin. Drug delivery can be modulated by altering alcohol : water or alcohol-polyol : water ratio. Some preferred phospholipids are soya phospholipids such as Phospholipon 90 (PL-90).

It is usually employed in a range of 0.5–10% w/w. Cholesterol at concentrations ranging between 0.1–1% can also be added to the preparation. Examples of alcohols, which can be used, include ethanol and isopropyl alcohol. Among glycols, propylene glycol and Transcutol are generally used. In addition, non-ionic surfactants (PEG-alkyl ethers) can be combined with the phospholipids in these preparations. Cationic lipids like cocoamide, POE alkyl amines, dodecylamine, cetrimide, etc. can be added too. The concentration of alcohol in the final product may range from 20 to 50%. The concentration of the non-aqueous phase (alcohol and glycol combination) may range between 22 to 70%.

In last decade lot of research has been carried out using ethosomes for effective topical delivery of various drugs like acyclovir, minoxidil, testosterone, bacitracin and cannabidol for topical gene delivery (Touitou, et al., 2000; Godin & Touitou, 2004; Lodzki, et al., 2004).

Niosomes are non-ionic surfactant vesicles and, like liposomes, are bilayered structures, which can entrap both hydrophilic and lipophilic drugs (Singh & Mezei, 1984). Niosomes are osmotically active and relatively stable (Baillie, et al., 1985). Niosomes in topical ocular delivery are preferred over other vesicular systems because they are chemically stable compared to liposomes; can entrap both lipophilic and hydrophilic drugs; have low toxicity because of their non-ionic nature; unlike phospholipids, handling of surfactants does not require special precautions and conditions; they exhibit flexibility in their structural characterization, for example in their composition, fluidity and size; can improve the performance of the drug via better availability and controlled delivery at a particular site; they are biodegradable, biocompatible, and non-immunogenic (Perini, 1996). The niosomes have been reported for effective topical delivery of dithranol (Agrawal, et al., 2001), ascorbyl palmitate (Gopinath, et al., 2004), acetazolamide (Aggarwal, et al., 2007), celecoxib (Kaur, et al., 2007) and minoxidil (Prabagar, et al., 2009).

Colloidal carrier in topical delivery of drug

The major limitations of use of vesicular carrier for topical delivery of drug are physical stability, drug leaking during storage and high cost of raw materials. To overcome the limitations of vesicular carrier, colloidal carrier like solid lipid nanoparticles (SLN), nanolipid structured carrier (NLC), microsphere and nanoparticles have been reported for topical delivery of drug. SLN are endowed with important features useful for safe drug delivery, such as good tolerability due to the use of physiological and biodegradable lipids with low systemic toxicity and cytotoxicity, high surface area, avoidance of potentially toxic additives during preparation process, possibility of large scale production by high pressure homogenization technique, wide potential application spectrum (dermal, peroral, intravenous), controlled drug release due to solid lipid matrix, successful incorporation of lipophilic as well as hydrophilic drugs besides protection of sensitive drug molecules from the environment (Siekmann & Westesen, 1992; Wang, et al., 2002; Chen, et al., 2006; Schwarz, et al., 1995).

However, there are some potential problems associated with the use of SLN as drug carrier. These include particle growth, particle aggregation, high water content of aqueous dispersions, unpredictable gelation tendency, burst drug release due to higher emulsifier concentration, limited drug loading capacity due to crystalline structure of solid lipid, and drug expulsion during storage due to polymorphic transformation of the lipid crystal (Muller, et al., 1995; Mehnert & Mader, 2001; Westesen & Siekmann, 1997).

NLC have received more attention over the last years and has been successfully tested for dermal application of different substances. They are characterized by a less ordered, less crystalline structure and have improved drug encapsulation efficiency and an ability to reduce drug leakage during storage (Radtke & Muller, 2001; Garcia-Fuentes, et al., 2005).

They are composed of physiological and biodegradable lipids. Most of the used lipids have an approved status for human use due to their low toxicity or are the excipients used in topical cosmetic or pharmaceutical preparations. Due to their small size they act as occlusives i.e. they form a film on the skin and thereby enhance the penetration of drugs through stratum corneum. Further, they have the potential to sustain the drug release which is very important for drugs that are irritating at high concentrations (Lippacher, et al., 2004; Radomska-Soukharev & Muller, 2006). When NLC dispersions are incorporated into hydrogels the nanoparticulate structure is maintained and aggregation and gel phenomenon of the particle generally observed in aqueous dispersions is avoided. The solid matrix of NLC further protects the incorporated chemically labile active compounds against chemical degradation. For this purpose xanthan gum, hydroxyethylcellulose, carbopol and chitosan are commonly used as gelling agents. The structure of the gel-forming polymer has a great impact on the application of semisolid nanostructured lipid carrier formulation and its performance on skin (Souto, et al., 2004).

Hydrogels in topical drug delivery

Hydrogels are three-dimensional, water-swollen structures composed of mainly hydrophilic homopolymers or copolymers. They are rendered insoluble due to cross-linking by chemical bonds, or other cohesion forces such as ionic interaction, hydrogen bonding, or hydrophobic interaction. Hydrogels are elastic solids in the sense that they exist as a reference configuration to which the system returns even after being deformed for a very long time.

Furthermore, because of their high water content, swollen hydrogels can provide a better feeling for the skin in comparison to conventional ointments and patches. Versatile hydrogel-based devices for topical delivery have been proposed so far. Sun, et al. (1997) devised composite membranes comprising of crosslinked poly(2-hydroxyethyl methacrylate (PHEMA) with a nonwoven polyester support. A Carbopol 934-based formulation containing phosphatidyl-choline liposomes (liposome-gel) was prepared by Kim, et al. (1997). In their study, the skin absorption behavior of hydrocortisone-containing liposome gel was assessed. Gayet & Fortier (1996) reported hydrogels obtained from the copolymerization of bovine serum albumin (BSA) and PEG. Due to their high water content over 96%, allowing the release of hydrophilic and hydrophobic drugs, their use as controlled-release devices in the yield of wound dressing was proposed as the potential application of the BSA-PEG hydrogels. Comprehensive studies on in situ photopolymerizable hydrogels made from terminally diacrylated ABA block copolymers of lactic acid oligomers (A) and PEG (B) for barriers and local drug delivery in the control of wound healing have been carried out by Hubbell (1996).

GUIDELINES RELATED TO DEVELOPMENT OF TOPICAL PRODUCTS

Topical drug products may be used for prophylaxis (e.g., sunscreens, astringents) or for treatment of skin conditions; such as bacterial, fungal and viral infections; inflammation; pruritis; corns; warts; and other dermatologic conditions. While the list of intended applications of dermatologic products may be limited, there is a multitude of over-the-counter (OTC) and prescription products available in a variety of formulations (e.g., gentamycin is available as an ointment and cream; benzoyl peroxide is available as a lotion, cream, and gel; and hydrocortisone is available as an ointment, cream, gel, and lotion). Add to this list numerous non-medicated dermatologics that are used to provide moisturizing, emollient, or protective effects. It is challenging for the pharmacist to remain aware of these products and provide suitable suggestions to the patient. However, following guidelines can be helpful during the development phase of products for topical drug delivery.

1. Creams provide an excellent emollient effect, have superior spreadability, and are less staining than oleaginous ointments. However, one needs to consider the skin condition and environmental factors when selecting a medicated or non-medicated cream or ointment. While both provide very good emollient effects, oleaginous ointments are preferred for dry, chapped skin in an environment of low humidity because of its occlusive properties. Creams are preferred for use over normal, healthy skin in more humid environments, as these permit some moisture evaporation from the skin and allow skin to 'breathe'.

2. Greasy products are less acceptable to patients, as these are greasy, may stain clothing, or are difficult to wash off, but are superior to water-soluble bases like polyethylene glycol in their emollient action. The latter may be attractive in term of ease of use, but are capable of irritating traumatized or broken skin.

3. Gel formulations generally provide faster drug release compared with ointments and creams, and may be suggested when available. These are superior in terms of use and patient acceptability. However, gels flow only if the container is shaken well each time one uses it, and this may cause an inconvenience to the elderly or weak patients.

4. When drug penetration into deeper skin layers is desired, oleaginous bases have proven superior to creams and water-soluble bases, which are attributable to their skin-hydrating properties. Steroids have been more effective topically when applied in a petrolatum base than when applied in a cream (o/w) vehicle.

5. The presence or absence of serious discharges from skin lesions will also dictate the best suited formulation for a dermatologic application. For example, zinc oxide has protective properties in minor skin irritations, burns, and abrasive lesions. Zinc Oxide Paste USP, which contains 25% zinc oxide and 25% starch in a hydrocarbon vehicle, is capable of absorbing the discharges because of its starch content. On the other hand, zinc oxide ointment, which is more readily available OTC, contains 20% zinc oxide in a vehicle similar to that of the paste, but it lacks starch, and, therefore, it has a poor capacity to absorb liquid.

6. Certain ointments and creams may be available in jars as well as tubes. In such cases, the pharmacist may want to evaluate the situation and discuss the advantages and disadvantages of using either packaging. While jars are economical when larger quantities are needed, a product is better protected from the environment and contamination when packaged in a tube. Besides, it may be more convenient for the patient to carry a tube rather than a jar.

7. Special precautions should be used in handling products that contain inflammable ingredients (collodions, tinctures, gels), and these should be stored in original containers with tight closures, away from heat and light. Direct skin contact with the collodion should be avoided except to the region of application, and it should be applied carefully with an applicator brush that is usually provided with the container. Disposal of unused product also requires special precautions that should be clearly explained to the patient.

8. Emulsions (creams, lotions) may break down if exposed to excessive heat or sudden changes in temperature.

9. Lotions should be shaken well prior to each use. While lotions are easier to apply, these do not remain on the skin as well and are generally less convenient to carry around compared with ointments, creams, or gels.

10. A topical product should never be applied over open wounds or broken skin unless it is labelled as a sterile product. Besides the risk of infection, such an application is often associated with problems of significant systemic drug absorption.

11. Care should also be exercised in applying any drug to inflamed skin. The integrity of inflamed skin is generally compromised, resulting in increased percutaneous migration and systemic absorption of most drugs.

12. The patient should be counselled on proper handling and storage of topical products, so as to avoid contaminating the product during use.

COSMETIC/ESTHETIC CRITERIA FOR DERMATOLOGICAL FORMULATIONS

Howsoever well we may design a topical vehicle to maximize drug bioavailability, it is still important to ensure that the preparation is esthetically acceptable to the patient. A poor product may mean that the treatment risks patient noncompliance or the transfer of allegiance to an alternative, competitor's product. Although a consumer may apply less astringent acceptability criteria to a dermatological than to, say, a cosmetic cream, patients still generally prefer a preparation, which is easy to remove from the container and, which spreads rapidly and smoothly yet adheres to the treated area while being neither tacky nor difficult to remove. For cosmetic emulsions, Clark (1983) summarized the possible interrelation between such properties as the appearance, feel, ease to use, and consistency in term of consumer requirement. Sherman (1981) developed a consistency profile for dermatologicals which takes into account product assessment prior to use, initial perception on the treatment area, application to the skin site, and residual impression

In simple terms, the general objective is to formulate a product that rubs into the skin to leave a residue which is undetectable to the eye and is neither tacky nor greasy. Stiff pastes may be difficult to rub into the skin or to apply an even film; application to damaged skin may be painful. However, it is often an advantage to leave a relatively thick layer of material on the skin to occlude the tissue or to protect it from mechanical, chemical or light damage. Ointments and pastes do this. The application procedure may loosen and dislodge scales, dead tissue, and remnants of previous doses, so that the medicament comes into more intimate contact with the diseased site; the stiff preparation also makes it easier to control the area of treatment. The recipe usually controls the consistency of an ointment by variation in the ratio of waxy components (structurally matrix agents) to the fluid fraction. For emulsions, the phase volume ratio is important; for self-bodied creams, the mixed emulsifier concentration is crucial. In gels, consistency control lies mainly in the concentration of the polymer or clay.

The tactile sensations of greasiness and tackiness arise from the properties of those vehicle constituents which form the film left on the skin. Particularly for creams, stearic acid and cetyl alcohol produce non-tacky films; hence the popularity of cosmetic vanishing creams composed of a suspension of stearic acid dispersed in a stearate soap gel. In such preparations the "oil" phase is wax-like and the microcrystals spread well on the skin without rolling. Formulations, which employ synthetic or natural gums as suspending agents should use the minimum amount, as these polymers tend to leave a tacky film on the skin.

Insoluble solids in a dermatological formulation leave the resultant film opaque, often with a powdery or crusty appearance. However, as the therapeutic treatment requires the presence of such solids in lotions and pastes, the formulator can do little to vary the nature of the film residue and patients accept the residue as an integral part of the treatment.

Table 7.2. Some cosmetic and usage criteria for topical vehicles

1. Visual appearance of product
2. Odor:
   (a) Development of pungent odor;
   (b) Loss of fragrance
3. Sampling characteristics of product, e.g., ease of removal from container
4. Application properties:
   (a) Hard, soft;
   (b) Spreads easily or with difficulty;
   (c) Softens when applied;
   (d) Creamy, watery (e.g., runs off skin), adheres, viscous;
   (e) Sticky, tacky, oily;
   (f) Pasty, lumpy, gritty, smooth, powdery;
   (g) Forms coherent film
5. Residual impression after application:
   (a) Oily, greasy, or sticky residue on treatment area;
   (b) Appearance of treatment area (e.g., dull, shiny, matt);
   (c) Irritation;
   (d) Odor on skin;
   (e) Ease of removal of residue

Table 7.3. Some physicochemical criteria for pharmaceutical semisolids

1. Stability of the active ingredients.
2. Stability of the adjuvant.
3. Rheological properties – consistency, extrudability, thixotropy, yield stress.
4. Loss of water and other volatile components.
5. Phase changes – homogeneity/phase separation, bleeding.
6. Particle size and particle size distribution of dispersed phase.
7. Apparent pH.
8. Particulate contamination.

PHYSICOCHEMICAL CRITERIA FOR DERMATOLOGICAL FORMULATIONS

The formulator of a topical dosage form, as for any other drug delivery system, must be aware of the physical and chemical behavior of the drug and the dosage form during preformulation studies; throughout bench-scale work, pilot plant studies, and batch processing; at the manufacturing level including filling, and during storage and use of the product. Many of the criteria that one uses to assess the dosage form are common to several types of pharmaceutical, but some standards are particularly relevant to topical semisolids. Table 7.3 presents a list of the general factors for a new semisolid, both during developmental studies and as a function of time on storage. The assessment procedure for the stability of a pharmaceutical examines the capability of a particular formulation, in a specific container, to remain within its physical, chemical, therapeutic, and toxicological specifications.

A general methodology for predicting chemical stability uses an accelerated stability test, which subjects the material to elevated temperatures and uses the Arrhenius relationship to establish a shelf-life (Rawlins, 1977). However, in a multiphase system, such as a cream, heat may alter the phase distribution and may even crack the emulsion, thus, having a limitation to assessing the preparation over a long time at the storage temperature. A related problem is that, because of the complexity of the vehicles, it may be difficult to separate the drug or labile adjuvant from the base so as to analyze it.

In addition to performing specific analytical tests, the pharmacist should note any qualitative changes in the product during storage; these changes are often apparent on inspection. The color may change e.g., natural fats, oils, and lanolin brown with age as they oxidize, becoming rancid with a disagreeable odor. The texture may alter as phase relationships vary.

One method which readily quantifies changes in the structure of a colloidal system uses a rheological assessment, preferably by developing multipoint rheograms.

Many dermatologicals contain water or other volatile solvents and batches may lose a proportion of the solvent either through the walls of unsuitable plastic containers or through faulty seams or ill-fitting caps. The product may lose weight and may shrink away from the container wall, becoming puffy and stiff so that its application properties suffer.

Dermatological formulations are often heterogeneous systems, which are susceptible to various phase changes when stored incorrectly. Emulsions may cream and crack, suspensions can agglomerate and cake, and ointments and gels may "bleed" as their matrices contract to squeeze out mobile constituents. High temperatures can produce or accelerate such adjustments.

For suspensions and emulsions, a stability protocol should monitor the particle/globule size distribution and note any changes on storage. A particle size analysis may often detect a potentially unstable formulation long before any other parameter changes markedly. Emulsion globules may grow as a gel network breaks down on storage, thus allowing Brownian motion to bring droplets into contact so that they coalesce. Crystals may enlarge, or change their habit, or revert to a more stable, less active, polymorphic form. Such alterations in crystal form may affect the therapeutic activity of the formulation.

The apparent pH of topical product may alter on storage. Although we cannot assign a fundamental meaning to a pH measurement in a complex dermatological vehicle, we can sometimes use a pH electrode as a tool to monitor variations in a formulation as it ages.

On the manufacturing scale, even with the most modern equipment and facilities, it can be difficult to produce creams and ointments completely free from foreign particles. Tin and aluminium tubes may contaminate a topical with "flashing" metal silvers and shavings formed during the manufacture of the containers. Their presence is particularly undesirable in ophthalmic ointments, and various pharmacopoeial tests limit the extent of such contamination.

EVALUATION OF TOPICAL DOSAGE FORMS

Evaluation of topical dosages form is carried out for following parameters:

A. Bioavailability and bioequivalence

As defined earlier, topical dosage forms are those designed for application to the skin for the treatment of local conditions. Some penetration below the stratum corneum may or may not occur, and may or may not be desirable. Unlike a transdermal formulation, topical products are not intended to result in any appreciable absorption into the systemic circulation. The ideal topical product is one that:

1. achieves a concentration in the target tissue that is sufficient to result in the desired pharmacological response;
2. has an acceptable systemic toxicity (preferably none); and
3. leaves the skin in an inactive form (e.g., as a metabolite) [Bodde et al. (1989)].

Evaluation of the bioavailability or bioequivalence of dosage forms applied to the skin is generally done for one of three reasons:

1. The manufacturer wishes to demonstrate that the dosage form proposed for marketing, and produced on a large scale, has an acceptable bioavailability when compared with the dosage form that was employed in the clinical trials conducted to support the New Drug Application (NDA);
2. The manufacturer wishes to demonstrate that a proposed change (e.g. manufacturing process, site of manufacturer, new source of raw material or other) will yield a product that can be expected to perform identically with the dosage form that was approved through the NDA process; or
3. A second manufacturer, through an Abbreviated New Drug Application (ANDA), wishes to gain approval to market a product that is a generic version of a product developed by the innovator or holder of the

NDA in each instance, the criteria applied to the determination of bioequivalance should be identical, regardless of the purpose for conducting the study (Potts, 1990).

Current regulation for the marketing of topical dosage forms in the United States depends on when the innovator's product was initially marketed. If the original product was approved before 1962, there are currently no requirements for *in vivo* bioavailablity or bioequivalance studies for generic versions of innovator products. Such products need only evaluation of skin irritation, cutaneous toxicity, and contact sensitivity (Potts, 1990). For post-1962 products, the 1984 Patent Term Restoration Act, or the Waxman-Hatch Amendments, make mandatory a bioequivalence study for all drug products approved through an ANDA. If we define bioequivalance in its broadest terms, one may state that two topical products are bioequivalent if they both result in equivalent clinical effectiveness and equivalent toxicity. This definition leads us to conclude that clinical

trials must be conducted for such dosage forms. However, it is also possible that other types of *in vivo* studies, or perhaps even *in vitro* methods, could serve as a surrogate for clinical trials, if acceptable correlations can be demonstrated (Woodford and Barry, 1982).

If one desires to evaluate the effectiveness of topical dosage form, several types of studies may be considered:

1. A well-controlled clinical trial
2. Measurement of a pharmacodynamic effect
3. Measurement of drug penetration into the skin
4. *In vitro* methods correlated with a clinical endpoint
5. Animal studies
6. Any other method that can be shown to be capable of measuring bioequivalence.

B. Evaluation of physical and chemical stability

General methods to determine the physical and chemical stability of topical dosage forms are summarized in Table 7.4.

Table 7.4. Evaluation of physical and chemical stability of topical products

Parameters	Characterization method
Stability of the active ingredients	Drug assay
Stability of color, odor	Reflectance spectrophotometry
Viscosity, extrudibility	Brookfield viscometer, utilitarian viscometer, penetrometer, extrusion rheometer
Loss of water and other volatile vehicle components	Gas chromatography
Phase distribution (homogeneity or phase separation, bleeding)	Manual observation, drug assay
Particle size distribution of dispersed phases	Dynamic light scattering methods
pH	pH meter
Texture, feel upon application (stiffness, grittiness, greasiness, tackiness)	Spreadometer, Extrusion rheometer
Particulate contamination	Optical microscopy
Microbial contamination and sterility	Sterility testing
In vitro drug release study	Side by side diffusion cell with artificial or biological membrane, dialysis bag diffusion
Skin permeation potential	Confocal light scattering method, fluorescence microscopy, transmission electron microscopy
Crystal habit	Optical microscopy, X-ray diffraction study

Semisolid systems provide us with two special problems here. First, semisolids are chemically complex, to the point that just separating drug and adjuvant from all other components is an analyst's nightmare. Many components interfere with standard assays and, therefore, difficult separations are the rule before anything can be analyzed. Also, since semisolids undergo phase changes on heating, one cannot use high-temperature kinetics for stability prediction. Thus, stability has to be evaluated at the storage temperature of the formulation, and this takes a long time. Under these circumstances, problematic stability may not be evident until studies have been in progress for a year or more. Be this as it may, stability details are worked out in the laboratories of industry, the pharmacist ordinarily accepting projected shelf lives as fact. Some qualitative indicators of chemical instability that the pharmacist might look for are the development of color (or a change in color or its intensity) and the development of an off odor. Often products yellow or brown with age as a result of oxidative reactions occurring in the base. Discolorations of this kind are commonly seen when natural fats and oils (e.g., lanolin) are used to build the vehicle. Extensive oxidation of natural fatty materials (rancidification) is accompanied by development of disagreeable odor. One may also notice phase and texture changes in a suspect product. Changes in product pH also indicate chemical decomposition, most probably of a hydrolytic nature (Goodman & Barry, 1989).

Time variable rhelogical behavior of a semisolid may also signal physical or chemical changes. However, manual measurements such as spreadability and feel on application are unreliable and most valid approach is to use the modern instrumentation techniques. These include extrusion rheometers, which measure the force it takes to extrude a semisolid through a narrow orifice; penetrometers, which characterize viscosity in terms of the penetration of a weighted cone into a semisolid; and Brookfield viscometers, with spindle and helipath attachments, which measure the force it takes to drive a spindle helically through a semisolid. As used with semisolids, the utilitarian rheometers provide only relative, although quite useful, measure of viscosity. Increase (or decrease) in viscosity by any of these measuring tools indicates changes in the structural elements of the formulation. The gradual transformations in semisolid structure that take place are more often than not impermanent, in which event, the systems are restored to their initial condition simply by mixing them. Substantial irreversible rheological changes are a sign of poor physical stability (Anderson, et al., 1988).

Change in the nature of individual phases of or phase separation may result from emulsion breakage, clearly a critical instability. More often, it appears more subtly as bleeding, the formation of visible droplets of an emulsion's internal phase in the continuum of the semisolid.

We should also take a dim view of changes in the particle size, size distribution or particulate nature of semisolid suspensions. They are the consequence of crystal growth, changes in crystalline habit, or the reversion of the crystalline materials to a more stable polymorphic form. Any crystalline alteration can lead to pronounced reduction in the drug delivery capabilities and therapeutic usefulness of a formulation.

A more commonly encountered change in formulations is the evaporative loss of water or other volatile phases from a preparation while it is in storage. This can occur as the result of inappropriate packaging or a flaw made in packaging. Some plastic collapsible tubes allow diffusive loss of volatile substances through the container walls. A bad seal may occur in any tube or jar, irrespective of its contents, with eventual loss of volatile ingredients around the cap or through the crimp. Such evaporative losses cause a formulation to stiffen and become puffy, and its application characteristics change noticeably (Hou & Flynn, 1986).

C. Evaluation of *in vitro* skin permeation

The use of topical/transdermal dosage forms to control drug permeation across the skin has seen extensive research in the past two decades. The permeation rate of the drug across the skin has been measured using several different kinds of *in vitro* skin permeation apparatus. A typical apparatus has three main components. The first is the donor compartment, where the formulation is applied uniformly. From the donor compartment, the drug passes through a permeation barrier or membrane (i.e. skin), which is the second compartment, into the receptor solution, which is the third compartment. Properties of the receptor solution, such as temperature and buffer composition, can have a significant effect on drug permeation through the skin. Typically, physiological saline or a phosphate-buffered solution maintained at 37°C is used. This will keep the skin surface at approximately 32°C, which simulates the temperature of the human skin. Generally, antibiotics and preservatives are added to the receptor solution to prevent microbial growth, enzymatic degradation, and to stabilize the skin. Drug permeation into and across the skin is evaluated using different *in vitro* models. These include horizontal-type skin permeation system, Franz diffusion cell and the flow-through diffusion cell.

Determination of amount of drug deposited into the skin

For determining the amount of drug deposited into the skin, El Maghraby, et al. (2001a) reported the modification of *in vitro* skin permeation method. In this method the *in vitro* drug release study is performed in two stages using a diffusion cell at $32 \pm 1°C$. In the first stage 10 ml of PBS (pH 6.5) is used as the receptor medium for 10 hr and *in vitro* skin permeation is carried out. At the end of 10 hr the donor compartment is washed five times with warm receptor fluid (45°C). The second stage uses 50% v/v ethanol as the receptor solution for a further period of 12 hr and performed without any donor phase. During this stage ethanolic receptor will diffuse into skin disrupting the carrier system, which may have penetrated, and deposited in the tissue and thus releasing both carrier-bound and free drug for collection to the receptor fluid. Use of 50% ethanol as a receptor fluid can slightly reduce the barrier nature of the stratum corneum hence the second stage should be performed after removal of the donor to avoid any excess permeation due to penetration enhancing activity of ethanol.

This design gave a more accurate comparative measure for the deposition of drug into deeper layer of skin, compared with determination of drug in skin using a washing protocol at room temperature. Thus, the problem of possible failure of washing procedure to remove carrier systems adhering to the stratum corneum surface is avoided.

Skin models used for evaluating the permeation and deposition of drug

During the preclinical development of topical formulation, it is difficult as well as unethical to test products in humans initially, owing to the potential toxicity of pharmaceutical agents. Therefore, traditional skin models from animals have been used for *in vitro* and *in vivo* studies. Practically, it would be advantageous to use human cadaver skin for permeation studies but, for most investigators, human cadaver skin is not readily available. Also, the skin samples are typically obtained from a variety of anatomical sites and after many different disease states, which might alter the percutaneous permeability of the drug (Costello, et al., 1995). Most topical/transdermal testing is performed using hairless mouse skin. However, other models are sometimes used including rat, guinea pig, rabbit and shed snake skin, artificial composite membranes, and, more recently, living skin equivalents [Kim, et al. (1993); Panchagnula, et al. (1997)]. Although there are many similar features between these models and human cadaver skin, no model has yet been tested that fully mimics the results obtained with human cadaver skin.

Hairless mouse skin

The hairless mouse is used predominantly because it is economical, attainable, easy to house and hairless [El-Kattan, et al. (2000)]. However, the permeability and lipid composition of hairless mouse skin are very different to those found in human cadaver skin. Hairless mouse skin tends to be very thin with a small stratum corneum and the permeability of hairless mouse skin in some studies has been found to be 30–40-fold higher than human cadaver skin [Ghosh & Bagherian (1996); Gorukanti, et al. (1999)].

Pig skin

Weanling pig skin (i.e. skin from a pig that has recently been weaned) is recognized as the closest alternative to human cadaver skin for its permeability and lipid composition. However, there are some slight structural differences between weanling pig and human skin, including bristles, more subcutaneous fat and less vasculature [Whyte, et al. (1996); Marekov, et al. (1998)].

Living skin equivalents

The skin equivalents used for permeation testing are typically epidermal or full-thickness skin. Full-thickness skin equivalents are composed of both dermal and epidermal tissues. These skin equivalents have many advantages, including the ability to eliminate animal experimentation. Also, they use human skin cells, which provide skin properties similar to those found in native human skin. In this context, it is interesting that all of the lipids found in the native human skin are found in skin equivalents, but in reduced quantities.

Polymeric and other artificial membranes have also been used for topical/transdermal experiments even though these membranes lack the complex histological structures present in the human skin. These membranes showed higher permeation relative to animal and human skin models.

D. Evaluation of skin sensitivities

One further problem of topical formulations associated with many ingredients, and of special concern with preservatives, is the development of skin sensitivities. The skin of some individuals is particularly susceptible to an allergic conditioning to chemicals that is known as type IV contact hypersensitivity. The evaluation of skin sensitivity of different topical products is carried out by following methods:

Draize test

The Draize sensitization test (DT) was the first predictive sensitization test accepted by regulatory agencies. One flank of 20 guinea pigs is shaved and 0.05 ml of 0.1% solution of test material in saline, paraffin oil or polyethylene glycol is injected into the anterior flank on day 0. Every other day through day 20, 0.1 ml of the test solution is injected into a new site on the same flank. After a 2-week rest period, the opposite untreated flank is shaved and 0.05 ml of test solution is injected into each animal (challenge). Twenty previously untreated controls are injected at the same time. The test site is visually evaluated after injection for 24 and 48 hr. A larger or more intensely erythematous response than that of controls is considered a positive response (Draize et al., 1944; Kleack, 1983)

Open epicutaneous test

The open epicutaneous test (OET) (Kero & Hannuksela, 1980) simulates the conditions of human use by utilizing topical application of the test material. The procedure determines the doses required to induce sensitization and to elicit a response in sensitized animals. The irritancy profile is determined by applying 0.025 ml of varying concentration to a 2 cm^2 area of the shaved flanks of six to eight guinea pigs. Test sites are visually evaluated 24 h after applications of test solutions to erythema. The dose not causing a reaction in 25% of the animals (minimal irritant concentration) is determined. During induction, test solution is applied to flank skin of six to eight guinea pigs for 3 weeks, or 5 times a week for 4 weeks. A control group is treated with vehicle only. The highest dose tested is usually the minimal irritant concentration and lower doses are based on usage concentration or a stepwise reduction. Twenty four to 72 hr after the last induction treatment, each animal is challenged on the untreated flank. The minimal irritant concentration, the maximum nonirritant concentration and five solutions of lower concentration are applied. Skin reactions are read on all-or-none basis at 24, 48 and 72 hr after application. The maximum non-irritating concentration in the vehicle treated group is calculated. Animals in test groups that develop inflammatory responses to lower concentrations are considered sensitized.

E. Evaluation of irritation potential of topical dosages form

Draize-type tests

Primary irritation and corrosion are most often evaluated by modifications of the method described by Draize (Draize et al., 1944). The Federal Hazardous Substance ACT (FHSA) adopted one modification as a standard procedure (Magee et al., 1994). The backs of six albino rabbits are clipped free of hair. Each undiluted material is tested on two 1-in^2 sites on the same animal (one site is intact and one is abraded in such a way that the stratum corneum is opened but no bleeding produced). Each test site is covered with two layers of 1-in^2 surgical gauze and secured in place. The entire trunk of the animal is then wrapped with rubberized cloth or other occlusive impervious material to retard evaporation of the substance and hold the patches

in position. After 28 and 48 h of application, the wrappings are removed and the test sites are evaluated for erythema and edema, using a prescribed scale. Modifications of the Draize procedure that have been proposed include changing the species tested, reduction of exposure period, use of fewer animals and testing on intact skin only (Guillot, et al., 1982). Several government bodies utilize their own modification of Draize procedure for regulatory decision. All Draize-type tests are used to evaluate corrosion as well as irritation. When severe reactions that may not be reversible are noted, test sites are observed for a longer period. Delayed evaluations are usually made on day 7 and 14, but may be as late as 35 days.

Non-Draize animal studies

Animal assays to evaluate the ability of chemicals to produce cumulative irritation have been developed (Phillips, et al., 1972). Those assays used often are not as well standardized as Draize-type tests and many variables have been introduced by multiple investigators.

Repeat application patch tests in which diluted materials are applied to the same site each day for 15 to 21 days have been reported using several species (the guinea pig or rabbit being most commonly used). Because the degree of occlusion is an important determinant of percutaneous penetration, the choice of covering materials may determine the sensitivity of a given test. A reference material of similar use or one that produces a known effect in humans is included in almost all replicate application procedures. Test sites are evaluated for erythema and edema, either using the scales of the Draize-type tests or more descriptive scales developed by the investigators.

Future prospects in dermatologicals

The dermatological pharmaceutical landscape is shifting. The changes in the industry have come relatively quickly, and the long-term repercussions are largely unknown. The challenge of developing New Chemical Entities (NCEs) in dermatology is that they take as much time and cost to develop as any other drugs for CVS or CNS.

Despite attention to finding NCEs, the recent trend of reformulating is likely to gain fire, as technological advancements permit the development of more patient-friendly and effective topical therapies. This trend is being fueled by demand from patients, prescribers and the economic pressures, which have forced the pharmaceuticals to pay special attention in this context. Thus, such breakthroughs in development of new entities and technologies are strictly needed to improve the market value and importance of dermatologicals

CONCLUSION

The major aim of topical applications is to induce a local, rather than systemic effect. Modern pharmaceutical industry uses different carrier systems that provide highly improved dosage forms for topical administration. In these types of dosage form the vehicle releases the active ingredients in an appropriate fashion so that percutaneous absorption can be controlled. Recent studies suggest the inherent potential of novel drug delivery systems for selective topical delivery, since the application of carrier system e.g. liposomes, transfersomes, microemulsion results in increased efficacy with decreased toxicity of drug, which could result from undesirable higher systemic absorption of the free drug. In future, we can expect different controlled-release dosage forms for topical delivery of different problematic molecules e.g. DNA delivery, gene delivery, antigen delivery. Undoubtedly, the novel drug delivery systems have a great promise in topical drug delivery to enhance the efficacy and safety of important but potentially toxic drugs. However, conventional topical drug delivery system would continue to be popular.

ACKNOWLEDGEMENTS

The authors are grateful to UGC, New Delhi for granting UPE status (University with potential for excellence) to University and providing the grant for establishment of centre of emerging life sciences (equipped with sophisticated instruments). One of the authors, Ms. Lakhvir Kaur, is thankful for DST, New Delhi, for providing DST-INSPIRE fellowship.

BIBLIOGRAPHY

- Agarwal, R., Katare, O.P., Vyas S.P. (2000). *Methods Find Exp Clin Pharmacol.*, 22(2): 129–133.
- Agarwal, R., Katare, O.P., Vyas, S.P. (2001). *Int. J. Pharm.*, 228: 43–52.
- Aggarwal, D., Pal, D., Mitra, A.K., Kaur, I.P. (2007). *Int. J. Pharm.*, 338: 21–26.
- Albery, W.J., Hadgraft, J. (1979). *J. Pharm. Pharmacol.*, 31: 129–139.
- Anderson, B.D., Higuchi, W.I., Raykar, P. (1988). *Pharm. Res.*, 5: 566–573.
- Baillie, A.J., Florence, A.T. (1985). *J. Pharm. Pharmacol.*, 37: 863–868.
- Baroli, B., Lopez-Quintela, M.A., Delgado-Charro, B., Fadda, A.M., Blanco-Mendez, J. (2000). *J. Control. Release*, 69: 209–218.
- Barry, B.W. (1973). *J. Pharm. Pharmacol.*, 25: 131.
- Barry, B.W. (1991). *J. Control. Rel.*, 15: 237–248.
- Barry, B.W. (Eds.) (1983). **Dermatological Formulation: Percutaneous Absorption**, Vol. 18, Marcel Dekker, Inc., New York.
- Bodde, H.E., Verhoeven, J., van Driel, L.M.J. (1989). *Crit. Rev. Ther. Drug Carr. Syst.*, 6: 87–115.
- Bohm, M., Luger, T.A. (1998). *Dermatology*, 196:75–79.
- Bolzinger, M.A., Thevenin, C., Poelman, M.C. (1998). *Int. J. Pharma.*, 176: 39–45.
- Ceglie, A., Das, K.P., Lindman, B. (1987). *Colloids Surf.*, 28: 29–40.
- Cevc, G., Blume G. (2001). *Biochim. Biophysic. Acta*, 1514: 191.
- Cevc, G., Blume, G., Schatzlein, A. (1997). *J. Control. Rel.*, 45: 211–226.

- Chen, H., Chang, X., Du, D., Liu, W., Liu, J., Weng, T., Yang, Y., Xu, H., Yang, X. (2006). *J. Control. Release*, 110(2): 296–306.
- Chowdary, K.P.R., Naidu, R.A.S. (1995). *Indian Drugs*, 32(9): 414–422.
- Costello, C.T., Jeske, A.H. (1995). *Phys. Ther.*, 75: 554–563.
- Dayan, N., Touitou E. (2000). *Biomaterials*, 21: 1879–1885.
- Delgado-Charro, M.B., Iglesias-Vilas, G., Blanco-Mendez, J., Lopez-Quintela, M.A.
- Dowton, S.M., Hu, Z., Ramachandran, C., Wallach, D.F.H., Weiner, N. (1993). *STP Pharma Sci.*, 3: 404–407.
- Draize, J.H., Woodard, G., Calvery, H.Q. (1944). *J. Pharmacol. Exp. Ther.*, 82: 377–390.
- Dubey, V., Mishra D., Asthana A., Jain N.K. (2006). *Biomaterials*, 27(18): 3491–3496.
- Dubey, V., Mishra, D., Jain, N.K. (2007). *Eur. J. Pharm. Biopharm.*, 67(2): 398–405.
- Egbaria, K., Weiner, N. (1991). *Cosmetic & Toiletries*, 106: 79–93.
- El Maghraby, G.M.M., Williams, A.C., Barry, B.W. (1999). *J. Pharm. Pharmacol.*, 51: 1123–1134.
- El Maghraby, G.M.M., Williams, A.C., Barry, B.W. (2000). *Int. J. Pharm.*, 196: 63–74.
- El Maghraby, G.M.M., Williams, A.C., Barry, B.W. (2001a). *J. Pharm. Pharmacol.*, 53: 1311–1322.
- El Maghraby, G.M.M., Williams, A.C., Barry, B.W. (2001b). *J. Pharm. Pharmacol.*, 53: 1069–1076.
- Elias, P.M. (1983). *J. Invest. Dermatol.*, 80: 44S–49S.
- El-Kattan, A., Asbill, C.S., Haidar, S. (2000). *Pharm. Sci. Technol. Today*, 12(3): 426–430.
- Elsayed, M.M., Abdallah, O.Y., Naggar, V.F., Khalafallah, N.M. (2007). *Pharmazie*, 62: 133–137.
- Essa, E.A., Bonner, M.C., Barry, B.W. (2002). *Int. J. Pharm.* 240: 55–66.
- Fang, J.Y., Hwang, T.L., Huang, Y.L., Fang, C.L. (2006). *Int. J. Pharm.*, 310: 131–138.
- Feldmann, R.J., Maibach, H.I. (1987). *J. Invest. Dermatol.*, 48, 181–183.
- Foldvari, M. (2000). *PSTI*, 3(12): 417–424.
- Foldvari, M., Moreland, A. (1997). *J. Liposome Res.*, 7: 115–126.
- Foldvari, M., Jarvis, B., Ogueijo, C.J.N. (1993). *J. Control. Release*, 27: 193–205.
- Fresta, M., Puglisi, G. (1997). *J. Control. Release*, 44: 141–151.
- Ganesan, M.G., Ho, N.F.H. (1985). *J. Control. Release*, 2: 61–65.
- Garcia-Fuentes, M., Alonso, M.J., Torres, D. (2005). *J. Colloid Interface Sci.*, 285(2): 590–598.
- Garg, T., Jain, S., Singh, H.P., Sharma, A., Tiwary, A.K. (2008). *Drug Develop. Ind. Pharm.*, 34(10): 1100–1110.
- Garnier, J.P. (1981a). *Clin. Trials J.*, 8: 55.
- Garnier, J.P. (1981b). *Pharm. J.*, 207: 475.
- Gayet, J.C., Fortier, G. (1996). *J. Control. Release*, 38: 177–184.
- Ghosh, T.K., Bagherian, A. (1996). *Pharm. Dev. Technol.*, 1: 285–291.
- Godin, B., Touitou, E. (2004). *J. Control. Release*, 81: 1–15.
- Godin, B., Touitou, E. (2005). *Current Drug Delivery*, 2(3): 265–275.
- Goodman, M., Barry, B.W. (1989). **Percutaneous Absorption**, IBC Technical Services, London, 567–593.
- Gopinath, D., Ravi, D., Karwa, R., Rao, B.R., Shashank, A., Rambhau, D. (2001). *Arzneimittel Forsch. Drug Res.*, 51: 924–930.
- Gorukanti, S.R., Li, L., Kim, K.H. (1999). *Int. J. Pharm.*, 192: 159–172.
- Guillot, J.P., Gopnnet, J,F., Clement, C., Caillard, L., Truhauk, R. (1982). *Food Chem. Toxicol.*, 20: 563–572.
- Guo, J., Ping, G., Sun, G., Jiao, C. (2000a). *Int. J. Pharm.*, 194: 201–207.
- Guo. J., Ping, G., Sun, G., Jiao, C. (2000b). *Drug Delivery*, 7: 113–116.
- Hadgraft, J. (1999). *Int. J. Pharm.*, 184(1): 1–6.
- Clark, E.W. (1983). *J. Soc. Cosmetic Chemists*, 26, 323.
- Hadgraft, J. (2001). *Int. J. Pharm.*, 224: 1–18.
- Hiruta, Y., Hattori, Y., Kawano, K., Obato, Y., Maitani, Y. (2006). *J. Control Release*, 113: 146–154.
- Hofer, C., Hartung, R., Gobel, R., Deering, P., Lehmer, A., Breul, J. (2000). *World J. Surgery*, 24: 1187–1189.
- Hofland, H.E.J., van der Geest, R., Bodde, H.E., Junginger, H.E., Bouwstra, J.A. (1994). *Pharm. Res.*, 11: 659–664.
- Honeywell-Nguyen, P.L., Frederik, P.M., Bomans P.H.H., Junginger, H.E., Bouwstra, J.A. (2002). *Pharma. Research*, 19(7): 991–997.

- Honeywell-Nguyen, P.L., Frederik, P.M., Bomans P.H.H., Junginger, H.E., Bouwstra, J.A. (2003). *J. Control. Rel.*, 86: 145–156.
- Horwitz, E., Pisanty, S., Czerninski, R., Helser, M., Eliav, E., Touitou, E. (1999). *Oral Surg. Oral Med. Oral Pathol. Oral Radiol. Endod.*, 87: 700–705.
- Hou, S.Y.E., Flynn, G.L. (1986). *Pharm. Res.*, 3: 525.
- Hubbell, J.A. (1996). *J. Control. Release*, 39: 305–313.
- Jain, S., Jain N.K. Transfersomes: A novel carrier for effective transdermal drug delivery, *In:* **Advances in Controlled and Novel Drug Delivery**, Ed., Prof. N.K. Jain, CBS Publishers & Distributors, Chapter 18, 426–451, 2001.
- Jain, S., Jain, N., Bhadra, D., Jain N.K. Sustained and targeted delivery of an analgesic agent using ultradeformable lipid vesicles. *Proceeding of the 54th Indian Pharmaceutical Conference*, Pune (India), Dec. 13–16, 2002a; I A-67.
- Jain, S., Jain, N., Tiwary, A.K., Jain, N.K. (2005b). *Current Drug Delivery*, 2(3): 223–233.
- Jain, S., Jain, N.K., Tiwary, A.K. (2008). *Current Drug Delivery*, 5: 275–281.
- Jain, S., Jain, P., Jain, N.K. (2003a). *Drug Dev. Ind. Pharm.*, 29(9): 1013–1026.
- Jain, S., Jain, S., Jain, N.K. (2002b). *Drug Delivery Tech.*, 2(3): 70.
- Jain, S., Sapre, R., Tiwary, A.K., Jain, N.K. (2005a). *AAPS Pharm. Sci. Tech.*, 6(3): Article 64. E513–E522.
- Jain, S., Sapre, R., Umamaheshwari, R.B., Jain, N.K. (2003b). *Ind. J. Pharm. Sci.*, 65(2): 152–161.
- Jain, S., Tiwary, A.K., Jain, N.K. (2006). *Current Drug Delivery*, 3(2): 157–166.
- Jain, S., Tiwary, A.K., Sapra, B., Jain, N.K. (2007). *AAPS Pharm. Sci. Tech.*, 8(4): Article 111. E1-E9.
- Jain, S.,; Umamaheshwari, R.B., Bhadra, D., Jain, N.K. (2004). *Ind. J. Pharm. Sci.*, 65(1): 72–81.
- Jain. N.K. (Eds.) (1997). **Controlled and Novel Drug Delivery**, CBS Publishers & Distributors, New Delhi.
- Jain. N.K. (Eds.) (2004). **Progress in Controlled and Novel Drug Delivery Systems**, CBS Publishers & Distributors, New Delhi.
- Jia, Y., Joly, H., Omri, A. (2008). *Int. J. Pharm.*, 359: 254–263.
- Joshi, M., Patravale, V. (2006). *Drug Dev. Ind. Pharm.*, 32(8): 911–918.
- Kaur, K., Sapra, B., Tiwary, A.K., Jain, S. (2007). *Current Drug Delivery*, 4(4): 276–282.
- Kero, M., Hannuksela, M. (1980). *Contact Derm.*, 6: 341–344.
- Kim, A., Lee, E.H., Choi, S.H., Kim, C.K. (2004). *Biomaterials*, 25: 305–313.
- Kim, C., Kim, J., Chi, S., Shim, C. (1993). *Int. J. Pharm.*, 99: 109–118.
- Kim, M.K., Chung, S.J., Lee, M.H., Cho, A.R., Shim, C.K. (1997). *J. Control. Release*, 46: 243-251.
- Klecak, G. (1983). **Dermatotoxicology**, 2nd ed., New York: Hemisphere, 193–236.
- Knepp, V.M., Szoka, F.C., Guy, R.H. (1990). *J. Control. Release*, 12: 25–30.
- Kreilgaard, M. (2001). *Pharm. Res.*, 18: 367–373.
- Kreilgaard, M. (2002). *Adv. Drug Deliv. Rev.*, 54: S77– S98.
- Lasch, J., Bouwstra, J.A. (1995). *J. Liposome Res.*, 5: 543–569.
- Lee, P.J., Langer, R., Shastri, V.P. (2003). *Pharm. Res.*, 20: 264–269.
- Lippacher, A., Muller, R.H., Mader, K. (2004). *Eur. J. Pharm. Biopharm.*, 58(3): 561–567.
- Lodzki, M., Godin, B., Rakou, L., Mechoulam, R., Gallily, R., Touitou, E. (2003). *J. Control. Release*, 93: 377–387.
- Longworth, A.R., French, J.D. (1990). *J. Pharm. Pharmacol.*, 21(S): 1S.
- Magee, P.S., Hostynek, J.J., Maibach, H.I. (1994). *Quant Struct Activity Relationship*, 13, 22–33.
- Manosrol, A., Kongkaneramit, L., Manosrol, O. (2004). *Int. J. Pharm.*, 270: 279–286.
- Marekov, L.N., Fesus, L., Steinert, P.M. (1998). *J. Biol. Chem.*, 273: 17763–17770.
- Mehnert, W., Mader, K. (2001). *Adv. Drug Deliv. Rev.*, 47(2): 165–196.
- Meuwissen, M.M., Mougin, L., Junginger, H.E., Bouwstra, J.A. (1996). *Proc. Int. Symp. Control. Release Bioact. Mater.*, 23: 303–304.
- Mezei, M., Gulasekharam, V. (1980). *Life Sci.*, 26: 1473–1477.
- Michaels, A.S., Chandrasekatan, S.K., Shaw, J.E. (1975). *Am. Inst. Chem. Eng. J.*, 21: 985–996.
- Mier, P., van den Hurk, J. (1977). *Br. J. Dermatol.*, 93, 509–517.
- Mishra, D., Dubey, V., Asthana, A., Saraf, D.K., Jain N.K. (2006). *Vaccine*, 24(22): 4847–4855.
- Müller, R.H., Keck, C.M. (2004). *J. Nanosci. Nanotechnol.*, 4(5): 471–483.

- Muller, R.H., Lucks, J.S., Schwarz, C., Zur Muhlen, A., Weyhers, H., Freitas, C., Ruhl, D. (1995). *Eur. J. Pharm. Biopham.*, 41(1): 62–69.
- Mura, P., Capasso, G., Maestrelli, F., Furlanetto, S. (2008). *J. Liposome Research*, 18(2): 113–125.
- Padamwar, M.N., Pokharkar, V.B. (2006). *Int. J. Pharm.*, 320: 37–44.
- Panchagnula, R., Stemmer, K., Ritschel, W.A. (1997). *Methods Find. Exp. Clin. Pharmacol.*, 19: 335–341.
- Paolino, D., Ventura, C.A., Steven N.S., Puglisi, G., Fresta, M. (2002). *Int. J. Pharma.*, 244: 21–31.
- Paul, A., Cevc, G. (1995a). *Vaccine Res.*, 4: 145–150.
- Paul, A., Cevc, G., Bachhawat, B.K. (1995b). *Eur. J. Immunol.*, 25, 3521–3524.
- Paul, A., Cevc, G., Bachhawat, B.K. (1998). *Vaccine*, 16(2/3): 188–195.
- Perini, G. (1996). *Boll. Chim. Farm.*, 135: 145–146.
- Phillips, L., Steinberg, M., Maibach, H.I., Akers, W.A. (1972). *Toxicol. Appl. Pharmacol.*, 21: 369–382.
- Pierre, M., Piemi, Y., Korner, D., Benita, S. (1999). *J. Control. Release*, 58: 177–187.
- Planas M.E., Gonzalez P., Rodriguez S., Sanchez, G., Cevc G. (1992). *Anesth. Analg.*, 95: 615–621.
- Potts, R.O. (1990). *In:* Topical products workshop notes. Sponsored by the AAPS and FDA, March 26-28, 1990, Arlington., 34–39.
- Potts, R.O., Francoeur, M.I. (1991). *J. Invest. Dermatol.*, 96, 495–499.
- Prabagar, B., Srinivasan, S., Won, L., Won, L., Jong, K., Dong, H., Dae, K., Jung, K., Bong, Y., Han, C., Jong, W., Chul, Y. (2009). *Int. J. Pharm.*, 377: 1–8.
- Puglia, C., Filosa, R., Peduto, A., Caprariis, P., Rizza, L., Bonina, F., Blasi, P. (2006). *AAPS Pharm. Sci Tech.*, 7(3): Article 64.
- Radomska-Soukharev, A., Muller, R.H. (2006). *Pharmazie*, 61(5): 425–430.
- Radtke, M., Muller, R.H. (2001). *New Drugs*, 2: 48–52.
- Rawlins, E.A. (Ed.) (1977). **Bentley's Textbook of Pharmaceutics**, 8th ed., Balliere Tindall, London, 256–351.
- Rhee, Y.S., Choi, J.G., Park, E.S., S.-C. Chi, Transdermal delivery of ketoprofen using microemulsions, *Int. J. Pharm.*, 228 (2001) 161–170.
- Ricci, M., Puglia, C., Bonina, F., Giovanni, C., Giovagnoli, S., Rossi, C. (2005). *J. Pharm. Sci.*, 94(5): 1149–1159.
- Schurer, N.Y. (1991). *Dermatolica*, 183: 77–94.
- Schwarz, C., Freitas, C., Mehnert, W., Muller, R.H. (1995). *Proc. Int. Symp. Control. Rel. Bioact. Mater.*, 22: 766–767.
- Sciarra, J.J. (1975). *Drug Cosmetic Ind.*, 116(6), 58.
- Sherman, P. (1981). *Rheol. Acta*, 10: 121.
- Siekmann, B., Westesen, K. (1992). *Pharma. Pharmacol. Lett.*, 1: 123–126.
- Singh, H.P., Jain, S., Tiwary, A.K. (2009). *AAPS J.*, 11(1): 54–64.
- Singh, K., Mezei, M. (1984). *Int. J. Pharm.* 19: 263–269.
- Sintov, A.C., Shapiro, L. (2004). *J. Controlled Release*, 95: 173–183.
- Sintov, A.C., Krymberk, I., Gavrilov, V., Gorodischer, R. (2003). *J. Pharm. Pharmacol.*, 55: 911–919.
- Song, Y.K., Kim, C.K. (2006). *Biomaterials*, 27: 271–280.
- Souto, E.B., Muller, R.H. (2006). *Pharmazie*, 61(5): 431–437.
- Souto, E.B., Muller, R.H. (2005). *J. Microencapsul.*, 22(5): 501–510.
- Souto, E.B., Wissing, S.A., Barbosa, C.M., Muller, R.H. (2004). *J. Cosmet. Sci.*, 55(5): 463–471.
- Spiclin, P.] Homara, M., Zupan¡ci¡c-Valant, A., Gašperlin, M. (2003). *Int. J. Pharm.* 256: 65–73.
- Sun, Y.M., Huang, J.J., Lin, F.C., Lai, J.Y. (1997). *Biomaterials*, 18: 527–533.
- Teeranachaideekul, V., Muller, R.H., Junyaprasert, V.B. (2007a). *Int. J. Pharm.*, 340: 198–206.
- Teeranachaideekul, V., Souto, E.B., Junyaprasert, V.B., Rainer H., Muller, R.H. (2007b). *Eur. J. Pharm. Biopahrm.*, 67: 141–148.
- Tojo, K., Valia, K.H., Chotani, G., Chien, Y.W. (1985). *Drug Dev. Ind. Pharm.*, 11: 1175–93.
- Touitou, E. Composition of applying active substance to or through the skin. **US patent, 5,716,638, 1996**.
- Touitou, E., Levi-Schaffer, F., Dayan, N., Alhaique, F., Riccieri, F. (1994). *Int. J. Pharm.*, 30: 131–136.
- Touitou, E., Dayan, N., Bergelson, L., Godin, B., Eliaz, M. (2000). *J. Control. Release*, 65: 403–418.
- Trotta, M., Peira, E., Carlotti, M.E., Gallarate, M. (2004). *Int. J. Pharm.*, 270: 119–125.

- Trotta, M., Peira, E., Debernadi, F., Gallarate, M. (2003). *Int. J. Pharm.*, 241:319–327.
- Trotta, M., Peira, E., Debernardi, F., Gallarate, M. (2002). *Int. J. Pharm.*, 241: 319–327.
- Uner, M., Wissing, S.A., Yener, G., Muller, R.H. (2005). *Pharmazie*, 60(8): 577–582.
- Valia, K.H., Tojo, K., Chien, Y.W. (1985). *Drug Dev. Ind. Pharm.*, 11: 1133–73.
- van Hal, D., van Rensen, A., Junginger, H., Bouwstra, J. (1996). *STP Pharma.*, 6: 72–78.
- van den Bergh, B.A.I., Wertz, P.W., Junginger, H.E., Bouwstra, J.A. (2001). *Int. J. Pharm.*, 217: 13–24.
- van den Bergh, B.A.I., Bouwstra, J.A., Junginger, H.E., Wertz, P.W. (1999a). *J. Control. Rel.*, 62: 367–379.
- van den Bergh, B.A.I., Vroom, J., Junginger, H.E., Bouwstra, J.A. (1999b). *Biochim. Biophys. Acta*, 146: 155–173.
- Villalobos-Hernandez, J.R., Muller-Goymann, C.C. (2007). *Eur. J. Pharma. Biopharm.*, 65: 122–125.
- Walters, K.A.J., Hadgraft, R.H., Guy (Eds.) (1989). **Transdermal Drug Delivery, Developmental Issues and Research Initiatives**, Marcel Dekker, New York, pp. 197–246.
- Wang, J.X., Sun, X., Zhang, Z.R. (2002). *Eur. J. Pharm. Biopharm.*, 54(3): 285–290.
- Wertz, P.W., Swartzendruber, D.C., Kitko, D.J., Madison, K.C., Downing, D.T. (1989). *J. Invest. Dermatol.*, 93: 169–172.
- Westesen, K., Siekmann, B. (1997). *Int. J. Pharm.*, 151: 35–45.
- Whyte, A., Ockleford, C.D., Byrne, S., Hubbard, A., Woolley, S.T. (1996). *J. Comp. Pathol.*, 115: 429–440.
- Williams, A.C., Barry B.W. (1992). *Crit. Rev. Ther. Drug Carr. Sys.*, 9: 305–53.
- Woodford, R., Barry, B.W. (1982). *J. Invest. Dermatol.*, 79: 388–391.
- Woodford, R., Barry, B.W. (1983). *Br. J. Dermatol.*, 89: 53–56.
- Yu, H.Y., Liao, H.M. (1996). *Int. J. Pharm.*, 127: 1–7.

8

Rectal Drug Delivery

Subheet Kumar Jain, A.K. Tiwary, Nikhil Sahajpal, Mohit Mahajan and N.K. Jain

INTRODUCTION

During the last 25 years great advancements have been made in drug formulations and innovative routes of administration have been reported. Our understanding of drug transport across tissues has increased. Although administration via the peroral route is the most commonly targeted goal of new drug and dosage form research and development, oral administration is not always feasible (from the formulation point of view) or desirable (for therapeutic reasons). The potential for oral dosage form development is severely limited for active agents that are poorly absorbed in the upper gastrointestinal (GI) tract and unstable to proteolytic enzymes. Some agents cause local stomach or upper GI irritation or require doses in excess of 500 mg. In some circumstances, oral drug delivery becomes impractical or even impossible (nausea, vomiting, convulsion, uncooperative or unconscious patients). Further, certain patient populations, notably children, the elderly, and those with swallowing problems, are often difficult to treat with oral tablets and capsules. Additionally, treatment of some diseases is best achieved by direct administration near the affected area, particularly with diseases involving ophthalmic, otic, dermal, oral cavity, and anorectal tissues. Although oral administration can be employed for drugs targeted for some of these diseased tissues, exposure of the entire body compartment to the administered drug is inefficient and can lead to undesired adverse effects. Rectal drug administration is amenable, however, to both local and systemic drug delivery. It has been effectively utilized to treat local diseases of the anorectal area as well as to deliver drugs systemically as an alternative to oral administration. Rectal administration provides rapid absorption of many drugs and may be an easy alternative to the intravenous route, having the advantage of being relatively painless, and have fast absorption of drugs (de Boer & Breimer, 1981).

RECTAL ROUTE OF DELIVERY

Administration of medicaments using rectal mucosa is called rectal drug delivery. The human rectum is the body cavity from which drugs can be easily administered either for local or systemic drug delivery. The feasibility and effectiveness of this route has been examined for the delivery of low as well as high molecular weight drugs. The main advantages of the rectal mucosal membrane are its thickness and vascularity in comparison with the colon. Another reason for preferring this route is that when drugs are delivered rectally, the liver can perhaps be avoided to some extent. The rectum's venous drainage is two-thirds systemic (middle and inferior rectal vein) and one-third portal (superior rectal vein), thus the rectal route bypasses around two-thirds of the first pass metabolism. Therefore, the drug reaches the circulatory system with significantly less alterations and in higher concentrations [Aulton, 2002]. However, one of the main problems with this route is patient acceptability. Rectal suppositories can be formulated by using a lipophilic or a hydrophilic base. These bases, along with other incorporated absorption promoters and enzyme inhibitors, help in improving the bioavailability of water-soluble compounds. The rectal dosage forms are prepared by considering all the major physical and chemical factors, including pKa, drug solubility, distribution coefficient and particle size. The rectal delivery route still lacks any significant progress or major breakthrough with regard to its application in humans (Morimoto et al., 1984, 1985; Hosny, 2001). Historically, the rectum also has fewer amounts of degradative enzymes in comparison with other traditional routes.

Advantages (Tramonte et al., 1997; Loyd & Allen, 2000)

A drug becomes a candidate for rectal administration when it is poorly absorbed from the upper (GI) tract, unstable to proteolytic enzymes, irritating to the stomach or upper GI tract, or difficult to be administered orally, such as with the very young or old patients. Depending upon formulation characteristics, suppositories or other rectal products can be used for localized or systemic drug delivery. Rectal dosage forms can deliver drug quantities greater than oral dosing allows in some cases. Of the types of rectal dosage forms, suppositories constitute

approximately 98% of current products administered rectally. The vehicle may be composed of one of the following: fatty bases with a low melting point; water-soluble (dissolving) components or glycerinated gelatin; or hydrogels (controlled release). The suppository can weigh up to 1 gram in pediatric and 2.5 grams in adult formulations. They are made to dissolve or melt at approximately 36–37°C. Solutions and suspensions are less frequently used because of inconvenience with administration, leakage, and in some instances, difficulties in long-term stability. Product spreading can be affected by viscosity and volume characteristics of the formulation. Drug absorption from solutions and suspensions can exceed that from suppositories in some cases (Shojaei, 1998; De Felippis, 2003; Song et al., 2004).

Although no doubt peroral route is the most preferred and targeted goal of new drugs and dosage forms yet rectal administration can be used as an alternative route in certain cases of therapeutic importance.

- In cases of nausea and vomiting, the act of taking medication orally may induce emesis so that drug is vomited before it is absorbed.
- Irritation to the stomach and small intestine associated with certain drugs can be avoided.
- Hepatic first pass elimination of high clearance drugs may be avoided partially (de Boer et al., 1979; de Boer and Breimer, 1997).
- Contact with digestive fluid is avoided, thereby preventing acidic and enzymatic degradation of some drugs.
- When oral intake is restricted, such as prior to X-ray studies, before surgery or in patients having disease of upper GI tract or when patient is unable to swallow.
- Useful in pediatric, geriatric and unconscious patients, severely debilitated patients, those who cannot take medications orally and those for whom the parenteral route might be unsuitable.
- Removing the dosage form can stop drug delivery and drug absorption can be easily

terminated in cases of accidental overdose or suicide attempts.

- Drugs, which traditionally are only given parenterally, may be administered rectally either as such or in combination with absorption promoting additives (Caldwell et al., 1983).
- Suppositories are used to administer drugs for either systemic or local application. Local applications include the treatment of hemorrhoids, itching and infections.
- Systemic application is used for a variety of drugs, including antinauseants, antiasthmatics, analgesics and hormones. For example, extemporaneously compounded suppositories containing metoclopramide, haloperidol, dexamethasone, diphenhydramine and benztropine can be administered prophylactically to effectively control severe nausea and vomiting, and a prolonged release morphine alkaloid suppository for chronic pain has been used.
- Overcome the first pass metabolism and improved bioavailability.
- In cases where rapid absorption of low molecular weight drugs is required.
- It offers to be a potential administrative site for drug delivery to lymphatic system.
- Large amount of drug can be administered, especially for rate-controlled drug delivery systems.

Disadvantages (Laxshmi et al., 2012)

- Many drugs are poorly or erratically absorbed across the rectal mucosa.
- Rectal administration offers a limited surface area for absorption.
- The formulation is subjected to dissolution problems due to the small fluid volume of the rectum.
- Drug metabolism in rectum may be altered due to varying microorganisms and mucosa.

ANATOMY AND PHYSIOLOGY OF RECTAL MUCOSA

Gastrointestinal research and training focuses upon digestive disease, with an almost complete avoidance of the sexual function and pathophysiology of the rectum. The upper GI tract is comparably more rugged as it is equipped to handle the wide variety of foods and substances ingested through the mouth. The colon/rectum is more fragile as it receives processed foods that have been broken down into simpler, more standardized components. It is a poor barrier to pathogens, while at the same time it hosts a variety of friendly bacteria that aid in the processes of digestion and maintenance of colonic health (de Boer et al., 1982; Song et al., 2004).

The layers of the colorectal wall, proceeding inward from the exterior, are a perirectal adipose (fatty) tissue supported by pelvic fascia, muscular propria, submucosa, and mucosa. The rectum is a reservoir 8–13 cm in length that ends with the voluntary muscles of the sphincter. It is a sensate organ that perceives its solid, liquid, and gaseous content and adjusts appropriately. Muscular control is both visceral and somatic. Signalling pathways of comfort and discomfort are closely associated with those of the genital and urinary muscular system, explaining the pleasure that many experience with anal sex (Swarbrick, 1987).

The submucosa can be compared to nylon; it is a web-like loose connective tissue capable of a great deal of stretch. The mucosa, comprising about 10% of the thickness of the rectal wall, is more like an accordion, expanding and contracting along its many folds. The mucosa in turn is divided into the epithelium, lamina propria and muscularis mucosa. The muscularis mucosa (not to be confused with the muscular propria) is smooth muscle tissue a few cell layers thick that lies at the base of the mucosa. The lamina propria is the structural network that connects the folds and crypts of the epithelium to the muscularis mucosa (Agra et al., 1998).

The single-cell thick rectal epithelium consists primarily of goblet cells and absorptive cells. Goblet cells contain mucus granules that are secreted as mucin to coat the tissue surface.

Absorptive cells are cone-like arrangements of microvilli that absorb water and some electrolytes. Epithelial crypts are tubular glands with a generative zone at the base; as cells mature they migrate to the surface. Thin strands of muscle help to provide structure to the crypts (Caldwell et al., 1983a-b).

The lamina propria is a structure of stromal cells that contain blood, lymphatic and nerve networks, as well as a resident population of inflammatory cells that include macrophages, lymphocytes, plasma cells and eosinophils. The real barrier to the outside world is a single layer of epithelial cells attached to a collagenous foundation. There may be spots in the rectum where the muscular mucosa is not complete, resulting in direct interaction between the crypt epithelium and lymphoid tissue in the sub-mucosa. These may be particularly vulnerable points for the entry of pathogens (Morimoto et al., 1985).

The mucosa is a delicate tissue that can be damaged by such relatively benign actions as oral cathartics, enemas, or hard stools. Thus, endoscopic examination and anal sex are likely to cause some degree of trauma. With trauma the secreted layer of mucin is depleted, as are the tall columnar cells of the crypts, and blood cells proliferate. Damage may consist of congestion and hemorrhage in the lamina propria, and may sometimes include detached

epithelium and inflammatory cell infiltration. The ano-rectal juncture brings a transition from glandular to squamous mucosal cell structure and a transition from smooth to voluntary muscles (Berko et al., 2002).

Rectal absorption

The absorption of drugs from the rectal epithelium involves the transcellular and the paracellular routes. The mechanism of uptake is dependent on the drug lipophilicity in the transcellular route, whereas drug diffusion through the spaces in the epithelial cells is the uptake mechanism in paracellular route [de Boer et al., 1992]. The absorption of systemically active drugs from rectal dosage forms involves release of drug in the rectum, diffusion to the rectal mucosa, absorption by the tissues and transport into general circulation. Depending on the height at which drug release occurs in the rectum and carried by the interior, middle or superior haemorrhoidal veins, drug carried by the inferior or middle veins goes directly into

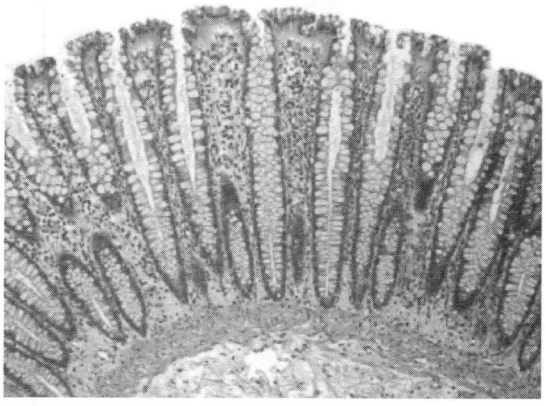

Fig. 8.1. Anatomy of rectal mucosa.

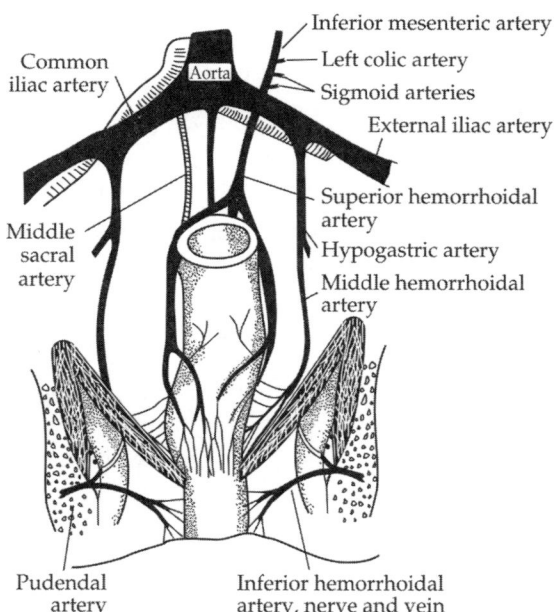

Fig. 8.2. Blood distribution pattern across the rectal mucosa.

the circulation (via the inferior vena cava) and bypasses the liver, to which the drug in the superior vein (and in the blood vessels from the large intestine in the case of orally administered drugs) is first transported (Moolennar & Schoonen, 1980).

It was once believed that medicaments from rectal dosage forms were largely transported by the inferior and middle hemorrhoid veins and, consequently, that rectal administration of drugs provided a means of avoiding degradation of drug by the liver and damage of the liver by the drug. However, it appears that a suppository may travel far enough into the rectum for much of its medicaments to be transported by the superior vein and, therefore, it is unwise to rely on these advantages (Klotz and Schwab, 2005).

Factors affecting rectal absorption

Rectal administration provides rapid absorption of many drugs and may be an easy alternative to the intravenous route, having the advantage of being relatively painless, and usually no more threatening to children. However, rectal administration of drugs should be avoided in immunosuppressed patients in whom even minimal trauma could lead to formation of an abscess (Ritschel et al., 1988).

The most important concern for the practitioner is irregular uptake due to clinically important patient-to-patient variability. The absorption of the drug may be delayed or prolonged, or uptake may be almost as rapid as if an intravenous bolus were administered, which may cause adverse cardiovascular or central nervous system effects. One reported death after rectal administration of multiple doses of morphine underscores the importance of being aware of this factor (Matsuda and Arima, 1999; Gourlay and Boas, 1992).

Factors affecting rectal transmucosal absorption

- Formulation (time to liquefaction of suppositories)
- Volume of liquid
- Concentration of drug
- Length of rectal catheter (site of drug delivery)
- Presence of stool in the rectal vault
- pH of the rectal contents
- Rectal retention of drug(s) administered
- Differences in venous drainage within the rectosigmoid region
- Partition coefficient of drug
- Physical state of medicament
- Presence of adjuncts in base

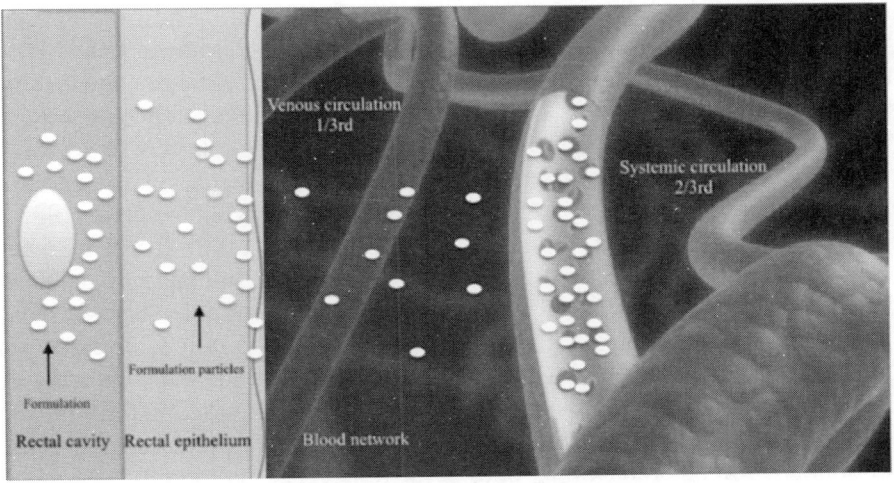

Fig. 8.3. Process of rectal absorption.

Anatomical differences in hemorrhoidal venous drainage of the rectum may substantially influence the systemic drug level achieved. Drugs administered high in the rectum (drained by the superior rectal veins) are usually carried directly to the liver and, thus, are subject to metabolism. Drugs administered low in the rectum are delivered systemically by the inferior and middle rectal veins before passing through the liver (van Hoogdalem et al., 1991a-b; Choonara, 1987; Khalil et al., 1990). Problems may occur with drugs that normally have a high hepatic extraction ratio. The clinical implications of rectal venous drainage for absorption and metabolism of most drugs are not well defined.

Diluent's volume is also an important determinant of rectal drug uptake, as demonstrated with methohexital administered rectally for pre-procedure sedation. Equivalent deep sedation was achieved with 25 mg/kg of a 10% solution (0.25 mL/kg) and with 15 mg/kg of a 2% solution (0.75 mL/kg). Peak blood levels of the drug, however, were significantly higher for a longer time in the children treated with the 2% solution. This finding could have important clinical implications for the depth and duration of sedation (Forbes and Vandewalker, 1988).

Rectal pH may also influence drug uptake by altering the amount of drug that is ionized. The greater lipid solubility of non-ionized drugs enhances their movement across biological membranes (van Hoogdalem et al., 1989, 1991a). The pH of the rectal vault in children ranges from 7.2 to 12.2 (Laub et al., 1990). This pH range favors absorption of the barbiturates that will remain in a non-ionized state because their pK_a is near the physiologic range (~7.6) (Stillwell, 1992).

Despite the limitations associated with drug absorption in the rectum, many drugs usually administered by the intravenous and orogastric routes have also been administered rectally. Sedatives commonly administered by this route include midazolam, diazepam, and ketamine (Laishley et al., 1986; Roelfse et al., 1990; Malinovsky et al., 1993; De Jong and Verburg, 1988). In children, the rectal route is convenient for the administration of benzodiazepines to treat status epilepticus because an intravenous line is not required (Gaudreault et al., 1988; Laub et al., 1990). The rectal dose generally must be higher than the dose administered intravenously or orally. The extent of the increase depends on the factors that affect absorption. The most important considerations are the slow onset of effect (minutes) and the prolonged duration of effect (hours). The peak blood levels vary considerably from patient to patient. The potential for rapid and almost complete absorption has serious implications when drugs with cardiac or pulmonary depressant effects are administered. Practitioners must be prepared to monitor the patient after drug administration and to manage an emergency should it occur; equipment suited to the size of the patient is required. The patient also may expel an immeasurable amount of the drug, which makes it difficult for the practitioner to decide how much more of the drug to administer.

Several drug characteristics are responsible for absorption of the drugs from the rectum. The partition coefficient, molecular weight, charge and hydrogen bond forming capacity play a crucial role in drug absorption. Small partition coefficient, high molecular weight, high charge and capacity to hydrogen bond formation are the factors associated with poor absorption of the drug. Further, the aqueous and alcoholic solutions are absorbed faster than the suspensions and suppositories [Moolner et al., 1985].

Drugs with a high fat to water partition coefficient are liberated relatively slowly from fatty bases. Partitioning between bases and rectal fluid is also affected by extremely variable volume of water in the rectum at different times and in different individuals; this volume is often very small. Formulation of a medicament in a different base may significantly alter release and absorption rates (Gourlay and Boas, 1992; Van

Hoogdalem et al., 1991b; Choonara, 1987; Khalil et al., 1990; Forbes and Vandewalker, 1988).

Rectal absorption of drug is significantly affected by the physical state of medicament e.g. the absorption of a medicament in suspension is limited by its dissolution rate and, therefore, when a drug is formulated as a suspension in suppository it is advantageous to use a fine powder to increase surface area.

Emulsifying agents (e.g. emulsifying wax, wool fat, wool alcohols, macrogol stearates and polysorbates) may be included in suppository bases to facilitate incorporation of aqueous solution or polar liquids, but they should be used with caution, as their effects on release and absorption are not always predictable. The presence of emulgents may complicate preparation of suppositories by causing foam in the base and bubble in the product. The possibility that inclusion of a powerful surface-active agent may cause greatly increased absorption of a medicament, with consequent toxic effects, must be borne in mind.

RECTAL PREPARATIONS

Rectal preparations are ideal for young infants, debilitated patients, or those who cannot tolerate oral intake. These preparations can be used for systemic or local administration. Local applications include the treatment of hemorrhoids, itching, inflammation, and infections. Systemic applications promote rapid onset of action for antinauseants, anti-asthmatics, antipyretics, analgesics, and hormones (Zempsky et al., 1998). The different dosage forms that are designed for rectal administration are:

- Suppositories
- Enema
- Ointment, cream and aerosol foams
- Jellies and gels
- Rectal capsules
- Contraceptive sponge
- Intrauterine progesterone drug delivery system
- Suspension

SUPPOSITORIES

The origin of the word suppositories is Latin, meaning 'to place under'. Suppositories are solid dosage forms intended to deliver medicine into the rectal, vaginal, or urethral orifice where they melt, soften or dissolve and exert localized or systemic action. Suppositories are commonly employed rectally, vaginally, and occasionally urethrally. They have various shapes and weights. The shape and size of a suppository must be such that it is capable of being easily inserted into the intended body orifice without causing undue distension, and once inserted, it must be retained for the appropriate period of time. Rectal suppositories are generally inserted with fingers, but certain vaginal suppositories, particularly the vaginal "inserts" or vaginal tablets prepared by compression may be inserted high in the vaginal tract with the aid of a special insertion appliance (Norton, 1996). The suppository types and their implications with respective drugs has been summarized in Table 8.1 (Gupta P.J., 2007).

Types of suppositories
(Ansel and Popovich, 1990)

Rectal suppositories

The USP describes rectal suppositories for adults as tapered at one or other ends and usually weighing about 2 g each. Infant rectal suppositories usually weigh about one-half that of adults suppositories. Drugs having systemic effects, such as sedatives, tranquilizers and analgesics, are administered by rectal suppository; however, the largest single use category is probably that of hemorrhoid remedies dispensed over the counter. The 2 g weight for adult rectal suppositories is based on use of cocoa butter as the base; when other bases are used the weights may be greater or less than 2 g (Table 8.2).

Vaginal suppositories

The USP describes vaginal suppositories as

Table 8.1. Different types of suppositories in clinical use

Suppository type	Drugs	Implications	Adverse effects
Local anesthetic	Lignocaine, cinchocaine	Anal pain due to strangulated hemorrhoids, anal fissure, post anal surgery	Local irritation and anal proctitis
Steroids	Hydrocortisone, prednisolone	Hemorrhoids, anal fissures, pruritus ani	Systemic absorption on prolonged use
Astringent	Zinc oxide, allantoin	Bleeding hemorrhoids, anal cryptitis	Local reaction
Antiseptic	Boric acid, benzalkonium chloride	Proctitis, fissures	Pruritus, local irritation

Table 8.2. Examples of rectal suppositories

Suppository	Commercial product	Suppliers	Strength (per suppository)	Type of effect	Category
Hydrocortisone acetate	Anusol-HC	Monarch Pharm, Bristol	20 mg	Local	Anti-inflammatory
Bisacodyl	Dulcolax suppositories	Boehringer Ingelheim	10 mg	Local	Cathartic
Chlorpromazine	Thorazine suppositories	Smith, Kline & French	25–100 mg	Systemic	Anti-emetic, tranquilizer
Ergotamine tartarate and caffeine	Cafergol suppositories	Sandoz	Ergotamine tartarate (2 mg); Caffeine (100 mg)	Systemic	Anti-adrenergic
Indomethacin	Indocin suppositories	Merck Sharp & Dohme	50 mg	Systemic	NSAID
Prochlorperazine	Compazine suppositories	Smith, Kline & French	2.5, 5.0 & 25 mg	Systemic	Anti-emetic
Promethazine HCl	Phenergan rectal suppositories	Wyeth-Ayerst	12.5, 25 & 50 mg	Systemic	Antihistaminic, anti-emetic, sedative

usually globular or oviform and weighing about 5 g each. Vaginal medications are available in a variety of physical forms e.g., creams, gels or liquids, which depart from the classical concept of suppositories. Vaginal tablets, however, do meet the definition, and represent convenience both of administration and manufacture (Table 8.3).

Urethral suppositories

Urethral suppositories (sometimes referred to as bougies) are not described specifically in the USP, either by weight or dimension. Traditional values, based on use of cocoa butter as base, for these cylindrical dosage forms are as follows: diameter, 5 mm; length, 50 mm female, 15 mm male; weight, 2 g female, 4 g male. Urethral suppositories are an unusual dosage form and are seldom encountered.

HISTORY

Suppositories, pessaries and bougies have been prescribed for the last 2000 years but their popularity as a medicinal form increased from around 1840. Suppositories for constipation, haemorrhoids and later as an alternative method

Table 8.3. Examples of vaginal suppositories

Active drug	Commercial product	Suppliers	Category and use
Sulfanilamide	AVC suppositories	Merrell Dow	Treatment of *Candida albicans* infections
Povidone-iodine	Betadine medicated vaginal suppositories	Purdue Federick	Relief of vaginitis due to *Candida albicans*, *Trichomonas*, and *Gardnerella vaginalis*
Clotrimazole	Gyne-Lotrimin vaginal tablets	Schering	Treatment of vulvovaginal candidiasis
Nystatin	Mycostatin vaginal tablets	Squibb	Local treatment of vulvovaginal candidiasis
Nonoxynol-9	Semicid vaginal contraceptive	Whitehall	Non-sysytemic reversible method of birth control
Sulfathiazole, sulfacetamide, sulfabenzamide and urea	Sultrin vaginal tablets	Ortho	Treatment of *Haemophilus vaginalis* vaginitis
Aminoacridine, polyoxyethylene nonyl phenol and docusate sodium	Vagisec plus suppositories	Schmid	Treatment of vaginitis caused by *T. vaginalis* and mixed infection

of drug administration, pessaries for vaginal infections and bougies for infections of the urethra, prostrate, bladder or nose (Taylor, 1990).

PRODUCT DEVELOPMENT

In general, when formulating suppositories, the pharmacist should consider whether the desired effect is to be systemic or local, the route of administration (rectal, vaginal or urethral) and whether a rapid or a slow and prolonged release of the medication is desired. A suppository that does not release its medication within six hours may not be completely utilized and may be expelled by the patient. The selection of a suppository base is dependent upon a number of physicochemical variables, including the solubility characteristics of the drug. To obtain maximum release of the drug from the base, a principle of opposite characteristics can be employed.

Fat-soluble bases, e.g., cocoa butter, *melt* quickly in the rectum to release the drug, whereas polyethylene glycol bases must *dissolve* in mucosal fluids, a process which may take longer. If higher molecular weight polyethylene glycols

are used, the time for dissolution is extended. Moistening with warm water immediately prior to insertion facilitates not only insertion but also dissolution. Drug release rate requirements are important in the selection of the suppository base. Factors such as the presence of water, hygroscopicity, viscosity, brittleness, density, volume contraction, special problems, incompatibilities, rate of drug release, pharmacokinetics and bioequivalence are important.

Presence of water

The presence of water, or using water to assist in incorporating an active drug, generally should be avoided in the preparation of suppositories. Water may accelerate the oxidation of fat, increase the degradation rate of many drugs, enhance reactions between the drug and other components in the suppository, support bacterial/fungal growth and require the addition of bacteriostatic agents. Further, if the water evaporates, the dissolved substances may crystallize.

Hygroscopicity

Polyethylene glycol-containing suppositories are

hygroscopic. The rate of moisture change is dependent on the chain length of the molecule, as well as on the temperature and humidity of the environment. Polyethylene glycols with molecular weight greater than 4,000 have lesser tendency to be hygroscopic than the lower weight PEGs.

Viscosity

Viscosity considerations are important in the preparation of the suppositories and the release of the drug. During preparation, if the viscosity of a base is low, it may be necessary to add a suspending agent such as silica gel to keep the drug uniformly dispersed until solidification. Also, the melt should be handled at the lowest temperature possible to maintain high viscosity and should be constantly stirred. If the viscosity of the base, after administration and when in the body, is very high, the release rate of the drug may be slowed due to a decrease in the diffusion of the drug through the base to reach the mucosal membrane for absorption. Approaches that have been utilized to increase viscosity would be to increase the fatty acid chain length of compounds in the base. For example, increased C-16 and C-18 mono- and di-glycerides can be added to the base. The addition of about 2% aluminum monostearate will also increase the viscosity of a fatty base; cety, stearyl and myristyl alcohols and stearic acid can also be used in concentrations of about 5% (Yamamoto & Muranishi, 1997).

Brittleness

Brittle suppositories can be difficult to handle, wrap and use. Cocoa butter suppositories generally are not brittle unless there is a high percentage of a solid present. When the percentage of nonbase materials exceeds about 30%, brittleness can result. Synthetic fat bases with high stearate concentrations or those that are highly hydrogenated are usually more brittle. Fracturing of fat and cocoa butter suppositories

may also result from shock cooling, which may be prevented by ensuring that the temperature of the mold is as close to the melted base temperature as possible. Placing suppositories in a freezer should be avoided, which would also cause shock cooling. Also, the addition of a small quantity (usually less than 2%) of Tween 80, Tween 85, fatty acid monoglycerides, castor oil, glycerin or propylene glycol will make these bases more pliable and less brittle.

Density

Density of the incorporated materials is important in the determination of the weight of the individual suppositories.

Volume contraction

Bases, excipients and active ingredients generally will occupy less space at lower temperatures than at higher temperatures. When a hot suppository melt is placed in a mold it usually will have a tendency to contract in size during cooling. This can result in a good release of the suppository from the mold but may also result in formation of such a cavity at the back, or open end, of the suppository mold. The presence of such a cavity is undesirable and can be corrected by allowing the melt to approach its congealing temperature immediately prior to pouring into the molds. It may be advisable to pour a small excess at the open end of the mold to accommodate slight contraction during cooling. Scraping with a blade or spatula will remove the excess after solidification.

Special problems

Vegetable extracts can be moistened by levigation with a small amount of melted base prior to incorporating. This will make it easier to distribute the active drug throughout the base. Hard, crystalline materials can be incorporated either by pulverizing to a very fine state of sub-division, or by dissolving in a small quantity of solvent and taking the solution up into the base.

If the material is water-soluble, an aqueous solvent and poly ethylene glycol base would be appropriate. Alternatively, if the material is oil-soluble and an oily solvent must be used, wool fat could be used to take up the solution for incorporation into the suppository base. Liquid ingredients, when mixed with an inert powder such as starch, will be less fluid, making them easier to handle, and the subsequent suppository will hold together better. Excess powder may be incorporated into a suppository base in different ways, depending upon the base used. For oil-miscible bases, a few drops of bland oil like mineral oil may be used. When incorporating excess powder into water-soluble bases, the ratio of low to high melting point ingredients may be varied. For example, since the addition of extra powders will make the suppository harder, a higher percentage of low molecular weight polyethylene glycols would help prepare a suppository of the proper density.

Incompatibilities

A number of ingredients are incompatible with polyethylene glycol bases, and include benzocaine, iodochlorhydroxyquin, sulfonamides, ichthammol, aspirin, silver salts and tannic acid. Other materials reported to have a tendency to crystallize out of polyethylene glycol include sodium barbital, salicylic acid and camphor.

Rate of drug release

The time for liquefaction of a hydrogenated vegetable oil or cocoa butter based suppository is approximately 3–7 minutes; for a glycerinated gelatin suppository about 30–40 minutes and for a polyethylene glycol suppository 30–50 minutes. The release of the drug and the onset of the drug action are dependent upon the liquefaction of the suppository base, dissolution of the active drug and diffusion of the drug through the mucosal layers. Table 8.4 provides a general summary of the relationship of drug release and the suppository base.

Table 8.4. Drug : Base release relationship

Drug : Base characteristic	Approximate drug release rate
Oil-soluble drug : oily base	Slow release
Water-soluble drug : oily base	Rapid release
Oil-soluble drug : water-miscible base	Moderate release rate
Water-miscible drug : water-miscible base	Moderate release based on diffusion

SUPPOSITORY BASES
(Thompson et al., 1992)

A suppository base should be stable, non-irritating, chemically and physiologically inert, compatible with a variety of drugs, melt or dissolve in rectal fluids, stable during storage, not bind or otherwise interfere with the release or absorption of drug substances and be aesthetically acceptable. Other desirable characteristics depend upon the drugs to be added. For example, higher melting point bases can be selected for incorporating drugs that generally lower the melting points of the base or when formulating suppositories for use in tropical climates. Lower melting point bases can be used when adding materials that will raise the melting points or if adding large amounts of solids (Table 8.4).

Oil-soluble bases

Cocoa butter, or theobroma oil, is an oleaginous base that softens at 30°C and melts at 34°C. It contains four different forms; alpha, beta, beta prime and gamma with melting points of 22°C, 34-35°C, 28°C and 18°C, respectively. The beta form is the most stable and is desired for suppositories. Cocoa butter will melt to form non-viscous, bland oil. However, it may leak from the body orifice, as it is immiscible with body fluids. The lower melting point polymorphs eventually will convert to the more stable form over time. Chloral hydrate will decrease the melting point of cocoa butter. Cocoa butter suppositories will release best from molds if the molds are absolutely clean and dry and the cocoa butter has not been overheated. Otherwise, mold sticking may be a problem.

Hydrogenated vegetable oil bases

Fattibase™ is a pre-blended suppository base that offers the advantages of a cocoa butter base with few of the drawbacks. It is composed of triglycerides derived from palm, palm kernel and coconut oils with self-emulsifying glyceryl monostearate and polyoxyl stearate used as emulsifying and suspending agents. It is stable with a low irritation profile, needs no special storage conditions, is uniform in composition and has a bland taste and controlled melting range. It exhibits excellent mold release characteristics and does not require mold lubrication. Fatty base is a solid, which has a melting point of 35–37°C and a specific gravity of 0.890 at 37°C; it is opaque-white and free of suspended matter.

Wecobee® bases are derived from palm kernel and coconut oils, and the incorporation of glyceryl monostearate and propylene glycol monostearate renders them emulsifiable. These bases exhibit most of the desirable features of cocoa butter but few of its shortcomings. They are stable and exhibit excellent mold release characteristics.

Witepsol® bases solidify rapidly in the mold and lubrication is not necessary as the suppositories contract nicely. High melting point Witepsol bases can be mixed with low melting point Witepsol bases to provide a wide range of possible melting ranges, i.e., 34–44°C. Since the Witepsol bases contain emulsifiers, they will absorb limited quantities of water.

Water-soluble bases

The use of water-soluble bases may result in some irritation because, as they take up water and dissolve, they may produce slight dehydration of the rectal mucosa. They are widely used, however, and release the drug by dissolving and mixing with the aqueous body fluids. Polyethylene glycol (PEG) suppository bases are the most popular in this class. They have the advantage in that the ratios of the low to the high molecular weight individual PEGs can be altered to prepare a base with a specific melting point, or one that will overcome the adverse characteristics of an excess of powder or liquid that must be incorporated into a suppository. PEG bases are listed as incompatible with silver salts, tannic acid, aminopyrine, quinine, ichthammol, aspirin, benzocaine, iodochlorhydroxyquin and sulfonamides. Sodium barbital, salicylic acid and camphor will crystallize out of PEG suppositories. High concentrations of salicylic acid will soften PEGs, and aspirin will complex with polyethylene glycols. PEG-based suppositories may be irritating to some patients. Suppositories prepared with PEG should not be stored or dispensed in a polystyrene prescription vial, as the PEG will adversely interact with polystyrene. All PEG suppositories should be dispensed in glass or cardboard containers. Polybase™ is a pre-blended suppository base that is a white solid consisting of a homogeneous mixture of PEGs and Polysorbate 80. It is a water-miscible base that is stable at room temperature, has a specific gravity of 1.177 at 25°C with an average molecular weight of 3440 and does not require mold lubrication.

MANUFACTURING PROCESS
(Petticrew et al., 1997)

The basic method of manufacture was the same for each preparation but the shape differed. Suppositories were 'bullet' or 'torpedo' shaped, pessaries 'bullet' shaped but larger and bougies long and thin, tapering slightly. A base was required that would melt at body temperature. Various oils and fats have been utilized but, until the advent of modern manufactured waxes, the substances of choice were theobroma oil (cocoa butter) and a glycerin-gelatin mixture.

The base was heated in a spouted pan over a water-bath until just melted. The medicament was rubbed into a little of the base (usually on a tile using a spatula) and then stirred into the rest. The melted mass was then poured into the relevant mould. Moulds were normally in two parts, made from stainless steel or brass (silver or electroplated to give a smooth surface). To facilitate removal, the moulds were treated with a lubricant such as oil or soap solution. To overcome the difficulty of pouring into the long, thin bougie mould, it was usual to make a larger quantity of base, to partially unscrew the mould, fill with base and then screw the two halves of the mould together thus forcing out the excess. When cool, any excess base was scraped from the top of the mould, the mould opened and the preparations removed, packed and labelled.

STABILITY (Stilwell, 1992)

The USP description of stability considerations for suppositories includes observations for excessive softening and evidence of oil stains on packaging materials. It may be necessary for the pharmacist to examine individual suppositories closely by removing any wrappers used for their packaging.

According to the USP, excessive softening is the major indication of instability in suppositories. Some suppositories may dry out, harden or shrivel. As a general rule, the USP recommends storage in a refrigerator, unless otherwise indicated. Cocoa butter instability during preparation may be manifest as the formation of polymorphs, which may be liquid at room temperature. This is most easily avoided by substituting an appropriate hydrogenated vegetable oil base for the cocoa butter. If necessary, fatty materials of higher melting points such as white wax or paraffin can be added to low melting point fatty bases or cocoa butter to increase formulation melting points. However, caution must be observed to prepare a suppository that will melt when administered. Melting point can be checked easily by placing a sample

suppository into a beaker of water that has been heated to 37°C. If it does not melt, the formulation should not be used for patient therapy. If water is incorporated into an oily base using an emulsifying agent (nonionic surfactant, wool fat, etc.), the product may become rancid and will not usually be as stable as the same drug added to a PEG-based suppository containing water.

QUALITY CONTROL

The BP includes standards for appearance, uniformity of weight, disintegration and content of active ingredients. A better appreciation of the significance of these tests is obtained by applying them to the products of dispensing.

Appearance

The BP states that, when cut longitudinally and examined with naked eye, the internal and external surface of the suppositories should be uniform in appearance. Compliance with this standard indicates satisfactory subdivision and dispersion of suspended material.

Uniformity of weight

Twenty suppositories are weighed individually and the average weight determined. No suppository must deviate from average weight by more than 5% except that two may deviate by not more than 7.5%.

Disintegration

The suppository is placed in a special container with perforated ends, which is immersed in a water bath maintained at 36–38°C and stirred slowly. The container is inverted below the surface every ten minutes. Disintegration is evident by:

- Complete solution except for insoluble powders, or
- Disintegration products that are small enough to sink or rise through the perforations, or
- Complete melting of any solid matter between the plates; no solid core must be detectable.

Three suppositories are tested and all must disintegrate within 30 min, unless otherwise specified in the monograph; e.g. for Glycerol Suppositories BP the time is 1 hr.

ENEMAS

These preparations are rectal injections employed to evacuate the bowel (evacuation enemas), influence the general system absorption (retention enemas) or to affect locally the set of disease. They may possess anthelmintic, nutritive, sedative or stimulating properties, or they may contain radiopaque substances for roentgenographic examination of lower bowel. Some official retention enemas are those of aminophylline, hydrocortisone and methylprednisolone acetate (Varela and Howland, 2004; Kot and Pettit-Young, 1992). Since they are to be retained in the intestine, they should not be used in larger quantities more than 150 ml for an adult. Usually the volume is considerably smaller, such as a few ml (Bateman & Smith, 1988).

A number of drugs such as valproic acid, indomethacin and metronidazole have been formulated as microenemas for the purpose of absorption. Sulfasalazine rectal enema has been administered for the treatment of ulcerative colitis. Starch enema may be used either by itself or as a vehicle for other forms of medication. Sodium chloride, sodium bicarbonate, sodium mono- and dihydrogen phosphate are used in enemas to evacuate the bowel. These substances may be used alone, in combination with each other or in combination with irritants such as soap. The absorption of large molecular weight drugs, such as insulin, is under current investigation.

A number of solutions are administered rectally for the local effects of the medication (e.g., hydrocortisone) or for systemic absorption (e.g., aminophylline). In the case of aminophylline, the rectal route of administration minimizes the undesirable gastrointestinal reaction associated with oral therapy. Clinically effective blood levels of the agents are usually obtained within 30 minutes following rectal instillation. Corticosteroids are administered as retention enemas or continuous drip as adjunctive treatment of some patients with ulcerative colitis.

Evacuation enemas

A cleansing or evacuation enema is the technique of introducing fluid into the rectum to remove feces and flatus (gas) from the colon and rectum. Commercially, many enemas are available in disposable plastic squeeze bottles containing a premeasured amount of enema solution. The agents present are solutions of sodium phosphate and sodium biphosphate, glycerin and docusate potassium, and light mineral oil. Some other functions of cleansing or evacuation edema are (Müller-Lissner, 1988):

* To aid illumination during X-rays.
* Before surgery.
* Before testing.
* During bowel retraining programs.
* To relieve constipation and impaction.
* To instill drugs.

Types of enema solutions
(Tramonte et al., 1997)

The only enemas that are completely safe for children are mineral oil and normal saline enemas. Normal saline enemas must be made at home. Mineral oil enemas can be purchased at local drug store or Pharmacy without a prescription. Fleet's Phosphate enemas (called saline enemas on the package) can also be purchased without a prescription. One must be careful while using a phosphate enema. The dosage of phosphate enemas must be accurate because they can cause serious side effects if given in too high a dose or given more than once per day. For all enemas, the amount of solution for child depends on the child's age or weight.

Mineral oil enema

Mineral oil enemas come in one size (4.5 oz). The amount of solution will be based on child's age: 2 to 6 years – 2.0 oz (1/2 enema); greater than 6 years old – 4.5 oz.

Homemade saline solution

To give a homemade enema, we require enema bag, an enema tube, a lubricant and distilled water. Another option is to use a rubber bulb syringe (De Leede et al., 1981).

We can make a homemade saline solution by adding 2 level teaspoons of table salt to a quart of lukewarm distilled water. Do not use soapsuds, hydrogen peroxide, or plain water as an enema. They can be dangerous (Tedesco and DiPiro, 1985).

The amount of normal saline solution to be given to children at various ages is: 2 to 6 years – 6 ounces, 6 to 12 years – 12 ounces; adolescents and adults – 16 ounces.

Phosphate solution

Sodium phosphate solution is used in Fleet's enemas. These enemas can be bought at pharmacies without a prescription. Often the pharmacy will also carry a store-brand enema containing the same ingredient. The advantage of phosphate enemas is that they come in a disposable squeeze bag with a soft-tipped nozzle. They also are the most powerful enema (Wynne & Edwards, 1992).

If healthcare provider recommends giving a phosphate enema, give 1 ounce for every 20 pounds child. Don't give any child more than 4.5 ounces of the enema. Phosphate enemas come in two sizes: children (2.25. oz) and adult (4.5 oz).

Children under 2 years old should not be given a phosphate enema. Dosage is based on child's weight: 20 pounds – 1 ounce, 40 pounds – 2 ounces, 60 pounds – 3 ounces, 80 pounds – 4 ounces, 90+ pounds – 4.5 ounces.

OINTMENTS, CREAMS AND AEROSOL FOAMS

Rectal and vaginal ointments and vaginal creams are in common use. Rectal ointments are used primarily to allay local conditions as pruritus ani and to relieve the pain and discomfort associated with hemorrhoids. The drugs present are generally the same as previously discussed for rectal suppositories, including local anesthetics, analgesics, protectives, and anti-inflammatory agents. To facilitate the insertion of ointment into the rectum, each rectal ointment tube is accompanied with a special rectal insertion and delivery tip. This tip replaces the ordinary ointment cap prior to use. After placement of the rectal tip on the ointment tube, the tip is slowly and carefully inserted into the anus. The ointment tube is depressed to release the medication through the rectal tip and into the anal canal. After use, the tip should be removed from the ointment tube and replaced with the original cap. The rectal tip should be thoroughly cleaned following each use. During the product selection process, either by the physician or the patient with assistance from the pharmacist, consideration should be given to the product formulation base. Water-soluble bases are easier and less messy to clean from applicator tips than oleaginous bases. Patients should be advised by the pharmacist not to interchange rectal tips from one product to another.

Vaginal ointments and creams are typically available containing anti-infective agents, estrogens, hormonal substances and contraceptive agents. Aerosol foams are commercially available containing estrogenic substances and contraceptive agents. The foams are generally oil-in-water emulsions, resembling light creams. They are water miscible and non-greasy (Ansel & Popovich, 1990).

Rectal capsules

Soft gelatin capsules may be used for rectal medications. They are often wider at one end and if this is inserted first, pressure from the anal sphincter will force the capsule into the rectum. Some have a water-soluble coating that acts as a lubricant when the capsule is moistened in water before use. The water and glycerol contents of the shell are critical, e.g., if the glycerol content is too high the capsules will be flabby in hot climates.

The vehicle for the medicament must be non-toxic, non-irritant, and compatible with the shell. For substances with high water solubility, which will leave the vehicle readily in the body, a water immiscible vehicle, e.g., paraffin or vegetable oil may be suitable. For other drugs, water-miscible vehicles are necessary, e.g., hydro-genated oils or their ethoxylated derivatives, with dispersing agents, such as lecithin, mono-glycerides or polysorbates (Senior, 1969a-b).

INTRAUTERINE PROGESTERONE DRUG DELIVERY SYSTEM

The Progestasert Intrauterine Contraceptive System (Alza Corporation, 1988) shown in Fig. 8.4 slowly releases progesterone for a period of 1 year after insertion. The continuous release of progesterone into the uterine cavity provides a local rather than a systemic action. Two hypo-theses for the contraceptive action have been offered: progesterone-induced inhibition of sperm capacity or survival; and, alteration of the uterine milieu so as to prevent nidation. The intrauterine device contains 38 mg of progesterone, a much smaller amount than would otherwise be taken by other routes over a year period for the same purpose. The intrauterine device is replaced annually for the maintenance of contraception.

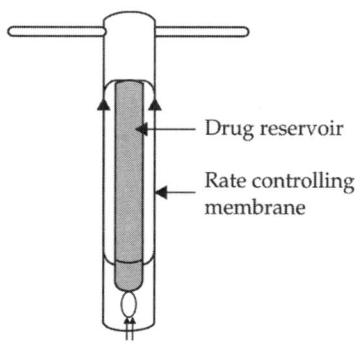

Fig. 8.4. Intrauterine progesterone pump for delivery of progesterone.

SUSPENSIONS

Barium sulfate suspension may be employed orally or rectally for the diagnostic visualization of the GI tract. Meselamine suspension was introduced onto the market in 1988 as Rowasa (Reid Rowell) for treatment of Crohn's disease, distal ulcerative colitis, proctosigmoiditis, and proctitis. Before its introduction, an extempo-raneous formulation of this suspension was necessary.

The impetus for the development of newer novel drug delivery system apart from thera-peutic efficiency is the cost. Different approaches for sustained delivery through the rectal route are summarized below (Table 8.5).

SUSTAINED RELEASE SUPPOSITORIES

The newer approach to drug delivery is to deliver drug into systemic circulation at a predetermined rate. The primary objectives of controlled drug delivery are to ensure safety and to improve efficacy of drugs as well as patient compliance. This is achieved by better control of plasma drug levels and less frequent dosing. The drug release or absorption from suppositories usually accompanies a lag time, which is generally not considered for calculation of pharmacokinetic parameters. The area under the curve (AUC), area under the first moment curve (AUMC), plasma concentration and time (*t*) plots of drugs from suppositories can be calculated using the difference in two exponentials.

$$C = Be^{-\lambda_2 t} - Ae^{-\lambda_1 t}$$

where A and B are the zero time intercepts corresponding to λ_1 and λ_2, which denote the apparent first order fast and slow disposition rate constants respectively, and time t [Kurosawa et al., 1985].

Soya lecithin is a phospholipid and with its emulsifying properties can act as a drug release modifier. Nishihata et al. (1985) demonstrated the usefulness of lecithin in preparation of

Table 8.5. Various recent approaches in rectal drug delivery

Approach	Drug	Results	Reference
Suppositories	Bisacodyl	Sustained drug release, required amount available in plasma	Tramonte et al. (1997)
Xyloglucan gels	Indomethacin, diltiazem	Sustained drug release, no first pass metabolism	Miyazaki et al. (1998)
Suppositories	Chloroquine	Surfactant enhances the absorption, significantly enhanced drug release	Onyeji et al. (1999)
Rectal gel	Insulin	Sustained release	Barichello et al. (1999)
Mucoadhesive suppositories	Propranolol	Increased bioavailability	Ryu et al. (1999)
Suppositories	Clomethiazole	Improved pharmacokinetics, increased bioavailability, improved pharmacodynamic effect	Rätz et al. (1999)
Double layer suppositories	Paracetamol	Increased drug absorption, longer retention, better *in vitro-in vivo* correlation	Chicco et al. (1999)
Suppositories	Clomethiazole	Similar pharmacokinetic profile with oral administration, used as alternative to oral and IV routes	Ratz et al. (1999)
Mucoadhesive liquid suppositories	Propranolol	No rectal mucosa irritation, complete avoidance of first pass metabolism, improved bioavailability	Ryo et al. (1999); Mackay et al. (1997)
Rectal gel	Insulin	Improved rectal absorption, better *in vivo* hypoglycemic activity	Borichello et al. (1999)
Bioadhesive gel	Insulin	No irritation, better absorption, sustained release	Yun et al. (1999)
PEG-suppositories	Chloroquine	Enhanced rectal absorption using surfactant, improved drug release, reduced drug irritation	Onyeji et al. (1999)
Thermo reversible suppositories	Insulin	Improved bioavailability, sustained release	Yun et al. (2000); Owens et al. (2000)
Submicron emulsion	Diazepam	Improved bioavailability, sustained release	Sznitowska et al. (2001)
Suppositories	Denaverine	Pharmacokinetic characterization of drug	Stabb et al. (2003)
Suppositories	Acetaminophen	Better absorption, sustained release	Varela & Howland (2004)

sustained-release diclofenac sodium suppositories. The initial studies in dogs showed that the effective plasma diclofenac sodium concentration was maintained for about 12 hr. It has been suggested that the lecithin can interact with anionic substance and form a relatively stable complex in an organic solvent and form micellar aggregate. An apparent slow release of diclofenac from lecithin suppositories may be due to the slow release of diclofenac sodium from micelles in the bulk triglycerides phase.

Nishihata et al. (1990) also prepared polymeric spheres of water-soluble polymer, Poys®, SA-20 and suspended in the melted triglycerides suppository base. The mean *in vitro* release time of diclofenac sodium from these suppositories was prolonged 5 times in comparison to that of conventional triglycerides suppositories. *In vivo* study in dogs showed apparent slow absorption rate with mean absorption time (MAT) of about 6.5 hr as compared to 1 hr for plain suppository.

Chicco et al. (1999) carried out an *in vivo* investigation of paracetamol availability using double-layered suppositories prepared using two different glyceride bases, a fast drug-releasing one

(Witepsol H15) and a slow drug-releasing one (Witepsol W35). The improved paracetamol availability could be ascribed to the absorption-enhancing effect of the monoglycerides. Moreover, the W35 has also a higher viscosity, which could possibly cause the suppository to be retained for a longer time in the lower part of the rectum, where the blood is drained directly to the systemic circulation. It was therefore hypothesized that the enhanced paracetamol availability could be also due to a liver bypass mechanism.

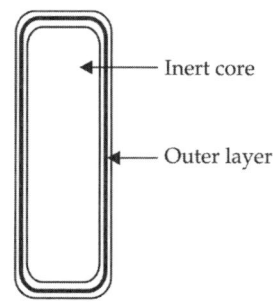

— Inert core

— Outer layer

Fig. 8.5. Schematic diagram of double layer suppository.

Samy et al. (2000) prepared the solid dispersion of a very slightly water-soluble drug, allopurinol using urea, sodium salicylate and β-cyclodextrin (β-CD) as carriers. Solid dispersion and crystallization of the drug with these carriers were used in suppository formulations to investigate their role in enhancement of drug release through the membrane barrier. The obtained data from these experiments proved the superiority of the PEG formulations containing co-evaporates of the drug to sodium salicylate, ratio 1 : 1, or of the drug to β-CD, ratio 1 : 2; $T_{90\%}$, 12 and 36 min, respectively.

Berko et al. (2002) formulated furosemide-containing rectal suppositories. The results of the *in vitro* drug release study showed increased drug liberation with the use of non-ionic surfactants incorporated in the suppository base in various concentrations. The comparison of the membrane diffusion examinations with the *in vivo* diuretic effect reveals that *in vitro* drug release and the pharmacological effect usually showed the same tendency, i.e., a greater extent of *in vitro* furosemide release was associated with a greater quantity of rat urine.

The neurotropic-musculotropic spasmolytic agent denaverine hydrochloride is used mainly in the treatment of smooth muscle spasms of the GI and urogenital tract. Despite its commercial availability as a solution for intravenous or intramuscular administration (ampoule), no pharmacokinetic data in man was available to date. Staab et al. (2003) described the use of rectal route for evaluating the pharmacokinetic parameters of denaverine.

Hanee et al. (2004) studied the role of various surfactants on the release of salbutamol from suppositories and demonstrated that Tween 80 may be added to the formulation to increase the dissolution rate of salbutamol. They further reported that the release rate of salbutamol altered linearly with the amount of Tween 80 in suppository formulations.

Phillips (2005) tested amphotericin B vaginal suppositories for the treatment of non-albicans *Candida* vaginitis. The experiment was performed in thirty-two patients and amphotericin B vaginal suppositories were found to be viable treatment option for refractory vaginitis caused by non-albicans *Candida*.

Uehara et al. (2006) in a prospective clinical study performed a pilot experiment to confirm the safety and effectiveness of *Lactobacillus* vaginal suppositories against the recurrence of bacterial urinary tract infection (UTI). A significant reduction in the number of recurrences was reported and no adverse complications were found. The administration of vaginal suppositories containing *L. crispatus* GAI 98332 was found to be safe and effective for the treatment and prevention of recurrent UTI.

Ray et al. (2007) observed the response of *Candida glabrata* to boric acid vaginal suppositories in comparison with oral fluconazole in patients with diabetes and vulvovaginal candidiasis, and found that diabetic women with *C. glabrata* VVC showed higher mycological cure with boric acid vaginal suppositories when administered for 14 days in comparison with single oral dose of 150-mg fluconazole.

Saleem et al. (2008) prepared the rectal suppositories of tramadol hydrochloride using different bases and polymers like PEG, cocoa butter, agar and the effect of different additives on *in vitro* release of tramadol hydrochloride was studied. The agar-based suppositories were found to be non-disintegrating/non-dissolving, whereas PEG-based were disintegrating/dissolving and cocoa butter-based were melting suppositories. These observations suggested that blends of PEG of low molecular weight (1000) with high molecular weight (4000 and 6000) in different percentages and agar in 10% w/w as base can be used to formulate rapid-release suppositories. The sustained-release suppositories could be prepared by addition of PVP, HPMC in agar-based suppositories and by the use of cocoa butter as base.

Moghimipour et al. (2009) carried out the *in vitro* evaluation and characterization of piroxicam suppositories and concluded that the combination of Witepsol and a propylene glycol is superior combination as compared to the lipophilic base alone, in terms of their ability to release the drug from the suppository formulations.

Ghorab et al. (2011) prepared suppositories by fusion method using different fatty bases as Witepsol H15, Witepsol E75, Suppocire AP and Suppocire BM, as well as with different hydrophilic bases as polyethylene glycol and poloxamer. Among the studied suppository bases polyethylene glycol was best suited for fast release of the drug and fatty and thermopile bases for sustained-release applications of fenoterol HBr.

Hargoli et al. (2013) used different bases for developing naproxen suppositories. The effects of different bases and surfactants on the physicochemical characteristics of the suppositories were determined by tests such as weight variation, melting point, assay, hardness, and release rate. Witepsol H15 with 0.5% w/w of Tween 80 and Witepsol W35 with 0.5% of cetyl-pyridinium chloride were found to be suitable and released nearly complete drug during 30 and 60 min, respectively.

Bendas and Basalious (2015) prepared vagina retentive cream suppositories (VRCS) of progesterone having rapid disintegration and good vaginal retention. VRCS of progesterone were prepared using oil in water (o/w) emulsion of mineral oil or theobroma oil in hard fat and compared it with conventional vaginal suppositories (CVS) prepared by hard fat. Their *in vivo* pharmacokinetic study suggested that VRCS of progesterone provided higher rate and extent of absorption compared to hard fat based suppositories.

HYDROGELS FOR RECTAL DELIVERY

The rectal route has been used to deliver many types of drugs, although patient acceptability is variable due to the discomfort arising from administered dosage forms. Its primary applications have been for local treatment of diseases associated with the rectum, such as hemorrhoids. Additionally, it is well known that drugs absorbed from the lower part of the rectum drain into the systemic circulation directly. Thus, the rectal route is a useful administration route for drugs suffering heavy first-pass metabolism. Conventional suppositories hitherto adapted as dosage forms for rectal administration are solids at room temperature, and melt or soften at body temperature. A problem associated with rectal administration using conventional suppositories is that drugs diffusing out of the suppositories in an uncontrolled manner are unable to be sufficiently retained at a specific position in the rectum, and sometimes migrate upwards to the colon. This often leads to a variation of the bioavailability of certain drugs, in particular, for drugs that undergo extensive first-pass elimination.

In this context, hydrogels may offer a valuable way to overcome the problem in conventional suppositories, provided that they are designed to exhibit a sufficient bioadhesive property following their rectal administration. For example, Ryu et al. (1999) reported that increased bioavailability of propranolol subject to extensive first-pass metabolism was observed by adding certain mucoadhesive polymeric compounds to poloxamer-based thermally gelling suppositories.

CONCLUSION

From the past many years interest in rectal drug delivery systems has been growing at an extensive pace. This chapter attempted to reveal the conventional strategies, their limitations and novel methods that have been used by explorers for improving the operation and acceptability of rectal-specific drug delivery systems. The rectal targeted drug delivery systems are aimed to enhance the therapeutic efficacy of the dosage form by increasing the amount of drug available at the targeted site. The formulations are intended for local as well as systemic effects. Recent research on targeted delivery systems for treatment of rectal-specific diseases has progressed from conventional system employing physiological properties of GIT to novel systems, which are significant in terms of decreasing the limitations associated with the conventional systems. Compared with conventional systems the rectal-based targeted drug delivery systems exhibit site-specific release, predetermined drug release properties, higher efficacy and prolonged retention in the inflamed tissue. However, the future of rectal-based drug delivery systems depends on how efficiently they will overcome the hurdles of regulatory requirements, scale-up, cost effectiveness and patient compliance.

ACKNOWLEDGEMENTS

The authors are grateful to UGC, New Delhi, for granting UPE status (University with potential for excellence) to University and providing the grant for establishment of centre of emerging life sciences (equipped with sophisticated instruments).

REFERENCES

- Agra, Y., Sacristan, A., Gonzalez, M. (1998). *J. Pain Symptom Manage.*, 15: 1–7.
- Anon, A. (1994). *MeReC Bulletin*, 5: 21–24.
- Ansel, H.C., Popovich, N.G. (1990). *In:* **Pharmaceutical Dosage Forms and Drug Delivery Systems**, Lea & Febiger, London, 373–389.
- Aulton, M.E. (2002). Harcourt Publishers; Churchill Livingstone, 2nd ed., pp. 535.
- Barichello, J.M., Morishita, M., Takayama, K., Chiba, Y., Tokiwa, S., Nagai, T. (1999). *Int. J. Pharm.*, 183(2): 125–132.
- Bateman, D.N., Smith, J.M. (1988). *B.M.J.*, 297: 1420–1421.
- Beebe, D.S., Belani, K.G., Chang, P.N. (1992). *Anesth. Analgesia.*, 75: 880–884.
- Bendas, E.R., Basalious, E.B. (2015). *Pharm. Dev. Technol.*, 8: 1–8.
- Berko, S., Regdon, J.G., Ducza, E., Falkay, G., István E. (2002). *Eur. J. Pharm. Biopharmaceutics*, 53(3): 311–315.
- Bjorkman, S., Gabrielsson, J., Quaynor, H., Corbey, M. (1987). *Br. J. Anaesth.*, 59: 1541–1547.
- Blom, H., Schmidt, J.F., Rytlander, M. (1984). *Acta Anaesthesiol. Scand.*, 28: 652–653.
- Caldwell, J.L., Nishihata, T., Ryttig, J., Higuchi, T. (1983a). *J. Pharm. Pharmacol.*, 34: 520.
- Caldwell, J.L., Nishihata, T., Higuchi, T. (1983b). *Pharm. Tech.*, 10: 50–55.
- Chicco, D., Grabnar, I., Kerjanec, A.S., Vojnovic, D., Maurich, V., Realdon, N., Ragazzi, E., Beli, A., Karba, R., Mrhar, A. (1999). *Int. J. Pharm.*, 189(2): 147–160.
- Choonara, I.A. (1987). *Arch. Dis. Child.*, 62: 771–772.
- Dange, S.V., Shah, K.U., Deshpande, A.S., Shrotri, D.S. (1987). *Indian Pediatr.*, 24: 331–332.
- de Boer, A.G., Hoogdalem E.J., Breimer D.D. (1992). *Advanced Drug Delivery Reviews*, 8(2/3): 237–253.
- de Boer, A.G., Breimer, D.D. (1997). *Adv. Drug Delivery Rev.* 28(2): 229–237.

- de Boer, A.G., Breimer, D.D. (1981). *In:* Prescott, L.F., Nimmo, W.S. (Eds.) **Drug Absorption**, ADIS Press, Sydney, 61–72.
- de Boer, A.G., Moolennar, F., De Leede, L.G.J., Breimer, D.D. (1982). *Clinical Pharmacokinetic*, 7: 285–311.
- de Bore, A.G., Breimer, D.D., Mattie, H., Pronk, J., Gubbens-Stibbe, J.M. (1979). *Clinical Pharmacology and Therapeutics*, 26: 701–709.
- De Felippis, M.R. (2003). *Am. Pharm. Rev.*, 6(4): 21–30.
- De Jong, P.C., Verburg, M.P. (1988). *Acta Anaesthesiol. Scand.*, 32: 485–489.
- De Leede, L.G.J., Breimer, D.D., de Boer, A.G. (1981). *Biopharm. and Drug Disp.*, 2: 131–136.
- Fallon, M., O'Neill, B. (1997). *B.M.J.*, 315: 1293–1296.
- Forbes, R.B., Vandewalker, G.E. (1988). *Can. J. Anaesth.*, 35: 345–349.
- Ghorab, D., Refai, H, Tag, R. (2011). *Drug Discov. Ther.*, 5(6): 311–8.
- Gupta, P.J. (2007). *Eur. Rev. Med. Pharmacol. Sci.*, 11: 165–170
- Gaudreault, P., Guay, J., Nicol, O., Dupuis, C. (1988). *Can. J. Anaesth.*, 35: 149–152.
- Gourlay, G.K., Boas, R.A. (1992). *Br. Med. J.*, 304: 766–767
- Graves, N.M., Kreil, R.L. (1987). *Pediatr. Neurol.*, 3: 321–326.
- Hanaee, J., Javadzadeh, Y., Taftachi, S., Farid, D., Nokhodchi, A. (2004). *Farmaco.*, 59(11): 903–6.
- Hamunen, K., Maunuksela, E.L., Seppälä, T., Olkkola, K.T. (1993). *Br. J. Anaesth.*, 71: 823–826.
- Hargoli, S., Farid, J., Azarmi, S.H., Ghanbarzadeh, S., Zakeri-Milani, P. (2013). *Indian J. Pharm. Sci.*, 75(2): 143–8.
- Hosny, E.A. (2001). *Drug Develop. Indus. Pharmacy*, 25(6): 745–752.
- Jantzen, J.P., Tzanova, I., Witton, P.K., Klein, A.M. (1989). *Can. J. Anaesth.*, 36: 665–667.
- Khalil, S.N., Florence, F.B., Van den Nieuwenhuyzen, M.C., Wu, A.H., Stanley, T.H. (1990). *Anesth. Analg.*,70: 645–649.
- Kot, T.V., Pettit-Young, N.A. (1992). *Ann. Pharmacother.*, 26: 1277–1282.
- Kurosawa, N., Owada, E., Ueda, K., Takahashi, A. (1985). *Int. J. Pharm.*, 27: 81–88.
- Laishley, R.S., O'Callaghan, A.C., Lerman, J. (1986). *Can. Anaesth. Soc. J.*, 33: 427–432.
- Lakshmi, P.J., Deepthi, B., Rama, R.N. (2012). *Asi. J. Res. Pharm. Sci.*, 4 (2): 143–149.
- Laub, M., Sjogren, P., Holm-Knudsen, R., Flachs, H., Christiansen, E. (1990). *Anaesthesia*, 45: 110–112.
- Loyd, V., Allen, J, **The Basics of Compounding: Compounding Suppositories: Part I - Theoretical Considerations**, 2004 (www.google.com)
- Mackay, M., Phillips, J., Hastewell, J. (1997). *Adv. Drug Delivery Rev.*, 28(2): 253–273.
- Malinovsky, J.M., Lejus, C., Servin, F. (1993). *Br. J. Anaesth.*, 70: 617–620.
- Matsuda, H., Arima, H. (1999). *Adv. Drug Deliv. Rev.*, 36(1): 81–99.
- Miyazaki, S., Suisha, F., Kawasaki, N., Shirakawa, M., Yamatoya, K., Attwood, D. (1998). *J. Contro. Release*, 56(1): 75–83.
- Moghimipour, E., Dabbagh, M.A., Zarif, F. (2009). *Asi. Jr. Pharm. Clin. Res.*, 2(3): 92–98.
- Moolennar, F., Schoonen, A.J.M. (1980). *Pharmacy International*, 1: 144–146.
- Moolenaar, F., Yska J.P., Visser J., Meijer D.K.F. (1985). *Eur. J. Clin. Pharmacol.*, 29(1): 119–121.
- Morimot, K., Lwamoto, T., Morisaka, K. (1984). *Pharm. Res.*, 73: 1366–1368.
- Morimoto, K., Akatsuchi, H., Morisaka, K., Kamada, A. (1985). *J. Pharm. Pharmacol.*, 37: 759–760.
- Muller-Lissner, S.A. (1988). *B.M.J.*, 296: 615–617.
- Nishihata, T., Tsutsumi, A., Ikawa, C., Sakai, K. (1990). *Drug Dev. Ind. Pharm.*, 16: 1675–1686.
- Nishihata, T., Wada, H., Kamada, A. (1985). *Int. J. Pharm.*, 27: 245–253.
- Norton, C. (1996). *British J. Nursing*, 5: 1252–1258.
- O'Brien, J.F., Falk, J.L., Carey, B.E., Malone, L.C. (1991). *Ann. Emerg. Med.*, 20: 644–647.
- Onyeji, C.O., Adebayo, A.S., Babalola, C.P. (1999). *Eur. J. Pharm. Science*, 9(2): 131–136.
- Owens, D.R., Zinman, B., Bolli, G. (2000). *Diabet. Med.*, 20: 886–898.
- Pannuti, F., Rossi, A.P., Iafelice, G. (1982). *Pharmacol. Res.*, 14: 369–380.
- Passmore, A.P., Wilson-Davies, K., Stoker, C., Scott, M.E. (1993). *B.M.J.*, 307: 769–771.
- Pedraz, J.L., Calvo, M.B., Lanao, J.M., Muriel, C., Santos L. J., Dominguez-Gil, A. (1989). *Br. J. Anaesth.*, 63: 671–674.

- Petticrew, M., Watt, I., Sheldon, T. (1997). *Health Technol. Assessment*, 1: 13.
- Phillips, A.J. (2005). *Am. J. Obstet. Gynecol.*, 192(6): 2009–12.
- Ratz, A.E., Schlienger, R.G., Linder, L., Langewitz, W., Haefeli, W.E. (1999). *Clinical Therapeutics*, 51(5): 829–840.
- Ray, D., Goswami, R., Banerjee, U., Dadhwal, V., Goswami, D., Mandal, P., Sreenivas, V., Kochupillai, N. (2007). *Diabetes Care*, 30(2): 312–7.
- Ritschel, W.A, Ritschel, G.B., Ritschel, B.E., Lucker, P.W. (1988). *Methods Find. Exp. Clin. Pharmacol.*, 10(10): 645–56.
- Roelfse, J.A., van der Bijl, P., Stegmann, D.H., Hartshorne, J.E. (1990). *Oral Maxillofac. Surg.*, 48: 791–797.
- Ryu, J.M., Chung, S.J., Lee, M.H., Kim, C.K., Shim, C.K. (1999). *J. Control. Release*, 59: 163–172.
- Saleem, M.A., Taher, M., Sanaullah, S., Najmuddin, M., Ali, J., Humaira, S., Roshan, S. (2008). *Indian J. Pharm. Sci.*, 70(5): 640–4.
- Samy, E.M., Hassan, M.A., Tous, S.S., Rhodes, C.T. (2000). *Eur. J. Pharm. Biopharmaceutics*, 49(2): 119–127.
- Senior, N. (1969a). *Pharm. J.*, 203: 703–706.
- Senior, N. (1969b). *Pharm. J.*, 203: 732–736.
- Shojaei, A.H. (1998). *J. Pharm. Pharmaceu. Sci.*, 1(1): 15–30.
- Song, Y., Wang, Y., Thakur, R., Meidan, V.M., Michniak, B. (2004). *Crit. Rev. Ther. Drug Carrier Syst.*, 21(3): 195–256.
- Staab, A., Schug, B.S., Larsimont, V., Elze, M. (2003). *Farmaco II*, 58(7): 509–512.
- Stilwell, B. (1992). *Community Outlook*, 26–27
- Swarbrick, J. (Ed.) (1987). *In:* **Encyclopedia of Pharmaceutical Technology**, Vol. 13.
- Sznitowska, M., Gajewska, M., Janicki, S., Radwanska, A., Lukowski, G. (2001). *Eur. J. Pharm. and Biopharmaceutics*, 52(2): 159–163.
- Taylor, R. (1990). *B.M.J.*, 300: 1063–1064.
- Tedesco, F.J., DiPiro, J.T. (1985). *Am. J. Gastroenterol.*, 80: 303–309
- Thompson, W.G., Creed, F., Drossman, D.A., Heaton, K.W., Mazzacca, G. (1992). *Gastroenterology International*, 5: 75–91.
- Thümmler, D., Mutschler, E., Blum, H. (2003). *Eur. J. Pharm. Sciences*, 18(2): 121–128.
- Tramonte, S.M., Brand, M.B., Mulrow, C.D. (1997). *J. Gen. Intern. Med.*, 12: 15–24.
- Uehara, S., Monden, K., Nomoto, K., Seno, Y., Kariyama, R., Kumon H. (2006). *Int. J. Antimicrob. Agent*, 28(1): 30–34.
- Ullyot, S.C. (1992). *Can. J. Anaesth.*, 39: 533–536.
- Uthman, B.M., Wilder, B.J. (1989). *Epilepsia.*, 30: S33–S37.
- van Hoogdalem, E., de Boer, A.G., Breimer, D.D. (1991a). *Clin. Pharmacokinet.*, 21: 11–26.
- Van Hoogdalem, E.J., de Boer, A.G., Breimer, D.D. (1991b). *Clin. Pharmacokinet.*, 21: 110–128.
- Van Hoogdalem, E.J., Wackwitz, A.T., de Boer A.G., Cohen, A.F., Breimer, D.D. (1989). *Br. J. Clin. Pharmacol.*, 27: 75–81.
- Varela, M.L., Howland, M.A. (2004). *Ann. Pharmacother,*, 38(11): 1935–1941.
- Watanabe, K., Yakou, S., Takayama, K., Isowa, K., Nagai, T. (2000). *Int. J. Pharm.*, 190(2): 122–128
- Wynne, H.A., Edwards, C. *Pharm. J.*, 248: 17–19.
- Yamamoto, A., Muranishi, S. (1997). *Adv. Drug Delivery Rev.*, 28(2): 275–299.
- Yun, M.O., Choi, H.G., Jung, J.H., Kim, C.K. (1999). *Int. J. Pharm.*, 189(2): 137–145
- Zempsky, W.T., Cote, C.J., Berlin, C.M. (1998). *Pediatrics*, 1001(4): 730.

9

Vaginal Drug Delivery Systems

V.R. Sinha, Amita Sarwal, Sandeep Kaur,
Harneet Kaur and Sumit Sharma

INTRODUCTION

Currently extensive efforts are being put forward for exploring the vaginal cavity as an alternative route of drug administration. Literature shows that over the last few decades, vagina remains to be a relatively unexplored route despite its potential as a noninvasive route of drug administration. Vaginal route offers some unique advantages for drug delivery such as bypassing first pass metabolism, large permeation area, relatively low enzyme activity, rich vascularization, ease of administration, and high permeability for low molecular weight drugs. These advantages have encouraged the use of vaginal route for local as well as systemic delivery of therapeutic agents. In spite of the various advantages associated with vaginal route, successful delivery of therapeutic agents remains a challenge due to unique physiological features of the vaginal route. Factors which generally pose barrier to drug delivery are thickness of vaginal epithelium, presence of thick layers of mucus, hormonal cyclic changes, vaginal pH, and vaginal microflora.

To be highly acceptable and to achieve good patient compliance and desired therapeutic benefit every delivery system should possess some user-friendly characteristics. For a vaginal delivery system, few characteristics are essential to be convenient for the patient such as maintenance of an optimal pH (3.5–4.5) in vaginal epithelium, ease of application, even distribution of drug, retention in vagina, compatibility with co-administered medicines, no adverse effect on coitus, odorless and colorless, can be applied several hours before intercourse, no leakage, messiness or feeling of fullness, no irritation, itching, burning or swelling; and convenient to insert and/or apply with or without an applicator.

Various dosage forms have been developed in the form of gels, creams, intravaginal rings, suppositories, vaginal tablets, etc. to achieve the therapeutic response through vaginal drug delivery. The disadvantage associated with this route is messiness, leakage and low residence time, leading to poor patient compliance. However, several systems have been developed to overcome these limitations by novel formulation approaches.

ANATOMY AND PHYSIOLOGY

The vagina (Fig. 9.1) is a fibromuscular, female reproductive organ, having slightly S-shape with

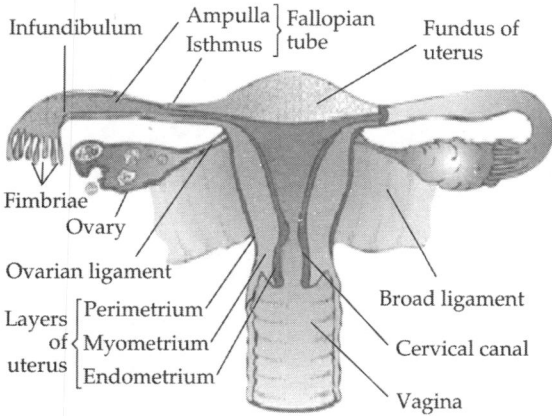

Fig. 9.1. Diagrammatic representation of female reproductive tract/system. (Reproduced with the permission of McGraw-Hill Companies, Inc.)

a length of 6–10 cm and extended from the cervix of the uterus to the vestibule. The vaginal wall consists of three layers: the epithelial layer, the muscular coat and tunica adventitia. The epithelium is a non-cornified, stratified squamous epithelium and its thickness is dependent on age. With hormonal activity the vaginal epithelium increases in thickness and is highest in the proliferative stage. Thickness of the vaginal epithelial cell layer varies with cyclic changes by approximately 200–300 Å.

Specific characteristics exhibited by vaginal wall like large surface area and its dispensability are attributed to the presence of numerous folds on vaginal surface, which are often called rugae. Smooth elastic fibers present in the muscular coat of vagina along with the loose connective tissue of tunica adventitia provide it with excellent elasticity. Arteries, blood vessels and lymphatic vessels are abundant in the walls of the vagina. A plexus of arteries extending from the internal iliac artery, uterine, middle rectal and internal pudendal arteries form network of blood vessels which supply blood to the vagina. Drugs absorbed from the vagina do not undergo first-pass metabolism because blood leaving the vagina enters the peripheral circulation via a rich venous plexus, which empties primarily into the internal iliac veins.

It has unique features in terms of secretion, pH and microflora, and these factors must be considered during the development and evaluation of vaginal dosage forms. The vaginal secretion is a mixture of several components such as proteins/peptides, glycoproteins, lactic acid, acetic acid, glycerol, urea, glycogen and ions such as Na^+, Ca^{++} and Cl^-. The composition of simulated vaginal fluid is given in Table 9.1.

Table 9.1. Composition of simulated vaginal fluid

Component	Quantity
Sodium chloride	3.51 g/L
Potassium hydroxide	1.40 g/L
Calcium hydroxide	0.222 g/L
Bovine serum albumin	0.018 g/L
Lactic acid	2.00 g/L
Acetic acid	1.00 g/L
Glycerol	0.16 g/L
Urea	0.4 g/L
Glucose	5 g/L

pH adjusted to 4.2 by using 1 mol HCl

The vaginal epithelium cells of fertile women release glycogen, which supplies nutrition to commensal bacteria *Lactobacillus* that further degrade glycogen to acid and thereby create acidic environment maintaining the pH around 3.5–4.5. The acidic environment restricts the growth of the pathogenic microorganisms. The vaginal pH changes with age, stages of the menstrual cycle, infections and sexual arousal.

The human vagina is inhabited by a range of microbes from a pool of over 50 species including both aerobic and anaerobic species such as *Lactobacillus*, *Candida albicans*, *Neisseria*, etc. The composition of the vaginal flora is not constant. Several factors lead to variation in the vaginal microbiota. These include different phases of menstrual cycle, gestation, use of contraceptives, frequency of sexual intercourse, use of showers or deodorant products, use of antibiotics or other medications with immune-suppressive properties.

ADVANTAGES OF VAGINAL DRUG DELIVERY

Vaginal route possesses some unique physiological features, which offer various advantages over other routes of drug administration:

1. Suitable for obnoxious agents that cannot be administered orally or otherwise may lead to emesis or gastric irritation.
2. Avoid hepatic first pass metabolism thus enhancing bioavailability. So, it is very effective alternative for those drugs, which undergo extensive first pass metabolism e.g., propranolol.
3. Help to decrease dose as well as dosing frequency by improving bioavailability and by sustaining drug action and thus improves patient compliance.
4. Help in reducing the fluctuations in plasma drug concentration such as in case of daily intake of drugs thereby lowering the incidence of side effects that usually occur due to high plasma concentrations of various drug molecules.
5. Vaginal route can be used for local as well as systemic effect.
6. Lesser number of metabolic enzymes may help to deliver the drugs that are metabolized or degraded in gastrointestinal tract before absorption.
7. Therapeutic action can be terminated by removing delivery device in case of need.
8. Vaginal administration is accompanied by rapid drug absorption resulting in quick onset of action.
9. In comparison to parenteral medication, vaginal route seems to be the convenient one for the patients on long-term therapy as it overcomes the discomfort caused by pain, tissue damage and probable infection through parenteral routes.
10. Exhibit good bioavailability for smaller drug molecules.
11. Approaches like addition of absorption enhancer can be used to improve the bio-availability of larger drug molecules.
12. Suitable choice for drugs those are not stable in gastrointestinal fluids.
13. Self-medication is possible with some of vaginal dosage forms.
14. Presence of mucus can be utilized for developing sustained-release mucoadhesive systems.
15. Some drugs, such as misoprostol used to induce labor, are also known to be more efficacious when administered vaginally compared with via other routes.

DISADVANTAGES ASSOCIATED WITH VAGINAL DRUG DELIVERY

1. It is associated with issues like cultural sensitivity, personal hygiene, and gender specificity.
2. May cause local irritation due to formulation ingredients or drug molecule itself.
3. Drug delivery characteristics of a specific formulation may get altered by sexual intercourse.
4. Less preferable in terms of convenience if other options are available.
5. Permeability of vaginal membrane changes with cyclic hormonal changes thus leading to changes in pharmacokinetics of drugs during different periods in the cycle.
6. Sensitivity of some drugs to acidic vaginal pH (3.5–4.5).
7. Leakage of drugs from the vagina leading to inconvenience.
8. The pH and volume of the vaginal fluid may affect the extent of drug absorption depending on degree of ionization as unionized forms are preferably absorbed.

FACTORS AFFECTING DRUG ABSORPTION FROM THE VAGINA

Various factors which are characteristic of this route (physiological) and factors which are characteristic of a particular dosage form and particular drug substance (pharmaceutical and physicochemical) affect the absorption of vaginally administered drugs. These factors are discussed in detail below.

1. Physiological factors

Vaginal physiology greatly affects the absorption of vaginally administered drugs. It includes the pH of vagina, thickness of mucosal epithelial membrane, microflora, cyclic hormonal changes, and presence of thick mucus.

1. Vaginal epithelium

Changes in the hormonal levels such as oestrogen, progesterone, luteinizing hormone, follicle-stimulating hormone, due to aging, biphasic menstrual cycling and pregnancy, etc. lead to changes in vaginal epithelium. The vaginal absorption of steroids is affected by the thickness of the vaginal epithelium. Steroids and local estrogen, e.g. oestrogen, appear to be better absorbed from thinner postmenopausal epithelium, whereas progesterone appears to be better absorbed from thicker, more vascularized epithelium. The biphasic cycle in humans consists of follicular and luteal phase. In the follicular phase, the epithelium is thick and cohesive in comparison to the luteal phase, where it becomes loose and porous with increased permeability with increased possibility of absorption of even high molecular weight hydrophilic drugs. In the post-menopausal phase, the vaginal epithelium becomes extremely thin, leading to a considerable increase in the permeability of this tissue because of reduced mitosis in the basal epithelial layers and the decline in small blood vessels.

2. Vaginal fluid

Vagina secretes copious amounts of fluid in spite of the fact that it does not possess any gland. Along with vaginal epithelium, vaginal secretions are also affected by changing hormonal levels such as oestrogen, progesterone, luteinizing hormone, follicle-stimulating hormone. Women of reproductive age produce fluid at a rate of 3–4 g/4 h, which is reduced by 50% in postmeno-

pausal women. Apart from hormonal changes vaginal secretions may also gets affected by sexual arousal which in turn may alter the drug release pattern from the vaginal delivery system. Drug absorption following vaginal administration is affected by the volume, viscosity and pH of vaginal fluid. Where the large volumes of vaginal fluid, on one hand, may dislodge the formulation from the vaginal cavity reducing drug absorption, on the other hand, may favor the absorption of poorly water-soluble drug. Moreover, drug absorption is hindered by the presence of excessively viscous cervical mucus.

3. Vaginal pH

Acidic vaginal pH is attributed to the presence of lactic acid which acts as a buffer to maintain the vaginal pH between 3.5 and 4.5. Lactic acid present in vaginal cavity produces *Lactobacillus acidophilus* by its action on glycogen. Factors like menstruation, frequent acts of coitus, presence of cervical mucus and the amount of vaginal transudate may cause an increase/decrease in vaginal pH which may lead to discomfort. During menopausal age, due to decreased production of glycogen and lactic acid, vaginal pH starts to fluctuate back and forth causing an imbalance.

Degree of ionization of drugs especially weak electrolytes, e.g., misoprostol and dinoprostone, is affected by the acidic vaginal pH, subsequently affecting the absorption of these molecules. This can be illustrated with the example of prostaglandins such as PGE_2. Prostaglandins being organic acids exhibit diminished aqueous solubility at low pH which also includes vaginal pH range, i.e., 3.5–4.5. So a change in vaginal pH (> 4.5) due to any of the reasons may lead to increase in the release rate from PGE_2 preparations because of increased solubility of the molecule which in turn may be attributed to the change in degree of ionization of drug molecule at elevated environmental pH.

4. Cyclic changes

The thickness of the vaginal epithelial cell layer,

width of intercellular channels, vaginal pH, vaginal secretions, and enzyme activity (endopeptidases and amino peptidases) within the vaginal cavity is altered with cyclic hormonal changes during menstruation which complicates the achievement of consistent drug delivery through vaginal administration.

5. Enzymatic activity

Enzymatic activity in vaginal cavity is less pronounced in comparison to gastrointestinal tract. Like other physiological parameters, enzymatic activity is also influenced by cyclic hormonal changes, e.g., the activity of beta-glucoronidase, acid phosphatase, alkaline phosphatase and esterase, varying in the vaginal tissue of premenopausal and postmenopausal women, which affects the vaginal drug delivery.

2. Physicochemical factors

Absorption characteristics of a drug molecule are partly dictated in terms of its physico-chemical properties like molecular weight, lipophilicity, ionization, surface charge, chemical nature, solubility, dissolution rate, pKa, chemical structure and chemical stability. Depending upon the pKa of the drug molecule, it may exist in unionized form or ionized form in the acidic vaginal environment. According to pH-partition hypothesis unionized form of the drug which is proposed to be more lipophilic in nature is able to cross the biological membrane. So as to get absorbed from vaginal membrane a drug molecule must remain unionized at the vaginal pH. Therefore, slightly acidic vaginal pH favors the greater absorption of acidic drugs (pH < pKa), while basic drugs are better absorbed when pH is slightly alkaline (pH > pKa). It is generally considered that low molecular weight lipophilic drugs are likely to be absorbed more than large molecular weight lipophilic or hydrophilic drugs.

Certain degree of water solubility is must for a drug to be vaginally administered as it has to be in contact with vaginal fluid which contains large amount of water. Solubility of drugs can be increased by reducing the particle size (by micronization) of the drug. Small particles exhibit greater effective surface area, thus, more intimate contact between solid surface and aqueous solvent resulting into higher dissolution rate which increases its absorption efficiency. The drug solubility is also a function of the geometric shape, the crystalline, hydrate, or salt form of the drug. In general, the amorphous form of the drugs is more soluble than the crystal form of same drug; the anhydrous forms are more soluble than hydrate forms and the salt form of lipophilic drug is more soluble than its free form.

3. Effect of excipients and type of dosage form

Type of dosage form dictates the type of therapeutic action the drug provides, i.e., local effect/systemic effect or immediate short term/sustained type of effect. Type of excipients used will affect the performance characteristics of the product such as dissolution of drug substance, the size of area over which the drug is deposited, the time for which the formulation remains in contact with the site of application. Good distribution and spreading characteristics of vaginal formulation are attributed to the hydrophilicity and rheological behavior of the formulation. Thus, the use of novel excipients may lead to improved retention and distribution of vaginal formulations.

Mucoadhesive agents promote the adherence of formulation with the vaginal mucosal surface, prolonging the residence time of the formulation. For example, xanthan gum and sodium alginate show site-specific bioadhesive properties in a simulated vaginal environment. Polycarbophil 934P exhibited pH-dependent bioadhesive properties.

Penetration enhancers act to promote drug absorption and penetration through vaginal mucosa by decreasing the penetration barrier. Chemical enhancers used commonly are bile salts, chelators, alcohols and fatty acids that may exert their effect by altering the rheological properties of the mucus layer; enhancing transcellular transport by interacting with phospholipids and/or proteins to increase membrane fluidity; inhibiting enzyme activity. With the addition of solubilizing agents and cosolvents, the aqueous solubility of drugs can be increased since water-soluble drugs are good candidates for vaginal drug delivery.

CHALLENGES TO VAGINAL DRUG DELIVERY

Therapeutically effective and constant vaginal drug delivery has always remained challenging because vaginal physiology is dependent on the hormonal changes including oestrogen, progesterone, luteinizing hormone, follicle-stimulating hormone, which may occur due to various factors like aging, biphasic menstrual cycling and pregnancy leading to alterations in the volume, viscosity and pH of vaginal fluid, thickness of vaginal epithelium, changes in enzymatic activity etc., which may alter the absorption of vaginally administered drug. Presence of vaginal fluid may have both positive and negative effects on the vaginal drug absorption. On one hand, it can improve the absorption of the drug by increasing the aqueous solubility of poorly water-soluble drug, on the other hand, it may pose barrier to drug absorption and sometimes may remove the drug from vaginal cavity, leading to decreased contact time of the formulation with the vaginal tissue. pH of vaginal fluid may have some affect depending on the acidic or basic nature of the drug. Since many of the drugs are weak electrolytes, acidic vaginal pH may change their degree of ionization and may affect the absorption of drug from vaginal epithelium.

VAGINA AS A SITE FOR DRUG DELIVERY

From the ancient times, due to the specific physiologic features exhibited by vagina, it has been used for the local delivery of drugs and since last few years it is being explored for systemic delivery of drugs because of its large surface area, high vascularity, and permeability to a wide range of compounds. Vaginal route has been used for local delivery of spermicidal, antifungal, labour-inducing agents, antibacterial, anti-protozoal, anti-viral, prostaglandins and steroids. It offers a favorable alterative for some drugs such as bromocriptine, propranolol, oxytocin, calcitonin, LHRH agonists, human growth hormone, insulin and steroids in comparison to parenteral route. Efforts are going on to exploit the vaginal route for the delivery of drugs for sexually transmitted diseases and for antiviral agents. Almost 50 microbicide drugs are in preclinical development for their utility as a microbicide for HIV prevention and 12 microbicides candidates are in various stages of clinical development. Focus is to develop a vaginal delivery system for these microbicides which is female controlled. It is proposed that such systems can provide better protection than standard prevention methods (e.g. condoms and behavioral modifications) against the transmission of sexually transmitted diseases by offering 'bidirectional' protection (i.e. protection to both partners). It is considered that a 'first uterine pass effect' occurs when drugs are delivered vaginally, thereby providing an explanation for the unexpectedly high uterine concentrations relative to the low serum concentration observed after vaginal administration. Hence, the vaginal route permits targeted drug delivery to the uterus, thereby maximizing the desired effects while minimizing the potential for adverse systemic effects.

Dosage forms

The most common generally used dosage forms for vaginal drug delivery includes creams, tablets, suppositories/pessaries, gels, bioadhesive systems, etc. whereas vaginal rings, inserts, films and tampons are recent systems. These systems can provide local effect such as antimicrobial or spermicidal as well as systemic delivery of drugs e.g. hormones, steroids. Various marketed vaginal preparations are listed in Table 9.2.

1. Suppositories/pessaries

The terms pessaries and suppositories are used interchangeably. Suppository is a general term which may be used for rectal, vaginal or urethral suppositories. But pessaries are specifically referred to those formulations which are intended to be inserted into the vagina. Vaginal suppositories or pessaries weigh about 3–5 gm and are molded in globular or oviform shape or compressed on a tablet press into conical shapes. These vaginal formulations are designed to melt in the vaginal cavity and are most commonly used to administer drugs for local infection, vaginal atrophy, cervical ripening prior to childbirth, contraceptive purpose and also for systemic delivery. Labour induction using vaginal suppository has been found recommendable in women. Moreover, to increase the residence time of suppositories in vagina, several bioadhesive polymers like HEC, sodium alginate, carbopol 934, etc. may be used.

Marketed vaginal pessaries include Gynostatum® VG which contains 100 mg clotrimazole and indicated for vulvovaginal candidiasis, trichomonas vaginitis, non-specific vaginitis, mixed vaginal infections. Gynazole-1® suppositories contain butoconazole and are indicated for vaginal yeast infections. It reduces vaginal burning, itching, and discharge that may occur with this condition. Hundred mg (one suppository) is to be inserted into the vagina at bedtime for three consecutive nights. Gynasaf® soft gelatin vaginal suppositories used to treat

Table 9.2. Marketed vaginal preparations

Preparation	API	Marketed by	Indication
Metrogel-vaginal	Metronidazole	Medicis Pharmaceuticals	Vaginal infections
Cleocin vaginal cream	Clindamycin phosphate	Pfizer	Vaginal bacterial infections
Cleocin vaginal ovules (suppositories)	Clindamycin phosphate	Pfizer	Vaginal bacterial infections
Lactal vaginal gel	Lactic acid and glycogen	Lavipharm	Maintaining and balancing normal vaginal pH
Blissel vaginal gel	Estriol		Vaginal dryness and vaginal atrophy in post-menopausal women
Conceptrol vaginal gel	Nonoxynol-9	Advance Care Product	For contraception
Cervidil suppositories	Dinoprostone	Controlled Therapeutics	Induction of labour
Trivagizole 3 vaginal cream	Tioconazole	Bristol Myers Squibb	Anti-fungal
Prochieve bioadhesive vaginal gel	Progesterone	Columbia Laboratories and Watson Pharmaceuticals	Infertility
Buffer gel	Hydrogen ion released from carbopol	ReProtect	Prevention of HIV transmission
Replens vaginal gel	Polycarbophil	Columbia Laboratories	Vaginal dryness and discomfort
Estring®	Estradiol	Pharmacia and Upjohn	Estrogen replacement therapy
Nuvaring®	Etonogestrel + Ethinyl estradiol	Merck	Contraception
Femring®	Estradiol acetate	Warner Chilcott	Estrogen replacement therapy

infective leucorrhoea, mixed infections and non-specific vaginitis, vaginal candidiasis, bacterial vaginosis and trichomonasis, contains clindamycin 100 mg, clotrimazole 200 mg. Suppositories should be inserted into the vagina for 3 consecutive nights, preferably before retiring to bed. Treatment should be timed so as to avoid the menstrual period.

Vaginal suppositories come in various shapes such as bullet, teardrop, long oval, tampon and round oval. The shape of suppositories is an important factor which women consider while buying them. Bullet and long oval are considered to be the most favored shapes among women. Various shapes of vaginal suppositories have been shown in Fig. 9.2.

2. Creams and gels

These are the most conventional systems for topical delivery of drugs. These are easy to manufacture and also have the advantage of spreading easily onto the surface and providing intimate contact with mucus. However, these dosage forms also have disadvantage of messiness, leakage and uneven drug distribution.

Marketed preparations of vaginal gels include Vagistat® antifungal vaginal cream which contains miconazole nitrate and helps in curing most vaginal yeast infections. It is a 3-day treatment pack. It gives relief from associated external itching and irritation.

Gynest® is an intravaginal cream (Fig. 9.3) preparation containing estriol 0.01% w/w

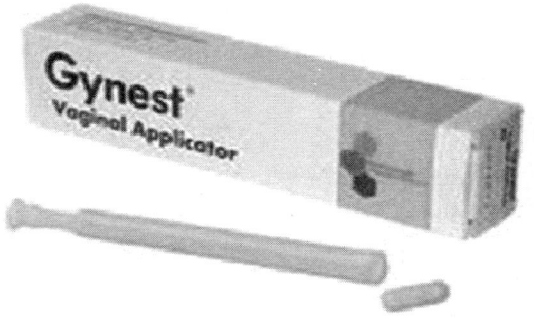

Fig. 9.3. Gynest vaginal cream.

indicated for the hormone replacement therapy for treatment of atrophic vaginitis and kraurosis in postmenopausal women. Also used for treatment of pruritus vulvae and dyspareunia associated with atrophic vaginal epithelium. The recommended initial daily dose is one applicator full per day. A maintenance dose of one applicator full twice a week may be used after restoration of the vaginal mucosa has been achieved.

Another example of vaginal gel is Prostin® E2 containing 1 mg/2 mg dinoprostone, indicated for induction of labour.

Vaginal® gels can be modified by the addition of thermosensitive and pH-sensitive in situ gelling agents and mucoadhesive agents which turns them into more smart systems that can function on the basis of specific physiological parameters such as temperature and pH. Muco-adhesive agents help in increasing the contact time of the formulation with the vaginal tissue

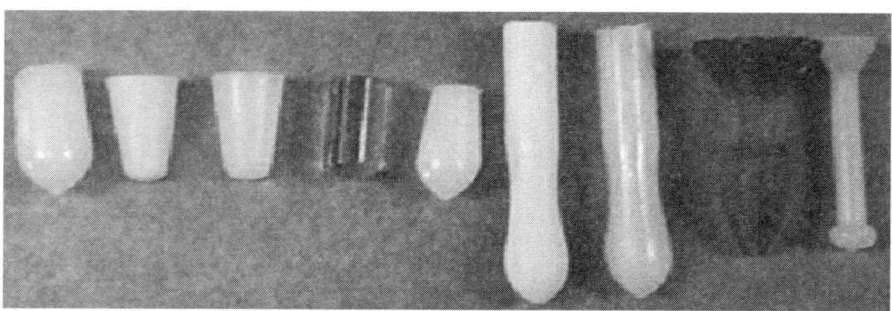

Fig. 9.2. Various types of vaginal suppositories with varying shapes and sizes. (Reproduced with permission from The University of North Carolina at Chapel Hill, North Carolina, United States)

by the formation of mucoadhesive bond between mucus and mucoadhesive agent present within the formulation.

3. Vaginal tablets

Vaginal tablets are similar to conventional oral tablets, contain similar components and can be manufactured easily by using standard tableting equipment. They are suitable for formulation of water-sensitive drugs and have long-term stability without cold-chain storage requirements. Candifem® vaginal tablet contains miconazole and ornidazole. Thus, it is a broad spectrum antifungal, antiprotozoal and antibacterial tablet. Hence, it is effective against vaginal infections caused by *Candida* species, *Trichomonas vaginalis* and certain Gram-positive and Gram-negative microorganisms.

Vagifem® is a vaginal tablet containing 10 µg estradiol and is used locally to treat menopausal changes in and around vagina (such as vaginal dryness/burning/itching). Candid® V1, V3 and V6 are vaginal tablets containing clotrimazole 500 mg, 200 mg, and 100 mg, respectively, to treat vaginal candidiasis commonly known as yeast infection. Numbers 1, 3 and 6 in the names indicate that Candid-V1 is used for one day, Candid-V3 is used for three days, and Candid V6 is used for six days. Canesten® vaginal tablets containing clotrimazole are available in different doses such as 100 mg (Fig. 9.4), 200 mg (CanestenComfortab 3), 500 mg (CanestenComfortab 1). These should be inserted high into the vagina once daily (preferably at bedtime) using the applicator(s) provided for 6, 3, or 1 days, respectively.

A conventional tablet has also been modified in various manners such as bioadhesive tablet to increase retention time in vagina. As ketoconazole shows concentration-dependent fungistatic effect, it has been formulated as bioadhesive tablet to increase the time of contact of drug with the vaginal mucosa using sodium carboxymethylcellulose or polyvinylpyrrolidone or hydroxypropylmethylcellulose (HPMC-E_{50}). Bioadhesive tablets containing 1:1 and 1:2 drug/polymer ratio using HPMC-E_{50} have shown *in vitro* a good sustained release action. A unique kind of system is osmotic pump tablets for the delivery of anti-retroviral to vaginal mucosa. Tablets can actively and in a controlled manner deliver topical anti-retrovirals for one to multiple days after a single intravaginal application. Drug release rate from these systems is typically a function of rate of water entry into the device due to an osmotic pressure gradient between the device core and the environment.

4. Vaginal films

Polymeric films are thin strips of polymeric water-soluble excipients which dissolve when placed on the vaginal mucosal surface to release the active ingredient. Polymeric films offer accurate dose administration and can be applied without an applicator. As films are solid dry drug delivery system, the "messy" discharge associated with product leakage is avoided. Once in contact with vaginal fluids, these films dissolve rapidly. As there is no introduction of additional fluids, this leads to reduced leakage. Additionally, their rapid dissolving nature ensures quick release once inserted. Other advantages include good portability, easy storage, discreet use, no product leakage, reduced cost, convenient application, prolonged retention time, even distribution and improved stability of drug at harsh conditions. Furthermore, vaginal polymeric thin films can be used to stabilize drugs susceptible to degradation in aqueous

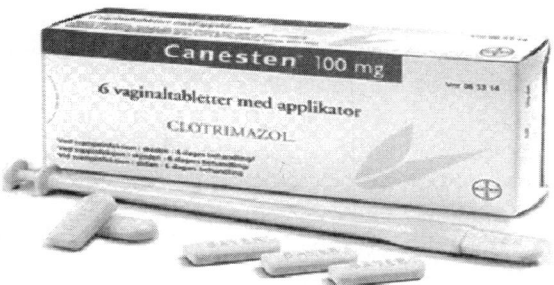

Fig. 9.4. Vaginal tablet – Canesten 100 mg.

condition. Additionally, results of published acceptability studies have shown that vaginal films were favorably accepted by women over other vaginal dosage forms such as gels, foams and tablets.

Polymers most commonly used in the preparation of polymeric vaginal films are hydroxypropylmethylcellulose (HPMC), sodium carboxymethylcellulose (SCMC), carbopol, chitosan etc. The commercially available vaginal films are vaginal contraceptive film (VCF), vaginal lubricating film and vaginal scented film.

Till now vaginal films containing contraceptives have been developed and marketed but having insight into the other vaginal problems like transmission of infections e.g. HIV, vaginitis, other fungal or viral infections there is a need to develop the vaginal films containing antifungal, antiviral agents for local treatment or prevention of transmission of infection during sexual contact. Various antimicrobial agents are suitable to be fabricated as film for vaginal administration. Nonoxynol-9 films have been formulated and studies have been done to assess the ability of a new contraceptive vaginal film containing two doses of nonoxynol-9 (N-9) to prevent the penetration of sperm into midcycle cervical mucus. Benzalkonium chloride (BZK) shows in *in vitro* and *in vivo* studies to immobilize sperm, to be active against STD-causing organisms and to penetrate and thicken cervical mucus. Mucoadhesive films and matrices based on chitosan and polyacrylic acid have been explored for vaginal delivery of drugs for local application.

5. Vaginal rings

Vaginal rings are circular polymeric rings designed to release the drug in a controlled fashion after the ring's insertion into the vagina. Their main use is for contraception. This technology can be used to prevent sexually transmitted infections. Since their first demonstration, they have been made from flexible polysiloxane and ethylene vinyl acetate copolymer. Contra-

ceptive rings have been used for years, both to deliver progesterone alone or in combination with estrogen. They act as chemical barriers to fertilization, as they are hormonal preparations. They release the hormones in a controlled manner which suppresses ovulation. These rings have to be inserted into vagina and they continue to release the hormones for few months. Different types of vaginal rings have been shown in Fig. 9.5.

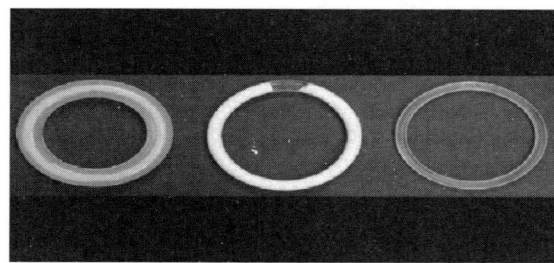

Fig. 9.5. Various types of vaginal rings. (Reproduced from the website of Northwestern University, Evanston, Illinois, USA with their permission)

NuvaRing®, a low dose contraceptive vaginal ring, releases ethynil estradiol and etonogestral for 3 weeks. It is a flexible, transparent ring made up of ethylene-vinyl acetate co-polymer, containing hormones that are dispersed throughout the ring's core and absorbed through the vaginal lining directly into the bloodstream, when inserted. NuvaRing® must be inserted and left in place for three consecutive weeks in order to prevent pregnancy for a month. Another ring should be inserted for continued contraceptive effect after giving a week's interval. NuvaRing® delivers 120 µg of etonogestrel (a progestin) and 15 µg of ethinyl estradiol (an estrogen) per day.

Estring®, a low dose estradiol ring, releases estradiol for 3 months. It is indicated for treatment of vaginal atrophy. It is a slightly opaque ring, made of a silicone elastomer, with a whitish core, containing a drug reservoir of estradiol hemihydrate. The outer diameter of the ring is 55 mm, cross-sectional diameter is 9 mm and core diameter is 2 mm. Each vaginal ring contains 2.0 mg of estradiol hemihydrate corresponding to 1.94 mg estradiol. It releases 7.5 microgram per 24 hours of estradiol (average) over a period of 90 days.

Femring® releases estradiol acetate to treat hot flashes and vaginal atrophy associated with menopause. It is made of cured silicone elastomer composed of dimethyl polysiloxanesilanol, silica (diatomaceous earth), normal propyl orthosilicate, stannous octoate; barium sulfate and estradiol acetate. Outer diameter of the ring is 56 mm with cross-sectional diameter 7.6 mm and core diameter 2 mm. It is available in two strengths. One contains 12.4 mg of estradiol acetate which releases at a rate equivalent to 0.05 mg of estradiol per day for 3 months. Second ring contains 24.8 mg of estradiol acetate, which releases at a rate equivalent to 0.10 mg of estradiol per day for 3 months.

From the past few decades research is also being going on the use of vaginal rings to prevent HIV infection. Antiretroviral drugs (dapavirine and maraviroc; tenofovir and dapivirine) incorporated in vaginal rings have been developed for the management of HIV infection.

6. Mucoadhesive delivery systems

Several drawbacks are associated with the conventional delivery systems (gels, tablets, foams, creams, irrigations) such as short residence time owing to self-cleaning property of vaginal tract, need for frequent and multiple daily dosing to achieve the desired therapeutic effects, etc. In this respect, mucoadhesive system seems a promising solution to the delivery system related problems and vaginal route appears highly appropriate for the mucoadhesive drug delivery system. Importance of mucoadhesive drug delivery systems lies in their ability to allow an intimate contact of the dosage form with the underlying absorption surface resulting in prolongation of residence time at the absorption site. Further, with increase in residence time, it is possible to achieve a decrease in dosing frequency and increase in patient compliance to the therapy. Therefore, such systems may prove helpful in improving the treatment of several diseases, by maintaining an effective concentration of the drug at the site of action for relatively longer period of time.

For vaginal route bioadhesive therapeutic systems have been developed in the form of semisolid and solid dosage forms. Various synthetic and natural polymers have been tried for mucoadhesive drug delivery systems. The most commonly used mucoadhesive polymers that are capable of forming hydrogels are synthetic polyacrylates, polycarbophil, chitosan, cellulose derivatives (hydroxyethylcellulose, hydroxypropylcellulose and hydroxypropyl-methylcellulose), hyaluronic acid derivatives, pectin, tragacanth, carrageenan and sodium alginate. Thiolated polymers have been explored as new mucoadhesive molecules. These mucoadhesive polymers are also classified according to their source of origin in Table 9.3. From the various mentioned bioadhesive polymers, polyacrylic acids have been extensively employed for vaginal applications. Among the polyacrylic acid polymers, polycarbophil, a polyacrylic acid cross-linked with divinylglycol, is most preferred. This water insoluble polymer has an apparent pKa of approximately 4.5 and picks up 60–100 times its weight in water. Marketed gel product Replens®, a bioadhesive polycarbophil gel, retains moisture and lubricates vagina for 3–4 days and maintains a healthy condition. Prochieve® 8% and Crinone® 8% are bioadhesive vaginal gel products of Columbia Laboratories used in hormone replacement therapy. Azidothymidine-loaded bioadhesive vaginal gel has been prepared successfully by using cold mechanical method with the aim of achieving controlled release with enhanced bioavailability over longer periods of time and has shown good extrudability, spreadability, and bioadhesive strength. An acid buffering gel, Acidform, forms a thin bioadhesive layer over the genital tract surface and is currently in Phase I clinical studies. Vaginal bioadhesive sustained-

Table 9.3. Different mucoadhesive polymers on the basis of their origin

Natural polymers	Protein-based	Collagen, albumin, gelatin
	Polysaccharides	Alginates, chitosan, dextran, starch, cellulose, agarose
Synthetic biodegradable polymers	Polyesters	Polylactic acid, polyglycolic acid, polycaprolactone
	Polyanhydride	Polyadipic acid, polysebacic acid
	Polyamides	Polyamino acids
	Phosphorous-based	Polyphosphates, polyphosphazenes
	Others	Polyurethanes, polycyanoacrylates
Synthetic non-biodegradable polymers	Cellulose derivatives	HPMC, ethyl cellulose, carboxymethylcellulose
	Silicone	Polydimethylsiloxane, colloidal silica, polymethacrylates
	Others	PVP, PVA, poloxamines

release tablet formulations may be developed using bioactives to increase the residence time of drugs in the vagina, thereby boosting the efficacy of the treatment, which may contain polymer like carbomer (Carbopol 974P, Carbopol 934P), hydroxypropylmethylcellulose (HPMC) and hydroxypropylcellulose (HPC). Liposome gel formulations containing antifungal drugs can reduce the toxicity of antifungal drugs and will provide longer duration of residence in presence of bioadhesive polymers. Bioadhesive tablets of ketoconazole, mucoadhesive polymer-coated curcumin liposomes have been found to increase their time of contact with the vaginal mucosa.

7. Electrospun fibers

Recently, a novel dosage form for intravaginal drug delivery has been developed using drug-eluting fibers fabricated by electrospinning, a technique that applies electrostatic forces to form polymeric fibers. Electrospinning is an elegant and facile method for formulating a solid-dosage form microbicide product. The process of electrospinning fibers is well-established, efficient and relatively inexpensive and, since most synthetic and many biological polymers can be electrospun, there is a wide array of possible formulations envisioned for diverse

antiretroviral drugs. Fibers are able to deliver a wide range of agents, incorporate multiple agents via composites, and facilitate controlled release over relevant time frames for pericoital and sustained (coitally-independent) use. Scale-up production of fiber-based microbicides is also technologically feasible. Hence, this novel system may lead to drug delivery through vaginal route to a new platform.

8. Nano-scale systems for vaginal drug delivery

Conventional vaginal drug delivery systems discussed so far (e.g. pessaries, foams, creams, gels and tablets) suffer from various disadvantages like low residence time, mucosal irritation, poor solubility of drug substance, high dosing frequency which contribute to poor subject or patient compliance. Nano systems may offer certain distinct advantages for vaginal drug delivery with respect to better bioavailability, improved safety and better drug utilization. It may modulate the pharmacokinetics of incorporated molecules because the properties that govern drug absorption, distribution, and elimination while in the human body are determined not by the drug properties, rather by the nanosystems' physical-chemical properties, particularly its interactions with biological barriers and modifiable parameters, such as composition, size, core properties, surface modifications (pegylation and surface charge), and ligand functionalization. Also, protein binding occurs when nanoparticles enter the physiological environment, modifying their biodistribution and biocompatibility characteristics but this can be controlled and manipulated by nanoparticle engineering for generating favorable biodistribution characteristics.

General properties of nanosystems that favor their use in drug delivery include versatility (virtually all drugs may be encapsulated), good toxicity profile (depending on used excipients), possibility of drug-release modulation, high drug payloads, easiness to produce and possible scale-up to mass production scale. Their ability to incorporate, protect and/or promote the absorption of non-orally administrable is of importance to improve the bioavailability of several molecules, protection of incorporated drugs from metabolism, allowing prolonged drug residence in the human body, thus reducing needed doses and prolonging time between administrations. The possibility of incorporating different drugs in the same delivery system and modulate their release individually is possible. This may contribute to simplify drug administration schedules, which is an important objective towards the reduction of drug administration errors.

Nanosystems seem to be able to reduce toxicity of drugs even if drug uptake is increased when encapsulated in nanocarriers, probably due to the slow-release properties of these systems and thus diminishing the achievement of prompt local high concentration of toxic drugs.

At present 40% of the drugs in the development pipelines and approximately 60% of the drugs coming directly from synthesis are poorly soluble. Nanosystems are gaining importance for the delivery of hydrophobic, poorly water-soluble drugs e.g. microemulsions are being used for solubilization of hydrophobic drugs.

Nanoparticles composed of degradable polymers can protect the payload from the harsh environment and allow for their sustained release within target cells in the epithelium. Drug encapsulated nanoparticles are solid colloidal particles, i.e., below 100 nm. Based on their size and polymeric composition, they are able to penetrate into the vaginal mucosa and have also shown potential for sustained drug delivery. Encapsulation of antiviral drugs into such systems may provide improved efficacy, decreased drug resistance, reduction in dosage, decrease in systemic toxicity and side effects, and improvement in patient compliance. Moreover these systems may be further incorporated into suitable inert vehicles like bioadhesive gels, to improve their application based on site of application. Also, biodegradability, biocompatibility and mucoadhesiveness may provide the added advantage.

Opsonization presents a major biological barrier to delivery of nanoparticles. After being absorbed systemically, opsonin proteins quickly bind to conventional non-stealth nanoparticles in the blood serum, due to which they are easily recognized by macrophages of the mononuclear phagocytic system and removed from the blood stream before fulfilling the desired functions. Several strategies are used to prevent the nanoparticles from being recognized by macrophages. The most preferred method is PEGylation, i.e., the adsorption of poly(ethylene glycol) to the surface of nanoparticles resulting in an increase in their blood circulation half-life by several orders of magnitude. It creates a hydrophilic protective layer around the nanoparticles thereby causing steric hindrance which is able to repel the absorption of opsonin proteins via steric repulsion forces, thereby preventing the attachment of opsonins and further removal by macrophages.

Mainly antifungal (clotrimazole, amphotericin-B), antibacterial (metronidazole), antiviral agents (tenofovir, aciclovir), curcumin, and interferon-α, etc. have been incorporated into nano systems for local as well as systemic delivery. These nano formulation systems include microemulsion, liposomes, nano-particles, solid lipid nanoparticles, nanofibres, etc. which can be used for vaginal drug delivery.

Microemulsions are thermodynamically stable and transparent dispersions of oil and water stabilized by an interfacial film of surfactant molecules. They are superior to other micellar systems in terms of solubilization potential and their thermodynamic stability offers advantages over unstable dispersions, such as emulsions and suspensions. They are also known to enhance drug solubility, stability and modify drug release. They are inherent permeation enhancers as surfactant is one of the components of the microemulsion. Micro-emulsion-based work has been reported in literature for the purpose of improving bio-availability of poorly soluble drugs and delivery of antifungal and microbicidal contraceptive bioactives. Moreover, microemulsion systems may be employed to decrease the cytotoxicity caused by active pharmaceutical agents such as nonoxynol-9, a spermicidal agent, when administered vaginally by incorporating into microemulsion does not exhibit cytotoxicity which it generally possesses when administered in solution form and it is not associated with local inflammation in rabbit model. Gel micro-emulsion systems for spermicidal agents, antiviral agents, antifungal agents and anti-bacterial agents have been studied for local as well as systemic delivery.

Self-microemulsifying drug delivery systems (SMEDDS) are the isotropic mixtures of oil, surfactant and hydrophilic solvent, having a unique ability of forming fine oil in water micro-emulsion upon mild agitation followed by dilution in aqueous media. SMEDDS have also been explored as a vaginal drug delivery system. SMEDDS enhance the water solubility and bio-availability of hydrophobic drugs. Antiretroviral UC-781, protease inhibitors for treatment of HIV, and progesterone to improve its bioavailability have been tried to be delivered through vaginal route.

Liposomes are small vesicular systems composed of cholesterol and other non-toxic phospholipids. Liposomal systems are bio-degradable, biocompatible, non-immunogenic, less toxic and can incorporate both hydrophilic and lipophilic drugs; thus, are also being explored as vaginal drug delivery system. The systemic toxicity of antifungal drugs is very high and liposomal formulation of such drugs can: (i) assure the high local drug concentration with concomitant avoidance of systemic absorption; and (ii) prevent recurrence of infection. Lipo-somal systems of clotrimazole, metronidazole, and chloramphenicol incorporated into bio-adhesive carbopol gels have shown potential for treatment of vaginal infections.

Nanoparticles are the particulate dispersions or solid particles in the size range of 10–1000 nm. Antiretroviral drugs can also be incorporated in nanoparticles for vaginal delivery. Among antimycotics, clotrimazole, is a poorly water-soluble drug used topically in the treatment of vulvovaginitis caused by *Candida albicans* which is generally associated with mucosal irritation, leakage of the formulation, and low residence time at the vaginal cavity. The nanocapsules intended for the vaginal delivery have improved the limitations of clotrimazole. Tenofovir or tenofovir disoproxil fumarate-loaded nanoparticles consisting of blend of poly(lactic-co-glycolic acid) (PLGA) and methacrylic acid copolymer (Eudragit-S-100, or S-100) has been found noncytotoxic and exhibited significant pH-responsive release of anti-HIV microbicides in the presence of human semen fluid simulant (SFS).

Solid lipid nanoparticles also have the potential to be considered as carriers for improved vaginal drug delivery due to numerous potential advantages, including the potential for sustained/controlled drug release and targeting, an increase in drug stability, the ability to incorporate a wide variety of drugs and their bio-compatibility. SLNs can be manufactured at the commercial scale more easily than liposomes.

Anti-HIV agent, tenofovir, loaded into poly-lysine-heparin functionalized solid lipid nanoparticles has been found non-cytotoxic to vaginal cells for 48 hours and with increased cellular uptake of tenofovir.

CONCLUSION

Vagina, because of its large surface area, high vascularity, and permeability to a wide range of compounds, has been explored as a potential route for delivery of a number of drugs both locally and systemically. Drugs can be delivered through incorporation in conventional dosage forms as well as in nano-sized delivery systems. Moreover, newly emerging systems provide better alternative for drug delivery by decreasing side effects as low doses may give rise to higher drug concentrations when administered vaginally and thus increase the efficiency of administration. Prolonged effects may also be obtained by using mucoadhesive delivery systems. Various new dosage forms like liposomal mucoadhesive gels, solid lipid nanoparticles, microemulsions, etc. can be used in order to improve the bioavailability and to modify the overall kinetics of the drug. Moreover, electrospun fibers are being explored for the delivery of various antiviral agents through vaginal route.

Thus, vaginal route may act as a good option for delivering local as well as systemically active agents with the potential availability of various types of dosage forms while increasing the bioavailability, decreasing the side effects, increasing efficiency of administration and also the patient compliance.

SUGGESTIVE READING

- S. Das, A. Choudhury, M. Kar. A Review on Novelty and Potentiality of Vaginal Drug Delivery. *Int. J. Pharm. Tech. Res*. (2011), 3: 1033–1044.
- L.M. Ensign, R. Cone, J. Hanes. Nanoparticle-based drug delivery to the vagina: A review. *J. Control Release* (2014), 190: 500–514.
- A. Deshpande, C.T. Rhodes, M. Danish. Intravaginal drug delivery. *Drug Dev. Ind. Pharm*. (1992), 18:1225–1279.
- A. Hussain, F. Ahmed. The vagina as a route for systemic drug delivery. *J. Control Release* (2005), 103: 301–313.
- K. Vermani, S. Garg. The scope and potential of vaginal drug delivery. *Pharm. Sci. Technolo. Today* (2000), 3: 359–364.
- V. Ashok, R.M. Kumar, D. Murali, A. Chatterjee. A review on vaginal route as a systemic drug delivery. *Crit. Rev. Pharm. Sci*. (2012), 1: 1–19.
- V.V. Kale, A. Ubgade. Vaginal mucosa – A promising site for drug therapy. *Br. J. Pharm. Res*. (2013), 3: 983–1000.

10

Stability Testing During Drug and Product Development

Saranjit Singh

INTRODUCTION

The purpose of product development is to prepare robust marketed formulations that maintain their quality within specifications till the end of the shelf life. The scope of product development encompasses new drugs, generics, value-added generics, line extensions, new drug delivery systems (NDDS) and reformulation activities, which include pack change and cost reduction. On the other hand, stability testing is defined as study of the influence of distribution and storage conditions on integrity of the drug or its product(s). The latter measures and documents the ability of a drug or product to retain its characteristics prior to the predicted retest period/expiry date. In fact, stability testing is a major procedural component during development of the drug and its products and is an indispensable activity.

Stability testing is practically initiated when the drug is still in the cradle stage and continues till the product remains in the market. Therefore, it is most time and money consuming. It focuses on the changes in physical (e.g., appearance, particle size, water content, etc.), chemical (e.g., integrity, assay, potency, degradation, etc.),

microbiological (e.g., level of microbial contamination) and functional properties (e.g., disintegration, dissolution, release, etc.). Stability data help to decide most suitable packaging, establish distribution/shipping conditions, and determine estimates of retest period/shelf life and storage directions.

Thus, stability testing is a key to establishing and sustaining a high quality product. However, the extensive exercise of stability testing and the huge expenditure involved in it gives no tangible benefit to the manufacturer, except providing confidence that the quality of a pharmaceutical will hold true until its shelf life. The latter is important for the manufacturer as there can be serious consequences, including loss of reputation and legal repercussions, if a product fails to comply with the specifications any time before the expiry date. However, more important is the concern for the patient, who must get an assured quality product when in need.

For the latter reason, the practice of stability testing is governed by regulatory requirements and guidelines, many of which have been issued at international, regional and local levels. The innovator industry, which is involved in new drug development, is primarily located in United States, Europe and Japan. Therefore, the focus of International Conference on Harmonisation (ICH, now International Council for Harmonisation) guidelines mainly has been on quality, safety and efficacy aspects of new drug substances and products. ICH had issued multiple guidelines on stability testing under codes Q1A-Q1F, with another guideline Q5C covering expectations for new biological/ biotechnological drugs and products (Table 10.1). Stability data requirements have also been laid down for Exploratory Investigational New

Drug and Investigational New Drug (IND) stages of new drug and product development by the United States Food and Drug Administration (USFDA) (USFDA, 1995; USFDA, 2006).

For existing drugs and related products, a guideline on stability testing has been issued by European Medicines Agency (EMEA) (EMEA, 2003). USFDA has also recently introduced guideline for stability testing of Abbreviated New Drug Applications (ANDAs) (USFDA, 2013) with almost the same provisions as of ICH Q1A-(R2) (ICH, 2003a), except 6 months long-

Table 10.1. ICH stability testing guidelines
http://www.ich.org/products/guidelines/quality/article/quality-guidelines.html
Accessed on 22.02.2017

ICH Code	Guideline Title	Remarks	Date of Finalization
Q1A (R2)	Stability Testing of New Drug Substances and Products (Second Revision)	This guideline provides recommendations on stability testing protocols including temperature, humidity and trial duration.	6 Feb 2003
Q1B	Stability Testing: Photostability Testing of New Drug Substances and Products	This forms an annex to the main stability guideline, and gives guidance on the basic testing protocol required to evaluate the light sensitivity and stability of new drugs and products.	5 Nov 1996
Q1C	Stability Testing for New Dosage Forms	It extends the main stability guideline for new formulations of already approved medicines and defines the circumstances under which reduced stability data can be accepted.	5 Nov 1996
Q1D	Bracketing and Matrixing Designs for Stability Testing of Drug Substances and Products	Describes general principles for reduced stability testing and provides examples of bracketing and matrixing designs.	5 Feb 2002
Q1E	Evaluation of Stability Data	Extends the main guideline by explaining possible situations where extrapolation of retest periods/shelf-lives beyond the real-time data may be appropriate. Furthermore, it provides examples of statistical approaches to stability data analysis.	5 Feb 2003
Q1F	Stability Data Package for Registration Applications in Climatic Zones III and IV	Provides guidance on specific stability testing requirements for Climatic Zones III and IV. Besides proposing acceptable storage conditions for long-term and accelerated studies, it gives guidance on data to cover situations of elevated temperature and/or extremes of humidity.	5 Feb 2003 (Withdrawn)
Q5C	Stability Testing of Biotechnological/Biological Products	Describes generation and submission of stability data of well-characterized proteins and peptides, their derivatives and products of which they are components.	30 Nov 1995

term and equal period accelerated testing at the time of submission. Primarily, issuance of guidances on generic product development and manufacture has been the focus of World Health Organization (WHO). WHO issued its first stability testing guideline in 1996 (WHO, 1996), just after introduction of ICH parent guideline Q1A in 1993 (ICH, 1993). It covered existing drugs in conventional dosage forms, which were in circulation in most countries under WHO's umbrella. At that time, ICH and WHO guidelines were modelled differently. Because ICH guidelines were more extensive and were revised from time to time (e.g., Q1A (1993) → Q1A(R) (2000) → Q1A(R2) (2003), the industry practices at global level in the last 20 years got aligned largely around these guidelines. This was also recognized by WHO, when it planned to revise its 1996 guideline. The latest 2009 WHO guideline (WHO, 2009) is modelled on ICH Q1A(R2) (ICH, 2003a), with even the language being similar at most places. There are a few differences, the first being that it covers stability testing of both new and existing drugs and products, against applicability of ICH guidelines to new drug substances and products only. Also, it covers due relaxations for existing drug substances and their products. In addition, it provides tables outlining long-term storage conditions for all the countries, and also separately lists test parameters for various dosage forms. The guideline was finalized after many years of effort and through a wide consultation process among the stakeholders, including those from ICH countries. In that sense, the present WHO guidance can be considered as a true 'global' guideline, which can be implemented for stability testing data generation that may be acceptable in large parts of the world. Of course, exceptions may exist of individual countries, where requirements might vary, like in number of batches, duration of testing, evaluation, etc.

STABILITY TESTING FROM DISCOVERY TO LAUNCH OF NEW DRUGS AND PRODUCTS

Overall product development and stability testing activities are most intricate in the case of new drugs. The development of new drug and its products, from discovery to launch, is distributed into different phases. The first is discovery phase, which is also called candidate optimization/confirmation stage. In this phase, the emphasis is on establishing physicochemical properties of the drug candidate. It is followed by early stage development, which extends till IND filing, where major task is pre-formulation, toxicology (TOX) formulation development, and pre-clinical studies. The late stage development covers clinical testing and NDA filing. The same involves dosage form selection, first-in-human (FIH) formulation development, and formulations developed and prepared in each subsequent clinical phase following current Good Manufacturing Practices (cGMP). Next is the patent exclusivity phase that encompasses cGMP formulation manufacturing.

The nature of stability testing intensifies parallel to discovery to launch phases for the new drug and its products (Fig. 10.1). Practically, stability data are required in all phases to demonstrate that the new drug and its dosage forms remain within acceptable chemical and physical limits, initially for the period of intended investigations and later during lifecycle of the drug and its products. All through this journey, modifications happen in the scale of preparation of the drug and its dosage forms, so it also becomes important to scale-up generation of the stability data at every step of discovery and development.

Usually, no experimental stability studies are suggested for the discovery phase. In early stage development, the studies are more basic and focus on intrinsic drug stability, solid/solution stability, drug degradation pathways, and stability testing of the TOX formulation. In the

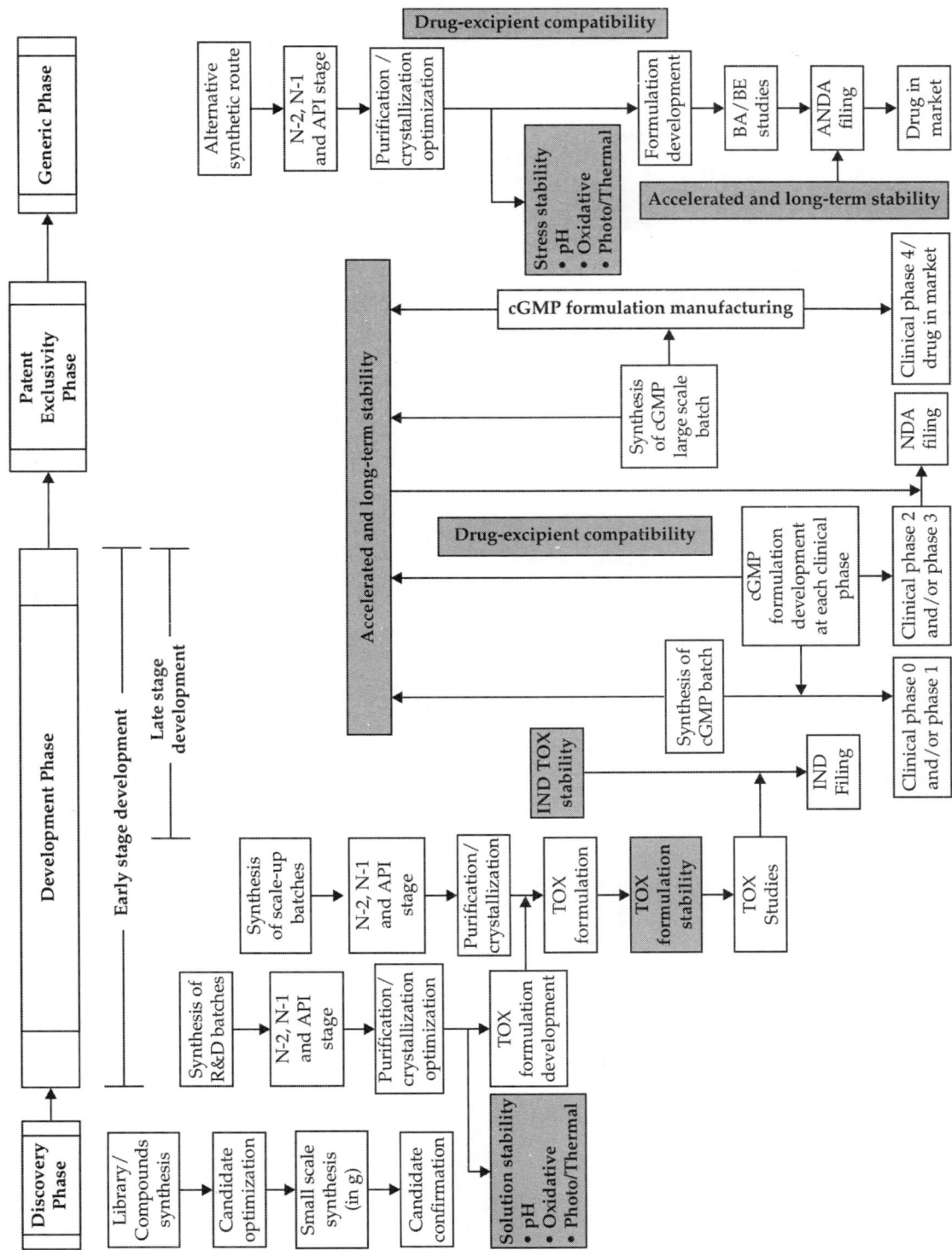

Fig. 10.1. Stability testing during discovery to launch phases of new drug and its products.

late stage development, emphasis is on stability testing of FIH and formulations for subsequent clinical phases manufactured under cGMP conditions; in-use stability testing, and stability testing of registration and commitment batches. During this period, companies also develop stability testing programs for distribution of drug substances and products, as the latter may encounter spikes in environment conditions during the period of distribution and shipment. Finally, on-going stability studies are carried out as a part of GMP requirement on marketed product(s) annually.

Much of the following discussion on analytical and stability studies during individual phases of drug and product development has genesis to the details provided by Ahuja and Scypinski (2001), and also USFDA draft stability testing guideline of 1998 (USFDA, 1998 Draft), which though withdrawn later, had clearly laid down a path for stability testing during IND, NDA and ANDA phases of drug development.

Stability studies during candidate optimization to early stage development

In the discovery phase, genomics, proteomics, combinatorial chemistry and high throughput screening yield mountain of new targets. However, the industry principle is: 'though study of more compounds improves chances of finding the right one, if you can eliminate the wrong compound quickly, you will find the right one rapidly and cost-effectively.' Very early in discovery, in silico studies are the main stay, and help in comparative evaluation of predicted physicochemical properties, activity and toxicity. Multiple software are available for the same, and several new ones are being developed, including those for prediction of drug degradation products. A key example is Zeneth by Lhasa Limited (http://www.lhasalimited.org/products/zeneth.htm, accessed on 22.02.2017).

Further, rank ordering of new chemical entities is done in early development stages. Initially, small quantities of potential candidates

are synthesized at R&D level. The available material is subjected to understanding of its chemistry, establishment of purity, determination of efficacy in animal models, screening of potential mutagenicity through Ames bacterial test, and evaluation of properties, like solubility, stability, permeability in caco-2 cells, preliminary pharmacokinetic profile, and potential for metabolic and toxicity liability. As 40% of molecules fail to reach the market because of poor biopharmaceutical properties, viz., solubility, permeability, dissolution rate, hygroscopicity, solid-state form and stability, therefore, early analytical activities also focus on them. Stability studies are usually restricted to short-term solid and solution state stability data generation on R&D and early scale-up batches, and assessment of stability of formulations required for efficacy, pharmacokinetics and toxicity studies on animals.

Clinical candidate selection

From the above candidate-screening phase, usually few compounds are selected that are further subjected to gross toxicity evaluation in at least one rodent and an equal number of non-rodent species, involving 7–14 days of dosing. The TOX formulation, which provides adequate exposure in animals, usually contains several times higher than the expected dose with respect to body weight in humans. A favourable safety profile of the selected new chemical entity from these short-term high dose animal studies helps in decision-making for favouring a compound to be taken forward. The analytical group supports the TOX program by multiple studies, viz., physicochemical characterization of the candidate compound, development of methods for its testing, preparation of certificates of analysis for drug substance and TOX test articles, establishment of impurity profiles in comparison to any previous batch(es) and additionally pre-formulation studies. Also, optimal solid-state (polymorphic) and chemical (salt) forms of the molecule are identified, targeted at selection of one that is most stable and bioavailable. The analytical methods for assay of the TOX formulations are developed and validated in preparation for the first Good Laboratory Practices (GLP) studies. Along with, release and stability testing of the TOX test articles are performed to support the suitability of the materials through their anticipated period of use. Typically, short-term accelerated stability studies are performed on the test formulations for at least 3 months to cover the time from date of manufacture through the last dose. At times, long-term studies are also initiated so that further information on stability behaviour of the drug under normative conditions is also available pre-hand.

Generally, stress (forced degradation) studies are initiated at this stage, which are meant to provoke a reaction or chemical change in the drug candidate (Singh and Bakshi, 2000; Singh et al., 2013). During stress studies on new drug substances, evaluation of solution stability extends to determining susceptibility to hydrolysis across a wide range of pH values; and examination of influence of oxidation, photolysis and thermal conditions. In the present times, good emphasis is also being paid to solid-state degradation behaviour of the drug substance, to mimic the degradation of the drug in solid dosage forms (Raijada et al., 2010). The studies are done using solid buffer salts, and exposure to combined conditions of temperature and humidity. Also, many studies in literature highlight that it is equally useful to detect and characterize volatile degradation products (Kurmi et al., 2015; Pravinchandra et al., 2015) for establishment of mass balance during drug degradation. Stress investigations in that way provide information on the drug's inherent instability and help identify major degradation products that are likely to be formed during manufacture, distribution and storage of the drug and products. They additionally allow development of stability-indicating assays (Singh and Bakshi, 2002), which have a role subsequently in the analysis of active(s) and degradation product(s). As these

studies are of short duration, they act as a rapid selection and elimination screen for drugs and their products, before lengthy and costly formal stability studies. The studies are often exploited to obtain pure degradation products, especially those formed in major percentage in any particular stress condition. The latter can then be used as test standards during analysis. The hydrolytic, oxidative and photolytic stress data provide information on the nature of degradation products likely to be formed and present in environment matrices (Singh et al., 2013; Narayanam et al., 2014). The forced degradation studies are conducted even subsequently in all stages of drug and product development (Alsante et al., 2007).

Toxicology formulation development and toxicity studies

In the next phase, gaining of knowledge on intrinsic stability of the new compound and support to ongoing TOX studies are continued. The toxicological investigations are conducted under GLP conditions with added species; and the exposure period is also enhanced to 2–4 weeks of dosing. Additional tests include: (1) GLP Ames test, (2) safety pharmacology, (3) genotoxicity profiling, and (4) pilot teratology studies (Ahuja and Scypinski, 2001). In parallel, the focus shifts to planning for development of FIH formulations for clinical studies. Analytical support teams undertake reference standard characterization; issue certificates of analysis for drug substance; develop new internal methods for cleaning validation, including stability-indicating methods for drug substance and TOX formulations; generate method validation summaries, including qualification of methods for GLP toxicological studies; study impurity profiles for new batches and compare with previous TOX batches; and generate analytical data for in-life toxicological study samples (homogeneity, periodic testing, and end-of-study). They also carry out excipient interaction studies and stability studies of prototype formulations. The selection of FIH formulation is usually based on satisfactory stability data and, preferably, a bioavailability study in a most suited animal species. The latter assists in predicting bioavailability profile of the prospective drug in humans. Additionally, data are compiled for establishing IND specifications for clinical materials. The stability study of TOX test articles is continued and investigation is extended to new TOX formulations, as may be necessary.

Exploratory investigational new drug Phase 0 studies

USFDA came out with a guideline in 2006 titled as 'Exploratory IND Studies', which offered non-binding recommendations targeted at planning of exploratory studies in humans under an IND application (USFDA, 2006). It was rather a new option for industry before conducting formal phase 1 clinical testing involving FIH formulation. While the traditional phase 1 studies sought to establish a maximally tolerated dose and looked for dose-limiting toxicities, exploratory IND studies were meant to administer either sub-pharmacologic doses of a product, or doses expected to produce a pharmacologic, but not a toxic effect. Thus, the new approach meant low potential risk to human subjects. Such limited exploratory IND investigations in humans could be initiated with less, or different, preclinical support than is required for traditional IND studies. The benefits outlined were that such studies could: (1) help determine whether a mechanism of action defined in experimental systems could also be observed in humans (e.g., a binding property or inhibition of an enzyme); (2) provide important information on pharmacokinetics (PK); (3) select the most promising lead product from a group of candidates designed to interact with a particular therapeutic target in humans based on PK or pharmacodynamic (PD) properties; and (4) help explore a product's biodistribution characteristics using various imaging technologies, as

the drug is administered in micro-dose. The studies were suggested to be done on limited number of subjects (healthy volunteers or patients), with the duration of dosing also limited to, say, 7 days. The guideline requires that sufficient information should be submitted to ensure proper identification, strength, quality, purity, and potency of the investigational candidate. Additionally, it recommends generation of 'information that demonstrates the stability of the product during TOX studies and an explanation of how stability will be evaluated during the clinical studies.'

First-in-Human Phase 1 studies

Phase 1 clinical studies mean first-time introduction of the investigational new drug into human subjects. The investigations, which are carried out mainly on healthy volunteers and in some cases directly on patients, are primarily targeted to reveal the side effects associated with increasing doses. The same may also provide early evidence of effectiveness and some clue to mechanism of action, when the study is done on patients. Phase 1 studies are also usually targeted to determine metabolism and pharmacokinetics of the drug of interest.

It is essential that animal to human migration during drug development is done as safely as possible. Therefore, before full-dose FIH studies, the available information should include salt selection, evaluation of results of forced degradation studies, drug degradation pathways, excipient compatibility studies, and all other efforts towards characterization of new drug substance. As clinical materials must have adequate quality, consistency, and stability, therefore, relevant documents proving the same shall be available. During this phase, usually a simple clinical formulation is developed, hence for phase 1, stability studies are short that focus on supporting the short-term clinical trials. Stability studies on such clinical formulation(s) involve accelerated and long-term testing relevant to duration of clinical trials. Usually, clinical trial phase 1 formulations need to have shelf-life of 3–6 months.

According to USFDA 1998 guideline (USFDA, 1998 Draft), information to support the stability of both the drug substance and the drug products during the proposed clinical study(ies) should include: (1) a brief description of the stability study, (2) description of the test methods used to monitor the stability of the drug substance and the drug product packaged in the proposed container/closure system, (3) data on monitoring of storage conditions, and (4) preliminary tabular data based on the representative material. The guideline explicitly states that neither detailed stability data nor the stability protocol according to ICH are needed to be submitted. Also, it makes clear that "when significant decomposition during storage cannot be prevented, the clinical trial batch of drug product should be retested prior to the initiation of the trial and information should be submitted to show that it will remain stable during the course of the trial. This information should be based on the limited stability data available when the trial starts. Impurities that increase during storage may be qualified by reference to prior human or animal data."

Clinical studies in Phase 2

The phase 2 activities, which in other way are also considered continuation of phase 1 studies, involve controlled clinical studies on the test drug on less than a few hundred patients having a particular indication. These studies are essentially meant to evaluate dose range, effectiveness, common short-term side effects and any other risks associated with the potential drug molecule. Simultaneous to these clinical studies, other aspects of development also continue like (1) drug substance characterization, (2) improvements in synthetic routes/processes, (3) identification of newer impurities and/or degradation products, (4) evaluation and control of stereochemistry (for stereoisomeric compounds) and/or potential solid-state forms

(e.g., hydrates, solvates, or polymorphs), (5) optimization of analytical methods, (6) revision of specifications, and (7) development of market image products. Also, phase 2 trials and the obtained results help the manufacturer to take decision on proceeding with full development of the new drug, which requires commitment of resources for large scale clinical trials and manufacturing of registration batches of both the drug substance and the drug product for eventual NDA submission.

With respect to stability evaluation, USFDA stability guideline (USFDA, 1998 Draft) adds that "development of drug product formulations during phase 2 should be based in part on the accumulating stability information gained from studies of the drug substance and its formulations. The objectives of stability testing during phases 1 and 2 are to evaluate the stability of the investigational formulations used in the initial clinical trials, to obtain the additional information needed to develop a final formulation, and to select the most appropriate container and closure (e.g., compatibility studies of potential interactive effects between the drug substance(s) and other components of the system). This information should be summarized and submitted to the IND during phase 2. Stability studies on these formulations should be well underway by the end of phase 2. At this point the stability protocol for study of both the drug substance and drug product should be defined, so that stability data generated during phase 3 studies will be appropriate for submission in the drug application."

Stability studies during phase 2, thus, run somewhat more than the duration of clinical studies, say at least 12–18 months. While the drug substance is continued to be monitored for long-term stability, information on stability of the finished product is collected in the proposed container/closure system till the clinical studies, and the same is continued further so as to gain information important for eventual market image products. For the latter, it is normal to prepare multiple formulations and screen out for the best package materials, for which a short-term stability study of 6 months is good enough, initially. The testing is even continued here under long-term storage conditions for 2–3 years. At this stage, protocol-based stability tests are initiated following the ICH parent guideline Q1A(R2) (ICH, 2003a). It may be reasonable to add here that if any comparator product has been used in the clinical trial, it might be good to carry out stability testing simultaneously on it also.

The developmental and stability studies on prospective final formulation involve compatibility studies between the drug and formulation excipients, and selection of the most appropriate container and closure systems. These investigations usually are conducted for short period under stress conditions such as 50°C or 60°C without and with humidity (usually 75% RH) for less than 3 months (more popular is 1 month). The data help to select excipients, primary package components, and storage conditions for the formulated product.

Clinical studies in Phase 3

Phase 3 studies are also known as pivotal efficacy trial(s) coupled with pre-NDA planning and development studies. These are carried out once enough evidence of efficacy of the new drug has been obtained in phase 2 clinical studies.

This particular subset of investigations involves the following: (1) expanded clinical trials on several hundred to several thousand patients, which are meant to provide confirmatory data on both safety and therapeutic efficacy of the new drug, and also assessment of the risk-benefit ratio; (2) evaluation of comparability of the proposed market formulation to the ones used in phase 1 and phase 2 studies through bioequivalence or bioavailability investigations; and (3) start of planning for NDA preparation, anticipating favorable results from this subset of clinical investigations.

During phase 3 activities, long-term stability testing of clinical formulations continues for minimum 24–36 months, while accelerated and long-term stability studies are initiated on the registration batches. Also, the analytical data for materials used in TOX studies, human dose confirmation, pivotal, and bioequivalency studies are reviewed and linked together, with specific emphasis on data on purity, impurities, stability, and *in vitro* product performance (e.g., dissolution), as these are critical from the perspectives of safety and equivalency. The same is echoed by USFDA (USFDA, 1998 Draft) explicitly through the following: the emphasis should be on testing final formulations in their proposed market packaging and manufacturing site. It is recommended that the final stability protocol be well defined prior to the initiation of phase 3 IND studies. In this regard, consideration should be given to establish appropriate linkage between the preclinical and clinical batches of the drug substance and drug product and those of the primary stability batches in support of the proposed expiration dating period. Factors to be considered may include, for example, source, quality and purity of various components of the drug product, manufacturing process of and facility for the drug substance and the drug product, and use of same containers and closures.

NDA submission and approval (Patent Phase)

Successful phase 3 on a new drug product is followed by submission of NDA to the regulatory agency for review. For the same, all types of available study data, whether preclinical, clinical, or technical, are compiled. During the filing of NDA, supporting 6-month accelerated and 12-month long-term stability data are generated. As usually 24 months shelf life is assigned based on satisfactory accelerated and long-term data, therefore, stability testing continues and updated reports, whenever available, can be submitted during the review period. In certain situations, prior agreement may be needed for submission of amendments during the review stage, but the same is usually not the case with respect to stability data, as they are covered under stability commitments filed as part of the NDA document.

The drug substance and formulation batches are scaled-up and the first pilot production batches are manufactured almost 15 months before NDA submission, and subjected to full-scale stability studies as per the protocol that meets the registration requirements of the pertinent licensing authorities. The protocol generally contains the following elements: (1) type, size and number of batches, (2) type of containers and closures, (3) container storage orientation, (4) test time points, (5) sampling plan, (6) test storage conditions, (7) test parameters, (8) test methods; (9) acceptance criteria, (10) evaluation, and (11) labelling. The parent ICH guideline Q1A(R2) (ICH, 2003a) covers the details of protocol for this phase.

The continued registration stability studies allow confirmation of the shelf life permitted at the time of the grant of marketing authorization and even for extension of the projected expiration period.

Where data on first production batches are not obtained initially, stability studies are carried out to fulfil the commitment to that respect made by the manufacturer to regulatory agency at the time of seeking marketing authorisation. The commitment stability studies are usually controlled by the same protocol, as employed for initial long-term stability study and submitted in the marketing authorization dossier. Any deviation (e.g., required for meeting revised recommendations) must be justified and documented. The results are formalized as a report. A summary of all the data generated, including any interim conclusions, is included. The summary is provided to the competent authorities as a part of the periodic review process.

The data are submitted at the time of registration according to ICH common technical document (ICH CTD) sections 2.3.S.7 and 2.3.P.8 (ICH, 2002a). These provide for nature of stability summaries, conclusions, post-approval stability protocol and stability commit-ment, and the manner in which stability data need to be submitted, for new drug substance and new drug product, respectively. For a drug substance, it is desired that summary of the types of studies conducted, protocols used, and the results obtained shall be presented. Also results from forced degradation studies under stress conditions shall be included. Conclusions with respect to storage conditions and retest date or shelf life, as appropriate, need to be added. Along with the same, post-approval stability protocol and stability commitment need to be filed, and results of the stability studies ought to be presented in an appropriate format such as tabular, graphical, and narrative. Information on analytical procedures used and their validation is also required. For drug products, usually no stress testing results are expected. For them, the conclusions include storage conditions and expiry period, and, if applicable, in-use storage conditions and relevant expiry period. Otherwise, stability commitment clause and manner of presentation of stability data remains the same, as for the drug substance.

Product launch and marketing in Phase 4

Phase 4 comes in picture after the product has been approved by the regulatory agency. It involves launching of the new drug and its products in the market. During this phase, stability studies are continued under the commit-ment (ICH, 2003a). From logistics point of view, the marketable products usually have a shelf life between 24–36 months. The products meant for export may bear a minimum life period of 36 months. Of course, extension of the period, generally to the maximum of 60 months, applies to all the cases, based on continuity of studies and generation of real time data. Whenever new dosage form, packages, or strength are developed and added as line extensions, stability studies on them are conducted by following ICH guidelines Q1C (ICH, 1996a) and/or Q1D (ICH, 2002b).

Guideline Q1C is just a half page recommendation advising on stability of a new dosage form intended to be introduced by the original applicant. The new dosage form is defined as "a drug product which is a different pharmaceutical product type, but contains the same active substance as included in the existing drug product approved by the pertinent regulatory authority". The guideline further suggests that: "Stability protocols for new dosage forms should follow the guidance in the parent stability guideline (ICH, 2003a) in principle. However, a reduced stability database at submission time (e.g., 6 months accelerated and 6 months long-term data from ongoing studies) may be acceptable in certain justified cases."

ICH Q1D was issued to assist those manufacturers who intended to bring out formulations with more than one drug strength, different sizes of the same container closure system, even different container closure systems, and/or secondary packaging systems. The guideline delves on reduced stability study designs covering two types, viz., bracketing and matrixing. The two have different principles. In bracketing, only samples on the extremes of certain design factors (e.g., strength, container size and/or fill) are tested at all time points, as in a full design. The design assumes that the stability of any intermediate levels is represented by the stability of the extremes tested, but is not considered appropriate if it cannot be demonstrated that the strengths or container sizes and/or fills selected for testing are indeed the extremes. On the other hand, in matrixing stability schedule, selected subset of the total number of possible samples for all factor combinations are tested at a specified time point. At a subsequent time point, another subset of samples for all factor combinations is tested. This design assumes that the stability of each subset of samples tested represents the stability of all samples at a given time point. The guidance provides sample designs for illustrative purposes (Table 10.2). The only problem with use of

reduced testing designs is the scientific justification that must precede every stage of their implementation.

STABILITY TESTING REQUIREMENTS DURING GENERIC PRODUCT DEVELOPMENT (ANDA FILING)

Once the patent phase is over, the innovator company continues with marketing of its drug and products. For such manufacturers, the requirement is only of on-going stability studies. Other companies, who are now free to develop and market generic drug and products, have the benefit that by this time significant knowledge about stability of the specific molecule and its products exists. A usual practice with the generic industry is to focus on a new drug and its products almost 6–8 years before the patent expiry. Thus, sufficient data, including stability information, is generated even during generic product development. The other gain for the generic companies is the availability of reference innovator product, which can be simultaneously subjected to stability testing for comparison purpose. The presence of stability test guidelines covering existing/generic drugs and products, with inherent flexibilities at places, is still another advantage.

The following are the salient relaxations in the requirements for stability testing of existing/generic drugs and products:

Drugs and products with monograph in pharmacopoeia

Usually, the term 'existing', as mentioned in some of the guidelines, covers compendial drugs and products. For them, the specifications defining their quality do exist. Specifically, the EMA guideline on stability testing of existing active substances and related finished products (EMEA, 2003) provides two options for drug substances covered by a pharmacopoeial monograph wherein suitable limits have been set

Table 10.2. Examples of bracketing and matrixing designs
http://www.ich.org/fileadmin/Public_Web_Site/ICH_Products/
Guidelines/Quality/Q1D/Step4/Q1D_Guideline.pdf
Accessed on 22.02.2017

Bracketing design

Strength		50 mg								
Batch		1	2	3	1	2	3	1	2	3
Container size	15 ml	x	x	x				x	x	x
	30 ml									
	60 ml	x	x	x				x	x	x

Matrixing design (one-half reduction)

Time points (months)			0	3	6	9	12	18	24	36
Strength	S1	Batch 1	x	x		x	x		x	x
		Batch 2	x	x		x	x	x		x
		Batch 3	x		x		x	x		x
	S2	Batch 1	x		x		x		x	x
		Batch 2	x	x		x	x	x		x
		Batch 3	x		x		x		x	x

Key: x = Sample tested

for the degradation products, but a re-test period is not defined. It states that: "(1) the applicant should specify that the drug complies with the pharmacopoeial monograph immediately prior to manufacture of the finished product, in which case no stability studies are required, provided that the suitability of the pharmacopoeial monograph has been demonstrated for the particular named source; or alternatively (2) the applicant should fix a re-test period based on the results of long-term testing, also considering results of testing under accelerated or, where applicable, intermediate storage conditions."

Stress testing of drug substance and products

With respect to stress testing, the same EMA guideline (EMEA, 2003) mentions that "when an active substance is described in an official pharmacopoeial monograph and fully meets its requirements, no data are required on the degradation products if they are named under the headings "purity test" and/or section on "impurities". Alternatively, for drugs not described in official compendia, one option is to provide the relevant data published in the literature to support the proposed degradation pathways, otherwise, stress testing should be performed". WHO guideline of 2009 (WHO, 2009), which also covers existing drug and products, suggests acceptance of relevant data published in the scientific literature to support the identified degradation products and pathways. It further suggests that stress testing should be performed only when no data are available. It means good scientific study published in the literature can be appended to the dossier, and the manufacturer can save itself from repeating these basic investigations. Again, stress testing of formulations, though not advised in ICH Q1A(R2) (ICH, 2003a) and WHO (WHO, 2009) guidelines, is a usual practice in industry. The studies on formulations yield valuable information on possible drug-drug, drug-excipient and formulation-packaging interactions. A protocol is proposed in the literature (Alsante et al., 2007).

Number of batches and duration of testing

For existing API, EMA guideline (EMEA, 2003) recommends two options: "(a) stability information from accelerated and long-term testing is to be provided on at least two production scale batches manufactured by the same manufacturing (synthetic) route and procedure described in part 3.2.S.2 of the application. The long-term testing and accelerated testing should cover a minimum of 6 months duration at the time of submission, or (b) stability information from accelerated and long-term testing is to be provided on at least three pilot scale batches manufactured by the same manufacturing (synthetic) route and procedure described in part 3.2.S.2 of the application. The long-term testing and accelerated testing should cover a minimum of 6 months duration at the time of submission."

The same guideline under section 2.2.3 'Selection of Batches' requires the following for existing drug products: "at the time of submission, data from stability studies should be provided for batches of the same formulation and dosage form in the container closure system proposed for marketing." It further suggests two options: (a) for conventional dosage forms (e.g. immediate release solid dosage forms, solutions) and when the active substances are known to be stable, stability data on at least two pilot scale batches are acceptable, or (b) for critical dosage forms or when the active substances are known

to be unstable, stability data on three primary batches are to be provided. Two of the three batches should be of at least pilot scale, the third batch may be smaller. The guideline even adds that "the manufacturing process used for primary batches should simulate that to be applied to production batches and should provide product of the same quality and meeting the same specification as that intended for marketing. Where possible, batches of the finished product should be manufactured by using different batches of the active substance. Stability studies should be performed on each individual strength and container size of the finished product unless bracketing or matrixing is applied. Other supporting data can be provided."

In the WHO guideline (WHO, 2009), the recommendation to test three primary batches extends to unstable existing/generic drugs and products. However, for established stable drug molecules and their products, the guideline provides relaxation in suggesting acceptance of data on two batches of production scale. Other provisions remain the same, as in EMA guideline (EMEA, 2003).

It may be reasonable to highlight here that, till recently, USFDA required only one batch data for generic drugs and products. Through a new notification (USFDA, 2013), it now requires three primary batch data on all the drugs and products in the ANDA. However, it gives the relaxation in the study duration by suggesting: "at the time of submission, provide 6 months of data that include accelerated and long-term conditions."

Test parameters

This heading in ICH, WHO and other guidelines is targeted to cover test attributes (list of tests, analytical procedures, and proposed acceptance criteria) for evaluation of stability test samples withdrawn at different times from the stability chambers. The ICH guideline Q1A(R2) (ICH, 2003a) does not directly provide any list of test parameters. It only mentions that those attributes shall be focused upon "that are susceptible to change during storage and are likely to influence quality, safety and/or efficacy", meaning that one need to set out shelf life specifications different from release specifications. It is also mentioned that "The testing should cover, as appropriate, the physical, chemical, biological and microbiological attributes." For dosage forms, additional mention exists with respect to preservative content (e.g., antioxidant, antimicrobial preservative), and functionality tests (e.g., for a dose delivery system). Specifically, for antimicrobial preservative, the directions are more explicit: "Any differences between the release and shelf life acceptance criteria for antimicrobial preservative content should be supported by a validated correlation of chemical content and preservative effectiveness demonstrated during drug development on the product in its final formulation (except for preservative concentration) intended for marketing. A single primary stability batch of the drug product should be tested for antimicrobial preservative effectiveness (in addition to preservative content) at the proposed shelf life for verification purposes, regardless of whether there is a difference between the release and shelf life acceptance criteria for preservative content." In difference to ICH, the WHO (2009) and ASEAN (2013) guidelines advantageously provide list of tests, both for active pharmaceutical ingredient and multiple types of dosage forms. A typical example is shown in Table 10.3.

Storage conditions

In total, three storage conditions are prescribed in the regulatory guidelines for formal stability testing. These are accelerated, intermediate and long-term. The accelerated storage condition in all guidelines is 40°C ± 2°C/75% RH ± 5% RH. For active pharmaceutical ingredients that fail to meet specifications on storage at 40°C/75% RH, and products like ointments, creams, gelatine capsules, etc., which may show physical changes under the same accelerated conditions, the storage is recommended under intermediate condition of 30°C ± 2°C/65% RH ± 5% RH. In comparison with these two fixed conditions, the long-term testing conditions are differentiated based on the classification of world into multiple zones. Zone I comprises the region with temperate environment; Zone II is Mediterranean (sub-tropical); Zone III encompasses countries having hot and dry environment; Zone IVA countries are hot and humid; while Zone IVB nations have hot and very humid climate. Since Zone II environment of ICH regions is more stringent than Zone I, hence for both Zones I and II, the long-term storage condition is 25°C ± 2°C/60% RH ± 5% RH. Zone III storage condition is 30°C ± 2°C/35% RH ± 5% RH, while the same for Zones IV and IVA are 30°C ± 2°C/65% RH ± 5% RH and 30°C ± 2°C/75% RH ± 5% RH, respectively. The long-term storage condition for each country in the world has been tabulated in the WHO guideline (WHO, 2009).

In particular, intermediate condition applies only to Zones I and II. As intermediate testing temperature matches the long-term test conditions for Zones III and IVA&B, therefore, there is no separate intermediate test condition for these.

It is now a general trend to carry out long-term stability studies at 30°C ± 2°C/75% RH ± 5% RH. The advantage is that it is most stringent out of all the conditions (except Zone III) and hence the data generated at this condition is accepted globally. Yet there is a requirement for the doers to check from regulatory of individual country, if they have any insistence on a different long-term storage condition. Like India has been established to have a long-term storage condition of 30°C ± 2°C /70% RH ± 5% RH (Singh et al., 2009, 2010), and the same is also indicated in the WHO list (WHO, 2009).

The regulatory guidelines also prescribe separate storage conditions for products packed in impermeable (25°C ± 2°C/any controlled condition or ambient humidity for Zones I/II and 30°C ± 2°C/any controlled condition or ambient

Table 10.3. Stability test parameters for various types of products (WHO, 2009)

Dosage form	Test parameters*
Tablets	Dissolution/disintegration, water content, moisture and friability/hardness.
Hard gelatin capsules	Brittleness, dissolution/disintegration, water content, and level of microbial contamination.
Soft gelatin capsules	Dissolution/disintegration, level of microbial contamination, pH, leakage and pellicle formation.
Oral solutions, suspensions and emulsions	Formation of precipitate, clarity (solutions), pH, viscosity, extractables, level of microbial contamination. For suspensions additional parameters are: dispersibility, rhelogical properties, mean size and distribution of particles. Also, polymorphic conversion, if applicable. Additionally for emulsions: phase separation, mean size and distribution of dispersed globules.
Powders and granules for oral solutions or suspensions	Water content and reconstitution time. Reconstituted products (solutions and suspensions) should be evaluated as described above under "Oral solutions, suspensions and emulsions", after preparation according to the recommended labelling, through the maximum intended use period.
Metered-dose inhalers and nasal aerosols	Dose content uniformity, labelled number of medication actuations per container meeting dose content uniformity, aerodynamic particle size distribution, microscopic evaluation, water content, leak rate, level of microbial contamination, valve delivery (shot weight), extractables/leachables from plastic and elastomeric components, weight loss, pump delivery, foreign particulate matter and extractables/leachables from plastic and elastomeric components of the container, closure and pump. Samples should be stored in upright and inverted/on-the-side orientations. For suspension-type aerosols, microscopic examination of appearance of the valve components and container's contents for large particles, changes in morphology of the active ingredient particles, extent of agglomerates, crystal growth, foreign particulate matter, corrosion of the inside of the container or deterioration of the gaskets.
Nasal sprays: solutions and suspensions	Clarity (for solution), level of microbial contamination, pH, particulate matter, unit spray medication content uniformity, number of actuations meeting unit spray content uniformity per container, droplet and/or particle size distribution, weight loss, pump delivery, microscopic evaluation (for suspensions), foreign particulate matter and extractables/leachables from plastic and elastomeric components of the container, closure and pump.
Topical, ophthalmic and otic preparations, including ointments, creams, lotions, paste, gel, solutions, eye drops and cutaneous sprays	Topical preparations should be evaluated for clarity, homogeneity, pH, suspendability (for lotions), consistency, viscosity, particle size distribution (for suspensions, when feasible), level of microbial contamination/sterility and weight loss (when appropriate). Evaluation of ophthalmic or otic products (e.g. creams, ointments, solutions and suspensions) should include the following additional attributes: sterility, particulate matter and extractable volume. Evaluation of cutaneous sprays should include: pressure, weight loss, net weight dispensed, delivery rate, level of microbial contamination, spray pattern, water content and particle size distribution (for suspensions).
Suppositories	Softening range, disintegration and dissolution (at 37°C).
Small volume parenterals (SVPs)	Colour, clarity (for solutions), particulate matter, pH, sterility, endotoxins. Stability studies for powders for injection solution should include monitoring for colour, reconstitution time and water content. Specific parameters to be examined at appropriate intervals throughout the maximum intended use period of the reconstituted drug product, stored under condition(s) recommended on the label, should include clarity, colour, pH, sterility, pyrogen/endotoxin and particulate matter. It may be appropriate to consider monitoring of sterility after reconstitution into a product, e.g. dual-chamber syringe, where it is claimed that reconstitution can be performed without compromising sterility.

(Contd.)

Dosage form	Test parameters*
	The stability studies for suspension for injection should include, in addition, particle size distribution, dispersibility and rheological properties. The stability studies for emulsion for injection should include, in addition, phase separation, viscosity, mean size and distribution of dispersed phase globules.
Large volume parenterals (LVPs)	Colour, clarity, particulate matter, pH, sterility, pyrogen/endotoxin and volume.
Transdermal patches	*In vitro* release rates, leakage, level of microbial contamination/sterility, peel and adhesive forces.

* Appearance, assay and degradation products are advised to be evaluated for all dosage forms, as well as preservative and antioxidant content, if applicable. The stability tests for sterile products include data from a sterility test of each batch at the beginning of the test period. Additional testing is recommended to demonstrate the maintenance of the integrity of the microbial barrier using an appropriately sensitive and adequately validated container and closure integrity test. The test is performed annually and at expiry. The test for pyrogens and endotoxins should be carried out at the time of release and at appropriate intervals during the stability period. For most parenteral products, testing at the beginning and the end of stability test period is adequate.

humidity for Zones III/IVA&B) and semi-permeable (25°C ± 2°C/40% RH ± 5% RH for Zones I/II and 30°C ± 2°C/35% RH ± 5% RH for Zones III and IVA/B). Storage conditions are even defined for products meant to be stored in a refrigerator (5°C ± 3°C, with monitoring, but not control of humidity) or in a freezer (–20°C ± 5°C).

Assignment of retest period/shelf life

The regulatory protocol of determination of retest period/shelf life from stability data is different from the Arrhenius plot extension method, usually covered in theory books. It is based on 95% confidence limit method (Fig. 10.2), which is discussed in sufficient details in ICH Q1A(R2) (ICH, 2003a), WHO (2009) and ASEAN (2013) guidelines. The same is applicable to retest/shelf life period determination of both new and generic drugs and products.

The regulatory agencies usually grant 2-year retest or shelf life period in the first instance, based on satisfactory 1 year long-term and 6 months accelerated stability data [if there is failure of drug or product to meet specifications before completion of these durations, the options are outlined in ICH guideline Q1E (ICH,

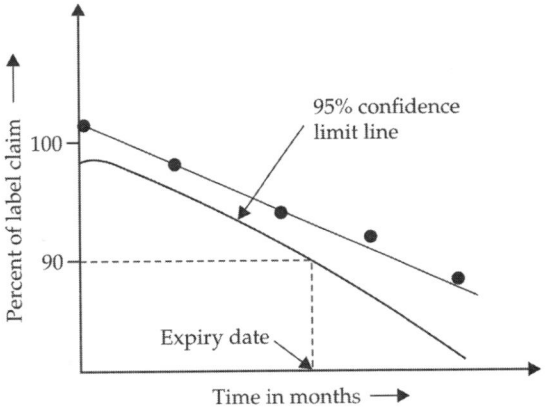

Fig. 10.2. Plot depicting 95% one-sided confidence limit method for determination of the expiry date. The expiry date is determined from 95% confidence limit line for the 5 points representing long-term data at 0, 3, 6, 9 and 12 months. The regression line represents only 50% confidence, so it is not taken for expiry date determination.

2003b)]. The shelf life for the third and subsequent years is allowed only on production of real-time satisfactory data for the later years. However, a somewhat flexible approach has been taken in the WHO guideline (WHO, 2009) for old and established stable products. A direct assignment of a 24 months shelf life is allowed provided that: (1) the active ingredient is known to be stable, (2) stability studies have been performed as per tabulated accelerated test conditions with no significant changes, (3) supporting data indicate that similar formulations have been assigned a shelf life of 24 months or more, and (4) the manufacturer continues to perform the real time studies until the proposed shelf life is covered. In general, for the situations where the stability data show very little change or no degradation, no formal statistical treatment is usually necessary, and only justification for the omission is to be included.

The requirement of mass balance

The ICH guideline Q1A(R2) (ICH, 2003a) has a requirement of establishment of mass balance during evaluation of stability samples for the new drugs. The guideline specifies that "any evaluation should consider not only the assay but also the degradation products and other appropriate attributes. Where appropriate, attention should be paid to reviewing the adequacy of the mass balance and different stability and degradation performance." The same sentence also exists in EMA guideline on stability testing of existing drug products (EMEA, 2003). This sentence in ICH guideline has been replaced in the WHO guideline (WHO, 2009) by the statement: "Any evaluation should cover not only the assay but also the levels of degradation products and other appropriate attributes. Where appropriate, attention should be paid to reviewing the adequacy of evaluation linked to finished pharmaceutical product stability and degradation "behaviour" during the testing." This somewhat diluted emphasis on mass balance requirement by WHO is due to extension of the guideline to existing and generic drugs and products, which are mostly required to meet compendial standards.

Yet, for those interested, the causes of mass balance issues and potential solutions have been summarized cogently by Baertschi et al. (2013).

SOME IMPORTANT STABILITY TESTING RELATED ASPECTS APPLICABLE TO BOTH NEW AND EXISTING DRUGS AND PRODUCTS

Retest period versus shelf life

Historically, drug substances and finished pharmaceutical products have been required by statute to bear an 'expiry date' on their labels. This expiry date means a period in which the drug substance or a product would retain its quality characteristics, specified either in the compendia, or set in-house by the manufacturer and approved by the regulatory agency. However, the labelling of 'expiry date' has been replaced by 'retest date', in particular for stable drug substances. This new concept was introduced in ICH guideline Q1A (ICH, 1993). There were two reasons for bringing this change: (1) stable drug substances were practically considered to have a very long expiry period, beyond maximum of 5 years, and hence labelling with an expiry date was considered unreal, and (2) as the drugs are very potent chemicals, discarding them even when they had not expired really, was considered unreasonable especially from the point of risk to the environment, unless sealed into leak-proof underground bunkers for rest of the life. The latter was followed by only few manufacturers worldwide, dependent upon strictness of the pollution laws in a country. The dumping of large quantity of expired bulk drugs in sewage or anywhere on the land meant their return to the water/food cycle, thus posing a serious threat to life on the planet. Hence, retest period determination and labelling with retest date was a very good scientific concept brought out by ICH.

Accordingly, pharmaceutical industry over the globe presently is supposed to determine retest period for stable drug substances, and expiry period for unstable drug substances and all finished pharmaceutical products. The same are then mentioned on the label. Of course, there are countries that have not yet shifted to retest date labelling, and incidentally India is one of them, where such labelling is allowed only for drug substance lots meant for export. The specific reason for the same is the skepticism of regulatory authorities in India about the absence of in-house facility in small or medium formulation companies to seal back the residual drug bulk in the same manner as was done by the original manufacturer. They are right as the retest period is anticipated to hold only if residual quantity is sealed back strictly, as was done by the manufacturer of the bulk drug substance, who determined the retest period in the first place and labelled the pack accordingly.

Stability testing protocol

Almost all guidelines covering stability testing of registration of both new and generic/existing drugs provide details of protocol supposed to be followed for stability testing. A nice example (500 mg paracetamol tablet packed in a PVC blister) can be found in the ASEAN guideline (ASEAN, 2013).

Presentation and recording of results

The stability data is supposed to be recorded in a proper format. A sample of the format provided by USFDA (USFDA, 1998 Draft) is shown in Table 10.4. Thus all-encompassing information

Table 10.4. Sample format for recording of stability data (USFDA, 1998 Draft)

STABILITY RAW DATA

Product name/Strength ....

Study number.. Date study started ....

Batch number .... Batch size ....

Date of manufacture .... Manufacturer/Site ....

Container/Size/Supplier..

Closure composition/Supplier .... Seal supplier ....

Date packaged .... Packager/Site ....

Storage condition .... Storage orientation ....

Chamber # ....　Shelf # ....　Location ....

Attribute	Method		Time (months)							
	SOP #	(Low/High)	0	3	6	9	12	18	24	etc.
Appearance										
Colour										
Odor										
Assay										
Disintegration										
Dissolution										
Water										
Hardness										
Friability										

on a batch is recorded at one place. Similar sheets are prepared for each batch.

Sampling and testing windows

When it is not possible to collect the sample from stability chamber at the designated time, the actual date of collection should be indicated in the format sheet. There is no regulatory mention on the issue of how early and late samples can be withdrawn from the stability chambers, in deviation to set schedule, and the time period that is allowed for sample analysis after withdrawal. Hence, various practices are followed by the industry. In general, less time window is given for the early time points and the same is increased as the study moves forward, e.g., 7 days for samples < 6 months, 10 days for 9–12 months, 14 days for 1–2 years, etc. The analysis is also required to be completed in shortest period of time (< 14 days), which is particularly true of accelerated testing as the pull points are close together. Another recommendation is to remove the samples from storage chambers ± 2 days of due date for accelerated studies, and ± 4 days of due date for long-term studies. The samples from accelerated tests are analyzed within ± 3 days, while samples from long-term testing stored till 12 months are tested within ± 2 weeks and above that ± 4 weeks.

Stability commitment

This concept was absent in original ICH guideline Q1A (ICH, 1993), but was introduced in the first revision Q1A(R) issued in 2000 (ICH, 2000). It required commitment from the manufacturer that it will come back to the regulatory agencies on its own with pending and annual stability data. Earlier, it was the regulatory agency which used to be after the manufacturers for pending data, but as the filings increased in numbers from the manufacturers from all over the world, regulatory agencies in ICH regions put the onus on the manufacturers to comply with this directive. The WHO guideline (WHO, 2009) also has this clause now.

In-use stability

This term is not found in ICH Q1A(R2) (ICH, 2003a). However, a complete guideline exists from EMA (EMEA, 2001). The topic is also mentioned in WHO guideline (WHO, 2009). The latter gives the purpose of in-use stability as "to provide information for the labelling on the preparation, storage conditions and utilization period of multi-dose products after opening, reconstitution or dilution of a solution, e.g., an antibiotic injection supplied as a powder for reconstitution." It clearly advises that the stability test should be designed to simulate the way the product is used in practice, including the filling volume of the container; dilution or reconstitution before use; and removal of appropriate quantities by the withdrawal methods used and described in the product literature. This testing is required to be performed on the reconstituted or diluted finished product throughout the proposed in-use period on primary batches as part of the stability studies at the initial and final time points; and if long-term data of full shelf life are not available before submission, at 12 months or the last time point at which data will be available. The testing may be performed at intermediate time points and at the end of the proposed in-use shelf life on the final amount of the product remaining in the container. In this specific case, a minimum of two batches, at least of pilot-scale, are subjected to the test. At least one of these batches should be chosen towards the end of its shelf life. If such results are not available, one batch should be tested at the final point of the submitted stability studies. The samples are evaluated for physical, chemical and microbial changes for the period of the proposed in-use. The testing is done using the same specific test parameters as employed for regular long-term and accelerated testing on the product. It is also mentioned that this testing is not repeated on commitment batches.

On-going stability testing

On-going stability testing means monitoring the stability of all future batches manufactured subsequent to first three production batches that are meant for registration and are covered under commitment. For this, one needs to have a continuous and appropriate program, which permits detection of any stability issue (e.g. changes in levels of the drug, rise in degradation products, or change in dissolution profile). A written protocol shall exist and the results must be presented in a formal report. A clear instruction in WHO guideline (WHO, 2009) is that "at least one production batch per year of active pharmaceutical ingredient (unless none is produced during that year) should be added to the stability monitoring program and tested at least annually to confirm the stability. In certain situations additional batches should be included in the ongoing stability program." Even for finished products, the instruction is nearly the same where also it is advised "at least one batch per year of product manufactured in every strength and every primary packaging type should be subjected to stability testing, unless none is produced during that year." However, a tagged condition is that the number of batches and frequency of testing should provide sufficient data to allow for the trend analysis. It is also directed that the protocol should extend to the end of the shelf life period and can be different from that of the initial long-term stability study submitted in the marketing authorization dossier. Of course, there has to be a reasonable justification for this deviation. Once out-of-specification results or significant atypical trends have been obtained during an on-going stability study, the same are required to be investigated and notified immediately to the relevant competent authorities. If the batch is already in the market, the possible impact and follow-up actions should be considered in consultation with the relevant regulatory agency.

The purpose here is to assure that all the future batches of drug substances and products continue to meet the stability requirement for the approved retest/expiration date. Therefore, these studies are conducted at the label storage conditions on representative production batches, with testing frequency of one batch per year (annual batch) for both drug substances and products.

Market surveillance and return sample stability testing are other two means to assure quality and confirm holding of the expiry dates. Evaluating them provides information to the manufacturers on the status of their products in the field and whether stability was being held till the expiry date.

Stability testing upon post-approval changes

Another critical aspect is the requirement to repeat the stability studies, whenever there are any types of post-approval changes. Subsequent to marketing authorization, there always exists possibility of variety of changes, e.g., in composition of the product, primary packaging, method of manufacture, etc. Such changes may be due to internal or external reasons. Internally driven changes include those in package design, addition of a new package, variation in shape and size of the dosage form, change in manufacturing process, etc. Examples of externally driven changes are regulatory restrictions on formulation ingredients, e.g., a flavouring agent or a dye.

These changes require stability re-work up from nil to complete, dependent upon the type of change to a marketing authorization. The design of the stability studies in such cases is based on the knowledge and experience acquired on active ingredients and the product. The information on such changes is provided to the competent authorities. Where strong influence is anticipated on the quality of the product, advance approval may be necessary. Whenever variations occur post approval, it becomes imperative that the impact of a particular variation is evaluated with respect to stability of the active pharmaceutical ingredient or the product. Good scientific insight on this is available in various guidelines (EMA, 2014; USFDA, 1998 Draft).

Labelling

The manufacturers are required to label drug substances and products with storage conditions and cautionary statements that are determined through formal stability studies. It is expected that the label storage conditions shall match the real storage conditions encountered by the drugs and products during distribution. However, in countries like India, where there is a big number of pharmaceutical manufacturers, unfortunately a large variety of storage conditions are put on the product labels, as listed in Table 10.5. The reading of the list clearly projects that not all storage conditions match with real conditions during transport and storage of products in wholesale and retail outlets in our country. In this context, the best option is to use labelling statements recommended by WHO in its current guideline (WHO, 2009) (Table 10.6), which exactly match the possible real distribution and storage conditions worldwide.

Specific stability program for distribution of drug products

As evident from the above-given discussion, stability testing during all phases, whether pre-clinical, clinical, registration and subsequent marketed batches, is carried out under relatively constant storage conditions. But practically, the environment during distribution and shipping is very variable. The variation might be lesser within the same climatic zone, but may be large if the products are to cross multiple climatic zones. The reasons may be seasonal changes, mode of transport, and the number of drop-off points (Lucas et al., 2004). Thus, the influence on stability, especially of unstable drugs and products, due to variation in supply chain conditions needs to be assessed, to complement stability data collected during the drug and product development. Of course, it is not possible to validate the shipping mode against all variations in the environmental conditions. Yet, the following are the best possible approaches:

Table 10.5. Labelling statements found on packaged products in India http://www.delhipharmtrust.org/ goodstoragepractice/introduction.html Accessed on 22.02.2017

1. Keep in a cool dry place.
2. Keep in a cool dark place.
3. Protect from heat and light.
4. Store below 25°C.
5. Store at +2° to 25°C.
6. Store below 20°C.
7. Store between 15° to 25°C.
8. Store in dark at 2° to 8°C.
9. Store away from sunlight.
10. Do not store above 25°C.
11. Store at room temperature.
12. Store in a dry place at 2–8°C.
13. Store below +4°C. Do not freeze.
14. Store below 30°C. Do not freeze.
15. Keep in a cool place. Do not freeze.
16. Store at a temperature between 2–10°C.
17. Store at controlled temperature 15–30°C.
18. Keep in a dry place, not exceeding 30°C.
19. Keep in a cool dry place protected from light.
20. Store below 30°C protected from 'moisture'.
21. Store at controlled room temperature (20–25°C).
22. Store in a cool place protected from frost.
23. To be preserved at temperature less than 22°C and sheltered from the light.

1. If results from routine studies indicate that the product stability profile is very stable, then one may decide that distribution studies are not warranted.
2. Distribution of drug and products requiring controlled-temperature storage is done in a manner to ensure that the product quality is not adversely affected during shipment.
3. Use stress tests and accelerated stability study data to evaluate the effect of short-term excursions higher or lower than label storage conditions that may occur during shipping of the drug and products.
4. Subject drug and products to thermal cycling under temperature conditions that simulate the changes likely to be encountered during distribution. Temperature cycling study for drug products that may be exposed to

Table 10.6. Label storage statements including additional labelling statements for use where the result of the stability testing demonstrates limiting factors (WHO, 2009)

Testing condition under which the stability of the product has been demonstrated	Recommended labelling statement
25°C/60% RH (long-term) 40°C/75% RH (accelerated)	"Do not store above 25°C"
25°C/60% RH (long-term) 30°C/65% RH (intermediate, failure of accelerated)	"Do not store above 25°C"[a]
30°C/65% RH (long-term) 40°C/75% RH (accelerated)	"Do not store above 30°C"[a]
30°C/75% RH (long-term) 40°C/75% RH (accelerated)	"Do not store above 30°C"
5°C ± 3°C	"Store in a refrigerator (2°C to 8°C)"
−20°C ± 5°C	"Store in freezer"

Limiting factors	Additional labelling statement, where relevant
Products that cannot tolerate refrigeration	"Do not refrigerate or freeze"[b]
Products that cannot tolerate freezing	"Do not freeze"[b]
Light-sensitive products	"Protect from light"
Products that cannot tolerate excessive heat, e.g. suppositories	"Store and transport not above 30°C"
Hygroscopic products	"Store in dry condition"

[a] "Protect from moisture" should be added as applicable.

[b] Depending on the pharmaceutical form and the properties of the finished products, there may be a risk of deterioration due to physical changes if subjected to low temperatures, e.g. liquids and semi-solids. Low temperatures may also have an effect on the packaging in certain cases. An additional statement may be necessary to take account of this possibility.

variations above freezing temperature may consist of 3 cycles of 2 days at refrigerated temperature (2–8°C), followed by 2 days under accelerated storage conditions (40°C). A temperature cycling study for drug products that may be exposed to sub-freezing temperatures may consist of 3 cycles of 2 days at freezer temperature (−10 to −20°C) followed by 2 days under accelerated storage conditions (40°C). For inhalation aerosols, the recommended cycle study consists of 3 or 4 six-hour cycles per day, between subfreezing temperature and 40°C (75–85% RH) for a period of up to 6 weeks. For frozen drug products, the cycle study should include an evaluation of effects due to accelerated thawing in a microwave or a hot water bath unless contraindicated in the labelling. Alternatives to these conditions may be acceptable with appropriate justification.

5. Select additional storage condition based on calculation of mean kinetic temperature (MKT), which is defined as: "single calculated temperature at which the total amount of degradation over a particular period is equal to the sum of the individual degradations that would occur at various temperatures" (USFDA, 1998 Draft).

Photostability testing

During development, along with temperature and humidity testing, it is important that photosensitivity of the products is established simultaneously, so that any unacceptable change that occurs upon exposure to light is known beforehand. For this, a systematic approach is used, as enshrined in ICH guideline Q1B (ICH, 1996b), wherein the development product is first exposed to light outside the immediate pack. The studies are discontinued if the formulations are found stable. Otherwise, the tests are continued with the drug product in the proposed immediate and/or the marketing pack. The trials are persisted till primary or a combination of primary and secondary pack is identified, which provides adequate protection to light.

The light stability tests are usually carried out on a single batch of products. The unpacked solid products are spread in a single or thin layer in a glass or plastic container (preferably a Petri plate). The depth of powders should not exceed 3 mm. Liquid samples may also be exposed similarly in chemically inert and transparent containers. The packed products are positioned in thin and single layer such that they get maximum exposure to the light source.

The total exposure of fluorescent light should not be less than 1.2 million lux hour and an integrated near UV energy of not less than 200 watt hour/square metre. Dark controls are run alongside during the testing.

Specific stability testing requirements for complex product categories

There are some categories of products, like fixed-dose combinations (FDCs), herbal drug preparations, drug delivery systems, and biological/biotechnological products, which offer typical challenges with respect to stability testing during development.

FDCs are defined as single products created by the combination of two or more active components, each of it contributing to the benefit of the new product. The definition covers the term 'polypill' that specifically contains three or more drugs in a single pill for the treatment of cardiovascular diseases. For combination formulations, pharmaceutical development issues are more in number (Kumar et al., 2008a). Their specific stability-related aspects include formation of drug–drug (Bhutani et al., 2005a; Bhutani et al., 2005b; Prasad et al., 2006; Kumar et al., 2008c) and drug–excipient (Kumar et al., 2009) interaction products; increase in levels of degradation products beyond thresholds; changes in formulation parameters, like disintegration, dissolution behavior, etc. There are also specific analytical issues, e.g., difficulty in the development of single analytical method for multiple drugs in the presence of excipients; problems in sample preparation for analysis, and the painful exercise of establishment of stability-indicating assays (Kumar et al., 2007; Kumar et al., 2008b). The expiry date for such products is based on the least stable drug. The testing protocol otherwise remains the same as with single-drug formulations.

The challenge of stability testing with herbal preparations is bigger, due to inherent complexity of the herbal drug material, and the multi-component nature of most herbal products. Generally, components in herbals are not fully characterised, and there is negligible information on their physicochemical properties and degradation chemistry. Even there exists increased possibility for the multiple interactions among the components. This not only makes establishment of assay procedures difficult, but the test parameters for evaluation of stability samples cannot be sometimes identified. In the latter situation, the best approach is to evaluate the stability samples through some sort of biological assay, may be *in vitro*. In case of these products, the stability test protocols remain the same as with conventional products, because they are manufactured, distributed and sold under similar conditions. Recently, herbal products have been mandated to bear an expiry date, meaning that they need to be characterised extensively before marketing.

Regarding drug delivery systems including nanopharmaceuticals, the main issues are the system integrity and maintenance of release characteristics of the drug till the last day of expiry. The delivery of drug from these systems is critically balanced and any influence on release profile during storage has to be established carefully. This is done through stringent evaluation parameters, focused on system's functionality, integrity, size of particulates, carrier material stability, drug stability, degradation products, etc. (Singh, 2016).

For biological and biotechnological products, the stability testing is treated differently than the conventional products, because of special characteristics of the products. In their case, stability evaluation necessitates complex analytical methodologies, which include physicochemical, biochemical and immuno-chemical methods of analysis. Also, biological activity generally forms part of pivotal stability studies, wherever applicable. The biological and biotechnological products are particularly sensitive to environmental factors, such as temperature changes, oxidation, light, ionic strength and shear. Therefore, primary data to support a requested storage period in their case is based on long-term, real time, real condition stability studies, and proper long-term stability program becomes critical to the successful development of a commercial product (ICH, 1995).

Stability testing laboratory and storage chambers

An essential component of the stability testing function in industry is the stability testing laboratory, which is required to be equipped with sufficient number and types of specialized environmental chambers that can simulate storage conditions listed in Table 10.7. The latter are expected to maintain the prescribed conditions (temperature/humidity/light) within

the acceptance criterion continuously for years and hence they must be robust for the purpose. They are either stand-alone or walk-in types (Fig. 10.3). The chambers shall be equipped with display, recording, safety, alarm and standby features (Fig. 10.4).

The WHO guideline (WHO, 2009) specifically states that: "short-term environ-mental changes due to opening of doors of the storage facility are accepted as unavoidable. The effect of excursions due to equipment failure are required to be assessed, addressed and reported if judged to affect stability results. Excursions that exceed the defined tolerances for more than 24 hours, and their effect, are to be described in the study report." The assessment of impact of excursion on the stored products is truly a big challenge as usually no guidance is available on this particular aspect. The impact of excursions can be justified if forced degradation data on formulations are available pre-hand. An alternative and better way is to have 24 hour vigil on the functioning of the chambers, training the in-house staff and making robust arrangements so that servicing and repairs of the affected chamber are completed within the stipulated time of 24 hours.

Like any other equipment, stability test chambers also need to be duly qualified, including Design (DQ), Installation (IQ), Operation (OQ), Calibration (CQ) and Performance (PQ) qualifications. Of course, the latter two need to be carried out at regular intervals. The measurement devices, viz. temperature controller, temperature sensor, thermometer, humidity controller, humidity probe, monitoring/display systems, chart recorders, data logger, etc. shall be calibrated at regular frequency. Some of the known problems with stability chambers are mechanical failure, power failure, temperature and humidity fluctuations, 24 hour monitoring system mal-functioning, water leakage, etc. These need to be given due attention. Emphasis must be paid on regular maintenance schedules to avoid major

Table 10.7. Recommended stability storage conditions for various products in Zones I–IV (WHO, 2009)

Product	Zone	Storage Condition (Minimum time period covered by data at submission)		
		Accelerated (6 months)	Intermediate (6 months)	Long-term* (12 months)**
General case: Solid oral dosage forms, solids for reconstitution, dry and lyophilised powders in glass vials	Zones I/II Zones III/IVA Zone IVB	40°C/75% RH 40°C/75% RH 40°C/75% RH	30°C/65% RH — —	25°C/60% RH 30°C/65% RH 30°C/75% RH
Drug products packaged in impermeable containers: Liquids in glass bottles, vials, or sealed glass ampoules, which provide an impermeable barrier to water loss	Zones I/II Zones III/IVA&B	40°C/any controlled condition or ambient humidity 40°C/any controlled condition or ambient humidity	30°C/any controlled condition or ambient humidity —	25°C/any controlled condition or ambient humidity 30°C/any controlled condition or ambient humidity
Drug products packaged in semi-permeable containers: Large volume parenterals (LVPs), small volume parenterals (SVPs), ophthalmics, otics, and nasal sprays packaged in semi-permeable containers, such as plastic bags, semi-rigid plastic containers, ampoules, vials and bottles with or without droppers/applicators, which may be susceptible to water loss	Zones I/II Zones III/IVA&B	40°C/not more than 25% RH 40°C/not more than 25% RH	30°C/65% RH***	25°C/40% RH 30°C/35% RH
Drug products intended for storage in a refrigerator	Zones I/II Zones III/IVA Zone IVB	25°C/60% RH 30°C/65% RH 30°C/75% RH		5°C ± 3°C, with monitoring, but not control of humidity
Drug products intended for storage in a freezer	All zones			−20°C ± 5°C

* Testing at more severe long-term condition is taken as an alternative to less stringent storage condition.
** 6 months for stable drugs in first two categories of products.
*** This intermediate condition is to evaluate the effect of temperature at 30°C.

downtime. Some of the vendors of stability test equipment these days provide risk management solutions for stability laboratory. Advantage can be taken of the same.

Attention is also required towards space management for storage of samples, sample tracking, disaster recovery plans, transfer of samples from one chamber to another, etc. It must be emphasized that stability chamber is a breathing equipment and those handling storage and withdrawal of samples from stability chambers must see that all samples have enough

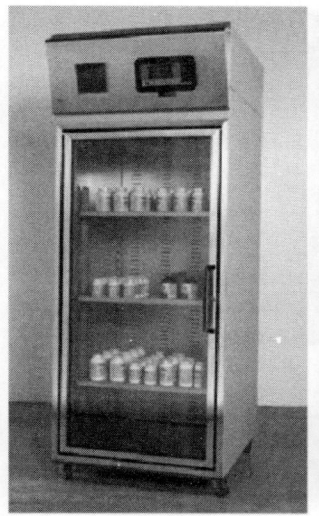 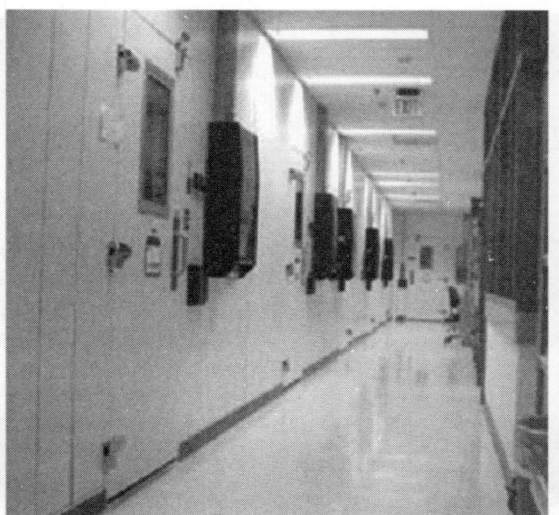 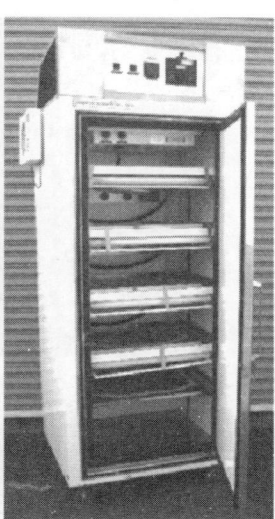

A   **B**   **C**

Fig. 10.3. Photographs showing reach-in stability chamber (A), walk-in corridor (B) and a photostability chamber (C). The walk-ins are found in companies that manufacture large number of products and have high volumes of production and sales.

space surrounding them so that there is smooth airflow around each.

THE INTRICACIES OF STABILITY TESTING PROGRAMS

Executing a stability testing program is no trivial task as the studies last for several years. The exercise is inherently painstaking, requiring meticulous planning. Considering that a typical stability protocol may include multiple product batches, dosage strengths and storage conditions, a large amount of data is generated during the course of a cGMP-regulated stability study. In managing a stability program, control of both the sample and its local environment is crucial. The sample and its package should not be compromised in any fashion during the study. Mishandling a project anytime into a study can prove very costly in terms of both money and time.

Therefore, the modern-day stability testing involves a large number of SOPs (Table 10.8), specialized tracking and management systems, apart from significant investment in the form of certified equipment, laboratory space, trained personnel, etc. An optimal workflow is developed for the lifecycle of stability samples, capitalizing on knowledge capturing, productivity, cost savings, and compliance. Commercial stability management software packages are available that offer facility of inventory management, resource scheduling, statistical analyses (shelf life projections, trend analysis, projections based on one-sided or two-sided confidence intervals, performing ANCOVA pooling of multiple studies, accelerated temperature shelf life calculations using the Arrhenius equation, etc.), and presentation of final data for submission to regulator. The software packages are usually validated and comply with USFDA 21 CFR Part 11 requirements of data security and provisions of electronic signatures and audit trails.

RECENT DEVELOPMENTS

There has been a change in the meaning of drug product stability in recent years. The emphasis and focus has shifted from assay of drug in a

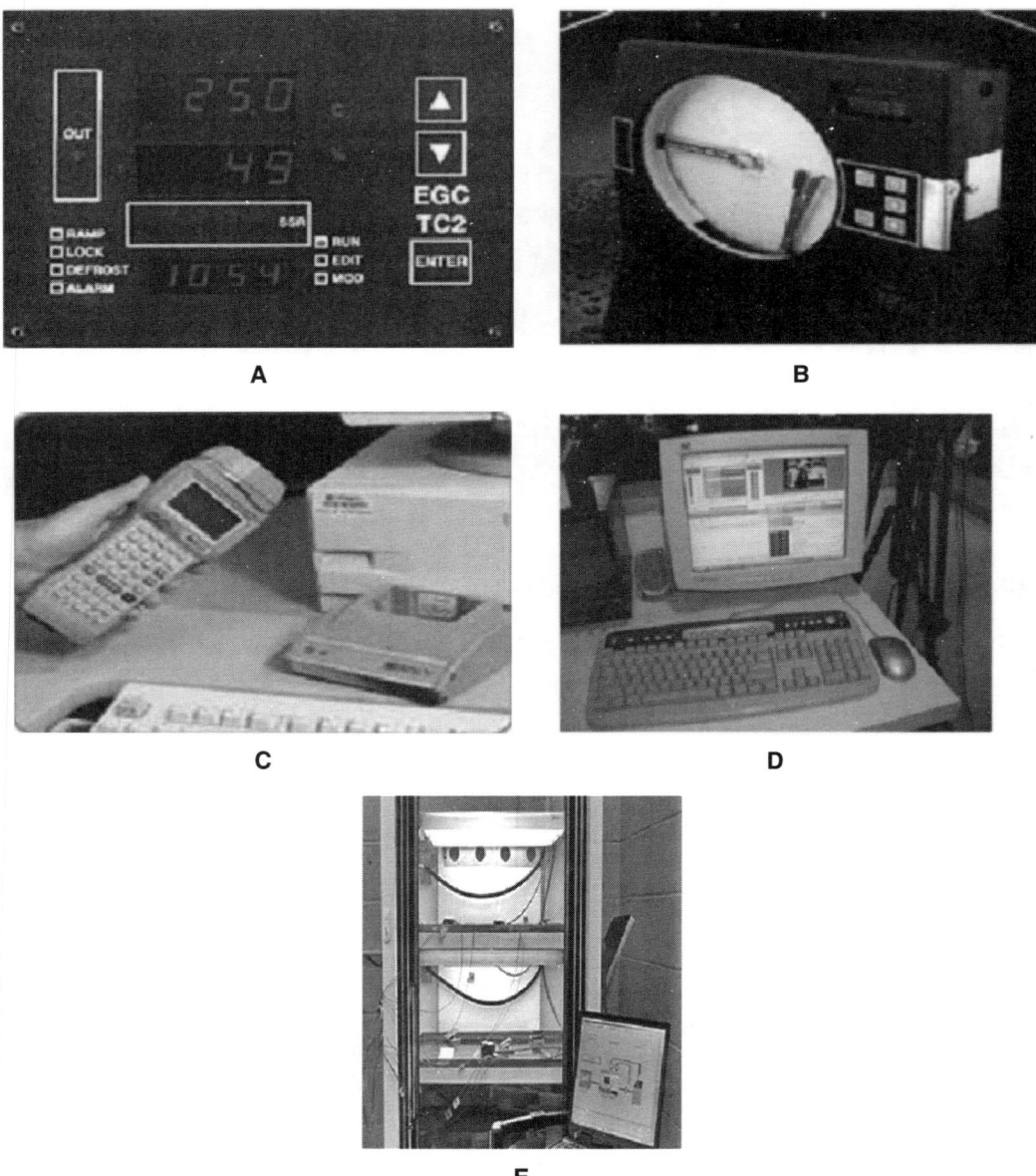

Fig. 10.4. Pictures showing display (A) and recording devices, viz. chart recorder (B), data logger (C) and computer system (D). Picture E shows computerized validation system for set conditions inside a stability chamber.

formulation to the levels of degradation products present. The ICH guideline Q3B on Impurities in New Drug Products (ICH, 2006) requires reporting, characterization and qualification (establishment of safety) of degradation products at levels $\geq 0.05\%$, $\geq 0.1\%$ and $\geq 0.15\%$, respectively. These requirements have been applied to generic drug products also (USFDA, 2005). Even the same standards are being extended to compendial products, an example

Table 10.8. List of typical SOPs required to run a successful stability program
http://www.locum.co.il/sops/sop_part4.php
Accessed on 22.02.2017

SOP Control
- Format and Layout of SOPs
- Index for Stability SOPs
- Indexing Procedure for Stability Studies

Starting a Study
- Initiating a Stability Study
- Contents of a Stability Protocol
- Setting the 'Start Date' for a Stability Study
- Determining the 'Due Dates' for a Stability Study Protocol
- The Initial Certificate of Analysis for a Stability Study

Study Parameters
- Setting Limits for Check Specifications in a Stability Study
- Number and Size of Batches for Stability Testing

Sampling
- Number of Samples Required for Performing Stability Tests
- Labelling of Stability Study Samples
- Storage Configuration of Samples in a Stability Environment
- Storing the Stability Study Samples under Controlled Conditions prior to Analysis

Active Drug
- Stress Testing the Bulk Drug Substance for Stability Analysis

Study Conditions
- Intervals and Climatic Conditions for a Development Stability Study
- Intervals and Climatic Conditions for a Pivotal/ Bioequivalence Stability Study
- Intervals and Climatic Conditions for a Validation/PM Stability Study
- Placing the Reference Listed Drug (RLD) on Stability

Packaging Procedures
- Packaging Procedures on Formulation Lots for a Stability Study
- Packaging Procedures on the Process Qualification Batch for a Stability Study
- Representative Sampling Procedures during Batch Packaging of Stability Samples

Container Systems
- Container-Liner-Closure Systems for a Stability Study
- Certification of a Container-Liner-Closure System

Test Results
- Reporting Test Results of a Stability Study
- Procedures for Handling Abnormal or Out-of- Specification (OOS) Results in a Stability Study

Test Methods
- The Control of Analytical Methods #'s and Edition #'s in Stability Documentation

Audit and Review Raw Data
- Auditing Stability Data in Laboratory Notebooks
- Cross-Referencing Laboratory Notebooks with Computerized Stability Documentation

Chart Control
- Recording Stability Study Climatic Conditions
- Review and Control of Temperature and Humidity Recording Charts

Validation and Sanitation
- Periodic Revalidation of Climatic Rooms and Chambers
- Sanitation and Housekeeping Requirements of Climatic Chambers
- Fault Correcting Procedures (after breakdowns) during a Stability Study
- Emergency Procedures during a Stability Study

In-House Methods
- Identifying other SOPs of Relevance to Stability Program

Stopping a Study
- Conditions for Stopping a Stability Study

Self Inspection
- Self Inspection Procedures in a Stability Department

Job Description and Training
- Job Description of Stability Department Personnel
- Using Stability SOPs and Compliance Program as Stability Training Tools
- The Do's and Don'ts of a Stability Study – a Department Training Tool
- Stability Department Compliance Staff Training

Reviewing Documentation
- Review and Auditing Stability Study Documentation
- The Layout and Format of a Regulatory Stability Report (a filed report)
- Documentation Requirements for a Stability Study – Contents of a Stability Dossier

Closing a Study
- Accepting and Signing off a Completed Stability Study

Table 10.9. Related compounds and their limits proposed for Donezepil hydrochloride tablets by USP
http://www.usp.org/sites/default/files/usp_pdf/EN/USPNF/
pendingStandards/donepezilHydrochlorideTablets_v1.pdf
Accessed on 22.02.2017

Related compound	Relative retention time (RRT)[*]	Relative response factor (F)	Limit (%)
DNP1[1]	0.23	1.5	NMT 0.15
DPMI[2]	0.49	1.9	NMT 0.15
Donepezibenzyl bromide[3]	0.68	0.73	NMT 0.15
Donepezil hydrochloride	1.0	1.0	—
Dehydrodeoxy donbepezil[4]	1.72	2.0	NMT 0.15
Deoxydonepezil[5]	2.12	0.67	NMT 0.15
Any individual unspecified impurity	—	1.0	NMT 0.1
Total impurities	—		NMT 0.75

[1] 2,3-Dihydro-5,6-dimethoxy-2-(4-piperidinyl)methyl-indan-1-one hydrochloride
[2] 5,6-Dimethoxy-2-(4-pyridyl)methyl-indan-1-one
[3] 1,1-Dibenzyl-4-[(5,6-dimethoxy-1-oxo-2,3-dihydro-1H-inden-2-yl)methyl]piperidinium bromide
[4] 1-Benzyl-4-[(5,6-dimethoxy-1H-inden-2-yl)methyl]piperidine hydrochloride
[5] 1-Benzyl-4-[(5,6-dimethoxy-2,3-dihydro-1H-inden-2-yl)methyl]piperidine hydrochloride
[*] RRT are based on the system having a dwell volume of 1 ml

of which is given in Table 10.9. Clearly, forensic analysis and control of minutea in pharmaceutical products is emerging as a big challenge for the analytical chemists and industry as a whole. The characterisation of degradation product impurities usually requires use of sophisticated and costly hyphenated analytical instruments like, LC-MS, LC-NMR, etc. (Bedse et al., 2009; Kumar et al., 2008; Narayanam et al., 2014, 2015; Shah et al., 2010; Singh et al., 2012). These are available in only few major companies and CROs around the world. To quantitate the degradation products at a level of ≤0.15%, one also has to buy their certified reference standards at a very high cost. The challenge is bigger for formulation scientists who need to stabilize their products so that the degradation product levels remain within the stringent specified limits even at the end of shelf life. There are several instances where increase in degradation product levels beyond the prescribed limits has led to product recalls and this is now happening throughout the world

(www.fda.gov/safety/recalls/default.htm; http://healthycanadians.gc.ca/recall-alert-rappel-avis/index-eng.php; https://www.gov.uk/drug-device-alerts, accessed on 22.02.2017).

A lot of attention is currently being paid also on out-of-trend (OOT) results in stability testing. OOT results mean that the profile of one of the batch falls apart in trend to other two batches. Statistical approaches to identify and confirm these OOT results have been proposed (PhRMA, 2003; PhRMA, 2005). Interestingly, the reason for their occurrence has also been put forth, and one cause identified is the storage of different batches of products at different locations within the chamber (Gaur et al., 2005a). The batches are manufactured at various times and are charged to the chamber at whatever shelf space is available. It was found that despite the temperature and humidity being the same at all the points within a chamber, the air velocity still varied at different locations, and this resulted in differential moisture pick up by a hygroscopic drug. Hence, it was advised that stability test chambers should be designed in a manner so that air velocity remains constant within the test chambers.

Although stability testing during product development and registration generally is focused towards selected markets or zones, yet, multinational companies, that market their drugs worldwide, are increasingly orienting their protocols to set of conditions that cover extreme environmental conditions. The specific changes for global testing include increase in duration of accelerated testing period from 6 to 12 months, and conduct of additional tests at 25°C/80% RH (higher humidity) and/or 50°C/75% RH (higher temperature) for 1–3 months.

A distinct advantage of these is the possibility of assessing any changes that can happen in the product due to spikes in environmental conditions during distribution across the world. A very interesting new observation, of typical relevance to marketing in tropical world, is that the combination of three environmental factors together, viz., temperature, humidity and light, results in more stronger deleterious effect on drug substances and products than temperature plus humidity conditions (Singh et al., 2002; Bhutani et al., 2003; Singh et al., 2003; Gaur et al., 2005b). It was found that hygroscopic drug substances and their packaged products gained moisture at a higher rate in the presence of light than in the dark. Perhaps this is the reason that stability studies in dark chambers sometimes do not divulge some of the problems observed practically but not revealed using the current stability test protocols. In tropical countries, light intensity is high throughout the year, and the fact is that one week of light in an Asian country equals total light in a year in a country in Europe.

Moreover, shops in developing tropical countries are usually unprotected from direct sunlight, and even the products are stored and sold outside their secondary packages. Therefore, developmental products containing hygroscopic drugs and excipients are advised to be tested in a photostability chamber, set at accelerated conditions of temperature and humidity (40°C/75% RH). Once the ICH dose of light is delivered, further testing can be continued in the dark conditions.

The concept of Quality-by-Design (QbD) can also be extended in some manner to stability testing. The first step involving 'product design' shall encompass understanding of the material properties and interactions that may affect chemical and physical stability of the drug in the formulation environment. In the second 'process design' step, one needs to understand and explore all processing parameters that could affect product purity and stability. Also important is to understand interactions between process parameters and material attributes, which are established in the design space using Design of Experiments (DoE) approach. Within this step, there should be endeavour to develop effective control strategies so that the same quality product is delivered batch after batch, which holds true even till the end of shelf life. In the third step of 'lifecycle management', the emphasis shall be to monitor the process performance, and also quality of the products through their whole lifecycle, i.e., till end of the shelf life. This last step also has in-built scope of process improvement, if feedback suggests need of improvement in any process parameter to obtain a yet better quality product.

One more recent development is the availability of ASAP software (http://www.freethinktech.com/ASAPprime.html#sthash.6Cp35o5o.dpuf, accessed on 22.02.2017), which is claimed to help in prediction of small-molecule drug product use periods, shelf lives and drug substance retest periods in as little as two weeks. It is said to carry out multidimensional analysis, which results in an accurate and comprehensive stability estimation with a quantitative assessment of the confidence intervals for the projected shelf life under any storage conditions. In addition, stability analysis using this software is claimed to provide a robust, science-based argument for choosing the optimal

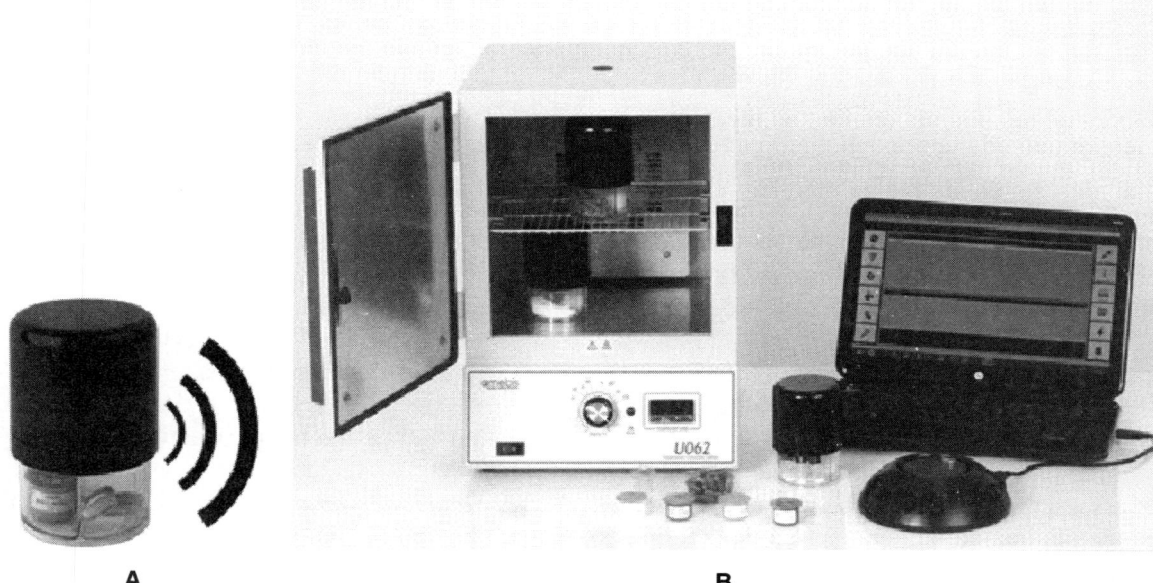

Fig. 10.5. Pictures showing the Amebis system that is used to perform the aging, while the ASAPprime® software builds the stability predictive model. The combined system is claimed to be useful to predict shelf life for changes in formulations and packaging during product development. The small container containing formulation and humidifying solution in separate compartments (A) is placed in an oven at desired temperature (B). The temperature and humidity values are picked up externally by the computer through wireless signalling. (http://amebisltd.com/)

combination of packaging, formulation, ingredient supplier and manufacturing process without the need for repeated and lengthy laboratory studies. The software has specific role in prediction of drug and product stability during their development. A small scale humidity chamber (Fig. 10.5) has also been introduced to generate stability data on developmental formulations, which are fed into the ASAP software to obtain relevant predictions.

CONCLUSIONS

Stability testing is an integral part of the drug and product development. It is only through stability studies on development, registration and marketed batches that absolute assurance is provided on drug and product integrity till the time of use. The stability tests ought to be carried out by following proper scientific principles and meeting regulatory requirements, as enshrined in multiple guidelines on both new and existing (generic) drugs and products.

REFERENCES

- Ahuja, S. and Scypinski, S. (2001). **Handbook of Modern Pharmaceutical Analysis**, Volume 3, Separation Science and Technology, Academic Press, San Diego, USA.
- Alsante, K.M., Ando, A., Brown, R., Ensing, J., Hatajik, T.D., Kong, W. and Tsuda, Y. (2007). The role of degradant profiling in active pharmaceutical ingredients and drug products, *Adv. Drug Del. Rev.*, 59, 29–37.
- Association of Southeast Asian Nations (2013). ASEAN Guideline on Stability Study of Drug Product, Indonesia (http://www.asean.org/storage/2012/10/ASEAN-Guideline-on-Stability-Study-of-

drug-Product-R1-2013.pdf. Accessed on 22.02.2017

- Baertschi, S.W., Pack, B.W., Hoaglund Hyzer, C.S. and Nussbaum, M.A. (2013). Assessing mass balance in pharmaceutical drug products: New insights into an old topic, *Trends Anal. Chem.*, 49, 126–136.

- Bedse, G., Kumar, V. and Singh, S. (2009). Study of forced decomposition behavior of lamivudine using LC, LC–MS/TOF and MS^n, *J. Pharm. Biomed. Anal.*, 49 (1), 55–63.

- Bhutani, H., Mariappan, T.T. and Singh, S. (2003). Behaviour of uptake of moisture by drugs and excipients under accelerated conditions of temperature and humidity in the absence and the presence of light, Part II: Packaged and un-packaged antituberculosis drug products, *Pharm. Technol.*, 27 (6), 44–52.

- Bhutani, H., Singh, S. and Jindal, K.C. (2005a). Drug-drug interaction studies on first-line anti-tuberculosis drugs, *Pharm. Develop. Technol.*, 10 (4) 517–523.

- Bhutani, H., Singh, S., Chakraborti, A.K. and Jindal, K.C. (2005b). Mechanistic explanation to the catalysis by pyrazinamide and ethambutol of reaction between rifampicin and isoniazid in anti-TB FDCs, *J. Pharm. Biomed. Anal.*, 39, 892–899.

- Gaur, A., Mariappan, T.T., Bhutani, H. and Singh, S. (2005a). A possible reason for the generation of out-of-trend stability results: Variable air velocity at different locations within the stability chamber, *Pharm. Technol.*, 29 (8) 44, 46–49.

- Gaur, A., Bhutani, H., Mariappan, T.T. and Singh, S. (2005b). Behaviour of marketed packaged formulations under accelerated conditions of temperature and humidity in the absence and the presence of light, *Ind. J. Pharm. Sci.* 67(4) 438–443.

- European Medicines Agency, Committee for Proprietary Medicinal Products (CPMP), (2001). Note for guidance on in-use stability testing of human medicinal products, London (http://www.ema.europa.eu/docs/en_GB/document_library/Scientific_guideline/2009/09/WC500003475.pdf, accessed on 22.02.2017).

- European Medicines Agency, Committee for Proprietary Medicinal Products (CPMP), (2003). Guideline on Stability Testing: Stability Testing of Existing Active Substances and Related Finished Products, London (http://www.ema.europa.eu/docs/en_GB/document_library/Scientific_guideline/2009/09/WC500003466.pdf, accessed on 22.02.2017).

- European Medicines Agency, Committee for Medicinal Products for Human Use (CHMP), (2014). Guideline on Stability Testing for Applications for Variations to a Marketing Authorisation, London (http://www.ema.europa.eu/docs/en_GB/document_library/Scientific_guideline/2014/04/WC500164972.pdf, accessed on 22.02.2017).

- International Conference on Harmonisation (1993). Stability Testing of New Drug Substances and Products, Q1A, Geneva (http://www.pharma.gally.ch/ich/q1a038095en.pdf; accessed on 22.02.2017).

- International Conference on Harmonisation (1995). Quality of Biotechnological Products: Stability Testing of Biotechnological/Biological Products, Q5C, Geneva ((http://www.ich.org/fileadmin/Public_Web_Site/ICH_Products/Guidelines/Quality/Q5C/Step4/Q5C_Guideline.pdf; accessed on 22.02.2017).

- International Conference on Harmonisation (1996a). Stability Testing for New Dosage Forms, Q1C, Geneva (http://www.ich.org/fileadmin/Public_Web_Site/ICH_Products/Guidelines/Quality/Q1C/Step4/Q1C_Guideline.pdf; accessed on 22.02.2017).

- International Conference on Harmonisation (1996b). Photostability Testing of New Drug Substances and Products, Q1B, Geneva (http://www.ich.org/fileadmin/Public_Web_Site/ICH_Products/Guidelines/Quality/Q1B/Step4/Q1B_Guideline.pdf; accessed on 22.02.2017).

- International Conference on Harmonisation (2000). Stability Testing of New Drug Substances and Products, Q1A(R), Geneva (http://www.caronproducts.com/lib/sitefiles/pdf/bulletins/Federal_register_Q1A(R).pdf; accessed on 22.02.2017).

- International Conference on Harmonisation (2002a). The Common Technical Document for the Registration of Pharmaceuticals for Human Use: Quality Overall Summary of Module 2 Module 3: Quality, M4Q(R1), Geneva (http://www.ich.org/fileadmin/Public_Web_Site/

ICH_Products/CTD/M4_R1_Quality/M4Q__R1_.pdf; accessed on 22.02.2017).

- International Conference on Harmonisation (2002b). Bracketing and Matrixing Designs for Stability Testing of New Drug Substances and Products, Q1D, Geneva (http://www.ich.org/fileadmin/Public_Web_Site/ICH_Products/Guidelines/Quality/Q1D/Step4/Q1D_Guideline.pdf; accessed on 22.02.2017).

- International Conference on Harmonisation (2003a). Stability Testing of New Drug Substances and Products, Q1A(R2), Geneva (http://www.ich.org/fileadmin/Public_Web_Site/ICH_Products/Guidelines/Quality/Q1A_R2/Step4/Q1A_R2__Guideline.pdf; accessed on 22.02.2017).

- International Conference on Harmonisation (2003b). Evaluation for Stability Data, Q1E, Geneva (http://www.ich.org/fileadmin/Public_Web_Site/ICH_Products/Guidelines/Quality/Q1E/Step4/Q1E__Guideline.pdf; accessed on 22.02.2017).

- International Conference on Harmonisation (2006). Impurities in New Drug Products, Q3B(R2), Geneva (http://www.ich.org/fileadmin/Public_Web_Site/ICH_Products/Guidelines/Quality/Q3B_R2/Step4/Q3B_R2__Guideline.pdf; accessed on 22.02.2017).

- Kumar, G., Singh, M., Jindal K.C. and Singh, S. (2008). LC and LC-MS study on establishment of degradation pathway of glipizide under forced decomposition conditions, *J. Chromatogr. Sci.*, 46, 510–517.

- Kumar, V., Bhutani, H. and Singh, S. (2007). ICH guidance in practice: Validated stability-indicating HPLC method for simultaneous determination of ampicillin and cloxacillin in combination drug products, *J. Pharm. Biomed. Anal.*, 43, 769–773.

- Kumar, V., Prasad, B. and Singh, S. (2008a). Pharmaceutical issues in the development of a polypill for the treatment of cardiovascular diseases, *Drug Discovery Today: Therapeutic Strategies*, 5(1), 63–71.

- Kumar, V., Shah, R.P. and Singh, S. (2008b). LC and LC-MS methods for the investigation of polypills for the treatment of cardiovascular diseases. Part 1: Separation of active components and classification of their interaction/degradation products, *J. Pharm. Biomed. Anal.*, 47(3), 508–515.

- Kumar, V., Malik, S. and Singh, S. (2008c). Polypill for the treatment of cardiovascular diseases. Part 2: LC-MS/TOF characterization of interaction/degradation products of atenolol/lisinopril and aspirin, and mechanism of formation thereof, *J. Pharm. Biomed. Anal.*, 48, 619–628.

- Kumar, V., Shah, R.P., Malik, S. and Singh, S. (2009). Compatibility of atenolol with excipients: LC-MS/TOF characterization of degradation/interaction products, and mechanisms of their formation, *J. Pharm. Biomed. Anal.*, 49 (4), 880–888.

- Kurmi, M., Golla, V.M., Kumar, S., Sahu, A. and Singh, S. (2015). Stability behaviour of antiretroviral drugs and their combinations. 1: Characterization of tenofovir disoproxil fumarate degradation products by mass spectrometry, *RSC Adv.*, 5, 96117–96129.

- Lucas, T.I., Bishara, R.H., and Seevers, R.H. (2004). A stability program for the distribution of drug products, *Pharm. Tech.*, 28 (7), 68–73.

- Narayanam, M. and Singh, S. (2014). Characterization of stress degradation products of fosinopril by using LC-MS/TOF, MS^n and on-line H/D exchange, *J. Pharm. Biomed. Anal.*, 92, 135–143.

- Narayanam, M., Sahu, A. and Singh, S. (2015). Use of LC–MS/TOF, LC–MS^n, NMR and LC–NMR in characterization of stress degradation products: Application to cilazapril, *J. Pharm. Biomed. Anal.*, 111, 190–203.

- Prasad, B., Bhutani, H and Singh, S. (2006). Study of the interaction between rifapentine and isoniazid under acid conditions, *J. Pharm. Biomed. Anal.*, 41, 1438–1441.

- Pravinchandra, S.K., Kurmi, M., Kumar, S. and Singh, S. (2015). Forced degradation of lafutidine and characterization of its non-volatile and volatile degradation products using LC-MS/TOF, LC-MS^n and HS-GC-MS, *New J. Chem.*, 39 (12), 9679–9692.

- PhRMA CMC Statistics and Stability Experts Team (2003). Identification of out-of-trend stability results: A review of the potential regulatory issue and various approaches, *Pharm. Technol.*, 27 (4), 38–52.

- PhRMA CMC Statistics and Stability Experts Team (2005). Identification of out-of-trend stability results, Part II, *Pharm. Technol.*, 29 (10), 66–79.

- Raijada, D.K., Prasad, B., Paudel, A., Shah, R.P. and Singh, S. (2010). Characterization of degradation products of amorphous and polymorphic forms of clopidogrel bisulphate under solid state stress conditions, *J. Pharm. Biomed. Anal.* 52, 332–344.
- Shah, R., Sahu, A. and Singh, S. (2010). Identification and characterization of degradation products of irbesartan using LC-MS/TOF, MS^n, on-line H/D exchange and LC-NMR studies, *J. Pharm. Biomed. Anal.*, 51, 1037–1046.
- Singh, S. and Bakshi, M. (2000). Guidance on conduct of stress tests to determine inherent stability of drugs, *Pharm. Technol. Asia*, Special issue, September/October 24–36.
- Singh S. and Bakshi, M. (2002). Development of validated stability-indicating assay methods: A critical review. *J. Pharm. Biomed. Anal.*, 28 (6), 1011–1040.
- Singh, S., Bhutani, H., Mariappan, T.T., Kaur, H., Bajaj, M. and Pakhale, S.P. (2002). Behaviour of uptake of moisture by drugs and excipients under accelerated conditions of temperature and humidity in the absence and the presence of light. 1. Pure anti-tuberculosis drugs and their combinations, *Int. J. Pharm.*, 245, 37–44.
- Singh, S., Mariappan, T.T. and Kaur, H. (2003). Behaviour of uptake of moisture by drugs and excipients under accelerated conditions of temperature and humidity in the absence and the presence of light. 3. Pure drugs and excipients, *Pharm. Technol.*, 27(12) 52–56.
- Singh, S., Paudel, A., Bedse, G., Thakare, R. and Kumar, V. (2009). Regional stability guidelines: India, Chapter 4: Global stability practices by M. Zahn, *in:* **Handbook of Stability Testing in Pharmaceutical Development Regulations, Methodologies, and Best Practices**, Springer New York, Kim Huynh-Ba (Ed.), pp. 66–69.
- Singh, S., Paudel, A., Bedse, G., Thakare, R. and Kumar, V. (2010). The challenge of diverse climates: Adequate stability testing conditions for India, Chapter 6, *in:* **Pharmaceutical Stability Testing to Support Global Markets**, Springer, New York, Kim Huynh-Ba (Ed.) pp. 37–44.
- Singh , S., Handa, T., Narayanam, M., Sahu, A., Junwal, M. and Shah, R.P. (2012). A critical review on the use of modern sophisticated hyphenated tools in the characterization of impurities and degradation products, *J. Pharm. Biomed. Anal.*, 69, 148–173.
- Singh, S., Junwal, M., Modhe, G., Tiwari, H., Kurmi, M., Parashar, N. and Sidduri, P. (2013). Forced degradation studies to assess the stability of drugs and products, *Trends Anal. Chem.*, 49, 71–88.
- Singh, S. (2016). Stability testing during development of nanopharmaceuticals, *Pharm. Nanotechnol.*, 3(4), 306–314.
- U.S. Department of Health and Human Services, Food and Drug Administration (1995). Content and Format of Investigational New Drug Applications (INDs) for Phase 1 Studies of Drugs, Including Well-Characterized, Therapeutic, Biotechnology-derived Products, Rockville, Md. (http://www.fda.gov/downloads/Drugs/GuidanceCompliance Regulatory Information/Guidances/UCM071597.pdf; accessed on 22.02.2017).
- U.S. Department of Health and Human Services, Food and Drug Administration (1998, draft). Stability Testing of Drug Substances and Drug Products, Rockville, Md. (http://www.fda.gov/ohrms/dockets/98fr/980362gd.pdf, accessed on 22.02.2017).
- U.S. Department of Health and Human Services, Food and Drug Administration (2005). ANDAs: Impurities in Drug Products, Rockville, Md. (www.fda.gov/downloads/Drugs/Guidance ComplianceRegulatory Information/Guidances/ucm072861.pdf; accessed on 22.02.2017).
- U.S. Department of Health and Human Services, Food and Drug Administration (2006). Exploratory IND Studies, Rockville, Md. (http://www.fda.gov/downloads/drugs/guidancecomplianceregulatory information/guidances/ucm078933.pdf; accessed on 22.02.2017).
- U.S. Department of Health and Human Services, Food and Drug Administration (2013). ANDAs: Stability Testing of Drug Substances and Products, Rockville, Md. (http://www.fda.gov/downloads/drugs/guidance complianceregulatoryinformation/guidances/ucm320590.pdf; accessed on 22.02.2017).
- World Health Organization (1996). Guideline for Stability Testing of Pharmaceutical Products Containing Well Established Drug Substances in Conventional Dosage Forms, Annex 5 to the thirty-fourth report of the WHO Expert Committee on

Specifications for Pharmaceutical Preparations, WHO Technical Report Series 863, Geneva (http://apps.who.int/medicinedocs/ pdf/s5516e/s5516e.pdf; accessed on 22.02.2017).

- World Health Organization (2009). Stability Testing of Active Pharmaceutical Ingredients and Finished Pharmaceutical Products, Annex 2 to the forty-third report of the WHO Expert Committee on Specifications for Pharmaceutical Preparations, WHO Technical Report Series 953, Geneva (http://apps.who.int/medicinedocs/documents/s19133en/s19133en.pdf, accessed on 22.02.2017).

11

Systematic Optimization of Pharmaceutical Products and Processes: Modern Approaches

Bhupinder Singh, Babita Garg, Premjeet Singh Sandhu, Ripandeep Kaur and Sumant Saini

INTRODUCTION

Design of an ideal pharmaceutical product invariably comprises multiple objectives. Such is particularly true for more intricate drug delivery systems (DDS) involving a variety of drugs, excipients, polymers and processes. For decades, this task has been conducted through trial and error, supplemented with the previous experience, knowledge, and wisdom of the formulator (Singh et al., 2008). The traditional approach of optimizing a formulation or process essentially entails studying the influence of the corresponding composition and process variables by changing One Variable at a Time (OVAT), while keeping others as constant. The technique, at times, is also referred to as Changing One Single Time (or Separate) variable or factor at a Time (COST) or OFAT (i.e., One Factor at a Time) or "shotgun" approach (Singh et al., 2005b). During the OVAT studies, the first variable is fixed at a favorable value, and the next is examined until no further improvement is attained in the response variable.

This approach can somehow achieve the solution of a specific problematic property, but attainment of the true optimum composition or process is never guaranteed. It may be ascribed to the presence of interaction(s), i.e., the synergistic or antagonistic influence of one or more variable(s) on others. During such inter-actions among variables, the OVAT approach gets stuck, usually far from optimum. Because there is no further improvement in the response, the experimenter may erroneously assume attainment of the optimum. The final product may be thought satisfactory but will really be sub-optimal, as a better formulation still exists, although unnoticed under the studied conditions. In a nutshell, the OVAT approach has proved to be not only too expensive in terms of time, money and effort, but also unfavorable to fix errors, unpredictable, and at times even un-successful. Overall, Box 11.1 enumerates various shortcomings of the traditional OVAT approach (Singh et al., 2008).

Systematic optimization techniques, on the other hand, have widely been practised to over-come such inconsistencies (Montgomery, 2001; Singh and Ahuja, 2004). Development of the principles behind such optimization techniques, now known as **Design of Experiments** (DoE), dates back to 1925, with its discovery by British

Box 11.1. Various limitations of OVAT approach
• Strenuous.
• Uneconomical.
• Time-consuming.
• Unsuitable to plug errors.
• Unsuitable to reveal interactions.
• Isolated and unconnected studies.
• Pseudo-convergent to untrue optimum.
• Result only in "just satisfactory" solutions.
• Detailed study of all variables is prohibitive.
• Prone to misinterpretation or faking of results.
• Futile when all variables change simultaneously.
• Unable to establish "cause and effect" relationship.
• Ineffective as it leads to unnecessary runs and batches.
• Irreproducible as infers randomly on the basis of origin.
• New product may retain defects inherent in the old one.

Box 11.2. Various meritorious features of systematic DoE optimization techniques
• Yield the "best solution" within the domain of study.
• Require fewer experiments to achieve an optimum formulation.
• Can trace and rectify a "problem" in a remarkably easier manner.
• Lead to comprehensive understanding of the formulation system.
• Help in finding the "important" and "unimportant" input variables.
• Tests and improves "robustness" amongst the experimental studies.
• Can change the formulation ingredients or processes independently.
• Aid in determining experimental error and detecting "bad data points".
• Can simulate the product or process behavior using model equation(s).
• Save a significant amount of resources viz. time, effort, materials and cost.
• Evaluate and improve the statistical significance of the proposed model(s).
• Can predict the performance of formulations even without preparing them.
• Detect and estimate the possible interactions and synergies among variables.
• Facilitate decision-making before next experimentation by response mapping.
• Provide reasonable flexibility in experimentation to assess the product system.
• Furnish ample information on formula behavior from one simultaneous study.
• Comprehend a process to aid in formulation development and later scale-up.

statistician, Sir Ronald Fisher (Fisher, 1925). The implementation of DoE optimization techniques invariably encompasses use of experimental designs and generation of mathematical equations and graphic outcomes, thus, depicting a complete picture of variation of the product/process response(s) as a function of the input variable(s) (Haaland, 1989; Singh et al., 2005b). Employing various rational combinations of formulation variables, DoE fits experimental data into statistical equations, uses these as the models to predict formulation performance, and optimizes the critical responses.

Of late, these modern DoE optimization techniques have become a regular practice globally, not only in the design and development of an assortment of new dosage forms, but also for modifying the existing ones. Be it in drug industry, institutional research or federal compliance with USFDA, ICH, NIH or ISO, DoE is being frequently sought-after in drug product/process development. Such systematic approaches are far more advantageous, as enlisted explicitly in Box 11.2.

The emerging domain of Quality by Design (QbD) also tends to employ DoE precepts in different quality procedures. QbD is another systematic approach to pharmaceutical development that begins with the predefined objectives of designing and developing formulations and manufacturing processes, emphasizing product and process understanding and process control, based on quality risk management and process analytical technology (PAT) (Lionberger et al., 2008). Realizing the significance of this minimization of variation, the pharmaceutical industry has recently focused its substantial efforts on improving its understanding of key unit operations and developing statistical, instrumental, and fundamental methods for characterizing and controlling various sources of variability in product performance. As a consequence, the industry is transitioning from the conventional approaches to multivariate QbD methods for assessing the effects of process variables on product quality. Beginning with the introduction of the PAT Guidance in 2003, a federal initiative on QbD has been drafted in ICH Q8 (R1), Q9, and Q10. The application of DoE methods during QbD is inherent during the entire product life cycle, right from variable screening to manufacturing.

BASIC TERMINOLOGY

Optimization

The word **optimize** simply means to make as perfect, effective or functional as possible (Schwartz and Connor, 1996). The term **optimized** has been used in the past to suggest that a product has been improved to accomplish the objectives of a development scientist (Singh and Ahuja, 2004). However, today the term implies that computers and statistics have been utilized to achieve the objective(s). With respect to drug formulations or pharmaceutical processes, **optimization** is a phenomenon of finding "**the best**" possible composition or operating conditions. Accordingly, **optimization** has been defined as the implementation of systematic approaches to achieve the best combination of product and/or process characteristics under a given set of conditions (Singh et al., 2008; Tye, 2004).

Variables

Design and development of drug formulation or pharmaceutical process usually involve several variables. The input variables, which are directly under the control of the product development scientist, are known as independent variables, e.g., compression force, excipient amount, mixing time, etc. Such variables can either be quantitative or qualitative. **Quantitative variables** are those that can take numeric values (e.g., amount of disintegrant, suspending agent, temperature, time, etc.), and are continuous. Instances of **qualitative variables**, on the other hand, include the type of emulgent, solubilizer or tabletting machine. Their influence can be evaluated by assigning dummy values to them. The independent variables, which influence the formulation characteristics or output of the process, are labelled as **factors**. The values assigned to the factors are termed as **levels**, e.g., 30° and 50° are the levels for the factor, i.e., temperature (Bolton, 1997; Schwartz and Connor, 1996; Singh et al., 2005b).

The characteristics of the finished drug product or the in-process material are known as dependent variables, e.g., drug release profile, friability, size of tablet granules, disintegration time, etc. (Doornbos and Haan, 1995; Montgomery, 2001). Popularly termed as **response variables**, these are the measured properties of the system to estimate the outcome of the experiment. Usually, these are direct function(s) of any change(s) in the independent variables.

Formulation system

Accordingly, a drug formulation, as depicted in Fig. 11.1, can be considered as a system consisting of input variables (X), the uncontrollable variables (U), a **transfer function** (T), and output (Y) (Singh et al., 2005b). The nomenclature of T depends upon the predictability of the output as an effect of change of the input variables. If the output is totally unpredictable from previous studies, T is termed as **black box**. The term **white box** is used for an empirical model with absolutely true predictability, while the term **gray box** is used for moderate predictability which usually is the case in the traditional studies. The entire DoE optimization endeavor aims at attaining a white box or nearly white box function from the erstwhile black or gray box status.

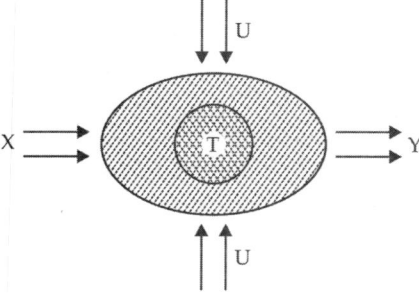

Fig. 11.1. A formulation system with controlled input variable(s) X, uncontrolled input variable(s) U, transfer function T, and output variable(s) Y (adapted from Singh et al., 2005b).

By and large, the more is the number of variables in a given system, the more complicated becomes the job of DoE optimization.

Effect and interaction

The magnitude of the change in response caused by varying the factor level(s) is termed as an **effect**. The main effect is the effect of a factor averaged over all the levels of other factors (Cochran and Cox, 1992). However, an **interaction** is said to occur when there is lack of additivity of factor effects. This implies that the effect is not directly proportional to the change in the factor levels. In other words, the influence of a factor on the response is nonlinear. Also, an interaction is said to take place when the effect of two or more factors is dependent on each other, e.g., effect of factor A depends on the level given to the factor B. The measured property of the interacting variables not only depends on their fundamental levels, but also on the degree of interaction between them (Singh et al., 2005b). Fig. 11.2 illustrates the concept of interaction graphically.

The term **orthogonality** is used if the estimated effects are independent of interactions and are due to the main factor of interest. Conversely, lack of orthogonality (i.e., independence) is termed as **confounding** or **aliasing**. An effect is confounded (or aliased) when one cannot assess how much of the observed effect

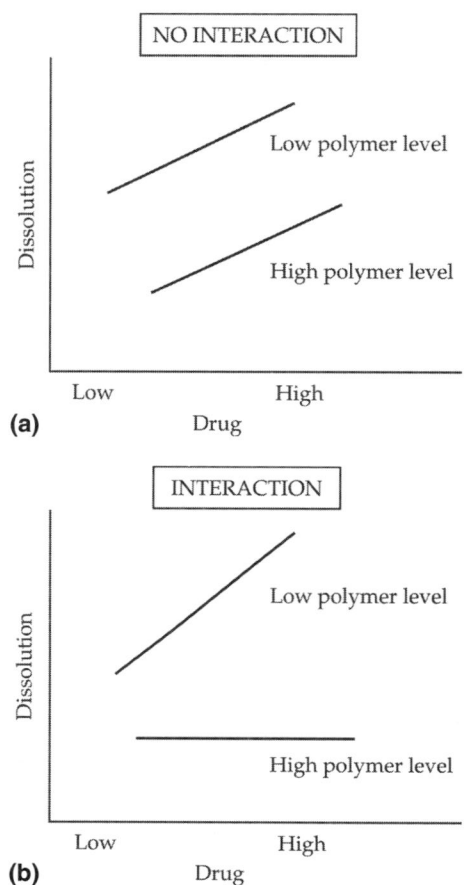

Fig. 11.2. Diagrammatic depiction of interaction. The unparallel lines (b) describe the phenomenon of interaction between drug and polymer levels affecting drug dissolution.

is due to the factor under consideration. The measure of the degree of confounding is known as **resolution** (Singh et al., 2005b). Confounding is a bias that must be controlled by suitable selection of the design and data analysis. Interaction, on the other hand, is an inherent quality of the data, which must be explored. Confounding must be assessed qualitatively, while interaction may be tested more quantitatively.

Coding

The process of denoting a natural variable into a dimensionless coded variable X_i such that the central value of experimental domain is zero is known as **coding** or **normalization**. Salient features of the coding process include depiction of effects and interaction using signs (+) or (−), allocation of equal significance to each axis, easier calculation of the coefficients, easier calculation of the coefficient variances, easier depiction of the response surfaces and ortho-gonality of the effects. Generally, various levels of a factor are designated as −1, 0 and +1, representing the lowest, intermediate (central) and the highest factor levels investigated, respectively. For instance, if starch, a disintegrating agent, is studied as a factor in the range of 5 to 10% (w/w), then codes −1 and +1 signify 5% and 10% concentrations, respectively. The code 0 would represent the central point at the mean of the two extremes, i.e., 7.5% w/w.

Factor space

The dimensional space defined by the coded variables is known as **factor space**. Fig. 11.3 illustrates the factor space for two factors on a bidimensional (2-D) plane during a typical tablet compression process. The part of the factor space that is investigated experimentally for optimization is the **experimental domain**. Also known

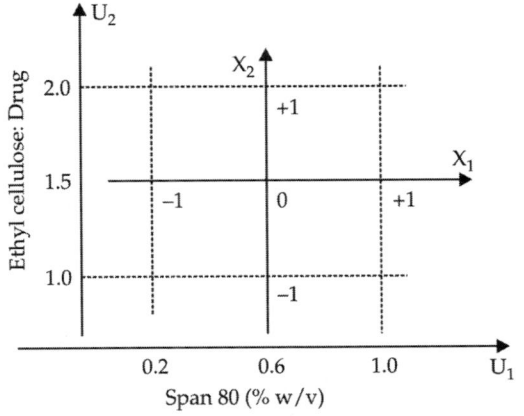

Fig. 11.3. Quantitative factors and the factor space. The axes for the natural variables, Ethyl cellulose: Drug and Span 80 are labelled as U_1 and U_2 and those of the corresponding coded variables as X_1 and X_2.

as the **region of interest**, it is enclosed by the upper and lower levels of the variables. The factor space covers the entire figure area and extends even beyond it, whereas the design space of the experimental domain is the square enclosed by $X_1 = \pm 1$, $X_2 = \pm 1$.

Experimental design

Conduct of an experiment and subsequent inter-pretation of its experimental outcome are the twin essential features of the general scientific methodology. This can be accomplished only if the experiments are carried out in a systematic way and the inferences are drawn accordingly. Required information is obtained as efficiently and precisely as possible. **Runs** or **trials** are the experiments conducted as per the selected experimental design (Singh et al., 2006b). Such DoE trials are so arranged in the design space that reliable and consistent information is achievable with minimum experimentation. The layout of the experimental runs in a matrix form, as per the experimental design, is known as **design matrix**. The choice of the design depends upon the proposed model, shape of the domain and the objective of the study. Primarily, the experimental (or statistical) designs are based on the principles of **randomization** (i.e., manner of allocation of treatments to the experimental units), **replication** (i.e., the number of units employed for each treatment) and **error control** or **local control** (i.e., grouping of specific type of experiments to increase the precision). These designs provide an idea of the (local) shape of the response surface (Fig. 11.4) being investigated, e.g., linear, quadratic, cubic and so on.

In each part of Fig. 11.4 (a, b and c), the value of the response increases from the bottom of the figure to the top, while those of the factor settings increase from left to right. If a response behaves as in Fig. 11.4a, the design matrix to quantify that behavior needs only to contain factors with two levels, low and high. If a response behaves as in Fig. 11.4b, the minimum number of levels required for a factor to quantify that behavior is

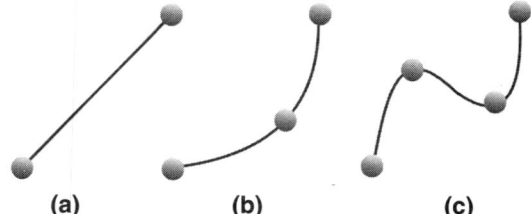

Fig. 11.4. Different types of responses as functions of factor settings: (a) linear; (b) quadratic; (c) cubic (adopted from Singh et al., 2005b).

three. Relatively more complicated cubic responses (Fig. 11.4c) are quite infrequent in pharmaceutical practice (Armstrong and James, 1990; Singh et al., 2005b).

Response surfaces

Conduct of DoE trials, as per the chosen statistical design, yields a series of data on response variables explored. Such data can be suitably modelled to generate mathematical relationship between the independent variables and the dependent variable. Graphical depiction of the mathematical relationship is known as response surface (Singh and Ahuja, 2004). A **response surface plot** is a 3-D graphical representation of a response plotted between two independent variables and one response variable. The use of 3-D response surface plots allows understanding of the behavior of the system by demonstrating the contribution of the independent variables.

The geometric illustration of a response, obtained by plotting one independent variable versus another, while holding the magnitude of response level and other variables as constant, is known as a **contour plot**. Such contour plots represent the 2-D slices of 3-D response surfaces. The resulting curves are called **contour lines**. Fig. 11.5 depicts a typical 3-D response surface and 2-D contour plot for the zeta potential as the response variable of the solid lipid nanoparticles of quercetin (Dhawan et al., 2010). For complete response depiction amongst 'n' independent variables, a total of $^{n}C_2$ number of response

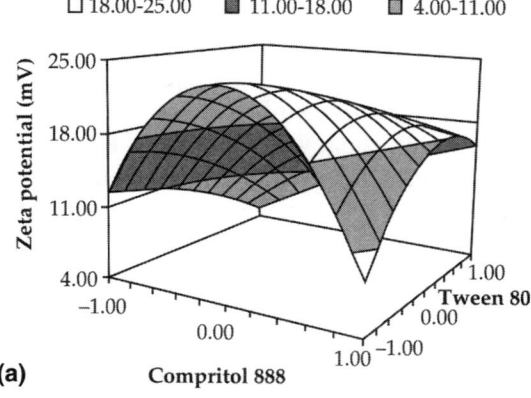

(a)

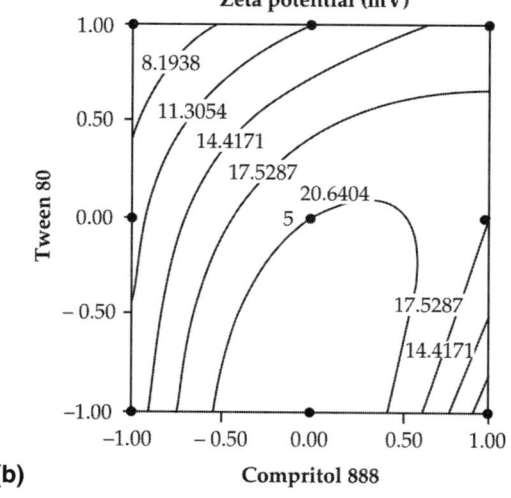

(b)

Fig. 11.5. (a) A typical response surface plotted between a response variable, i.e., zeta potential (mV), and two factors viz. Compritol 888 and Tween 80, in case of solid lipid nanoparticles; (b) the corresponding contour plot (Dhawan et al., 2010).

surfaces and contour plots may be required. In other words, 1, 3, 6 or 10 number of 3-D and 2-D plots is needed to provide depiction of each response for 2, 3, 4 or 5 number of variables, respectively.

Mathematical models

Mathematical model, simply referred to as the **model**, is an algebraic expression defining the dependence of a response variable on the independent variable(s). Mathematical models can either be empirical or theoretical. An empirical model provides a way to describe the factor-response relationship. It is most frequently, but not invariably, a set of polynomial equations of a given order. Most commonly used linear models are shown in Equations (1–3):

$$\varepsilon(y) = \beta_0 + \beta_1 X_1 + \beta_2 X_2 \qquad ...(1)$$

$$\varepsilon(y) = \beta_0 + \beta_1 X_1 + \beta_2 X_2 + \beta_{12} X_1 X_2 \qquad ...(2)$$

$$\varepsilon(y) = \beta_0 + \beta_1 X_1 + \beta_2 X_2 + \beta_{12} X_1 X_2 + \beta_{11} X_1^2 + \beta_{22} X_2^2 \qquad ...(3)$$

where, $\varepsilon(y)$ represents the measured response, X_1, the value of the factors, and are the constants representing the intercept, coefficients of first-order terms, coefficients of second-order quadratic terms and coefficients of second-order interaction terms, respectively. Equations (1) and (2) are linear in variables, representing a flat surface and a twisted plane in 3-D space, respectively. Equation 3 represents a linear second-order model that describes a twisted plane with curvature, arising from the quadratic terms.

Factor studies

Systematic screening and factor influence studies are usually carried out as a prelude to DoE optimization. These are often sequential stages in the development process. Screening methods are used to identify important and critical effects. Factor studies aim at quantitative determination of the effects as a result of a change in the potentially critical formulation or process parameter(s). Such factor studies usually involve statistical experimental designs, and the results so obtained provide useful leads for further response optimization studies. Factor studies include **screening of influential factors** and **factor influence studies**.

As the term suggests, "screening" is analogous to separating "rice" from "rice husk", where "rice" is a group of factors with significant influence as response, and "husk" is a group of the rest of the non-influential factors (Singh et al., 2006b). A product development scientist normally has numerous possible input variables to be investigated for their impact on the response variables. During initial stages of optimization, such input variables are explored for their influence on the outcome of the finished product to see if they are factors. The process, called as screening of influential variables, is a paramount step. An input variable, identified as a factor increases the chance of success, while an input variable that is not a factor has no consequence. Further, an input variable falsely identified as a factor unduly increases the effort and cost, while an unrecognized factor leads to wrong picture and a true optimum may be missed. The entire exercise aims at selecting the active factors and excluding the unnecessary variables, but not at obtaining complete and exact numerical data on the system properties.

Having screened the influential variables, a more comprehensive study, i.e., **factor influence study**, is subsequently undertaken to quantify the effect of factors, and to determine the interactions, if any (Singh et al., 2006b). Herein, the studied experimental domain is less extensive, as fewer active factors are studied. The models used for this study are neither predictive nor capable of generating a response surface. The number of levels is usually limited to two (i.e., at the extremes). However, sufficient experimentation is carried out to allow for the detection of interactions amongst factors. The experiments conducted at this step may often be reused during optimization or response modelling phase by augmenting with additional design points. Central points (i.e., at the intermediate level), if added at this stage, may prove to be useful in identifying the curvature in the response, in allowing the reuse of the experiments at various stages; and if replicated, in validating the reproducibility of the experimental study.

Of the numerous technical terms employed during DoE optimization, the vital ones are summarized in Box 11.3.

Box 11.3. Key terms used in DoE optimization

- **Optimize:** Make as perfect, effective, or functional as possible

- **Optimization:** Implementation of systematic approaches to achieve "the best" combination of product and/or process characteristics under a given set of conditions using QbD and computers

- **Factors:** Experimentally controlled independent variables affecting the performance of a product or process

- **Signal factors:** Controllable input variables influencing a response

- **Independent variables:** Input variables, which are directly under the control of product development scientist

- **Quantitative factors:** Input variables with continuous numeric values

- **Categorical variables:** Qualitative variables which cannot be quantified, e.g., type of polymer, tablet machine, etc.

- **Response variables:** Measured system property to estimate experimental outcome

- **Nuisance factors:** Uncontrollable factors which complicate the estimation of effects and interactions

- **Robust:** A product or process which is less variable to external uncontrollable influences

- **Levels:** Values assigned to the independent factors

- **Constraints:** Restrictions imposed on levels of a factor

- **Effect:** Magnitude of change in response by varying factor level(s)

- **Main effects:** Factor effects averaged at all other factor levels

- **Interactions:** Lack of additivity of factor effects

- **Orthogonality:** Sole dependence on main factor(s) and independence from interactions

- **Confounding:** Aliasing, equaling or lack of orthogonality or independence of variables

- **Empirical model:** Mathematical model describing factor-response relation using polynomial equations

- **Response surface plot:** A 3-D graphical representation of a response plotted between two independent variables and one response variable

- **Contour plot:** Geometric illustration of a response obtained by plotting one independent variable against

- another, holding the magnitude of response and other variables as constant

- **Contour lines:** Curves drawn on a contour plot corresponding to a response value

- **Factor space:** Dimensional space defined by the coded variables

- **Experimental domain:** Part of the factor space, investigated experimentally for optimization

- **Randomization:** An unbiased way of treatment allocation to experimental units

- **Replication:** Number of units employed for each treatment

- **Error control:** Grouping of specific type of experiments to increase experimental precision

- **Runs:** Experiments conducted according to the selected experimental design

- **Design matrix:** Layout of experimental runs in matrix form, as per the experimental design

- **Design augmentation:** Enhancement, extension and reuse of a primitive experimental design to a more advanced one

- **Antagonism:** Overall, negative change due to interaction among factors

- **Synergism:** Overall, positive change due to interaction between factors

- **Coding (or normalization):** Process of transforming a natural variable into a non-dimensional coded variable

- **Blocks:** Sets of relatively homogeneous experimental conditions, wherein every level of the primary factor occurs the same number of times with each level of nuisance factor

- **Response surface designs:** Designs facilitating response surfaces by allowing estimation of main effect, interaction and even quadratic effects

- **Screening designs:** Experimental designs employed for the purpose of factor screening

- **Rotatable design:** Experimental design where prediction ability of a response is constant in all directions at a given distance from the centre point of the domain

- **Residual:** Quantitative difference between the observed value of a variable and the value predicted using the proposed model

- **Outlier:** An unusually different response value as compared to the predicted values

Overall methodology

The theme of DoE optimization methodology provides comprehensive information on diverse DoE aspects organized in a seven-step sequence (Singh et al., 2005b), as illustrated in Fig. 11.6.

The optimization study begins with **Step I**, where an endeavor is made to ascertain the initial drug product development objective(s) in an explicit manner. Various main response parameters, which closely epitomize the objective(s), are chosen for the purpose.

In **Step II**, the experimenter has several potential independent product and/or process variables to choose from. By executing a set of suitable screening techniques and designs, the formulator selects the "vital few" influential factors among the possible "so many" input variables. Following selection of these factors,

a factor influence study is carried out to quantitatively estimate the main effects and interactions. Experimental studies are undertaken to define the broad range of factor levels as well.

During **Step III**, an appropriate experimental design is worked out on the basis of the study objective(s), the number and the type of factors, factor levels, and responses being explored. Working details on various aspects of the experimental designs, normally required to implement DoE optimization, have been elucidated in the subsequent section. Afterwards, response surface modelling (RSM) is characteristically employed to relate a response variable to the levels of input variables, and a design matrix is generated to guide the drug delivery scientist to choose optimal formulations.

In **Step IV**, the drug products and/or processes are experimentally executed according to the

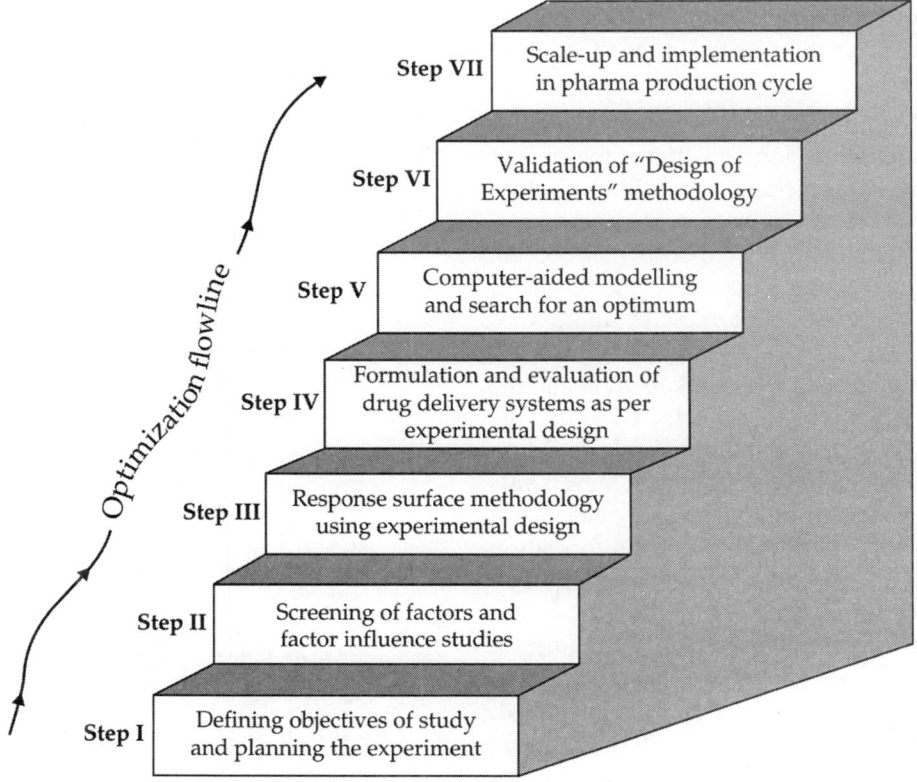

Fig. 11.6. Seven-step ladder for optimizing drug delivery systems (adopted from Singh et al., 2005b).

approved experimental design, and the chosen responses are evaluated.

Later, in **Step V**, a suitable mathematical model for the objective(s) under exploration is proposed; the experimental data, thus obtained, are analyzed accordingly, and the statistical significance of the proposed model is discerned. Optimal formulation compositions are searched within the experimental domain, employing graphical or numerical techniques. This entire exercise is invariably executed with the help of pertinent computer software.

Step VI is the penultimate phase of the optimization exercise, involving validation of response prognostic ability of the model put forward. Drug formulation performance of some studies, taken as the checkpoints, is assessed vis-à-vis that predicted using RSM, and the results are critically compared.

Finally, during **Step VII**, which is carried out in the industrial milieu, the process is scaled up and set forth ultimately for the production cycle.

Classes of experimental designs

An experimental design constitutes the pith of entire DoE exercise (Singh et al., 2008). Before the selection of an experimental design, it is essential to demarcate the experimental domain (i.e., the area to be investigated) within the factor space (i.e., the broad range of factor studies). To accomplish this task, first a pragmatic range of experimental domain is embarked upon and the levels and their numbers are selected so that the optimum lies within its realm. While selecting the levels, one must see that the increments between them should be realistic. Too wide increments may miss finding the useful information between the levels, while a too narrow range may not yield accurate results.

There are numerous types of experimental designs to choose from. Various commonly employed experimental designs for RSM, screening and factor-influence studies during pharmaceutical product/process development include:

> A. Factorial designs
> B. Fractional factorial designs
> C. Plackett-Burman designs
> D. Central composite designs
> E. Box-Behnken designs
> F. Equiradial designs
> G. Mixture designs
> H. Taguchi designs
> I. Optimal designs
> J. Split-Plot designs

A. Factorial designs

The most frequently employed experimental design, factorial design (FD), is the one in which all levels of a given factor are combined with all levels of every other factor in the experiment (Li, 2003). Full FDs involve studying the effect of all the factors (k) at various levels (x), including the interactions among them, with the total number of experiments being x^k.

An FD can be termed as 'symmetric', if the number of levels is the same for each factor, and 'asymmetric' in cases of a different number of levels for different factors (Lewis et al., 1999). Fig. 11.7 portrays a 2^3 FD, in which each point represents an individual experiment.

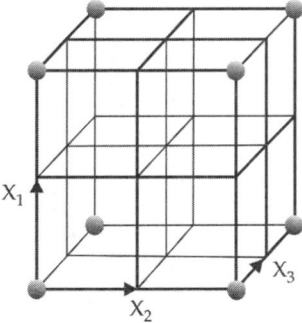

Fig. 11.7. Diagrammatic representation of a 2^3 factorial design (adopted from Singh et al., 2005b).

B. Fractional factorial designs

A fractional factorial design (FFD) is a finite fraction ($1/x^r$) of a complete or full FD, where r

is the degree of fractionation and x^{k-r} is the total number of experiments required (Doornbos and Haan, 1995). This design is particularly preferred over FD when the number of required experiments exceeds the manageable levels due to an increase in the number of factors or factor levels (Singh et al., 2005b). Fig. 11.8 graphically represents an FFD as a hypercube, with its corners represented by spheres, depicting the experiments studied.

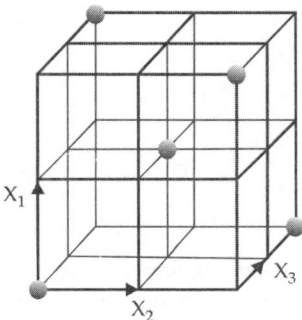

Fig. 11.8. Diagrammatic representation of a 2^{3-1} fractional factorial design (adopted from Singh et al., 2005b).

For a two-level, three-factor design, a full FD will require 2^3, i.e., eight experiments, where seven effects are determined. Out of these seven effects, there are three main effects, and the other four effects are due to the interactions among the three factors. An FFD with $r = 1$, on the other hand, will require only 2^{3-1}, i.e., four experiments, estimating a total of three effects (Singh et al., 2005b).

C. Plackett-Burman designs

The Plackett-Burman designs (PBDs) are specialized two-level FFDs used generally for screening of K, i.e., $N - 1$ factors, where N is a multiple of 4 (Plackett and Burman, 1946). Also known as **Hadamard designs** or **symmetrically reduced 2^{k-r} FDs**, the designs can easily be constructed employing a minimum number of trials (Loukas, 2001). Because these designs cannot be represented as cubes, they are sometimes called **non-geometric designs**. PBDs are

quite favorably employed during the screening processes.

D. Central composite designs

Also known as **Box-Wilson design**, the **central composite design** (CCD) is the most often used design for quadratic models (Singh and Ahuja, 2002; Singh et al., 2009b). The design comprises of a combination of a two-level factorial points $(2n)$, axial or star points $(2n)$ and a central point (Box and Wilson, 1951). Thus, the total number of factor combinations in a CCD is given by $2^n + 2n + 1$. The axial points for a two-factor problem include, $(\pm \alpha, 0)$ and $(0 \pm \alpha)$, where 'α' is the distance of the axial points from the center. A two-factor CCD is identical to a 3^2 FD with square experimental domain with α as ± 1, as shown in Fig. 11.9(a). On the other hand, when 'α' is $\sqrt{2} = 1.414$, the experimental domain is spherical in shape, as shown in Fig. 11.9(b).

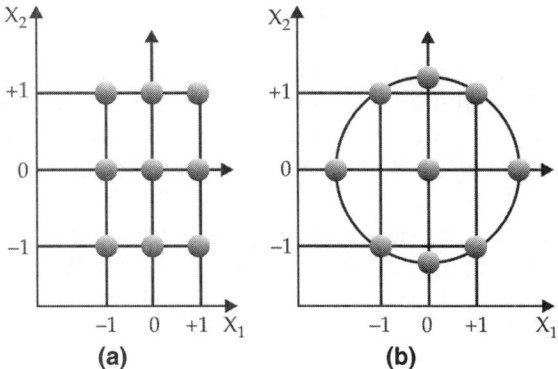

Fig. 11.9. Diagrammatic representation of (a) central composite design (rectangular domain) with $\alpha = 1$; (b) central composite design (spherical domain) with $\alpha = 1.414$ (adopted from Singh et al., 2005b).

E. Box-Behnken designs

Box-Behnken Design (BBD) is a specially made design that requires only 3 levels (-1, 0, 1) (Box and Behnken, 1960). It overcomes the inherent pitfalls of CCD, where each factor has to be studied at 5 levels, thus, increasing the number of experiments with a rise in the number of factors. Thus, a BBD is an economical alternative to CCD (Bodea and Leucuta, 1998; Myers, 2003). The design is rotatable (or nearly rotatable), and the proposed experimental runs are located at the midpoints of edges and the center of the experimental domain, as portrayed in Fig. 11.10.

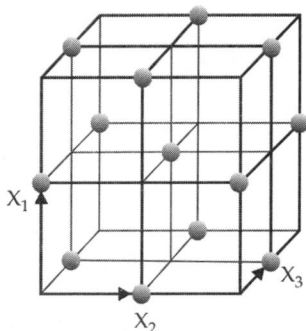

Fig. 11.10. Diagrammatic representation of a Box-Behnken design for three factors (adopted from Singh et al., 2005b).

F. Equiradial designs

These designs consist of N points on a circle about the centre of interest in the form of a regular polygon (Singh et al., 2005b). Taking into account the limited number of parameters ($p =$ 3) in the model, only 3- to 6-sided polygons are used. The design takes into account all the experiments, as numerically expressed in Eq. (4).

$$x_1 = \sin\frac{2i\pi}{N}; \; x_2 = \cos\frac{2i\pi}{N} \qquad \dots (4)$$

where i takes all integral values between 0 and $N-1$. The designs may be rotated by any angle and still retain the same properties. Fig. 11.11 explicitly illustrates several important cases of equiradial designs.

G. Mixture designs

Simultaneously varying all the factors under consideration at all levels may not be possible under many situations. Particularly in DDS with multiple excipients, the characteristics of the finished product usually depend not so much on the quantity of each substance present, but on

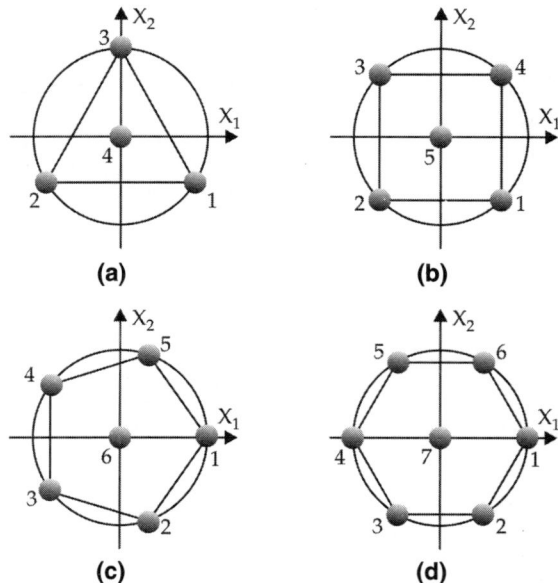

Fig. 11.11. Diagrammatic representation of a two-factor equiradial designs; (a) triangular four-run design; (b) square five-run design; (c) pentagonal six-run design; (d) Doehlert hexagonal seven-run design (adopted from Singh et al., 2005b).

their proportions. Here, the sum total of the proportions of all the excipients is unity, and none of the fractions can be negative. Therefore, the levels of different components can be varied with the restriction that the sum total should not exceed one. Mixture designs are highly recommended in such cases (Singh et al., 2005b). The design region for mixture proportions is a simplex, a regularly-sided figure of $k - 1$ dimensions with k vertices. The technique consists of first generating data from $n + 1$ experiments, where n is the number of factors (Araujo and Brereton, 1996). Based on $n + 1$ responses and predetermined rules, one result is eliminated and a new experiment is performed. For instance, with two factors, the simplex is the line segment from $(0, 1)$ to $(1, 0)$. With three factors, the simplex would have vertices at $(1, 0, 0)$, $(0, 1, 0)$ and $(0, 0, 1)$.

Simplex mixture designs (SMD), also at times referred as **Scheffé's designs**, can either be centroid or lattice designs (SLD) (Scheffe,

1958). Both of these are identical for first- and second-order models, but differ from third-order onwards. The design points are uniformly distributed over the factor space and form the lattice. The design point layout for three factors using various models is shown in Fig. 11.12, where each point refers to an individual experiment. A simple instance of product development exercise using simplex design has been illustrated quite explicitly in a standard pharmaceutical treatise (Lachman et al., 1989).

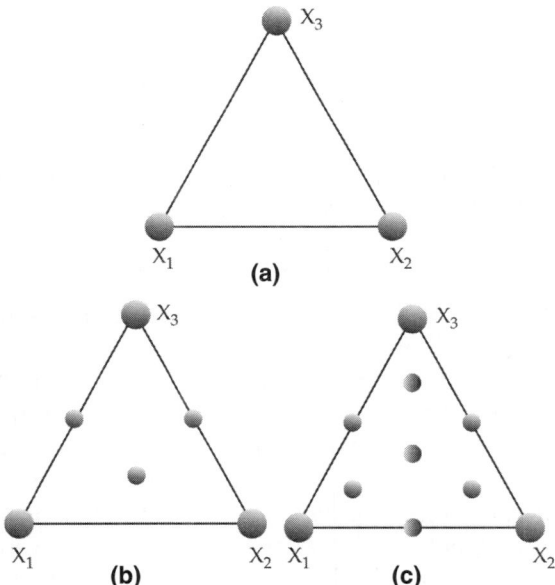

Fig. 11.12. Diagrammatic representation of simplex mixture designs: (a) linear model; (b) quadratic model; (c) special cubic model (adopted from Singh et al., 2005b).

H. Taguchi designs

Genichi Taguchi, a Japanese engineer, proposed several approaches to experimental designs that are sometimes called "Taguchi Methods" (Taguchi, 1986). These methods utilize two-, three-, and mixed-level fractional factorial designs. Large screening designs seem to be particularly favored by Taguchi adherents. Taguchi referred an experimental design as "off-line quality control", as it is a method to ensure good performance in the design stage of products or processes. The aim here is to make a product or process less variable (i.e., more robust) in the face of variation over which we have little or no control. The response variable in Taguchi data analysis is not the usual raw response or quality characteristic, but the signal-to-noise ratio (S/N ratio). The S/N ratio is a performance statistic, calculated across the entire outer array for each inner run, which becomes the response for a fit across the inner design runs. Pictorially, we can view this design as being a conventional design in the inner array factors (Fig. 11.13) with the addition of a "small" outer array factorial design at each corner of the "inner array" box.

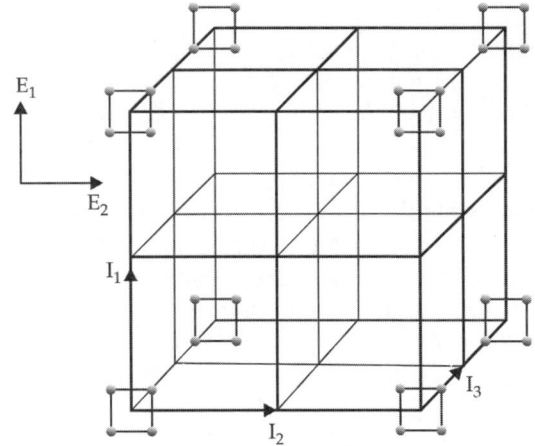

Fig. 11.13. Diagrammatic representation of inner 2^3 and outer 2^2 arrays for Taguchi robust design with "I" as the inner array and "E" as the outer array (adopted from Singh et al., 2005b).

I. Optimal designs

Optimal designs are a type of computer-aided designs, particularly useful where the classical designs do not apply. Unlike standard classical designs such as factorials and fractional factorials, optimal design matrices are usually not orthogonal and effect estimates are correlated. In general, such custom designs are generated based upon a specific **optimality criterion**, such as D-, A-, G-, I-, and V-optimality criteria (Singh et al., 2005b). The most popular criterion in the custom designs is D-optimality. This optimality criterion results in minimizing the generalized variance of the parameter estimates for a pre-specified model. As a result, the 'optimality' of the given design is model-dependent, i.e., the experimenter must specify a model for the design before a computer can generate the specific treatment combinations. D-optimal designs are based on the principle of minimization of parameter variance and co-variance.

J. Split-Plot designs

The **split-plot design**, also termed as "randomized complete block design", involves blocked experiments, where the number of experiments tend to block themselves, and serve as experimental units for a subset of the factors. Thus, these designs involve two levels of experimental units. The blocks are referred to as whole plots, while the experimental units within blocks are called split plots, strip plots, subplots or split units. Corresponding to the two levels of experimental units are two levels of randomization. One randomization is conducted to determine the assignment of block-level treatments to whole plots. Then, as always in a blocked experiment, randomization of treatments to split-plot experimental units occurs within each block or whole plot. This design can be portrayed as a flow diagram containing total area (i.e., whole plot) divided in the form of sectors, or as being a conventional design in the inner array factors (Fig. 11.14).

Besides the above, the experimental designs like **Star designs**, **Rechtschaffner designs**, **Extreme Vertices designs**, **Centre of Gravity designs** (Podczeck, 1995) and **Cotter designs** are also popular in the development of pharmaceutical products and processes, and in their factor screening. Table 11.1 gives a comparative account of important experimental designs employed for RSM, listing their advantages and disadvantages.

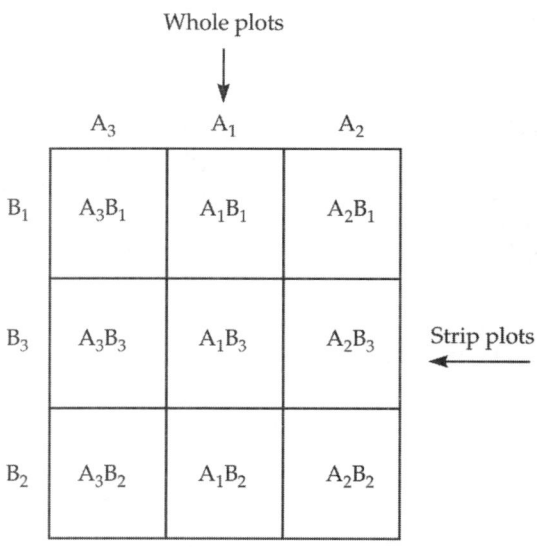

Fig. 11.14. Diagrammatic representation of a general layout of split-plot design.

Selection of experimental design

Choice of a design amongst the various types of available options depends upon the amount of resources available and the degree of control over making wrong decisions (i.e., Type I and Type II errors for testing hypotheses) that the experimenter desires. It is a good idea to choose a design that requires somewhat fewer runs than the budget permits, so that center point runs can be added to check for curvature in a 2-level screening design and backup resources are available to re-do runs that have processing mishaps. By and large, low-resolution designs like FDs (full or fractional), PBDs suffice the purpose of simpler screening of a large number of experimental parameters. Screening designs support only the linear responses. Thus, if a nonlinear response is detected, or a more accurate picture of the response surface is required, a more complex design type is necessary. Hence, when the investigator is interested in estimating interaction and even quadratic effects, or intends to have an idea of the local shape of the response surface, the response surface designs, capable of detecting curvatures, are used (Singh et al.,

Design	Description
Table 11.1. Merits and demerits of various experimental designs	
A: SCREENING DESIGNS	
Fractional factorial designs	The erstwhile high number of experiments in an FD can be significantly reduced in a systematic way in an FFD. An FFD is a finite fraction ($1/x^r$) of a complete or full FD, where r is the degree of fractionation and x^{k-r} is the total number of experiments required. *Merits:* • Suitable for large number of factors or factor levels. *Demerits:* • Difficult to construct. • Effects are confounded with interaction terms.
Plackett-Burman designs	PBDs are special two-level FFDs used generally for screening of K factors, i.e., $N-1$ factors, where N is a multiple of 4. Also known as Hadamard designs or symmetrically reduced 2^{k-r} FDs, the designs can easily be constructed employing a minimum number of trials. *Merits:* • Suitable for very large number of factors, where even FFDs require a large number of experiments. *Demerits:* • Design structure is complex. • Results in confounding of effects, as number of experiments is quite less.
Taguchi designs	Employed to develop the products or processes as robust amidst natural variability. Also referred to as "off-line quality control" experimental designs, the TgDs ensure good performance in the development of products or processes. Based upon the magnitude of signal-to-noise ratio, the TgDs can be used especially in factor screening for maximization or minimization of responses, or matching to a targeted value. *Merits:* • Suitable for both factor screening and optimization studies. • Use of arrays provides better precision and suitability for usage in robustness testing. *Demerits:* • Requires critical understanding of the aliases or confounding during robustness experiment.
B: RESPONSE SURFACE DESIGNS	
Factorial designs	A factorial experiment is one wherein all levels (x) of a given factor (k) are combined with all levels of every other factor in the experiment, with the total number of experiments being x^k. *Merits:* • Efficient in estimating main effects and interactions. • Used for screening of factors, factor influence studies. • Maximum usage of data. *Demerits:* • Reflection of curvature not possible in a 2-level design. • More experimental runs are required with addition of center points. • Prediction outside the region is not advisable.
Central composite designs	For non-linear responses requiring second-order models, CCDs are most frequently employed. The total number of factor combinations in a CCD is given by $2^k + 2k + 1$. *Merits:* • Combines the advantages of FDs and star designs.

(Contd.)

Design	Description
	• Allows the work to proceed in stages while augmenting the FD by adding a centre point. • Requires fewer experiments. *Demerits:* • Difficult to practice with fractional values of rotatability α.
Box-Behnken designs	A specially made design requires only three levels for each factor, i.e., –1, 0 and +1. A BBD is an economical alternative to CCD. *Merits:* • Requires fewer experimental runs and considered to be highly economical over the composite designs. • High resolution property in attaining solutions with better precision. *Demerits:* • Do not require axial points, thus, poses difficulty in predicting the points outside the region of interest.
Mixture designs	In DDS with multiple excipients, the characteristics of the finished drug product usually depend not so much on the quantity of each substance present but on their proportions. Simplex mixture designs (SMDs) are highly recommended in such cases. In a two-component mixture, only one factor level can be independently varied, while in a three-component mixture, only two factor levels can be independently varied. *Merits:* • Suitable for formulations wherein a constraint is imposed on some combination of factor levels. *Demerits:* • Difficulty in comprehending the polynomials generated. • Interactions and quadratic effects are not estimated.
Optimal designs	When the domain is irregular in shape, optimal designs can be used. These are the non-classic custom designs generated by exchange algorithm using computer. In general, such custom designs are generated based on a specific optimality criterion such as D-, A-, G-, I-, and V-optimality criteria. *Merits:* • Can be employed even if the value of experimental domain is either irregular or unknown. *Demerits:* • Involves a relatively complex model.

2005b). The compilation in Table 11.2 acts as a help guide while selecting an experimental design, based upon the desired motive of the study.

MODELIZATION

Following choice and implementation of an apt experimental design, apt models need to be generated. Generally, the polynomial mathematical equations are obtained, their statistical significance determined and the choice of the apt model made taking the help of model diagnostic plots.

A. Calculation of coefficients of polynomial equations

Regression is the most widely used method for quantitative factors. It cannot be used for qualitative factors, because interpolation between discrete (i.e., categorical) factor values is meaningless. In ordinary least-squares regression (OLS), a linear model, expressed as Eq. (5), is fitted to the experimental data such that the sum of squared differences between predicted and observed responses is minimized.

$$Y = \beta_0 + \beta_1 X_1 \text{ or } Y = \beta_0 + \beta_1 X_1 + \beta_{11} X_1^2 \quad \ldots (5)$$

Table 11.2. Application of important experimental designs depending upon the nature of factor, models and strategies

	2^k FD	x^k FD	FFD	PBD	CCD	BBD	EQD	SMD	TgD	DOD
Factor type										
Formulation	✓	✓	✓	✓	✓	✓	✓	✓	✓	✓
Process	✓	✓	✓	✓	✓	✓	✓	—	✓	✓
Both	✓	✓	✓	✓	✓	✓	✓	—	✓	✓
Number of factors										
≤ 3	✓	✓	✓		✓	✓	✓	✓	✓	✓
4–6	✓	✓	✓	✓	✓	✓	✓		✓	✓
> 6			✓	✓					✓	
Factor level										
2	✓	—	✓	✓	—			✓	✓	✓
≥ 3	—	✓			✓	✓	✓	✓	✓	✓
Model proposed										
Linear model	✓	✓	✓	✓				—	✓	
Interaction model	✓	✓	✓	✓	✓	✓	✓	✓	✓	
Quadratic model	—	✓	—		✓	✓	✓	—		
Mixture model	—	—	—	—	—	—	—	✓	—	
Custom made model	—	—	—	—	—	—	—	—	—	✓
Screening and factor influence study	✓	✓	✓	✓	—	—	—	✓	✓	✓
Response surface mapping	✓	✓			✓	✓	✓	✓	✓	✓

FD: Factorial Design; FFD: Fractional Factorial Design; PBD: Plackett-Burman Design; CCD: Central Composite Design; BBD: Box-Behnken Design; EQD: Equiradial Design; SMD: Simplex Mixture Design; TgD: Taguchi Design; DOD: D-Optimal Design

Multiple linear regression analysis (MLRA) can be performed for more factors, interactions, and higher order terms. In certain situations, where the factor-response relationship is non-linear, multiple non-linear regression analysis (MNLRA) may also be performed. In situations, where there are large numbers of variables, such as in multivariate studies, the methods of partial least squares (PLS) or principal component analysis (PCA) can also be employed for regression (Westerhuis and Coenegracht, 1997). PLS is an extension of MLRA and is used when there are fewer observations than the number of predictor variables.

B. Estimation of the significance of coefficients and model

Significance of coefficients can be determined using ANOVA, followed by Student's t test (Bolton, 1997). The values of Pearsonian coefficient of determination (r^2) and that adjusted for degrees of freedom ($r_{adj}{}^2$) of the polynomial equation are also compared. The value of r^2 is the proportion of variance explained by the regression according to the model and is the ratio of the explained sum of squares to that of the total sum of squares (SS), as explained in Eq. (6).

$$r^2 = \frac{SS_{\text{Total}} - SS_{\text{Residuals}}}{SS_{\text{Total}}} \qquad \ldots (6)$$

The closer the value of r^2 to unity, the better is the fit and more suitable, apparently, is the model.

Predicted residual sum of squares (PRESS) is the sum of squared differences leave-one-out method, as explained in Eq. (7). Ideally, the value should be zero or close to it.

$$PRESS = \sum (Y_i - Y_j)^2 \qquad \dots (7)$$

C. Model diagnostic plots

The goodness of fit of a model can be investigated using one or more of the plots illustrated in Fig. 11.15.

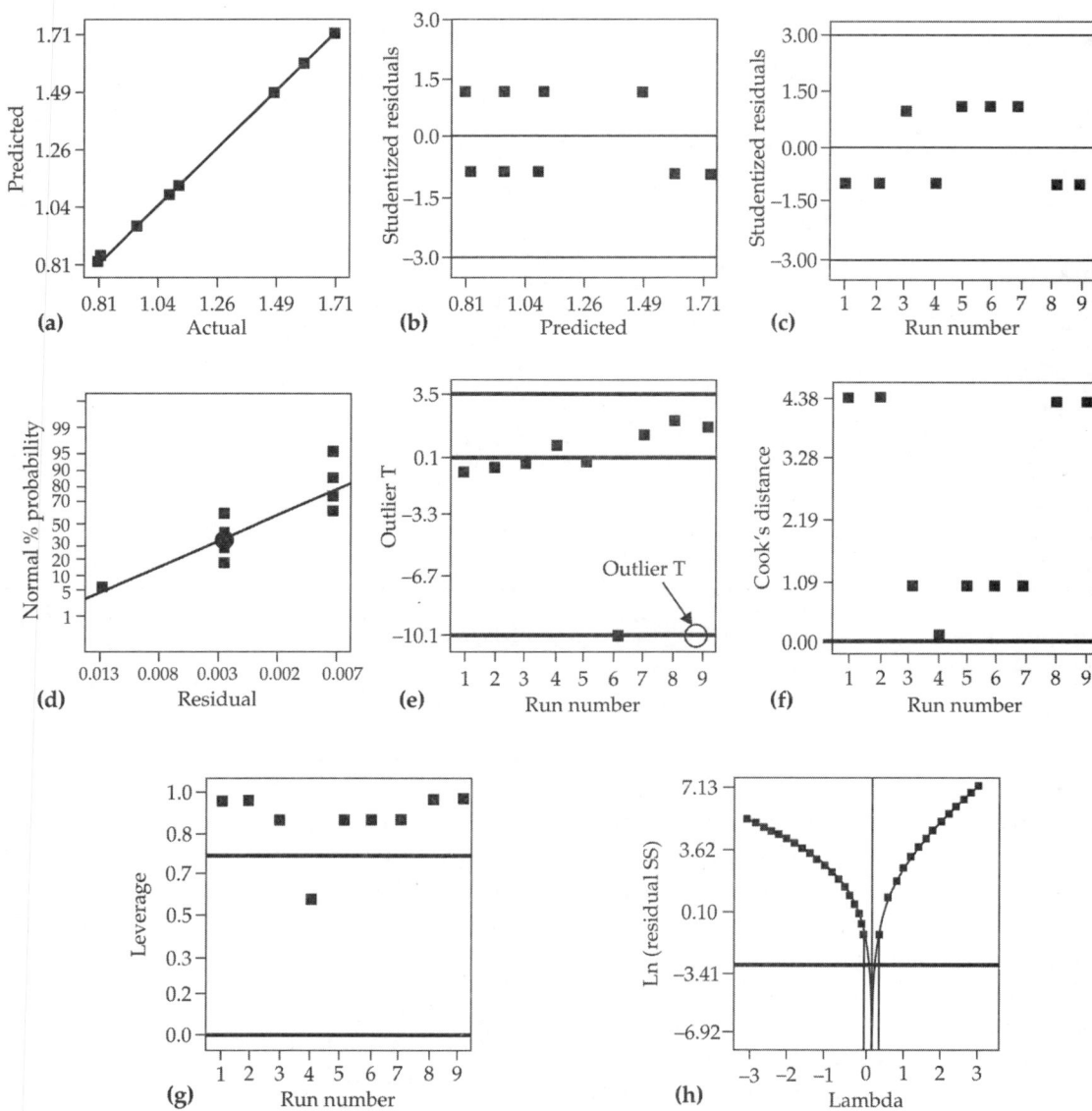

Fig. 11.15. Model diagnostic plots to investigate the goodness of fit of the proposed model(s). (a) predicted vs. actual; (b) studentized residuals vs. predicted; (c) studentized residuals vs. run; (d) normal probability plots; (e) outlier T plot; (f) Cook's distance plot; (g) leverage plot; (h) Box-Cox plot (adopted from Singh et al., 2005b).

- **Actual vs. predicted:** A graph is plotted between the actual and the predicted response values (Montgomery, 2001; Singh and Ahuja, 2002; Singh et al., 2005c). This helps in detecting a value or a group of values that are not easily predicted by the model.
- **Residuals vs. predicted:** Residuals (or error) is the quantitative difference between the observed and the predicted response(s). Studentized residuals are the residuals converted to their standard deviation units.
- **Residuals vs. run:** This is a plot of the residuals versus the order of the experimental runs. It checks for the "lurking variables" that may have influenced the response during the experiment.
- **Residuals vs. factor:** This is a plot of the residuals versus any selected factor. It checks whether the variance, not accounted for by the model, is different for different levels of a factor.
- **Normal probability plot:** It investigates the normal probability distribution of residuals, as judged from the linear trend of the points, when plotted on a probit scale.
- **Outlier T plot:** This is a measure of, by how many standard deviations, the actual value deviates from the value predicted after deleting the point in question.
- **Cook's distance plot:** This provides measures of the influence, potential or actual, of the individual runs (Cook, 1977).
- **Leverage plot:** This is a measure of degree of influence of each point on the model fit.
- **Box-Cox plot:** The Box-Cox plot is a tool to help in determining the most appropriate power transformation for application to response data (Box and Cox, 1964).

OPTIMUM SEARCH

From the models, thus selected, optimization of one response or the simultaneous optimization of multiple responses needs to be accomplished graphically and/or numerically.

A. Graphical optimization

Known popularly as response surface analysis, graphical optimization displays the area of feasible response values in the factor space (Myers, 2003; Schwartz and Connor, 1996; Singh and Ahuja, 2004). The experimenter has to make a choice, "trading off" one objective for other(s), according to the relative importance of the objectives considered. The success in locating an optimum lies in the judicious interpretation and/or comparison of the resulting plots, leading to attainment of the best compromise. One or more of the following techniques may be employed for this purpose.

Location of the stationary point

After completing the experimental work, often the goal of the formulation scientist is to locate the optimum. The nature of the response surface is interpreted graphically, and a **stationary point** is located, which may be maximum, minimum, or a target value. At this point, the partial derivatives of the response with respect to the design variable are all zeroes. Fig. 11.16a & b show the location of stationary points in case of a maximum and minimum, respectively. The case in which the stationary point is neither a maximum nor a minimum is known as the **saddle point**, as shown in Fig. 11.16c.

Search methods

Search methods are employed for choosing the upper and lower limits of the responses of interest. The response surfaces in these search methods, as defined by the appropriate equations, are searched to find the combination of independent variables yielding the optimum. Two major steps, viz. **feasibility search** and **grid search** are used. Together, these techniques are also referred to as the **brute force method**. The feasibility search method is used to locate a set of response constraints that are just at the limit of possibility. One selects several values for the responses of interest, and a search of the response surface is made to determine whether a solution

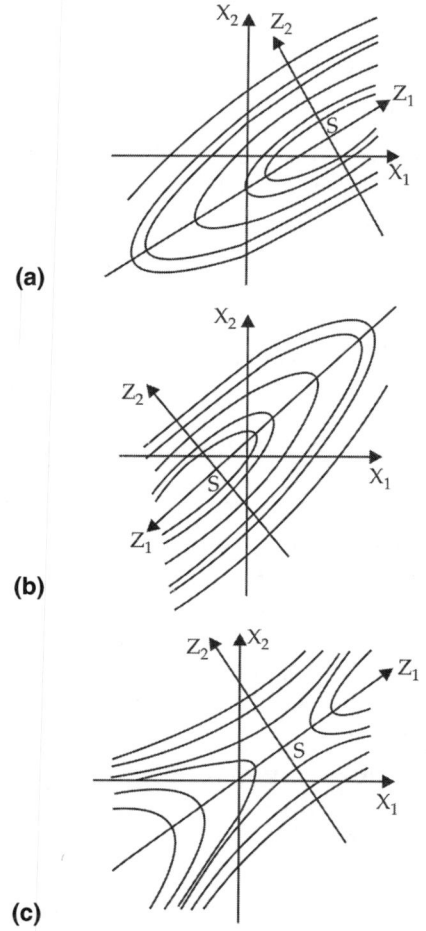

(a)

(b)

(c)

Fig. 11.16. Diagrammatic representation of contour lines for location of the stationary point: (a) maximum; (b) minimum; (c) saddle point (adopted from Singh et al., 2005b).

is feasible. Subsequently, the exhaustive grid search is applied, wherein the feasible experimental range is divided into a grid of smaller specific sizes and searched methodically (Singh et al., 2006a; Singh et al., 2009b).

Overlay plots

The response surfaces or contour plots are superimposed over each other to search for the best compromise visually. Minimum and maximum boundaries are set for acceptable objective values. The region is highlighted

wherein all the responses are acceptable. This is termed as an overlay plot or a combined contour plot. Within this area, an optimum is located, trading off different responses. Fig. 11.17 illustrates the overlay plot generated during formulation optimization of floating-bioadhesive tablet formulation of cefuroxime axetil in our laboratories (Bansal et al., 2015).

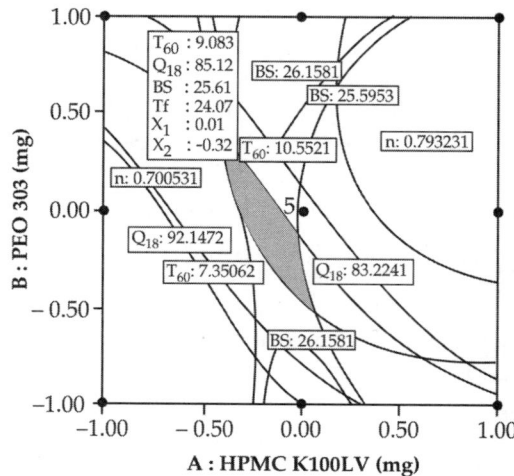

Fig. 11.17. Overlay plots showing the location of the optimized floating-bioadhesive matrix tablets of cefuroxime axetil.

Besides, there are other vital methods used for graphically searching the optimum formulation like Pareto-optimality charts.

B. Mathematical optimization

Graphical analysis is usually preferred in the case of single response. However, in cases of multiple responses, it is usually advisable to conduct numerical or mathematical optimization first to uncover a feasible region.

Desirability function

Desirability function is a way of overcoming the difficulty of multiple, sometimes opposing responses (Singh et al., 2005b). In this method, each response is associated with its own partial desirability function. The optimum is the point with the highest value for desirability. The experimenter should study the contour plot of desirability surface around the optimum and combine this with contour plots of the most important responses. A large area or volume of high desirability will indicate a robust formulation or set of processing conditions. Although the method requires appropriate computer software, yet it is a highly useful and pragmatic method of optimization.

Objective functions

These methods are used to seek an optimum formulation by solving the objective function either for a maximum or a minimum in the presence of equality and/or inequality constraints. This approach is also known as classical optimization and is applicable only to unconstrained problems. These techniques, however, find relatively limited use in optimization of pharmaceutical drug formulations and delivery systems, where the problems are generally the constrained ones.

C. Sequential search methods

Despite the numerous merits of simultaneous approaches, there are situations where there is hardly any *a priori* knowledge about the effects of variables (Doornbos and Haan, 1995; Schwartz and Connor, 1996). Such situations arise when choosing a very extensive experimental domain is difficult or the possible experimental domain is not known at the beginning of the study, thus, calling for the application of the sequential optimization methods. In sequential approach, optimization is attempted in a stepwise fashion. Experimentation is started at an arbitrary point in the experimental domain and responses are evaluated.

The inherent advantages of these methods are:

- No need to plan all the experiments simultaneously.
- *A priori* knowledge of the response surface is not essential.
- Interactive.

However, various disadvantages encompass:

- Number of experiments to reach an optimum cannot be predicted.
- Optimum found may not be the global optimum.
- Robustness is not known.
- Unsuitable for multiple objective problems.
- Attainment of optimum is judged only by the expert developmental scientist(s).
- Mathematical model and complete response surface is not generated.
- Yields unreliable results when multiple optima exist.
- Applicable only when response surface is continuous.

Steepest ascent (or descent) methods are direct optimization methods for first-order designs (Lewis et al., 1999), especially when the optimum is outside the domain and is to be arrived at rapidly. Optimum path method is just analogous to steepest ascent method and is employed where the optimum is searched outside the experimental domain by extrapolation. The technique of Evolutionary Operations (EVOP), wherein the production procedure (formulation and process) is allowed to evolve to the optimum by careful planning and constant repetition, is quite popular in several industrial processes.

D. Artificial neural networks

In the last decade, the application of artificial neural networks (ANNs) in the field of pharmaceutical development and optimization of dosage forms has become a blown-out topic of discussion in the pharmaceutical literature (Amani et al., 2008; Djekic et al., 2008; Rizkalla and Hildgen, 2005; Takayama et al., 1999). The ANNs are model-independent computational paradigms that can simulate the neurological processing ability of the human brain. The neural networks, consisting of inter-connected adaptive processing units, so-called neurons, are able to discern complex and latent patterns in the information presented to them. ANN is a computer-based learning system that can be applied to quantify a non-linear relationship between causal factors and pharmaceutical responses by means of iterative training of data obtained from a designed experiment. The results obtained from implementation of an experimental design are used as input information for learning. Once trained, the neurons of an ANN may be used to forecast outputs from new sets of input conditions.

A typical ANN must have one input layer and one output layer, and may contain one or more hidden layers, as depicted in Fig. 11.18. The information is passed from input layer to the output layer through hidden layer(s) by the network connections or synapses. Modelling starts with a random set of synaptic weights and proceeds in iterations. During each of iterations, connection weights are adapted via selected modelling. The basis of such modelling technique is to minimize the "δ error", i.e., the difference between the momentary network signal and the aimed signal based on the experimental results. When the minimal "δ error" is obtained, learning is completed and connection weights become the memory units. After this, the test set of values can be applied on a learned ANN to evaluate it. Subsequently, it can be used for output prediction on the basis of the new input values. The modelling is invariably done via suitable computer software.

Selection of an optimization methodology

In case of single response, graphical analysis is often opted for (Lewis et al., 1999). However, in case of multiple response variables, certain responses can oppose one another. Accordingly,

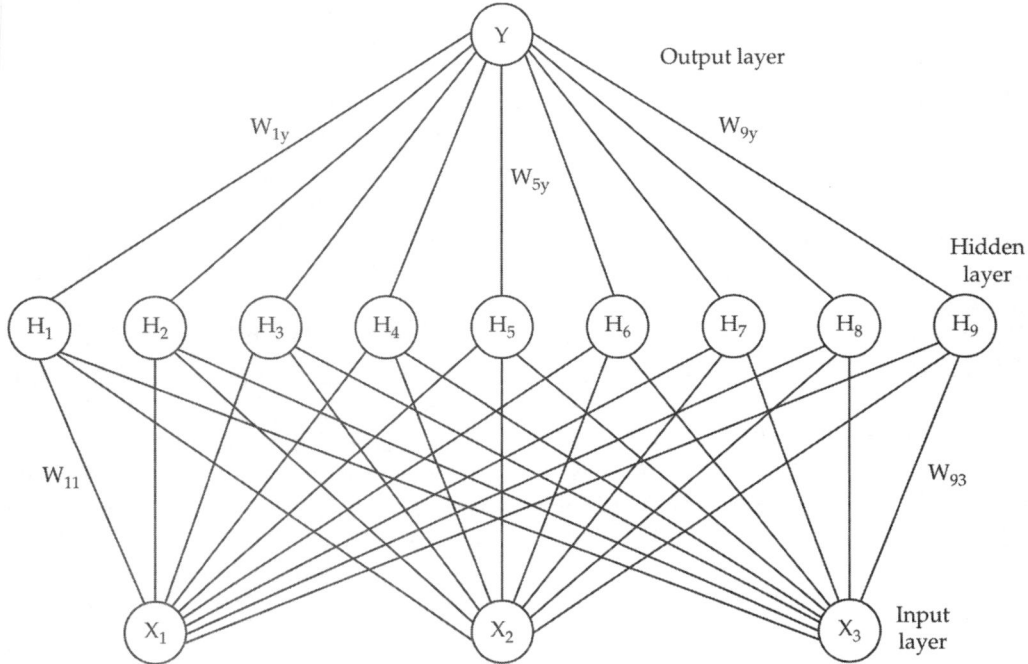

Fig. 11.18. Schematic diagram illustrating various parts of an artificial neural network. X_1-X_3 represent the input factors; Y is the response variable connected to the input layer via various nodes of hidden layer (H_1-H_9). W_{11} and W_{93} represent the connections between the corresponding input factors and the nodes of the hidden layer while W_{1y}, W_{5y}, and W_{9y} denote the connections between the respective hidden nodes and output layer, Y (adopted from Singh et al., 2005b).

changes in a factor that improve one response may have a negative effect on another. Since it is not usually possible to obtain the best values for all the responses, optimization principally embarks upon finding experimental conditions where different responses are most satisfactory, over all. Nevertheless, there is a certain degree of subjectivity in weighing up their relative importance. Table 11.3 provides a ready reference for suitability of various optimization methods for different experimental conditions.

COMPUTER USE IN DoE OPTIMIZATION

The merits of DoE optimization techniques are galore and their acceptability upbeat. Putting such rational approaches into practice, however, usually involves a great deal of mathematical and statistical intricacies. Today, with the availability of powerful and economical hardware and that of the comprehensive DoE software the erstwhile computational hiccups have been greatly simplified and streamlined. Computer software have been used almost at every step during the entire optimization cycle ranging from selection of design, screening of factors, use of response surface designs, generation of the design matrix, plotting of 3-D response surfaces and 2-D contour plots, application of optimum search methods, interpretation of the results, and finally, the validation of the methodology. Hence,

when selecting a DoE software package, it is important to look for not only a statistical engine that is fast and accurate, but also the following:

- A simple graphic user interface (GUI) that is intuitive and easy-to-use.
- A well-written working manual with tutorials to get off to a quick start.
- A wide selection of designs for screening and optimizing processes or product formulations.
- A spreadsheet flexible enough for data entry as well as dealing with missing data and changed factor levels.
- Graphic tools displaying the rotatable 3-D response surfaces, 2-D contour plots, inter-action plots and the plots revealing model diagnostics.
- Facility to randomize the order of experimental runs.
- Design evaluation tools that will reveal aliases (i.e., confounded or equal effects) and other potential pitfalls.
- After-sales technical support, online help and training offered by manufacturing vendors.

Box 11.4 lists some commonly used computer software packages for DoE optimization, especially in pharma circles, along with their respective web sources.

With the easy availability and affordability of the DoE software, these powerful tools can be implemented with the simple click of a mouse. However, there are some key issues that depend

Table 11.3. Suitability of various optimization methods under variegated situations

Optimization method	Model situations for use
Graphical analysis	Mathematical model of any order, normally not more than 4 factors, preferably in single response
Desirability function	Mathematical model of any order, number of factors between 2 and 6, multiple responses
Steepest ascent	First-order model, optimum outside the domain, single response
Optimum path	Second-order model, optimum outside the domain, single response
Sequential simplex	No mathematical model, direct optimization, single or multiple responses
Evolutionary operations	Industrial situation, little variation possible
Artificial neural networks	High levels of predictability obtained, model becomes complicated beyond 3–4 factors

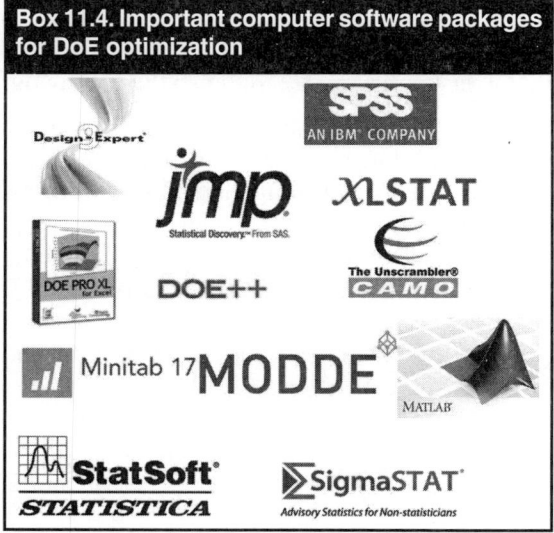

Box 11.4. Important computer software packages for DoE optimization

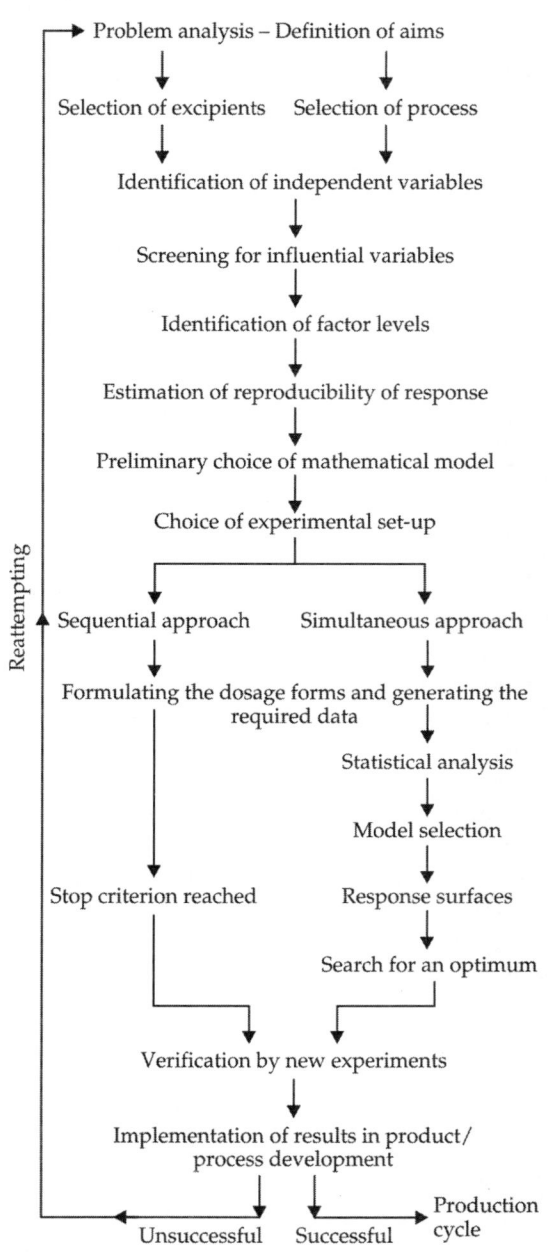

Fig. 11.19. Schematic flow diagram of the overall strategy for optimization of drug formulations (adopted from Singh & Ahuja, 2004).

upon the experimenter but not upon the software. These include choosing suitable responses (output variables) and factors (input variables), setting appropriate factor ranges or levels, managing the experimentation, interpreting numeric outcomes and graphic manifestations of the findings, presenting the results, and finally deciding whether to continue further with process optimization or just run confirmatory experiment(s) to validate DoE.

OVERALL OPTIMIZATION STRATEGY

The overall approach for conduct of optimization studies in pharmaceutical dosage forms can be described by an optimization plan (Myers, 2003; Singh and Ahuja, 2004). The salient steps involved in an optimization strategy include (Fig. 11.19).

Problem definition: The optimization problem (e.g., release of a drug from dosage form) should be clearly understood and defined.

Selection of factors and levels: The independent variables selected should be quantifiable and easily controllable. The levels of each variable are either established from the prior experience or pilot studies. If a large number of independent variables are involved, a preliminary screening study for the influential variables should be carried out.

DoE OPTIMIZATION OF PHARMA-CEUTICAL PRODUCTS AND PROCESSES: A LITERATURE INSIGHT

Optimization employing various experimental designs has been used for a long time like, the FDs since 1926, the screening designs since 1946, the CCDs since 1951 and mixture designs since 1958 (Box and Wilson, 1951; Fisher, 1935; Plackett and Burman, 1946; Scheffe, 1958). The use of DoE optimization techniques, however, permeated into the field of pharmaceutical product development around four decades ago. The first literature report on the rational use of optimization appeared in 1967, when a tablet of sodium salicylate was optimized using an FD (Marlowe and Shangraw, 1967). Since then, these systematic approaches have been put into practice in routine drug product/process development at steady pace (Singh et al., 2005a).

A quick glance at the chronological bar chart (Fig. 11.20) reveals that since 1990, there has been a sudden spurt in the number of published work on the use of rational optimization in drug product development. This may largely be attributed to the realization of significant benefits of systematic DoE techniques, coupled with the ready accessibility of effective and cost-effective computational tools in the armamentarium of a formulator. Amongst the products optimized, the major proportion constitutes the relatively intricate novel DDS, as shown in Fig. 11.20, obviously where the benefits of DoE optimization can be better realized. In contrast, hardly any study has been reported on the DoE optimization of conventional drug formulations in the last few years.

A product development scientist has to handle a heterogeneous group of formulations, including uncoated or coated tablets, controlled release tablets, effervescent tablets, soluble tablets, dispersible tablets, capsules, microspheres, granules, pellets, etc. amongst the solid dosage forms; gels, ointments, creams and suppositories amongst semisolids; solutions, emulsions, suspensions, lotions, inhalations, etc., amongst the liquid dosage forms; and aerosols, patches, films, plasters amongst the others. The characteristics of these dosage forms vary markedly from immediate release (fast disintegration, fast dissolution) to (very) slow release matrix tablets. Extensive literature search carried out in pharmaceutical journals and texts till date reveals that the DoE optimization techniques have been employed for almost all of these dosage forms, ranging from the simple conventional ones to that of the most intricate novel DDS. Fig. 11.21 presents a pictorial depiction of the proportion of various kinds of dosage forms formulated using DoE approach.

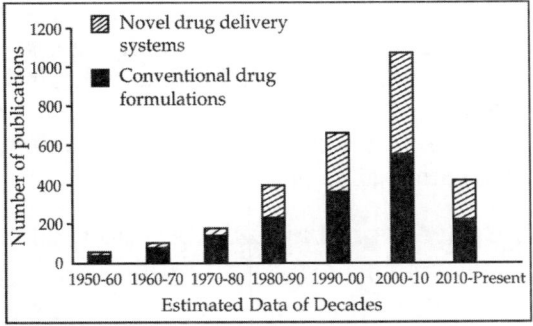

Fig. 11.20. Bar diagram portraying the chronological development in the number of research publications on use of systematic DoE optimization techniques.

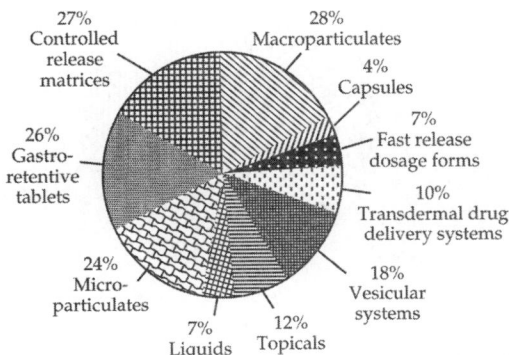

Fig. 11.21. Pie chart showing the proportion of various pharmaceutical dosage forms optimized using DoE.

Diverse experimental designs have been employed for optimization of DDS. Overall, Fig. 11.22 shows that FD and its modifications (FFD, PBD, and Taguchi) occupy significant slice of the pie chart, almost one half of the entire chart, indicating their distinct popularity while optimizing the varied kind of DDS. The FDs are verily the orthogonal designs allowing independent estimation of main effects and interactions among various factors. Higher-level FDs have been found to be quite efficient in determining the quadratic effects too. The experimental designs, next in popularity, are the composite designs (CCD, BBD, and CGD) and mixture designs. Composite designs have particularly been quite preferred for investigating second-order effects in drug delivery development. A brief account of optimization of diverse type of drug formulations and processes is being presented as under with select literature instances of each type.

A. Solid oral dosage forms

The optimization of tablet(s), the most popular solid oral dosage form, has been carried out since 1967 (Marlowe and Shangraw, 1967). Amongst the conventional tablet dosage forms, the targeted responses for optimization include weight uniformity, disintegration time, crushing strength, physicochemical stability, thickness, content uniformity and *in vitro* dissolution profile. Various tablet constituents have been most frequently investigated as the independent variables. The number of investigated independent variables generally range between 2 and 6, while the optimized responses between 1 and 4, the broader range being 1 to 10.

Relatively limited reports are available on the optimization of relatively simpler capsule dosage form. The independent variables, which have been considered for optimizing capsules, encompass quantities of the ingredients, capsule size, operating rate of semi-automatic filling machine, etc., for responses like, powder blend homogeneity, flow, weight, dissolution rate, etc. Apart from the tablets and capsules, the macro-particulates including pellets, beads and micro-granules prepared usually by the process of extrusion spheronization have also been optimized for yield, mean particle size, size distribution, granulate hardness, granule friability, porosity, flow rate, etc. Table 11.4 provides selected literature instances on formulation optimization of solid oral dosage forms.

B. Conventional Liquid Formulations

There are several reports on optimization of diverse liquid formulations, viz. emulsions, solutions, suspensions, lotions, etc. Amongst the ophthalmic and parenteral formulations, solubility, chemical stability and viscosity have

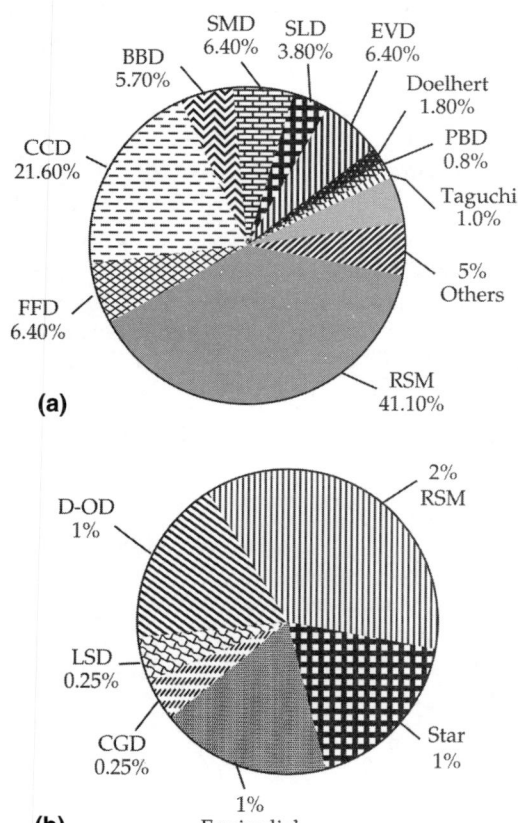

Fig. 11.22. Pie chart showing proportion of the individual experimental design application in (a) pharmaceutical formulations, and (b) processes.

Table 11.4. Selected systematic optimization reports on solid oral dosage forms

Drug	Design	IV	RV	Reference(s)
TABLET DOSAGE FORMS				
Torsemide	BBD	3	2	Shenawy et al., 2017
Chlorphenaramine	BBD	2	4	Dave et al., 2016
Quetiapine	FD	2	3	Kalyankar et al., 2015
Itraconazole	CCD	2	2	Sun et al., 2014
Troxipide	CCD	4	2	Gao et al., 2014
Pyridostigmine	CCD	2	2	Tan et al., 2013
Carvedilol	CCD	2	2	Aktas et al., 2013
Lamivudine	CCD	2	4	Singh et al., 2012
Domperidone	CCD	2	4	Arora et al., 2011
Sinomenine	CCD	2	2	Zhang and Geng, 2010
Tramadol	CCD	2	3	Singh et al., 2010
Azithromycin	CCD	2	4	Zhang et al., 2010
Acetaminophen	CCD	2	2	Cantor et al., 2009
Metoclopramide	CCD	3	4	Vora and Rana, 2008
Artemisinin	FD	3	2	Ngo et al., 1997
Vitamin C	BBD	3	4	Chang, 1994
Pyridoxal HCl	FD	6	2	Durig and Fassihi, 1993
Aspirin	FD	4	3	Devay et al., 1988b
CAPSULE DOSAGE FORMS				
Nifedipine	FFD	4	1	Mercuri et al., 2017
Propranolol	CCD	3	2	Zhang et al., 2015
Montelukast sodium	CCD	4	2	Ranjan et al., 2014
Gliclazide	CCD	2	2	Pal and Nayak, 2011
Famotidine	CCD	2	2	Guan et al., 2010
Berberine	CCD	3	2	Chen et al., 2008
α-Methyl dopa	SMD	7	1	Saavedra and Cuadra, 2001
MICROPARTICULATE BEADS				
Finasteride	BBD	3	4	Ahmed et al., 2016
Lycopene	BBD	3	2	Celli et al., 2016
Tizanidine HCl	CCD	3	2	El Mahrouk et al., 2014
Glibenclamide	CCD	2	2	Nayak et al., 2012
Tramadol	CCD	2	2	Singh and Kumar, 2012
Caffeine	CCD	5	5	Mallipeddi et al., 2010
Neutrase	CCD	4	2	Ortega et al., 2009
PELLETS				
Naproxen	MD	4	3	Shah et al., 2016
Ethyl cellulose	CCD	5	5	Mallipeddi et al., 2014
Sirolimus	CCD	2	2	Hu et al., 2012

FD: Factorial Design; BBD: Box-Benkhen Design; CCD: Central Composite Design; SMD: Simplex Mixture Design; IV: Independent Variables; RV: Response Variables been optimized by varying the formulation composition. Table 11.5 enlists some literature reports on the use of optimization techniques in the development of liquid formulations. Emulsions, microemulsions, solutions, lotions or suspensions have been optimized for responses as turbidity, cloud point, physical stability, preservative efficacy, etc., primarily by altering the levels of the ingredients. The FD, CCD or SMD have been utilized as the experimental designs, with the number of independent variables ranging between 2 and 8, and responses between 1 and 5.

C. Process optimization of conventional dosage forms

Optimization techniques have also been successfully applied since 1975 to the process of pre-tabletting granulation, using wet or dry method, to produce optimum granules for compression (Malinowski & Smith, 1975). The responses taken into consideration for optimization have primarily been the physical properties of granules, i.e., geometric mean diameter, particle size distribution, bulk and tap densities, friability, flow rate, compactibility index, recompressibility of roller compacted dry granules, etc. The main independent variables for wet granulation pertain to the composition

of the binder solution, i.e., percentage of binder, total amount, amount of alcohol in a hydro-alcoholic binder solution, etc. The process variables, which usually have been investigated include impeller speed, kneading time, time for granulation, etc. In the process of dry granulation using roll compactor, the roll speed, horizontal feed speed and vertical feed speed have been the key input variables.

Tablet coating operations are considered to be critical and intricate processes involving stringent control of variables (Banker & Anderson, 1987). Optimization of variegated coating processes has been carried out since 1977 (Dincer & Ozdurmus, 1977), which includes aqueous-, non-aqueous- and enteric-film coating. Important independent variables studied comprise, film former concentration, plasticizer concentration, viscosity of the solution, spraying time, length of drying interval, pan speed, bed temperature, etc. In some instances (Hutchings et al., 1994; Alkhatib & Sakr, 2003), curing time and curing temperature have also been evaluated. The responses optimized for all type of coating processes are principally the defects in the physical appearance of coating viz. mottling, picking, peeling, cracking, pitting and pin-hole formation. Literature indicates that the number of independent variables has ranged between 3

Table 11.5. Systematic optimization reports on liquid dosage forms					
Formulation	**Drug**	**Design**	**IV**	**RV**	**Reference**
Nanosuspension	Gefitinib	FD	3	3	Srinivas et al., 2016
Nanosuspension	Valsartan	CCD	5	3	Sowmya, et al., 2015
Microemulsion	Econazole	CCD	2	2	Sunmara et al., 2014
Emulsion	Cetearyl glucoside	DOD	4	2	Djuris et al., 2014
Syrup	Acetaminophen	RSM	4	2	Worakul et al., 2002
Emulsion	Oxybenzone	SMD	3	3	Marti-Mestres et al., 2000
Suspension	Erythromycin	FD	3	4	Elkheshen et al., 1997
Oral solution	Lamivudine	CCD	5	2	Nguyen et al., 1995
Parenteral nutrition	Nutrient mixtures	PBD	5	1	Ozil and Rochat et al., 1988

RSM: Response Surface Methodology; SMD: Simplex Mixture Design; FD: Factorial Design; PBD: Plackett-Burman Design; CCD: Central Composite Design; IV: Independent Variables; RV: Response Variables to 6, and the response variables between 1 and 6. Factorial designs (full and fractional) appear to be more suitable for this purpose. The process of manufacture of beads and granules has also been optimized for extrusion-spheronization, fluidized bed granulation, etc., utilizing a variety of designs. Table 11.6 summarizes the selected process optimization reports on conventional dosage forms.

A brief account of various factors and responses used during optimization of conventional dosage forms is abridged as Table 11.7.

D. Oral controlled-release compressed formulations

Compared to the conventional formulations, application of systematic DoE techniques in optimizing the controlled-release (CR) dosage forms has relatively been a recent phenomenon, though the first report appeared in 1985 (Harris et al., 1985). The studied CR dosage forms encompass the compressed matrices (hydrophilic/hydrocolloid, inert silicone elastomers and wax matrices), osmotic drug delivery systems (Singh et al., 2007) and macroparticulate systems. Sustained-release compressed matrices have been used since long to provide a constant therapeutic plasma level of drug. Amongst gastroretentive systems, the floating and mucoadhesive DDS are the most popular (Arza et al., 2009; Singh et al., 2009b). This is particularly true for drugs exhibiting a narrow therapeutic window in the gastrointestinal (GI) tract. The common independent variables for all of these DDS have been the quantities of the ingredients, and the optimized response variable has invariably been the *in vitro* dissolution profile. Other responses specific to a particular type of gastroretentive system include bioadhesive strength, floating time, gastric residence time, etc. Osmotic drug delivery systems, designed

Table 11.6. Process optimization of conventional dosage forms

Process	Design	IV	RV	Reference
Tablet formulation	SMD	2	5	Chavez et al., 2015
Hot melt extrusion	RSM	2	3	Baronsky-Probst et al., 2015
Crystallo-coagglomeration	FD	2	1	Garala et al., 2013
Tablet formulation	FD	2	3	Charoo et al., 2012
Blend homogeneity	CCD	2	1	Puchert et al., 2011
Film coating	FD	2	1	Prpich et al., 2010
Capsule filling	DOD	4	3	Klous et al., 2004
Emulsification	BBD	2	2	Lemaitre-Aghazarian et al., 2004
Aqueous film coating	FD	2	1	Alkhatib and Sakr, 2003
Fluidized bed granulation	MLRA	4	2	Rambali et al., 2003
Extrusion-spheronization	FD	3	3	Santos et al., 2002
Pre-tablet granulation	FD	8	2	Vojnovic et al., 1999
Spheronization	RSM	2	2	Heng et al., 1996
Pre-tablet granulation	SMD	3	3	Vojnovic et al., 1994
Film coating	CCD	2	1	Hutchings et al., 1994
Granule coating	BBD	3	2	Turkoglu and Sakr, 1992
Enteric film coating	FD	2	1	Devay et al., 1982

FD: Factorial Design; SMD: Simplex Mixture Design; BBD: Box-Benkhen Design; CCD: Central Composite Design; DOD: D-Optimal Design; RSM: Response Surface Methodology; MLRA: Multiple Linear Regression Analysis; IV: Independent Variables; RV: Response Variables

Table 11.7. List of various independent variables and response variables chosen for systematic optimization of conventional dosage forms

Delivery system(s)	Factors	Response variables
Tablets	Drug loading, polymer, ratio of polymer to filler, binder, lubricant, type of granulation	Disintegration time, hardness, drug release, weight variation, thickness
Coated tablets	Type of coating material, type of coating equipments, thickness of coating, rate of spray drying, duration of coating	Disintegration time, hardness, drug release, weight variation, thickness, taste masking, percentage degradation
Capsules	Particle size, Carr's index, Hausner's ratio, moisture content	Lag time, flow properties, drug release characteristics
Parenterals	Droplet size, phase ratio, osmotic pressure, cosolvent ratio, internal diameter of vial, drug concentration in solution, isotonicity, nature of the solvent (aqueous/oily)	Percent release, droplet size, stability, drug solubility, reconstitution time, clarity
Liquids (solutions, suspensions, emulsions)	Percent electrolyte, surfactant, thickner, cosolvent, mixing rate and time, homogenization time, concentration and nature of emulsifier, suspending agent	Percent sediment volume, viscosity, redispersibiliy, electrophoretic mobility, flowability, bulk density, droplet size, phase volume ratio, thermodynamic stability
Topicals (gels, creams, ointments, etc.)	Type and concentration of gelling agent, drug loading, drug-gelator ratio	Irritation potential, release and permeation profile, surface hydrophilicity, grittiness, spreadability, extrudibility, viscosity

especially for zero-order release, have been optimized for their drug release profiles using amount of polymers and orifice size as the independent factors. The optimization methodology of choice has been the FD and the FFD with some reports on use of CCD, BBD and others as well. The independent variables have ranged between 2 to 7 and the response variables between 1 and 6. Table 11.8 provides selected literature instances on formulation optimization of oral CR DDS.

E. Microparticulate systems

Microparticulate systems, including microcapsules and microspheres, have been employed extensively as novel DDS because of their stellar advantages over the unit dosage forms. These advantages comprise the reduced risk of systemic toxicity and local irritation, predictable gastric emptying rate, less variable absorption profiles, high bioavailability with minimum plasma fluctuations of drugs, and reduced side effects. However, microparticulate systems have

also some limitations, as they require specialized processing equipment and have high production costs involving a large number of processing variables. Though the first report appeared in 1982 (El-Banna and Efimova, 1982), yet the major work on optimization of different microparticulate DDS have been reported only in the last decade. The optimized micro/nanoparticulates include those prepared using either biodegradable polymers like albumin, gelatin, polyisobutyl cyanoacrylate, polycaprolactone, polylactide-co-glycolide and chitosan, or non-biodegradable polymers, like ethylcellulose, Eudragits, etc. The optimized formulation variables have been the emulsifier concentration, pH, drug/polymer ratio, composition of the internal phase of the emulsion, etc. in case of microcapsules, microspheres and nanoparticles; and phospholipid and cholesterol levels in case of the vesicular DDS. The process variables that have been studied are the nature of mixing pattern in the baffled/non-baffled container, homogenization pressure, stirring rate and time,

Table 11.8. Systematic optimization of oral CR drug delivery systems

Drug	Design	IV	RV	Reference
MUCOADHESIVE TABLETS				
Fluconazole	FD	2	3	Pathak et al., 2016
Troxipide	RSM	4	2	Gao et al., 2014
Baclofen	CCD	2	5	Jivani et al., 2012
Domperidone	CCD	2	4	Arora et al., 2011
Hydralazine	CCD	2	4	Singh et al., 2009
Atenolol	FD	2	5	Singh et al., 2006
Diltiazem	CCD	2	4	Singh and Ahuja, 2002
FLOATING TABLETS				
Metformin HCl	RSM	3	3	Senjoti et al., 2016
Rifampicin	BBD	3	4	Vora et al., 2013
Ranitidine	RSM	4	3	Hooda et al., 2012
Nimodipine	SMD	5	4	Barmpalexis et al., 2011
Ranitidine	FD	2	2	Dave et al., 2004
Calcium	FD	2	3	Li et al., 2003
GRANULES/BEADS/PELLETS				
Cefdinir	BBD	3	5	Radhakrishnan et al., 2016
Naproxen	BBD	3	2	Kan et al., 2014
Valsartan	FD	2	3	Shrivastava et al., 2009
Prednisolone	DOD	2	3	Mennini et al., 2008
Omeprazole	ANN	2	3	Turkoglu et al., 2004
Diclofenac Na	BBD	2	2	Kramar et al., 2003
SUSTAINED-RELEASE TABLETS				
Pentoprazole	BBD	3	3	Tak et al., 2016
Captopril	FD	2	7	Sauri et al., 2014
Metoprolol succinate	CCD	2	4	Li et al., 2013
Gliclazide	DOD	2	4	Jin et al., 2008
Metformin HCl	CCD	2	2	Mandal et al., 2007
Nicardipine HCl	SMD	3	4	Huang et al., 2005
Sodium fluoride	SLD	3	2	Tillotson and Sakr, 2004
Theophylline	FD	2	1	Alkhatib and Sakr, 2003
Didanosine	Doehlert	2	1	Sanchez-Lafuente et al., 2002
Naproxen	BBD	2	3	Zaghloul et al., 2001
OSMOTICALLY-CONTROLLED SYSTEMS				
Metaprolol succinate	BBD	3	5	Bannerjee et al., 2016
Atenolol	RSM	3	2	Xue et al., 2014
Ambroxol hydrochloride	CCD	2	2	Zhao et al., 2011
Dipyridamole	CCD	2	2	Zhang et al., 2009

(Contd.)

Drug	Design	IV	RV	Reference
		MICROPARTICLES		
Ibuprofen	FD	4	1	Azouz et al., 2016
Gentamicin	FD	3	2	Dorati et al., 2016
Cefpodoxime proxetil	BBD	3	3	Mujtaba et al., 2014
Albendazole	CCD	2	4	Leonardi et al., 2008

FD: Factorial Design; RSM: Response Surface Methodology; SMD: Simplex Mixture Design; ANN: Artificial Neural Networks; BBD: Box-Benkhen Design; CCD: Central Composite Design; D-OD: D-Optimal Design; IV: Independent Variable; RV: Response Variable

duration of cross-linking process, needle gauge, injection rate, etc. The response variables of interest for optimization have been the characteristics of the particulate system in the resulting formulation, *in vitro* drug release, entrapment efficiency, percentage yield, percentage of loose surface crystals, etc. The drugs explored include anticarcinogens, NSAIDs, vitamins, peptides, bronchodilators, antibacterials, etc.

Now-a-days, nanoparticles employing various biodegradable and synthetic polymers are becoming popular for successfully providing various benefits like site-specificity, enhancement in bioavailability, controlled release of various drugs, etc. Such systems can either be implanted as depot preparations or applied with site-specificity (ophthalmic, nasal, pulmonary, etc.). A brief account of independent factors and experimental designs employed for systematic optimization of microparticulate and nanoparticulate systems is provided in Table 11.9.

F. Formulation with enhanced bioavailability potential

Several reports are available on optimization of diverse kinds of DDS with enhanced bioavailability potential. The optimized systems encompass solid dispersions, inclusion complexes, fast release tablets, mouth dissolving tablets and self-emulsified drug delivery

Table 11.9. Selected literature instances on formulation optimization of microparticulate systems

Drug	Design	IV	RV	Reference
Laccase	BBD	4	2	Mansor et al., 2016
Vitamin C	FD	4	5	Ripoll and Clement et al., 2016
Prochlorperazine	FD	3	2	Shah et al., 2015
Cinnarizine	FD	3	4	Reham et al., 2015
Almotriptan	FD	3	2	Zaheer and Marihal, 2014
Rifampicin	BBD	4	2	Maurya et al., 2012
Insulin	BBD	2	3	Ubaidulla et al., 2009
Seratiopeptidase	FFD	2	1	Rawat and Saraf, 2008
Carvedilol	FD	2	3	Patil and Sawant, 2008
Guaifenesin	FD	2	2	Mani et al., 2004
Diltiazem HCl	FD	2	3	Singh and Agarwal, 2002

FD: Factorial Design; FFD: Fractional Factorial Design; BBD: Box-Benkhen Design; IV: Independent Variable; RV: Response Variable systems. The number of independent variables broadly ranged between 2 and 6, and the response variables between 1 and 6. The factors have been the quantity of ingredients and the solvent used for the preparation, while the response variables included drug release profile, bioavailability, etc. Table 11.10 comprises the selected literature instances of optimized DDS with enhanced bioavailability potential.

G. Nanostructured drug delivery systems

Pharmaceutical nanotechnology has witnessed a recent upsurge due to several advantages of nano-particles over other drug delivery systems. Their size allows them to be administered intravenously via injection unlike other colloidal systems which occlude both needles and capillaries. Due to their small size, they can pass through the sinusoidal spaces in the bone marrow and spleen more efficiently vis-à-vis other systems like microspheres. Also, due to their large surface area, they have higher loading capacity too. Nanoparticles used in the drug delivery include polymeric nanoparticles, solid lipid nanoparticles (SLNs) and nanostructured lipid carriers (NLCs). Besides these, vesicular systems are considered as a novel means of drug delivery that can enhance bioavailability of encapsulated drug and provide therapeutic activity in a controlled manner for a prolonged period of time. Such systems invariably contain phospholipids as the integral part of the carrier along with cholesterol and surfactants for vesicle stabilization.

Table 11.10. Select optimization reports on DDS with enhanced bioavailability potential

Drug	Design	IV	RV	Reference
SOLID DISPERSIONS AND INCLUSION COMPLEXES				
Clove oil	BBD	3	3	Ganesh et al., 2016
Glimepiride	FD	2	1	Harish and Shiva, 2015
Nimodipine	DOD	5	4	Panagiotis et al., 2011
Meloxicam	FD	2	3	Pathak et al., 2008
Etodolac	CCD	2	4	Singh et al., 2007
Nimesulide	FD	2	4	Gohel and Patel, 2003
COEVAPORATES AND CO-PRECIPITATES				
GWX (coded drug)	CCD	2	4	Sertsou et al., 2002
Prochlorpearazine	FD	2	2	Nagarsenker and Garad, 1998
MOUTH DISSOLVING AND FAST-RELEASE TABLETS				
Chlorpheniramine maleate	BBD	2	4	Dave et al., 2016
Jiawei Qinge	CCD	3	2	Zhang et al., 2013
Granisetron HCl	BBD	2	3	Hema et al., 2013
Clonazepam	FD	2	1	Shirsand et al., 2011
Lorazepam	FD	2	3	Shirsand et al., 2010
Rofecoxib	FFD	2	2	Sammour et al., 2006
Captopril	BBD	2	4	Lee et al., 2003

FD: Factorial Design; FFD: Fractional Factorial Design; BBD: Box-Benkhen Design; CCD: Central Composite Design; D-OD: D-Optimal Design; IV: Independent Variable; RV: Response Variable

Liposomes are the most promisingly used vesicular carriers made of lipidic bilayer. These can be prepared by disrupting biological membranes, for example, naturally-derived phospholipids with mixed lipid chains (e.g., egg phosphatidylethanolamine) or other surfactants by sonication. These can be filled with drugs to deliver them at the desired site of action for treatment of cancer and other diseases. Self-nanoemulsifying drug delivery systems (SNEDDS) possess unparalleled potential in improving oral bioavailability of poorly water-soluble drugs. Following their oral adminis-tration, these systems rapidly disperse in GI fluids, yielding micro- or nanoemulsions containing the solubilized drug. Owing to their miniscule globule size, the micro/nanoemulsified drug can easily be absorbed through lymphatic pathways, bypassing the hepatic first-pass effect and P-gp efflux. Table 11.11 provides a terse account on key instances of various nano-structured systems optimized using experimental designs.

H. Transdermal and topical therapeutic systems

Various studies have demonstrated that the trans-dermal route is a better alternative to the oral route in the administration of drugs for systemic delivery. The potential meritorious features associated with transdermal drug delivery are well documented (Wester and Maibach, 1992). These include avoidance of first-pass effect, administration of lower doses, potentially decreased side effects, constant plasma levels and improved patient compliance. In the development of a transdermal drug delivery system (TDDS), skin penetration enhancement of the drug is a key factor because of the barrier properties of the stratum corneum. Several optimization studies on TDDS have been carried out generally using 2 to 4 input variables and 1 to 4 response variables. Principally, the TDDS have been optimized for *in situ* penetration rate and lag time using type and concentration of penetration enhancer, and vehicle composition as the controllable factors. Literature findings reveal that CCD, FD and ANN have been employed as the popular designs for the TDDS. Over the past two decades, the transdermal patch has become a proven technology that offers a variety of significant clinical benefits over other dosage forms. In addition, transdermal patches being user-friendly, convenient and painless, offer multi-day dosing and improved patient compliance (Wolff, 2000). These matrix types of TDDS have been optimized for concentration of solvents by studying the influence of drying conditions, taking drying time and temperature as controllable independent variables.

Topical semisolid formulations have been optimized for percutaneous absorption, spread-ability, chemical stability, appearance, skin irritation, etc., by monitoring the formulation composition using varied kind of experimental designs. The number of independent variables ranged between 2 and 3, while the response variables between 1 and 4. Table 11.12 provides a selective list of optimization reports on TDDS and topical formulations.

I. Other Drug Delivery Systems

Apart from the above-mentioned DDS, several other therapeutic systems like nasal, pulmonary, vaginal and rectal DDS have been successfully optimized using modern systematic optimization techniques, as exemplified in Table 11.13.

J. Process Optimization of DDS

There are numerous reports on use of experi-mental designs solely in the optimization of formulation process of various DDS. The processes, generally, involve temperature diffe-rence between inlet and outlet of spray drier, homogenization speed, stirring rate, etc., for microparticles; emulsification time, homogeni-zation pressure, etc., for nanoparticles. Table 11.14 enlists the selected reports on process optimization of various drug delivery systems.

Table 11.11. Selected literature instances on formulation optimization of nanostructured systems

Drug	Design	IV	RV	Reference
NANOPARTICULATE SYSTEMS				
Efavirenz	FD	2	2	Gupta et al., 2017
Risperidone	BBD	3	3	Alzubaidi et al., 2017
Bicalutamide	BBD	3	3	Dhas et al., 2015
Ciprofloxacin HCl	BBD	3	2	Dizaj et al., 2015
Quercetin	FD	2	3	Kumar et al., 2015
Bicalutamide	BBD	3	2	Kudarha et al., 2014
Curcumin	FD	2	4	Kasinathan et al., 2014
Dutasteride	CCD	2	3	Park et al., 2013
Paclitaxel	BBD	3	2	Yerlikaya et al., 2013
Isotretinoin	FCCD	2	4	Raza et al., 2013
Haloperidol	BBD	3	3	Yasira and Sara, 2013
Triptolide	CCD	3	3	Zhang et al., 2013
Etoprofen	MD	2	2	Shah et al., 2012
siRNA	FFD	5	3	Cun et al., 2010
Chloramphenicol	BBD	3	3	Hao et al., 2011
Dithranol	FD	2	2	Gambhire et al., 2011
Simvastatin	FFD	3	3	Shah and Pathak, 2010
Antisense oligonucleotides	BBD	3	2	Gazori et al., 2009
9-Nitrocamptothecin	FD	4	1	Derakhshandeh et al., 2007
Ciprofloxacin	FFD	2	3	Dillen et al., 2004
Acyclovir	FD	2	3	Devi et al., 2003
Aceclofenac	CCD	2	1	Alonso et al., 2000
LIPOSOMAL SYSTEMS				
Prednisolone	D-OD	2	3	Sylvester et al., 2016
Alendronate	BBD	3	2	Ailiesei et al., 2014
Bovine lactoferrin	FD	4	2	Yao et al., 2014
Tenofovir	CCD	2	1	Xu et al., 2011
Nobiliside A	CCD	2	4	Xiong et al., 2009
Benzocaine	D-OD	2	4	Mura et al., 2008
Finasteride	CCD	2	2	Kumar et al., 2007
Coenzyme Q10	FD	4	4	Xia et al., 2006
Nimesulide	FD	2	3	Singh et al., 2005
Idoxuridine	FD	2	2	Seth et al., 2004
SELF-EMULSIFYING DRUG DELIVERY SYSTEMS				
Lopinavir	D-OD	3	3	Garg et al., 2016
Docetaxel	D-OD	4	2	Valicherla et al., 2016
Olmesartan	MD	3	3	Beg et al., 2015
Valsartan	CCD	4	3	Bandyopadhyay et al., 2015
Glipizide	CCD	3	3	Dash et al., 2015

(Contd.)

Drug	Design	IV	RV	Reference
Embelin	BBD	3	2	Parmar et al., 2015
Candesartan cilexetil	MD	3	2	Sharma et al., 2015
Lovastatin	FCCD	2	6	Beg et al., 2014
Trans-resveratrol	CCD	2	3	Singh and Pai, 2014
Irbesartan	FD	2	5	Patel et al., 2013
Ezetimibe	CCD	2	3	Bandyopadhyay et al., 2012
Oridonin	CCD	3	3	Liu et al., 2009
Lovastatin	CCD	2	6	Singh et al., 2008
Cyclosporine A	BBD	2	1	Zidan et al., 2007
Simvastatin	SMD	2	3	Meng and Zheng, 2007
Ketoprofen	FD	2	3	Patil et al., 2004
Fluticasone propionate	CCD	2	2	Magee et al., 2003
Ubiquinone	BBD	2	4	Nazzal et al., 2002

FD: Factorial Design; FFD: Fractional Factorial Design; BBD: Box-Benkhen Design; CCD: Central Composite Design; D-OD: D-Optimal Design; SMD: Simplex Mixture Design; IV: Independent Variable; RV: Response Variable

Table 11.12. Formulation optimization reports on transdermal and topical drug delivery systems

Formulation	Drug	Design	IV	RV	Reference
TRANSDERMAL DRUG DELIVERY SYSTEMS					
Transdermal patch	Simvastatin	BBD	3	2	Parhi et al., 2016
Transdermal patches	Risperidone	ANN	2	3	Siafaka et al., 2015
Nanoethosomes transgel	Tramadol	BBD	3	3	Ahmed et al., 2015
Topical microemulsion	Itraconazole	DOD	3	4	Kumar and Shishu, 2014
Transdermal microemulsion	Diflunisal	SMD	3	5	Sallam, 2013
Transdermal system	Furosemide	FD	2	2	Agyralides et al., 2004
SR matrices	Didanosine	DOD	4	5	Sanchez-Lafuente et al., 2002
Transdermal patches	Terbutaline sulfate	FD	3	1	Manna et al., 2000
Tranasdermal patch	Melatonin	ANN	3	3	Kandimalla et al., 1999

FD: Factorial Design; BBD: Box-Benkhen Design; CCD: Central Composite Design; SMD: Simplex Mixture Design; ANN: Artificial Neural Networks; DOD: D-Optimal Designs; IV: Independent Variables; RV: Response Variables

A brief account of various factors and response variables used during optimization of various DDS is compiled as Table 11.15.

K. Screening of influential variables

Albeit the experimental designs have frequently been employed for optimization of DDS, their use for screening of influential factors has been reported relatively sparsely. Plausibly, screening of the factors, carried out as a prelude to drug delivery development and optimization, may have been left unreported. Alternatively, the factors may have been selected on the basis of empiricism or the previous literature findings. Various reports appearing in literature on the use of screening designs for identifying the influential variables during development of diverse DDS have been compiled as Table 11.16.

Table 11.13. Selected optimization reports on nasal/pulmonary/vaginal/rectal DDS

Route	Drug	Design	IV	RV	Reference
Intranasal	Timolol maleate	FD	2	2	Jagdale et al., 2016
Intranasal	Selegiline	MVT	4	4	Kumar et al., 2016
Intranasal	Meloxicam	FD	4	9	Pallagi et al., 2015
Intranasal	Rivastigmine	FD	3	3	Shah et al., 2015
Intranasal	Midazolam	FD	2	5	Patel et al., 2015
Intranasal	Zolmitriptam, Ketorolac tromethamine	BBD	3	3	Kumar et al., 2015
Inhalation	Rifapentine	FD	2	5	Patil-Gadhe and Pokharkar, 2014
Inhalation	Amiloride HCl	FFD	3	5	Amaro et al., 2011
Inhalation	Salvianolic acids	CCD	2	3	Fang et al., 2011
Inhalation	Insulin	CCD	5	12	Maltesen et al., 2008
Inhalation	Salbutamol sulphate, Terbutaline sulphate	FD	2	3	Mendes et al., 2004
Inhalation	Insulin	FD	2	3	Stahl et al., 2002
Vaginal suppository	Progesterone	RSM	2	2	Iwata et al., 1995
Intranasal	Propranolol HCl	SMD	2	2	Chu et al., 1991
Rectal suppository	Theophylline	FD	2	1	Devay et al., 1988

FD: Factorial Design; CCD: Central Composite Design; BBD: Box-Behnken Design; RSM: Response Surface Methodology; SMD: Simplex Mixture Design; IV: Independent Variables; RV: Response Variables

Table 11.14. Process optimization reports on various drug delivery systems

Drug delivery system	Design	IV	RV	Reference
Drug extraction	CCD	5	1	Seifollah et al., 2017
Solid dispersion	CCD	4	3	Roosta et al., 2015
Microballons	BBD	3	4	Bansal et al., 2015
Nanoparticles	RSM	3	2	Kasinathan et al., 2014
Microspheres	CCD	3	3	Nandy et al., 2014
Pellets	CCD	5	5	Mallipeddi et al., 2014
Microspheres	CCD	3	3	Elsaid Ali et al., 2013
Floating microballoons	CCD	3	4	Awasthi et al., 2012
Microspheres	CCD	2	4	Kumar and Bhatia, 2010
Pellets	CCD	2	2	Lai et al., 2009
Phospholipid complex	CCD	2	3	Yue et al., 2008
Solid dispersion	FFD	2	1	Shah et al., 2007
SR matrices	PBD	2	3	Furlanetto et al., 2003
Nanoparticles	CCD	2	2	Marengo et al., 2003
Pellets	FD	2	2	Santos et al., 2002
Microspheres	FD	2	3	Narayan et al., 2001
Spheroids	FFD	2	3	Abuzarur-Aloul et al., 1998

FD: Factorial Design; FFD: Fractional Factorial Design; PBD: Plackett Burman Design; CCD: Central Composite Design; BBD: Box-Benkhen Design; RSM: Response Surface Methodology; IV: Independent Variables; RV: Response Variables

Table 11.15. List of various independent variables and response variables chosen for optimizing DDS

Drug delivery system	Factors	Response variables
Oral SR matrices	Polymer content, coating dispersion, plasticizer, curing time, lubricant	Dissolution profile, *in vivo* plasma profile, lag time, moisture uptake, tapped density of granules
Gastroretentive floating and bioadhesive tablets	Polymer-drug ratio, polymer grades, ratio of polymers, ratio of diluents	Dissolution kinetics, duration of buoyancy, detachment force, tensile strength, shear force, tablet density
Osmotic tablets	Orifice size, content of pore former, polymer content, coat weight, plasticizer type and content	Drug release profile, lag time, burst strength
Macroparticulates	Drug content, surfactant content, water content, impeller speed, polymer coating load, extruder speed and screen size, spheronizer speed and load	Pellet yield, dissolution time, percentage of stuck pellets, steady state extrusion force, bulk density, flowability, pellet size
Microparticulates	Polymer type and content, amount of cross-linking agent, cross-linking time, solvent, pH, phase volume ratio, stirring speed, surfactant, emulsifier, injection rate	Dissolution kinetics, yield, particle size, loose surface crystals, drug entrapping efficiency
Solid dispersions, inclusion complexes, co-evaporates and co-precipitates	Carrier, polymer, lubricant, solvent, spray feeding volume, polymer to drug ratio, diluent	Drug release profile, dissolution efficiency, weight variation, hardness, friability, disintegration
Fast-disintegrating tablets	Drying time, compression force, particle size, moisture content of wet granules	Disintegration time, tensile strength, tablet porosity
SEDDS	Amount of lipid, surfactant, cosolvent	Drug release profile, surface length diameter, zeta potential, liquefaction time, emulsification time
Nanoparticles	Polymer, surfactant, stabilizer, pH, stirring speed	Percent yield, drug loading, drug release profile, polydispersity index, particle diameter, zeta potential
Liposomal drug delivery systems	Phospholipid, stabilizers, lipid charge, sonication time, pH, cosolvent, surfactant	Percent encapsulation, average amount of polymer adsorbed per lipid, entrapment volume, size of vesicles, drug leakage, stabilization ratio
Transdermal patches	Solvent concentration and proportion, polymer, permeation enhancers, oven temperature and drying time, adhesive type, membrane thickness	Drug release parameters, flux, lag time, penetration rate, and total irritation score, mechanical properties of adhesives
Gels	Type and content of penetration enhancers, gelling agent, cosolvent ratio, polymer, drug content	Permeation enhancement, drug release kinetics
Iontophoretic drug delivery	Drug content, pH, osmolarity, ionic strength, current density	Flux, lag time, cumulative amount permeated
Inhalation drug delivery	Surfactant, suspending agent, vacuum, pre-sonication hydration, purification, lamellae composition, cryoprotectants (in case of lyophilization)	Effective particle size, encapsulation efficiency, efficiency of lyophilization, and respirable fraction

Table 11.16. Optimization reports on use of screening designs in various DDS

Type of DDS	Drug(s)	Factors	Response(s)	Design	Reference
Osmotic pump	Dicloxacillin sodium and amoxicillin trihydrate	Osmotic agent, pore forming agents, and coating agents	Drug release profile	PBD	Patel et al., 2016
Transdermal patch	Jackfruit mucilage	Amount of jackfruit mucilage, amount of plasticizer	Thickness, folding endurance, % drug release	FD	Bhoyar et al., 2016
Transdermal films	Simavastatin	Amount of film forming polymer, percentage of skin permeation enhancer	Amount of drug released in 12 h	FFD	El-Say et al., 2014
Microspheres	Diclofenac	Amount of PVA, amount of Eudragit	Encapsulation efficiency, drug loading	FFD	Deshmukh and Jitendra, 2013
Niosomes	Sumatriptan succinate	Sumatriptan amount, surfactant type, surfactant–cholesterol ratio, hydration time	Particle size, Zeta potential, % EE	TgD	González-Rodríguez et al., 2012
Transdermal system	Furosemide	Type of permeation enhancer, conc. of permeation enhancer, conc. of gelling agent	Cumulative amount of drug permeated	FD	Agyralides et al., 2004
Gastric floating drug delivery system	Calcium carbonate	HPMC; HPMC/carbopol ratio, magnesium stearate	Floating force, time to reach the maximum floating, area under the floating kinetics	TgD	Li et al., 2002
SR matrices	Didanosine	Eudragit RS-PM : Ethocel 100 ratio, compression force	Particle size, drug content	D-OD	Sanchez-Lafuente et al., 2002

FD: Factorial Design; FFD: Fractional Factorial Design; D-OD: D-Optimal Design; PBD: Plackett Burman Design; TgD: Taguchi Design

A CASE STUDY ON GASTRORETENTIVE FLOATING-BIOADHESIVE DRUG DELIVERY SYSTEMS OF RIVASTIGMINE

Rivastigmine is a cholinesterase inhibitor extensively prescribed for the treatment of mild-to-moderate Alzheimer's disease. Being an inhibitor of both acetylcholinesterase and butyrylcholinesterase, it has recently been recommended for the treatment of mild-to-moderate dementia associated with Parkinson's disease too. The efficacy of rivastigmine is dose-related, with total oral dose ranging between 6 mg and 12 mg administered 2 to 3 times a day. Rivastigmine, however, is associated with severe central cholinergic GI side effects. A rapid increase in brain acetylcholine levels after effective inhibition of target enzymes has been believed to precipitate these side effects. Besides, the twice or thrice daily dosage regimen associated with a drug like rivastigmine tends to reduce its patient compliance.

Pharmacokinetically, the side effects of rivastigmine are most likely related to the large fluctuations in the plasma levels, high values of maximal plasma concentration (i.e., C_{max}), and short values of time to reach C_{max} (i.e., t_{max}).

Thus, the strategies that prolong t_{max} and reduce the fluctuations in plasma drug levels have been shown to reduce the incidence of GI adverse events of oral rivastigmine dosage forms. Development of oral conventional CR products, in this regard, however, is precluded by their inability to retain and localize the DDS within the desired region of GI tract. The gastroretentive DDS can improve the CR characteristics of the formulation by continuously releasing the drug for prolonged periods of time in the stomach region before it reaches the absorption site, thus, ensuring its optimal bioavailability too. Amongst the myriad approaches used to improve the gastric residence time of DDS, the vital ones include floating DDS (FDDS), bioadhesive systems, swelling and expanding systems, and high density systems. The most widely employed system among them is FDDS.

Nevertheless, it is effective only when the fluid level in the stomach is sufficiently high. As the stomach empties and the tablet is at the pylorus, the buoyancy of the dosage form may be impeded. This serious limitation can largely be overcome by enabling the FDDS to adhere to the mucous lining of stomach wall. Floating and bioadhesive DDS, therefore, greatly improve the possibility of increasing the residence time of DDS in the stomach, resulting in more effective absorption and increased bioavailability of drugs. A combination of ionic polymers (like carbomers) and non-ionic polymers (like celluloses), in this regard, has extensively been employed to attain desired sustained drug release and/or gastroretention characteristics. Accordingly, it is a challenging task to attain the desired floating-bioadhesive potential and sustained-release characteristic to the DDS using a blend of these diversely behaving polymers.

Systematic studies using DoE could efficiently surmount this hiccup of balancing floatation and bioadhesion employing optimized polymer blends. DoE optimization is well-documented to develop "the best possible" formulation under a given set of conditions circumventing unnecessary experimentation and, thus, saving considerable time, money and effort. Application of such DoE techniques for the development of optimized drug delivery products is known to provide an in-depth understanding and ability to explore and defend the ranges for varied formulation and processing factors.

The objectives of the current studies, accordingly, was to develop optimized CR floating-bioadhesive tablets of rivastigmine, which provides a sustained release of the drug at the preferred GI site and also reduce the frequency of dosing, thereby increasing the patient compliance.

A. Formulation of floating-bioadhesive tablets

Effervescent floating-bioadhesive tablets were prepared by direct compression method. Rivastigmine, Carbopol and HPMC were sieved through #30 sieve and Avicel PH 101 (filler), sodium bicarbonate (1.2%) and magnesium stearate (1%) were sieved through #60 sieve prior to use. The amount of rivastigmine hydrogen tartarate (equivalent to 12 mg base) was kept as constant. All the materials were accurately weighed and blended by gentle trituration and, subsequently, compressed into tablets using flat-faced, round punches of 8 mm diameter.

B. Factor screening studies

Taguchi orthogonal array design was employed for screening of formulation and process variables involved in the development of gastrointestinal retentive tablets. A total of eight tablet formulations were prepared and evaluated for bioadhesive strength (BS) and percent drug release in 12 h (Q_{12},%) as the key response variables. Table 11.17 depicts the experimental runs as per the Taguchi screening design adopted for the current studies along with the formulation and process variables investigated for the purpose.

Table 11.17. Design matrix as per the Taguchi orthogonal array design

Trials	A: Carbopol	B: HPMC	C: MST	D: NaHCO$_3$	E: BT	F: CP type	G: HPMC type
1	+1	+1	−1	−1	+1	+1	−1
2	−1	−1	−1	−1	−1	−1	−1
3	−1	+1	+1	+1	+1	−1	−1
4	+1	−1	+1	−1	+1	−1	+1
5	+1	−1	+1	+1	−1	+1	−1
6	−1	−1	−1	+1	+1	+1	+1
7	−1	+1	+1	−1	−1	+1	+1
8	+1	+1	−1	+1	−1	−1	+1

Factors	Levels Low (−1)	High (+1)
Carbopol (mg)	20	35
HPMC (mg)	15	30
Magnesium stearate (MST, mg)	1	3
NaHCO$_3$ (mg)	10	20
Blending time (BT, min)	10	20
Carbopol type	CP 971P	CP 974P
HPMC type	Methocel K4M CR	Methocel K15M CR

C. Model generation and screening of influential variables

Screening presumes considerable approximation of additivity and absence of any interactions. Therefore, the first-order designs like TgD were employed for the purpose and the interaction terms were ignored. The design has specific advantage of requiring minimal (i.e., 8) runs for large number (i.e., 7) of independent variables. Seven coefficients (β_1 to β_7) were calculated with β_0 as the intercept, as shown in the general polynomial equation (Eq. 8)

$$Y = \beta_0 + \beta_1 X_1 + \beta_2 X_2 + \beta_3 X_3 + \beta_4 X_4 + \beta_5 X_5 \quad ...(8)$$

The first-order equations generated for the studied response variables viz. bioadhesive strength and Q_{12} are compiled in the form of equations in Table 11.18, along with their coefficients. The first-order mathematical model generated for each response variables were found to be statistically significant ($p < 0.05$). As shown in the table, only two coefficients in case of bioadhesive strength and only two coefficients in case of Q_{12} were found to be statistically significant.

Fig. 11.23 shows the bar chart presenting the influence of each factor on various response variables individually. Based on comprehensive analysis of the first-order equations and the relative importance of each response variable, five factors, i.e. MST, NaHCO$_3$, blend time, CP type and HPMC type were found to be least influential among the independent variables, though these are important for tablet formulation. The two factors, CP and HPMC, were found to have significant role on both the response variables. Higher amount of CP coupled with

Table 11.18. Coefficient values and statistical parameters obtained for first-order equations of the studied response variables

Coefficient code	First-order polynomial coefficients for response variables	
	Bioadhesive strength (BS)	**Q_{12}**
β_0	+89.45	+80.13
β_1	+72.80 (P = 0.0029)	+2.87 (P = 0.0277)
β_2	+5.42 (P = 0.0392)	−8.13 (P = 0.0098)
β_3	−2.83 (P = 0.0746)	−2.13 (P = 0.0374)
β_4	−0.33 (P = 0.5697)	+0.37 (P = 0.2048)
β_5	+0.42 (P = 0.4303)	−0.13 (P = 0.7952)
β_6	+1.30 (P = 0.1595)	−1.13 (P = 0.0704)
β_7	−0.45 (P = 0.4088)	−0.63 (P = 0.1257)
r^2	1.0000	0.9998
Model	P = 0.0086	P = 0.0261

$$BS = 1.55 + 1.51X_1 + 0.25X_2 - 0.068X_3 + 0.13X_4 + 0.018X_5$$
$$Q_{12} = 77.42 - 8.58X_1 - 9.42X_2 + 0.58X_3 - 3.08X_4 - 0.58X_5$$

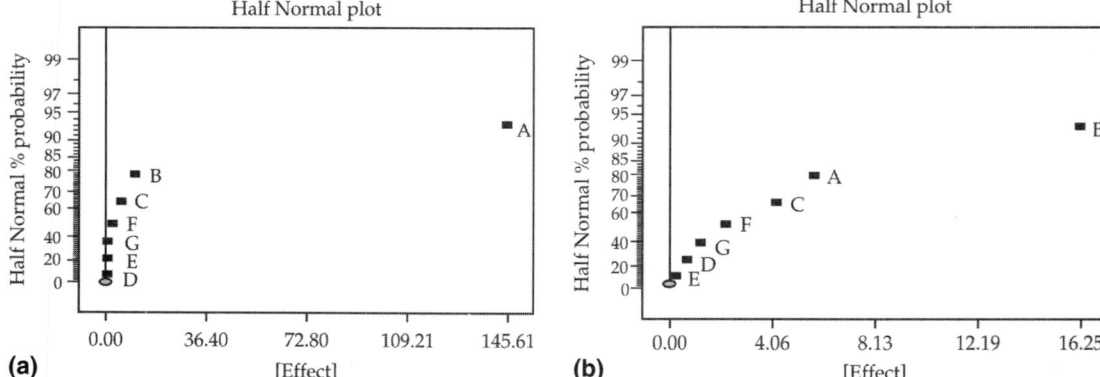

Fig. 11.23. Bar chart depicting the effect of each factor on the studied response variables, (a) BS, (b) Q_{12}.

lower amounts of HPMC leads to a system with good bioadhesive properties but with inefficient drug release control. On the other hand, low amounts of CP coupled with high amounts of HPMC leads to insufficient bioadhesion and inability of the formulation to release the drug completely. Hence, it was decided to formulate CR GI retentive tablets by systematically optimizing the amounts of CP and HPMC employing a 3^2 CCD.

D. Optimization of effervescent floating-bioadhesive tablets of rivastigmine employing face-centered cubic design

A face-centered cubic design, FCCD (with $\alpha = 1$), using three levels each of the two factors, viz. polymer X_1 (i.e. Carbopol 971P) and polymer X_2 (i.e. HPMC), was adopted for further investigations as required by the design, and the factor levels were suitably coded. Table 11.19

Table 11.19. Composition of various effervescent floating-bioadhesive formulations prepared as per the experimental design

Formulation code	Trial No.	Coded factor levels	
		X_1	X_2
TA	1	−1	−1
TB	2	−1	0
TC	3	−1	1
TD	4	0	−1
TE	5	0	0
TF	6	0	1
TG	7	1	−1
TH	8	1	0
TI	9	1	1

Translation of coded levels in actual units

Coded level	−1	0	1
X_1: Carbopol (mg)	15	25	35
X_2: HPMC (mg)	10	20	30

summarizes an account of the 13 experimental runs studied employing a total of nine formulations. All the studies were conducted in triplicate, and the formulation at central point (0, 0) was studied in quintuplicate.

E. Characterization of the prepared formulations

E1. Determination of bioadhesive strength

Goat gastric mucosa was used for evaluating the bioadhesion strength. Before testing, the mucosa was kept in SGF for 12 h. The mucosa was then placed on the base of texture analyzer. The tablet was attached to the stainless steel probe (using adhesive) fixed to the mobile arm of the texture analyzer. The area of contact of mucosa was moistened with 50 µl of SGF. The mobile arm was lowered at a rate of 0.5 mm.s^{-1} until contact with the membrane. A contact force of 10 g was maintained for 300 s, after which the probe was withdrawn from the membrane. The peak detachment force was recorded as the mucoadhesive strength.

Fig. 11.24 depicts the *ex vivo* bioadhesive strength of all formulations prepared as per the experimental design. As depicted in the figure, formulations TA, TB, TC and TD possessed very low bioadhesive strength primarily attributable to the low levels of CP in these formulations. HPMC alone does not seem to play a significant role in imparting bioadhesive potential to the formulation. However, it acts synergistically with CP, which is evident from the fact that formulation TI (high levels of HPMC and high levels of CP) possesses better bioadhesion as compared to TG (low levels of HPMC and high levels of CP). A more detailed study of the individual and combined effect of these polymers was conducted by plotting response surfaces and contour plots which will be dealt in subsequent sections.

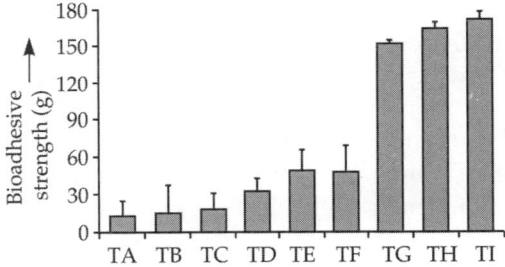

Fig. 11.24. *Ex vivo* bioadhesive strength of all formulations prepared as per the experimental design.

E2. In vitro drug release studies

Dissolution studies were carried out for all the formulations prepared as per the experimental design employing paddle type (USP apparatus II) dissolution tester as described previously. The raw data obtained from *in vitro* drug release studies were analyzed using the ZOREL software with in-built provisions for applying the correction factor for volume and drug losses during sampling, calculating the values of percent drug released, rate of drug release and log fraction released at varied times. Using the software, the values of kinetic constant (k), Fickian diffusion coefficient (k_1), polymer relaxation coefficient (k_2) and diffusional release exponent (n) were also determined. Based on the phenomenological analysis, the type of release, whether Fickian, non-Fickian (anomalous) or zero-order, was predicted. The values of percentage of drug released in 16 h (Q_{16}) were computed from the drug release profile and the time taken to release 60% of drug (T_{60}) for all the formulations was computed using the Stineman interpolation option of Graph software (Micromath Inc, USA).

Fig. 11.25 depicts the dissolution profile of all formulations prepared as per the experimental design. The inset shows the corresponding drug release rate profile at the mid points of time intervals. As depicted in the figure, the drug release profile of formulations TA, TG and TD is relatively less regulated than the other six formulations. This can be attributed to the low levels of HPMC in these formulations which is majorly responsible for controlling the release. Following the attempts to fit in the respective dissolution data to Korsmeyer-Peppas model in all the studies, excellent degree of statistical significance (p < 0.001) in all cases and phenomenally high values of r^2, AOEV, F ratio and negligible values of standard error of estimation (SEOE) were obtained.

Evaluation of the diffusional release constant, n, showed values ranging between 0.5109 and 0.6209, indicating non-Fickian drug release behavior. The results are in consonance with earlier literature reports, where non-Fickian behavior has been proposed for release of drugs from GR tablets. The values of kinetic constant, k, showed a declining trend with an increase in the concentration of HPMC at all the levels of CP, indicating a significant change in the polymer characteristics with change in their relative amount. Maximum extent of drug release was observed at the lowest levels of both the ingredients.

E3. Buoyancy time

The duration (T_b) for which the formulation floats in the dissolution medium in the upper one-third of the dissolution vessel (USP apparatus II, paddle type), was visually observed periodically after every 15 min. Sodium bicarbonate induced CO_2 generation in the presence of dissolution medium resulted in immediate tablet floatation with almost zero-lag time. Buoyancy time (T_b) evaluation of the tablets showed an increasing trend in a quite significant manner with increase in HPMC content, ostensibly owing to swelling (hydration) of the hydrocolloid

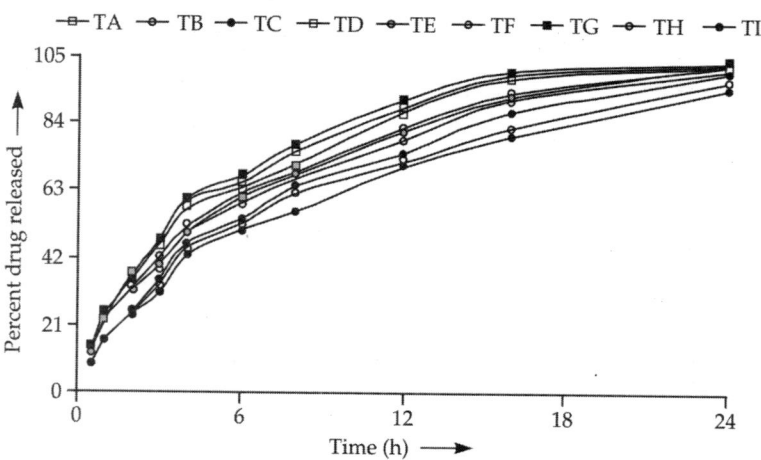

Fig. 11.25. *In vitro* drug release profiles of the floating-bioadhesive tablet formulations prepared as per the FCCD.

particles on the tablet surface, which, in turn, results in an increase in the bulk volume. It has already been documented in literature that the balance between polymer swelling and water acceptance are vital factors to ensure floatation. The gas-generating agent, sodium bicarbonate, induces CO_2 generation in the presence of the acidic dissolution medium, thereby increasing the polymer hydration and decreasing tablet density. Fig. 11.26 depicts the buoyancy time of various formulations prepared as per the experimental design.

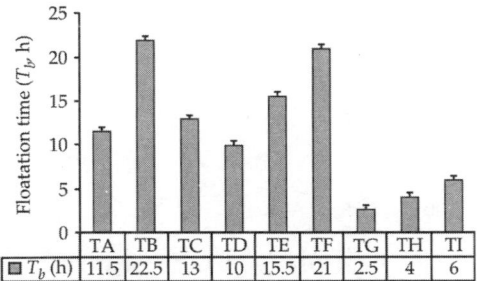

Fig. 11.26. Buoyancy time of all effervescent floating-bioadhesive tablet formulations prepared as per the experimental design.

The air entrapped in the swollen polymer maintains a density less than unity and confers buoyancy to these dosage forms, as is vivid from the data in the table. However, with an increase in CP 971P content, buoyancy time rather tended to decrease, which may be due to higher density of CP (1.76 g/cc) than HPMC (1.30 g/cc). Hence, increasing concentration of CP 971P has a distinct negative effect on the floating behavior of the delivery system.

F. Optimization data analysis

The response variables considered for systematic optimization were T_b, BS, Q_{16} and T_{60}. Design Expert® software ver. 6.0 (Stat-Ease, USA) was employed to fit full second-order polynomial equations with added interaction terms to correlate the studied responses with the examined variables. The polynomial regression results were demonstrated using perturbation charts, 3-D response curves and contour plots. Finally, the prognosis of optimum formulations was conducted in two stages; first, a feasible space was located and second, an exhaustive grid search was conducted to predict the possible solutions. The optimized formulation was also located by overlay plot option and desirability function option of the Design Expert® software, while "trading off" of the responses.

F1. Model generation and calculation of coefficients

Seven coefficients were calculated with β_0 as the intercept, as shown in Eqn. 9, which indicated the model terms for the purpose.

$$Y = \beta_0 + \beta_1 X_1 + \beta_2 X_2 + \beta_3 X_1^2 + \beta_4 X_2^2 + \beta_5 X_1 X_2 + \beta_6 X_1^2 X_2 + \beta_7 X_1 X_2^2 \qquad ...(9)$$

All the coefficients of quadratic polynomials were found to be quite statistically significant. Also, the models for all response variables were found to be highly significant ($p < 0.0001$). The values of r^2 for these models ranged between 0.9951 and 0.9994, indicating excellent fit of the RSM polynomials to the response variable data. The closeness of adjusted r^2 (i.e. Adj. r^2) and predicted r^2 (i.e. Pred. r^2) to the actual r^2 also suggested goodness of fit to the data.

F2. Response surface mapping

The response surface diagrams, constructed to map the response over the entire experimental domain, are known to facilitate the understanding of the variables and their interactions. The 3-D response surfaces and their 2-D contour plots, constructed for various response variables, viz. T_b, T_{60}, Q_{16}, and BS, are depicted in Figs. 11.27–11.30.

As depicted in Fig. 11.27, both CP and HPMC exhibit a significant and opposite effect on T_b of tablets. The values of T_b show a curvilinear decline with increasing the levels of CP at all levels of HPMC. This can be attributed to the high density of CP making it difficult to float. On the other hand, increasing the levels of

HPMC exhibits a significant positive effect on T_b of tablets at all levels of CP. This can be attributed to the lower density and higher swelling properties of HPMC making the tablet easier to float. The corresponding contour plot also depicts maximum value of T_b at high levels of HPMC and low levels of CP.

Fig. 11.28 depicts a nearly linear increasing trend in the values of T_{60} with increasing the levels of HPMC at all levels of CP. On the other hand, increasing the levels of CP exhibited a negative effect on the values of T_{60} at higher levels of HPMC, the effect being insignificant at lower levels. The corresponding contour plot also depicts maximum value of T_{60} at high levels of HPMC and low levels of CP.

As depicted in Fig. 11.29, Q_{16} exhibits a curvilinear and linear decreasing trend with increasing the levels of HPMC at low and high levels of CP, respectively. Increasing the levels of CP, conversely, also exerts a positive effect on the values of Q_{16} at higher levels of HPMC, the effect being negligible at lower levels of HPMC. The curved and linear lines of the corresponding contour plot also depict the same.

Fig. 11.30 clearly depicts the significant influence of CP in imparting bioadhesive properties to the tablets. As shown in the figure, the values of BS increase considerably on increasing the levels of CP from low to intermediate, after which a steep rise is observed with increasing the levels of CP from intermediate to

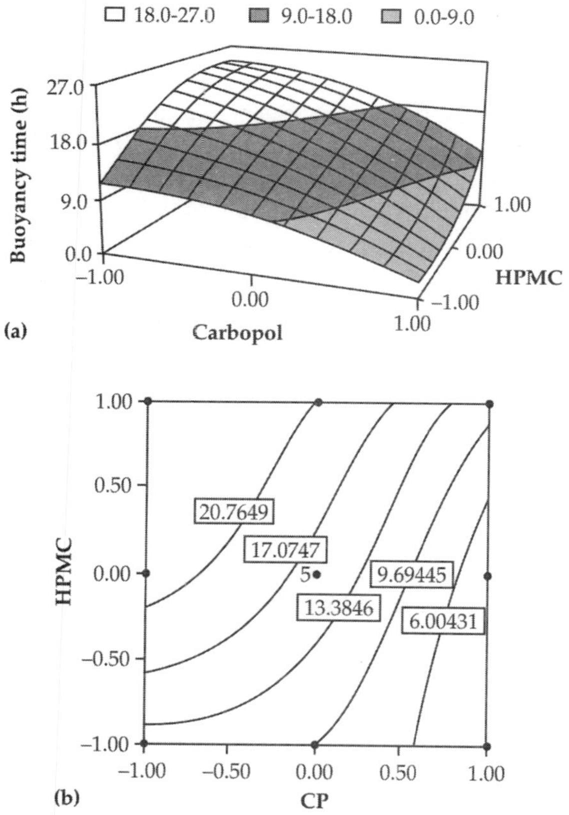

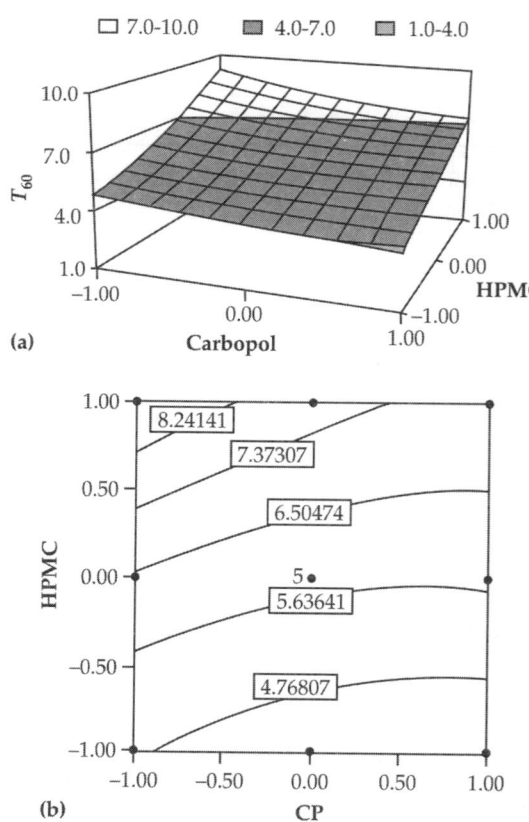

Fig. 11.27. Response surface (a) and contour (b) plots showing the influence of CP and HPMC on T_b of gastroretentive tablets.

Fig. 11.28. Response surface (a) and contour (b) plots showing the influence of CP and HPMC on T_{60} of gastroretentive tablets.

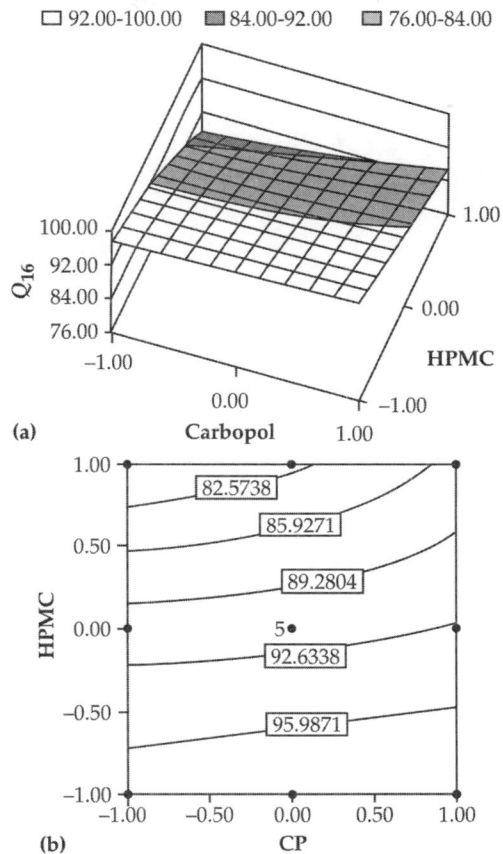

Fig. 11.29. Response surface (a) and contour (b) plots showing the influence of CP and HPMC on Q_{16} of gastroretentive tablets.

high levels. Increasing or decreasing levels of HPMC do not seem to exert any significant effect (as compared to CP) on the values of BS. The corresponding contour plot also depicts maximum value of BS at highest levels of CP.

In a nutshell, comprehensive analysis of the response surfaces and contour plots suggested the need of appropriate balancing between the two factors, i.e. CP and HPMC.

G. Search for the optimum formulation

The optimum formulation within the entire experimental domain was searched by brute-force methodology and graphical optimization method.

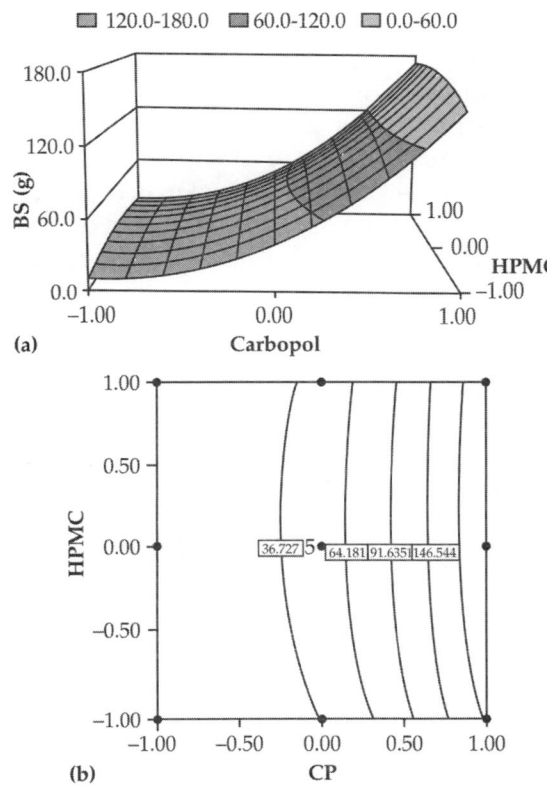

Fig. 11.30. Response surface (a) and contour (b) plots showing the influence of CP and HPMC on BS of gastroretentive tablets.

Brute-force methodology

Herein, optimum search was attempted by feasibility search followed by exhaustive grid search respectively. The criterion adopted for feasibility search was:

$$T_b > 7 \text{ h}; \ T_{60} > 4.5 \text{ h}; \ Q_{16} > 89\%; \ BS > 66 \text{ g}$$

A desired region, for each response variable, was selected from the feasibility search table. The feasible region was further expanded to conduct grid search. Exhaustive grid search was conducted by adopting a more stringent criterion:

$$T_b > 8 \text{ h}; \ T_{60} > 5 \text{ h}; \ Q_{16} > 93\%; \ BS > 100 \text{ g}$$

Based on the final grid search, the formulation corresponding to the coded levels, HPMC: 0.56 and CP: –0.36 (i.e. containing 30.6 mg of

CP and 16.4 mg of HPMC) was selected as the optimal gastroretentive tablet formulation. The selection of the optimum formulation (shown in thick border area in all grid search tables) was based on maximization of all response variables, viz. T_b (to maintain floatation of tablets), BS (to aid in bioadhesion), T_{60} (for extension of drug release) and Q_{16} (to ensure complete drug release). The said formulation exhibited a T_b of 8.08 h, T_{60} of 5.11 h, Q_{16} of 94.72% and BS of 104.91 g.

As per the graphical optimization method, the desirable region was also selected using overlay plotting, wherein the constraints for choosing an optimum formulation were selected, as indicated in Fig. 11.31.

Also the numeric optimization was explored through numeric optimization. The desirability function was assigned to the constraints set for the desired goal and the whole experimental domain was searched for the compositions, wherein the set constraints were met to be optimum. Table 11.20 presents the constraints set for numeric optimization, formulation

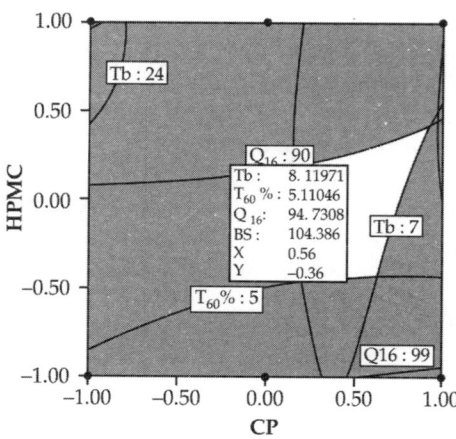

Fig. 11.31. Overlay plot depicting the location of optimized effervescent floating-bioadhesive tablet formulation.

compositions for various formulations and the corresponding desirability values. The results of Table 11.18 show that the formulations meeting the criteria lie within the specific region of the experimental domain. Finally, the formulation corresponding to solution 3, as indicated in the table, was chosen as the optimum formulation.

Table 11.20. Results of numeric optimization for rivastigmine loaded effervescent floating-bioadhesive tablets

CONSTRAINTS				
Variable	**Goal**	**Lower limit**	**Upper limit**	
A	In range	−1	+1	***
B	In range	−1	+1	***
T_b	In range	7.5 h	24 h	***
T_{60}	In range	4.5 h	9.0 h	***
Q_{16}	In range	90%	99%	***
BS	In range	75 g	170 g	***

SOLUTIONS						
A	**B**	**T_b**	**T_{60}**	**Q_{16}**	**BS**	**Desirability**
0.30	−0.11	12.11 h	5.56 h	92.62%	78.45 g	1.00
0.53	−0.23	9.00 h	5.33 h	93.74%	102.49 g	1.00
0.56	**−0.36**	**8.11 h**	**5.11 h**	**94.73%**	**104.38 g**	**1.00**

No. of asterisks (*) designate the level of significance.

In the current studies, the optimized formulation chosen by Brute-force methodology, overlay plots and numeric optimization, came out to be identical, thus, vouching the accuracy of the applied DoE methodology.

H. Validation of optimization analysis

Six formulations, including the optimized formulation, were selected as check points to validate the DoE methodology. The effervescent floating-bioadhesive tablets were formulated (as described in section, "Formulation of floating-bioadhesive tablets") using the chosen composition and evaluated for T_b, BS, Q_{16} and T_{60} in the manner described earlier. The observed and predicted responses for six check point formulation were critically compared and the percent error calculated with respect to the observed responses. Linear correlation plots between predicted and observed responses of the check-point formulation were constructed and the residual graphs plotted. The linear correlation plots between observed and predicted values, and residual plots for all the six check-point formulations (T-VAL1 – T-VAL5) and the optimized formulation T-OPT, are depicted in Figs. 11.32–11.35. All the correlation plots were found to be quite linear (as r^2 values ranged between 0.9186 and 0.9956), corroborating "sameness" between the observed and the predicted responses, thus indicating high degree of prognostic ability of the developed polynomial models. The prediction error for the response variables ranged between -4.43% and 4.55%, while the magnitude of overall percent prediction error was observed to be miniscule, i.e. 0.138 ± 3.47, indicating extremely high degree of RSM prognosis. The corresponding residual plots were also found to be quite regulated with uniform, relatively narrow and random scatter around zero-axis.

Overall, all the above results demonstrate unambiguous accuracy, validity and finally, high prognostic ability of the proposed RSM model in the optimization of the drug delivery system and prediction of studied response variables.

CONCLUSIONS

Today, in the globally competitive world, a product development scientist always remains in a dynamic environment, taking numerous challenges in his stride. These challenges invariably arise as a result of increasing quality consciousness among physicians as well as patients, escalating toil of manufacturers to improve efficacy and cost-efficacy of their products, and rapidly changing compendial and regulatory specifications. Needless to mention, there has always been a constraint on time, resources, and materials. Hence, it is important for a pharmaceutical scientist to use effective methodology to develop products in a timely manner without sacrificing the quality. However, despite applying the best knowledge, skills, and wisdom to achieve the said goal using OVAT approaches, the outcome is not easily ascertainable. The formulator may either hit the "bull's eye" quickly or miss the target altogether. Employing modern DoE optimization techniques can make it much simpler to modify the existing formulations and meet the redefined objectives. With the rising awareness on the utility and knowledge of these modern systematic approaches, the science of DoE has permeated actually into several disciplines of medicine, dentistry, engineering, technology, and biomedical sciences too.

Defining the relationship between the variables and quality traits of a formulation or a process, without the application of an apt design model, is almost an impossible task. Trial and error OVAT methods, in this regard, can never allow the formulator to know how close any particular formulation is to an optimal drug delivery solution. A formulation scientist should, therefore, sincerely consider the use of optimization studies especially when finding the correct compromise is not simple and straightforward. Besides helping him in selecting a true optimum for the objectives, these DoE techniques tend to reveal the degree of improvement in the formulation characteristics as well.

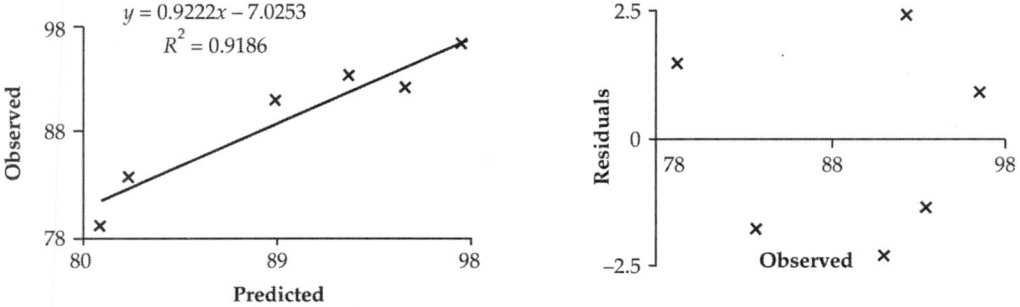

Fig. 11.32. Linear correlation plot and residual plot for Q_{16}.

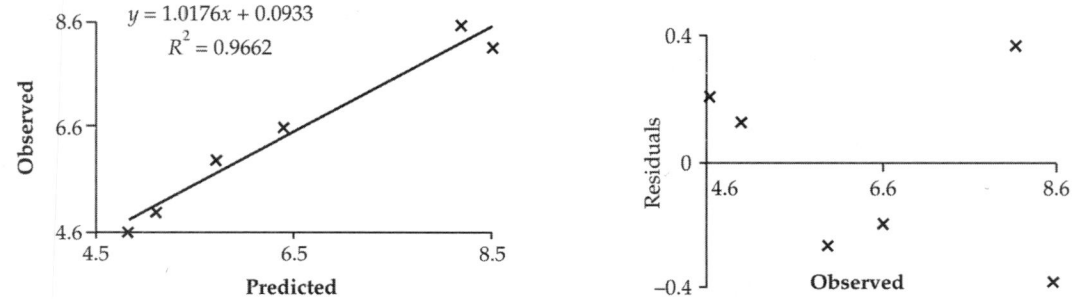

Fig. 11.33. Linear correlation plot and residual plot for T_{60}.

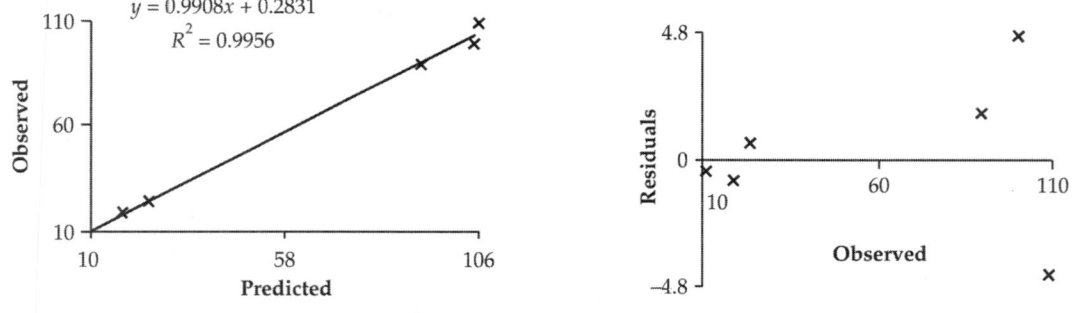

Fig. 11.34. Linear correlation plot and residual plot for BS.

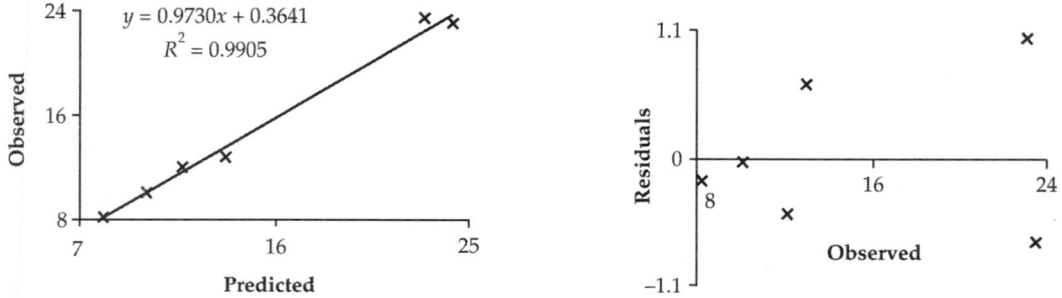

Fig. 11.35. Linear correlation plot and residual plot for T_b.

Such systematic experimental studies can also prove to be instrumental in the product and/or process validation and subsequent scale-up operations. Owing to the involvement of fairly small volume of materials, money, men and machination in this development cycle, the payoffs of this modern approach are phenomenal in drug industry. Accordingly, the key Federal and Regulatory Agencies like ISO, USFDA, ICH, NIH and EMEA have been pressing upon the judicious use of experimental designs, not only in optimizing drug formulations and processes, but also for assessing the product quality using the principles of QbD.

Despite the well-established applications of DoE in predicting responses, its reliability of prognosis can vary. Keeping in mind the famous adage, garbage-in-garbage-out (GIGO), the degree of predictability will depend largely upon the accuracy and abundance of the input data and the choice of appropriate procedures. For successful implementation of a DoE exercise, the choice of suitable experimental design and experimental domain are the twin prerequisites. An incorrect experimental design can adversely affect the predictive ability, while an unsuitable experimental range may either miss the optimum or require much greater experimentation. Simple experimental designs coupled with rational optimization procedures can furnish vast amount of information about the system from small experimentation. However, an inappropriate DoE may generate insufficient data from a limited number of experiments, eventually leading only to "half-baked delicacy" products and processes. Unquestionably, the formulator can attain "the best" drug formulation only using DoE but within the experimental domain studied.

Nevertheless, we should not consider DoE as either a magic wand or a panacea for all product development problems. In fact, DoE and product knowledge tend to complement each other. A "designed" product or process should enhance system information instead of acting as a surrogate to the experience. At times, the wise scientist can even choose the influential variables through empiricism and observation, bypassing the rigors of screening and factor influence studies. In fact, the more the formulator knows about the system, the better he can define it, and the higher precision he can monitor it with. Thus, DoE tends to expedite the formulation process by augmenting (rather than replacing) the much-needed formulation skills, creativity and product knowledge.

Regardless of a spurt of literature reports and publications, we have yet to make the most of this revolutionary practice for optimizing the drug products and processes routinely. The major impediment is our traditional stance of sticking to the established OVAT norms. The difficulty in optimizing a pharmaceutical formulation systematically is due to the difficulty in understanding the real factor-response relationship. Once this empirical "cause-effect" relationship is unearthed, the developmental or post-developmental thoughts can be realized quite rapidly and rationally. Thus, the need of the hour today is to persuade our fellow researchers to adopt this cutting edge paradigm of DoE methods and challenge the old weary ones. This shift in paradigm can provide astute insight for future improvements, leading to newer opportunities in the form of next-generation product launches. A journey of thousand miles always begins with a single step. It is the most opportune time to get started first with full patience, perseverance and passion. Eventually, the day would not be far when the benefits of DoE would be harvested by drug industry and research groups to their fullest advantage. Certainly, adopting newer "attitudes" and "aptitudes" can only lead to attaining higher "altitudes".

SUGGESTED FURTHER READINGS

- Amani, A., York, P., Chrystyn, H., Clark, B.J., Do, D.Q., 2008. Determination of factors controlling the particle size in nanoemulsions using artificial neural networks. *Eur. J. Pharm. Sci.*, 35, 42–51.

- Araujo, P.W., Brereton, R.G., 1996. Experimental design II- Optimization. *Trends Anal. Chem.*, 15, 63–70.
- Armstrong, N.A., James, K.C., 1990. **Understanding Experimental Designs and Interpretation in Pharmaceutics**. Ellis Horwood, London.
- Arza, R.A., Gonugunta, C.S., Veerareddy, P.R., 2009. Formulation and evaluation of swellable and floating gastroretentive ciprofloxacin hydrochloride tablets. *AAPS PharmSciTech*, 10, 220–226.
- Bansal, S., Beg, S., Garg, B., Asthana, A., Asthana, G.S., Singh, B., 2015. QbD-oriented development and characterization of effervescent floating-bioadhesive tablets of cefuroxime axetil. *AAPS PharmSciTech*.
- Bodea, A., Leucuta, S.E., 1998. Optimization of propranolol hydrochloride sustained release pellets using Box-Behnken design and desirability function. *Drug Dev. Ind. Pharm.*, 24, 145–155.
- Bolton, S., 1997. **Factorial designs, Pharmaceutical Statistics: Practical and Clinical Applications**. 3rd edn. Marcel Dekker, New York.
- Box, G.E.P., Behnken, D.W., 1960. Some new three-level designs for the study of quantitative variables. *Technometrics*, 2, 455–475.
- Box, G.E.P., Cox, D.R., 1964. An analysis of transformations. *J. Royal Stat. Soc. Ser. B*. 26, 211–243.
- Box, G.E.P., Wilson, K.B., 1951. On the experimental attainment of optimum conditions. *J. Royal Stat. Soc. Ser.*, B 13, 1–45.
- Cochran, W.C., Cox, G.M., 1992. **Experimental Design**, 2nd edn. Wiley, New York.
- Cook, D.R., 1977. Detection of influential observations in linear regression. *Technometrics*, 19, 15–18.
- Dhawan, S., Kapil, R., Singh, B., 2010. Formulation development and systematic optimization of solid lipid nanoparticles of quercetin for improved brain delivery. *J. Pharm. Pharmacol.*, 63, 342–351.
- Djekic, L., Ibric, S., Primorac, M., 2008. The application of artificial neural networks in the prediction of microemulsion phase boundaries in PEG-8 caprylic/capric glycerides based systems. *Int. J. Pharm.*, 361, 41–46.
- Doornbos, D.A., Haan, P., 1995. Optimization Techniques in Formulation and Processing. *In:*

Swarbrick, J., Boylan, J. C. (Ed.), **Encyclopedia of Pharmaceutical Technology**. Marcel Dekker, New York, pp. 77–160.
- El-Banna, H.M., Efimova, L.S., 1982. Construction and use of factorial design in fluidized bed microencapsulation. *Pharm. Ind.*, 44, 641–645.
- Fisher, R.A., 1925. **Statistical Methods for Research Workers**. Oliver and Boyd, Edinburgh.
- Fisher, R.A., 1935. **The Design of Experiments**. 1st edn. Oliver and Boyd, Edinburgh.
- Garg, B., Katare, O.P., Beg, S., Lohan, S., Singh, B., 2016. Systematic development of solid self-nanoemulsifying oily formulations (S-SNEOFs) for enhancing the oral bioavailability and intestinal lymphatic uptake of lopinavir. *Colloids Surf. B.*, 141, 611–22.
- Gupta, S., Kesarla, R., Chotai, N., Misra, A., Omri, A., 2017. Systematic approach for the formulation and optimization of solid lipid nanoparticles of efavirenz by high pressure homogenization using design of experiments for brain targeting and enhanced bioavailability. *Biomed. Res. Int.*, 2017, 1–18.
- Haaland, P.D., 1989. **Experimental Design in Biotechnology**. Marcel Dekker, New York.
- Lachman, L., Lieberman, H.A., Kanig, J.L., 1989. **The Theory and Practice of Industrial Pharmacy**, 3rd ed. Varghese Publishing House, Hind Rajasthan Building, Dadar, Bombay.
- Lewis, G.A., Mathieu, D., Phan-Tan-Luu, R., 1999. **Pharmaceutical Experimental Design**. 1st ed. Marcel Dekker, Singh, B.; Ahuja, N. (2000) Book Review on "Pharmaceutical Experimental Design" *Int. J. Pharm.* 195, 247–248, New York.
- Li, J., 2003. Factorial designs, *In:* Chow, S.C. (Ed.), **Encyclopedia of Biopharmaceutical Statistics**. Marcel Dekker, New York, pp. 233–256.
- Lionberger, R.A., Lee, S.L., Lee, L., Raw, A., Yu, L.X., 2008. Quality by design: concepts for ANDAs. *AAPS J.*, 10, 268–276.
- Loukas, Y.L., 2001. A Plackett-Burman screening design directs the efficient formulation of multicomponent DRV liposomes. *J. Pharm. Biomed. Anal.*, 26, 255–263.
- Marlowe, E., Shangraw, R.F., 1967. Dissolution of sodium salicylate from tablet matrices prepared by wet granulation and direct compression. *J. Pharm. Sci.*, 56, 498–504.

- Montgomery, D.C., 2001. **Design and Analysis of Experiments**. 5th edn. Wiley, New York.
- Myers, W.R., 2003. Response surface methodology. *In:* Chow, S.C. (Ed.), **Encyclopedia of Biopharmaceutical Statistics**. Marcel Dekker, New York.
- Plackett, R.L., Burman, J.P., 1946. The design of optimum multifactorial experiments. *Biometrica*, 33, 305–325.
- Podczeck, F., 1995. The development and optimization of tablet formulations using mathematical methods. *In:* Alderborn, G., Nystrom, C. (Eds.), **Pharmaceutical Powder Compaction Technology**. Marcel Dekker, New York, pp. 276–298.
- Rizkalla, N., Hildgen, P., 2005. Artificial neural networks: comparison of two programs for modelling a process of nanoparticle preparation. *Drug. Dev. Ind. Pharm.*, 31, 1019–1033.
- Scheffe, H., 1958. Experiments with mixtures. *J. Royal Stat. Soc. Ser., B.* 20, 344–360.
- Schwartz, J.B., Connor, R.E., 1996. Optimization techniques in pharmaceutical formulation and processing. *In:* Banker, G.S., Rhodes, C.T. (Eds.), **Modern Pharmaceutics**. Marcel Dekker, New York.
- Singh, B., Ahuja, N., 2002. Development of controlled-release buccoadhesive hydrophilic matrices of diltiazem hydrochloride: optimization of bioadhesion, dissolution, and diffusion parameters. *Drug Dev. Ind. Pharm.*, 28, 431–442.
- Singh, B., Ahuja, N., 2004. Response surface optimization of drug delivery systems, *in:* Jain, N.K. (Ed.), **Progress in Controlled and Novel Drug Delivery Systems**, 1st edn. CBS Publishers & Distributors, New Delhi, pp. 470–509.
- Singh, B., Arora, S., Singh, R., 2007. Osmotically controlled oral drug delivery systems. *Pharma. Buzz*, 2, 20–28.
- Singh, B., Bandopadhyay, S., Kapil, R., Ahuja, N., 2008. Systematic optimization of drug delivery systems: An insight. *The Pharm. Rev.*, 7, 146–186.
- Singh, B., Bandopadhyay, S., Kapil, R., Katare, O.P., 2009a. Novel nanostructured lipidic drug delivery systems. *The Pharma. Rev.*, 7, 118–122.
- Singh, B., Chakkal, S.K., Ahuja, N., 2006a. Formulation and optimization of controlled release mucoadhesive tablets of atenolol using response surface methodology. *AAPS PharmSciTech*, 7, E1-E10.
- Singh, B., Dahiya, M., Saharan, V., Ahuja, N., 2005a. Optimizing drug delivery systems using "Design of Experiments". Part II: Retrospect and Prospects. *Crit. Rev. Ther. Drug Carrier Syst.*, 22, 215–292.
- Singh, B., Gupta, R.K., Ahuja, N., 2006b. Computer assisted optimization of pharmaceutical formulations and processes, 10th chapter. *In:* **Pharmaceutical Product Development**, N.K. Jain. ed., CBS Publishers & Distributors, New Delhi. pp. 273–318.
- Singh, B., Kumar, R., Ahuja, N., 2005b. Optimizing drug delivery systems using "Design of Experiments". Part 1: Fundamental aspects. *Crit. Rev. Ther. Drug Carrier Syst.*, 22, 27–106.
- Singh, B., Mehta, G., Kumar, R., Bhatia, A., Ahuja, N., Katare, O.P., 2005c. Design, development and optimization of nimesulide-loaded liposomal systems for topical application. *Current Drug Deliv.*, 2, 143–153.
- Singh, B., Pahuja, S., Kapil, R., Ahuja, N., 2009b. Formulation development of oral controlled release tablets of hydralazine: optimization of drug release and bioadhesive characteristics. *Acta Pharm.*, 59, 1–13.
- Taguchi, G., 1986. **Introduction to Quality Engineering**. UNIPUB/Krauss International, New York.
- Takayama, K., Takahara, J., Fujikawa, M., Ichikawa, H., Nagai, T., 1999. Formula optimization based on artificial neural networks in transdermal drug delivery. *J. Control Release*, 62, 161–170.
- Tye, H., 2004. Application of statistical "design of experiments" methods in drug discovery. *Drug Discov. Today*, 9, 485–491.
- Wester, R.C., Maibach, H.I., 1992. Percutaneous absorption of drugs. *Clin. Pharmacokinet.*, 23, 235–266.
- Westerhuis, J.A., Coenegracht, P.M.J., 1997. Multivariate modelling of the pharmaceutical two step process of wet granulation and tabletting with multiblock partial least squares. *Chemometrics*, 11, 372–392.
- Wolff, H.M., 2000. Optimal process design for the manufacture of transdermal drug delivery systems. *Pharm. Sci. Technol. Today*, 3, 173–181.

12

Drug Release Kinetic Modelling of Extended Release Drug Delivery Systems

Bhupinder Singh, Babita Garg, Shikha Lohan, Atul Jain and Sarwar Beg

INTRODUCTION

Advances in the field of drug delivery have endowed the pharmaceutical scientists to look towards drug formulation development and subsequent patient therapy. During the last couple of decades, the science of formulation development has undertaken remarkable strides for developing diverse types of newer drug delivery systems (DDS). Despite enormous innovations in novel DDS through alternative routes of administration, oral drug delivery has unambiguously been the most sought after by the patients and manufacturers alike (Gupta et al., 2009). From the patients' perspective, its status is primarily a consequent of the wide acceptability of this "natural" route, better safety vis-à-vis the parenteral route, low cost of therapy, ease of administration, and improved patient compliance (Singh et al., 2009).

The term "drug release" most often refers to a complex phenomenon, one part of which is "drug dissolution" in case the drug is initially present in the solid state. Being rate governing step, drug release is usually a pivotal step in the development of extended release drug delivery systems. Fig. 12.1 schematically illustrates 5

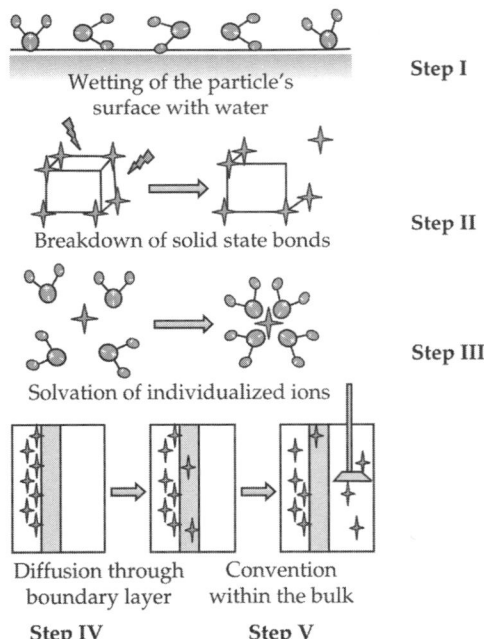

Fig. 12.1. Major steps involved in the dissolution of a solid drug particle in a well-stirred aqueous liquid.

major steps, which are generally involved in the dissolution of a solid drug particle in a well-stirred aqueous liquid. Simultaneously, mathematical modelling of such DDS and predictability of drug release is a field marked with enormous future potential. Mathematical modelling of drug release can be very helpful not only to speed-up the product development, but also to improve understanding of the mechanisms of controlling drug release from advanced delivery systems. This chapter furnishes an overview on the current status of mathematical modelling of drug release kinetics, different mechanisms of the respective models, and vital applications towards developing robust extended release (ER) formulations with desired *in vitro* and *in vivo* temporal profiles.

EXTENDED RELEASE DRUG DELIVERY SYSTEMS

Extended release drug delivery systems (ER-DDS) are designed to extend constant plasma levels within the therapeutic window, diminishing the "saw-tooth" fluctuations that accompany periodic dosing of conventional drug formulations (Tae et al., 2017; Wahlgren et al.,

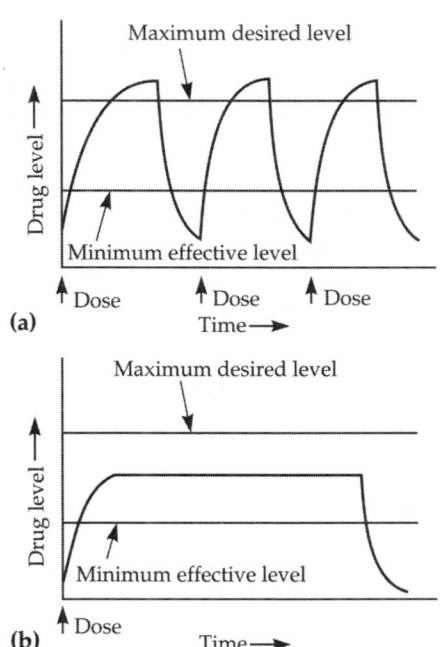

Fig. 12.2. Plasma level profiles following (a) conventional, and (b) extended release dosing.

2009; Lee and Robinson, 2000), as illustrated in Fig. 12.2.

Principal meritorious visages of ER-DDS encompass fewer administrations, better patient compliance, reduced potential of over- and under-dosing, superior efficiency upon treatment, optimal drug usage, enhancement of bioavailability particularly for drugs absorbed by active transport, and the overall economy (Zhao et al., 2009; Robinson and Lee, 1987; Nahar and Jain, 2011). Together with extensive and intensive research in the realm, the ER-DDS market has been expanding phenomenally with an alarming increase in the regulatory approvals in the last few years (Olkkola and Hagelberg, 2009). Amongst the prevalent ER-DDS, the key approaches encompass matrices (insoluble, soluble or biodegradable) (Gonzalez and Ghaly, 2010; Chi et al., 2010), microcapsules, osmotic pumps (Yakubu et al., 2009), coated beads (Basu and Rajendran, 2008), ion-exchange resins (Akkaramongkolporn et al., 2008), etc. A convenient classification of ER systems is based on the major rate controlling mechanisms of active drug substance (i.e., through diffusion, swelling, erosion or osmosis), which is dependent upon the nature of interaction between the polymer and the environmental fluids (Hiremath and Saha, 2008; Nokhodchi et al., 2008; Weiser and Saltzman, 2014), as depicted in Fig. 12.3.

Diffusion-controlled systems

Usually, the ER systems are diffusion-regulated DDS, wherein drug release rate is determined by its diffusion through the water-insoluble polymer. Among the wide spectrum of ER-DDS technologies, diffusion devices are the simplest to adapt for large-scale manufacturing (Pillai et al., 2001; Robinson and Lee, 1987; Salsa et al., 1997). Such systems are of two types, viz. reservoir devices and matrix devices.

Reservoir devices

These devices consist of active ingredient contained in core, surrounded by an inert

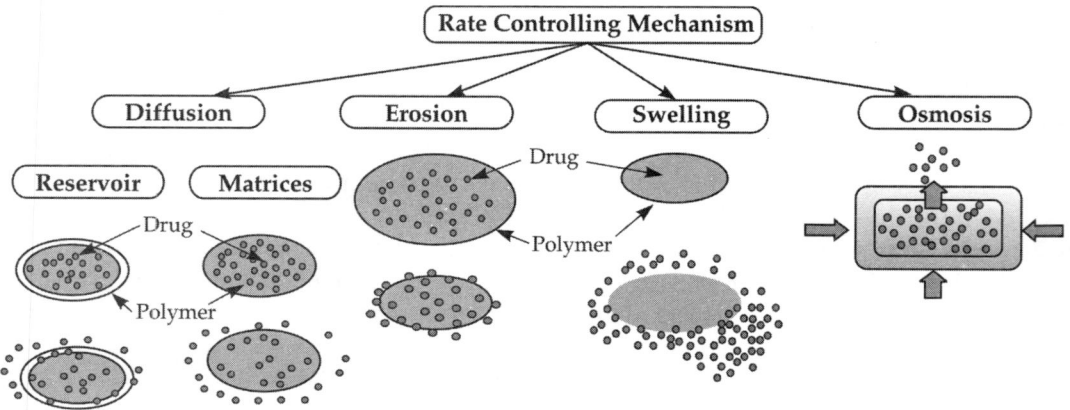

Fig. 12.3. Rate controlling mechanisms involved in ER systems.

polymeric membrane; the rate-limiting step for drug release being diffusion through the polymer. Drug release from a reservoir is governed by a blend of dissolution and diffusion, with latter controlling the release rate after proper selection of the coating membrane (Chein, 1992; Deshpande et al., 2010; Ruozi et al., 2016). These systems include membranes, capsules, microcapsules, liposomes and hollow fibers. Drug release rate in reservoir systems can remain fairly constant and is determined by apt choice of polymer and its consequent effect on drug diffusion and partition (Pillai et al., 2001; Johannes et al., 2009; Weiss et al., 2014).

Matrix devices

These are monolithic diffusion-controlled devices, wherein the active agent is homogeneously distributed in a polymeric matrix (Fig. 12.3), dispersed as a separate phase or dissolved in the polymer (Mittal et al., 2009b; Lee and Robinson, 2000). Albeit drug release occurs primarily by diffusion through the polymer, the environmental fluids may leach the drug out of the polymer, if the latter is permeable to fluids (Varma et al., 2004; Baker, 1987). Such devices can be conveniently prepared by using a simple polymer fabrication technique involving physical blending of the active agent with matrix formers, followed by compaction, extrusion, or solvent casting. When the diffusion rate and the polymer dissolution rate are equally balanced, drug dissolution becomes fairly constant until the polymer core completely dissolves, and diffusion reaches a steady state. However, when drug dissolution rate is slower than its diffusion rate, the former controls the drug release. The diffusion rate is a two step process. The drug first dissolves in the solvent penetrating the matrix and subsequently diffuses out of the matrix.

In fact, the relative proportion of the two processes of dissolution and diffusion controls the release kinetics (Varma et al., 2004). As drug release continues, its rate normally decreases, since the active agent has a progressively longer distance to travel, and therefore, requires a longer diffusion time to release. In addition to polymer and drug, other formulation components and the geometry of the system may also influence drug release kinetics. Nevertheless, it is easier to control release kinetics of matrix-type systems than those of coating systems. Based on the nature of the matrix-forming material, five major types of matrix systems can be differentiated, viz. hydrophilic, plastic, lipidic, resin, and biodegradable matrices (Fuertes et al., 2010; Heredia et al., 2009). Emphasis is placed on hydrophilic matrices as they are suitable for a wide range of drugs and offer many distinct advantages over the hydrophobic matrices. A large number of simple monolithic and sophisticated matrix systems are available commercially too (Pascoal et al., 2015).

Erosion-controlled systems

Herein, drug release occurs through either 'bulk erosion' of the material or 'surface erosion' of the polymer (Heller and Hoffman, 2004; Escudero et al., 2010). In bulk erosion, the rate of water penetration into the solid device exceeds the rate at which the polymer transforms into water-soluble materials. As water enters the polymer, erosion transpires throughout the whole volume. Cracks and crevices form in the polymer, and it rapidly disintegrates. On the other hand, in surface erosion, the rate at which water enters the polymer device is less than the rate of polymer transformation to water-soluble materials. The surface area of the polymer matrix limits the process. With time, the device becomes thinner while maintaining its structural integrity.

For bulk erosion, two mechanistic stages are encountered during drug release (Burkersoda et al., 2002). The first stage is dictated by the hydrolysis of the drug or how much water is diffusing into the polymeric device. The second stage involves the diffusion of the drug through the polymeric matrix (Fig. 12.4a). For surface erosion, the device erodes like a bar of soap (Fig. 12.4b). The release rate is influenced by the degradation of the polymeric material and is therefore proportional to the surface area of the system. The release mechanism is directly related to how the polymer degrades.

In most of the biodegradable hydrophilic matrix systems, the matrix slowly erodes in the body fluids (Franco-Marques et al., 2009; Burkersoda et al., 2002). Such a phenomenon of conversion of an erstwhile water-insoluble polymer into soluble one is termed as 'bioerosion' and such a polymer is referred to as 'bioerodible'. Water diffuses into the bioerodible matrix tablet, the gel layer increases, followed by continuous diffusion of the drug. The fully hydrated outer layer erodes from the core and a mechanism involving erosion and diffusion appears to be operative. Slow polymer hydration may cause premature drug diffusion and disintegration of the tablet due to fast water penetration. These bioerodible (or bio-degradable) systems, wherein drug is uniformly distributed throughout a polymer, as in a monolithic system, are eventually absorbed by the body (Sangoia et al., 2014). As the polymer surrounding the drug is eroded, the drug escapes (Fig. 12.4a & b).

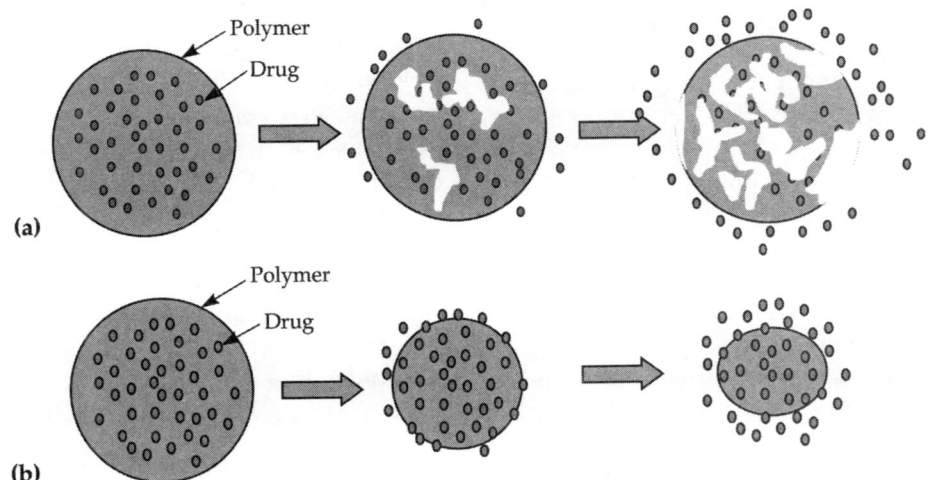

(a)

(b)

Fig. 12.4. Drug release from (a) bulk-eroding, or (b) surface-eroding biodegradable devices.

Drug molecules initially dispersed in the polymer are released as the polymer starts eroding or degrading. Most commonly used bio-degradable polymers in oral drug delivery are poly(lactic acid) (PLA), poly(lactic-co-glycolic acid) (PLGA), polyanhydrides, polyorthoesters, and polyphosphoesters. Being hydrophilic, PLGA polymers essentially erode by bulk erosion. Polyanhydrides and polyorthoesters, on the other hand, are hydrophobic, and degrade by surface erosion. Besides bioerodible matrices, the reservoir systems with drug-loaded cores surrounded by polymer coatings also erode, combining advantage of long-term constant rate drug release with bioerodibility. In the 'pendant-chain systems' (Fig. 12.5), drug molecules are covalently attached to main polymer chain via degradable linkages. Hence, as the polymer is exposed to water, linkages break down releasing the drug.

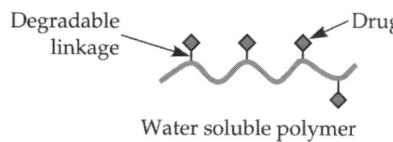

Fig. 12.5. Pendant-chain system with biodegradable linkage for drug release.

Swelling-controlled systems

Such devices are designed using water as the main agent controlling the drug release, as the drug molecules cannot physically diffuse out of the device. Swelling ER devices usually incorporate drugs in a hydrophilic polymer that is stiff (or glassy) when initially dry, but swells when placed in body fluids or aqueous dissolution media (Kamenska et al., 2009; Tahara et al., 1995). The soluble drug dissolves and diffuses out of swollen polymer matrix network into the external environment.

Associated with the swelling process is an abrupt change from a 'glassy to rubbery' state (Gazzaniga et al., 2008; Ferrero et al., 2010). Most materials used in swelling systems are hydrogel polymers that swell without dissolving,

when placed in water. These hydrogels can absorb a great deal of fluid and, at equilibrium, typically comprise 60–90% fluid and only 10–30% polymer. One of the most remarkable and useful features of a polymer manifests itself when swelling is triggered by a change in environment (e.g., pH, temperature, or ionic strength) surrounding a DDS. The mechanism of drug release that dominates in hydrophilic matrices is related to hydrosolubility of active principle. When this is very low, possibility of release by diffusion is nearly zero and drug release is almost by surface erosion, giving characteristic zero-order profile. Else, if drug is moderately or highly hydrosoluble, the mechanism governing release is diffusion (Vazquaz et al., 1992).

In general, the two major factors controlling drug release from swelling ER matrix systems are: (i) the rate of aqueous medium infiltration into the matrix, followed by a relaxation process (hydration, gelation, or swelling); and (ii) the rate of matrix erosion. As a result of these simultaneous processes, two fronts are evident – a swelling front, where the polymer gets hydrated; and an eroding front. The distance between the two fronts, i.e. diffusion layer thickness depends on the relative rates at which swelling and eroding fronts move relative to each other (Fyfe and Blazek-Welsh, 2000). The profile of the gel layer thickness versus time consists of three stages: (i) initial increase due to polymer swelling, (ii) maintenance of constant gel layer thickness, and (iii) reduction of gel layer thickness as the glassy core depletes. The growth of the hydrophilic polymer gel depends on the swelling rate at the water penetration front and erosion rate at the outer surface of the gel. Optimized interplay of swelling-based relaxation and erosion mechanisms has yielded constant zero-order drug release rates with fruition (Suja-Areevath et al., 1998; Lu et al., 2010).

Osmotic-controlled systems

The osmotic pump is similar to a reservoir device

but contains an osmotic agent (e.g., the active agent in salt form), which acts to imbibe water from the surrounding medium via a semi-permeable membrane (Verma et al., 2002; Singh et al., 2003b; Singh et al., 2007a). Pressure is generated within the device, which forces the active agent out of the device via an orifice. Whilst the internal volume of the device remains constant, and there is an excess of solid (saturated solution) in the device, the release rate remains constant delivering a volume equal to the volume of solvent uptake. In the osmotic systems, osmotic pressure is the driving force that generates constant drug release. Osmotically-controlled ER systems are mainly classified as elementary osmotic pump, push-pull osmotic pump, osmotic pump with non-expanding second chamber, besides the specific types (Kumar et al., 2009; Singh et al., 2003a; Wang et al., 2009; Guan et al., 2010). Fig. 12.3 schematically represents a typical elementary osmotically-controlled delivery device.

MODELLING OF DRUG RELEASE KINETICS

Invariably, it may be desired to design an effectual and cost-effectual oral DDS capable of delivering a drug in the systemic circulation at a slow release rate over extended periods. Essential to the development of successful controlled delivery systems is comprehension of interaction of various design parameters, like physical properties, and geometry with the actual diffusion process (Heller and Hoffman, 2004). The objective can essentially be accomplished by regulating drug release kinetics from its device. The quintessence of ER drug delivery, therefore, is modulation and modelling of its drug release kinetic potential eventually to yield an impeccable pharmacokinetic profile and pharmacodynamic effect (Ritschel, 1989). Mathematical modelling, coupled with numerical simulation of drug release kinetics can be very helpful to accelerate the process of drug

product development, and to better understand the mechanisms of controlling drug release from such ER-DDS (Jiang et al., 2010).

A number of mathematical theories and kinetic models have been put forth by diverse researchers in the last few decades to analyze drug release from different types of immediate and modified release dosage forms (Korsmeyer et al., 1983a; Higuchi, 1963). Professor Takeru Higuchi, in this context, is considered as the "father" of mathematical modelling of drug delivery. The quantitative interpretation of the values obtained in the dissolution assay is facilitated by the usage of a generic equation that mathematically translates the dissolution curve in function of some parameters related with the pharmaceutical dosage forms. The kind of drug, its polymorphic form, crystallinity, particle size, solubility and amount in the dosage form can influence the release kinetics (Grassi and Grassi, 2005).

However, some key aspects should be taken into consideration while using and/or developing mathematical theories to quantify drug release from pharmaceutical dosage forms:

- When developing a new mathematical theory for a particular ER-DDS, the physical, chemical and/or biological processes must be taken into consideration. Also, the accuracy of a mathematical theory generally increases with increasing model complexity. The slowest process involved in the mass transport step must also be taken into contemplation while fitting the same into a mathematical equation.
- A single mathematical theory cannot be applied to all types of drug delivery systems.
- A theoretical prediction may or may not hold well when the actual experimental results are deduced.

Zero-order kinetic model

Drug dissolution from ER-DDS that do not disaggregate and release the drug slowly can be represented by the following zero-order kinetic equation:

$$W_0 - W_t = K_0^*.t \qquad \qquad ...(1)$$

where, W_o and W_t are the amounts of drug in the pharmaceutical dosage form initially and at time t, respectively, and $K^*{}_0$ is a proportionality constant. Dividing this equation by W_o and simplifying, Eqn. 2 is obtained:

$$\frac{M_t}{M_\infty} = K_0.t \qquad \qquad ...(2)$$

where, $M_t/M_\infty = 1 - (W_t/W_o)$, represents the fraction of drug dissolved in time t and K_o is the apparent zero-order release rate constant. This linear graphic relation between the drug-dissolved fraction and time can be used to describe the drug release of several types of ER dosage forms like some matrix tablets with low soluble drugs, coated forms, osmotic systems, etc. (Nagaraju et al., 2009; Guan et al., 2010; Su et al., 2009; Cheng et al., 2010).

The following relation can, in a simple way, express this model:

$$M_t = M_0 + K_0.t \qquad \qquad ...(3)$$

where, M_o is the initial amount of drug in the solution (most of the times, $M_0 = 0$) and K_0 is the zero-order release equation. Hence, linear regression analysis is conducted between M_t/M_∞ and time (t) after forcing the line through origin. The magnitude of the zero-order kinetic rate constant, K_0, is resolved from the gradient (slope) of linear relationship.

First-order kinetic model

The application of first-order kinetic model to drug dissolution studies was first proposed by Gibaldi and Feldman (1967), and later by Wagner (1969). Although its mechanism is difficult to conceptualize theoretically, yet this model has been also used to describe absorption and/or elimination of most drugs (Lo et al., 2009; Mittal et al., 2009a; Hassan et al., 2010; Costa-Balogh et al., 2009). The dissolution phenomenon of a solid particle in liquid medium implies surface action, as seen by the classical equation proposed

by Noyes and Whitney (Noyes and Whitney, 1897a & 1897b).

$$\frac{dC}{dt} = K(C_s - C_t) \qquad \qquad ...(4)$$

where, C_t is the concentration of the solute in time t, C_s is the solubility in the equilibrium at experimental temperature and K is a first-order proportionality constant. Proposing the formation of a stagnant layer around the dissolving particle through which the diffusion of the solute into the bulk takes place, this equation was altered by Brunner and Tolloczko (1900) to incorporate the value of the solid area accessible to dissolution, S, getting a new proportionality constant, K_1 as:

$$\frac{dC}{dt} = K_1 S(C_s - C_t) \qquad \qquad ...(5)$$

and using the Fick's first law, they established the following relation among the constant K_1 and D, the solute diffusion coefficient in the dissolution media, V, the liquid dissolution volume and h, the width of the diffusion layer:

$$K_1 = \frac{D}{Vh} \qquad \qquad ...(6)$$

And the ultimate model was proposed by Nernst (1904) and Brunner (1904) as:

$$\frac{dC}{dt} = \frac{D}{V.h}.S.(C_s - C_t) \qquad \qquad ...(7)$$

With poorly soluble drugs, e.g., when $C_t \ll C_s$ (i.e. <10%), it is reduced to Eqn. 8:

$$\frac{dC}{dt} = \frac{D}{V.h}.S.C_s \qquad \qquad ...(8)$$

To apply the model to drug release kinetics, linear regression analysis is conducted between log (percent release) as the dependent variable and time as the independent variable. The value of the first-order kinetic rate constant, K_1, is estimated as the slope of the line. The amount of drug released in this manner in a unit time is proportional to the amount of drug remaining in its interior.

Second-order kinetic model

Typically, the second-order rate equation (Abdou, 2000) is given as:

$$\frac{W_t}{W_\infty(W_\infty - W_t)} = K_2.t \qquad ...(9)$$

where, K_2 is the apparent second-order drug release constant of the solute drug. Expressing in the terms of M_t and M_∞:

$$\frac{M_t}{M_\infty(M_\infty - M_t)} = K_2.t \qquad ...(10)$$

Accordingly, linear regression analysis is conducted between $M_t/M_\infty(M_\infty - M_t)$ and time after forcing the line through zero intercept, and values of the second-order kinetic rate constant, K_2, as the slope and other regression parameters are found.

Higuchian model

Higuchian model describes the release of poorly water-soluble drugs from surface of a planar tablet. The very first attempts were made by Wignand and Taylor (1959) and Wagner (1959) when they observed that the ER preparations yielded near pseudo-first-order rates over the terminal portion of percent drug release-time data. However, the first mathematical equation to describe drug release from the oral homogeneous and heterogeneous matrix systems was described by Higuchi (1963).

$$Q = \sqrt{D.\varepsilon/\tau.(2A - \varepsilon.C_s).C_s.t} \qquad ...(11)$$

where, Q is the total amount of drug released per unit surface in time t, D is the apparent diffusion coefficient of the drug in the hydrated matrix, τ is the tortuosity of the matrix, ε is the porosity of the hydrated matrix, C_s is the solubility of the drug in the release medium, and A is the loading dose of drug in the matrix. Eqn.

11 is simplified to Eqn. 12, when A is quite large in relation to C_s.

$$Q = K_H.\sqrt{t} \qquad ...(12)$$

Here, K_H is the Higuchi dissolution constant treated in diverse manner by diverse authors using diverse theories.

Higuchi describes drug release as a diffusion process based on Fick's law, originating in a linear relationship with square root of time (Langer, 1980). This relation can be used to describe the drug dissolution from several types of modified-release DDS, as in the case of matrix tablets with water-soluble drugs (Schwartz et al., 1968; Gayakwad et al., 2009; Tang et al., 2009). Eqn. 12 is alternatively described as:

$$\frac{M_t}{M_\infty} = K_H.\sqrt{t} \qquad ...(13)$$

where, M_t is the amount of drug released at time t and M_∞ is the amount of drug released at an infinite time when the pharmaceutical dosage form is exhausted, and M_t/M_∞ is the fractional release of drug at time t (Weiss, 2015).

To apply this model to drug release kinetics, linear regression analysis is performed between the fractional release of drug, M_t/M_∞ and square root of time ($\sqrt{t}$). Mean percent drug released data are regressed against "p" number of values of $\sqrt{t}$, third reading onwards. The regression line is forced to zero as the Higuchian model has no provision for the intercept. Various regression parameters including coefficient of determination (r_p^2), standard error of estimate (SE), the significance of regression or variance ratio ($F_{1,p-2}$) and amount of explained variance (AOEV) can be determined.

Peppas and related models

In a still more general form, Eqn. 13 is expressed as a semi-empirical equation (Eqn. 14), known popularly as **power law** to analyze dissolution data under perfect sink conditions, rating drug release exponentially to the elapsed time (t), as proposed by Korsmeyer et al. (1983a).

$$\frac{M_t}{M_\infty} = k.t^n \qquad \ldots(14)$$

To bring about the computation of the kinetic constant (k) and release exponent (n) values for each dosage form unit pertaining to Eqn. 14, regression analysis is accomplished between the logarithm of fractional drug released versus logarithm of time data, as in the Eqn. 15.

$$\log\frac{M_t}{M_\infty} = \log k + n.\log t \qquad \ldots(15)$$

The slope of this log-log relationship fetched the value of n, while the antilogarithm of its intercept yielded the value of k.

The **kinetic constant**, k, defines the structural and geometric characteristics of the ER delivery device. The value of n represents the 'drug release exponent' characterizing different release mechanisms (Peppas, 1985; Korsmeyer et al., 1983b). The value of $n = 0.5$ (Eqn. 15) is representative of a system where release is controlled entirely by Fickian diffusion mechanism and rate of drug transport from the system is proportional to $t_{1/2}$. The equation could be used to determine the "n" value from the portion of the release curve where $M_t/M_\infty < 0.6$, provided drug release occurs in a uni-dimensional way and the width-thickness or length-thickness ratio of the formulation matrix system is numerically at least 10. This model has generally been employed to analyze drug release from pharmaceutical polymeric dosage forms, when the release mechanism is not well known or when more than one type of release phenomena could be involved (Ritger and Peppas, 1987a; Ritger and Peppas, 1987b; Peppas and Narasimhand, 2014). The release can also be characterized through mean dissolution time (MDT), a parameter obtainable from k and n values through mathematical relationship (Eqn. 16) among them (Korsmeyer et al., 1983b, Harland et al., 1988).

$$MDT = \frac{n}{(n+1)}.k^{1/n} \qquad \ldots(16)$$

In addition, based upon the log-log relationship between percent drug release and time at varied times, the values of $t_{q\%}$ viz. $t_{50\%}$, $t_{60\%}$, $t_{70\%}$, $t_{80\%}$ and $t_{90\%}$ of drug release were also interpolated from the drug release data as in the Eqn. 17.

$$t_{q\%} = 10^{\left(\log\left[\frac{q\%}{100}\right] - \log k_r\right)/n_r} \qquad \ldots(17)$$

A modified form of the power law equation has also been developed to accommodate the lag time (t) in the beginning of the drug release from the pharmaceutical dosage form (El-Arini and Leuenberger, 1995; Pillay and Fassihi, 1999).

$$\frac{M_{(t-1)}}{M_\infty} = a(t-1)^n \qquad \ldots(18)$$

Expressing Eqn. 9 in its logarithmic version:

$$\log\frac{M_{(t-1)}}{M_\infty} = \log a + n\log(t-1) \qquad \ldots(19)$$

When there is possibility of a burst effect, b, this equation becomes:

$$\frac{M_t}{M_\infty} = at^{1/2} + b \qquad \ldots(20)$$

In the absence of burst effect, however, the "b" values would be zero. This mathematical model, also known as the Power Law, has been used very frequently to describe the drug release from DDS (Garg and Gupta, 2009; Nagda et al., 2009; Zugasti et al., 2009; Ahuja et al., 2007). For some swellable matrices, departure from Fickian mechanism is seen and the behavior of drug release is termed as non-Fickian. It arises from coupling of the diffusion (Case I) and molecular relaxation (Case II) phenomena (Peppas and Sahlin, 1989). Case II transport is characterized by the zero-order release kinetics and a unity value of "n". Accordingly, the non-Fickian release behavior of swellable matrices is further analyzed using an equation wherein the diffusion and relaxation mechanisms of transport are considered simultaneously:

$$\frac{M_t}{M_\infty} = k_1 . t^n + k_2 . t^{2n} \qquad ...(21)$$

where, the first term on the right hand side is the Fickian contribution and the second term is the Case II relaxation contribution. The constants, k_1 and k_2, express the respective contributions of the diffusion and the polymer relaxation mechanisms, allowing quantitative evaluation of their importance on overall release. The co-efficient M is purely Fickian diffusion coefficient for device of any shape and its determination is based on the aspect ratio, $2a/l$, where a is the radius and l is the thickness of the device (Peppas and Sahlin, 1989). The percentages of Fickian and relaxational drug release can also be determined from the values of k_1 and k_2. These semi-empirical equations are applied to phenomenological analysis of release behavior from matrix systems and hence are advantageously used to approach the constant release of the drug during development of ER matrix formulations. Numerous reports cite the use of these equations for evaluation of drug release of systems where drug diffusion occurs through the polymeric network, yet these can successfully be employed for spheres and cylinders too. However, use of these equations for analysis of drug release data has to be done judiciously, since such

mathematical relationships are used only for systems where the drug diffusion coefficient is clearly concentration independent (Peppas, 1985). Table 12.1 enlists values of "n" for varied device geometries indicating the transport mechanism (Ritger and Peppas, 1987b; Rinaki et al., 2003; Peppas et al., 2000).

In applying Eqn. 13, drug release data (mass or percent dissolved) are plotted as a function of $t^{1/2}$. If a linear relationship over a given time interval is obtained, it can safely be inferred that diffusion is the sole mechanism for drug release (Ford et al., 1987). The slope of a plot between percent released versus $t^{1/2}$ has the units of $t^{-1/2}$ and the quantity is referred to as Drug Release Rate (DRR; Eqn. 22).

$$DRR = \frac{M_t}{M_0 \sqrt{t}} = \frac{S}{V}\sqrt{\frac{D'}{\pi}} \qquad ...(22)$$

Thus, for a purely diffusional release mechanism and for a formulation in which the drug solubility exceeds that of the initial tablet dose, Eqn. 13 predicts that the drug release can be computed from the knowledge of the surface area (S) by volume (V) ratio of the dry tablet and the effective drug diffusion coefficient (D) in the hydrated matrix tablet (Gao and Meury, 1996). As the dissolution medium penetrates the polymeric matrix of diffusion ER-DDS, rate of drug release increases in the initial stages due to polymer swelling and erosion, remains constant as a result of synchronization between swelling,

Table 12.1. Release exponent and mechanism of drug release from various swellable oral drug delivery systems (Langer and Peppas, 1983; Ritger and Peppas, 1987a; Harland et al., 1988; Peppas et al., 2000)

Values of diffusional release exponent (n) for varied device shapes			Drug transport mechanism	Rate as a function of time
Thin films	**Cylinders**	**Spheres**		
0.50	0.45	0.43	Fickian diffusion	$t^{-0.5}$
$0.50 < n < 1.00$	$0.45 < n < 0.89$	$0.43 < n < 0.85$	Anomalous case II, non-Fickian transport	t^{n-1}
1.00	0.89	0.85	Case II transport	Zero-order
$n > 1.00$	—	—	Super case II transport	t^{n-1}

drug diffusion and dissolution, and finally decreases as dissolution takes over (Peppas and Franson, 1983). Drug-release kinetics associated with popular gel-layer dynamics of hydrophilic matrices generally range initially from Fickian to anomalous (non-Fickian), and from quasi-constant (near zero-order) to constant. In a nutshell, the model can be described in its 'explicative' form as Fig. 12.6.

To examine the physical conditions, which determine mechanism of diffusional drug release from a polymer matrix, a dimensionless 'Swelling Interface Number', S_w, was also proposed by Peppas and co-workers (Peppas and Franson, 1983; Korsmeyer and Peppas, 1983) as defined by Eqn. 23:

$$S_w = \frac{v\delta(t)}{D} \qquad ...(23)$$

where v is the velocity of the moving solvent front, $\delta(t)$ is the time dependent thickness of the swollen phase, and D is the drug diffusion coefficient in the swollen phase. S_w is also known as the pseudo-Peclet number, which compares the relative mobility of the penetrating solvent and the drug, in the presence of macromolecular relaxation in the polymer. For $S_w \ll 1$, rate of drug diffusion through swollen polymer is much

faster than the rate at which the glassy/rubbery front advances and a zero-order release kinetic for the drug is anticipated. On the other hand, when $S_w \gg 1$, the swelling front advances faster than the diffusion of the drug thereby resulting in Fickian release. However, for $S_w \approx 1$, a non-Fickian drug release behavior is anticipated.

In diffusional ER system, the drug gets uniformly dissolved or dispersed in polymer matrix exhibiting release rates continuously diminishing with time. This is the result of increasing diffusional resistance and decreasing area at penetrating diffusion front. Fig. 12.7 illustrates the characteristics of drug release from spherical matrices as a function of initial drug distribution. These theoretical curves show that both the uniform and parabolic initial drug level distribution results in initially high release rate followed by a rapid decline; the latter phase exhibiting reduced initial release rate when compared to the former. In contrast, a sigmoidal initial distribution is capable of introducing a characteristic inflection point and, thus, consider-able linearity into cumulative release curve. As a result, a prolonged constant release rate, similar to a membrane reservoir system, is obtained. The parabolic type of concentration distribution is characteristic of a glassy polymer, partially

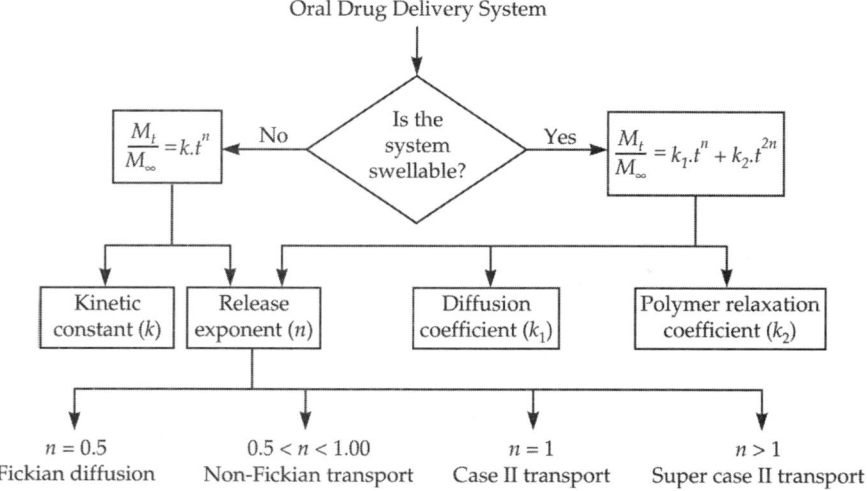

Fig. 12.6. Explicative representation of Korsmeyer-Peppas model.

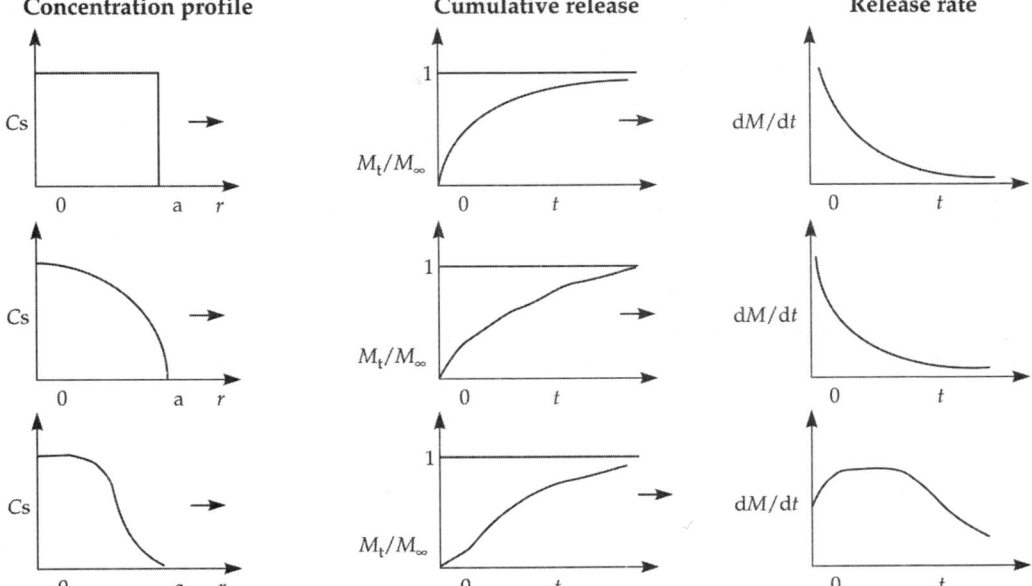

Fig. 12.7. Theoretical profiles illustrating the effect of initial drug concentration and distribution on the characteristics of drug release.

penetrated by solvent undergoing non-Fickian diffusion (Peppas and Franson, 1983). In case of diffusion ER DDS, a phase erosion of the polymeric carrier occurs that may be associated with fast or slow dissolution of the macromolecular chains. As the dissolution medium penetrates the polymeric matrix, it swells leading to the formation of a thin layer of polymer in the rubbery state (Olkkola and Hagelberg, 2009). Drug diffusion through this gel layer is relatively very fast and is governed by the thickness of this layer.

Cube root and related models

Three classical diffusion-controlled kinetic models have been reported for describing the drug release of single spherical particle under the sink conditions (Hixson and Crowell, 1931; Niebergall et al., 1963; Higuchi and Hiestand, 1963). The models have been summarized in Table 12.2.

Here, W_t and W_o are the particle weights (or amounts of drug in the pharmaceutical dosage

Table 12.2. Diffusion-controlled models for spherical particle dissolution conditions

Main model	Supplementary model	Reference	Eqn. no.
$W_t^{1/3} = W_0^{1/3} - K_{1/3}.t$	$K_{1/3} = \left(\dfrac{4\pi\rho}{3}\right)^{1/3} \dfrac{DC_s}{\rho h}$	Hixson & Crowell, 1931	24
$W_t^{1/2} = W_0^{1/2} - K_{1/2}.t$	$K_{1/2} = \left(\dfrac{3\pi\rho}{2}\right)^{1/2} \dfrac{DC_s}{k'\rho}$	Niebergall et al., 1963	25
$W_t^{2/3} = W_0^{2/3} - K_{2/3}.t$	$K_{2/3} = \left(\dfrac{4\pi\rho}{3}\right)^{2/3} \dfrac{2DC_s}{\rho}$	Higuchi & Hiestand, 1963	26

form) remaining at time t and initially at start of dissolution of study; $K_{1/3}$, $K_{1/2}$ and $K_{2/3}$ are the respective composite rate constants; ρ is the density of the particle; D is the diffusion coefficient; C_s is solubility; h is the diffusion layer thickness; and k' is a constant. Eqn. 24–26 have respectively, the cube root, square root and two-thirds root dependency on particle weight. A particular dissolution profile can often be fitted by at least two of these equations almost equally well (Veng-Pedersen and Brown, 1976). Thus, it seems that the dissolution behavior of spherical particles is still not theoretically well-defined, calling for an integrated equation valid for all powders. Nevertheless, among these models, Eqn. 24 (i.e., cube-root law) is the most widely used relationship (Liu et al., 2008; Garg et al., 2009), assuming proportionality between the dissolution rate and the particle surface area as a function of the cubic root of its volume.

Generalizing Eqn. 24 in a simplistic manner by integrating all the constant terms together in terms of a single Hixson-Crowell coefficient (K_{HC}) and expressing in the terms of M_t and M_∞, Eqn. 27 is obtained as:

$$(M_\infty)^{1/3} - (M_t)^{1/3} = K_{HC}.t \qquad ...(27)$$

Accordingly, linear regression analysis is performed between the difference of the cube roots of M_∞ and M_t as the dependent variable and time (t) as the independent variable. After forcing the regression line through origin, the regression parameters, viz., r^2, s_E, $F_{1,m-2}$ and $AOEV_m$ are also determined for various dosage form units.

Originally developed for single particles, the cube-root law has been extended to multiparticulate systems too. Cube root constant, $K_{1/3}$ or K_s, incorporates surface-volume relation, as cube root law kinetic model applies more aptly to the geometric shapes of drug formulations with release rate limited by diminishing surface of the drug particles in planes parallel to drug surface. Hence, it is more relevant to the dissolution from tablets where dimensions

diminish proportionally keeping initial geometry invariant, rather than to swelling or eroding polymeric matrices.

Weibull model

The general Weibull function (Weibull, 1951; Langenbucher, 1972; Carvalho et al., 2010; Li et al., 2010) is expressed as Eqn. 28:

$$m_W = 1 - e^{\left[-(t-T_i)^b(1/a)\right]} \qquad ...(28)$$

where m_W is the accumulated fraction of the material (drug) in solution at time t, a is the scale parameter defining the time scale of the process, T_i is the location parameter that represents the time lag between the onset of dissolution, and b is the shape parameter that characterizes the curve in the form of a more useful relationship as being non-linear upwards. Weibull distribution function is arranged as:

$$(1 - m_W) = e^{\left[-(t-T_i)^b(1/a)\right]} \qquad ...(29)$$

Taking negative logarithms of both sides, Eqn. 30 is attained:

$$-\ln(1 - m_W) = (t - T_i)^b(1/a) \qquad ...(30)$$

Taking further the positive common logarithms of both the sides:

$$\log[-\ln(1 - m_W)] = b\log(t - T_i)^b - \log a \quad ...(31)$$

Putting across m_W in terms of fraction drug released, M_t/M_∞, however:

$$\log\left[-\ln\left(1 - \frac{M_t}{M_\infty}\right)\right] = b\log(t - T_i) - \log a \qquad ...(32)$$

Assuming there is no lag time, T_i:

$$\log\left[-\ln\left(1 - \frac{M_t}{M_\infty}\right)\right] = b.\log t - \log a \qquad ...(33)$$

Else, the lag time, T_i, is identified as the time associated with first perceptible drug concentration, and the value is substituted in Eqn. 32.

Thus, least square linear regression analysis is acted upon between log $[- \ln (1 - M_t/M_\infty)]$ as the dependent variable and time (t) as the independent variable, and various regression parameters determined for various dosage forms. From the values of scale parameter (a) and shape parameter (b), the magnitude of dissolution time (T_d) is also computed as:

$$T_d = a^{1/b} \qquad \ldots(34)$$

Cooney model

Cooney presented a detailed analysis for spheres and cylinders undergoing surface erosion (Cooney, 1972). His model is based on the assumption that there is one single zero-order kinetic process, which is confined to the surface of the drug delivery system. For a cylinder with the initial length L_0 and initial diameter D_0, the following equation was derived quantifying the drug release rate f as a function of time t (Eqn. 35).

$$f = \frac{(D_0 - 2Kt)^2 + 2(D_0 - 2Kt)(L_0 - 2Kt)}{D_0^2 + 2D_0 L_0} \qquad \ldots(35)$$

where K is a constant. When L_0/D_0 approaches zero (film geometry) the curves transform into a horizontal line with a constant relative drug release rate of 1. It is interesting to note that for disc-like cylinders (ratios of $L_0/D_0 < 1$, curves numbered 0.1, 0.2 and 0.5), the relative drug release rate remains finite up to complete drug release. In contrast, for rod-like cylinders ($L_0/D_0 > 1$, curves numbered 1, 2, 5 and infinity), the relative drug release rate approaches zero at late time points.

ARTIFICIAL NEURAL NETWORKS

Lately, artificial neural networks (ANNs) can be used to model drug delivery (Takayama et al., 1999; Takahara et al., 1997) and first time used by Takahara et al. (1997). An ANN consists of one input layer, one output layer and one or more hidden intermediate layers. Each layer is composed of several units, corresponding to "neurons". The input layer encompasses n input values of causal factors, e.g. the drug loading, compression force or excipient content. The output layer can, for instance, consist of constants describing the drug release profile. The information is passed from input layer to the output layer through hidden layer(s) by the network connections or synapses as illustrated in Fig. 12.8. The strength of these links can vary; they are also called "weights". Thus, ANNs can be considered as non-linear regression analysis tool. Once the system is "trained", it can be used to make quantitative predictions for the output values based on new input values.

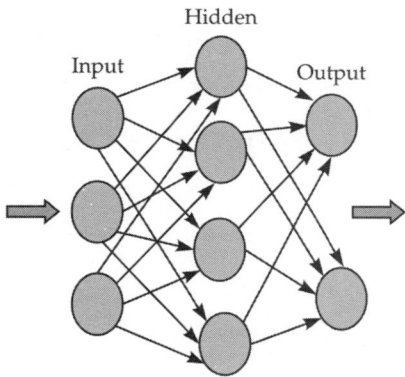

Fig. 12.8. Arrangement of artificial neural networks.

OTHER EMPIRICAL MODELS

By and large, since 1963, when Higuchi gave the first mathematical model to describe ER, fitting *in vitro* drug release data from oral DDS to mathematical expressions has formed the basis of several research reports and reviews. Accordingly, besides the aforesaid models, there have been numerous other kinetic models postulated in drug release literature (Flynn et al., 1974; Grassi et al., 1997; Siepmann and Gopferich, 2001; Karasulu et al., 2000; Narasimhan, 2001; Siepmann et al., 2002). Mathematical models described to analyze drug release from ER formulations have primarily been based upon drug dissolution and diffusion from the matrix as a result of liquid penetration, and at times, on the swelling and erosion of the components. Table 12.3 succinctly enlists various other popular empirical models employed for kinetic modelling briefly outlining their respective applicability.

Table 12.3. Mathematical equations related with various drug release and dissolution theories (Kitazawa et al., 1975; Tsong et al., 2003; Goldberg et al., 1967)

Theory	Equation	No.	Associated characteristics
Fick's 1st law of diffusion	$J_{ix} = -D_i \left(\dfrac{\partial C}{\partial x} \right)$	36	This classical theory assumes diffusion of a solute under steady-state conditions only.
Fick's 2nd law of diffusion	$\dfrac{\partial c}{\partial t} = D_i \left(\dfrac{\partial^2 c}{\partial x^2} \right)$	37	It considers non-steady conditions, and is applied when drug concentration tends to decrease with time.
Kitazawa theory	$\ln \dfrac{w^\infty}{w^\infty - w} = k't$	38	It assumes constant surface area under sink conditions.
Goldberg limited solvation	$\theta = k_1 (C_s - C_t)$	39	It assumes drug concentration less than saturation drug concentration at solid-solvent interface.
Probit model	$\dfrac{M_t}{M_\infty} = A.\phi(\alpha + \beta.A.\log t)$	40	These empirical physicochemical models are applied to mathematically describe the course of dissolution of an ER or immediate-release product especially following sigmoid dissolution curves.
Gompertz model	$\dfrac{M_t}{M_\infty} = e^{-\alpha.e^{\beta.\log t}}$	41	
Logistic model	$\dfrac{M_t}{M_\infty} = \dfrac{A.e^{(\alpha+\beta.A.\log t)}}{1 + e^{(\alpha+\beta.A.\log t)}}$	42	
Baker & Lonsdale model	$\dfrac{2}{3}\left[1 - \left(1 - \dfrac{M_t}{M_\infty}\right)^{2/3}\right] - \dfrac{M_t}{M_\infty} = K_b.t$	43	It describes the drug release from a ER spherical matrix and has been used for the linearization of drug release profiles from a variety of DDS.
Flanagan model	$\dfrac{DC_s t}{\rho h} = \left(\dfrac{3W_o}{4N\pi\rho}\right)^{1/3} - \left(\dfrac{3W}{4N\pi\rho}\right)^{1/3}$ $-h\ln \dfrac{h + \left(\dfrac{3W_o}{4N\pi\rho}\right)^{1/3}}{h + \left(\dfrac{3W_t}{4N\pi\rho}\right)^{1/3}}$	44	It is applicable to all the diffusion-based particle dissolution processes.
Convective-Diffusion model	$-\dfrac{da}{dt} = \dfrac{DC_s F}{a\rho}$	45	It assumes that the dissolution rate is diffusion-rate controlled. The effective diffusion layer thickness is the same for all particles of the same size and is equal to or greater than the particle radius, particles are dissolving under sink conditions, and the particles are spherical.

(Contd.)

Theory	Equation	No.	Associated characteristics
Hopfenberg model	$$\frac{M_t}{M_\infty} = 1 - [1 - k_t t(t-1)]^n$$	46	It assumes that the drug diffusion coefficient, D, increases exponentially with time while the polymer chain cleavage follows first-order kinetics.
Deborah model	$$(DEB)_D = \frac{\lambda_m}{\theta_D}$$	47	If $(DEB)_D \ll 1$ or $(DEB)_D \gg 1$, it indicates Fickian diffusion either in the rubbery or glassy state. However, for $(DEB)_D \approx 1$, non-Fickian (anomalous) diffusion including special case I transport is anticipated depending on the relative importance of the Fickian diffusion and polymer relaxation processes.

J_{ix}: flux (mg/cm^2.s^{-1}); D_i: diffusion coefficient; $\partial c/\partial x$: concentration gradient; $\partial c/\partial t$: drug dissolution rate; K: first-order dissolution constant; C_s: equilibrium drug concentration; C_t: drug concentration at time t; θ: dissolution rate per unit area; k_1: effective interfacial transport constant; w^∞: amount of drug in solution at infinite time; $(w^\infty - w)$: amount of undissolved drug; C_s: aqueous solubility of drug; M_t: drug released at time t; M_∞: total amount of dissolvable drug; A: relational model constant; α: location or scale parameter; β: acceleration or shape parameter

SOFTWARE FOR DRUG RELEASE KINETICS

Computers are finding increasing application in handling and treatment of data generated during pharmaceutical research. Numerous computer programs with diverse pharmaceutical applications have been developed by different workers. However, only a couple of these software are meant to evaluate drug release from different oral dosage forms (Vigoreaux and Ghaly, 1994; Sande and Karlsen, 1989; Lu et al., 1996). Owing to ever-increasing complexity of the pharmaceutical professional's work patterns, the need for newer user-interactive software, however, remains.

Accordingly, Singh et al. (1998) prepared a software, ZOREL for studying drug release kinetics from diverse drug delivery systems. The program, written in FORTRAN, uses raw dissolution data as the input. It initially corrects the dissolution data for drug and/or volume losses using WR and/or WOR sampling algorithms (Singh et al., 1997) occurring at the time of sampling and on the basis of the weight of the dosage form and the drug content, estimates the values of amount and percent drug released at various times for each formulation unit. The

values of log mean fraction released are computed and regressed against log time to yield the values of kinetic constant (k) and release exponent (n) as per Peppas and Higuchi and subsequently calculations are made for mean dissolution time (MDT) using Korsmeyer-Peppas relationship propounded for swelling matrices, the respective contributions of the diffusion and the polymer relaxation along with the constants of k_1 and k_2, are also computed. Based on the phenomenological analysis, the software predicts the type of release viz. Fickian, non-Fickian (anomalous) or zero-order. In addition, the values of mean ($\pm$SD) percent released are calculated and regressed against square root of time up to various observations. The values of rate of drug release and $t_{50\%}$, $t_{60\%}$ up to $t_{90\%}$ of the drug release are computed using the program.

A wide variety of other mathematical models has been developed to fit the drug release data, most of which are presented as non-linear equations. Only one special program MSFIT has been reported for fitting dissolution data, and only five release models have been implemented, and these could be applied only over a limited range (Lu et al., 1996). Alternatively, the non-linear fitting of dissolution data can be performed using other professional statistical software packages such as MicroMath Scientist (Phaechamud, 2008), GraphPad Prism (Di Colo et al., 2006), SigmaPlot (Papadopoulou et al., 2006), or SYSTAT (von Orelli and Leuenberger, 2004). However, these programs require the user to define the equation manually and to provide an initial value for each parameter. On the other hand, DDSolver is a menu-driven add-in program for Microsoft Excel spreadsheet package written in Visual Basic for Applications. This program can be used to

- facilitate the modelling of dissolution data using non-linear optimization methods based on a built-in model library containing 40 dissolution models;
- simplify the task of assessing the similarity between dissolution profiles using various popular approaches; and
- speed-up the calculation, reduce user errors, and provide a convenient way to report dissolution data quickly and easily.

DISSOLUTION PROFILE COMPARISONS

Invariably, the drug release profile of an oral DDS needs to be evaluated vis-à-vis a reference or another test product. To accomplish the same, dissolution profiles may be considered similar by virtue of overall profile similarity and/or similarity at every dissolution sample time point. From computational perspective, it is more intricate to compare complete multiple-point dissolution profiles than a single-point test. Several methods have been proposed in literature for comparison of dissolution profiles (Hurtado et al., 2003; Chow and Ki, 1997; Gohel et al., 2009; Maggio et al., 2008; Sathe et al., 1996). Each method is based on a distinct kinetic model describing drug dissolution from conventional immediate release (IR) formulation or ER dosage form. Quantitative interpretation of dissolution curve is facilitated by use of a generic equation on the cumulative drug release profile of the drug products.

Polli et al. (1996) divided these techniques as model-independent, model-dependent, and ANOVA-based approaches. Different results can be discerned depending on the method used for the comparison. Important model-independent approaches encompass the ratio-test procedures and pairwise procedures.

Ratio-test procedures

These approaches compare dissolution profiles of drug formulations furnishing tangible basis to formulate dissolution specifications. Of the various types of test procedures performed, 90% confidence interval for mean ratio percent dissolved, percent dissolution efficiency (% DE), and mean dissolution time (MDT) are the popular ones (Gohel et al., 2009). Use of percent dissolved data is mostly preferable as it is the simplest and most natural calculation of three approaches. In addition, it allows the establishment of criteria at any time point, unlike mean time, which could be calculated only after nearly the entire drug is dissolved.

Mean dissolution time (MDT)

MDT is estimated using Eqn. 48:

$$MDT = \frac{\int_0^\infty t.W_d(t).dt}{\int_0^\infty W_d(t).dt} = \frac{ABC}{W_0} \qquad ...(48)$$

where ABC (area between curve) is the shaded area as in Fig. 12.9, $W_d(t)$ is cumulative drug amount dissolved at any time, and W_0 is the actual (not labelled) quantity of drug available for dissolution (Tsong et al., 2003). ABC can be estimated arithmatically using trapezoidal rule.

Alternatively, MDT can also be calculated using Eqn. 49:

$$MDT_{in\,vitro} = \frac{\sum_{i=1}^n t_{mid}.\Delta M}{\sum_{i=1}^n \Delta M} \qquad ...(49)$$

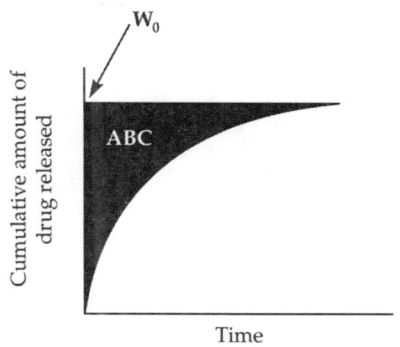

Fig. 12.9. Graphical estimation of mean dissolution time and dissolution efficiency.

where "i" is the sample dissolution number from a possible "n" number, ΔM is the additional drug amount dissolved between i and $i-1$, and t_{mid} is the corresponding midpoint. MDT is computable by other graphical means too (Podczek, 1993). Estimation of MDT in any case needs knowledge of time at which the dissolution process is complete.

Dissolution efficiency (DE%)

$DE_\%$ is another vital parameter suitable for the evaluation of *in vitro* dissolution, as suggested by Khan (1975).

$$DE_\% = \left(\frac{\int_0^t Y.\mathrm{d}t}{Y_{100}.t} \right) \times 100 \qquad ...(50)$$

Verily, $DE_\%$ represents the proportion of the area under the dissolution curve (AUC$_t$) up to a certain time "t", expressed as a percentage of the area of the rectangle described by 100% dissolution in the same time, inclusive of AUC_t and ABC_t both, as depicted in Fig. 12.9. Accordingly,

$$DE_\% = \frac{AUC_t}{\text{Area}_{rectangle}.Y_{100}.t} \times 100$$

$$= \frac{AUC_t}{AUC_t + ABC_t} \times 100 \qquad ...(51)$$

Pairwise procedures

Several measures have been propounded and used for dissolution comparison amongst the paired data using either similarity or dissimilarity criteria (Gohel et al., 2009; Maggio et al., 2008; Costa and Lobo, 2001; Polli et al., 1996). Important ones encompass difference factor (f_1), similarity factor (f_2), Rescigno indices (ξ_i), Mean square-distance (D_2), Mahalanobis distance, etc.

Difference factor (f_1)

First proposed by Moore and Flanner (1996), f_1 is ratio of absolute difference of the test (T_i) and reference (R_i), normalized with respect to the sum of the mean percent dissolutions of the reference lot.

$$f_1 = \left(\frac{\sum_{i=1}^{P} \mu_{R_i} - \mu_{T_i}}{\sum_{i=1}^{P} \mu_{R_i}} \right) \times 100 \qquad ...(52)$$

where the corresponding μ values represent the respective means, and W_i can be an optional weight factor. This measure is therefore a scaled difference of the two profiles. As it is normalized with respect to reference means, it is sensitive to reference product profile. In other words, with exactly the same size of difference between two profiles, the measure can furnish different values when the reference profiles are different.

Similarity factor (f_2)

Similarity factor is a logarithmic transformation of reciprocal of square-root transformation of one plus mean squared difference between dissolution values of test T_i and reference products R_i over all time points, P (Maggio et al., 2008; Gohel et al., 2009; Ma et al., 2000).

$$f_2 = 50.\log\left\{ \left[1 + \frac{1}{P}.\sum_{i=1}^{P} \left| \mu_{R_i} - \mu_{T_i} \right|^2 \right]^{-0.5} \times 100 \right\} \qquad ...(53)$$

The f_2 value fits the dissolution comparison results between 0 and 100; it is 100 when the test and reference profiles are identical and approach 0 as dissimilarity increases. This method is more adequate to compare dissolution profile when more than three or four dissolution time points are available. However, if the average difference between R_i and T_i is higher than 100, normalization of the data is required (Moore and Flanner, 1996, Shah et al., 1998a, Shah et al., 1998b). The f_2 has been adopted by US FDA and European Agency for the Evaluation of Medicinal Products (EMEA), as a similarity criterion between two *in vitro* dissolution profiles (FDA, 1997b, Shah et al., 1998a, FDA, 1997a). It is quite insensitive to the shape of the dissolution profiles and does not take into account unequal spacing between sampling time points. The sample statistic of f_2 cannot be used to formulate a statistical hypothesis for assessment of dissolution similarity, and, therefore, is impossible to furnish false positive and false negative decisions for approval of drug products. Simulation results, however, indicate that the similarity factor is too liberal in concluding similarity between dissolution profiles (Liu et al., 1997).

Rescigno indices (ξ_i)

These were initially proposed as dissimilarity measures between reference and test products, based on plasma level time profiles (Rescigno, 1992). Dissolution based first-order index (ξ_1), however, is more frequently referenced in literature:

$$\xi_1 = \left(\frac{\sum_{i=1}^{P} \left| \mu_{R_i} - \mu_{T_i} \right|}{\sum_{i=1}^{P} i \left| \mu_{R_i} - \mu_{T_i} \right|} \right) \quad \ldots(54)$$

Likewise, the second-order (ξ_2) Rescigno index can be computed as:

$$\xi_2 = \left(\frac{\sum_{i=1}^{P} \left\{ \left| \mu_{R_i} - \mu_{T_i} \right| \right\}^2}{\sum_{i=1}^{P} \left\{ \left| \mu_{R_i} + \mu_{T_i} \right| \right\}^2} \right) \quad \ldots(55)$$

where R_i and T_i are the values of percent dissolved amount at each sample time point for reference and test product, respectively, and i is the positive integer number. This dimensional index always presents values between 0 and 1 and inclusive measuring differences between two dissolution profiles. Both the indices are 0 when the two release profiles are identical and 1 when drug from either of the formulation (test or reference) is not released at all.

Besides, several other measures of difference or similarity of two profiles have been propounded in the last decade (Veng-Pedersen et al., 2000; Tsong et al., 1997; Saradansa, 2001). Notable amongst them are enumerated as:

Maximum distance (D_{Max})

Maximum distance, i.e. the magnitude of the maximum difference of two curves, is a measure of uniform similarity.

$$D_{\max} = Max_{i=1}^{P} \{D_i\} \quad \ldots(56)$$

Difference of area under the profiles (D_{AUC})

D_{AUC} is an insensitive global measure of the difference between the two mean dissolution profiles at individual time points:

$$D_{AUC} = 0.5 \times \sum_{i=1}^{P} \left[\left(\mu_{T_i} + \mu_{T_{i-1}} \right) - \left(\mu_{R_i} + \mu_{R_{i-1}} \right) \right]$$

$$\times (t_i - t_{i-1}) \quad \ldots(57)$$

Other measurements defined as functions of the difference at each time point are either derived or modified from the following two basic metrices of difference between two mean dissolution curves.

Mean distance (D^1)

D^1, in the generalized form, can be written as:

$$D^1 = \sum_{i=1}^{P}\left\{\left|\mu_{R_i} - \mu_{T_i}\right|\right\}/P \qquad ...(58)$$

Area between the profiles (D_{ABC})

D_{ABC}, on similar heels (Tsong et al., 2003), can be computed as:

$$D_{ABC} = 0.5 \times \sum_{i=1}^{P-1}\left|\mu_{T_i} - \mu_{T_{i-1}}\right| \times [(t_{i+1}+t_i)-(t_i+t_{i-1})] \qquad ...(59)$$

It may employ the optional weight, w_i as $[(t_{i+1}+t_i)/2 - (t_i + t_{i-1})/2]$. In fact, D_{ABC} is insensitive if the point of cross of the two dissolution profiles cannot be identified.

Mean squared distance (D^2)

D^2, involving squared terms, is more sensitive to large difference at a time-point compared to measure that uses absolute value terms:

$$D^2 = \left(\sum_{i=1}^{P}\left\{\left|\mu_{R_i} - \mu_{T_i}\right|\right\}^2/P\right)^{0.5} \qquad ...(60)$$

Model-dependent techniques

These techniques, employing one or more of the afore-discussed diverse generic numerical relationships can also be successfully used to accomplish dissolution comparisons, besides the model-independent methods.

ANOVA methods

These methods can be further differentiated into multivariate ANOVA, multiple univariate ANOVA, and the level and shape approach (Yuksel et al., 2000). These methods are usually overly discriminating and investigating statistical rather than pharmaceutical equivalence (FDA, 1997a & 1997b).

These methods are routinely utilized for comparison of drug release profiles of numerous IR and extended release (ER) formulations. Table 12.4 portrays the computation of various model-independent and ANOVA-based comparative parameters using experimental data obtained in

Table 12.4. Dissolution profile comparisons between optimized and marketed ER formulations of tramadol hydrochloride using varied approaches

PERCENT DRUG DISSOLVED				
Time (h)	Formulation A*		Formulation B#	
	Mean	SD	Mean	SD
0.25	19.07	0.48	13.37	0.58
0.50	25.93	0.21	21.76	0.54
01.0	33.18	0.56	29.47	0.27
02.0	38.87	0.26	35.72	0.26
03.0	49.96	0.09	46.23	0.47
04.0	58.6	0.96	55.89	0.61
05.0	67.24	0.35	65.56	0.25
06.0	70.89	0.14	72.46	0.30
08.0	78.39	0.04	75.36	0.11
10.0	86.06	0.22	83.38	0.45
12.0	88.15	1.57	88.41	0.15
18.0	91.71	0.94	94.82	0.24
24.0	100.47	0.50	100.91	0.14

RATIO TEST PROCEDURES		
Mean dissolution time, MDT (h)	5.03	5.16
Dissolution efficiency, $DE_\%$ (12 h)	64.79	62.63
Dissolution efficiency, $DE_\%$ (24 h)	78.90	78.69

PAIR-WISE PROCEDURES	
Difference factor, f_1	4.59
Similarity factor f_2	74.24
Rescigno index, ξ_1	0.0225
Rescigno index, ξ_2	0.0233
Area difference, D_{AUC}	5.03
Mean difference, D^1	2.76
Squared difference, D^2	3.12

MULTIVARIATE ANOVA-BASED METHODS		
1-way ANOVA	F-ratio = 0.78934	No significant difference

* Marketed once-a-day ER tramadol formulation (Tramzac-TC,™ Zydus-Alidac, Ahmedabad, India)
# Optimized hydrodynamically balanced bioadhesive formulation containing CP 971 & HPMC K100 LV

our laboratories on gastroretentive drug delivery systems of tramadol hydrochloride (Singh et al., 2007b).

DISSOLUTION CORRECTION FORMULAE

All the official compendia require solid IR oral drug formulations to pass the official test(s) for dissolution rate using one-time point dissolution, wherein the dosage form is expected to release and dissolve in a specified time period. In case of ER preparations, multiple samples are drawn using:

(i) With replacement (WR) technique, wherein the aliquot of withdrawn sample is replaced with an equal volume of fresh dissolution medium.

(ii) Without replacement (WOR) technique, wherein the aliquot of sample withdrawn is not replaced back.

(iii) Automatic continuous withdrawal and replacement using the automated sipper system consisting of flow-through cell, fraction collector and peristaltic system.

In the first case of WR sampling, there is drug loss and dilution of dissolution medium with fresh medium, and consequently, there is under-reporting of drug concentration. A gradual fall, therefore, is observed following the time at which the dissolution profile becomes asymptotic, i.e., the maximum of drug is released. In the second case of WOR sampling, loss of both volume and drug levels takes place simultaneously, leading eventually to less change in resultant drug concentration in the medium. Hence, the maximum is slightly higher than the actual values, albeit no fall is observed after reaching the maximum. In the last case, however, as very small volume is withdrawn and returned almost immediately to the reservoir of dissolution medium, no correction whatsoever is required. Compensation is ought to be made by calculation in the former two cases. Haplessly, no official compendium has mentioned any tangible corrections to account for these. Since such correction factors need to be applied to the voluminous dissolution data generated during product development and formulation

evaluation, application of these correction factors manually or using calculators would not only be tedious and time-consuming but error-prone too. It explains the need to define the mathematics and nature of these correction factors, and encompassing the consequent algorithms in the development of computer software for evaluation of drug release kinetics.

To enquire about the same, correspondence was initiated with the offices of USP and BP. In response, the office of United States Pharmacopoeia stated, "the assumption is that the analyst will correct for the volume loss mathematically when the loss significantly affects the results." The experts in B.P. committee, however, were a little more emphatic in their response. They wrote:

(i) No compensation is required when the volume of dissolution medium equal to the volume of the samples withdrawn is replaced or when single sampling occurs.

(ii) Compensation by calculation is only required when the volume of dissolution medium equal to the volume of the samples withdrawn is not replaced.

Thus, it could be easily inferred from these communications with official agencies that no correction is assumed to be required in the first case of WR sampling, while in the second case of WOR sampling an appropriate correction is advisable. Nonetheless, it is obvious from the above discussion that correction needs to be applied in both of these cases. Aronson in 1993 postulated some proposals to correct for loss of the drug from dissolution medium due to sampling during drug release studies. However, the formulae proposed by him were applicable indirectly to percent drug release data only, but not to the raw dissolution data. Based on the indirect formula proposed by Aronson, Singh et al. (1997) subsequently derived, validated and reported such corrections germane to the absorbance or concentration data. Several scientists have been benefitted from this revelation including over a score of the members of dissolution discussion group (DDG), who requested and received the reprints of the published report for successful implementation at their respective ends.

The formula for calculation of corrected amount of drug dissolved, after the nth sample (Aronson, 1993) is computed from the total amount of drug in the system, is given by the following relationship (Eqn. 61).

$$C_n \times V_n + \sum_{i=1}^{n-1} C_i \times V_s \qquad \text{...(61)}$$

where, C_n and V_n are the drug concentration and volume of dissolution medium, respectively, at the nth sample, C_i is the concentration at the ith time point and V_s is the sample volume.

The factors for correction of the raw concentration data are derived from Eqn. 61 by substituting volume of dissolution medium present in the chamber (i.e., V_n) at the nth sampling by $[V_t - \{(n-1) \times V_s\}]$ where V_t is the total volume of dissolution medium employed in the beginning of the dissolution run. This equation, on division by V_t throughout and rearrangement, results in Eqn. 62:

$$Conc_{corr} = C_n + \frac{V_s}{V_t}\left[\sum_{i=1}^{n-1} C_i - (n-1).C_n\right] \text{...(62)}$$

A more simplified form is achieved on addition of C_n to the first term in brackets and on subtracting the same from the second term:

$$Conc_{corr} = C_n + \frac{V_s}{V_t}\left[\sum_{i=1}^{n} C_i - n.C_n\right] \qquad \text{...(63)}$$

In accordance with this relationship, the addition of $V_s/V_t [\sum C_i - n \times C_n]$ to the observed data (C_n) results in the corrected concentration values. These equations, in the form given, are applicable directly only to WOR (without replacement) studies, where an aliquot of dissolution medium equal to the volume of sample withdrawn is not replaced. A similar set of equations is derived for WR (with replace-

ment) studies by substituting the parameter V_n in Eqn. 61 by V_t, which is possible in this case, as the total medium remains unchanged during the entire dissolution run. This simple substitution yields Eqn. 64 that is applied to correction of drug levels dissolved after the nth WR sample.

$$Conc_{corr} = C_n + \frac{V_s}{V_t}.\sum_{i=1}^{n-1} C_i \qquad \text{...(64)}$$

Validation of correction factors

The proposed algorithms for WR and WOR sampling were validated using the aptness of the formulae and using theoretical data simulated for the purpose. Subsequent validation was carried out using the experimental data obtained in our laboratory using 16-hour dissolution run on the ER formulations of diclofenac sodium. As the outcome of the proposed formulae had important bearing, the studies were carried with $n = 10$ in each dissolution study.

EPILOGUE

Thousands of drug molecules are available commercially today to combat a gamut of diseases, especially the chronic ones. Nevertheless, none of these drug candidates fulfills all the objectives of efficacy and safety. Accordingly, the research to explore new drugs and newer delivery systems of old drugs has been continuing unabated. As a convention, drugs are administered at frequent time intervals in order to provide the desired effect for prolonged periods. This type of dosing regimen, however, results in a temporal drug profile in the body characterized by recurrent peaks and troughs. Attention, therefore, has been focussed on achieving the desirable drug release profiles by formulating these drugs as their ER systems. These systems initially release a part of the drug dose to rapidly attain its effective therapeutic levels. Subsequently, drug release kinetics tends to follow a well-defined behavior in order to maintain those desired drug levels. This step becomes further convoluted owing to various physicochemical and physiological factors influencing drug release.

Use of mathematical modelling is indispensible to understand and interpret such kinetics of drug release from ER formulations. A model, in this case, can simply be thought as a "mathematical metaphor of some aspects of reality" that ensembles phenomena governing drug release kinetics. Often termed as 'empirical models', such mathematical models are aided by their flow-chart descriptions usually called as 'explicative models'. The major driving forces for the use of mathematical modelling in drug delivery are saving time and resources. Given the desired route of drug administration, drug dose and target release profile, mathematical predictions allow good estimates of the optimal composition, geometry and formulation procedure of the respective dosage form. The quantitative analysis of the physical, chemical and biological phenomena involved in drug release control offers another fundamental advantage. This knowledge is not only of academic interest but a pre-requisite for efficient improvement of drug efficacy and safety. This is particularly true for highly potent drugs with narrow therapeutic window between the therapeutic and toxic drug levels.

Till date, numerous mathematical theories have been reported in literature to decipher drug release kinetics. Besides providing an understanding of phenomena underlying release of drug, these kinetic models present a holistic account of formulation design to attain the desired drug release profile. This improved drug release mechanistics can eventually lead to comprehensive product and process behavior, the essence of implementing Quality by Design (QbD) paradigms. Often, the drug dissolution profile of a product also needs to be evaluated vis-à-vis a reference or another test product during pharmaceutical product development. Also, the development of algorithms of the dissolution correction formulae has also been the shot in the arm of a development pharmacist. Solving the numeric intricacies during implementation of such kinetic procedures of drug release from a formulation after applying suitable dissolution corrections customarily calls for an apt computer interface.

The current book chapter is a humble endeavor to examine, from a pharmaceutical and mathematical viewpoint, the mechanisms underlying the release of drugs from their respective DDS, to compare the drug dissolution profiles with the existing ones and to highlight and surmount various pertinent issues, hitherto overlooked.

REFERENCES

- Abdou, H.A. (2000). Dissolution. *In:* Gennaro, A.R. (Ed.) **Remington: The Science and Practice of Pharmacy**. Philadelphia, Lippincott Williams & Wilkinson.
- Ahuja, N., Katare, O.P., Singh, B. (2007). Studies on dissolution enhancement and mathematical modelling of drug release of a poorly water-soluble drug using water-soluble carriers. *Eur. J. Pharm. Biopharm.*, 65, 26–38.
- Akkaramongkolporn, P., Ngawhirunpat, T., Nunthanid, J., Opanasopit, P. (2008). Effect of a pharmaceutical cationic exchange resin on the properties of controlled release diphenhydramine hydrochloride matrices using Methocel K4M or Ethocel 7cP as matrix formers. *AAPS PharmSciTech*, 9, 899–908.
- Aronson, H. (1993). Correction factor for dissolution profile calculation. *J. Pharm. Sci.*, 82, 1190–1191.
- Baker, R. (1987). Diffusion-controlled systems. *In:* Baker, R. (Ed.) **Controlled Release of Biologically Active Agents**. New York, John Wiley & Sons.
- Basu, S.K., Rajendran, A. (2008). Studies in the development of nateglinide loaded calcium alginate and chitosan coated calcium alginate beads. *Chem. Pharm. Bull.* (Tokyo), 56, 1077–84.
- Brunner, E. (1904). Reaktion geschwindigkeit in heterogenen systemen. *Z. Physik Chem.*, 47, 56–102.

- Brunner, E., Tollockzo, S. (1900). Uber die auflosungs geswindigkeit fester korper. *Z. Physik Chem.*, 35, 283–290.
- Burkersoda, F.V., Schedl, L., Gopferich, A. (2002). Why degradable polymers undergo surface erosion or bulk erosion? *Biomaterials*, 23, 4221–4231.
- Carvalho, F.C., Sarmento, V.H., Chiavacci, L.A., Barbi, M.S., Gremiao, M.P. (2010). Development and *in vitro* evaluation of surfactant systems for controlled release of zidovudine. *J. Pharm. Sci.*, 99, 2367–74.
- Chein, Y.W. (1992). Oral Drug Delivery and Delivery Systems. **Novel Drug Delivery Systems**. Marcel Dekker, New York.
- Cheng, L., Lei, L., Guo, S. (2010). *In vitro* and *in vivo* evaluation of praziquantel loaded implants based on PEG/PCL blends. *Int. J. Pharm.*, 15, 129–38.
- Chi, N., Guo, J.H., Zhang, Y., Zhang, W., Tang, X. (2010). An oral controlled release system for amroxol hydrochloride containing a wax and a water insoluble polymer. *Pharm. Dev. Technol.*, 15, 97–104.
- Chow, S.C., Ki, F.Y.C. (1997). Statistical comparison between dissolution profiles of drug products. *J. Biopharm. Stat.*, 7, 241–258.
- Cooney, D.O. (1972). Effect of geometry on the dissolution of pharmaceutical tablets and other solids: surface detachment kinetics controlling. *AIChE J.*, 18, 446–449.
- Costa-Balogh, F.O., Sparr, E., Sousa, J.J., Pais, A.C. (2009). Drug release from lipid liquid crystalline phases: Relation with phase behavior. *Drug Dev. Ind. Pharm.*, 36, 470–81.
- Costa, P., Lobo, J.M.S. (2001). Modelling and comparison of dissolution profiles. *Eur. J. Pharm. Sci.*, 13, 123–133.
- Deshpande, P.B., Dandagi, P., Udupa, N., Gopal, S.V., Jain, S.S., Vasanth, S.G. (2010). Controlled release polymeric ocular delivery of acyclovir. *Pharm. Dev. Technol.*, 15, 369–78.
- Di Colo, G., Baggiani, A., Zambito, Y., Mollica, G., Geppi, M., Serafini, M.F. (2006). A new hydrogel for the extended and complete prednisolone release in the GI tract. *Int. J. Pharm.*, 310, 154–61. Epub 2006 Jan 18.
- El-Arini, S.K., Leuenberger, H. (1995). Modelling of drug release to polymer matrices: Effect of drug loading. *Int. J. Pharm.*, 121, 141–148.
- Escudero, J.J., Ferrero, C., Jimenez-Castellanos, M.R. (2010). Compaction properties, drug release kinetics and fronts movement studies from matrices combining mixtures of swellable and inert polymers. II. Effect of HPMC with different degrees of methoxy/hydroxypropyl substitution. *Int. J. Pharm.*, 15, 56–64.
- FDA (1997a). **Guidance for Industry on Dissolution Testing of Immediate Release Solid Oral Dosage Forms**. Center for Drug Evaluation and Research, Rockville.
- FDA (1997b). **Guidance for Industry on Extended Release Oral Dosage Forms: Development, Evaluation and Application of *in vitro/in vivo* Correlations**. Center for Drug Evaluation and Research, Rockville.
- Ferrero, C., Massuelle, D., Doelker, E. (2010). Towards elucidation of the drug release mechanism from compressed hydrophilic matrices made of cellulose ethers. II. Evaluation of a possible swelling-controlled drug release mechanism using dimensionless analysis. *J. Control Release*, 141, 223–33.
- Flynn, G.L., Yalkowsky, S.H., Roseman, T.J. (1974). Mass transport phenomena and models: Theoretical concepts. *J. Pharm. Sci.*, 63, 479–510.
- Ford, J.L., Rubinstein, M.H., Mccaul, F., Hogan, J.E., Edgar, P.J. (1987). Importance of drug type, tablet shape and added diluents on drug release kinetics from hydroxypropyl methylcellulose matrix tablets. *Int. J. Pharm.*, 40, 223–234.
- Franco-Marques, E., Mendez, J.A., Girones, J., Ginebra, M.P., Pelach, M.A. (2009). Evaluation of the influence of the addition of biodegradable polymer matrices in the formulation of self-curing polymer systems for biomedical purposes. *Acta Biomater*, 5, 2953–62.
- Fuertes, I., Caraballo, I., Miranda, A., Millan, M. (2010). Study of critical points of drugs with different solubilities in hydrophilic matrices. *Int. J. Pharm.*, 383, 138–46.
- Fyfe, C.A., Blazek-Welsh, A.I. (2000). Quantitative NMR imaging study of mechanism of drug release from swelling hydroxypropyl methylcellulose tablets. *J. Control Release*, 68, 313–333.
- Gao, P., Meury, R.H. (1996). Swelling of hydroxypropyl methylcellulose matrix tablets. (I): Characterization of swelling using novel optical imaging method. *J. Pharm. Sci.*, 85, 725–731.

- Garg, A., Singh, S., Rao, V.U., Bindu, K., Balasubramaniam, J. (2009). Solid state interaction of raloxifene HCl with different hydrophilic carriers during co-grinding and its effect on dissolution rate. *Drug Dev. Ind. Pharm.*, 35, 455–70.
- Garg, R., Gupta, G.D. (2009). Preparation and evaluation of gastroretentive floating tablets of acyclovir. *Curr. Drug Deliv.*, 6, 437–43.
- Gayakwad, S.G., Bejugam, N.K., Akhavein, N., Uddin, N.A., Oettinger, C.E., D'souza, M.J. (2009). Formulation and *in vitro* characterization of spray-dried antisense oligonucleotide to NF-kappa B encapsulated albumin microspheres. *J. Micro-encapsul.*, 26, 692–700.
- Gazzaniga, A., Palugan, L., Foppoli, A., Sangalli, M.E. (2008). Oral pulsatile delivery systems based on swellable hydrophilic polymers. *Eur. J. Pharm. Biopharm.*, 68, 11–8.
- Gibaldi, M., Feldman, S. (1967). Establishment of sink conditions in dissolution rate determinations: Theoretical considerations and application to non-disintegrating dosage forms. *J. Pharm. Sci.*, 56, 1238–1242.
- Gohel, M.C., Parikh, R.K., Nagori, S.A., Jena, D.G. (2009). Fabrication of modified release tablet formulation of metoprolol succinate using hydroxypropyl methylcellulose and xanthan gum. *AAPS PharmSciTech*, 10, 62–8.
- Goldberg, A.H., Higuchi, W.I., Ho, N.F., Zographi, G. (1967). Mechanism of interphase transport. I. Theoretical considerations of diffusion and interfacial barriers in transport of solubilized systems. *J. Pharm. Sci.*, 56, 1432–1437.
- Gonzalez, Y.M., Ghaly, E.S. (2010). Modified drug release of poloxamer matrix by including water-soluble and water-insoluble polymer. *Drug Dev. Ind. Pharm.*, 36, 64–71.
- Grassi, M., Grassi, G. (2005). Mathematical modelling and controlled drug delivery: matrix systems. *Curr. Drug Deliv.*, 2, 97–116.
- Grassi, M., Lapasin, R., Price, S., Colombo, I., Carli, F. (1997). Modelling of drug release from a polymeric matrix. *Proc. Int. Symp. Control Rel. Bioact Mater.*, 48, 503–504.
- Guan, J., Zhou, L., Nie, S., Yan, T., Tang, X., Pan, W. (2010). A novel gastric-resident osmotic pump tablet: *in vitro* and *in vivo* evaluation. *Int. J. Pharm.*, 383, 30–6.
- Gupta, H., Bhandari, D., Sharma, A. (2009). Recent trends in oral drug delivery: a review. *Recent Pat. Drug Deliv. Formul.*, 3, 162–73.
- Harland, R.S., Gazzaniga, A., Sangalli, M.E., Colombo, P., Peppas, N.A. (1988). Drug/polymer matrix swelling and dissolution. *Pharm. Res.*, 5, 488–494.
- Hassan, N., Ali, M., Ali, J. (2010). Novel buccal adhesive system for anti-hypertensive agent Nimodipine. *Pharm. Dev. Technol.*, 15, 124–30.
- Heller, J., Hoffman, A.S. (2004). Drug delivery systems. *In:* Ratner, B.D., Hoffman, A.S., Schoen, F.J. & Lemons, J.E. (Eds.) **Biomaterials Science: An Introduction to Materials in Medicine**. San Francisco, CA, Elsevier Academic Press.
- Heredia, V., Bianco, I.D., Tribulo, H., Tribulo, R., Seoane, M.F., Faudone, S., Cuffini, S.L., Demichelis, N.A., Schalliol, H., Beltramo, D.M. (2009). Polyisoprene matrix for progesterone release: *in vitro* and *in vivo* studies. *Int. J. Pharm.*, 382, 98–103.
- Higuchi, T. (1963). Mechanism of sustained action medication: Theoretical analysis of rate of release of solid drugs dispensed in solid matrices. *J. Pharm. Sci.*, 52, 1145–1149.
- Higuchi, W.I., Hiestand, E.N. (1963). Dissolution rates of finely divided powders. I: Effect of a distribution of particle size in a diffusion-controlled process. *J. Pharm. Sci.*, 52, 67–71.
- Hiremath, P.S., Saha, R.N. (2008). Oral matrix tablet formulations for concomitant controlled release of anti-tubercular drugs: design and *in vitro* evaluations. *Int. J. Pharm.*, 362, 118–25.
- Hixson, A.W., Crowell, J.H. (1931). Dependence of reaction velocity upon surface and agitation: Theoretical consideration. *Ind. Eng. Chem.*, 23, 923–931.
- Hurtado, P.M., Vargas Alvarado, Y., Dominguez-Ramirez, A.M., Cortes Arroyo, A.R. (2003). Comparison of dissolution profiles for albendazole tablets using USP apparatus 2 and 4. *Drug Dev. Ind. Pharm.*, 29, 777–84.
- Jiang, P.J., Patel, S., Gbureck, U., Caley, R., Grover, L.M. (2010). Comparing the efficacy of three bioceramic matrices for the release of vancomycin hydrochloride. *J. Biomed. Mater. Res. B. Appl. Biomater.*, 93, 51–8.
- Johannes, L.T., Mikael Laaksonen, H., Tapio Hirvonen, J., Murtomaki, L. (2009). Cellular

automata model for drug release from binary matrix and reservoir polymeric devices. *Biomaterials*, 30, 1978–87.

- Kamenska, E., Kostova, B., Ivanov, I., Rachev, D., Georgiev, G. (2009). Synthesis and characterization of Zwitterionic co-polymers as matrices for sustained metoprolol tartrate delivery. *J. Biomater. Sci. Polym. Ed.*, 20, 181–97.
- Karasulu, H.Y., Ertan, G., Kose, T. (2000). Modelling of theophylline release from different geometrical erodible tablets. *Eur. J. Pharm. Biopharm.*, 49, 177–182.
- Khan, K.A. (1975). The concept of dissolution efficiency. *J. Pharm. Parmacol.*, 27, 48–49.
- Kitazawa, S., Johno, I., Ito, Y., Teramura, S., Okada, J. (1975). Effects of hardness on the disintegration time and the dissolution rate of uncoated caffeine tablets. *J. Pharm. Parmacol.*, 27, 765–770.
- Korsmeyer, R.W., Gurny, R., Doelker, E., Buri, P., Peppas, N.A. (1983a). Mechanism of solute release from porous hydrophilic polymers. *Int. J. Pharm.*, 15, 25–35.
- Korsmeyer, R.W., Gurny, R., Doelker, E., Buri, P., Peppas, N.A. (1983b). Mechanisms of potassium chloride release from compressed hydrophilic, polymeric matrices: Effect of entrapped air. *J. Pharm. Sci.*, 72, 1189–1191.
- Korsmeyer, R.W., Peppas, N.A. (1983). Macromolecular and modelling aspects of swelling-controlled systems. *In:* Roseman, T.J. & Mandsorf, S.Z. (Eds.) **Controlled Release Delivery Systems**. New York, Marcel Dekker.
- Kumar, P., Singh, S., Mishra, B. (2009). Development and evaluation of elementary osmotic pump of highly water soluble drug: tramadol hydrochloride. *Curr. Drug Deliv.*, 6, 130–9.
- Langenbucher, F. (1972). Linearization of dissolution rate curves by the Weibull distribution. *J. Pharm. Pharmacol.*, 24, 979–981.
- Langer, R., Peppas, N.A. (1983). Chemical and physical structure of polymers as carriers for controlled drug delivery of bioactive agents: A review. *J. Macromol. Sci.*, 23, 61–126.
- Langer, R. (1980). Polymeric delivery systems for controlled drug release. *Chem. Engg. Commun.*, 6, 1–48.
- Lee, T.W.-Y., Robinson, J.R. (2000). Controlled release drug delivery systems. *In:* Gennaro, A.R.

(Ed.) Remington: **The Science and Practice of Pharmacy**. 20th ed. Philadelphia, Lippincott Williams & Wilkinson.

- Li, F., Wang, Y., Liu, Z., Lin, X., He, H., Tang, X. (2010). Formulation and characterization of bufadienolides-loaded nanostructured lipid carriers. *Drug Dev. Ind. Pharm.*, 36, 508–17.
- Liu, J.P., Ma, M.C., Chow, S.C. (1997). Statistical evaluation of similarity factor f_2 as a criterion for assessment of similarity between dissolution profiles. *Drug Inf. J.*, 31, 1255–1271.
- Liu, Y., Zhang, P., Feng, N.P., Zhang, X., Xu, J. (2008). Release kinetics of oridonin self-microemulsifying drug delivery system *in vitro*. *Zhongguo Zhong Yao Za Zhi*, 33, 2049–52.
- Lo, J.B., Appel, L.E., Herbig, S.M., Mccray, S.B., Thombre, A.G. (2009). Formulation design and pharmaceutical development of a novel controlled release form of azithromycin for single-dose therapy. *Drug Dev. Ind. Pharm.*, 35, 1522–9.
- Lu, D.R., Abu-Izza, K., Mao, F. (1996). Non-linear data fitting for controlled release devices: An integrated computer program. *Int. J. Pharm.*, 129, 243–251.
- Lu, Z., Chen, W., Hamman, J.H. (2010). Chitosan-polycarbophil interpolyelectrolyte complex as a matrix former for controlled release of poorly water-soluble drugs. I: *in vitro* evaluation. *Drug Dev. Ind. Pharm.*, 36, 539–46.
- Ma, M.C., Wang, B.B., Liu, J.P., Tsong, Y. (2000). Assessment of similarity between dissolution profiles. *J. Biopharm. Stat.*, 10, 229–249.
- Maggio, R.M., Castellano, P.M., Kaufman, T.S. (2008). A new principal component analysis-based approach for testing "similarity" of drug dissolution profiles. *Eur. J. Pharm. Sci.*, 34, 66–77.
- Mittal, A., Parmar, S., Singh, B. (2009a). *In vitro* and *in vivo* assessment of matrix type transdermal therapeutic system of labetalol hydrochloride. *Curr. Drug Deliv.*, 6, 511–9.
- Mittal, A., Sara, U.V., Ali, A. (2009b). Formulation and evaluation of monolithic matrix polymer films for transdermal delivery of nitrendipine. *Acta Pharm.*, 59, 383–93.
- Moore, J.W., Flanner, H.H. (1996). Mathematical comparison of dissolution profiles. *Pharm. Tech.*, 19, 64–74.
- Nagaraju, R., Meera, D.S., Kaza, R., Arvind, V.V., Venkateswarlu, V. (2009). Core-in-cup tablet

design of metoprolol succinate and its evaluation for controlled release. *Curr. Drug Discov. Technol.*, 6, 299–305.

- Nagda, C., Chotai, N.P., Patel, U., Patel, S., Soni, T., Patel, P., Hingorani, L. (2009). Preparation and characterization of spray-dried mucoadhesive microspheres of aceclofenac. *Drug Dev. Ind. Pharm.*, 35, 1155–66.
- Nahar, M., Jain, N.K. (2011). Conrolled and novel drug delivery systems. *In:* Jain, N.K. (Ed.) **Pharmaceutical Product Development**. CBS Publishers & Distributors, New Delhi.
- Narasimhan, B. (2001). Mathematical models describing polymer dissolution: Consequences for drug delivery. *Adv. Drug Del. Rev.*, 48, 195–201.
- Nernst, W. (1904). Theorie de reaktions geschwindigkeit in heterogenen systemen. *Z. Phyik Chem.*, 47, 52–55.
- Niebergall, P.J., Milosovich, G., Goyan, J.E. (1963). Dissolution rate studies. II: Dissolution of particles under conditions of rapid agitation. *J. Pharm. Sci.*, 52, 236–241.
- Nokhodchi, A., Momin, M.N., Shokri, J., Shahsavari, M., Rashidi, P.A. (2008). Factors affecting the release of nifedipine from a swellable elementary osmotic pump. *Drug Deliv.*, 15, 43–8.
- Noyes, A.A., Whitney, W.R. (1897a). The rate of solution of solid substances in their own solutions. *J. Am. Chem. Soc.*, 19, 930–934.
- Noyes, A.A., Whitney, W.R. (1897b). Uber die auflosungs geswindigkeit festen stiffen in inhren eigning losungen. *Z. Physik Chem.*, 23, 684–692.
- Olkkola, K.T., Hagelberg, N.M. (2009). Oxycodone: new 'old' drug. *Curr. Opin. Anaesthesiol.*, 22, 459–62.
- Papadopoulou, V., Kosmidis, K., Vlachou, M., Macheras, P. (2006). On the use of the Weibull function for the discernment of drug release mechanisms. *Int. J. Pharm.*, 309, 44–50. Epub 2005 Dec 20.
- Pascoal, A.D.S.M.R., Da Silva, P.M., Coelho Pinheiro, M.N. (2015). Drug dissolution profiles from polymeric matrices: Data versus numerical solution of the diffusion problem and kinetic models. *Int. Comm. Heat and Mass Transfer*, 61, 118–127.
- Peppas, N.A. (1985). Analysis of Fickian and non-Fickian drug release from polymers. *Pharm. Acta Helv.*, 60, 110–111.

- Peppas, N.A., Bures, P., Leobundung, W., Ichikawa, H. (2000). Hydrogels in pharmaceutical formulations. *Eur. J. Pharm. Biopharm.*, 40, 223–234.
- Peppas, N.A., Franson, N.M. (1983). The swelling interface number as a criterion for prediction of diffusional solute release mechanism in swellable polymers. *J. Polym. Sci. Phys. Ed.*, 21, 983–997.
- Peppas, N.A., Narasimhan, B. (2014). Mathematical models in drug delivery: How modelling has shaped the way we design new drug delivery systems. *J. Control Release*, 190, 75–81.
- Peppas, N.A., Sahlin, J.J. (1989). A simple equation for the description of solute release. (III): Coupling of diffusion and relaxation. *Int. J. Pharm.*, 57, 169–172.
- Phaechamud, T. (2008). Variables influencing drug release from layered matrix system comprising hydroxypropyl methylcellulose. *AAPS PharmSciTech*, 9, 668–74.
- Pillai, O., Dhanikula, A.B., Panchagnula, R. (2001). Drug delivery: an odyssey of 100 years. *Curr. Opin. Chem. Biol.*, 5, 439–46.
- Pillay, V., Fassihi, R. (1999). Unconventional dissolution methodologies. *J. Pharm. Sci.*, 88, 843–851.
- Podczek, F. (1993). Comparison of *in vitro* dissolution profiles by calculating mean dissolution time (MDT) or mean residence time (MRT). *Int. J. Pharm.*, 97, 93–100.
- Polli, J.E., Rekhi, G.S., Shah, V.P. (1996). Methods to compare dissolution profiles. *Drug Inf. J.*, 30, 1113–1120.
- Rescigno, A. (1992). Bioequivalence. *Pharm. Res.*, 9, 925–928.
- Rinaki, E., Valsami, G., Macheras, P. (2003). The power law can describe the entire drug release from HPMC-based matrix tablets: A hypothesis. *Int. J. Pharm.*, 255, 199–207.
- Ritger, P.L., Peppas, N.A. (1987a). A simple equation for description of solute release. I: Polymers in Fickian and non-Fickian release from non-swellable devices in the form of spheres, cylinders or discs. *J. Control Release*, 5, 23–36.
- Ritger, P.L., Peppas, N.A. (1987b). A simple equation for description of solute release. II: Fickian and anomalous release from swellable devices. *J. Control Release*, 5, 37–42.

- Ritschel, W.A. (1989). Biopharmaceutics and pharmacokinetic aspects in the design of controlled release peroral drug delivery systems. *Drug Dev. Ind. Pharm.*, 15, 1073–1103.
- Robinson, J.R., Lee, V.H.L. (1987). **Controlled Drug Delivery: Fundamentals and Applications**, New York, Marcel Dekker.
- Ruozi, B., Veratti, P., Vandelli M.A., Tombesi, A., Tonelli, M., Forni F., Pederzoli, F., Belletti, D., Tosi, G. (2017). Apoferritin nanocage as strepto-mycin drug reservoir: Technological optimization of a new drug delivery system. *Int. J. Pharm.*, 518, 281–288.
- Salsa, T., Veiga, F., Pina, M.E. (1997). Oral controlled release dosage forms. (I): Cellulose ether hydrophilic matrices. *Drug Dev. Ind. Pharm.*, 23, 929–938.
- Sande, S.A., Karlsen, J. (1989). Curve fitting of dissolution data by personal computer. *Int. J. Pharm.*, 55, 193–198.
- Sangoia, M.S., Todeschinia, V., Stepp, M. (2014). Monolithic LC method applied to fesoterodine fumarate low dose extended-release tablets: Dissolution and release kinetics. *J. Pharm. Anal.*, In Press.
- Saradansa, H. (2001). Defining similarity of dissolution profiles through Hotelling's T^2 statistics. *Pharm. Tech.*, 24, 46–54.
- Sathe, P.M., Tsong, Y., Shah, V.P. (1996). *In vitro* dissolution profile comparison: Statistics and analysis. Model-dependent approach. *Pharm. Res.*, 13, 1799–1803.
- Schwartz, J.B., Simonelli, A.P., Higuchi, W. (1968). Drug release from wax matrices: Analysis of data with first-order kinetics and with diffusion-controlled model. *J. Pharm. Sci.*, 57, 274–277.
- Shah, V.P., Tsong, Y., Sathe, P.M., Williams, R.L. (1998a). Dissolution profile comparison using similarity factor, f_2. *Dissolution Technol.*, 6, 15.
- Shah, V.P., Tsong, Y., Sathe, P.M., Liu, J.P. (1998b). *In vitro* dissolution profile comparison: Statistics and analysis of the similarity factor f_2. *Pharm. Res.*, 15, 889–896.
- Siepmann, J., Gopferich, A. (2001). Mathematical modelling of bioerodible, polymeric drug delivery systems. *Adv. Drug Del. Rev.*, 48, 229–247.
- Siepmann, J., Streubel, A., Peppas, N.A. (2002). Understanding and predicting drug delivery using the sequential layer model from hydrophilic matrix tablets. *Pharm. Res.*, 19, 306–314.
- Singh, B., Arora, S., Singh, R. (2007a). Osmotically controlled oral drug delivery systems. *Pharma Buzz*, 2, 20–28.
- Singh, B., Chakkal, S.K., Dhiman, A. (2003a). Osmotically controlled drug delivery systems: Need of the hour. Part I: Basic concepts. *Express Pharma Pulse*, 9, 2–3.
- Singh, B., Chakkal, S.K., Dhiman, A. (2003b). Osmotically controlled drug delivery systems: Need of the hour. Part II: Technology. *Express Pharma Pulse*, 9, 25–26.
- Singh, B., Kaur, T., Singh, S. (1997). Correction of raw dissolution data for loss of drug during sampling. *Indian J. Pharm. Sci.*, 59, 196–199.
- Singh, B., Pahuja, S., Kapil, R., Ahuja, N. (2009). Formulation development of oral controlled release tablets of hydralazine: optimization of drug release and bioadhesive characteristics. *Acta Pharm.*, 59, 1–13.
- Singh, B., Rani, A., Ahuja, N., Dhar, D., Arora, S. (2007b). Development and Optimization of Hydro-dynamically Balanced Gastroretentive Drug Delivery Systems of Tramadol Hydrochloride, *Proc. 1st Chandigarh Science Congress on Science and Technology for the Emerging Needs of Society,* Panjab University, 10–11 March, Abstract No. 251.
- Singh, B., Singh, S. (1998). A comprehensive computer program for study of drug release kinetics from compressed matrices. *Indian J. Pharm. Sci.*, 60, 313–316.
- Su, Z., Sun, F., Shi, Y., Jiang, C., Meng, Q., Teng, L., Li, Y. (2009). Effects of formulation parameters on encapsulation efficiency and release behavior of risperidone poly(D,L-lactide-co-glycolide) microsphere. *Chem. Pharm. Bull.* (Tokyo), 57, 1251–6.
- Suja-Areevath, J., Munday, D.L., Cox, P.J. (1998). Relationship between swelling, erosion and drug release in hydrophilic natural gum mini-matrix formulations. *Eur. J. Pharm. Sci.*, 6, 207–217.
- Tae, H.K., Shin, S., Bulitt, J.B., Youn,Y.S., Yoo, S.D., Shin, B.S. (2017). Development of a physiologically relevant population pharmaco-kinetic *in vitro–in vivo* correlation approach for designing extended-release oral dosage formulation. *Mol. Pharmaceutics*,14, 53–65
- Tahara, K., Yamamoto, K., Nishihata, T. (1995). Overall mechanism behind matrix sustained release tablets prepared from hydroxypropyl methyl-cellulose 2910. *J. Control Release*, 25, 59–66.

- Takahara, J., Takayama, K., Nagai, T. (1997). Multi-objective simultaneous optimization technique based on an artificial neural network in sustained release formulations. *J. Controlled Release*, 49, 11–20.
- Takayama, K., Fujikawa, M., Nagai, T. (1999). Artificial neural network as a novel method to optimize pharmaceutical formulations. *Pharm. Res.*, 16, 1–6.
- Tang, Y., Zhou, W., He, F., Liu, C., Yang, D. (2009). Release mechanism of huperzine-A swelling sustained-release tablets. *Zhongguo Zhong Yao Za Zhi*, 34, 1795–8.
- Tsong, Y., Hammerstrom, T., Chen, J.J. (1997). Multipoint dissolution specification and acceptance sampling rule based on profile modelling and principal component analysis. *J. Biopharm. Stat.*, 7, 423–39.
- Tsong, Y., Sathe, P.M., Shah, V.P. (2003). *In vitro* dissolution profile comparison. **Encyclopedia of Biopharmaceutical Statistics**.
- Varma, M.V.S., Kaushal, A.M., Garg, A., Garg, S. (2004). Factors affecting mechanism and kinetics of drug release from matrix-based oral controlled drug delivery systems. *Am. J. Drug Deliv.*, 2, 43–57.
- Veng-Pedersen, P., Gobburu, J.V., Meyer, M.C., Straughn, A.B. (2000). Carbamazepine level-A *in vivo-in vitro* correlation (IVIVC): a scaled convolution based predictive approach. *Biopharm. Drug Dispos.*, 21, 1–6.
- Veng-Pedersen, P., Brown, K.F. (1976). Experimental evaluations of three single particle dissolution models. *J. Pharm. Sci.*, 65, 1442–1447.
- Verma, R.K., Krishna, D.M., Garg, S. (2002). Formulation aspects in the development of osmotically controlled oral drug delivery systems. *J. Control Release*, 79, 7–27.
- Vigoreaux, V., Ghaly, E.S. (1994). Fickian and relaxational contribution quantification of drug release in a swellable hydrophillic polymer matrix. *Drug Dev. Ind. Pharm.*, 20, 2519–2526.
- Von Orelli, J., Leuenberger, H. (2004). Search for technological reasons to develop a capsule or a tablet formulation with respect to wettability and dissolution. *Int. J. Pharm.*, 287, 135–45.
- Wagner, J.G. (1959). Sustained action oral medication. II: The kinetics of release of drug *in vitro*. *Drug Standards*, 27, 178–186.
- Wagner, J.G. (1969). Interpretation of percent dissolved-time plots derived from *in vitro* testing of conventional tablets and capsules. *J. Pharm. Sci.*, 58, 1253–1257.
- Wahlgren, M., Christensen, K.L., Jorgensen, E.V., Svensson, A., Ulvenlund, S. (2009). Oral-based controlled release formulations using poly(acrylic acid) microgels. *Drug Dev. Ind. Pharm.*, 35, 922–9.
- Wang, W., Xie, X., Yang, D., Chen, X. (2009). Swelling property of common hydrophilic polymers and their use in push-pull osmotic-pump tablets. *Zhongguo Zhong Yao Za Zhi*, 34, 2319–21.
- Weibull, W. (1951). Statistical distribution function of wide applicability. *J. Appl. Mech.*, 18.
- Weiser, J.R., Saltzman, W.M. (2014). Controlled release for local delivery of drugs: barriers and models. *J. Controlled Release*, 190, 664–673.
- Weiss, M. (2015) Modelling accelerated and decelerated drug release in terms of fractional release rate. *Eur. J. Pharm. Sci.*, 68, 51–55.
- Weiss, M., Kriangkrai, W., Sungthongjeen, S. (2014). An empirical model for dissolution profile and its application to floating dosage forms. *Eur. J. Pharm. Biopharm.*, 56, 87–91.
- Wignand, R.G., Taylor, J.D. (1959). Exponential expression for *in vitro* release of drug from sustained release preparations. *Drug Standards*, 27, 165–171.
- Yakubu, R., Peh, K.K., Tan, Y.T. (2009). Design of a 24-hour controlled porosity osmotic pump system containing PVP: formulation variables. *Drug Dev. Ind. Pharm.*, 35, 1430–8.
- Yuksel, N., Kanik, A.E., Baykara, T. (2000). Comparison of *in vitro* dissolution profiles by ANOVA-based, model-dependent and -independent methods. *Int. J. Pharm.*, 209, 57–67.
- Zhao, L., Yang, X., Xu, R., Wu, J., Gu, S., Zhang, L., Gong, P., Chen, H., Zeng, F. (2009). Safety, tolerability and pharmacokinetics of phenoprolamine hydrochloride floating sustained-release tablets in healthy Chinese subjects. *Int. J. Pharm.*, 377, 99–104.
- Zugasti, M.E., Zornoza, A., Goni Mdel, M., Isasi, J. R., Velaz, I., Martin, C., Sanchez, M., Martinez-Oharriz, M.C. (2009). Influence of soluble and insoluble cyclodextrin polymers on drug release from hydroxypropyl methylcellulose tablets. *Drug Dev. Ind. Pharm.*, 35, 1264–70.

13

In Vitro/In Vivo Correlations (IVIVC) As A Vital Tool in Pharmaceutical Product Development and Federal Biowaivers

Bhupinder Singh, Sumant Saini, Sarwar Beg,
Ranjot Kaur and Rajneet Kaur Khurana

INTRODUCTION

Despite the tremendous strides in the field of diverse non-oral drug delivery systems, most of the pharmaceutical products in the commercial circulation are meant only for oral intake owing to apparent benefits of better patient compliance and safety, low cost and ease of manufacturing. Development of such oral drug products and their subsequent regulatory approval is a fastidious process (Singh, 2012). As per the federal requirements, all oral pharmaceutical products need to be thoroughly evaluated for their *in vivo* bioavailability, whether immediate release or extended release. The manufacturers have to evaluate the efficacy of formulations employing bioavailability studies through oral route to establish the theoretical drug release profile for the formulations based on the desired plasma level-drug profile. The manufacturers must submit a detailed report on the bio-availability studies performed for comparing their products with the reference product. Among the multiple quality traits demanded by the federal regulatory agencies to evaluate the product performance and therapeutic capability of the test formulations, the bioavailability-bioequivalence (BA-BE) studies remain the most vital prerequisite and requisite parameters for approval (Singh et al., 2010a; Singh and Beg, 2012). Demonstration of bioequivalence for any generic product compared to the reference listed drug (RLD) product being mandatory regulatory prerequisite within the acceptable limits, the manufacturers have to essentially undertake the comprehensive *in vivo* human bioavailability trials under medical supervision.

BIOAVAILABILITY AND BIOEQUIVALENCE ISSUES

For the first time, it was Oser and coworkers (1945) who described the concept of oral bio-availability as physiological availability of the drugs in the systemic milieu. Ideally, it reflects the concentration of active moiety in the biological fluids, and measurement of both true rate and total amount of drug that reaches the systemic circulation from an administered dosage form. Thus, bioavailability, in general, determines the therapeutic effectiveness of a drug, which further depends upon the ability of the dosage form to deliver the medicament to the desired site of action to obtain the desired pharmacodynamic response (Dressman and Lennernas, 2000). As per the USFDA, bioavailability of drug is a function of "rate and extent at which the drug reaches into the systemic circulation". This definition is most widely accepted and used globally.

Comparing the drug bioavailability by various routes of administration, it is found to be higher with the parenteral route, followed by the most popular oral route, whereas the topical route displays minimum bioavailability. Orally administered drugs pass through the intestinal wall and enter into the liver through portal vein where first-pass metabolism of the drug takes place, eventually leading to reduced bioavailability. Fig. 13.1 depicts the biofate of the drugs upon oral administration involving various physiological processes.

The rate and extent to which drug molecules absorb into the systemic circulation ultimately affect the bioavailability of drugs and their elicited pharmacodynamic response. Fig. 13.2 pictographically portrays the effect of different rates and extent of absorption on oral bioavailability of drugs. The inset (Fig. 13.2) clearly explains that if the rate of absorption is very slow (case B), the levels may not be pharmaco-

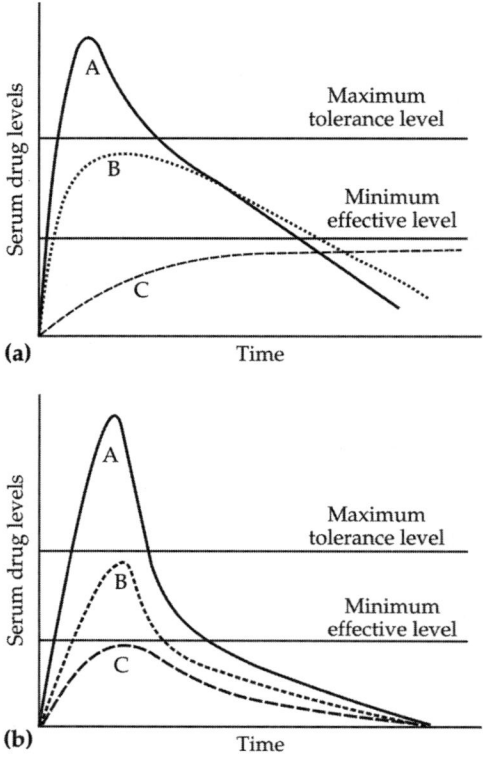

Fig. 13.2. Pictographic illustration of serum drug levels of three different formulations with (a) same extent but different rate of absorption; and (b) same rate but different extent of absorption.

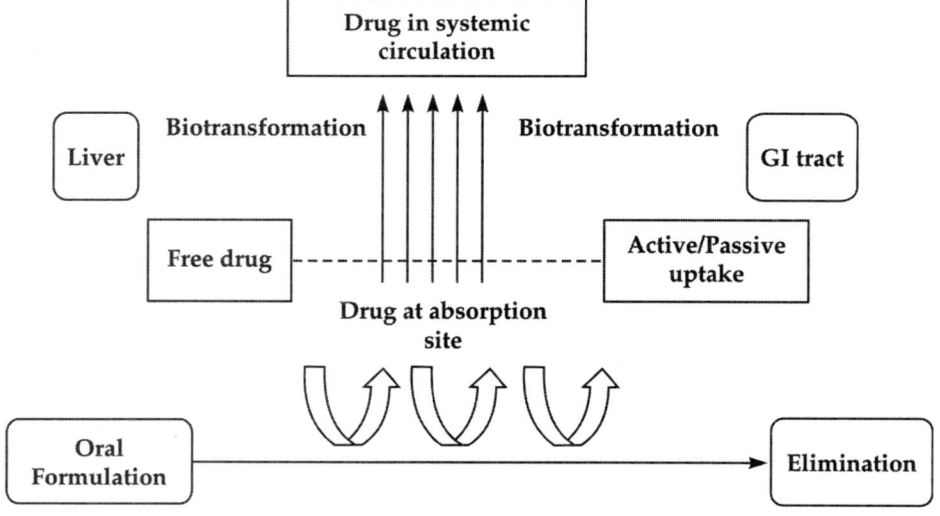

Fig. 13.1. Various factors limiting oral absorption of many drugs.

dynamically productive, as the minimum effective level is not reached. Further, extremely fast absorption (case C) also, at times, is unwelcome, as the levels are likely to cross minimum toxic level and exhibit signs of drug overdosage. Hence, a plasma concentration time profile should behave in an ideal manner, with moderate fast absorption rate (case A). Herein, in case A, the levels tend to remain in the therapeutic window for a sizable duration, thus attaining optimal therapeutic effects with minimal toxicity. The extent of absorption, on the other hand, is usually more important factor for the drugs that are administered repetitively for the treatment of only chronic conditions, such as infection, asthma, arthritis, diabetes, hypertension or epilepsy.

Thus, by and large, bioavailability of a drug from its respective drug formulation is controlled by three principal factors, namely:

1. Rate and extent of release of the drug from the dosage form;
2. Subsequent absorption from the solution state; and
3. Biotransformation during the process of absorption.

Assessment of bioavailability from plasma concentration-time data usually involves determining the maximum plasma drug concentration (C_{max}, peak drug level), the time at which maximum plasma drug concentration occurs (t_{max}, peak time), and the area under the plasma concentration-time curve (AUC). C_{max}, t_{max} and AUC are the three indispensible parameters, which provide clairvoyant understanding of the plasma level time data.

The plasma drug concentration increases with the extent of absorption and the C_{max} is reached when elimination rate of drug equals its absorption rate. Nevertheless, bioavailability determinations based on the C_{max} values can be misleading, as drug elimination begins as soon as the drug enters the bloodstream. The most widely used general index of absorption rate is

t_{max}; the slower the absorption, the later the t_{max}. However, t_{max} is often not a good biopharmaceutical measure, as it is a discrete value depending upon frequency of blood sampling and, in case of relatively flat concentrations near the peak, depends on assay reproducibility. The C_{max}/AUC metric is also employed to indicate rate of absorption. AUC is the most reliable measure of bioavailability. It is directly proportional to the total amount of unchanged drug that reaches the systemic circulation. For an accurate measurement, blood must be sampled frequently over a long enough time period to observe virtually complete drug elimination. Drug products may be considered bioequivalent in extent and rate of absorption, if their plasma level curves are essentially superimposable. Drug products that exhibit similar AUC values but differently shaped plasma level curves are equivalent in extent but differ in their absorption rate-time profiles. Nevertheless, for the drugs with long biological half-life, it is rather impractical and uneconomical to determine the total AUC. The promising concept of partial area analysis, that compares the AUC until the t_{max} of the reference formulation vis-à-vis the test formulation, comes to the rescue in such cases (Sakore and Chakraborty, 2011).

STATISTICAL APPROACHES FOR BIOEQUIVALENCE

The general objective in assessing bioequivalence is to compare the log-transformed bioavailability measure after administration of the T (test) and R (reference) products. The values and distribution among various subject groups of pharmacokinetic parameters in terms of rate and extent of drug absorption like AUC and C_{max} tend to involve vital metrics as **average bioequivalence**, **individual bioequivalence** and **population bioequivalence**. In this regard, the population and individual approaches are based upon the comparison of an expected squared distance between the T and R formulations to the expected squared distance between two of the R formulations. An acceptable T formulation, therefore, is the one where the T-R distance is not substantially greater than the R-R distance. In both of these population and individual bioequivalence approaches, this comparison appears as a comparison to the reference variance, referred to as "scaling to the reference variability".

Among these three bioequivalence metrics, most federal agencies require average bioequivalence as the obligatory requirement for regulatory approval of drug products which tends to compare population mean between the test and reference products. Bioequivalence is usually claimed if the ratio of average bioequivalence between test and reference products is within 80 to 125% with 90% assurance (log-transformed data). However, average bioequivalence has several limitations as it focuses only on population mean, ignoring the distribution of metrics and subject by formulation interaction. To circumvent such limitations, individual bioequivalence has lately been proposed by USFDA as an improvement on the study design, informativeness and method of analysis used in the bioequivalence studies. Population bioequivalence, a relatively newer paradigm with limited federal acceptance, takes into account the population means and variances in logarithmic scale.

Besides selection of right method for establishment of bioequivalence, one of the major problems encountered during bioavailability studies is high variability in results within the same dosage form. This variability may be due to differences in treatments, intra- and/or inter-subject variations, environment-related differences in the subject population, and the subjects within a population or residuals error, which cannot be ascribed to any of aforesaid variability. To alleviate the hassles of variability, experiments have to be statistically designed in such a manner that one may be able to analyze the split-up of the total variability to various possible causes. In order to have a perfect prediction of bioequivalence, decision rules are the valuable analytical tools based on the truth tables. True bioavailability results have to be arrived accurately and casualness can let the manufacturer and/or consumer patient suffer as is indicated in the truth table (Table 13.1).

BIOWAIVERS: NEED OF THE HOUR

Generic drugs are considered as the customized preparations comparable to their branded counterparts in dosage form, strength, quality, efficacy, performance, intended use, and above all, in BA-BE studies (i.e., biostudies). All the generic drug formulations intended to reach the market need to demonstrate bioequivalence with the corresponding innovator's reference product(s). Establishment of bioequivalence through biostudies in humans is usually a colossal task, involving numerous difficulties, some of which are enlisted in Box 13.1. In order to demonstrate therapeutic equivalence, one must satiate the desirable clinical attributes of *prescribability*, i.e., physician's choice for prescribing an appropriate

Table 13.1. Truth table for declaring bioequivalence during BA-BE studies

Arrived outcome	Existing truth	
	Bioequivalent	**Bioinequivalent**
Bioequivalent	Correct decision Everybody gains	Incorrect decision Consumer loses
Bioinequivalent	Incorrect decision Manufacturer loses	Correct decision Consumer gains

Box 13.1. Major hitches involved during bio-studies in human

- Highly expensive
- Quite time-consuming
- Involvement of usually large number of normal, healthy, adult, drug-free and overnight-fasted human subjects
- Mandatory federal compliance· Inaccessibility of sophisticated analytical methodology
- Scarcity of pharmacokinetic expertise
- Non-availability of pharmacokinetic software tools
- Intricacies of biopharmaceutical and statistical data analysis
- Involvement of numerous ethical issues
- Mandatory medical intervention

drug product between the brand-name product and its generic copies, *switchability*, i.e., switching from one drug product (e.g., a brand-name product) to another (e.g., a generic product) within the same patient, and *interchangeability*, i.e., to exhibit pharmaceutical equivalence and bioequivalence between more than one product for generic substation (Singh and Beg, 2012).

Taking USFDA as the pivotal regulatory agency, waiver from a biostudy (i.e., biowaiver) can be granted for special categories of drug product as:

- A parenteral solution intended solely for administration by injection, or an ophthalmic or otic solution containing the same active and inactive ingredients in the same concentration as a drug product that is the subject of an approved full NDA or ANDA.

- Administered by inhalation as a gas, e.g., a medicinal or an inhalation anaesthetic; and contains an active ingredient in the same dosage form as a drug product that is the subject of an approved full NDA or abbreviated NDA.

- A solution intended for application to the skin, or a solution, elixir, syrup, tincture for external application.

- A solution for aerosolization or nebulization through oral and nasal route.

For drugs or drug formulations, not falling in any of the above-mentioned categories, bio-equivalence studies are mandatory from federal perspectives. Accordingly, every pharma house endeavors to circumnavigate these hitches by seeking respite in the requisite biowaivers. And to accomplish the said task, a biopharmaceutical scientist invariably draws the maximum out of the most valuable tools like Biopharmaceutics Classification System (BCS) and *In vitro/In vivo* Correlations (IVIVC) (Singh et al., 2010b).

BIOPHARMACEUTICS CLASSIFICATION SYSTEM (BCS)

The BCS is a scientific framework for classifying a drug substance based on its aqueous solubility and intestinal permeability. When combined with the *in vitro* dissolution characteristics of the drug product, the BCS takes into account three major factors such as solubility, permeability and dissolution rate.

A classification of drugs based on the above mentioned criteria as per the BCS is shown in Fig. 13.3.

Fig. 13.4 depicts the sequential events associated with oral administration of solid dosage forms including drug dissolution in the GI (gastrointestinal) tract, absorption into the systemic circulation, and transit of unabsorbed fraction. Thus, in order to be absorbed into systemic circulation, the drug(s) must be hydrophilic enough to be dissolved (i.e., soluble), yet lipophilic enough to get across the GI membrane (i.e., permeable). The drug in the dosage form is released and dissolved in the surrounding GI fluid to form a solution. Once the drug reaches into the solution form, it passes across the membranes of the GI tract. Then onwards, the drug is absorbed into systemic circulation (Singh et al., 2010b).

Thus, solubility, dissolution and permeability are considered as the rate-limiting factors for governing the biopharmaceutical performance of the drugs. Fig. 13.5 pictorially illustrates the significance of solubility, permeability and

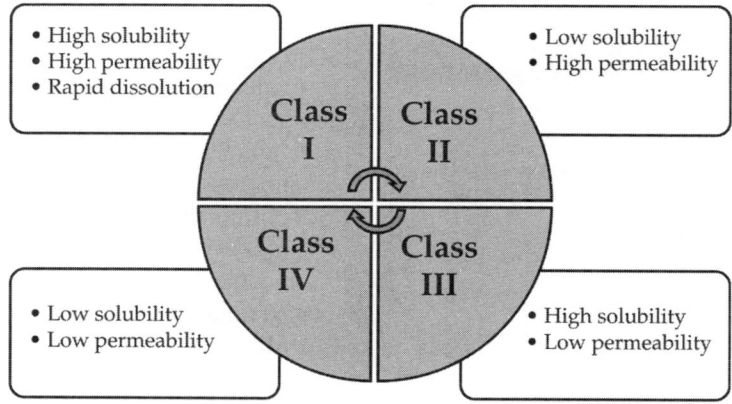

Fig. 13.3. Overview of Biopharmaceutical Classification System (BCS).

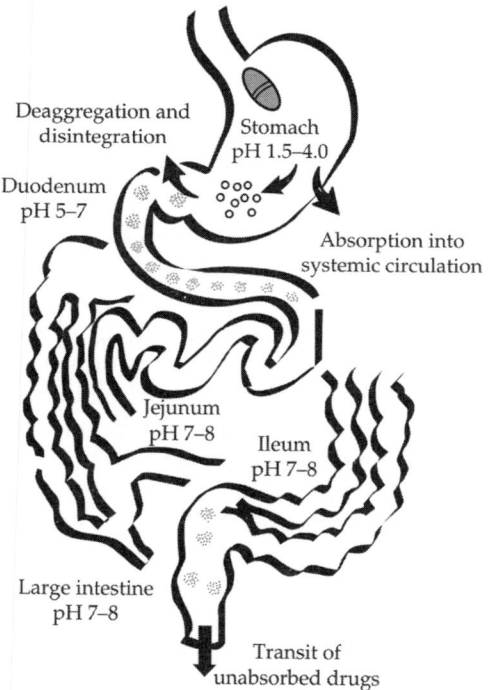

Fig. 13.4. Sojourn of a typical oral formulation in human gastrointestinal tract.

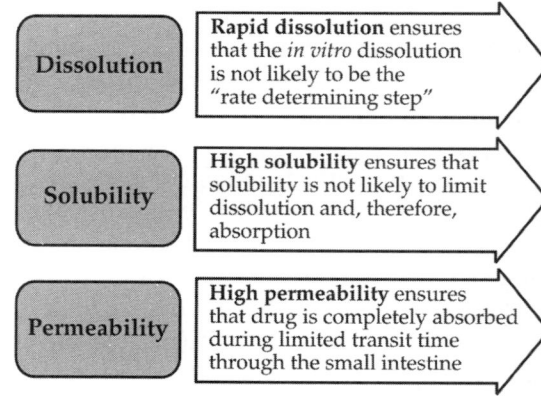

Fig. 13.5. Three vital factors influencing the BCS classification of drugs.

dissolution as the key limiting factors for establishing IVIVC in the light of BCS.

Solubility

The solubility substance may be defined as the amount of substance that has passed into solution when equilibrium is attained between the solution and excess (i.e., undissolved) substance, at a given temperature and pressure. A drug substance is considered "highly soluble" when the highest dose strength is soluble in ≤ 250 ml water over a pH range of 1 to 7.5 wherein the volume estimate of 250 ml is derived from the typical volume of water consumed during the oral administration of dosage form, which is about a glassful, or 8 ounces of water.

The pH-solubility profile of the drug substance is determined at 37 ± 1°C in aqueous medium with pH in the range of 1–7.5. Standard buffer solutions described in pharmacopoeias are considered appropriate for use in solubility studies. The concentration of drug substance in selected buffers or pH conditions should be determined using a validated solubility-indicating assay that can distinguish between the drug substances and their degradation products. If degradation of drug is observed as a function of buffer composition and/or pH, it should also be taken into consideration. A sufficient number of pH conditions should be evaluated to accurately define the pH-solubility profile. The number of pH conditions for a solubility determination depends upon ionization characteristics of the test drug substance. Methods other than shake flask method are used to predict equilibrium solubility of test drug substance.

Permeability

Permeability may be defined as the ability of a drug molecule to permeate through the biological membrane into the systemic circulation. A drug substance is considered "highly permeable" when the extent of absorption in humans is determined to be ≥ 90% of an administered dose, based on mass-balance or in comparison to an intravenous reference dose. A compound may traverse the biological barrier by a variety of routes, i.e., passive transcellular transport, paracellular route or a carrier-mediated transmembrane transport. The methods that are routinely used for determination of permeability include *in vivo* or *in situ* intestinal perfusion in a suitable animal model, *in vitro* permeability methods using excised intestinal tissues, monolayer of suitable epithelial cells, e.g., Caco-2 cells or TC-7 cells. Intestinal perfusion models and *in vitro* methods are recommended for passively transported drugs. The observed low permeability of some drug substances in humans could be attributed to the efflux of drug by various membrane transporters like glycoprotein-P. This leads to misinterpretation of the permeability of drug substance. An alternative to intestinal tissue models is the use of well-established *in vitro* systems based on the human adenocarcinoma cell line, i.e., Caco-2 cell lines.

These cell lines serve as a model of small intestinal tissue. The differentiated cells exhibit the microvilli typical of the small intestinal mucosa and the integral membrane proteins of the brush-border enzymes. In addition, they also form the fluid-filled domes typical of a permeable epithelium.

Dissolution

Drug dissolution is the process by virtue of which drug is released, dissolved and becomes available for absorption. It is directly proportional to the solubility of the drug and this can be explained on the basis of a mathematical relationship, proposed by Noyes and Whitney in 1897 (Eq. 1).

$$\frac{dC}{dT} = K(C_s - C_b) \qquad \ldots (1)$$

where, dC/dT is the rate of dissolution, K is the first-order dissolution rate constant, C_s is the concentration of drug in the stagnant water layer (also called as the equilibrium solubility, saturation solubility, or maximum solubility) and C_b is the concentration of drug in the bulk of the solution as a function of time, t. A drug product is considered to be "rapidly dissolving" when ≥ 85% of the labelled amount of drug substance dissolves within 30 minutes using USP apparatus I or II in a volume of ≤ 900 ml buffer solutions (USP, 1995).

Pragmatically, the dissolution rate of a drug can be enhanced by altering its surface area and/or solubility. The diffusion and partition behavior of a drug remaining invariant, all other parameters cannot be significantly influenced looking into the simulation of GI conditions *in vivo*. Whereas the diffusion coefficient is inversely related to medium viscosity, the degree of agitation can diminish the thickness of the diffusion layer and hasten the process of dissolution. Further, it is impossible to modify the film thickness or diffusion coefficient in an *in vivo* environment.

BCS AND DISSOLUTION SPECIFICATIONS

The absorption of drug into systemic circulation depends upon the release of the drug substance from the drug product, the dissolution or solubilization of the drug under physiological conditions, and the permeability across the GI tract, as shown in Fig. 13.6.

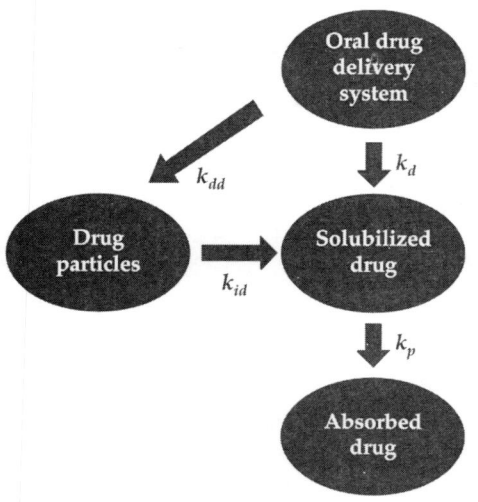

Fig. 13.6. Various steps involved during drug dissolution and absorption of an orally administered drug.

The term "k_d" in Fig. 13.6 represents the dissolution rate and is a function of solubility of drug and nature of the formulation; "k_{dd}" represents disintegration rate and is dependent upon the formulation characteristics; "k_{id}" represents solubilization rate and is dependent on the solubility of API; "k_p" represents permeability rate which depends upon the molecular structure and nature of API and excipients. In case of Class I drugs, both k_d and k_p are high, whereas for Class II and IV drugs, $k_d \gg k_p$. On the other hand, if $k_d \ll k_p$, the absorption of drug becomes dissolution controlled. The dissolution controlled absorption can be intrinsic dissolution controlled if $k_{dd} \gg k_{id}$, and disintegration controlled if $k_{dd} \ll k_{id}$.

An orally administered drug product has to pass through a variety of physiological environments of GI tract before it gets absorbed. BCS, in conjunction with the numerous compendial and physiological media available, can be employed as a fundamental guidance for designing appropriate biorelevant dissolution conditions, leading to a more meaningful prediction of *in vivo* performance.

For Class I drugs, simple and mild aqueous dissolution media, such as SGF without pepsin is suitable, while milk as dissolution medium might be appropriate for specific food/formulation interaction. For neutral Class II drugs, simulated intestinal fluid (SIF) in fasted state (i.e., FaSSIF), reflects the dissolution in the upper GI tract under fasted conditions. If a Class II drug is a weak base, SGF could be used to assess the dissolution of the drug in the stomach under fasted state conditions. To verify the possibility of drug precipitation under intestinal conditions, performing dissolution in FaSSIF may be appropriate. Comparison of dissolution results obtained under pre-prandial (FaSSIF) to that of fed state SIF (i.e., FeSSIF) could be a good indicative of whether the formulation should be administered before or after meals. In case of Class II weak acids, dissolution could be performed in FaSSIF as a suitable representative of intestinal fasted state conditions. Milk with its composition of lipids and proteins or FeSSIF containing high bile salt/lecithin levels can be employed to simulate the fed state conditions (Klein, 2010).

The BCS is associated with drug dissolution and absorption model, which identifies the key parameters controlling drug absorption as a set of dimensionless numbers, namely the absorption number, dissolution time, the dissolution number, dose number, absorbable dose and dose volume. The absorption number (A_n) is the ratio of the mean residence time (T_{res}) to the mean absorption time (T_{abs}), and is calculated as:

$$A_n = \frac{T_{res}}{T_{abs}} = \frac{\dfrac{\pi R^2 L}{Q}}{\dfrac{R}{P_{eff}}} \qquad \ldots (2)$$

Dissolution time (T_{diss}) is the theoretical time taken by a drug particle to dissolve.

$$T_{diss} = \frac{phr_0}{3DC_s} \qquad \ldots (3)$$

The dissolution number (D_n) is a ratio of mean residence time (T_{res}) to mean dissolution time (T_{diss}) and could be estimated as:

$$D_n = \frac{T_{res}}{T_{diss}} = \frac{\dfrac{\pi R^2 L}{Q}}{\dfrac{\rho r_0^2}{3DC_{s\,min}}} \qquad \ldots (4)$$

The dose number (D_0) is the dose divided by an uptake volume of 250 ml and the drug's solubility, expressed as:

$$D_0 = \frac{Dose}{V_0 \times C_{s\,min}} \qquad \ldots (5)$$

Absorbable dose (D_{abs}) is the maximum amount of drug that can be absorbed.

$$D_{abs} = P_{eff} C_s A(T_{si}) \qquad \ldots (6)$$

where, L = tube length, R = tube radius, Q = fluid flow rate, r_0 = initial particle radius, V_0 = gastric volume (250 ml), ρ = particle density, h = thickness of the diffusion layer, P_{eff} = effective permeability, T_{si} = mean small intestine transit time and $C_{s\,min}$ = minimum aqueous solubility in the physiological pH range 1–8. The mean residence time (T_{res}) is the average of residence time in the stomach, small intestine and the colon.

The dose volume (V_{dose}) is the ratio of the amount of dose (M_0) and the drug solubility (C_s)

$$V_{dose} = \frac{M_0}{C_s} \qquad \ldots (7)$$

BIOPHARMACEUTICAL DRUG DISPOSITION CLASSIFICATION SYSTEM (BDDCS)

The concept of BDDCS was initially derived from the observations that the great majority of BCS Class I and II compounds (high permeability) are primarily eliminated by metabolism, whereas the great majority of BCS Class III and IV compounds (low permeability) are primarily eliminated unchanged into the urine and/or bile. In conjunction with the findings of transporter-enzyme interplay from several cellular and animal studies, the BDDCS classifies drug substances into four classes based on their aqueous solubility and extent of metabolism: Class I (high solubility, extensive metabolism), Class II (low solubility, extensive metabolism), Class III (high solubility, poor metabolism) and Class IV (low solubility, poor metabolism) (Fig. 13.7).

BDDCS		
	HIGH SOLUBILITY	LOW SOLUBILITY
EXTENSIVE METABOLISM	**Class 1** Transporter effects minimal	**Class 2** Efflux transporter effects predominate in the gut, while the absorptive and efflux transporter effects occur in the liver
POOR METABOLISM	**Class 3** Absorptive transporter effects predominate (but may be modulated by efflux transporters)	**Class 4** Absorptive and efflux transporter effects could be important

Fig. 13.7. Overview of Biopharmaceutical Drug Disposition Classification System (BDDCS).

The primary purpose of BDDCS was to predict drug disposition of new molecular entities and the importance of transporters in drug absorption and elimination. However, since there appeared to be a very good correlation between high metabolism and high permeability (hence extensive absorption), it has been recommended that the extent of drug metabolism (i.e., ≥ 90% metabolized) be added as an alternative method for the extent of drug absorption (i.e., ≥ 90% absorbed) in defining BCS Class I drugs for biowaivers. This may be rationalized by the lipophilic nature of a number of drugs, which is not only important in facilitating the permeation of these compounds into the intestinal membrane, but also critical in allowing their access to the metabolizing enzymes. Indeed, many drugs with a fair degree of lipophilicity have been found to be highly permeable and also extensively metabolized in the intestine and/or liver. It is noteworthy that the matrix of drug metabolism in BDDCS is limited to the metabolic processes involving CYP450 and Phase 2 enzymes (such as glucuronidation and sulfation) that occur after drug absorption. There may be other enzymes that are not localized in the liver or intestinal mucosa, e.g., hydrolytic enzymes, such as esterases, and gut bacteria that are responsible for reduction of some compounds.

IN VITRO/IN VIVO CORRELATIONS (IVIVC)

The term IVIVC first appeared in pharmaceutical literature as a result of awareness of concept of *in vivo* bioavailability and *in vitro* dissolution rate determination. Verily, an endeavor to relate *in vitro* dissolution and *in vivo* pharmacokinetic results is referred to as IVIVC analysis.

As per United States Pharmacopoeia (USP, 1995), IVIVC is "the establishment of a rational relationship (quantitative) between a biological property (e.g., C_{max}, AUC or t_{max}), or a parameter derived from a biological property produced by a dosage form and a physicochemical property or characteristic of same dosage form (e.g., extent of release at various time points, MDT)". USFDA, however, describes IVIVC as "a predictive mathematical model describing the relationship between an *in vitro* property of a dosage form and a relevant *in vivo* response." Generally, the *in vitro* property is the rate or

extent of drug dissolution or release, while the *in vivo* response parameter is the plasma drug concentration or amount of drug absorbed.

Over past few decades, IVIVC has gained unique importance in pharmaceutical formulation development by providing better insight for predicting the *in vivo* bio-pharmaceutical performance of the product from the *in vitro* drug release data. As time is considered to be a highly important factor during product development, the use of such rational technique is considered to be a vital tool in this direction. Lately, the concept of IVIVC has extensively been discussed by pharmaceutical scientists, particularly for extended release (ER) drug products. The ability to predict the expected bioavailability characteristics accurately and precisely through dissolution profile characteristics is a long sought-after goal of the pharmaceutical scientists. An acceptable IVIVC requires that the *in vitro* dissolution and *in vivo* release or dissolution behavior of a dosage form should be either similar or have a scalable relationship to each other. IVIVC could only be established when the factor controlling the appearance of the drug in the blood flow is linked with the formulation (e.g., sustained release (SR) formulation for Class I drug) or the characteristics of the active pharmaceutical ingredient (e.g., slow dissolution for Class II drug) presented as an immediate release (IR) formulation *in vivo* and not with any physiological limiting factor (for example rate limited permeation). In practice, the formulations with release from the dosage form slower than the dissolution of the drug and marked with high permeability characteristics (SR formulations of Class I and II) are the best candidates. In IVIVC, the pharmacokinetic (PK) absorption or *in vivo* release parameters are related to the *in vitro* dissolution, which reflects a global performance of the drug product.

During IVIVC establishment, variability in dissolution performance reflects the difference in drug release behavior from the drug dosage form plausibly owing to diverse factors such as alteration in the polymer grade or concentration, difference in the physicochemical characteristics of the drug substance or difference in the manufacturing process. When correlation is established and validated, prediction of *in vivo* profile can be made reliably on the basis of *in vitro* dissolution profile.

Significance of IVIVC

The concept of IVIVC has gained tremendous attention recently in pharmaceutical industry, academia, and regulatory sector. It acts as a tool to reliably correlate *in vitro* drug dissolution data and *in vivo* drug absorbed. Such a tool shortens the drug development period, economizes the resources and leads to improved product quality.

The main objective of establishing IVIVC is to facilitate *in vitro* dissolution studies to serve as surrogate for *in vivo* bioequivalence testing, thus supporting biowaiver, especially during scale-up and post-approval changes (SUPAC). Understanding and controlling the relationship between *in vitro* release and *in vivo* response in a compound plays a critical role in development of modified release formulations, generics, fixed dose combination products and drug delivery systems. During the manufacturing and marketing of any therapeutic agent, development and optimization of formulation are integral parts, which are indeed time-consuming and costly procedures. Optimization process may require alteration in formulation composition, manufacturing process, equipment and batch sizes. If these types of changes are applied to a formulation, studies in healthy human volunteers may be required to prove that the new formulation is bioequivalent with the old one. The implementation of these requirements not only halts the marketing of the new formulation but also increases the cost of the optimization processes. A validated IVIVC can be used to predict *in vivo* behavior of the formulation to assess likelihood of success before entering it in a biostudy, thus, eliminating many biostudies that are unnecessary.

With increasing introduction of modified release and novel drug delivery systems, it is obligatory to understand the concept of IVIVC in greater depth. Conducting dissolution analysis with IVIVC is a fast and inexpensive method for obtaining optimal formulations as opposed to slow and expensive bioavailability or bioequivalence studies that provide "hit or miss" results. Earlier the IVIVC is implemented in the drug development process, easier and more cost-effective is its implementation for all the future changes in the formulation. Box 13.2, in a nutshell, summarizes the key advantages of IVIVC in a typical pharmaceutical product development set-up.

Box 13.2. Key advantages of IVIVC

- Bypasses the hassles of biostudies by serving as a surrogate for human bioequivalence studies
- Helps to reduce costs by obviating the need to perform expensive BA/BE human trials
- Speeds up the product development process
- Demonstrates bioequivalence when certain pre-approval changes are made in formulation, equipment, manufacturing process or in manufacturing site
- Improves product quality using more meaningful dissolution specifications
- Reduces "regulatory burden" due to biostudies

IVIVC methodology

A typical IVIVC model tends to involve two essential elements viz. model development and model validation. Developing a predictable IVIVC depends upon the complexity of the delivery system, its formulation composition, method of manufacture, physicochemical properties of the drug and the dissolution method.

Model development

In the process of IVIVC development, the *in vitro* drug release parameters, which resemble *in vivo* drug performance, are identified. The appropriate design of *in vitro* dissolution tests, capable of discriminating between the formulations with different bioavailabilities, plays a major role in the ability of the IVIVC predictability. Therefore, it is essential that *in vitro* dissolution tests closely reflect *in vivo* situations, when they are used to establish an IVIVC. Thus, for all categories, it is anticipated that well-designed dissolution test is a key prognostic tool in the assessment of both, the drug's potential for oral absorption and the bioequivalence of its formulations (Qureshi, 2010).

There could be four different types of federally acceptable correlations, viz. level A, level B, level C and multiple level C, and level D. The concept of correlation level is based upon the ability of the correlation to reflect the complete plasma drug level–time profile which results from administration of given dosage form (FDA Guidance, 1997a & 1997b).

Level A IVIVC

It is considered to be the most useful and popular correlation from regulatory perspectives. It is the highest category of correlation, where a point-to-point correlation exists between the entire *in vitro* dissolution (or drug release) time course and the entire *in vivo* response time course, e.g., the time course of plasma drug concentration or amount of drug absorbed, or *in vivo* dissolution of the drug from the dosage form. This estimation of *in vivo* absorption profile from the concentration-time data can be achieved through the one-stage or two-stage convolution/deconvolution methods employing Wagner-Nelson or Loo-Riegelman approach (Veng-Pederson, 1980). Subsequent to the estimation of *in vivo* absorption profile, the relationship with *in vitro* dissolution is evaluated. An instance of establishing "level A" IVIVC is illustrated in Fig. 13.8.

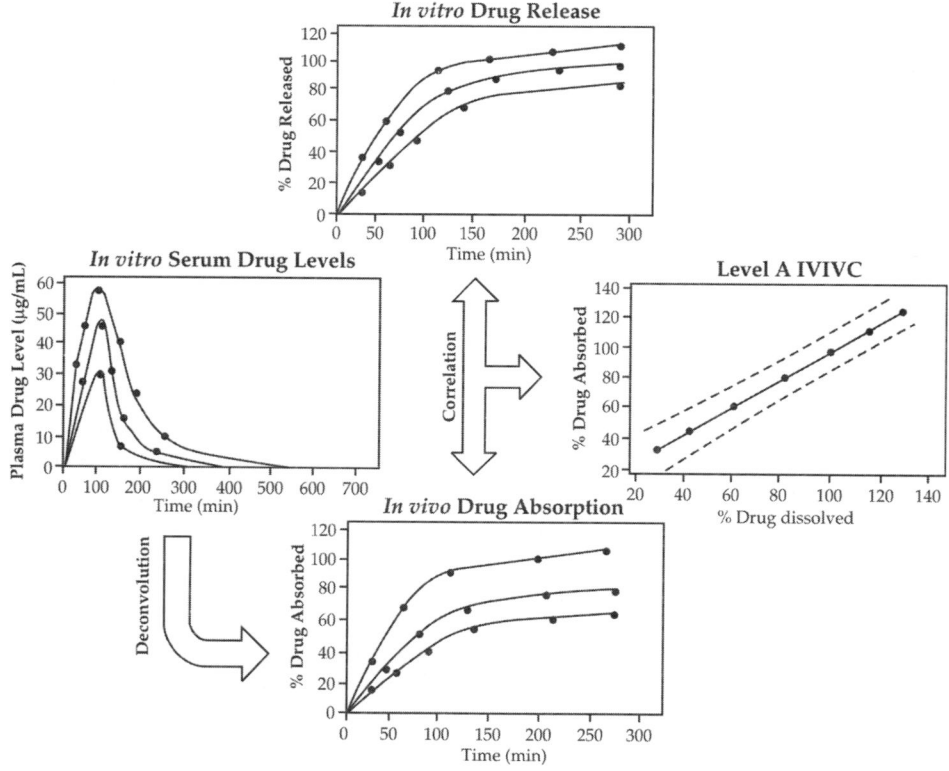

Fig. 13.8. Step-wise establishment of "Level A" IVIVC.

The one-stage convolution methods compute the *in vivo* absorption and simultaneously model the *in vitro-in vivo* data, obviating the need for the administration of an intravenous, oral solution or immediate-release bolus dose. This system employs the response mapping operator (RMO) approach. While the two-stage "system-deconvolution" method allows for systematic model development, the best IVIVC is explored through the application of numeric deconvolution method which predicts plasma drug concentration using a mathematical model, stated in Eq. 8, based on convolution integral (Veng-Pedersen et al., 2000). Fig. 13.9 portrays the one-step deconvolution method employing model-independent approach.

$$C_t = \int C_\delta(t-\mu).r_{abs}(\mu).du \qquad \dots (8)$$

where, C_δ = concentration-time course that would result from the instantaneous absorption of unit amount of drug; C_t = plasma drug concentration at time 't'; r_{abs} = drug input rate of dosage form; μ = variable of integration.

Overall, the schematic representation of convolution and deconvolution approaches used for holistic development of IVIVC is illustrated in Fig. 13.10. As per federal guidelines, the manufacturers have to establish IVIVC model at least in three different formulations varying release profiles (i.e., slow, medium and fast) for development of a meaningful model correlation. An example of establishing "level A" IVIVC in case of slow, medium and fast dissolution is depicted in Fig. 13.11.

Apart from the convolution technique, alternative methods like Bayesian or artificial neural network approaches have also been used for mathematical modelization of the data in single algorithm. This approach needs perfect comprehension of all the calculations and the covariates to be included in the programming part.

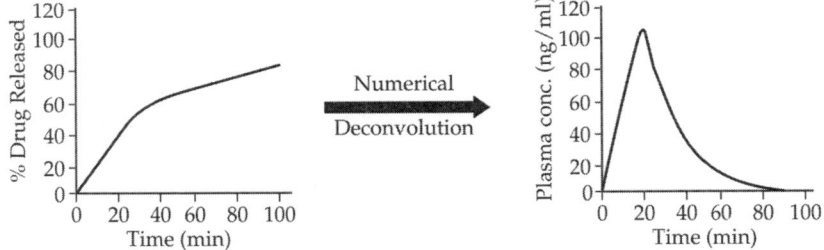

Fig. 13.9. One-step numerical deconvolution employing model-independent approach.

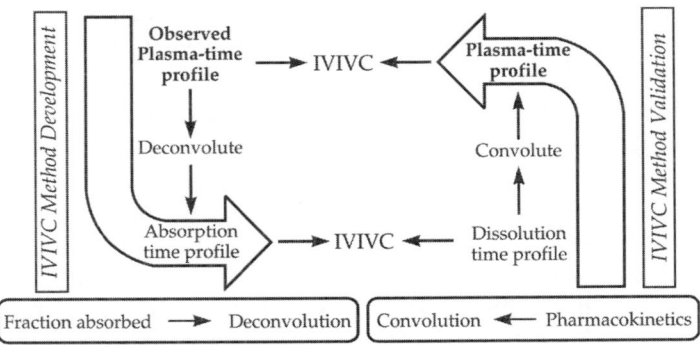

Fig. 13.10. Schematic presentation of the two key steps of convolution and deconvolution employed during establishment of IVIVC.

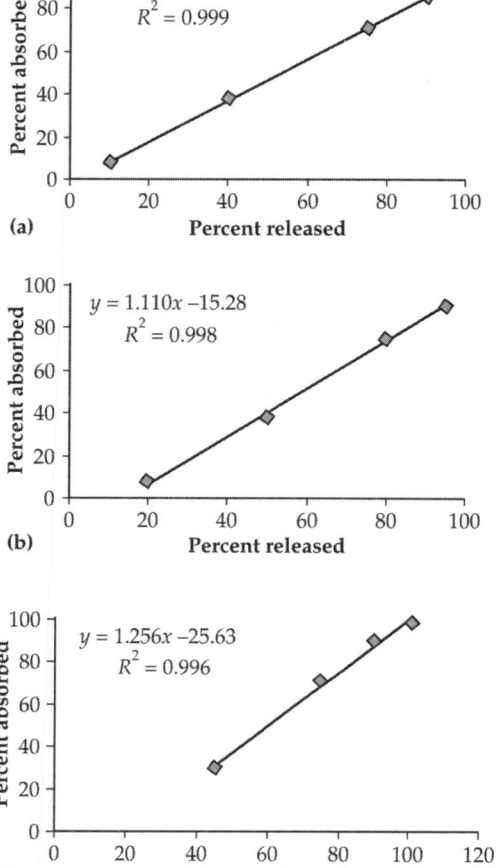

Fig. 13.11. "Level A" IVIVC in case of (a) fast dissolution, (b) medium dissolution, and (c) slow dissolution conditions.

Level B IVIVC

Level B correlation is based upon mean time parameters computed using statistical moment analysis. Typically, mean residence time (MRT) *in vivo* or mean dissolution time (MDT) *in vivo* is compared with the MDT *in vitro*. Level B correlation utilizes all of the *in vitro* and *in vivo* data but is not considered to be a point-to-point correlation because it does not uniquely reflect the actual *in vivo* plasma level curve, since there are a number of different *in vivo* curves that produce similar mean residence time values.

The term MRT describes the average time for which the drug molecules reside in the body. The residence time for the drug molecules in the body may be sorted according to their residence time into groups. The total residence time is the summation of the number of molecules in each group multiplied by their residence times. Thus, MRT is the ratio of sum of the residence times of all the drug molecules divided by total number of such molecules. To accomplish this, the drug dose may be converted to number of moles by dividing the dose in grams by molecular weight. Multiplying the number of moles by the Avogadro's number (6.023×10^{23}) yields the number of molecules, which turns out to the tune of 10^{20}. Hence, for estimation of pharmacokinetic parameters, one needs to determine residence times of each of such 10^{20} molecules and eventually calculate their mean and variance as MRT and variance of residence time (VRT), respectively.

Level C IVIVC

It establishes a single point relationship between *in vitro* dissolution parameter (e.g., $t_{50\%}$ or percent dissolved in 4 h) and a pharmacokinetic parameter (AUC, t_{max} or C_{max}). One dissolution time point (like $t_{50\%}$, $t_{90\%}$, etc.) is usually compared to one pharmacokinetic parameter (like AUC, t_{max}, C_{max}, etc.). Level C is the weakest level of correlation, as the partial relationship between absorption and dissolution is only established. Because of its obvious limitations, a level C correlation has limited usefulness in predicting *in vivo* drug performance and is subject to the same caveats as a Level B correlation in its ability to support product and site changes as well as justification of quality control standard extremes. Level C correlations can be useful in the early stages of formulation development when pilot formulations are being selected. While the information may be useful in formulation development, waiver of an *in vivo* bioequivalence study (biowaiver) is generally not possible.

Multiple level C IVIVC

It relates one or more pharmacokinetic parameters of interest (like C_{max}, AUC, or any other suitable metrics) to the amount of drug dissolved at various time points. It can be employed to justify biowaiver(s) provided that the correlation has been established over the entire dissolution profile with one or more pharmacokinetic parameters of interest. A relationship should be demonstrated at each time point at the same parameter such that the effect on the *in vivo* performance of any change in dissolution can be assessed, at least three dissolution time points covering the early, middle, and late stages of the dissolution profile are required. If such a multiple level C correlation is achievable, then the development of a "level A" correlation is also likely.

Level D IVIVC

It is a non-parametric rank order correlation between the *in vitro* dissolution parameter and an *in vivo* pharmacokinetic parameter. It is usually based on ordinal (but not quantitative) data, thus, considered to be a weaker correlation.

IVIVC has been observed to furnish invaluable information as plausible pharmacokinetic and pharmacodynamic performance of an archetypical drug delivery system. Level A correlation, in particular, has been employed for in-house ratification of *in vivo* drug delivery efficacy. There are umpteen instances in literature too which indicate the utility of IVIVC in development of ominous drug delivery systems. Table 13.2 enlists select literature instances on establishment of various levels of IVIVC in drug delivery systems.

IVIVC versus BCS

Class I compounds like metoprolol, propranolol, labetolol, diltiazem, verapamil, enalapril, phenylalanine and caffeine possess high permeability and solubility. These are expected to be well-absorbed owing to their high A_n and high D_n, unless they are unstable, form insoluble complexes, are secreted directly from gut wall, or undergo first pass metabolism. When a Class I drug is formulated as an ER product in which the release profile controls the rate of absorption, and the solubility and permeability of the drug is site independent, a level A correlation is most likely. However, once the permeability is site dependent a level C correlation is expected. The major challenge in development of drug delivery system for Class I drugs is to achieve a target release profile associated with a particular pharmacokinetic and/or pharmacodynamic profile. Formulation approaches include both control of release rate and certain physicochemical properties of drugs like pH-solubility profile of drugs.

Class II compounds like phenytoin, danazol, ketoconazole, mefenamic acid, nifedipine, flurbiprofen, diclofenac, naproxen, piroxicam and ketoprofen tend to exhibit high permeability and low solubility. These have a high A_n but low D_n, which means absorption rate is faster than dissolution rate, i.e., drug is absorbed quickly after dissolution, thus, dissolution is the rate limiting step. For Class II drugs, therefore, a strong correlation between dissolution rate and the *in vivo* performance can be established. When a Class II drug is formulated as an ER product, and the solubility and permeability of the drug are site independent, a level A correlation is expected. However, once the permeability is site dependent little or no IVIVC is expected. The systems that are developed for Class II drugs are based on their solubility enhancement. The key techniques include micronization, lyophilization, and addition of surfactants, emulsion formulations, microemulsion systems, and use of complexing agents like cyclodextrins.

Class III drugs, like cimetidine, acyclovir, neomycin, famotidine, nadolol, atenolol, and ranitidine possess low permeability and high solubility. They are rapidly dissolving but permeability is the rate-controlling step in drug absorption. Furthermore, Class III drugs exhibit a high variability in rate and extent of absorption,

Table 13.2. Select literature instances on establishment of various levels of IVIVC for diverse pharmaceutical products

Dosage form	Drug	Disease	Level of IVIVC	Reference
Extended release tablet	Veliparib (ABT-888)	Cancer	Level A	Mittapalli et al., 2017
Transdermal patch	Lidocaine	Neuralgia	Level A	Kondamudi et al., 2016
Solid dispersions	Silybin	Hepatotoxicity	Level A	Cao et al., 2013
Transdermal patch	Bufalin	Cancer	Level A	Yanga et al., 2013
Gastroretentive tablets	Rivastigmine	Alzheimer's disease	Level A, B, multiple level C	Kapil et al., 2013
	Lamivudine	AIDS		Singh et al., 2012
Transdermal patch	Azasetron	Chemotherapy-induced nausea and vomiting	Level B	Sun et al., 2012
PLGA implants	Risperidone	Schizophrenia	Level B	Amann et al., 2011
Immediate release tablets	Isosorbide mononitrate	Angina pectoris	Level A	Qiang et al., 2011
SR matrix tablets	Theophylline	Bronchial asthma	Level A	Ochoa et al., 2010
Immediate release tablets	Etoricoxib	Rheumatoid arthritis	Level A	Okumua et al., 2009
SR matrix tablets	Glipizide	Diabetes	Level A	Sankaliya et al., 2008
Polymeric microspheres	Vapreotide	Esophageal bleeding, cirrhotic disease	Level B	Souza and De Lucca, 2006
Biodegradable implants	Buserelin	Prostate cancer, breast cancer	Level A Level B Level C	Schlieckera et al., 2004

but if dissolution is fast such that 85% of drug dissolves in 15 minutes, the variation could be attributed to GI transit, luminal contents, and membrane permeation rather than dosage form factors. As drug permeation is rate controlling, limited or no IVIVC is expected. Class III drugs require the technologies that address to fundamental limitations of absolute or regional permeability. Peptides and proteins constitute the part of Class III and the technologies handling such materials are on rise now-a-days.

Class IV drugs like taxol, furosemide, cyclosporine and terfenedine possess low permeability and solubility. This class of drugs exhibits signi-ficant problems for effective oral delivery; no IVIVC is expected. Class IV drugs present a major challenge for development of drug delivery system and the route of choice for administering such drugs is parenteral with the formulation containing solubility enhancers.

Table 13.3 illustrates the select literature instances on the federal recommendations of bio-waivers of drug delivery products.

Recent modifications in the BCS proposed by FDA, i.e., Biopharmaceutics Drug Disposition Classification System (BDDCS), holds good in regulating the role of solubility and metabolism (instead of intestinal perme-

Table 13.3. Select federal biowaiver recommendations for various drug products from the BCS prospective

Drug	Biowaiver recommendations	Comments
BCS Class I		
Stavudine	Positive	Rapid dissolution/excipients similar to approved product
Metronidazole	Positive	Dissolution similar to reference product
BCS Class II		
Diclofenac salt	Positive	Dissolution similar to reference product
Rifampicin	Negative	Reported BE failures for unknown reasons
BCS Class III		
Acetaminophen Cimetidine	Positive	Rapid dissolution, excipients similar to reference product
Ranitidine HCl	Positive	Wide TI, rapid dissolution, excipients similar to reference product
BCS Class IV		
Furosemide	Negative	Possible excipient interactions and pharmacokinetic data
Ciprofloxacin	Negative	Reported BA-BE data, possible excipient interactions

TI: Therapeutic index

ability in case of BCS) on the plausibility of IVIVC establishment and potential biowaivers. It has been proved to be a useful tool in predicting the overall drug disposition and routes of drug elimination, following oral and intravenous dosing. A substantial difference between BDDCS and BCS is that the highly soluble and poorly metabolized drugs (BDDCS Class III) could be BCS Class I when their absorption is mediated by uptake transporters or paracellular passage. Thus, making the BCS prediction of *in vivo* drug performance is relatively less accurate. Further, it elaborates the effect of efflux and absorption transporters in governing the oral drug absorption process too (Benet et al., 2011).

IVIVC model validation

The objective of IVIVC is to successfully predict the outcome (*in vivo* profile) with a given model and test condition (*in vitro* profile). Thus, an IVIVC model evaluation should be carried out to demonstrate predictability of the *in vivo* performance of a drug product, from the *in vitro* dissolution characteristics. The focus is on predictive performance of the model, and therefore, the prediction error is evaluated. Depending on the intended application of an IVIVC and the therapeutic index of the drug, evaluation of predictability internally and/or externally may be appropriate (Ghosh et al., 2008). Evaluation of internal predictability is preferred for narrow therapeutic index drugs and is based on the initial data sets used to define the IVIVC model. Evaluation of external predictability is recommended for non-narrow therapeutic index drugs and is based on additional test data sets obtained from a different or a new formulation. Fig. 13.12 illustrates the typical instance of the validation of IVIVC model employed during practice.

Internal validation

Evaluation of internal predictability is based upon the initial data used to define the IVIVC model. Internal predictability is applied to IVIVC established using formulations with three or more release rates for wide therapeutic index drug exhibiting conclusive prediction error. If

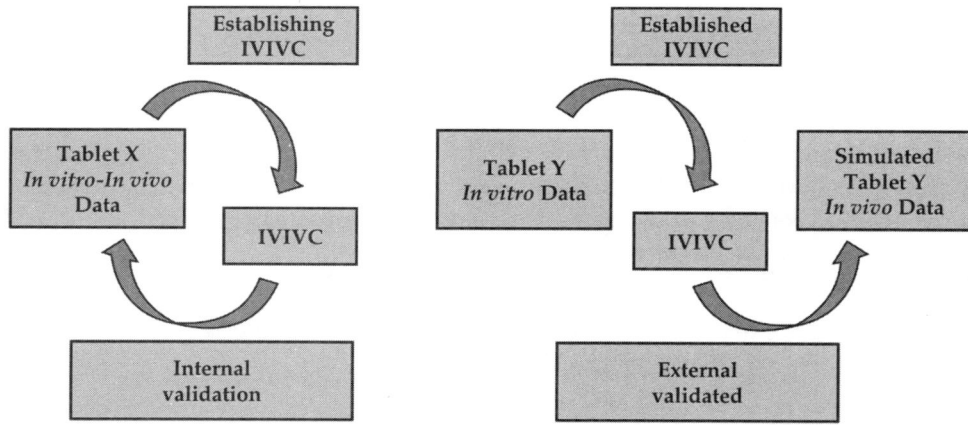

Fig. 13.12. Internal and external model validation flowchart employed during IVIVC.

formulations with three or more release rates are used to develop the IVIVC model, no further evaluation beyond this initial estimation of prediction error may be necessary for non-narrow therapeutic index drugs. All IVIVCs should be studied regarding internal predictability. One recommended approach involves the use of the IVIVC model to predict each formulation's plasma concentration profile (or C_{max} and/or AUC for a multiple level C IVIVC) dissolution data of respective formulations. This is performed for each formulation employed to develop the IVIVC model. Practically, *in vitro* dissolution rate is first estimated from dissolution data and is converted to *in vivo* dissolution rates by using the IVIVC model generated slope and intercept. If the cumulative drug release profile is sigmoid, then the Hill equation (Eq. 9) could be used to parameterize the *in vitro* drug release (Emami, 2006).

$$\text{Percentage dissolved} = \frac{D_{max} \times t^\gamma}{D_{50}^\gamma + t^\gamma} \quad \text{.... (9)}$$

where, %D is the percent drug dissolved at time 't', D_{max} is the maximum percentage of drug dissolved, D_{50} is the time required for dissolution of 50% of the drug, γ is the sigmoidicity factor.

The prediction of plasma concentration from the corresponding *in vivo* dissolution profiles is then accomplished by convolution of the *in vivo*

dissolution rates and pharmacokinetic model for response results from i.v. bolus data, oral solution or rapidly releasing (*in vivo*) immediate release dosage form. The model predicted bioavailability is then compared to the observed bioavailability for each formulation. The percent prediction errors (%PE) for C_t, C_{max} or AUC could be determined as described in Eq. 10.

$$\%\text{PE} = \frac{\text{Observed} - \text{Predicted}}{\text{Predicted parameter}} \times 100 \quad \text{...(10)}$$

Average absolute percent prediction error (%PE) of 10% or less for C_{max} and AUC establishes the predictability of the IVIVC. In addition, the %PE for each formulation should not exceed 15%. If these criteria are not met, evaluation of external predictability of the IVIVC should be performed as a final determination of the ability of the IVIVC to be used as a surrogate for bioequivalence.

External validation

External predictability evaluation is not necessary unless the drug has a narrow therapeutic index, only two release rates are used to develop the IVIVC, or if the internal predictability criteria are not met. Evaluation of external predictability is based on additional test data sets. These data sets may have several differing characteristics compared to the data sets used in IVIVC development. The formulations with different release rates provide the optimal test of an IVIVC's predictability. In the absence of such a formulation, data from other types of formulations may be considered. In each case, bioavailability data should be available for the data set under consideration.

The %PE of 10% or less for C_{max} and AUC establishes the external predictability of an IVIVC. %PE between 10–20% indicates inconclusive predictability and the need for further study using additional data sets. Results of estimation of PE from all such data sets should be evaluated for consistency of predictability. %PE greater than 20% generally indicates inadequate predictability, unless otherwise justified.

IN VITRO/IN VIVO RELATIONSHIP (IVIVR)

IVIVR is a relatively broad-based predictive mathematical model also outlined in the FDA guidance as a prelude to the traditional IVIVC approach. At times, it implies a semi-quantitative association between *in vitro* metrics and *in vivo* data. IVIVR also encompasses the advantages of IVIVC in introducing the non-linear modelling when classical linear IVIVC relationships are not sufficient or are not applicable. As the classical IVIVC approach has limitations with respect to accomplishment of linearity between the *in vitro* fraction of drug absorbed (F_a) and *in vivo* fraction of drug dissolved (F_d) in case of immediate release drug products, IVIVR holds good in exploring plausible degree of coherence in the data for exploring the IVIVC in later stages (Polli, 2013). Postulation of a generalized IVIVR model, in this regard, significantly helps during early phase of development of a drug product, where no *in vivo* data are yet available, thus, making it impossible to establish a classical IVIVC/IVIVR model (Liu

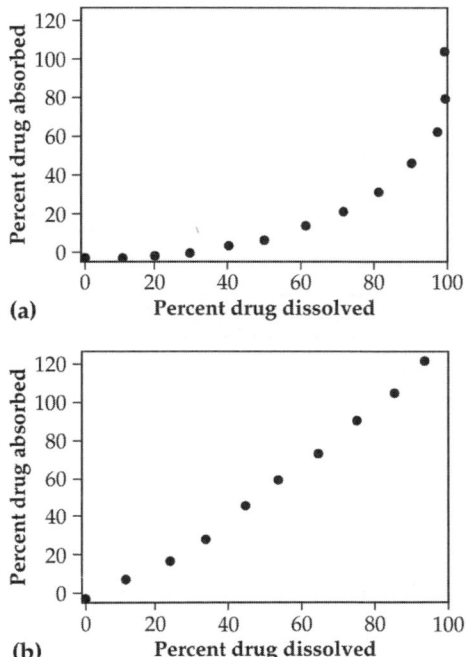

Fig. 13.13. Apparent differences between the IVIVR (a), and IVIVC (b).

et al., 1996; Mauger and Chinchilli, 1997). Fig. 13.13 illustrates the instance of a generalized IVIVR and classical IVIVC phenomena during immediate release drug product development.

IVIVC FOR DRUG PRODUCT DEVELOPMENT IN THE INDUSTRIAL SCENARIO

The IVIVC for drug product development in an industrial milieu can be accomplished in different stages. The initial phase starts with development of an IVIVR, which, in the later stages, is explored for the possibility of a perfect IVIVC model establishment (Emami, 2006). The flow chart portrayed in Fig. 13.14 provides a detailed account of the steps involved during establishment of IVIVC.

Stage 1

It is often referred as "**assumed IVIVR**", which involves defining the objectives and goals of the

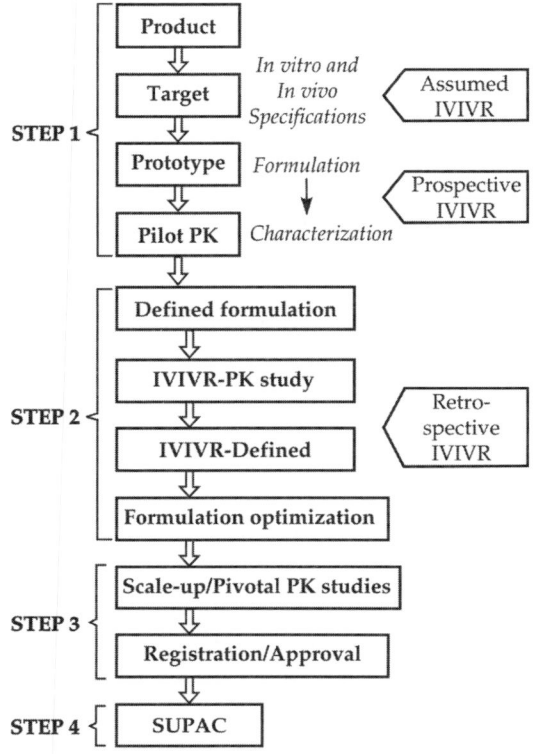

Fig. 13.14. Critical steps involved in establishment of IVIVR in an industrial set-up.

product. Essentially, at this stage, a level A correlation is assumed and the formulation strategy is initiated with the objective of achieving the target *in vitro* profile. This work is usually conducted at the laboratory level with the simplest dissolution methodology that seems appropriate. It tends to provide initial guidance and direction for the early formulation development activity. Thus, during stage 1 and with a particular product concept in mind, appropriate *in vitro* targets are established to meet the desired *in vivo* specifications. This assumed model can be the subject of revision as the prototype formulations are developed and characterized *in vivo*, with the results often leading to a further cycle of prototype formulation and *in vivo* characterization. Out of this cycle and *in vivo* characterization, extensive *in vitro* testing is often performed for establishing the **retrospective**

IVIVR. To understand how an IVIVR is used throughout the product development cycle, it is useful to understand the physicochemical characteristics of the drug substance itself, in context to the relevance of dissolution testing at diverse gastrointestinal physiological conditions. Based on this information, *in vitro* methods are usually developed *a priori* and a theoretical *in vitro* target is established for achieving the desired drug absorption profile.

Stage 2

In this stage, a defined formulation that meets the *in vivo* targets is aimed to progress through the normal formulation optimization process. Based on this prior understanding, and a sort of retrospective data generated during stage 1, an empirical basis exists for determining the primary formulation-related rate controlling variables. For extended-release products, prior understanding is usually more obvious than might be the case for immediate-release products. Based on this information, a number of products with different release rates are usually manufactured by varying the primary rate controlling variables but within the same qualitative formulation. Extensive *in vitro* characterization is again performed across pH, media and apparatus, followed by their correlation with the pilot *in vivo* pharmacokinetic studies, which rationally provide meaningful execution of the **prospective IVIVR** model.

Stage 3

At this stage, after attaining a complete experimental model of the IVIVR, the validation studies are carried out on the formulations under scale-up via pivotal pharmacokinetic and clinical studies for final approval through regulatory filing.

Stage 4

The end phase involves formulation of control strategy, where necessary modification in the approved formulation is taken under the criterion of scale-up and post-approval changes.

NEWER PARADIGMS IN IVIVC

Lately, paradigms like *In Vitro/In Vivo* Matching (IVIVM) and *In Vitro/In Vivo* Profiling (IVIVP) have also been used for predicting *in vivo* behavior of the formulations by examining their *in vitro* release profiles. However, such newer approaches have limited federal importance, as these do not provide highly predictable outcomes, thereby limiting their utility in determining the quality of a test product. The key details regarding these newer paradigms in IVIVC are as follows:

In Vitro/In Vivo Matching (IVIVM)

IVIVM reflects an unconvincing interpretation and practice of IVIVC. This would require one or more products having different *in vivo* (plasma concentration-time) profiles and *in vitro* dissolution profiles (Saeed, 2011). If one set of experimental conditions provides a matched ranking between *in vitro* dissolution and *in vivo* absorption profiles, it is considered as achieving IVIVM. If none of the prior dissolution methods provide such matching, then a new set of experimental conditions may also be developed to match the ranking. This helps in providing initial inkling for providing correlation between the *in vitro* and *in vivo* dissolution profiles.

In Vitro/In Vivo Profiling (IVIVP)

Considering limitations in defining or interpreting IVIVC, a more appropriate and direct definition and interpretation is highly desirable to link or relate the *in vitro* (dissolution) and *in vivo* (blood drug concentration-time) profiles (Saeed, 2011). In this regard, the main purpose to conduct a dissolution test is to establish a dissolution profile and then predict a *C-t* profile from it to assess the potential *in vivo* characteristics of the test product. Therefore, it can be said that, in reality, the purpose of commonly referred practices of IVIVC is to transfer a dissolution data (*in vitro*) to a *C-t* (*in vivo*) profile, or simply referred as "*In vitro/In vivo* Profiling (IVIVP)". Fig. 13.15 pictorially depicts the establishment of IVIVP for immediate and extended release drug products.

IVIVC APPLICATIONS

Development of oral drug delivery systems

The pharmaceutical applications of IVIVC have greatly benefitted the researchers from academia as well as industry for developing novel oral drug products of diverse kinds, generic as well as innovators (Mario et al., 2012; Cao et al., 2013).

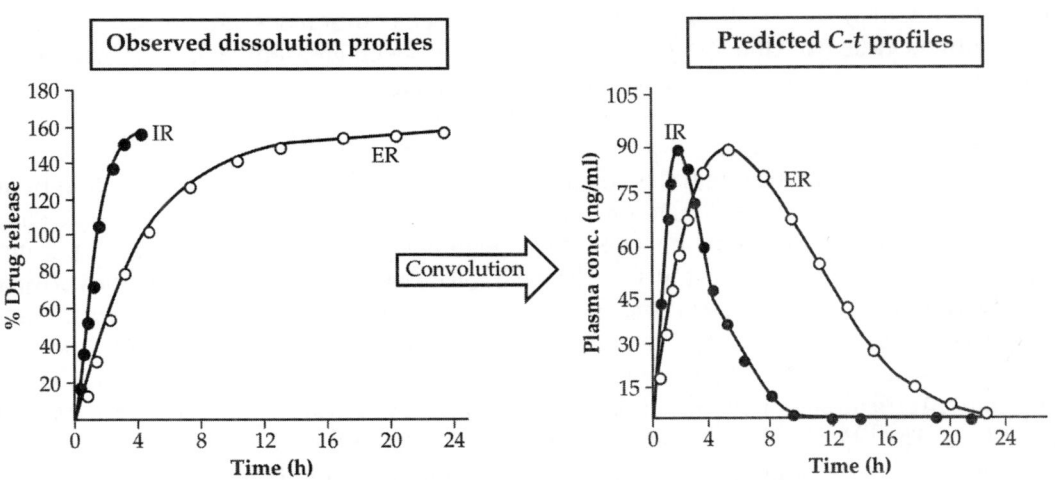

Fig. 13.15. Establishment of *in vitro/in vivo* profiling (IVIVP).

Establishment of IVIVC model helps the formulator in providing a wealth of information for systematic development of robust drug delivery products by predicting their likely *in vivo* product performance directly from their corresponding *in vitro* dissolution profile. On industrial fronts, IVIVC can be well-utilized at various stages of product development resulting in the formulation of more valuable and impeccable robust formulations. Lately, diverse oral drug delivery technologies have been investigated for establishing the IVIVC as a pivotal tool for product development and attaining federal biowaiver (Okumua et al., 2009; Dutta et al., 2006; Sankaliya et al., 2008; Ochoa et al., 2010).

Setting-up the dissolution specifications

In vitro dissolution specifications should generally be based on the performance of the clinical/bioavailability lots. These specifications may sometimes be widened, so that scale-up lots, as well as stability lots, meet the specifications associated with the clinical/bioavailability lots. This approach is based on the use of the *in vitro* dissolution test as a quality control test without any *in vivo* significance, even though in certain cases (e.g., ER formulations), the rate limiting step in the absorption of the drug is the dissolution of the drug from the formulation. An IVIVC adds *in vivo* relevance to *in vitro* dissolution specifications, beyond batch-to-batch quality control. In this approach, the *in vitro* dissolution test becomes a meaningful predictor of *in vivo* performance of the formulation, and dissolution specifications may be used to minimize the possibility of releasing lots that would be different in *in vivo* performance (FDA PQRI Workshop, 2012).

It is relatively easier to establish a multipoint dissolution specification for modified-release dosage forms. The FDA guidance describes the procedures of setting dissolution specifications in cases of level A, multiple level C and level C

correlation and where there is no IVIVC (Singh et al., 2012; Kapil et al., 2013; Cao et al., 2013). Once an IVIVC is developed, it should be used to set specifications in such a way that the fastest and lowest release rates allowed by the upper and lower dissolution specifications result in a maximum difference of 20% in the predicted C_{max} and AUC. Predicted plasma concentration, and the consequent AUC and C_{max}, can be calculated using convolution or any other appropriate modelling techniques, described earlier.

IVIVC for non-oral drug delivery systems

Till the last decade or so, the concept of IVIVC remained restricted only to the realm of oral drug delivery systems. Though the principles of IVIVC have mostly been applied to oral products, yet introduction of many new dosage forms administered through somewhat analogous non-instantaneous routes calls for methodologies and standards for non-oral systems too. IVIVC has also been developed and applied to topical, transdermal, ocular, nasal, inhalational products, etc. (Sun et al., 2012; Yanga et al., 2013; Schlieckera et al., 2004; Amann et al., 2011). Nevertheless, there is limited fruition in the development of IVIVC for such non-oral dosage forms, which could be due to several reasons, a few of these have been discussed above.

IVIVC for topical drug products

Application of IVIVC for topical drug products has been explored quite recently. The key parameters employed for such IVIVC models include establishment of correlation between the *in vitro* drug release and *in vivo* pharmaco-dynamic response. The *in vitro* release can be assessed using a Franz-diffusion cell assembly, which acts as a surrogate for *ex vivo* permeation studies by reducing the hassles associated with it, along with significant savings of the time and resources (Ambulgekar, 2013).

IVIVC for transdermal drug products

IVIVC in case of transdermal drug delivery systems is somewhat different compared to the oral route of administration. In most instances, steady state flux has been extrapolated to determine the *in vivo* plasma concentrations using pharmacokinetic modelling approaches (Vanal Buskirk et al., 2012; Yanga et al., 2013). IVIVC can be helpful to achieve mechanistic understanding of the transdermal system and helps in simulating/predicting the plasma concentration-time profile of the drugs recommended for prolonged therapy (e.g., hormones, cortico-steroids). Despite advancements in this area, the successful establishment of an IVIVC model for transdermal drug products remains quite challenging owing to the selection of ideal dissolution specifications along with for the purpose. Besides, the complex mechanism of drug permeation across human epidermis is considered to be highly intriguing for replicating the *in vitro* dissolution (Chaturvedula and Banga, 2007).

IVIVC for parenteral drug products

In general, several parenteral drug delivery systems are developed for potent drugs, like hormones, growth factors, antibiotics, etc., for long-term delivery, ranging widely from a day to a few weeks to several months. Design of such systems is quite complex and involves multistep processes to achieve defined product quality. In addition, establishing the relationship between plasma drug concentrations to the *in vitro* drug release for these systems would be difficult due to the limited volume of tissue fluids and area of absorption at the site of administration, unlike following the oral route of administration (Zolnik and Burgess, 2008). Therefore, it is very difficult to specify the *in vitro* dissolution conditions that reflect the observed differences in the *in vivo* plasma profiles corresponding to the *in vitro* release profiles. To establish a good IVIVC model in such instances, the *in vivo* drug concen-trations should be monitored in the tissue fluids at the site of administration by sophisticated techniques such as microdialysis, followed by attempts to establish the correlation with the *in vitro* drug release profile.

IVIVC for ocular drug delivery systems

Exploration of IVIVC has now been practised for performance evaluation of ocular drug products. The recent literature reports have demonstrated that the exploration of IVIVC for ocular drug products particularly meant for drug delivery to the posterior segment of the eye. In such cases, the correlation can be established between the *in vitro* % drug released with the *in vivo* % drug permeated through the corneal section of the eye (Paul et al., 2010). Multiple factors viz. molecular weight, log permeability coefficients and/or degree of ionization tend to influence the *in vitro* and *in vivo* parameters employed for performance evaluation of such drug products. The % drug released *in vitro* from the dosage form can be estimated in simulated artificial tear fluid, while the % drug absorbed *in vivo* can be accessed from animal models like rabbit. Besides the usefulness of isolated rabbit corneal or scleral membrane using two-chamber glass diffusion cell system, ARPE19 cell line models, human retinal pigmented epithelium cells have demonstrated better prediction of the performance over the *in vitro* dissolution studies.

IVIVC for inhalational drug products

Investigation of IVIVC for inhalational products involves establishment of correlation between the total lethal dose administered *in vivo* ($TLD_{in\,vivo}$) versus total lethal dose administered *in vitro* ($TLD_{in\,vitro}$). Existence of good correlation demonstrates the efficacy of inhalational drug therapy with respect to the particle size and particle density, along with the suitability of delivery device, precision in dose monitoring and specificity of the particles to the lung alveoli for the purpose (Newman et al., 2010).

Accomplishing biowaivers

Biowaivers upon changing the manufacturing site

A biowaiver, using an IVIVC developed with two formulations/release rates, for a non-narrow therapeutic index drug will likely be granted for an ER drug product for level 3 manufacturing and non-release controlling excipient changes as defined in SUPAC-MR (FDA, 1997C).

Biowaivers for lower strengths

If an IVIVC is developed with the highest strength, waivers for changes made on the highest strength and any lower strength may be granted if these strengths are compositionally proportional or qualitatively the same, the *in vitro* dissolution profiles of all the strengths are similar, and all strengths have the same release mechanism.

Table 13.4 enlists the important requirements in terms of solubility, permeability and potency of the drug for establishing IVIVC and subsequently seeking federal biowaivers from regulatory agencies like USFDA, EMEA and WHO.

Biowaivers of newer strengths

This biowaiver is applicable to strengths lower than the highest strength, within the dosing range that has been established to be safe and effective, if the new strengths are compositionally proportional or qualitatively the same; have the same release mechanism; have similar *in vitro* dissolution profiles; and are manufactured using the same type of equipment and the same process at the same site as other strengths that have bioavailability data available.

Inapplicability of BCS-based biowaiver

Narrow therapeutic range drugs

Narrow therapeutic range drug products containing certain drug substances (examples include digoxin, lithium, phenytoin, theophylline and warfarin) are subject to therapeutic drug concentration or pharmacodynamic monitoring, and/or where product labelling indicates a narrow therapeutic range designation. Because not all drugs are subject to therapeutic drug concentration or pharmacodynamic monitoring due to narrow therapeutic index, sponsors should contact the appropriate review division to determine whether a drug should be considered to have a narrow therapeutic range. If external predictability of an IVIVC is established, the following waivers will likely be granted if at least two formulations/release rates have been studied for the development of the IVIVC. A biowaiver will likely be granted for an ER drug product using an IVIVC for level 3 changes in process or release controlling excipients, or complete removal or replacement of non-release controlling excipients, as defined in SUPAC-MR.

Products designed to be absorbed in the oral cavity

A request for a waiver of *in vivo* BA/BE studies based on the BCS is not appropriate for dosage

Table 13.4. Comparative federal requirements of IVIVC for biowaivers

Parameter	USFDA	EMEA	WHO
Solubility (Soluble)	Solubility at pH 1–7.5	Solubility at pH 1–6.8	Solubility at pH 1.2–6.8
Permeability (Permeable)	If extent of absorption in humans is 90% or more	No specific criterion	If extent of absorption in humans is 85% or more
Dose proportionality for high potency APIs	5 mg API per dosage unit		10 mg API per dosage unit

USFDA: US Food & Drug Administration; EMEA: European Medicines Agency; WHO: World Health Organization forms intended for absorption in the oral cavity (e.g., sublingual or buccal tablets).

CONCLUSION

The unparalleled utility of IVIVC in successful grant of biowaivers has already been proven as a major rational and economic respite for the pharma companies. However, equally vital is the significance of IVIVC in the development of an effective, cost-effective and robust IR or ER drug products. The contribution of IVIVC in judicious selection of most successful and discriminating dissolution apparatus and media is highly warranted. Albeit the correlation, in practice, implies a linear relationship (i.e. IVIVC). Several authors have suggested exploring non-linear relationships (i.e. IVIVR) too, particularly for IR products. The principles of IVIVC model development have been successfully applied to oral dosage forms. Nevertheless, much needs to be done to explore the ground rules for developing and validating IVIVC models for novel and non-oral DDS like microspheres, nanoparticles and liposomes. IVIVC is undoubtedly a highly useful tool in the armamentarium of a pharmaceutical scientist for biowaivers and product development. Much needs to be done, however, to harp its immense benefits in the systematic development of diverse drug delivery systems especially in the industrial milieu.

REFERENCES

- Amann, L.C., Gandal, M.J., Lin, R., Liang, Y., Siegel, S.J. *In vitro-in vivo* correlations of scalable PLGA-risperidone implants for the treatment of schizophrenia. *Pharm. Res.*, 2011; 27(8): 1730–1737.
- Ambulgekar, S. *In vitro* and *in vivo* investigation of topical formulations of erythromycin. *Int. J. Biopharm.*, 2013; 4(2): 135–139.
- Benet, L.Z., Broccatelli, F., Oprea, T.I. BDDCS applied to over 900 drugs. *AAPS J.* 2011; 13: 519–547.

- Chaturvedula, A., Banga, A.K. *In vitro-in vivo* correlation: Transdermal drug delivery systems. **Pharmaceutical Product Development:** *In vitro-in vivo* **Correlation**, 1st ed. Informa Healthcare, UK, pp.153–176.
- Dressman, J.B., Lennernas H. Solubility and drug dissolution. *In:* **Oral Drug Absorption: Prediction and Assessment** (Ed.), Drugs and pharmaceutical sciences. New York: Marcel Dekker Inc. 2000: 137–229.
- Dutta, S., Qiu, Y., Samara, E., Cao, G., Granneman G.R. Once-a-day extended-release dosage form of divalproex sodium III: Development and validation of a level A *in vitro–in vivo* correlation (IVIVC). *J. Pharm. Sci.*, 2006; 94(9): 1949–1956.
- Emami, J. *In vitro-in vivo* correlation: From theory to applications. *J. Pharm. Pharm. Sci.*, 2006; 9(2): 169–189.
- FDA's Experience on IVIVC – Generic Drugs. PQRI Workshop on Application of IVIVC in Formulation Development Co-sponsored with FDA/FIP/AAPS/USP. September 5–6, 2012 Bethesda, MD, USA.
- Ghosh, A., Bhaumik, U.K., Bose, A., Mandal, U., Gowda, V., Chatterjee, B., Chakrabarty, U.S., Pal, T.K. Extended release dosage form of glipizide: Development and validation of a level A *in vitro-in vivo* correlation. *Biol. Pharm. Bull.*, 2008; 31: 1946–1951.
- Guidance for industry: Dissolution testing of immediate release solid oral dosage forms. U.S. Department of Health and Human Services, Food and Drug Administration, Center for Drug Evaluation and Research (CDER), U.S. Government Printing Office: Washington DC, Sept. 1997a.
- Guidance for industry: Extended release oral dosage forms: Development, evaluation and application of *in vitro/in vivo* correlations. U.S. Department of Health and Human Services, Food and Drug Administration, Center for Drug Evaluation and Research (CDER), U.S. Government Printing Office: Washington DC, September 1997b.
- Guidance for industry: SUPAC-MR: Modified release solid oral dosage forms. U.S. Department of Health and Human Services, Food and Drug Administration, Center for Drug Evaluation and Research (CDER), U.S. Government Printing Office: Washington DC, September 1997c.

- Kapil, R., Dhawan, S., Beg, S., Singh, B. Bucco-adhesive films for once-a-day administration of rivastigmine: systematic formulation development and pharmacokinetic evaluation. *Drug Dev. Ind. Pharm.*, 2013; 39(3): 466–80.

- Klein, S. The use of biorelevant dissolution media to forecast the *in vivo* performance of a drug. *AAPS J.* 2010; 12(3): 397–406.

- Kondamudi, PK., Tirumalasetty, P., Malayandi, R., Mutalik, S. and Pillai, R. Lidocaine Transdermal Patch: Pharmacokinetic Modeling and *In Vitro-In Vivo* Correlation (IVIVC). *AAPS PharmSciTech.*, 2016; 17: 588–596.

- Liu, F.Y., Sambol, N.C., Giannini, R.P., Liu, C.Y. *In vitro-in vivo* relationship of oral extended-release dosage forms. *Pharm. Res.*, 1996; 13(10): 1501–1506.

- Mauger, D.T., Chinchilli V.M. *In vitro-in vivo* relationships of oral extended-release drug products. *J. Biopharm. Stat.*, 1997; 7(4): 565–578.

- Mittapalli, RK., Nuthalapati, S., DeBord , AED., Xiong, H. Development of a Level A *In Vitro-In Vivo* Correlation for Veliparib (ABT-888) Extended Release Tablet Formulation. *Pharm. Res.*, 2017; 1–6.

- Newman, S.P., Pitcairn, G.R., Hirst, P.H., Bacon, R.E., O'Keefe, E., Reiners, M., Hermann, R. Scintigraphic comparison of budesonide deposition from two dry powder inhalers. *Eur. Respir. J.*, 2000; 16: 178–183.

- Ochoa, L., Igartua, M., Hernández, R.M., Solinís, M.A., Gascón, A.R., Pedraz, J.L. *In vivo* evaluations of two new sustained release formulations elaborated by one-step melt granulation: Level A *in vitro-in vivo* correlation. *Eur. J. Pharm. Biopharm.*, 2010; 75: 232–237.

- Okumua, A., DiMaso, M., Löbenberg, R. Computer simulations using GastroPlus to justify a biowaiver for etoricoxib solid oral drug products. *Eur. J. Pharm. Biopharm.*, 2009; 72: 91–98.

- Oser, B.L., Melnick, D., Hochberg, M. Physiological availability of the vitamins. Comparison of various techniques for determining vitamin availability in pharmaceutical products. *J. Nutr.*, 1945; 30: 67–69.

- Paul, S., Mondol, R., Ranjit, S., Maiti, S. Anti-glaucomatic niosomal system: Recent trend in ocular drug delivery research. *Int. J. Pharm. Pharm. Sci.*, 2010; 2: 15–18.

- Qiang, L., He, X., Gao, X., Xu, Y.Y., Wang, Y.F., Gu, H., Ji, R.F., Sun, S.J. Study on dissolution and absorption of four dosage forms of isosorbide mononitrate: Level A *in vitro-in vivo* correlation. *Eur. J. Pharm. Biopharm.*, 2011; 79: 364–371.

- Qureshi, S. *In vitro/in vivo* correlation (IVIVC) and determining drug concentrations in blood from dissolution testing – A simple and practical approach. *The Open Drug Deliv. Journal*, 2010; 4: 38–47.

- Qureshi, S. Different IVIV relationship terminologies. Drug dissolution testing: For simple and practical ideas. http://www.drug-dissolution-testing.com/?p=1106 (Accessed on 6 March 2017)

- Sakore, S., Chakraborty, B. *In vitro-in vivo* correlation (IVIVC): A Strategic Tool in Drug Development. *J. Bioequiv. Availab.*, 2011; S3: 2-12.

- Sankaliya, J.M., Sankalia, M.G., Mashru, R.C. Drug release and swelling kinetics of directly compressed glipizide sustained-release matrices: Establishment of level A IVIVC. *J. Control Release*, 2008: 129; 49–58.

- Schlieckera, G., Schmidtb, C., Fuchsb, S., Ehingerb A., Sandowc, J., Kissela, T. *In vitro* and *in vivo* correlation of buserelin release from biodegradable implants using statistical moment analysis. *J. Control Release*, 2004; 94: 25–37.

- Singh, B., Beg, S. Obtaining federal biowaivers employing IVIVC. *Chronicle Pharmabiz*, 2012; 34: 34–48.

- Singh, B., Garg, B., Chaturvedi, S.C., Arora, S., Mandsaurwale, R., Kapil, R. Formulation development of gastroretentive tablets of lamivudine using the floating-bioadhesive potential of optimized polymer blends. *J. Pharm. Pharmacol.*, 2012; 64(5): 654–69.

- Singh, B., Dehal, S., Kapil, R. *In vitro/in vivo* correlations (IVIVC): Role in biowaivers and product development of drug delivery systems. *In:* **Nanocolloidal Carriers: Site-Specific and Controlled Drug Delivery**, Vyas S.P. (Ed.), CBS Publishers & Distributors, New Delhi. 2010a: 275–319.

- Singh, B., Mohapatra, A., Bandyopadhyay, S., Kapil, R. Endeavoring biowaivers using BCS and IVIVC. *The Pharma Rev.*, 2010b; 8: 87–93.

- Singh, B. Biowaivers and biosimilars: Reinforcing intent and content of researchers and regulators. *J. Bioequival. Bioavail.*, 2012; 4(5): 15–16.

- Souza, S.D., DeLuca P.P. Methods to assess *in vitro* drug release from injectable polymeric particulate systems. *Pharm. Res.*, 2006; 23(3): 460–474.
- Sun, L., Cun, D., Yuan, B., Cui, H., Xi, H., Mu, L., Chen, Y., Liu, C., Wang, Z., Fang, L. Formulation and *in vitro/in vivo* correlation of a drug-in-adhesive transdermal patch containing azasetron. *Eur. J. Pharm. Sci.*, 2012; 101(12): 4540–4548.
- USP. "*In vitro* and *in vivo* evaluation of dosage form < 1088>". Rockville, Maryland. 1995 (23rd ed.): 1824–1929.
- Van Buskirk, G.A., Arsulowicz, D., Basu, P., Block, L., Cai, B., Cleary, G.W., Ghosh, T., González, M.A., Kanios, D., Marques, M., Noonan, P.K., Ocheltree, T., Schwartz, P., Shah, V., Spencer, T.S., Tavares, L., Ulman, K., Uppoor, R., Yeoh, T. Passive transdermal systems whitepaper incorporating current chemistry, manufacturing and controls (CMC) development principles. *AAPS PharmSciTech*, 2012; 13: 218–230.
- Veng-Pedersen, P. An algorithm and computer program for deconvolution in linear pharmaco-kinetics. *J. Pharmacokinet. Biopharm.*, 1980; 8: 463–81.
- Veng-Pedersen, P., Gobburu, J.V., Meyer, M.C., Straughn, A.B. Carbamazepine level A *in vivo-in vitro* correlation (IVIVC): A scaled convolution based predictive approach. *Biopharm. Drug Dispos.*, 2000; 21: 1–6.
- Zolnik, B.S., Burgess D.J. *In vitro-in vivo* correlation on parenteral dosage forms. *In:* **Biopharmaceutics Applications in Drug Development**, Krishna R and Yu L (Editor). Springer-Verlag, USA, pp. 336–358.

14

Quality by Design (QbD) and its Role in Pharma Product Development

Bhupinder Singh, Rajneet Kaur Khurana, Teenu, Rishi Kapil and Naveen Ahuja

INTRODUCTION

The pharmaceutical industry is highly regulated across the globe. While drug products have been instrumental in reducing the patient mortality and morbidity rates, there has always been a tangible element of risk associated with their usage by the patients. Primarily, this has been attributed to inadequate or inconsistent quality of the drug products. Hence, regulating pharmaceutical quality has always been a vital concern to the regulatory agencies (Singh, 2014). The major hiccups in accomplishing quality in a product can be attributed to the cumulative variability in drug substance(s), excipients, process(es), packaging material(s), and so on, as illustrated in Fig. 14.1.

Since decades, adoption of systematic approaches for developing the products with robust quality, enhanced resource economics and improved process capability has yielded high fruition in several technology-driven industries. The pharma industry, however, has harvested its immense potential relatively quite lately. A thought provoking article that appeared in The Wall Street Journal more than a decade back (i.e., September 2002) was considered an eye opener for the Federal agencies (Lionberger et al. 2008;

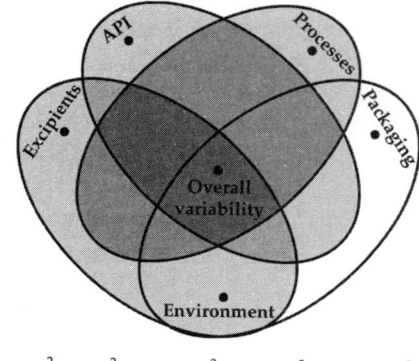

$$\sigma^2_{Product} = \sigma^2_{API} + \sigma^2_{Excipient} + \sigma^2_{Process} + \sigma^2_{Packaging} + \sigma^2_{Interactions}$$

Fig. 14.1. Plausible sources of variability during drug product development.

Ferreira and Tobyn, 2014). It stated, "although the pharmaceutical industry has a little secret even as it invents futuristic new drugs, yet its manufacturing standards lag far behind the potato chips and laundry soap makers". With the consequent growing concern and criticism, in this regard, the ICH instituted a series of quality guidances like Q8, Q9, Q10 and Q11, all emphasizing the adoption of systematic principles of Quality by Design (QbD) and Process Analytical Techniques (PAT) (Singh et al., 2013; ICH Q8, Q9, Q10). Endorsement of such rational paradigms by key global regulatory agencies including FDA (USA), EMEA (Europe), MHRA (UK), Health Canada, TGA (Australia), MCC (South Africa), ENVISA (Brazil), PMDA (Japan) and many others is unequivocal testimony to their immense significance it seems to hold for all the potential stake holders, viz. patients, industrial scientists and regulators. Table 14.1 provides a chronological account on the evolution of regulatory guidances on QbD by various federal agencies and other related activities like publication of instances on QbD-based filing, discussion reports, question and answers, etc.

Based upon quality philosophy QbD embarks upon systematic development of drug products and pharmaceutical processes. The philosophy primarily focuses on developing drug products with improved safety, efficacy and quality with reduced manufacturing cost envisioned by J.M. Juran by planning quality at first place to avoid quality crisis (Juran, 1992). Beginning with predefined objectives, QbD emphasizes on product and process understanding on the basis of sound science and risk management (Lionberger et al., 2008; Yu et al., 2014). Adoption of QbD principles, in particular, tends to unearth scientific minutiae during systematic product development and manufacturing process(es). For pharma-

Table 14.1. Chronological account of evolution of regulatory guidances by federal agencies and other QbD related activities

Agency	Guidelines/Activities	Month-Year
USFDA	Pharmaceutical cGMP for the 21st Century – A Risk-Based Approach: Second Progress Report and Implementation Plan	Sep 2003
USFDA	Guidance for Industry: PAT - A Framework for Innovative Pharmaceutical Development, Manufacturing, and Quality Assurance	Sep 2004
USFDA	Pharmaceutical cGMP for the 21st Century - A Risk-Based Approach: Final Report	Sep 2004
EMA	The European Medicines Agency Road Map to 2010	March 2005
ICH	Pharmaceutical Development (Q8) & Quality Risk Management (Q9)	Nov 2005
ICH	Pharmaceutical Quality System (Q10)	May 2007
ICH	Pharmaceutical Development (Q8(R2))	Aug 2009
WHO	Quality Risk Management	Aug 2010
EMA	Road Map to 2015	Dec 2010
USFDA	Guidance for Industry: Process Validation: General Principles and Practices	Jan 2011
EMA-FDA	EMA-FDA Pilot Program for Parallel Assessment of Quality by Design Applications	March 2011
ICH	Development and Manufacture of Drug Substances (Q11)	May 2011
ICH	ICH-Endorsed Guide for ICH Q8/Q9/Q10 Implementation	Dec 2011
EMA	ICH Quality IWG Points to consider for ICH Q8/Q9/Q10 guidelines	Feb 2012
EMA	Guideline on Real Time Release Testing (formerly Guideline on Parametric Release)	March 2012
EMA	Guideline on Process Validation (Draft)	March 2012
USFDA	Quality by Design for ANDAs: An Example for Immediate-Release Dosage Forms	April 2012
ICH	Development and Manufacture of Drug Substances	May 2012
EMA-FDA	EMA-FDA Pilot Program for Parallel Assessment of QbD Applications and Q&A	Aug 2013
EMA	Guideline on process validation for finished products	Feb 2014
ICH	Pharmaceutical Product Lifecycle Management (Q12)	Sept 2014
FDA	Submission of Quality Metrics Data (Draft Guidance)	Nov 2016

ceutical industry in particular, QbD execution leads to improved time to market, enhanced knowledge sharing, limited product recalls and rejects, reduced consumer skepticism towards generics, decreased post-approval changes and efficient regulatory oversight (Sangshetti et al., 2014; Kannissery et al., 2016). Box 14.1 illustrates the key benefits of QbD in robust understanding of the product and process.

The regulatory agencies are now-a-days emphasizing on the approaches based on QbD,

rather than merely relying upon "Quality by Testing (QbT)", "Quality by Chance" or "Quality by Inspection" (Singh and Beg, 2013; Singh, 2014). Box 14.2 enlists the key differences between the traditional QbT and modern QbD approaches for developing drug products. One of the integral tools in the QbD armamentarium while developing optimized products and processes has been "Design of Experiments (DoE)" employing apt usage of experimental designs (Singh et al., 2011a). Amidst a multitude of plausible interactions of the drug substance with a plethora of functional and non-functional excipients and processes, the DoE methodology targets to produce the breakthrough systems with minimal expenditure of time, developmental effort and cost. With the objective of developing impeccable products or processes, earlier this task used to be attempted through trial and error, supplemented with the previous knowledge, wisdom and experience of the formulator, termed as 'one factor at a time' (OFAT) approach (Singh and Ahuja, 2004). Using this methodology, the solution of a specific problematic product or process characteristic could be achieved, but attainment of the true optimal solution was never guaranteed. However, the DoE-based approach usually provides systematic development of drug product or process leading to the best solutions with minimal expenditure of time, money and effort (Singh et al., 2005). This modern approach

---

Box 14.1. Phenomenal benefits of implementing QbD approach during drug product development

Benefits of QbD implementation in product development

- Development of high quality drug products
- Thorough understanding of product(s) and process(es)
- Enhanced knowledge sharing
- Reduced consumer-generic skepticism
- Excellent returns on investment
- Improved time to reach market
- Dynamic control strategy leading to greater operational flexibility
- Limited product recalls and rejects
- Decreased post-approval changes
- Efficient regulatory oversight
- Regulatory filing based on science and mechanistic rationale
- Significant savings on resources as testing is only real-time

---

Box 14.2. Comparison of QbT and QbD

Quality by Testing (QbT)	Quality by Design (QbD)
• Current state of manufacturing	• Desired state of manufacturing
• Relies on end-product testing	• End-product testing is for validation only
• Testing outweighs the design	• Testing balances with the design
• Quality attainment is never guaranteed	• Quality is always accomplished
• Doesn't get much along with Federal QbR*	• Complements well with Federal QbR
• Time, effort and money consuming	• Reduced expenditure of resources
• Indecisiveness due to siloed conditions	• Judicious planning using team approach
• Narrower operating ranges	• Wider operating ranges
* QbR – Question based Review	

of formulation development furnishes thorough and thought-through understanding of the products and process(es) (Fig. 14.2) (Yu, 2008). Such approaches are far more advantageous, because they require fewer experiments to achieve an optimum formulation, make problem tracing and rectification quite easier, reveal interaction among drugs, excipients and processes, simulate the product performance, and comprehend the process to assist in better formulation development and subsequent scale-up (Myers, 2003; Riley and Li, 2010). As DoE has much wider domain of application beyond even the pharma sector, a terser jargon on the heels of QbD paradigm, viz. "Formulation by Design (FbD)", was recently proposed by us, applicable to the integrated use of DoE and other QbD principles, specifically in the rational development of pharmaceutical dosage forms (Singh et al., 2011a; Singh and Beg, 2013).

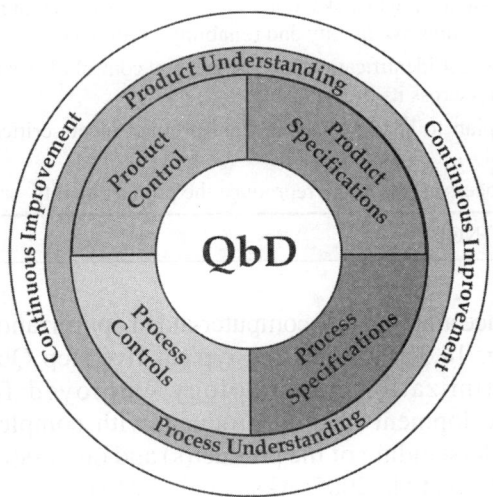

Fig. 14.2. QbD leads to product and process understanding, and continual improvement.

The holistic QbD-based philosophy of product development revolves around the key elements viz. meticulous drug product development by initially defining the quality target product profile (QTPP), identification of critical quality attributes (CQAs), critical formulation

attributes (CFAs) and critical process parameters (CPPs), apt choice of experimental designs, precise definition of design and control spaces, and subsequently embarking upon the optimum formulation (Lionberger et al., 2008; Rathore and Winkle, 2009).

QbD Terminology

Specific terminology, both technical and otherwise, is usually employed during QbD practice. To facilitate better understanding of precepts of QbD of DDS, important terms have been compiled in Box 14.3 (Singh et al., 2011a; Singh et al., 2014).

As a prelude to the application of QbD, it is essential to have the awareness of the QbD terminology and prior multi-disciplinary knowledge on various possible product and process variables ahead (Yu, 2008). A "knowledge space", i.e., entire worth-exploring realm, therefore, has to be identified from the possible vast ocean of scientific information based upon prior knowledge. A "knowledge space", thereby, encompasses information on all those product and process variables that may even minutely affect the overall product quality. A "design space" has to be demarcated as a subset construct of "knowledge space" ensuring optimal product quality or process performance involving "selected few" influential variables. "Control space" is further deduced from this "design space" as the experimental domain earmarked for the detailed in-house studies especially in an industrial set-up within the refined ranges of input variables. "Design space" applies systematic approach on archival data to convert the "knowledge space" to "control space"(Singh et al., 2011a,b). Extensive experimentation may be necessary for relatively intricate drug delivery systems in order to reduce uncertainty and justify a design space than that required for conventional formulation systems like tablets. Working within the design space is not considered as a "change", and it would not initiate any post-approval changes as per the federal guidelines by ICH and

Box 14.3. Vital terminology employed during QbD optimization of drug delivery systems	
Term	**Definition**
Quality Target Product Profile	Prospective and dynamic summary of the quality characteristics of a drug product that would ideally be achieved to ensure its quality, safety and efficacy
Critical Quality Attributes	Parameters ranging within appropriate limits, which ensure the desired product quality
Critical Process Parameters	Independent process parameters most likely to affect the quality attributes of a product or intermediates
Critical Formulation Attributes	Formulation parameters affecting critical quality attributes
Failure Mode & Effect Analysis (FMEA)	Systematic method to enhance safety and customer satisfaction by identifying failure modes or potential risks based upon severity, likelihood and/or detectability of the plausible failures
Explorable Space	Dimensional space defined by coded variables for the factors being investigated
Knowledge Space	Scientific elements to be considered and explored on the basis of previous knowledge as product attributes and process parameters
Design Space*	Multidimensional combination and interaction of input variables and process parameters, demonstrated to provide quality assurance
Control Space**	Domain of design space selected for detailed controlled strategy
Risk Assessment	Process to identify and mitigate risks, find root causes of process failure, prevent problems to improve quality and reliability of product
Quality Risk Management	Systematic process for identification, assessment and control of risk to the product quality across its lifecycle
Control Strategy	Comprehensive plan to ensure that the final product meets critical requirements
Continuous Improvement	Monitoring of process capability to reproduce the product quality
* Proven Acceptable Range (PAR); ** Normal Operating Range (NOR)	

USFDA. The enhanced understanding of the formula components and process(es) enables the scientists to strategize rationally to control the entire formulation system. The entire plan, by and large, is at times referred to as "Control Strategy" (Sangshetti et al., 2014).

QbD Methodology

QbD hits the bull's eye using five vital strengths, viz. (i) meticulous drug product development, (ii) apt choice of experimental designs, (iii) identification of critical quality attributes (CQAs), (iv) critical formulation attributes (CFAs) and critical process parameters (CPPs), and (v) precise definition of design and control space and accurate computer-aided optimization. Fig. 14.3 illustrates the typical five-step QbD optimization methodology employed for development of drug products with complete understanding of the product(s) and process(es) (Singh et al., 2005; Aksu et al., 2014).

Step I: Ascertaining Drug Product Objective(s)

The quality target product profile (QTPP) is a prospective summary of quality characteristics of the drug delivery product ideally achieved to ensure the desired quality, taking into account the safety and efficacy of the drug product. During drug product development, QTPP is embarked

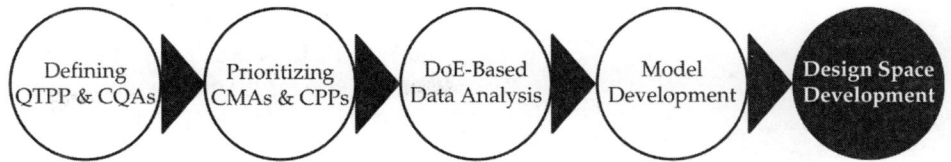

Fig. 14.3. Flow diagram depicting the five-step QbD methodology.

upon through brainstorming among the team members cutting across multiple disciplines in the industry. QTPP includes concepts that are required on the label of the pharmaceutical product (FDA and CDER 2007). It is a patient and labelling-based concept and can be considered as the "user interface" of the ready-made pharmaceutical product. Therefore, QTPP is expected to be the same for a generic and the reference product. A generic product may use a different formulation or design for applying the QTPP. Many features of QTPP are restricting or determining works of formulation and process development researchers. Instances of QTPP elements include route of administration, form and amount of dosage, maximum and minimum doses, presentation of pharmaceutical product and target patient population (Lionberger et al., 2008).

Critical quality attributes (CQAs) are the physical, chemical, biological or microbiological characteristics of the product that should be within an appropriate limit, range or distribution to ensure the desired product quality. CQAs can be of various types such as related to drug substance and excipients, intermediate products, finished products, etc. The differentiation of CQAs from the QTPP is based on the severity of harm a patient may get plausibly owing to the product failure. Thus, after defining the QTPP, the CQAs which pragmatically epitomize the objective(s) are earmarked for the purpose.

Step II: Prioritizing Input Variables for Optimization

Material attributes (MAs) and process para-meters (PPs) are considered as the independent input variables associated with a product and/or process, which directly influence the CQAs of

the drug product. Ishikawa-fish bone diagram is used to establish the cause-effect relationship among the input variables affecting the quality traits of the drug product. Fig. 14.4 illustrates a typical cause-effect diagram highlighting the plausible causes of product variability and their impact on drug product CQAs.

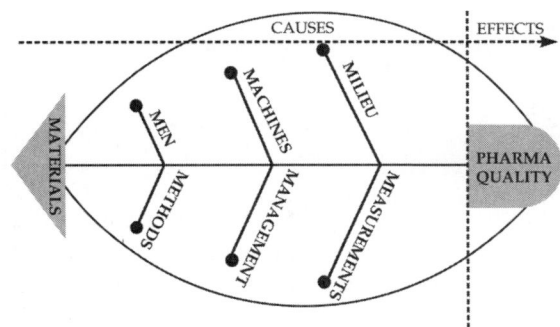

Fig. 14.4. A typical Ishikawa-fish bone diagram depicting sources of variability in pharmaceutical product development.

Prioritization exercise is carried out employing initial risk assessment and quality risk management (QRM) techniques for identifying the "prominent few" input variables, termed as CMAs and CPPs from the "plausible so many" through factor screening studies. QRM is rational approach, which not only provides holistic understanding of the risks associated with each stages of product development, but also facilitates mitigation of risks too. Fig. 14.5 depicts the flow layout of prioritization strategy employed for identifying the highly influential factors during product and/or process optimization. Beyond prioritization, the formal practice of risk assessment is considered to be highly useful for identifying the CMAs/CPPs

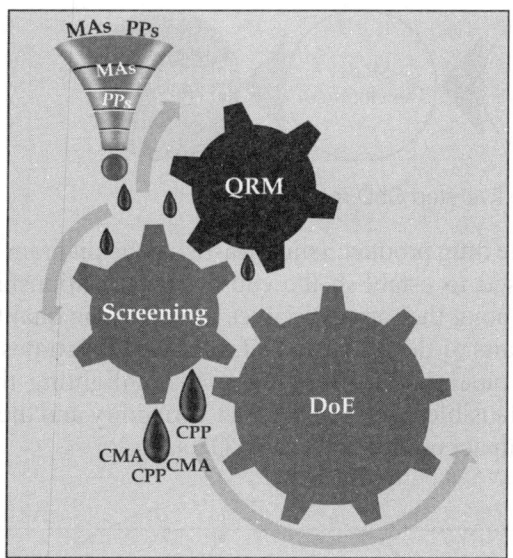

Fig. 14.5. Prioritization using QRM and factor screening is necessary to identify CMAs and CPPs as a prelude to DoE optimization.

with potential risk(s) based on the prior art and knowledge to assess the criticality associated with the product and process. Fig. 14.6 portrays the four steps QRM strategy involving risk assessment and risk management for identifying the potential CMAs, along with a prototype risk evaluation chart.

Diverse risk assessment techniques have been published in literature during drug delivery practice. Comparison Matrix, Risk Estimation Matrix (REM), Failure Mode and Effects Analysis (FMEA), Hazard Analysis and Critical Control Points (HACCP) and Hazard Operability Analysis (HAZOP) are the examples of commonly employed risk assessment techniques (Guebitz et al., 2012). Using these techniques, various MAs and PPs are assigned with different risk levels viz. low, medium and high risk based on their severity and likelihood of occurrence. The moderate to high risk factors are chosen from patient perspectives through brainstorming among the team members for judicious selection of CMAs. Before venturing into product or process optimization, prioritization of CMAs/CPPs using risk assessment is not considered to be obligatory, but at times facilitate ease in identifying the right factors with minimal usage of time.

Step III: Design-Guided Factor Screening and Optimization Data Analysis

The design-guided experimental strategy primarily embarks upon usage of select experimental designs for accomplishing the goals of both factor screening and optimization. The low-resolution first-order experimental designs are highly helpful in screening and factor influence studies, while response surface designs are employed for factor optimization studies. Response surface methodology (RSM) is considered a pivotal part of the

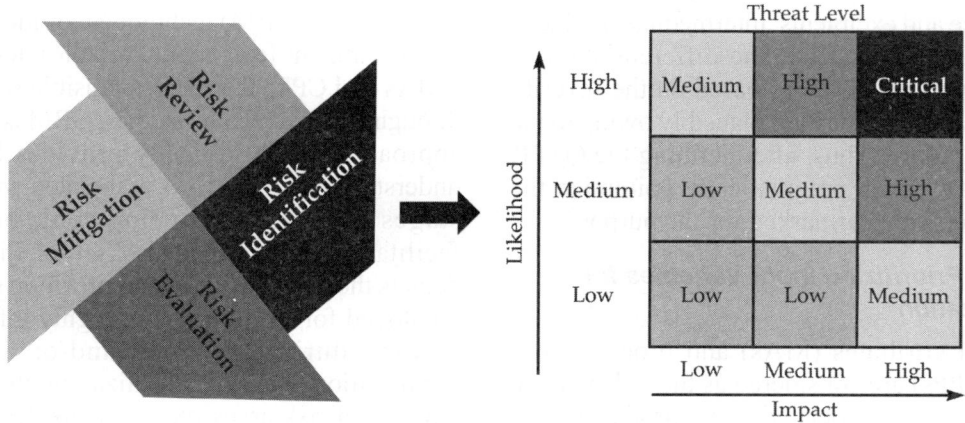

Fig. 14.6. Layout of risk management strategy employing a typical risk estimation matrix.

entire QbD exercise for optimization of product and/or process variables discerned from the risk assessment and screening studies. The response surface experimental designs particularly help in mapping the responses on the basis of the studied objective(s), CQAs being explored at high, medium or low levels of CMAs. During design-guided experimental analysis, the experimental designs generate a layout of experimental runs in matrix form. The drug formulations are experimentally prepared as per the design matrix and chosen response variables are evaluated meticulously.

Step IV: Modelization and Search for Optimum

Modelization is carried out by selection of apt mathematical models like linear, quadratic and cubic to generate the 2D and 3D-response surface to relate the response variables or CQAs with the input variables or CMAs/CPPs for identifying underlying interaction(s) among them. Multiple linear regression analysis (MLRA), partial least squares (PLS) analysis and principal component analysis (PCA), are some of the key multivariate chemometric techniques employed for modelization to discern the factor-response

relationship (Ferreira and Tobyn, 2014). Besides, the model diagnostic plots like perturbation charts, outlier plot, leverage plot, Cook's distance plot and Box-Cox plot are also helpful in unearthing the pertinent scientific minutiae and interactions among the CMAs. The search for optimum solution is accomplished through numerical and graphical optimization techniques like desirability function, canonical analysis, artificial neural network, brute-force methodology and overlay plot. Subsequent to the optimum search, the optimized formulation is located in the design and control spaces. Design space is a multi-dimensional combination of input variables (i.e., CMAs/CPPs) and output variable (i.e., CQAs) to discern the optimal solution with assurance of quality. Fig. 14.7 illustrates the interrelationship among various spaces like, explorable, knowledge, design and control spaces. Usually in industrial milieu, a narrower domain of control space is construed from the design space for further implicit and explicit studies.

Step V: QbD Validation, Scale-up and Production

Validation of the QbD methodology is a crucial step that forecasts the prognostic ability of the

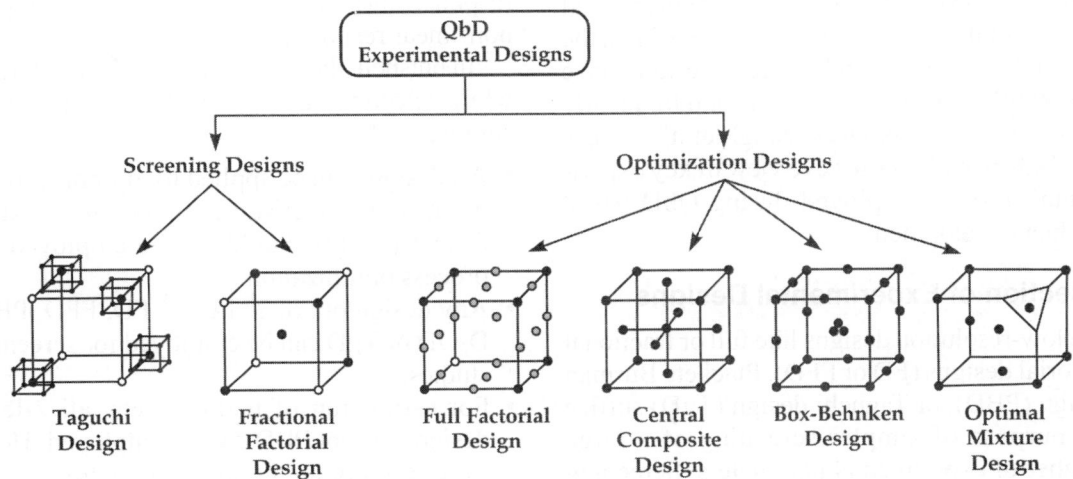

Fig. 14.7. Key instances of experimental designs used during QbD-based optimization along with their diagrammatic representations.

studied polynomial models. Various product and process parameters are selected from the experimental domain and evaluated as per the standard operating conditions laid down for the desired product and process related conditions carried out earlier, commonly termed as checkpoints or confirmatory runs. The results obtained from these checkpoints are then compared with the predicted ones through linear correlation plots and the residual plots to check any typical pattern like ascending or descending lines, cycles, etc. To corroborate QbD performance, the product or process is scaled-up through pilot-plant, exhibit and production scale, in an industrial milieu to ensure the reproducibility and robustness. A holistic and versatile "control strategy" is meticulously postulated for "continuous improvement" in accomplishing better quality of the finished product.

EXPERIMENTAL DESIGNS EMPLOYED DURING QbD OPTIMIZATION OF DDS

An experimental design constitutes the gist of the entire QbD exercise. Systematic QbD optimization of a DDS includes a careful "screening" of influential variables and subsequent RSM analysis using experimental designs. Out of all the experimental designs, the factorial, composite and mixture designs have been employed most extensively and frequently to optimize various DDS (Singh et al., 2005). Fig. 14.8 provides bird's eye view of key experimental designs employed during QbD-based product development.

Selection of Experimental Designs

The low-resolution designs like full or fractional factorial designs (FD or FFD), Plackett-Burman design (PBD), or Taguchi design (TgD) suffice the purpose of simpler screening of a large number of experimental parameters. Screening designs support only the linear responses (Singh et al., 2005; Singh et al., 2011b). Thus, if a non-

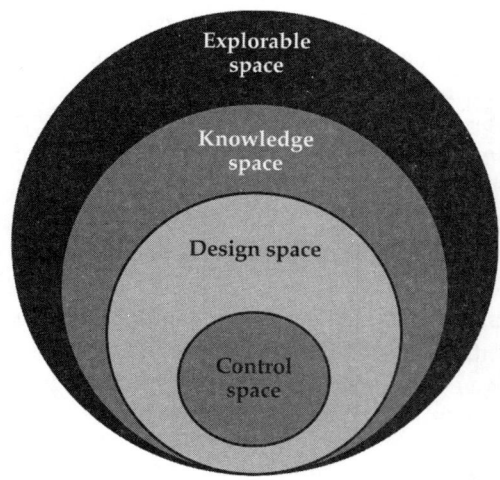

Fig. 14.8. Interplay of knowledge, design and control spaces during QbD-based drug product development.

linear response is detected, or a more accurate picture of the response surface is required, a more complex design type is necessary. In this context, factorial, Box-Behnken, composite, optimal and mixture designs are commonly used as the high resolution second-order designs for drug product optimization. Hence, when the investigator is interested in estimating interaction and even quadratic effects, or intends to have an idea of the local shape of the response surface, the response surface designs, capable of mapping non-linear responses, are used.

In nutshell, the major aspects to be considered while selecting an experimental design can be summarized as:

- All designs can be applied for optimization of product characteristics, but simplex-mixture design (SMD) should not be employed for process optimization.
- Any design out of 2^k FD, x^k FD, FFD, PBD, D-OD or TgD can be employed for screening studies.
- For estimation of main effects, all 2-level designs except PBD can be employed. However, for higher number of factors (> 6), screening should first be employed using FFD, PBD or TgD.

- If there are only two factor levels, any design out of 2^k FD, FFD or mixture design can be employed. However, in case of > 3 factor levels, CCD, BBD, mixture, simplex and optimal designs are preferred.
- For quadratic models, x^k FD, CCD, BBD or EqD are preferred for process optimization.

QbD-based Model Development and Optimization Data Analysis

A model is a mathematical or graphical expression defining the quantitative dependence of a response variable on the independent variables. Numeric models can either be empirical or theoretical. An empirical model provides a way to describe the factor-response relationship. Usually, it is a set of polynomials of a given order or degree. The models mostly employed to describe the response(s) are first, second and very occasionally, third order polynomials (Box et al., 1978). A first-order model is postulated in the first instance. In case a simple model is found to be inadequate for describing the phenomenon, the higher order models are followed.

The coefficients for quantitative factors can be estimated using regression analysis. However, in case of the qualitative factors, as interpolation between discrete (i.e., categorical) factor values is meaningless, regression analysis is not employed. For more factors, interactions and higher order terms, multiple linear regression analysis (MLRA) is usually preferred. For a combination of categorical and continuous variables, polynomial equations between response and the continuous variable are generated for each level of categorical variable. Multiple non-linear regression analysis (MNLRA) should be preferred when the factor-response relationship is non-linear. In multivariate studies, where there are large number of variables, the chemometric methods like partial least squares (PLS) or principal component analysis (PCA) can also be employed for

regression (Box and Draper, 1987). PLS, an extension of MLRA, is used when there are fewer observations than the number of predictor variables. In general, model analysis is conducted considering statistical tools like ANOVA, MANOVA, Student's t-test, predicted residual sum of squares (PRESS) and Pearsonian coefficient of determination (r^2).

Multiple Linear Regression Analysis (MLRA)

In case of the experiments involving qualitative factors, the interpolation between the discrete (i.e., categorical) factor values has been found to be meaningless and does not allow the application of simple regression analysis techniques for the purpose. Thus, for more factors, interactions and higher order terms, multiple linear regression analysis (MLRA) are usually preferred. In MLRA technique, polynomial equations between the responses and the continuous variables are generated for each level of categorical variables.

Principal Component Analysis (PCA)

PCA is a mathematical procedure that transforms a large set of variables into a lower dimensional set of new variables designated as principal components. This is an exploratory analysis technique that depends on the analysis objective and can be used to observe patterns/clusters in the data. The purpose of PCA is to express the latent information contained in the data set using a lower number of variables, also called as principal components (PC) (Ferreira and Tobyn, 2014). In PCA, data is transformed to describe the amount of variability in the data set in three-dimensional axial projections. The first axis depicts the total possible variance whereas the second axis depicts the remaining possible variance (without correlating with the first axis) and the third axis depicts the total variance remaining after accounting for the earlier two axes without correlating with either of the axes.

Partial Least Square (PLS) Analysis

PLS is a bilinear statistical technique widely accepted for modelling the relations between different sets of observed variables. It is considered as an extension of MLRA, and preferably used when there are fewer observations than the number of predictor variables. The basic assumption of the PLS is that it modifies relations between sets of the observed variables by a small number of latent variables (not directly observed or measured) by incorporating regression, dimension reduction techniques, and modelling tools (Ferreira and Tobyn, 2014). A PLS model tends to identify the multidimensional direction in the X space that explains the maximum multidimensional variance direction in the Y space.

Model Diagnostic Plots in QbD Optimization

Model diagnostic plots tend to identify the distribution of data and facilitate enhanced understanding of the cause-effect relationship among the studied variables with the responses. One or more diagnostic plots are usually employed during QbD optimization as tools for analyzing the factor sparsity and at times to investigate the goodness of fit of the proposed QbD model. The diagnostic plots employed during MLRA are quite different from those used for PCA and PLS models.

Model diagnostic plots during MLRA

Instances of model diagnostic plots employed during MLRA-based optimization data analysis include half-normal plots, Pareto charts, actual vs. predicted plot, Outlier-T plot, Cook's distance plot, Leverage plot, Box–Cox plot, etc. (Ferreira and Tobyn, 2014). Fig. 14.9 illustrates various model diagnostic plots used during MLRA modelling.

Model diagnostic plots during PCA

Fig. 14.10 illustrates the model diagnostic plots employed during PCA-based data analysis.

Instances of various model diagnostic plots like biplot, scree plot, score plot, loading plot, scatter plot and their significance have been given in the following section (Ferreira and Tobyn, 2014).

Validation of QbD Models

The major graphical tools employed for testing and revising QbD model encompass linear correlation plots, normal probability plot of residuals, response vs. prediction plot, residual lag plot, residuals histogram, etc. These model validation plots furnish information on the location, spread, skewness, outliers and multiple nodes of the data.

OPTIMUM SEARCH METHODOLOGY

From the models thus selected, optimization of one response or the simultaneous optimization of multiple responses needs to be accomplished graphically, numerically or using artificial neural networks (ANN) (Schwartz et al., 1973). A pictographic account on various modelling approaches used for the optimum search in the QbD methodology is depicted in Fig. 14.11.

Graphical optimization

Graphical optimization deals with selecting the best possible formulation out of a feasible factor space region (Lewis et al. 1999). The desirable limits of response variables are set and the factor levels are screened accordingly. Graphical optimization can be accomplished through one or more of the following methodologies.

Brute-force search

Brute-force search, also known as exhaustive search, is the simplest and most accurate of all possible optimization search methods, as it implies checking every single point in the function space (Singh et al., 2005). Herein, the formulations that can be prepared by almost every possible combination of independent factors are screened for their response variables.

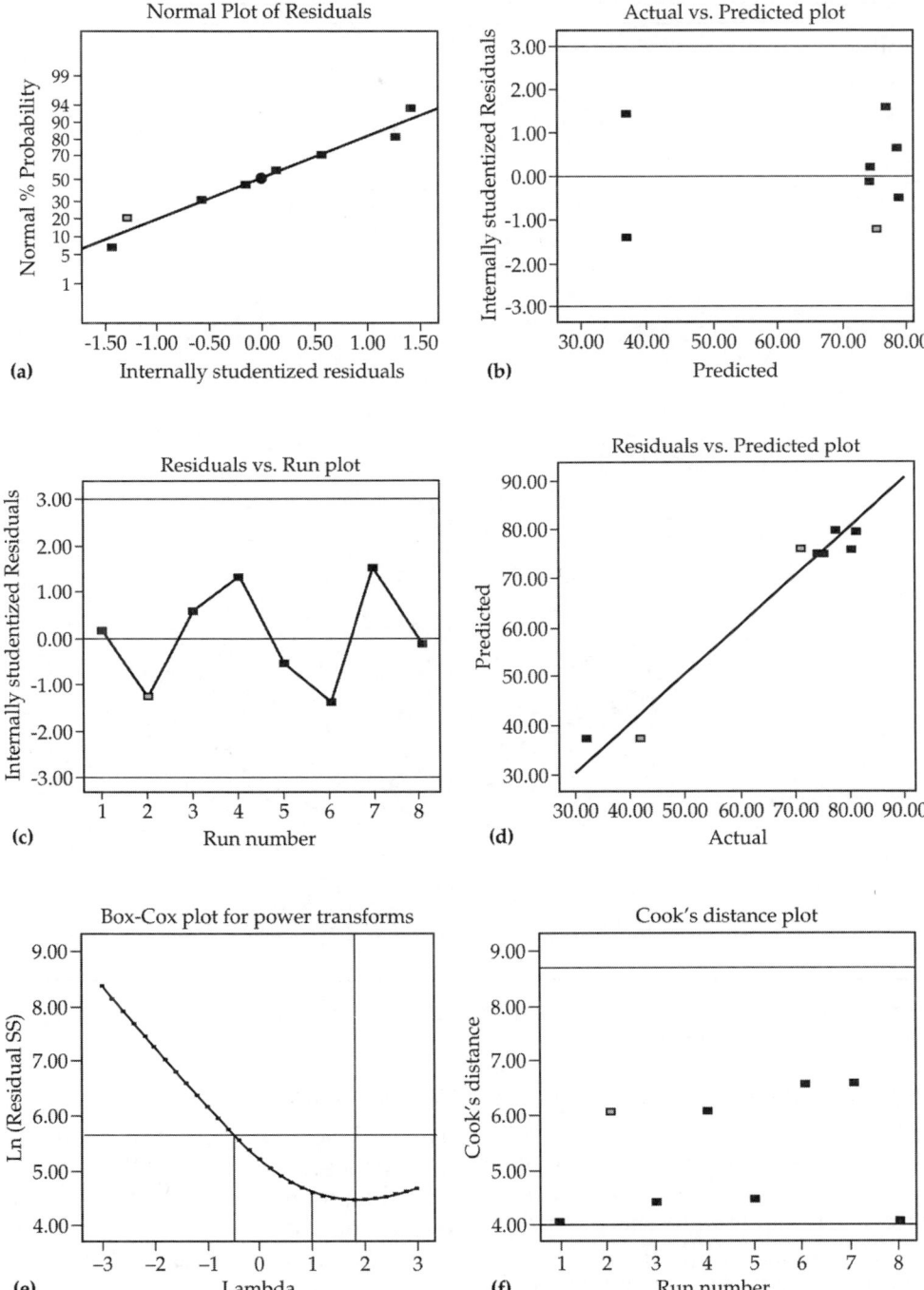

Fig. 14.9. MLR-based model diagnostic plots during DoE optimization, (a) Normal plot of residuals, (b) Actual vs. predicted plot, (c) Residual vs. run plot, (d) Residual vs. predicted plot, (e) Box-Cox plot for power transforms, (f) Cook's distance plot.

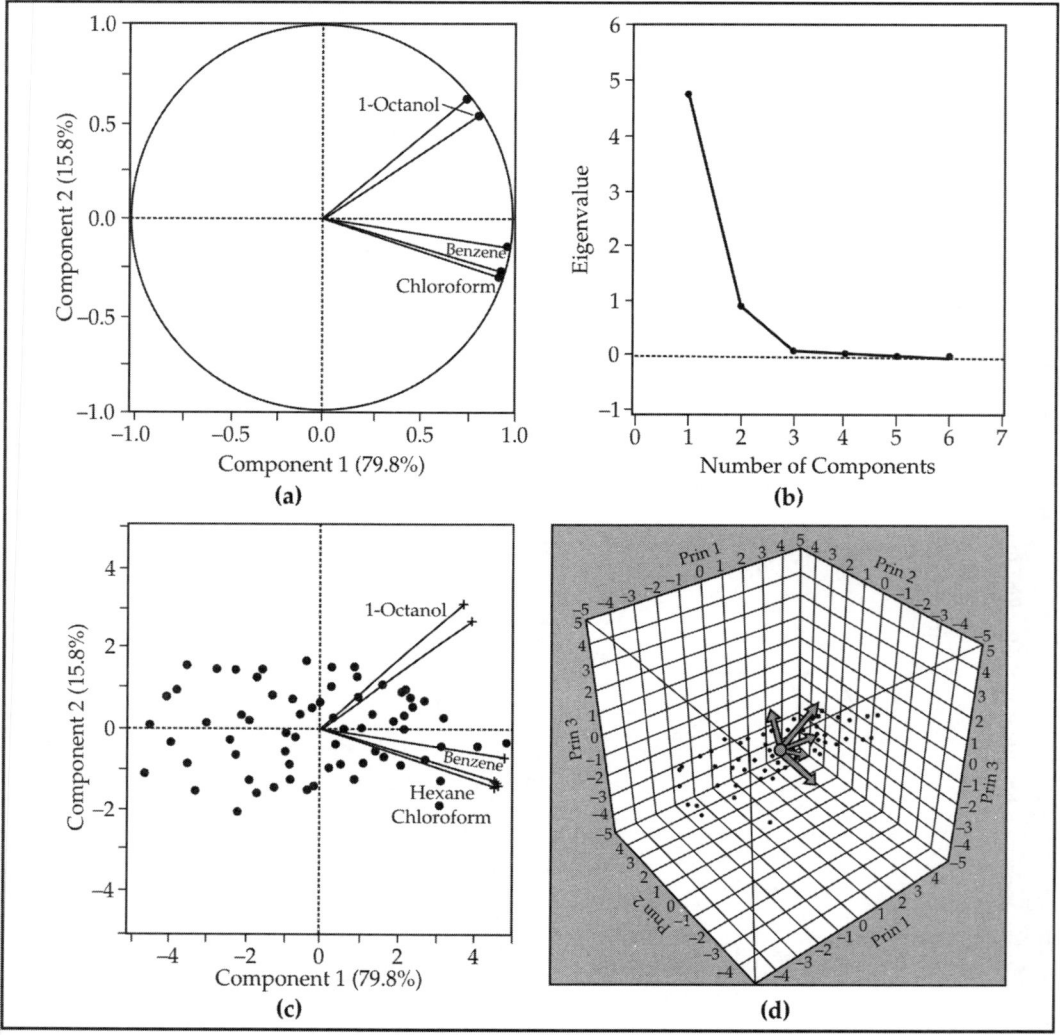

Fig. 14.10. Model diagnostic plots during PCA-based multivariate statistical optimization. (a) Biplot, (b) Eigenvalue plot, (c) Summary plot, (d) Scatter plot.

Subsequently, the acceptable limits are set for these responses, and an exhaustive search is again conducted by further narrowing down the feasible region. The optimized formulation is searched from the final feasible space (termed as grid search), which fulfills the maximum number of criteria set during experimentation. The advantage of this exhaustive method is that the chances of missing the true optimum formulation are only miniscule.

Overlay plots

The bi-dimensional response contour plots are superimposed over each other to search for the best compromise visually. This is termed as an overlay plot or a combined contour plot. Most often, this overlay plot as a whole signifies the "knowledge space" and considered as the best option to present the "design space" or "proven acceptable range (PAR)" for assuring desired quality levels and regulatory purpose (Yu et al.,

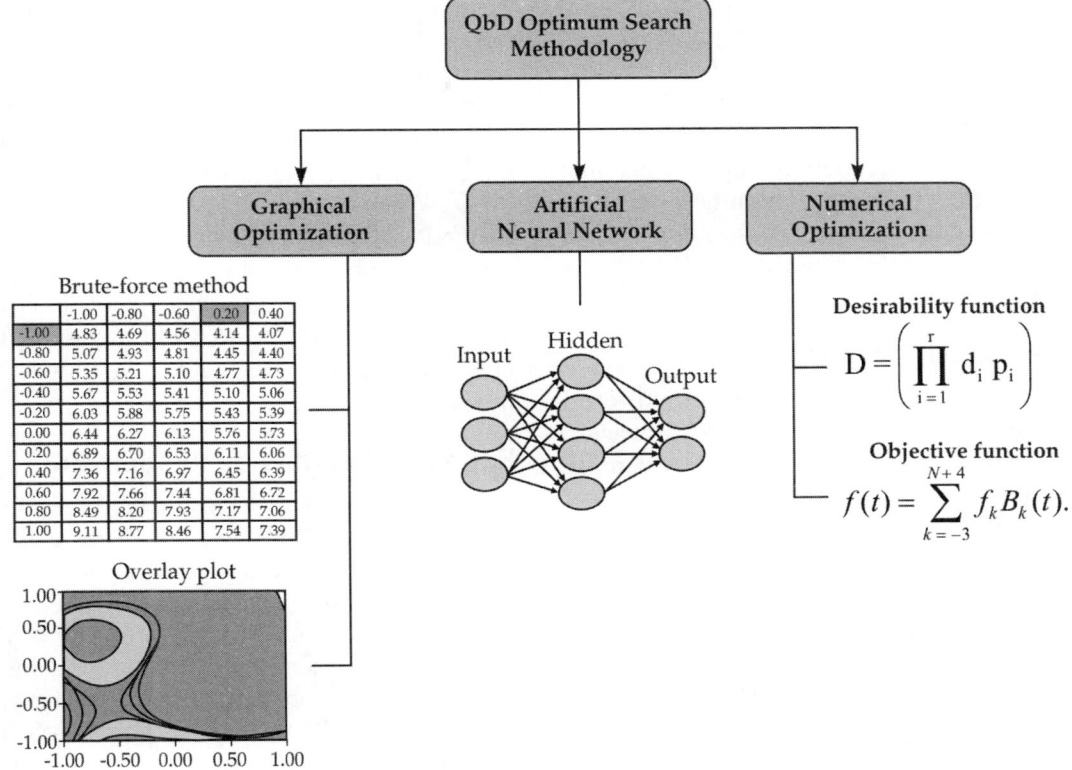

Fig. 14.11. Optimum search methodology during QbD-based optimization.

2014). Minimum and maximum boundaries are set for acceptable objective values. The region is highlighted as the design space wherein all the responses are within the acceptable range. In this region, the optimum formulation is located by "trading off" different responses. Besides, it is ideal in industrial practices to identify a region termed as "control space" or "normal operating range (NOR)" within the PAR for setting in-house specifications. Fig. 14.12 illustrates the knowledge space demarcating the location of PAR and NOR regions.

Canonical analysis

Canonical analysis indicates the predictability of each of the components of the criterion set of variables from the corresponding components, extracted from the predictor set of variables. The technique can only be employed for single

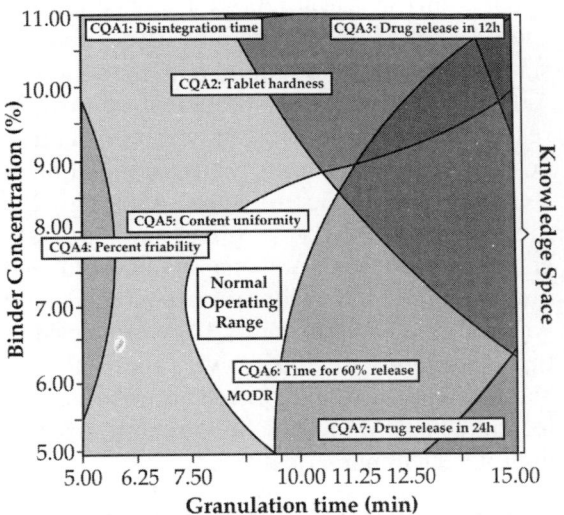

Fig. 14.12. Typical instance of design space overlay plot for process optimization of wet granulation process employed during tablet manufacturing.

response optimization. A saddle point is a point in the domain of a function of two variables which is a stationary point but not a local extremum (Singh et al., 2005). At such a point, in general, the surface resembles a saddle that curves up in one direction, or curves down in a different direction (like a mountain pass). In terms of contour lines, a saddle point can be recognized, in general, by a contour that appears to intersect itself.

Mathematical optimization

Graphical analysis is usually considered adequate in case of single response. However, in cases of multiple responses, it is usually advisable to conduct mathematical or numerical optimization first to uncover a feasible region.

Desirability function

Desirability function is a way to overcome the difficulty of multiple, sometimes opposing responses. In this method, each response is associated with its own partial desirability function (Gohel et al., 2009; Vaghani et al., 2012). The point possessing the highest value for desirability, usually 1 or close to 1, is termed as optimum (Shah et al., 2008). The experimenter should study the contour plot of desirability surface around the optimum and combine this with contour plots of the most important responses. A large area or volume of high desirability will indicate a robust formulation or set of processing conditions. Although the method essentially requires appropriate computer software, yet it is a highly useful and pragmatic method of optimization, especially when the number of factors is 3 or more. Besides, the techniques of "objective function" and "sequential unconstrained minimization technique (SUMT)" have also been utilized to optimize DDS numerically.

Artificial Neural Networks (ANNs)

ANNs are the machine-based computational techniques that attempt to simulate some of the neurological processing abilities of the human brain. The ANNs offer unique advantages of non-linear processing capacity and the ability to model poorly understood systems (Miyazaki et al., 2008; Gohel and Nagori, 2009; Leonardi et al., 2009; Zhang et al., 2009; Barmpalexis et al., 2010). When compared with other optimization methods, the results are comparable with better prognostic abilities. However, they are quite difficult to implement at higher number of factors and/or levels, and fail to yield any statistical criterion to declare the degree of aptness of the model.

Extrapolation outside the domain

Steepest ascent (or descent) methods are direct optimization methods for first-order designs, especially when the optimum is outside the domain and is to be arrived at rapidly (Lewis et al., 1999). Optimum path method is just analogous to steepest ascent method, but is employed where the optimum is searched outside the experimental domain by extrapolation. The technique of evolutionary operations, wherein the production procedure (formulation and process) is allowed to evolve to the optimum by careful planning and constant repetition, is quite popular in several industrial processes.

OVERALL QbD STRATEGY FOR DEVELOPMENT OF DDS

The overall approach for conduct of an QbD study in nanostructured DDS can be described by a holistic plan (Myers, 2003; Singh and Ahuja, 2004).

The salient steps involved in the QbD strategy include:

- *Problem definition:* The QbD problem is clearly comprehended, QTPP vividly defined and possible responses (CQAs) ascertained.
- *Selection of factors and factor levels:* The independent factors (i.e., CMAs, CFAs and/ or CPPs) are identified amongst the quantifiable and easily controllable variables.

- *Design of experimental protocol:* Based on the choice of independent factors and the response variables (i.e., CQAs), a suitable experimental design is selected and the number of experimental runs are determined.
- *Formulating and evaluating the dosage form:* Various drug delivery formulations are prepared as per the chosen design and evaluated for the desired response(s).
- *Selection of design space and optimum formulation:* The experimental data are used for generation of a mathematical model and an optimum formulation is located using suitable graphical and/or numerical methods.
- *Validation of QbD optimization:* The predicted optimal formulation is prepared and the responses evaluated. Results, if validated, are carried further to the production cycle via pilot plant operations and scale-up techniques.
- *Control strategy and continuous improvement:* At the end of QbD-based product development, the control strategy need be formulated for continuous improvement even after regulatory approval.

SOFTWARE USAGE DURING QbD

The merits of QbD techniques are galore and their acceptability upbeat. Putting such rational approaches into practice, however, usually involves a great deal of mathematical and statistical intricacies. Today, with the availability of powerful and economical hardware and that of the comprehensive QbD software, the erstwhile computational hiccups have been overcome and streamlined (Singh, 2014). Pertinent computer software available for DoE optimization include Design-Expert®, MODDE®, Unscrambler®, JMP®, Statistica®, Minitab®, etc., are at the rescue, which usually provide interface guide at every step during the entire product development cycle. Software provide support for chemometric analysis through multivariate techniques like MNLRA, PCA, PLS, etc. encompass MODDE®, Unscrambler®, SIMCA®, CODDESA®. For QRM execution using Fish-bone diagrams, REM and FMEA matrices during risk assessment studies, etc., software like, Minitab®, Risk®, Statgraphics, FMEA-Pro, iGrafx, etc., can be made use of.

QbD APPLICATIONS IN PRODUCT DEVELOPMENT LIFECYCLE

Beyond any cynicism, QbD has been an inimitable quality-targeted approach for attaining excellence while developing efficacious and inexpensive safe and robust drug products. Besides, it facilitates macroscopic and microscopic comprehension of products or processes, and helps in accomplishing federal compliance with phenomenal ease and economy, whether for generics or innovators (Singh and Beg, 2013). Today, pharmaceutical scientists on industrial fronts have not only been deriving its stellar benefits during entire product development lifecycle, but even beyond. The other key domain where QbD principles are being frequently used encompasses the analytical method development. In addition, QbD has slowly been percolating into several other interdisciplinary areas like API development, dissolution testing, manufacturing, bioequivalence studies and stability testing (Fig. 14.13). The pictorial flow layout of the application of strategic principles of QbD during diverse phases of drug product development cycle is illustrated in Fig. 14.14.

Generic product and new product development

Since 1st January 2013, USFDA has mandated the QbD implementation for all the generic products entering into the US market. In this regard, an ANDA application must include four key elements such as defined QTPP (as it relates to the quality, safety and efficacy of the product to make them pharmaceutical equivalent with the innovator product) and patient-centric CQAs, the product CMAs primarily influencing the CQAs, appropriate manufacturing process(es) followed by the design space and control strategy

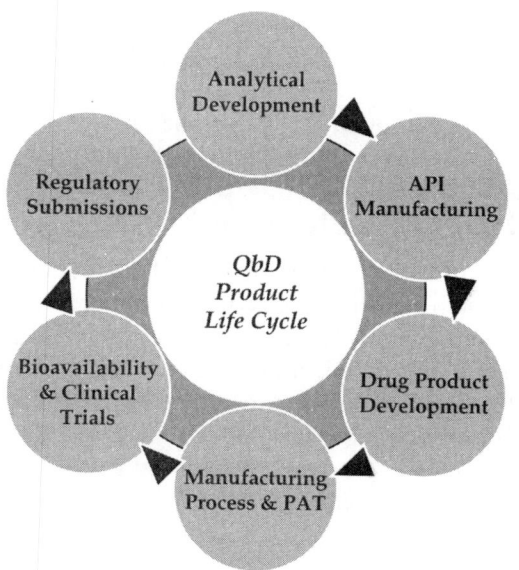

Fig. 14.13. QbD is useful overall product development even after the product launch.

(Lionberger et al., 2008). Unlike the generic products, QbD implementation for manufacturing of the new drug products is not mandatory for marketing in US. The key difference between QbD applications for NDA and ANDA products is most apparent at the first step of the process, but so far no specifications have been posted for defining the target product profile for NDA products. The applicant, however, may include other vital elements of QbD for generic product development for demonstrating the product and process understanding.

Existing product development

Application of QbD principles to the drug product(s) already commercialized in the market is referred as retrospective QbD, which involves critical analysis of the prior development report and manufacturing history of the product to assess its quality, efficacy and safety by mitigating potential risk(s) (Singh and Beg, 2013). In addition, retrospective QbD helps in reviewing the product and/or process(es) related attributes for identification of the CQAs, assess-

for the entire product including input material controls, process controls and monitors. Utility of vital tools like risk assessment, DoE and PAT, though not mandatory requirements, yet can be used with advantage(s) when appropriate

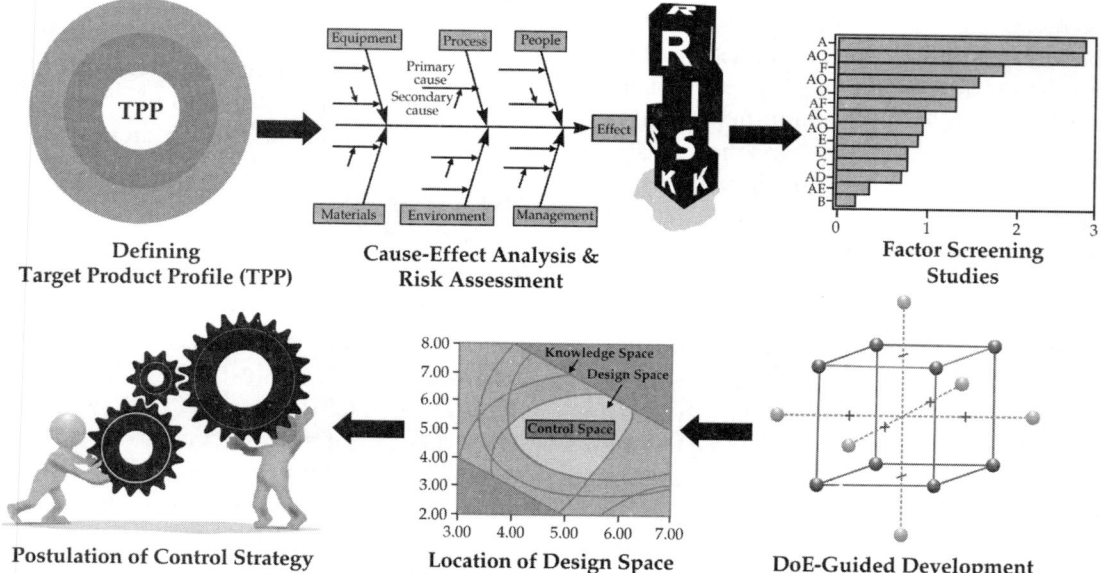

Fig. 14.14. Application of strategic QbD principles in pharmaceutical product development.

ment of raw material attribute(s), construction of process flow diagram(s) and risk assessment to review the process parameters, generation of design and control spaces, and formulation of the control strategy for continual improvement, thus, facilitating overall product quality and process performance.

Analytical method development

Analytical Quality by Design (AQbD), on the heels of QbD, endeavours at understanding the predefined analytical objectives. These comprise quality target method profile (QTMP) of an analytical method, and identifying the critical method variables (CMVs) affecting the critical analytical attributes (CAAs) for attaining enhanced method performance, like high robustness, ruggedness and flexibility for continual improvement within the ambit of design space (Reid et al., 2013). Besides, AQbD helps in reducing and controlling the source of variability to gain in-process information for taking control decisions in a timely manner. This facilitates attaining flexibility in analysis of API and impurities in dosage forms, stability samples and biological samples, and to go beyond traditional ICH procedure of method validation. Like FbD, the AQbD also embarks upon risk-assessment studies through REM/FMEA, and DoE-guided factor screening and optimization studies for improving the method performance. Instances of CMVs during AQbD optimization include mobile phase composition, flow rate, gradient time, column oven temperature, pH, while CAAs include peak area, retention time, theoretical plates, asymmetry factor and capacity factor (Bhutani et al., 2014). Box 14.4 illustrates the list of CMVs and CAAs employed during AQbD approach of method development.

According to the USFDA report on establishment of analytical method, AQbD execution involves three different phases, viz. procedure design (i.e., method development and understanding), procedure performance qualification (i.e., method analysis and optimization), and

Box 14.4. Instances of commonly used critical method parameters (CMPs) and critical analytical attributes (CAAs) used during analytical quality by design (AQbD)	
List of vital CMPs	**List of vital CAAs**
• Stationary phase	• Peak area
• Gradient time	• Assay recovery
• Oven temperature	• Retention time
• Mobile phase pH	• Peak resolution
• Buffer strength	• Theoretical plates
• Flow rate	• Tailing factor
• Injection volume	• Assymetry factor
• Column dimension	• Capacity factor

continued procedure performance verification (i.e., method validation and transfer) (Martin et al., 2015). Implementation of AQbD in an industrial milieu encompasses postulation of an analytical target profile (ATP), identification of CMVs and CAAs, design-guided method development and analysis, establishment of method operable design region (MODR), and formulation of control strategy for continual improvement in the method performance.

Drug substance development

Developing drug substances employing the systematic QbD-based paradigm has been recently popularized to accomplish the desired objective of producing drug substance with reduced variability, high purity and yield. ICH Q11 guidance, in this regard, provides detailed understanding of the key principles of manufacturing drug substance employing rational paradigms. As per the QbD approach, the quality defined target profile include molecular, physiochemical and biological properties, pharmacokinetics, storage and packaging conditions, etc. (Rossi and Braggio, 2011). The concentrations of reactants, solvents, initiators, stabilizers employed during synthesis of drug substance are mainly used as the CMAs, which are subsequently optimized for their impact on CQAs like API particle size and size distribution, polymorphism, hygroscopicity, density, flow property, aqueous solubility, etc.

Dissolution testing

Dissolution testing is primarily considered as one of the most important quality control tests for preparing the release specification for any pharmaceutical dosage form. The QbD approach helps in optimizing the drug product composition for accomplishing drug release profile analogous to that of the reference listed product. Important examples of CQAs, which determine the product quality include amount of drug released at specified time intervals, mean dissolution time, dissolution efficiency, release exponent, etc., whereas the concentration of polymers, disintegrants, type of medium are used as CMAs, which tend to affect the dissolution profile of drug products (Dickinson et al., 2008).

Bioequivalence testing

Implementation of QbD during bioequivalence study helps in optimizing the drug products (i.e., generics) in obtaining desired pharmacokinetic profile matched with that of the reference listed product. Important pharmacokinetic metrics like, C_{max}, t_{max}, AUC, AUC_{0-t}, $AUC_{0-\infty}$, are considered as the critical quality traits for optimizing the formulation variables like concentration of release controlling polymer, coating and coating percentage, etc.

Biologicals and herbal products

Most often, QbD has been applied to the development of processes and products of small molecules only. Though quite disparate from each other, the biologicals and herbals both, on the other hand, are relatively more intricate, multi-component and heterogeneous systems, which are not precisely defined, analyzed or characterized (Rathore and Winkle, 2009; Elliott et al., 2013). Hence, scrupulous understanding of the relationships between process variables, and product CQAs is obligatory for such

products (Das et al., 2014). Several attempts have lately been made to apply chemometric multivariate tools and DoE to develop optimized processes yielding robust biosimilars, improved yield of production of proteins, enzyme, etc., and upgraded efficiency of herbal extraction procedures.

Stability testing

QbD approach in stability testing furnishes better understanding of the product stability and shelf-life, information on degradation products, and compatibility of container(s)/closure(s) with packaging materials (Krumenaker, 2015). This helps in preparing the specifications related to safety and efficacy of finished product(s) with respect to the concentration of degradants and their final qualifications for marketing approval.

QbD APPLICATIONS IN PRODUCT LIFECYCLE MANAGEMENT

In fact, the utility of versatile QbD approach is not only restricted to various stages of product development of small molecules as well as bigger biological macromolecules, but also extends to the entire product lifespan (McCurdy, 2011). Application of QbD at various stages of product lifespan, starting from the early developmental phase to even after the post-approval commercial launch and post-marketing surveillance stage, is spelled out as:

Pre-clinical developmental phase

The ability to use prior knowledge from previous products, prior published or patent literature and prior experience is helpful in applying QbD during early stages of developing the lead molecule. Prior knowledge of patient needs helps in meeting the requirement of desired quality characteristics in the new drug product.

Non-clinical and clinical phase

To meet the predefined specifications, the experiments conducted at pre-clinical and non-clinical stages are used to meet the requirements of the target product. This includes the *in vitro* and *in vivo* tests, depending upon the type of product, feasibility experiments, toxicology tests or clinical study details. Under the ambit of QbD-based approach of product development, clinical studies help in providing thought-through information on the quality attributes of the product and in micro-refinement of the product and manufacturing process(es).

Scale-up phase

QbD tends to provide a great deal of understanding during scale-up phase. This allows to document changes and rationalization during changeover from small pilot scale to the full-scale commercial manufacturing. Further, the information extracted at this stage is useful in designing the control strategy for continuous improvement.

Marketing approval phase

Submissions based on QbD provide more scientific information on the product, processes and change controls employed during optimization. This helps in improving the quality of submissions and ultimately provides regulatory flexibility for faster approval from the regulatory agencies.

QbD-BASED UNDERSTANDING OF PRODUCT AND PROCESS

The objective of pharmaceutical QbD is to increase process capability and reduce product variability that often reduces the product defects, rejections, and recalls. Achieving this objective requires robustly designed product and process (Huang et al., 2009). Albeit diverse QbD tools like cause-effect diagrams, Pareto charts, risk assessment tools, factor screening and optimization employing experimental designs have been considered to be pivotal, yet the implementation of other vital techniques have been popularized for improving the product and process understanding. These include chemometry, drug release kinetic modelling, *in vitro/in vivo* correlations, pharmacokinetic simulation, toxicity prediction, which tend to provide the minute details on the product behavior. Beyond this, utilization of process controls, process engineering, process capability tools, extensometry and real time release testing (RTRT) furnishes understanding on the process behavior, respectively. The improved understanding on the product and process behavior facilitates the identification and control of factors influencing the drug product quality. This ultimately facilitates regulatory flexibility by reducing the product variability, defects, rejections and recalls.

EPILOGUE

A formulation scientist can derive unique benefits of QbD employing multivariate DoE approaches for rational development and formulation optimization of various drug products and processes associated with them. It has been proved to be useful even if the primary aim is not the selection of the optimum formulation, as it tends to divulge the degree of improvement in the product characteristics as a function of change in (any) excipient or process parameter(s). Today, the federal agencies in terms of QbD need the "in-built product quality" rather than testing the quality of the finished product. Comprehending the formulation or process variables rationally using QbD not only would help in attaining product development excellence with phenomenal ease at low cost but also in federal compliance. As a rule, when finding the correct solution is not simple, a pharmaceutical scientist should mandatorily consider the use of QbD for developing novel and nanostructured drug products, wherein the variability and vulnerability of the systems make them ultra-sensitive to diverse formulation factors and processes these systems tend to undergo. QbD is a quality-centric approach, which provides enormous benefits to meet the unmet needs of patients as well as pharmaceutical manufacturers for development of efficacious, cost-effective, safe and stable drug products. Notwithstanding the immense vitality of this QbD philosophy in industrial milieu, its importance is enormous in diverse fields beyond the formulation development such as in analytical method development, pharmaceutical manufacturing, and stability studies too. This approach not only helps in developing optimal solutions, but also in permeating rational research mindsets towards evolving "out-of-box" strategies. Apt implementation of QbD paradigm, accordingly, would be pivotal in achieving a "win-win situation" not only for patients, drug industry, and regulators, but for the whole gamut of drug delivery scientists too.

REFERENCES

- Aksu, B., Beg, S., Garg, B., Kapil, R., Singh, B. Quality by Design (QbD) and its applications. *In:* Development of Nanostructured Drug Delivery Systems: pp: 1-30, Vol. 4: Nanostructured Drug Delivery (ISBN: 1-626990-54-9) Nanobiomedicine (Series ISBN: 1-626990-50-6), 2015, Singh, B. Vyas, S.P., Kaur, I.P. (Ed.). Studium Press LLC, Houston, USA.
- Barmpalexis, P., Kanaze, F.I., Kachrimanis, K., Georgarakis, E. Artificial neural networks in the optimization of a nimodipine controlled release tablet formulation. *Eur. J. Pharm. Biopharm.*, 2010; 74: 316–23.
- Bhutani, H., Kurmi, M., Singh, S., Beg, S., Singh, B. Quality by Design (QbD) in analytical sciences: An Overview. *Pharma Times*, 2014; 46: 71–75.
- Box, G.E.P., Draper, N.R. Empirical Model-Building and Response Surfaces, 1st ed. 1987, Wiley Interscience, New York, USA.
- Box, G.E.P., Hunter, WG, Hunter, JS. Statistics for Experimenters, 1978, Wiley Interscience, New York, USA.
- Das, A.K., Mandal, S.C., Mandal. V., Beg. S., Singh, B. QbD as an emerging paradigm in extraction technology for developing optimized bioactives. *Pharma Times*, 2014; 46: 50–56.
- Dickinson, P.A., Lee, W.W., Stott, P.W., Townsend, A.I., Smart, J.P., Ghahramani, P., Hammett, T., Billett, L., Behn, S., Gibb, R.C., Abrahamsson, B. Clinical relevance of dissolution testing in quality by design. *AAPS J.*, 2008; 10: 208–211.
- Elliott, P., Billingham, S., Bi, J., Zhang, H. Quality by design for biopharmaceuticals: A historical review and guide for implementation. *Pharm. Bioprocess*, 2013; 1: 105–122.
- Guidance for industry and review staff target product profile – A strategic development process tool, FDA CDER, Maryland, USA, 2007.
- Ferreira, A.P., Tobyn, M. Multivariate analysis in the pharmaceutical industry: Enabling process understanding and improvement in the PAT and QbD era. *Pharm. Dev. Technol.*, 2015;20: 513-27.
- Gohel, M., Nagori, S.A. Fabrication and evaluation of captopril modified-release oral formulation. *Pharm. Dev. Technol.*, 2009; 14: 679–86.
- Gohel, M., Parikh, R.K., Aghara, P.Y., Nagori, S.A., Delvadia, R.R., Dabhi, M.R. Application of simplex lattice design and desirability function for the formulation development of mouth dissolving film of salbutamol sulphate. *Curr. Drug Deliv.*, 2009; 6: 486–94.
- Guebitz, B., Schnedl, H., Khinast, J.G. A risk management ontology for Quality-by-Design based on a new development approach according GAMP 5.0. *Expert Sys. Appl.*, 2012; 39: 7291–7301.
- Huang, J., Kaul, G., Cai, C., Chatlapalli, R., Hernandez-Abad, P., Ghosh, K., Nagi, A. Quality by design case study: An integrated multivariate approach to drug product and process development. *Int. J. Pharm.*, 2009; 382: 23–32.
- ICH Harmonised Tripartite Guideline: Pharmaceutical Development Q8(R2). http://www.ich.org/fileadmin/Public_Web_Site/ICH_Products/Guidelines/Quality/Q8_R1/Step4/Q8_R2_Guideline.pdf. (Accessed on 27 September 2016)
- ICH Harmonised Tripartite Guideline: Pharmaceutical Quality System (Q10). http://www.ich.org/fileadmin/Public_Web_Site/ICH_Products/Guidelines/Quality/Q10/Step4/Q10_Guideline.pdf. (Accessed on 28 February 2017)
- ICH Harmonised Tripartite Guideline: Quality Risk Management (Q9). http://www.ich.org/fileadmin/Public_Web_Site/ICH_Products/Guidelines/Quality/Q9/Step4/Q9_Guideline.pdf. (Accessed on 13 March 2017)

- Kannissery, P., M. Abu T., Naseem, A.C., Shahid H.A., Javed A. Pharmaceutical product development: A quality by design approach. *Int. J. Pharm. Investig.*, 2016, 6:129–138.
- Krumenaker, A. 6 considerations for QbD use in stability studies. IVT Network: Institute of Validation Technology. http://www.ivtnetwork.com/article/6-considerations-qbd-use-stability-studies. (Accessed on 26 August 2016)
- Juran, J.M. Juran on Quality by Design: The new steps for planning quality into goods and services. Juran Institute Inc. Press, USA 1992.
- Leonardi, D., Salomon, C.J., Lamas, M.C., Olivieri, A.C. Development of novel formulations for Chagas disease: Optimization of benznidazole chitosan microparticles based on artificial neural networks. *Int. J. Pharm.*, 2009; 367: 140–7.
- Lewis, G.A., Mathieu, D., Phan-Tan-Luu, R. Pharmaceutical experimental design. 1st ed. 1999, New York, Marcel Dekker.
- Lionberger, R.A., Lee, S.L., Lee, L., Raw, A., Yu, L.X. Quality by Design: Concepts for ANDAs. *AAPS J.*, 2008; 10: 268–76.
- Martin, G.P., Barnett, K.L., Burgess, C., Curry, P.D., Ermer, J., Gratzl, G.S., Hammond, J.P., Herrmann, J., Kovacs, E., LeBlond, D., LoBrutto, R., McCasland-Keller, A., McGregor, P.L., Nethercote, P., Templeton, A., Thomas, D., Weitzel, M.L.J. Lifecycle management of analytical procedures: Method development, procedure performance qualification, and procedure performance verification. www.usp.org/sites/default/files/usp_pdf/EN/USPNF/.../lifecycle_pdf. (Accessed on 13 March 2017)
- McCurdy, V. Quality by Design. Process Understanding: For Scale-Up and Manufacture of Active Ingredients. I. Houson. Wiley-VCH Verlag GmbH, Germany, 2011.
- Miyazaki, Y., Yakou, S., Yanagawa, F., Takayama, K. Evaluation and optimization of preparative variables for controlled-release floatable microspheres prepared by poor solvent addition method. *Drug Dev. Ind. Pharm.*, 2008; 34: 1238–45.
- Myers, W.R. Response Surface Methodology. Encyclopedia of Biopharmaceutical Statistics. Chow, S.C. Marcel Dekker, New York, 2003.
- Rathore, A.S., Winkle, H. Quality by design for biopharmaceuticals. *Nat. Biotechnol.*, 2009; 27: 26–34.
- Reid, G.L., Morgado, J., Barnett, K., Harrington, B., Wang, J., Harwood, J., Fortin, D. Analytical Quality by Design (AQbD) in Pharmaceutical Development. http://www.americanpharmaceuticalreview.com/Featured-Articles/144191-Analytical-Quality-by-Design-AQbD-in-Pharmaceutical-Development/. 2013. (Accessed on 25 April 2016)
- Riley, B.S., Li, X. Quality by design and process analytical technology for sterile products – Where are we now? *AAPS PharmSciTech*, 2010; 12: 114–8.
- Rossi, T., Braggio, S. Quality by Design in lead optimization: a new strategy to address productivity in drug discovery. *Curr. Opin. Pharmacol.*, 2011; 11: 515–520.
- Sangshetti, J.N., Deshpandea, M., Zaheera, Z., Shindeb, D.B., Arote, R. Quality by Design approach: Regulatory need. *Arabian J. Chem.*, 2014; http://dx.doi.org/10.1016/j.arabjc.2014.01.025
- Schwartz, J.B., Flamholz, J.R., Press, R.H. Computer optimization of pharmaceutical formulations. I. General procedure. *J. Pharm. Sci.*, 1973; 62: 1165–70.
- Shah, P.P., Mashru, R.C., Rane, Y.M., Badhan, A.C. Design and optimization of artemether microparticles for bitter taste masking. *Acta Pharm.*, 2008; 58: 379–92.
- Singh, B. Quality by Design (QbD) for Holistic Pharma Excellence and Regulatory Compliance. *Pharma Times*, 2014; 46: 1–18.
- Singh, B., Ahuja, N. Response surface optimization of drug delivery systems. Progress in Controlled and Novel Drug Delivery Systems. 1st ed. Jain, N.K. CBS Publishers, New Delhi, 2004.
- Singh, B., Beg, S. Quality by Design in product development life cycle. *Chron. Pharmabiz*, 2013; 22: 72–79.
- Singh, B., Kapil, R., Nandi, M., Ahuja, N. Developing oral drug delivery systems using formulation by design: Vital precepts, retrospect and prospects. *Expert Opin. Drug Deliv.*, 2011a; 8: 1341–60.
- Singh, B., Bhatowa, R., Tripathi, C.B., Kapil, R. Developing micro-/nanoparticulate drug delivery systems using "design of experiments". *Int. J. Pharm. Investig.*, 2011b; 1: 75–87.
- Singh, B., Khurana, R.K., Lohan, S., Sandhu, P.S., Beg, S., Naveen, A. Developing optimized nano-

pharmaceuticals employing rational use of systematic multivariate techniques. NanoPharmaceuticals (ISBN: 1-626990-52-2) NanoBioMedicine (Series ISBN: 1-626990-50-6), 2015, Singh, B., Singh, K.K., Rekhi, G.S., (Ed.). Studium Press LLC, Houston, USA.

- Singh, B., Kumar, R., Ahuja, N. Optimizing drug delivery systems using systematic "Design of Experiments." Part I: Fundamental aspects. *Crit. Rev. Ther. Drug Carrier Syst.*, 2005; 22: 27–105.
- Singh, B., Raza, K., Beg, S. Developing "Optimized" drug products employing "Designed" experiments. *Chem. Ind. Digest*, 2013; 12: 1–7.
- Vaghani, S.S., Patel, S.G., Jivani, R.R., Jivani, N.P., Patel, M.M., Borda, R. Design and optimization of a stomach-specific drug delivery system of repaglinide: Application of simplex lattice design. *Pharm. Dev. Technol.*, 2012; 17: 55–65.
- Yu, L.X. Pharmaceutical quality by design: Product and process development, understanding, and control. *Pharm. Res.*, 2008; 25: 781–91.
- Yu, L.X., Amidon, G., Khan, M.A., Hoag, S.W., Polli, J., Raju, G.K., Woodcock, J. Understanding pharmaceutical quality by design. *AAPS J.*, 2014; 16: 771–83.
- Zhang, X.Y., Chen, D.W., Jin, J., Lu, W. Artificial neural network parameters optimization software and its application in the design of sustained release tablets. *Yao Xue Xue Bao*, 2009; 44: 1159–64.

15

Pharmaceutical Packaging

V.R. Sinha, R. Kumria, O.P. Katare, Harneet Kaur,
Sandeep Kaur and Amita Sarwal

INTRODUCTION

Packaging of pharmaceuticals is required not only for the protection of the product but also to ensure the product stability during the period of shelf-life. Any fault in the package can adversely affect the product. A thorough investigation and evaluation of the package ingredients that are in immediate contact with the product need to be done. Two attributes are most important with regard to the package; one is the expectation from the package to provide protection to the product from temperature, moisture, light, oxygen, etc., while the other is the being inert in itself. WHO guidelines define packaging as a process that a bulk material must undergo to become a finished product.

The essential elements of pharmaceutical packaging are providing protection, presentation, identification, information, convenience, compliance and compatible unit, which maintain the integrity and stability of the product (Table 15.1). Additionally, it should be economical and disposable. Package provides protection against climatic conditions (temperature, moisture, atmospheric gases, pressure, particulate matter and light), microbes (bacteria, fungi, yeast, etc.),

Table 15.1. Role of packaging
• Protection against
– Light
– Reactive gases
– Moisture
– Microbes
– Physical damage
– Pilferage and adulteration
• Presentation
• Identification
• Information
• Compatibility
• Convenience

mechanical stress (during packaging operations, transportation, accidental drops and carriage), chemicals and misuse. Presentation helps in building the image of a product. Packaging helps in identification of the product and various desired information are displayed as per the label requirement of the product. It should be convenient to use or to administer the product e.g. eye drops, collapsible tubes, metered dose inhalers (MDI). It should be compatible with product and should neither contaminate the product nor be adversely affected by the product. After exhaustion of the product, it should be easily disposed (recyclable or biodegradable). It should also take care of pilferage and adulteration risks.

The packaging process includes filling and assembling, sterilization in the final container, if applicable, and placing labels on the container and storage at the manufacturing and shipping sites.

Packs are known to affect the shelf-life of all the pharmaceutical products including ethical, semi-ethical and proprietary. Transparent packaging is specially being encouraged to replace the opaque packaging as it allows streamline quality control, simplification of labelling, extended shelf-life and even enhanced product aesthetics. Additionally, the packaging should be economical and should provide information regarding the product and should also be compliant with the regulatory requirements.

Packaging design takes into account the needs of the product, manufacturing and the distribution system. The fundamental functions of packaging are to provide protection thereby not to allow leak, diffusion and permeation of the product; to be strong enough to hold the contents during normal handling and storage; not to be altered by the ingredients of the formulation in its final form. Some of the definitions regarding nature of the pack given in USP 37 are enlisted in Table 15.2.

Innovation in packaging warrants the development of safe, convenient, sturdy elegant packaging for newer pharmaceutical product. Newer polymers in plastics, newer low permeability films and foils, improvement in glass (e.g. coated glass) provide novel properties to the packaging. Just over half of medicines (51%) are taken orally as tablets and capsules that are packed in blister/strip packs or fed into plastic bottles. Powders, pastilles and liquids also make up part of the oral medicine intake. Other medicines include parenterals (29%), inhalation (17%) and transdermal (3%) preparations. Dosage forms are available in a variety of different shapes and sizes

Table 15.2. Definitions (USP 37)

- **Well closed container:** A well-closed container protects the contents from extraneous solids and from loss of the article under the ordinary or customary conditions of handling, shipment, storage and distribution.
- **Tight container:** A tight container protects the articles from contamination by extraneous liquids, solids, or vapors, from loss of the article, and from efflorescence, deliquescence or evaporation under the ordinary or customary conditions of handling, shipment, storage, and distribution and is capable of tight re-closure.
- **Hermetic container:** A hermetic container is impervious to air or any other gas under the ordinary or customary conditions of handling, shipment, storage, and distribution.
- **Light-resistant container:** A light resistant container protects the contents from the effects of light by virtue of the specific properties of the material of which it is composed, including any coating applied to it.

  Alternatively, a clear and colorless or a translucent container may be made light-resistant by means of an opaque covering or by use of secondary packaging, in which case the label of the container bears a statement that opaque covering or secondary packaging is needed until the articles are to be used or administered.
- **Tamper-resistant container:** A packaging system that may not be accessed without obvious destruction of the seal or some portion of the packaging system.

(e.g. tablets). These changes in dosage forms have an impact on packaging with an increasing need to provide tailored, individual packaging solution, to maintain the quality, aesthetics and effectiveness of the dosage form. Need for specialized packages including child-resistant, senior-friendly has further increased expectations from the packaging industry.

The pharmaceutical packaging comprises of primary packaging, secondary packaging and accessories. These include primary packaging material, secondary packaging material and accessories (Table 15.3). The **primary pack** consists of those packaging components that form the part of the pack, which contains the product and are in direct contact of the product e.g. bottle, cap, liner, etc. The main function of the primary pack is to contain or restrict the

Table 15.3. Primary, secondary packaging material and accessories

Primary	Secondary	Accessories
• Glass bottles and jars	• Cartons (paperboard boxes)	• Pharmaceutical closures
• Plastic bottles	• Prescription dispensing containers	• Dispensing closures
• Strip packs	• Corrugated boxes	• Rubber stoppers
• Blister packs	• Paper drums	• Paper, foil laminated lids
• Pouches	• Shipping containers	• Leaflets
• Ointment tubes	• Injection trays	• Labels
• Vials and ampoules		• Shrink wrap and bands
• IV containers		• Wrappers
• Pre-filled syringes		• Inner seals
• Aerosol containers		• Gum tapes
• Pre-filled inhalers		• BOPP tapes
• Paperboard containers		

product and to provide protection to the product. All other packaging materials used external to the primary pack are known as the **secondary packaging** materials. These provide physical protection to ensure safe warehousing and mechanical protection required in shipment and transport. These include cartons, corrugated boxes, shipment containers, etc. There may be some associated components in packaging, e.g. dosing dropper, calibrated spoon.

Primary packaging materials should not:
(a) have adverse effect on product due to chemical reaction, leaching, absorption or adsorption, particulate contamination;
(b) be adversely affected by product;
(c) be influenced by adverse manufacturing conditions (e.g. sterilization, freezing).

Functions of secondary packaging are depicted in Table 15.4.

UNIT-DOSE PACKAGING

Unit-dose packaging is defined as a single unit container for administration as a single dose, direct from the container. In this a single item or a specific quantity (dose) is enclosed within a disposable pack. These dosage units guarantee safer medication, are more practical, improve patient compliance and are more useful for less stable products. **Device packaging** comprises of

Table 15.4. Secondary packaging component function

• Protection from excessive
  – Transmission of reactive gases
  – Moisture
  – Light
  – Microbes
• Protection to flexible containers
• Protection from rough handling during transportation

packaging along with an administration device. This is user-friendly and improves patient compliance. This allows an easier administration by means of devices such as prefilled syringes, droppers, transdermal delivery systems, pumps and aerosol sprays. These devices ensure that the product is administered correctly and in the right amount. There are a number of packaging materials used for primary as well as secondary packaging (Table 15.5). The choice of packaging material will depend upon:

(a) the dosage form desired,
(b) the degree of protection required,
(c) compatibility with the dosage form,
(d) presentation and aesthetics,
(e) customer convenience e.g. size, weight of dosage form,
(f) filling method,
(g) sterilization method to be employed, and
(h) cost.

Table 15.5. Types of raw materials used for pharmaceutical packaging

Type	Use
Glass	Bottles, Vials, Ampoules, Syringes, Cartridges, IV containers, Aerosol containers
Plastics	Bottles, Syringes, IV containers, Tubes, Bags, Laminates, Pouches, Lids, Tapes, Aerosol containers (dip tube, gasket housing, actuator buttons, stems)
Rubbers	Closures, Vial wrappers, Caps, Plungers
Paper/cardboards	Labels, Inserts, Display units, Pouches, Laminates, Cartons, Corrugated boxes, Foils, Gum tapes, Paper drums
Metals	Collapsible tubes, Foils, Needles, Aerosol containers, Cans

Apart from packaging material, the selection of pack is important. While selecting the package for a medication one must realize that the main object is to deliver a drug to a specific site of effective activity in the patient and the packaging must contribute to this end. The product/pack couple is designed as one unit to achieve the above objective. The choice of packaging for a specific pharmaceutical product is dependent upon:

(a) the nature of product and its compatibility with the material;
(b) the type of patient – whether child, elderly, adult;
(c) the type of dose – granules, tablet, ointment;
(d) method and site of administration – dispensing device, etc.;
(e) method of distribution – through hospital, pharmacy, retailer;
(f) capacity of the packaging needed – small bulk for pharmacies, OPD; and
(g) required shelf-life and likely sales area.

PACKAGING MATERIALS

Packing materials are critical to the stability of the finished product, and hence various criteria are to be considered before the selection of pharmaceutical packing system and these include:

1. Type of raw material to be used for a particular product.
2. Relative barrier properties and inertness of the pack with reference to those required by the product during the shelf-life.
3. The type of exposure that the product is expected to go through, e.g. mechanical, climatic, etc.
4. The control and test procedures that are required to be carried out to ensure reproducibility in quality of material used.
5. Any contribution of packaging component to the product.

A number of different packaging materials are available for primary and secondary packing purpose.

Primary packaging material

Though all the aspects for the selection of packaging material have their own importance, protection is invariably the most critical factor as it determines the shelf-life of a product including mechanical, climatic and biological protection. The various packaging materials used include plastics, glass, metals, films, foils, and laminates.

Plastics

Use of plastics for pharmaceutical containers evolved steadily in the late twentieth century. Plastics are durable, easily molded into a variety of shapes, flexible, often unbreakable and biocompatible in many applications. Plastics are robust, strong, light, aesthetic, pilfer-proof, protective, easy to carry; convenient to open, use or administer, close, dispose; and tamper evident. They are capable of being used in high speed automated processing (machinability). Plastic containers can be produced easily at economical cost. These can form child-resistant and sterilizable packs. Due to availability of variety of polymers, plastics can satisfy these different requirements. These can be used as homo- or co-polymer or in combination with aluminium and board material. The advantages and limitations offered by plastics as packaging material are listed in Table 15.6. The examples of additives present in plastics are listed in Table 15.7.

Table 15.6. Properties of plastics used as packaging materials

Advantages
- Variety of plastic material available, which may satisfy requirement of the pharmaceutical packaging.
- Low freight cost due to its less weight.
- Available in versatile design.
- Poor conductor of heat.
- Very good mechanical strength.
- Non-breakable.

Disadvantages
- Permeated by vapor.
- Drug–plastic interaction may occur due to presence of many additives.
- Most are sensitive to heat.

Table 15.7. Additives, processing aids and residues that may be extracted from plastic containers

• Accelerators	• Flame retardants
• Antiblocking agent	• Lubricants
• Antioxidants	• Light excluders
• Antislip additives	• Modifiers
• Anti-static agents	• Mould release agents
• Catalyst	• Opacifiers
• Colorant	• Plasticizers
• Emulsifier	• Stabilizers
• Extenders	• UV absorbers
• Fillers	

Plastics are a group of substances of natural or synthetic origin consisting chiefly of polymers of high melting point that can be molded into a shape or form by application of heat or pressure. These consist of molecules called the monomers and these monomers undergo a process of polymerization forming a plastic. The process of polymerization may involve various chemicals,

which assist in polymerization such as accelerators, initiators, solvents, catalysts, etc.

Plastics may be amorphous or crystalline. Amorphous materials give good clarity, transparency, and hardness with possible brittleness and are more permeable to gases and moisture but are less inert. Crystalline materials are opaque or translucent, more flexible, with low permeability to gases and moisture and are more inert. The polymers used in pharmaceutical packaging are listed in Table 15.8.

Table 15.8. Polymers as packaging materials

- Polyethylene (PE)
  - Low density polyethylene (LDPE)
  - High density polyethylene (HDPE)
- Polypropylene (PP)
- Polystyrene (PS)
- Polycarbonate (PC)
- Polyvinyl chloride (PVC)
- Nylon (Polyamide) (PA)
- Polyacrylonitrile polymers
- Polyethylene terephthalate (PET)
- Cellulose acetate
- Ethylene, vinyl alcohol (EVOH)
- Polychlorotrifluoroethylene (PCTFE)
- Polyvinylidene chloride (PVdC)
- Styrene acrylonitrile (SAN)
- Polytetrafluoroethylene (PTFE)
- Acrylonitrile butadiene styrene (ABS)

Plastic polymers can be divided into two categories: (i) thermosetting polymers, and (ii) thermoplastics. A polymerization process involving a curing or vulcanization stage during which the material becomes "set" to a permanent state by heat or pressure produces thermoset polymers. These include phenolics, melamine, urea, epoxies, certain polyesters and polyurethanes. Thermoplastic polymers are heat-softening materials, which can be repeatedly heated, made mobile and then reset to a solid state by cooling. These include more number of polymers e.g. polyethylene, polyvinyl chloride, polystyrene, polypropylene, nylon, polyester, polyvinylidene chloride, polycarbonate. Plastics may also be divided into categories, such as, homopolymer, copolymers, terpolymers depending upon whether polymerization involves one, two or more types of monomers, respectively.

Plastics have found immense application in the pharmaceutical industry and the demand is ever increasing. This may be attributed to the ease of formation of plastic containers, light-weight, availability of high quality plastic container, resistance to breakage and freedom to design the container in any shape and size. A great benefit of working with plastic material is the numerous possibilities of creating innovative designs. All manufacturers of glass containers are well aware of the limitations in designing complex glass designs and costs associated with it. However, migration/leaching of components from plastic containers to product may pose problems. This issue can be resolved using well-known medical grade polymers for the preparation of plastic containers.

Sterilization of plastics: Sterilization processes can be carried out on plastic containers. The general methods of sterilization, which can be applied on plastics together with the conditions of sterilization, have been outlined in Table 15.9.

The plastic containers used in pharmaceutical products are primarily made up of the following polymers: low, medium and high density polyethylene (PE), plasticized and unplasticized polyvinyl chloride (PVC), homopolymer and copolymer of polypropylene (PP) and polystyrene (PS). Other plastics used in pharmaceuticals include polymethyl methacrylates (PMM), polytrifluoroethylene; some materials also include nylon (PA), acrylonitrile butadiene styrene (ABS), styrene acrylonitrile (SAN), polycarbonate (PC), etc.

Plastic pharmaceutical containers include plastic bags for parenterals, plastic trays for tablets and capsules, tubes for creams and ointments, jars, boxes for powder, etc. A number of different plastics and their blends are used for this purpose, including the following main polymers.

Polyethylene

Polyethylene is available in three different grades: low (LDPE), medium (MDPE) and high (HDPE) density (according to the density of the PE ranging from 0.91 to 0.96 g/cm^3). As the

Table 15.9. General methods of sterilization of plastics

Method of sterilization	Sterilization conditions	Plastics suitable for the process
Autoclaving (moist heat)	121°C for 15 min or 115°C for 30 min	HDPE, PP, PC, PMP, ETFE, Teflon, FEP, PFA; and under certain conditions, plasticized PVC
Dry heat	160–180°C for 1–3 h	ECTFE, Tefzel, ETFE, Teflon, FEP, PFA, PMP, PSF, TFE
Gaseous sterilization	100% ethylene oxide under negative pressure/10–15% ethylene oxide with an inert gas/formaldehyde	HDPE, PP, PC, PMP, ETFE, Teflon, FEP, PFA, PPCO, PE, PVC, PS
Gamma irradiation/ accelerated electrons	25l Gy/2.5 Mrad	High molecular weight, amorphous, low-density materials are most resistant to radiations
Chemical disinfectants	Formalin/iodophors, quaternary ammonium compounds/benzalkonium chloride	Generally suitable for all plastics, surface attack may be seen when applied on chemically less resistant plastics (e.g. acrylic, PS, PC, PVC)

$$\left[\begin{array}{ccc} & H & H \\ & | & | \\ -\!\!\!\!&C\!-\!C\!&\!-\!\!\!\! \\ & | & | \\ & H & H \end{array}\right]_n$$

Polyethylene (PE)

$$\left[\begin{array}{ccc} & H & CH_3 \\ & | & | \\ -\!\!\!\!&C\!-\!C\!&\!-\!\!\!\! \\ & | & | \\ & H & H \end{array}\right]_n$$

Polypropylene (PP)

density of PE increases both physical and chemical properties vary. An increase in polymer density makes the material more rigid, less impact resistant, less translucent, stronger, less flexible with an increase in melting point. The clarity and translucency also depend upon the density of PE. The low, medium and high density PE has oxygen transmission of 500, 250–535 and 185, respectively. Antioxidants and antistatic additives are used in bottle grades of polyethylene.

High-density polyethylene (HDPE) is the most crystalline material and is most widely used for containers by the pharmaceutical industry. It offers a good barrier against moisture but a relatively poor one against oxygen and other gases. Most of the solvents do not react with PE and it is unaffected by strong acids and alkalis. HDPE generates most applications in standard rigid containers for solid oral medications.

Polyethylene is a material of choice along with polypropylene (PP) as a polymeric material used for on-line blow-fill-seal (BFS) technology. These are inert and give a good balance of properties for BFS technology including ease of forming, opening and handling of the finished containers.

Linear low-density polyethylene (LLDPE) is a relatively newer material, which is receiving a lot of interest as a film forming material. LLDPE is being used for plastic tubes and as a seal ply to provide high mechanical strength.

Polypropylene (PP)

Polypropylene is somewhat similar to HDPE, has a remarkably low density and so is able to produce more finished products than a similar weight of any other thermoplastic resin. This offsets its slightly high cost. It also has an excellent resistance to almost all types of

chemicals, including acids, and most organic materials. This polymer does not crack under any circumstance and provides almost complete barrier against gas and vapor. It has a high melting point and this makes it suitable for sterilizable products. It, however, suffers from a drawback of being brittle at low temperature. Though it has good impact strength and impact durability, improvement in low temperature impact strength is required in most cases. This improvement is generally achieved through the use of an elastomer.

Polystyrene

Polystyrene is a clear rigid hard material with good tensile strength but is one of the most brittle plastics when dropped. It is resistant to mineral oils, water and alkali but is soluble in organic solvents. It is fairly permeable to moisture and is generally not a suitable packaging material for pharmaceutical products.

$$\left[\begin{array}{cc} H & H \\ | & | \\ C\!-\!C \\ | & | \\ H & \bigcirc \end{array}\right]_n$$

Polystyrene (PS)

Polycarbonate (PC)

This plastic material has good impact resistance with excellent dimensional stability. It has a low

$$H\!\!-\!\!\left[\!O\!-\!\!\bigcirc\!\!-\!\!\overset{\overset{\displaystyle CH_3}{|}}{\underset{\underset{\displaystyle CH_3}{|}}{C}}\!\!-\!\!\bigcirc\!\!-\!\!O\!-\!\overset{\overset{\displaystyle O}{\|}}{C}\!\right]_n\!\!-\!\!OH$$

Polycarbonate (PC)

water absorption capacity and is heat resistant. PC is used to make membrane filters, reusable bottles and sterilizable medical packaging.

Polyvinyl chloride (PVC)

Among the vinyl polymers including polyvinyl chloride (PVC), polyvinylidene chloride (PVdC), polyvinyl acetate (PVAc) and polyvinyl alcohol (PVA); PVC finds maximum application. PVC is an inexpensive, tough, clear material that is relatively easily processed. Polyvinyl chloride is available as unplasticized PVC (UPVC), plasticized PVC or as an impact modified PVC. PVC may show some deterioration upon ageing; therefore, stabilizers are invariably added into these to improve stability. The amount of plasticizer in PVC may be greater than the amount of PVC. This may lead to reduced chemical resistance and increased gas/moisture permeation. Plasticized PVC is soft and flexible.

$$\left[\begin{array}{c} H \quad H \\ | \quad \quad | \\ -C-C- \\ | \quad \quad | \\ H \quad Cl \end{array} \right]_n$$

Polyvinyl chloride (PVC)

PVC bottles of crystal clarity, fairly good oxygen barrier, and greater stiffness can be produced. In its purest form PVC is crystal clear and stiff with poor impact resistance. It can be softened with the help of plasticizers. Stabilizers, modifiers, monomer residues, fillers, anti-oxidants, colorants can be added into PVC to impart the desired attributes. It can be plasticized to produce articles, which range in flexibility from soft to hard. It has a good resistance to chemicals and water permeation and has an excellent elasticity.

PVC and HDPE account for the largest volume of raw materials employed in the production of pharmaceutical bottles. PVC is employed extensively in the production of semi-rigid and flexible bottles for low barrier liquid pharmaceuticals such as contact lens solutions and laxatives. Rigid PVC has been used for many

years for providing protection to the pharmaceuticals.

PVdC (polyvinylidene chloride) has an excellent resistance to permeability by moisture and gases, very good chemical resistance plus toughness, flexibility and heat sealability. PVdC, although existing as a film, is more usually found in aqueous dispersion or a solvent coating. Polyvinyl acetate and copolymers find use as an adhesive and a heat sensitive base. Polyvinyl alcohol has excellent grease resistance and good gas barrier properties when dry. It has been used to produce water-soluble sachets.

Polyesters or polyethylene terephthalate (PET)

The most commonly used film for tape is formed by the reaction of dimethylterephthalic acid and ethylene glycol to give polyethylene (glycol) terephthalate. PET films are tough and highly tear-resistant. PET is used for preparation of stretch blown containers and pharmaceutical usage as a small molding.

$$HO-\begin{array}{c} H \quad H \\ | \quad \ | \\ C-C \\ | \quad \ | \\ H \quad H \end{array}\left[\begin{array}{c} \ \\ O-C \\ \| \\ O \end{array} \right. \bigcirc \left. \begin{array}{c} \quad \ \\ C-C \\ \| \quad | \\ O \quad H \end{array} \begin{array}{c} H \\ | \\ C \\ | \\ H \end{array} \right]_n OH$$

Polyethylene terephthalate (PET)

Advanced olefin copolymer (COC)

The polyolefin group includes ultra and very low-density polyethylene, low-density polyethylene (LDPE) and linear low-density polyethylene (LLDPE), medium density polyethylene (MDPE), high-density polyethylene (HDPE), polypropylene (homopolymer/co-polymer). Also included are ultra high molecular weight grades of HDPE. Advanced olefin co-polymer, the cycloolefin copolymer (COC), is new, high barrier, thermoforming plastic suitable for pharmaceutical and cosmetic packaging with excellent moisture barrier properties, outstanding transparency and good rigidity. Vials made of high purity COC polymer offer transparency as compared to glass. This polymer provides excellent barrier properties, high chemical resistance and breakage resistance. These attributes make this polymer ideal for primary packaging of pharmaceuticals. A summary of salient properties of various plastics used in pharmaceutical packaging is presented in Table 15.10.

The European Pharmacopoeia provides a list of plastics that are permitted for use in pharmaceutical containers. These are:

1. PVC for containers for human blood, blood components and aqueous solutions for IV infusion.
2. PVC for components used in blood transfusion.
3. Polyolefin.
4. LDPE for parenteral and ophthalmic preparations.
5. HDPE for parenteral preparations.

6. PP for parenteral preparations.
7. Ethylene-vinyl acetate copolymer (EVAc) for total parenteral nutritional (TPN) products.
8. Silicone oil as lubricant.
9. Silicone elastomer for closures and tubing.

The list of approved additives includes antioxidants, stabilizers, plasticizers, lubricants, colour and impact modifiers. Antistatic and mould release agents can be used only for containers for oral and external preparations. For selection of appropriate polymer material, the key aspects are that the drug is not absorbed; it does not migrate through the material, and does not yield any material in a quantity sufficient to alter the stability or the toxicity of the product. Tests of compatibility include physical changes, permeation, pH change, effect of light and chemicals, and biological testing. BP categorises plastic containers into three different types:

Table 15.10. Salient properties of various plastics used in pharmaceutical packaging

Plastic types / Properties	PE	HDPE	PVC	PP	PS	PA	PC	Polymethyl methacrylate	Phenol formaldehyde	Urea formaldehyde
Light-sensitive	✓		✓							
Rigid		✓	✓							
Flexible	✓									
Non-toxic	✓		✓							
Air impermeable	✓	✓	✓	✓			✓			
Moisture impermeable	✓			✓	✓	✓	✓		✓	✓
Autoclavable		✓		✓		✓		✓	✓	
Electrostatic	✓	✓	✓							
Oil-resistant		✓								
Translucent		✓		✓		✓				
Transparent			✓		✓		✓	✓		
Heat-resistant	✓			✓		✓	✓		✓	✓
Impact-resistant						✓	✓	✓		

1. Plastic containers for aqueous solutions for parenteral infusion. The most commonly used polymers in this case include polyethylene, polypropylene and polyvinyl chloride. They may be in shapes of bags or bottles. These must withstand the sterilization conditions to which the containers are submitted, should be impermeable to microorganisms, and should be sufficiently transparent to allow visual inspection.
2. Sterile plastic containers for blood and blood components.
3. Empty sterile containers of plasticized PVC for blood and blood components.

Plastics form a very significant part of the packaging industry. There are several procedures and processes, which would never have been possible but for plastics. These include prostate devices, catheters, tracheotomy tubes, and blood collection containers, to name a few. These also form secondary packaging containers. Wide ranges of plastics are available for these purposes. A careful selection of the material is required with regard to the customer usage, manufacturability, sterility, barrier properties, etc. Depending upon the target material properties, likely material candidates are determined by comparing their properties with the property profile derived from the functional requirements. There are various material properties which affect the functional performance of plastics, including mechanical, optical, and electrical properties. Electrical properties may cause hazard to electronic instruments and may attract dirt whereas the mechanical and optical properties have more relevance.

The various mechanical properties tested in case of plastics include the following:

- **Impact strength:** This gives a measure of the ability to withstand shock loading. The test material may receive a blow from a swinging pendulum. The material will fracture if the impact force exceeds the limit of elasticity of the material. Glass has much lower impact strength as compared to plastics.
- **Tensile strength:** This gives a measure of the maximum force needed to pull apart a specimen of a material per unit area. Elongation measures the ability of the material to stretch.
- **Stiffness:** This gives a measure of resistance of bending against a load.
- **Tear strength:** This gives the measure of force required to tear a plastic and also the force required to propagate the tear. While this property is undesirable in case of shipping sacks yet it is desirable in case of tear tapes.
- **Flex resistance:** This gives a measure of the resistance to develop pinholes or fracture, when subjected to repeat flexing.
- **Coefficient of friction or slip:** This property has more relevance to form-fill-seal (FFS) operations. This property of plastics depicts the ease of sliding of one material film over the other that is required in packaging machinery. Reverse of this is **blocking**, which gives the tendency of different films to stick together.
- **Fatigue resistance:** This gives the ability of a plastic to withstand repeated short time stress/deformation without cracking.

In addition to the above general tests, some other tests, which are specific to the product requirements e.g. behavior at low temperature, melting point, heat sealability, sterilizability, etc., are also performed. The optical properties of importance in case of plastics include:

- **Light transmission:** It gives the measure of light transmission through a film.
- **Clarity:** This gives an indication of degree of distortion of an object seen through the film of the material under test.
- **Haze:** This gives a measure of haziness caused during product inspection through a film of the material.
- **Gloss:** It is indicative of how well a plastic surface reflects light and is important for visual appearance of an object.

- **Cavitation/panelling:** Plastics are prone to distortion, partial collapse, swelling or dimpling.
- **Stress cracking:** Low-density plastics are also prone to cracking under stress.
- **Crazing:** This happens particularly in case of polystyrene (PS) and some other substances where a surface reticulation occurs, which may grow and lead to disintegration.
- **Poor printability:** Plastics such as polyolefins need particular pretreatment before ink may be applied on them.
- **Poor impact resistance:** Some plastics have a poor impact resistance e.g. polystyrene, PVC, etc.

Majority of these limitations can be overcome by using combination of plastics with additives, other plastic materials, films, foils, laminates, etc.

Glass

Glass has been the container of choice for pharmaceutical dosage form as it has high barrier qualities. Things started to change with the advent of plastics, which offer a tough competition to glass. However, for sensitive products, glass still forms a very desirable and cost effective option. The many advantages that glass offers have enabled it to exist in the pharmaceutical packaging till date (Table 15.11). Glass offers superior quality protection. It is economical, chemically inert, impermeable with no diffusion or leakage (for good quality glass), strong and rigid, recyclable, hygienic, sterilizable, easily washable, resistant to high temperature, compatible and transparent. Another particular advantage of glass is that it is resistant to decomposition by atmospheric conditions or by solid or liquid contents of different chemical composition. Variation in chemical composition of glass can make changes in chemical behavior and radiation protective properties of glass.

Recently the advantages of both the containers have been put together made in union in the form of plastic coated glass. Advanced

Table 15.11. Glass as packaging material

Advantages
- Chemically inert
- Imparts no odor and taste to the product
- Non-corrosive
- Strong and rigid
- Impermeable
- Transparent and sparkle
- No change on aging
- FDA approved

Disadvantages
- Fragile
- Less pressure safety and impact resistance (aerosol containers can withstand pressure below 25 psig and use of less than 50% propellant is quite safe)
- High freight cost due to its weight

glass containers are light weight with surface treatment. A number of glass containers used in pharmaceutical industry include ampoules, bottles, vials, syringes and cartridges.

Colorless white flint soda glass is made of silica, calcium oxide, sodium oxide, alumina and small quantities of ferric oxide, titanium dioxide, potassium and magnesium oxide. Several types of glass are available. These have been categorized as per USP into four different types (Table 15.12). **Type I** glass is borosilicate glass and has high hydrolytic resistance and a high thermal shock resistance due to chemical composition of the glass itself. **Type II** glass is a soda-lime-silica glass, which has had a surface treatment by sulphuring or sulphating, forming a coating of sodium sulphate, which is soluble in water, neutralizes the excessive surface alkalinity. Glasses are being given different treatments in order to improve their surface lubricity, increasing impact resistance and aesthetic appearance. Surface treated glass finds wide application in pharmaceutical industry.

Type III glass is the regular soda lime glass in which the containers are untreated and have an average chemical resistance. It contains alkaline metal oxides and alkaline earth oxides and has a limited alkalinity.

Table 15.12. Types of glass (USP-37)

Type	General description	Properties	Suitability
I	Highly resistant, borosilicate glass	Alkalinity is removed by using boric oxide to neutralize the oxides of potassium and sodium	Preparations for parenteral and non-parenteral administration
II	Treated soda-lime glass	Obtained by treating the hot surface of type III glass by sulphur dioxide/ammonium sulphate/ammonium chloride	Preparations for most acidic and neutral products for parenteral and non-parenteral administration
III	Soda-lime glass	It is an alkaline glass having high percentage of lime and soda and no boric oxide as compared to type I glass	Not used for parenteral products or for powders for parenteral use, except where suitable stability test data indicate that type III glass is satisfactory
NP	General purpose soda-lime glass	It has similar compositions to that of type III glass but there is no guarantee of similar properties	Non-parenteral products (oral or topical use)

The British Pharmacopoeia, 2012 categorizes the glass containers according to hydrolytic resistance into 4 types. **Type I**, neutral glass, with high hydrolytic resistance, suitable for most preparations whether or not for parenteral use. **Type II**, soda lime silica glass, high hydrolytic resistance glass suitable for acidic and neutral aqueous preparations whether or not for parenteral use. **Type III** is soda lime glass with moderate hydrolytic resistance suitable for non-aqueous preparations for parenteral use, powders for parenteral use (except for freeze dried preparations) and for non-parenteral preparations.

Glass is used for different containers ranging from ampoules, vials (Figs. 15.1, 15.2 and 15.3),

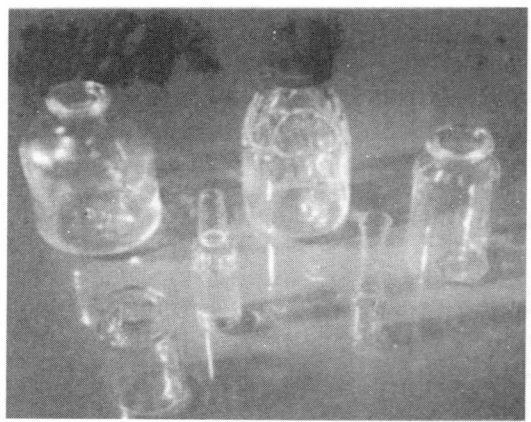

Fig. 15.2. Vials and ampoules.

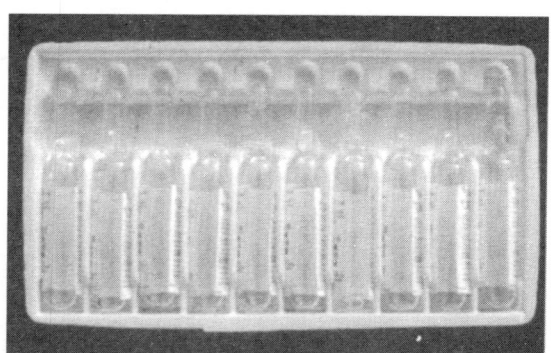

Fig. 15.1. Sealed ampoules in a tray.

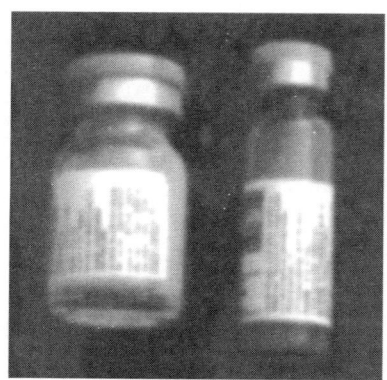

Fig. 15.3. Sealed vials.

cartridge tubes, disposable syringes and aerosols. Ampoules are generally made up of neutral glass. These were one of the first unit dose containers but are increasingly being replaced by cartridge tubes and pre-filled syringes. Vials on the other hand are produced by soda glass, when used for tablets and capsules. Injection vials can still be obtained in either neutral or soda glass or occasionally in treated soda glass. Glass disposable syringes have been replaced by plastic syringes. Glass containers for aerosol purposes present risk of breakage as compared to the metal containers. Metal containers on the other side do not offer flexibility in design. Glass is being used for aerosol purposes making use of good bottle strength. Alternatively adequate bottle strength may be provided with an external coating of a flexible plastic (e.g. PVC) on the glass container. Uncoated bottles are used for keeping low-pressure aerosols.

Except for the breakage risk, glass offers the best product protection with distinct advantages. This is testified also with the fact that FDA acceptance of glass rarely presents any problem. Lightweight coated glass with improved color range and strength seem to be very promising for pharmaceutical packaging in the future.

Films/foils and laminates

Films, foils and laminates perform different roles, such as supportive, barrier, heat seal and decorative. Paper is usually used as a supportive ply, which can be readily printed to give a decorative appeal. Aluminium, on the other hand, is used for its barrier properties and a decorative appeal. Metallization is another relatively new process wherein particles of metal are laid down to a surface under vacuum to alter the surface properties of materials. However, this is not able to provide as good barrier properties as achieved by aluminium. Plastics as film or coating can be used for decoration, flexibility, barrier purpose, heat sealability, transparency, and to protect the other plies within the lamination.

Films, foils or laminates are made up of a single layer, multi-layers or a combination of materials. Single ply materials include paper and plastics, which do not require an additional coating to achieve heat seal or can be employed as a direct wrap (polyethylene and plasticized PVC).

- **Single ply materials:** These including LDPE, LLDPE, or a mixture of blend involving combination of LDPE, MDPE, HDPE, EVAc (ethylene vinyl acetate), etc. find a wide range of applications for the formation of bags, sacks, sachets, overwraps, shrink-wraps, stretch wraps, etc. Deep freeze packs make use of LDPE, LDPE mixtures. Single ply plastics are also used in window cartons (cellulose acetate, polyester, regenerated cellulose) and in plastic cartons (PVC).

- **Shrink-wraps:** Shrink-wrap utilizes a plastic which, when placed around an object, makes a tight wrap around the object (Fig. 15.4). LDPE, PP, PVC, EVAc have been used for this purpose.

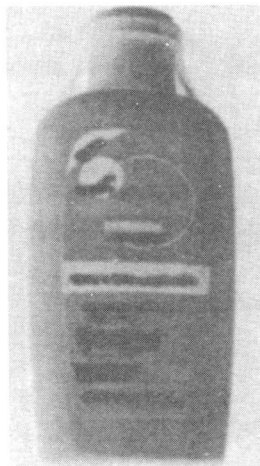

Fig. 15.4. Shrink-wrap.

- **Stretch wraps:** These films must be elastic in nature, once in position must not relax and lose tension. LLDPE is the main material used for this purpose. LDPE, EVAc and unplasticized PVC films may be used in combination.

- **Cling films:** These are an elastic-type material that undergoes stretch. PVC and PVdC were earlier used as cling films but recently LLDPE and LDPE mixtures are being used for the purpose.

PVC is used in overwrap films, shrink films, shrink sleeving, and thermoforming for blisters and for bubble packs. PVC films may be plasticized or unplasticized PVC films. The former types are used for forming pillow pack, as these are highly permeable to moisture. Unplasticized PVC films have low permeability to oxygen but are moderately permeable to moisture. PVdC films are soft but very strong and are difficult to handle. They provide an excellent barrier to moisture and gases. Polyvinylidene fluoride (PVdF) is more inert as compared to PVdC but is more expensive. Polyvinyl fluoride (PVF) offers a high weather resistance but is again very expensive. Polystyrene (PS) is used for blister-type packs. It is highly permeable to moisture and fairly permeable to gases.

Films

- **Regenerated cellulose film (RCF):** These films, though continuous, resemble paper in its properties, are moisture sensitive and not heat sealable, and may be coated with nitrocellulose or PVdC on one or both the sides. Even after coating these films remain moisture sensitive and need storage under controlled conditions.
- **Films and coatings based on plastics:** These films are from organic origin and may be continuous, clear, colored or opaque with a glossy surface. They are flexible, strong and sealable. They resist water and form effective barrier against water vapor depending upon their caliper, area, gradient, temperature, etc.
- **Special films:** The polyolefins include LDPE, MDPE, HDPE, LLDPE etc., and are used for formation of bags and to form heat seal inner ply in laminations, sacks, shrink and stretch films. LDPE films are frequently used as a lamination ply to bond two materials together.

HDPE films are employed in boil-in-the-bag applications.

PVdC films are soft cling films but are very strong and have excellent barrier properties. Polystyrene films lack barrier properties and may be used in blister-type packs for non-barrier usage. Aclar® films are polymonochlorotrifluoroethylene (PCTFE) films that offer high inertness and excellent barrier properties. Polytetrafluoroethylene (PTFE) is used as a coating for closures. Polyvinylidene fluoride (PVdF) and polyvinyl fluoride (PVF) are high barrier films but they are very expensive. Polyester (PET) films form good barrier against gases but only fair to moisture. It may be used as an outer ply to laminates.

Foils

Aluminium foils: Aluminium foil is the material most widely used for packaging of tablets and capsules though it is the most expensive constituent of the laminate. Aluminium foil is made from the metal that has 99% purity and the gauge of the foil may vary from 0.006 to 0.040 mm. Aluminium foil offers excellent barrier properties to moisture, gases and light, and gives the pack brightness and an attractive look. The foil provides hygienic, tamper evident pack, which is odorless, tasteless and non-toxic. It provides a convenient, safe and versatile packaging for tablets, capsules, liquids and powders.

Aluminium foil is strong and can be laminated. It can form push-through lids or preformed trays for tablets. When used as collapsible tube these do not draw air into them (forming dead ends), which may contaminate the product.

Aluminium foil is particularly suitable for blister packs. The tray of the blister may be made of PVC/PVdC while the lidding is done with the help of aluminium foil. Aluminium foil can be made into alloy, which can alter its properties like brittleness, toughness and ductility. Aluminium foil is also used for forming strip packs. Strip packs provide economical high barrier performance pack and can be filled at high speed on modern, sterile filling lines. In case of sachets and pouches aluminium packs are robust and keep the product in good condition. These can withstand rigorous "burst" tests and are convenient and economical.

Aluminium foil laminated with paper or plastic is frequently used as a heat-sealed membrane hermetically closing the container under a plastic screw cap. The resulting aluminium membrane provides excellent barrier properties preventing moisture or gas transmission and tamper-evident seal.

Laminates

Laminates are combination of different plies put together to get some desired properties. These form thin films using minimum material and are cost effective. These however, are not eco-friendly as they make recycling very difficult. Any laminate may consist of a number of plies selected from paper, cellulose, films, foils, coatings, etc. depending upon:

(a) Availability of the material.
(b) Technical requirements.
(c) Cost of base material.
(d) Cost of lamination process, printing and the yield.

These may include paper/PVdC/paper/PVdC, paper/LDPE/Surlyn, regenerated cellulose/LDPE, etc. Two laminations, which are widely used, include paper/foil/polythene and paper/foil/Surlyn. In this lamination the easy printability, strength and brilliance of paper (outer ply) are put together with the barrier properties of foil (center ply) and heat sealability of Surlyn (inner ply). These are used for strip and sachet packaging.

The main pharmaceutical applications of laminations include strip packaging, blister packaging and sachet packaging. Films, foils or laminates are flexible, tamper-evident and encourage the unit-dose packaging. These packs, including the blister and strip packs, are reasonably child-resistant. The demand for blister packs in particular is shooting up and there is a great potential of growth in this particular area.

Metals

Metal containers are strong, relatively unbreakable, opaque, and impervious to water vapor, gases, odor and bacteria. They are resistant to high and low temperatures. Due to their chemical reactivity, metals require the application of coatings and lacquers to prevent chemical reaction and corrosion. Special coatings and coating techniques are being developed for this purpose. Metal containers being used in the pharmaceutical industry include small-elongated collapsible tubes and shallow drums. Metal containers have dominated themselves in the field of aerosols. Though glass, plastic and plastic coated glass aerosols are finding their own specialized application, metal aerosols are likely to retain the bulk of the market as long as cost advantages are offered. Aluminium foil is another metal extensively used in the pharmaceutical industry. It has been dealt with under foils heading in this chapter.

Metals are also used for the formation of closures. Some of these closures are similar to those used on glass and plastic containers, e.g., plastic and metal screw closures and friction closures such as plug or slip lids. Other metal closures include lever lids and permanent mechanically seamed-on closures.

Tin plate was once used for pastille tins, ointment tins and various build-up containers for powders, tablets, capsules, etc. These were followed by the use of aluminium. The use of metals is declining, as they cannot compete with the cost of plastic and glass. Some metals currently in use in the pharmaceutical packaging include tin plate, tin-free steel, aluminium, alloy of aluminium and stainless steel. Aluminium and its alloys are used for aerosol containers, rigid and collapsible tubes, shallow drawn containers, blisters and sachet packaging. Tin plate containers are used for the formation of built-up containers and shallow drawn containers. Stainless steel is widely used in pharmaceuticals for mixing vessels and manufacturing equipment. It is also used for packaging of high-pressure aerosols. Tin is occasionally used for collapsible tubes. Metal containers still play a very important role in packaging, accounting for one-quarter of the total sales of all packaging materials.

Closures

Closures form a very critical component of the containers. Pharmaceutical closures are essentially elastomeric closures. The selection of elastomer involves consideration of chemical, physical and biological properties, with emphasis on the stability profile of drug/container system. Primarily the function of the closure system is to retain the contents safely and prevent hazards resulting in leakage, seepage, spillage, pilferage, loss of quality, purity, etc. by some source of contamination, impurity, etc. Additionally, the containers should not give rise to undesirable interactions between the contents and the outside environment. Closures must allow the easy and safe administration of drugs. Closures may be required to be pierced with a needle as in the case of multidose parenterals. There are four main types of rubber, which are used in pharmaceuticals:

1. Butyl rubbers (co-polymers of isobutylene and isoprene or butadiene).
2. Nitrile rubbers (butadiene-acrylonitrile co-polymers).
3. Chloroprene rubbers (neoprene; polymers of 1:4 chloroprene).
4. Silicon rubbers.

Butyl rubbers are ecomomical, chemically resistant, with desired aging properties and low water vapor/air permeability. It is not good for oils. Nitrile rubbers are resistant to oil, heat treatment, vapor absorption and permeability but leaching and bactericide absorption is high. Neoprene rubbers are resistant to heat and oil with low water absorption and permeability as compared to natural rubbers. Silicon rubbers are costly but most heat resistant (about 250°C) with very low water absorption and permeability, strength and aging properties. When piercing is not required, the containers are made from plastics such as polyethylene or polypropylene. An aluminium cap may secure the rubber closures.

Closures may be achieved by a number of basic means or a combination of these including pressure, temperature and adhesion. Pressure type closures make use of mechanical pressure or atmospheric pressure. Mechanical pressure is utilized in screw closure, plug seal, lever lid, etc., whereas atmospheric pressure is utilized in vacuum-sealed tin. Use of temperature is made in case of closures e.g. welding, heat sealing or electrical heat sealing. Adhesion is made use of in closures in the form of solvents, adhesives, cold seal material, etc.

The materials employed for the formation of closures include:

1. Metals like aluminium, aluminium alloys, tinplate, tin-free steel, stainless steel.
2. Glass for formation of stoppers.
3. Rubbers and plastics (thermosetting or thermoplastic type).

Plastics may be modified by use of coatings/lacquers. Thermosetting plastics include phenol formaldehyde (PF), bakelite and urea formaldehyde (UF). Thermoplastic-based containers may be made from PS, LDPE, LLDPE, PP, and polythene of medium or high density.

Liners are generally used in the inner side of the containers. These are made from aluminium foil, tin foil, polythene, expanded polyethylene (EPE), Saran (PVdC) film, PVdC coating, PET film, solid polythene, solid PVC and PTFE, etc. The closures used in pharmaceuticals include rubber closures, caps or overseals, and some special type of closures.

(a) **Rubber closures:** Rubbers used in pharmaceutical packaging contain only limited number of ingredients, which are difficult to extract. These closures do not pose a problem and can be used in contact with a large number of drug preparations.

Rubber closures for containers for aqueous parenteral preparations have been classified into two types, according to B.P. 2016, **Type I** closures are those which meet the strictest requirements and which are to be preferred; **Type II** closures are those, having mechanical properties suitable for special use (e.g. multiple piercing), cannot meet the requirements as severe as those for the first category because of their chemical composition. Rubber closures for vials are shown in Fig. 15.5. Fragmentation test and self-sealability of closures of parenteral preparation are examined in Tables 15.13, 15.14 and 15.15, respectively.

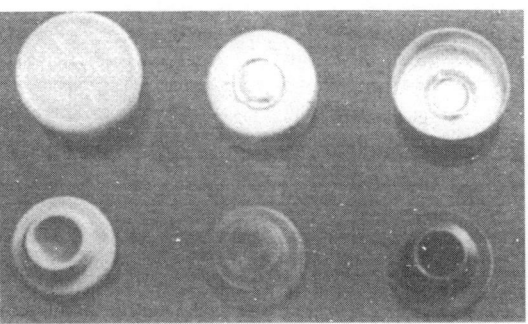

Fig. 15.5. Closures, caps and overseal for vials.

(b) **Caps and overseals:** Caps or overseals are used to secure the rubber closure to the container in order to maintain the integrity of the seal under normal conditions of handling and storage (Fig. 15.5). These caps are usually made of aluminium and may be equipped with a plastic top to facilitate opening. These form tamper-evident packs. Aluminium caps form secondary packaging material, as these are not in direct contact with the product.

(c) **Special types of closures:** Child-resistant closures safeguard children against drug intoxication, opening such packaging may prove to be difficult for the increasing number of elderly persons in the population.

Tamper-evident closures

Tampering includes three aspects, namely altering, pilfering and falsifying the pharmaceutical product. Tamper-evident closures are designed to prevent accidents and malicious tampering to create safe packaging. The concept of tamper-evident packaging is increasingly being recognized in pharmacopoeias. These include products ranging from OTC drugs, toothpaste, topical and dermatological products, oral cosmetic liquids, contact lens solutions and tablets. Various types of tamper-evident packaging are listed in Table 15.16.

Child-resistant closures

Tragic accidents involving the drug intoxication of children has led to new legislation making it

Table 15.13. Fragmentation test (IP, 2014) for rubber closures (aqueous preparation)

Place a volume of water corresponding to nominal volume minus 4 ml in each of 12 clean vials

↓

Close vial with closure and secure caps for 16 hours

↓

Pierce each closure with 21 SWG hypodermic needle (bevel angle of 10° to 14°) and inject 1 ml water and remove 1 ml air

↓

Repeat the above operation 4 times for each closure (use new needle for each closure)

↓

Pass the liquid in the vials through a filter with a pore size of 0.5 μm

↓

Count the number of fragments visible to the naked eye

↓

Total number of fragments should not be more than 10 except butyl rubber where the fragment should not exceed 15

Table 15.14. Fragmentation test (IP, 2014) for rubber closures (dry preparation)

Close 12 clean vials with the closures

Pierce each closure with 21 SWG hypodermic needle (bevel angle of 10° to 14°) and inject 1 ml water and remove 1 ml air

Repeat the above operation 4 times for each closure (use new needle for each closure)

Pass the liquid in the vials through a filter with a pore size of 0.5 μm

Count the number of fragments visible to the naked eye

Total number of fragments should not be more than 10 except butyl rubber where the fragment should not exceed 15

Table 15.15. Self-sealability (IP, 2014) test for rubber closures

Fill separately 10 vials with water to nominal volume and close the vials with closure and secure the cap

Pierce each cap 10 times at different sites with 21 SWG hypodermic needle

Immerse the vials in 0.1% w/v solution of methylene blue under reduced external pressure (27 kPa) for 10 minutes

Restore the normal pressure and keep the vials immersed for 30 minutes

Wash the vials

None of the vials should contain trace of colored solution

SWG = Standard wire gauge
Note: Test is applicable to multidose containers *only.*

Table 15.16. Tamper-evident packaging

- Film wrappers
- Blister packs
- Bubble packs
- Heat shrunk bands or wrappers
- Paper foil for plastic packs
- Bottles with inner mouth seals
- Tape seals
- Breakable cap ring systems
- Sealed tubes
- Plastic blind end heat sealed tubes
- Sealed cartons
- Aerosol containers
- Metal and composite cans

---

difficult for drug packaging to be opened by young children, while being easier for the adults to open. These are termed as child-resistant closures. These have proved effective in reducing child mortality from intoxication by oral prescription drugs. International standards have been laid down by ISO and ECN (European Committee for Standardization for child-resistant closures). Poison Prevention Packaging Act of 1970 (PPPA) has been enforced by U.S. Consumer Product Safety Commission (CPSC) which requires special packaging of hazardous household substances to protect children from serious personal injury or serious illness from handling, using, or ingesting. The three most common reclosable child-resistant closures are press-turn, squeeze-turn and a combination lock. Drug products containing controlled substances, most human oral prescription drug products (including oral investigational drugs used in outpatient trials), and OTC drug preparations containing aspirin, acetaminophen, diphenhydramine, liquid methyl salicylate, ibuprofen, loperamide, lidocaine, dibucaine, naproxen, iron, or ketoprofen, require special packaging.

Closure efficiency

The ability of a closure to prevent the exchange between a product and the atmosphere outside is determined by keeping the pack with the closure under varying temperature and humidity conditions and evaluating the system. These include:

1. Placing a desiccant in a pack stored under high RH and evaluating the moisture gain.
2. Putting liquid in the pack, placing it under high temperature and low relative humidity (RH) and then detecting the moisture loss.
3. Holding pack under water with vacuum applied on the pack and observing the water ingress into the container.
4. Checking a poor seal by applying vacuum on inverted pack and looking for seepage.
5. Cap removal torque is checked on time-temperature related basis.
6. Checking the compression ring seal in a cap liner.

Secondary packaging materials

Paper and board packaging materials

Paper and board are broadly cellulose/natural fiber materials. They find more diverse applications when compared with primary packaging materials. Cartons/corrugated board made from these materials is relatively recent invention.

Paper

Paper is widely used in pharmaceutical industry primarily due to the advantages like low cost, wide availability, non-toxic origin, availability in a variety of range, ease of printing, coating, lamination, opening, use, modification by addition of additives, good rigidity, strength, bio-degradability and disposal.

It suffers from some drawbacks of being moisture sensitive, needs modification in permeability to moisture and gases, is porous and is unable to form a barrier. However, advantages of paper outweigh its limitations and it is used widely for formation of labels, leaflets, etc. Strength of paper depends on its GSM (gram per square meter), which serves as an important parameter for its quality control.

Paper and board may be used for applications such as wrapping materials, labels, patient package inserts, bags and sacks, corrugated boxes, cartons, shipment containers, gummed tape, fitment for cases, paper liners, linings and lamination. Without these, packaging of products would be more expensive and difficult.

Labels are slips made generally of paper and are attached to a container bearing name, description and other details regarding the product. Another feature being introduced into the pharmaceutical label is bar coding. European Article Numbering bar coding has become an integral part of products sold globally. This coding is a facilitation tool to track the products effectively at any point of time to ensure effective supply chain management and speedy product recall if needed. There is an increasing trend of including information leaflets into products. Patient package inserts (PPI) are such leaflets, which are inserted into the product package. These contain non-technical explanation informing patients about the medicine in the package.

Paper and board containers include:

1. Fiber board kegs and drums, which are used for solid bulk drugs, bulk tablets or bulk excipient containment and transport.
2. Paper and composite open mouth sacks used for bulk excipients where there is no risk to or from the environment.
3. Composite containers that can be used as tubes for protection or for small powder drums.

Paper board and other cellulosic material have a major future in pharmaceutical industry. These are renewable and economical alternative to petroleum-based materials.

PHARMACEUTICAL PACKS

Out of the various pharmaceutical containers, blisters form the largest segment of the market, followed by blow-molded plastic containers, ampoules and vials, caps and closures, tubes, accessories, and glass. Other products include flexible bags, pouches, and prefilled syringes.

Blister packs

Unit dosage pack offers individual protection until the dose is removed, provides personal dosage, is tamper-evident, has no risk of cross-contamination, and no opening or reclosing problems, etc. Unit dose packaging is a major trend and has a strong influence on blister packaging. Blister pack consists of a thermoformed plastic tray with a lidding material made from plastic, paper, foil or a combination of these (Fig. 15.6). These may be made up of cold forming plastic and foil combination with topical lidding.

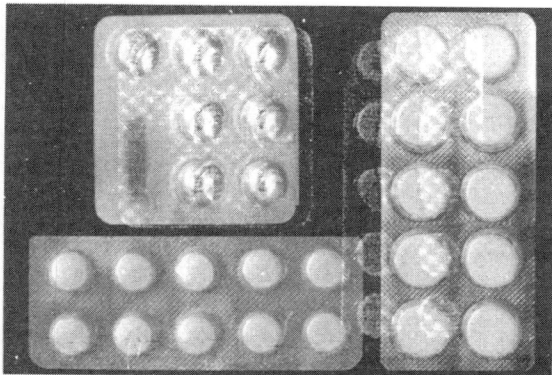

Fig. 15.6. Blisters.

The basic components of pharmaceutical blister packages are forming films (80–85% of weight), lidding material (15–20% of weight), heat seal coating and printing ink. The blister package is formed by a series of steps. A thermoplastic polymer is softened by application of heat. Vacuum drawing the softened polymer follows this into a contoured mould. The polymer sheet is released from the mould after cooling. This then proceeds to the filling station of the packaging machine where the semi-rigid blister is filled with the product and lidded with heat sealable material. This material may be push-through or peelable type. Majority of packs these days are push-through types.

The various types of forming films used for blister packs include:

1. Rigid PVC films
2. PVdC coated PVC
3. Polypropylene
4. PET
5. Polystyrene
6. CTFE homopolymer
7. Cyclo-olefin copolymers (COC)
8. Combinations

PVC without softening agents is called rigid PVC. It is clear, has a high flexural strength, good chemical resistance, and low permeability. As such it dominates the market share being economical. PVdC coating reduces the moisture permeability of PVC blister package by a factor of 5–10 and hence is very useful for moisture sensitive drugs/combinations. Polypropylene has a low water vapor permeability and easy recyclability. So it was thought of being a good substitute for PVC. But during blistering operations PP requires a very precise temperature control during thermoforming, cooling, wrapping and also encounters post-processing shrinkage. It is difficult to run PP on the blister machine and so is not a polymer of choice for the purpose. PET and polystyrene are not much in use due to their high vapor permeability. Chlorotrifluoroethylene (CTFE homopolymer) thermoforms easily, has high moisture barrier and exhibits crystal clarity. It is more stable to ageing when compared to PVdC but its high cost renders its use disadvantageous. COC also has high clarity and stiffness and is compatible with thermoforming. It is used in combination with layers of PVC, PE, PP, but this increases the cost of packaging.

Lidding material provides the base or main structural component upon which the final blister package is built. The most popular caliper or thickness of lidding material ranges from 0.46–0.61 mm. Lidding material should have good printability and be compatible with heat seal coating process. Generally clay coatings are added to the lidding material to enhance printing. Some of the lidding materials used in pharmaceutical packaging include:

1. Hard aluminium
2. Soft aluminium
3. Paper/aluminium
4. Paper/PET/aluminium

Hard aluminium is the most widely used push-through lidding material. One side of the hard aluminium is coated with print primer while the other side is coated with heat-sealing coating. Soft aluminium is used for child-resistant push-through foils. This material is also supplied with perforated sealed seams to inhibit easy peel-off. Paper-aluminium combinations are used for child-resistant push-through packages in Europe; hence the aluminium foil in this case is relatively thin. When same combination is used in US, the aluminium foil is relatively thick, to provide an effective peeling. Paper/PET/aluminium laminate is used for peel-off-push-through foil. This laminate is meant to first peel off the paper/ PET laminate from the aluminium and then to push the tablet through the aluminium.

Blister pack is the best form of unit dosage packing in pharmaceutical industry. It is considered to be one of the most convenient forms of packaging keeping in view the ease of dispensation and tamper resistance. For the peeling off kind of backing material, usually a lamination of polyester, usually PVC (polyvinyl chloride) or its combinations with polystyrene and polypropylene, is used. Depending upon the need for better moisture protection, laminations with lower water vapor transmission rate (WVTR) are preferred. Such lamination is usually PVC with polychlorotrifluoroethylene or PVC coated with polyvinylidene chloride.

A novel blister pack has been developed for moisture sensitive drugs in which each blister-containing tablet is connected to a bigger blister-containing desiccant through channels (Fig. 15.7).

Strip package

These packs consist of one or two plies, made from regenerated cellulose, paper, plastic, foil

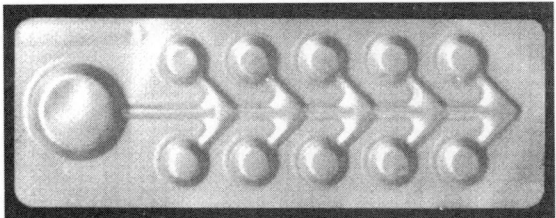

Fig. 15.7. Blister with a desiccant.

or a combination of these (Fig. 15.8). The dosage form is inserted into a pocket area against a recess in a heated platen (or roller) or may be inserted in preformed pockets. This form of packaging is used for packaging of tablets and capsules. Two sheets of film are used for making a strip package and the sheets are fed through heated crimping roller. Continuous strip of pockets are formed and cut as required. The product is sealed between the two sheets of film along with a seal around each tablet/capsule and perforations for easy cutting.

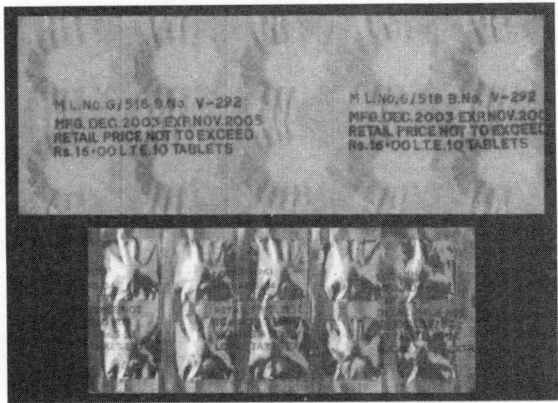

Fig. 15.8. Strip pack.

The use of high barrier material like foil, or saran-coated film together with excellent seal formation, enables this packaging suitable for moisture-sensitive products. Other lamination found suitable for strip packaging is a four fold one consisting of paper/polyethylene/foil/ polyethylene. Usually a cellophane film, on account of its heat sealable nature and transparency is also used, especially when the product is to be very visible and the visibility of the product is important.

Bubble pack

A bubble pack consists of a heat shrinkable plastic film used along with a rigid backing material (Fig. 15.9). The film is heat softened and vacuum drawn to make a pocket. The product is then dropped into the pocket formed in the film as above. The pocket is then heat sealed with the rigid backing material to form a bubble pack. In case of a heat-shrinkable material, the package (product covered with film) is passed through a heated tunnel, whereby the film shrinks to form a cover over the product.

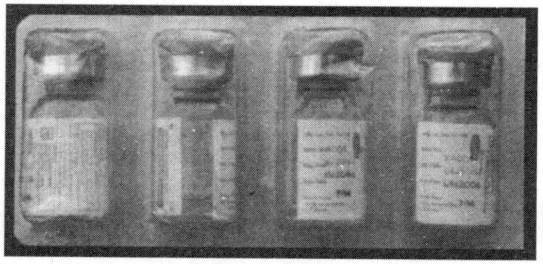

Fig. 15.9. Bubble pack.

Shrink banding

Shrink banding is based on the property of polymer which shrinks on heating. The PVC/polymer used is extruded like a tube of a diameter slightly more than the diameter of the bottle, which is to be shrunk banded. The required length of the polymer is cut and is slid over the bottle, which is then passed through a heat tunnel and the application of the heat makes the polymer shrink around the cap of the bottle as a seal. Such a seal may be perforated for easy-to-cut-off mode.

Foil, Paper, Plastic Pouches

A flexible pouch is made in form-fill-seal machine, popularly known as FFS machines, and the pouch is formed during the product filling. It may be by vertical or horizontal forming. The film is drawn over a metal collar and around a vertical tube from which the product is filled into the tube. Since the film is wrapped around the tube, the filling tube determines the circumference of the pouch. A longitudinal seal is made, which can be a fin seal or overlap one (Fig. 15.10a). The reciprocating sealers crimp the bottom of the packaging film and provide a base seal to the pouch. The filling tube dispenses measured volume of the product into the bottom sealed pouch and with the help of the reciprocating sealer a final seal of the package is provided. Since it is a continuous process the top seal of the package will become the bottom seal of the subsequent package and so on. Such vertical form-fill process is suitable for liquids, granules and powders on account of gravity flow.

A horizontal FFS is more suitable for small volumes as the package formed is flatter. As compared to the vertical FFS, where the film is wrapped around a vertical tube, a horizontal system involves folding the film upon itself as a result of which a pocket is created in the film. The product is then placed in the pocket and top sealed (Fig. 15.10b). The packages made by such

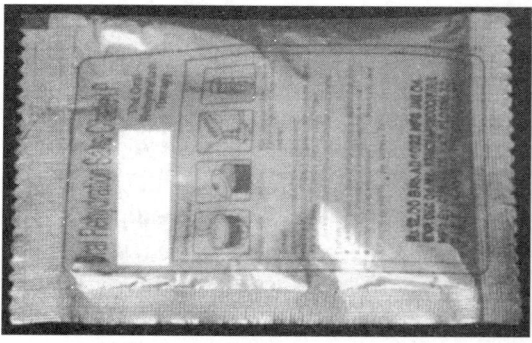

Fig. 15.10a. Fin seal pouch.

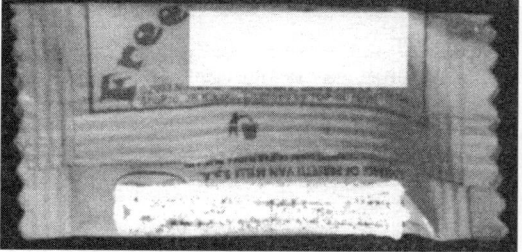

Fig. 15.10b. Top seal pouch.

vertical and horizontal equipment can be made tamper-proof by ensuring surface-to-surface seals by using proper sealants in the lamination. Such a lamination can be used for a good printed exterior surface of the package. Paper is the most common part of the outer surface of the lamination and depending upon the degree of gloss, etc. required in the final package, other variations in the outermost surface of the lamination can be made of cellophane, polyester, nylon, etc.

For better cover against moisture, in case of moisture-sensitive products, aluminium foil is used between the outermost layer and the heat seal layer. With improvements in packaging technology the laminations are also improving and metalized laminations are being used for high barrier applications and appearance.

Aerosol containers

The aerosol containers are made from glass and drawn aluminium (Fig. 15.11). Usually for pharmaceutical product it is made up of drawn aluminium. A hydrocarbon is used as a propellant. If there are compatibility problems between the product and the container, the inner side of the container may be coated. On the upper top side of the container is fixed a spray nozzle, attached to a dip tube, which touches the product.

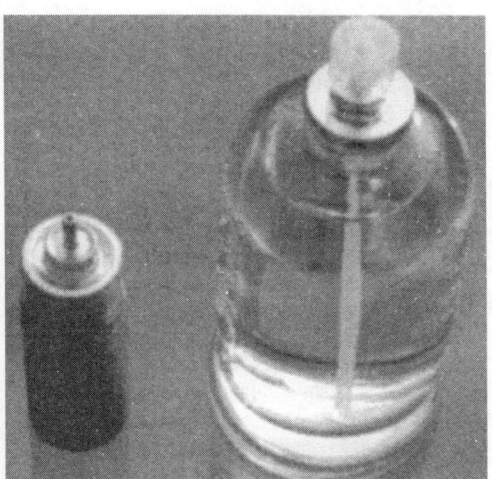

Fig. 15.11. Aerosols.

The spray nozzle is usually metered to allow a specific dose to be dispensed with each spray. These are used for inhalers, etc.

Bottle Seals

Bottle seals, which are tamper-resistant, use an inner seal that is bonded to the neck of the bottle and will get destroyed once the bottle is opened. Several variants of such inner and tamper-proof seals have been developed over the time. Usually a lamination, which is twin layered, is bonded together with an adhesive. Such a lamination is inserted over the bottle cap using wax or glue applied to the rim of the bottle. The application of the cap forces the inner seal into contact with the glued rim of the bottle. Inner seals can be pressure sensitive also and during capping the adhesive bonds inner seal to the rim of the bottle. Apart from this heat-sensitive adhesives can also be used for the purpose of tamper-proofing, which is activated when the bottle is passed under a heating induction coil. Usually aluminium foil is used for this kind of sealing and plastic caps are preferred over metal caps, which can rupture the foil.

Breakable Caps

Breakable closures are being used for alcoholic beverages like beer, etc., where an aluminium foil shell is placed over the bottle neck and passes over the bottle closure to the neck of the bottle and is pressure sealed. To remove the closure the bottom portion of the closure will have to be torn off. These are used for solvents, etc. For pharmaceutical purpose roll-on-pilfer-proof (ROPP) caps are mostly used (Fig. 15.12).

Sealed Tubes

Collapsible plastic, metal or laminated tubes are used for packaging. Metal tubes are used where the product is moisture-sensitive and needs a high degree of barrier. These are usually made of aluminium. Inserts are used to seal the tube and make it puncture-resistant (Fig. 15.13). If

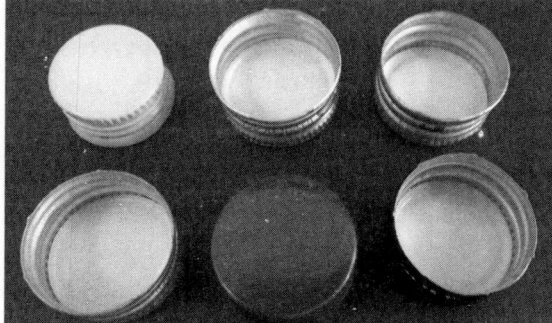

Fig. 15.12. ROPP cap.

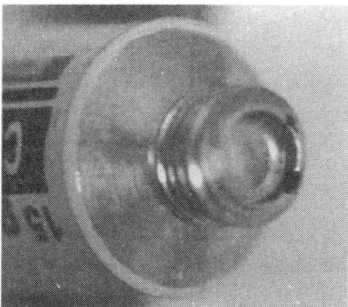

Fig. 15.13. Sealed tube.

any attempt is made to tamper with such a product the inserts will be punctured and pierced open. Extruded plastic tubes are also used. They are filled from the other end and are sealed by crimping the ends in the case of metal tubes or by induction sealing in case of laminated or plastic tubes.

Tape Seals

This type of sealing requires the application of a pressure-sensitive tape over the package closure, which will be ruptured off when the package is opened. High-density lightweight paper is usually used for this purpose as these have poor tear strength and cannot survive any attempt at removal once they are applied.

Cartons and corrugated boxes

Cartons are secondary pack made up of thick paper in which the filled bottles, vials, ointment

tubes etc. are placed as these are made up of paper and relevant information can be printed over it. It provides strength and opaqueness to primary package. Leaflets containing detailed information regarding the product can also be inserted into it. It is usually of two types – tuck-in (Fig. 15.14a) and sealed (Fig. 15.14b). The latter is a tamper-evident packaging. These cartons are finally placed in a bigger container (corrugated boxes) for final shipment, which is sealed with a gum tape. The strength of a corrugated box depends upon the GSM (gram per square meter) of the paper used and the number of ply used to make it.

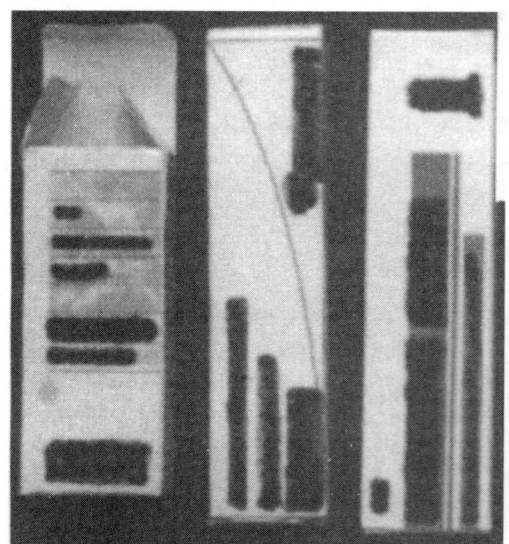

Fig. 15.14a. Tuck-in cartons.

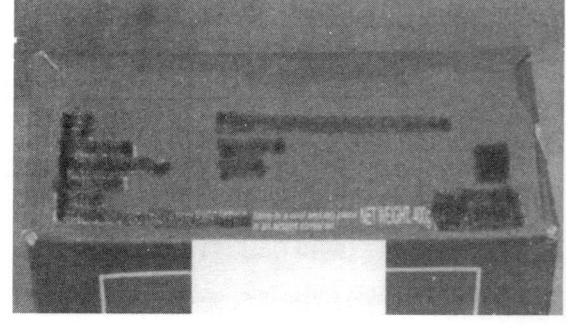

Fig. 15.14b. Sealed carton.

QUALITY ASSURANCE FOR PACKAGING

Quality assurance comprises an important concept of the total approach to GMP. To ensure high quality of drugs, the quality management system must take into consideration the requirements of the local authorities and the legislation, the product, the production process, and the policy of the manufacturer.

Deficiencies in the quality assurance system can have serious implications and packaging defects that may have a deleterious affect on the dosage form. Quality assurance (QA) encompasses all activities and functions concerned with the attainment of quality, including packaging.

Designing

The foremost requirement for packaging must be a good design as relevant to the need of the product, product-pack stability, compatibility, manufacturing and distribution system, the patient, and the legislation.

Product/component stability and compatibility parameters to be studied include moisture and gas protection, light and temperature protection, microbiological integrity, pH stability, and the migration of components from the medicines to the packaging components including preservatives, volatile actives, stabilizers, plasticizers, antioxidants, etc. The QA team needs to stress on the physical aspect of production and marketing e.g. component dimensions (compatibility with machines), machinery (line speed, etc.), stock policy (batch sizes, etc.), distribution system (domestic or export, weight, friability, etc.), legislation (fill weight, labelling, etc.), aesthetic aspect and supplier (limitations, requirements, etc.).

Quality control

The quality control (QC) test specifications must be built around the component specifications and should be designed to achieve consistency through identifying the product, market and production requirements, defining and rating the acceptable quality levels, ensuring relevant sampling, and making a realistic test regime.

The QC testing programme depends upon the company policy, type of material/container, the market use, and the supplier confidence and production requirements. The laboratory routine analysis should include identification, visual inspection, quantity, dimension test, physical test, chemical tests, microbiological test, component and performance measurements, defect classification and action plans and records.

Sampling

Sampling is used to check the correctness of the label, packaging material container reference, acceptance of consignments, detecting adulteration of the medicinal product, obtaining a sample for retention, etc. Effective sampling must take into account the homogeneity and uniformity of the material so as to ensure that the sample is representative of the entire batch.

Inspection and audit of suppliers

The primary goal of inspection is to ascertain the quality of the packaging. These include documentation, storage of starting material and finished product, validation of programmes, production and in-process controls, calibration of instruments and measurement systems, control of labels, etc. National/international authorities audit pharmaceutical manufacturers. All suppliers of pharmaceuticals and packaging materials play an important role in the chain of quality assurance of the final medicinal product.

ADDITIONAL REQUIREMENTS FOR COMMONLY USED DOSAGE FORMS

The package must also contain relevant information regarding the product, storage condition, administration and use, warning along with other information required by the regulatory

Table 15.17. Labeling requirement of a drug product

- Name of product
- Quantity
- Content
- Batch No.
- Mfg. date
- Exp. date
- Mfg. licence number
- Directions for use
- Storage conditions
- Special instructions
- Name and address of manufacturer

authorities. General labelling information for a product is shown in Table 15.17.

Tablets

The following are the labelling requirements for tablets:

1. Store in well closed containers protected from light, moisture, crushing and mechanical shock.
2. Special tablets e.g. effervescent tablets should be stored in tightly closed containers/ moisture-proof packs.
3. Effervescent tablets should be labelled, "Not to be swallowed".

Capsules

Capsules must comply with the labelling requirements as under:

1. Store/pack in a manner that protects them from microbial contamination.
2. Keep in well closed containers.
3. Protect from light, excessive moisture, or dryness.
4. Do not store above 30°C.

Parenteral preparations

Unless specified otherwise these should be stored in containers with sufficient transparency to allow visual inspection:

1. Containers should not adversely affect the quality of the product by either leaching or extracting product components.

2. Closures for parenterals should have firm seals to avoid contamination/entry of microbes.
3. Closures should be inert.
4. Elastomer of the closure should allow piercing of needle through it with least shedding.
5. For multidose containers, the closure should be sufficiently elastic to allow resealing after the needle is withdrawn.

Topical semi-solid forms

Containers for these preparations should be made of material:

1. Which does not adversely affect the quality of the preparation.
2. Does not allow diffusion of any kind into or across the container.
3. Closures for such preparations should be designed to minimize microbial contamination.
4. Closure should be tamper-evident.
5. Container should protect the preparation from light, moisture, damage during handling and transportation.
6. Preparations for nasal, aural, vaginal or rectal use should be supplied in containers adapted for the appropriate delivery of the product to the site of application, or should be supplied with an applicator.

These preparations should be stored in well-closed containers. The preparation should maintain its integrity throughout the shelf-life and should be stored at temperature not exceeding 25°C.

Aerosols

USP specifies certain warning(s), which should appear on the aerosol containers:

1. Avoid inhaling. Keep away from eyes or other mucous membrane.
2. Contents under pressure. Do not puncture or incinerate container. Do not expose to heat. Store at temperature not above 12°C. Keep out of reach of children.

3. Do not inhale directly; deliberate inhalation of contents can cause death.

4. Use only as directed; intentional misuse by deliberately concentrating and inhaling the contents can be harmful or fatal.

Packaging of blood and related products

Special consideration has to be given for packaging of blood and its related products. Some of the salient points mentioned in the USP are listed below:

1. Plastic containers for the collection, storage, processing and administration of blood and its components should be sterile.

2. In normal conditions of use, the materials of the different parts of the containers should not release monomers or other substances in amounts likely to be harmful and should not lead to any abnormal modifications of the blood. The containers may contain anti-coagulant solutions depending on their intended use.

3. The container may be in the form of a single unit or the collecting container may be connected by one or more tubes to one or more secondary containers to allow separation of the blood components to be effected within a closed system.

4. The outlets are of a shape and size allowing for adequate connection of the container with the blood transfusion equipment.

5. The protective coverings on the blood-taking needle and on the appendages should be designed to ensure that sterility is maintained. They are easily removable but are tamper-evident.

6. The containers should be fitted with a suitable device for suspending or fixing, which does not hinder the collection, storage, processing or administration of blood.

7. The containers should be shaped in such a manner that when filled they may be centrifuged.

8. The container should be sufficiently transparent to allow adequate visual examination of its contents before and after taking the blood. It should also be sufficiently flexible to offer minimal resistance during filling and emptying under normal conditions of use.

9. The container should contain not more than 5 ml of air.

10. It should be resistant to centrifugation and stretch.

11. It should not show any leakage.

12. Vapor permeability should be very less.

13. It should empty under pressure in less than 2 minutes.

14. It should be resistant to temperature variations.

15. It should comply with sterility and pyrogen tests.

16. Sterile plastic containers for human blood and blood components are packed in protective tamper-evident envelopes. The protective envelopes should be suffi- ciently robust to withstand normal handling. On removal from its protective envelope the container should show no signs of leakage and no growth of microorganisms.

The labelling requirements for blood and plasma products are depicted in Table 15.18.

TESTS ON CONTAINERS

USP has prescribed various tests on the unit as well as multiple dose containers such as hydrolytic resistance test, permeation test, light transmission test, etc.

Glass containers

Generally hydrolytic resistance and chemical resistance tests are carried out on glass containers. According to USP 37, glass grains test, surface glass test, surface etching test and test for arsenic are carried out on glass containers. The European Pharmacopoeia (EP) provides tests for glass containers including hydrolytic resistance, arsenic, hydrolytic resistance for powdered glass

Table 15.18. Labeling requirements for blood and plasma products

Whole human blood	Plasma
• ABO and Rh groups • Volumes of blood and anticoagulant present • Date on which blood was collected • Expiry date • Required storage conditions • Contents must not be used if there is any visible sign of deterioration • Number or code by which history of the preparation can be traced back to the original donor	• Name of the patient • Identifying batch No. • Information concerning potency or concentration • Name and address of manufacturer • Date of manufacturer • Expiry date • Storage conditions • Nature and concentration of any added bacteriostatic agent • Names and percentages of anticoagulant and other added substances • Quantity of WFI required to reconstitute the original volume • Protein content of reconstituted liquid • Contents must not be used more than 3 h after reconstitution

and hydrolytic resistance of etched glass. However, the Japanese Pharmacopoeia prescribes test for visual inspection, soluble iron, light transmission and soluble alkali.

Glass grains test

The step-wise procedure of test and sample preparation and test is depicted in Tables 15.19 and 15.20. In this test the containers are washed, dried, and crushed, sieved and again crushed through a nest of sieves. Iron particles are removed from the sample, which is then washed with acetone and dried. 10 g of this crushed glass is mixed with high purity water in a conical flask and exposed to standard regimen of autoclaving at 121°C for 30 minutes. The water is then separated in another container; to it are added washings of the specimens made using purified water. The pooled sample is titrated with 0.02 M HCl using methyl red solution as indicator. The volume of acid used should be in accordance with the values given in Table 15.21.

Surface glass test

The procedure for Surface glass test is given in Table 15.22 and limit test values are given in Table 15.23.

Surface etching test

It is used in addition to the Surface glass test when it is necessary to determine whether a container has been surface treated and/or to distinguish between type I and type II glass containers. Alternatively, the Glass grains test and Surface glass test may be carried out either on unused samples or on samples used in the Surface glass test. The procedure for the test is given in Table 15.24.

The results obtained from the Surface etching test are compared to those obtained from Surface glass test. For type I glass containers, the values obtained are close to those found in Surface glass test. For type II glass containers, the values obtained greatly exceed those found in the Surface glass test; and they are similar to, but not larger than, those obtained for type III glass containers of the same filling volume.

Plastic containers

Some of the important tests prescribed in IP, 2014 are shown in Tables 15.25, 15.26 and 15.27.

Physicochemical tests

The USP physicochemical tests are designed to determine physical and chemical properties of plastics and their extracts, based on the extraction of plastic material, and it is essential that the designated amount of plastic be used. USP 37 specifies surface area that must be available for extraction at the designated temperature. The extracting medium, unless specified otherwise,

Table 15.19. Glass grains test (USP 37) – Specimen preparation

Rinse the containers
↓
Dry them
↓
Crush into fragments
↓
Crush to produce two equal parts of 100 g each
↓
Place 30–40 g in a mortar
↓
Crush further by striking with single blow with hammer
↓
Nest the sieves
↓
Empty the mortar into 25# sieve (repeat on remaining portions of glass emptying each time in 25# sieve)
↓
Shake the sieves
↓
Remove the glass from 25# and 40#
↓
Shake on shaker for 5 min
↓
Spread the specimen on glazed paper and remove iron particles with the help of a magnet
↓
Transfer the specimen to a 250 mL conical flask of resistant glass
↓
Wash with three 30 mL portions of acetone, decant acetone
↓
Dry the contents for 20 min at 140°C
↓
Transfer to weighing bottle
↓
Final specimen for powdered glass test

Table 15.20. Glass grains test (USP 37)

10.0 g of prepared specimen
↓
Add to conical flask containing 50 ml of high purity water
↓
Cap all the flasks
↓
Autoclave (for 10 min)
↓
Close vent cock
↓
Adjust temp to 121°C
↓
Hold the temp (121 ± 1°C for 30 min.)
↓
Reduce the heat and wait and allow autoclave to cool to atmospheric pressure
↓
Cool the flask in running water
↓
Decant water
↓
Wash the residual powdered glass (3 times with 15 mL high purity water)
↓
Add the decanted washings to main portion
↓
Add 0.05 mL of methyl red solution
↓
Titrate immediately with 0.02 M HCl
↓
Record the volume of 0.02 M HCl
↓
Volume doesn't exceed that indicated in table for the type of glass concerned

1. **Nonvolatile residue (NVR):** NVR measures organic/inorganic residue soluble in extraction media [limit – not more than (NMT) 15 mg].
2. **Residue on ignition:** This test is performed when the NVR is greater than 15 mg (limit – NMT 5 mg).

is purified water and is maintained at 70°C during extraction. The current minimum surface area is 120 cm^2. After the extraction process has taken place, the following checks are performed:

Table 15.21. Types of glass and their test limits

Type of glass	General description of glass[a]	Type of test	Limits	
			Size[b], mL	mL of 0.02 N acid
I	Highly resistant, borosilicate glass	Powdered glass	All	1.0
II	Treated soda-lime glass	Water attack	100 or less	0.7
			Over 100	0.2
III	Soda-lime glass	Powdered glass	All	8.5
NP	General purpose soda-lime glass	Powdered glass	All	15.0

[a] The description applies to containers of this type of glass usually available.
[b] Size indicates the overflow capacity of the container.

Table 15.22. Procedure for surface glass test (USP 37)

Rinse the containers twice with purified water
↓
Fill the containers with CO_2-free water up to filling volume
↓
Cap the containers and autoclave as described for glass grains test
↓
Remove the containers from autoclave and cool them
↓
Combine the liquids of all containers into a conical flask
↓
Add 0.05 mL of methyl red solution to each 25 mL of test liquid
↓
Titrate with 0.01 M HCl

Table 15.23. Limit values for Surface glass test (USP 37)

Filling volume (mL)	Maximum volume of 0.01 M HCl per 100 mL of test liquid (mL)	
	Types I and II	Type III
Upto 1	2.0	20.0
Above 1 and upto 2	1.8	17.6
Above 2 and upto 5	1.3	13.2
Above 5 and upto 10	1.0	10.2
Above 10 and upto 20	0.80	8.1
Above 20 and upto 50	0.60	6.1
Above 50 and upto 100	0.50	4.8
Above 100 and upto 200	0.40	3.8
Above 200 and upto 500	0.30	2.9
Above 500	0.20	2.2

Table 15.24. Procedure for Surface etching test (USP 37)

Rinse the containers twice with high purity water
↓
Fill each container to brimful point with a mixture of HF and HCl (1 : 9)
↓
Allow to stand for 10 minutes and then empty them
↓
Rinse with purified water and repeat the rest procedure as described under Surface glass test

3. **Heavy metals:** This detects the presence of metals such as lead, tin, zinc, etc.
4. **Buffering capacity:** This measures the alkalinity/acidity of the extract.

Primary container/closure system may interact with the dosage form. Extractable and bleachable matter may be generated and may contaminate the product. An **extractable** is a chemical species that can be released from a

Table 15.25. Leakage test for plastic containers (non-injectables and injectables) (IP, 2014)

Fill 10 containers with water and fit the closure
↓
Keep them inverted at RT for 24 hrs
↓
No sign of leakage from any container

Table 15.26. Water vapor permeability test for plastic containers used in blood and blood components (IP, 2014)

Fill empty container with the same mixture of anticoagulant solution and NaCl injection
↓
Close the container and weigh it
↓
Store the container at 5°C in an atmosphere with a RH of 50% for 21 days
↓
At the end, loss in weight should be not more than 1%

Table 15.27. Collapsibility test for plastic containers (non-injectables and injectables) (IP, 2014)

This test is applicable for those containers which have to be squeezed for the withdrawal of the product. A container by collapsing inwards during use yields at least 90% of its nominal content at required flow rate at ambient temperature.

container or closure material of construction that has the potential for contaminating the dosage form. Under certain stress conditions this may be generated through an interaction with the closure system. Whereas **leachable** is a chemical species that has migrated from packaging component, or any other component, of the product into the dosage form, under normal conditions of use or under stability studies. The chemicals that can migrate from the container/closure system include stabilizer, contaminant, lubricant, antioxidant, plasticizer and monomer. The US FDA has been and continues to be the driving force behind the safety evaluation of

materials and container closure system. Establishing the safety of container system is of great importance to the medical and pharmaceutical industry. The FDA's guidance document requires the evaluation of four attributes to establish suitability, protection, compatibility, safety and performance/drug delivery.

Protection

A container intended to provide protection from light, or offered as a light-resistant container, must meet the requirements of the USP (2014) Light transmission test. The ability of a container to protect against moisture can be ascertained by performing the USP (2014) Water vapor permeation test. Integrity of the container can be evaluated using dye penetration test, microbial ingress test, gas detection test, etc.

Compatibility

Compatible components will not interact with the dosage form and may not show leaching. Regular screening of the product using Liquid Chromatography (LC)/Mass Spectrometry (MS), GC/MS, etc. would detect and quantitate the elements. Other changes such as pH shift, precipitation, discoloration, which may cause degradation of the drug, should also be evaluated.

Safety

Packaging components should be constructed of materials that will not leach harmful or undesirable amounts of substances. This is difficult to determine. An extraction study with sample including preparation of sample, followed by incubation in solvents at well-defined and well-controlled times and temperatures is carried out. The USP physicochemical tests (mentioned earlier) for extraction are relevant, sensitive and inexpensive.

Elastomeric container closure used in pharmaceuticals, for injections, fall into this test class. Two extraction media are used, purified water and isopropyl alcohol. The extraction is performed at a specific temperature and time period. The tests performed are turbidity, pH change, reducing agent, heavy metals, total extractable zinc, ammonium, etc.

Performance

The container/closure system should have the ability to function in an intended manner so as to improve patient compliance. Also, it should have the ability to deliver the right amount or the right rate e.g. the prefilled syringes, transdermal patches, dropper or spray bottles, metered dose inhalers (MDI).

BRIEF REGULATORY ASPECT OF PHARMACEUTICAL PACKAGING

The pharmaceutical industry is one of the most regulated industries with control on various aspects implemented through:

1. Good laboratory practice (GLP)
2. Good clinical practice (GCP)
3. Good manufacturing practice (GMP)
4. Labelling instructions
5. Control on how the product is advertised (mainly prevalent in the regulated market)
6. Product disposal regulations

The regulatory agencies require that the pack have the following characteristics:

- Containing the product
  (a) protection of the product
  (b) protection of the consumer
  (c) dosage control
- Carrying the label
  (a) information to the recipient
  (b) legal control of the product
- Contaminating the environment
  (a) packaging wastage
  (b) ozone depletion
- Protection of the consumer
  (a) child-resistant closures
  (b) tamper-evident packaging

Glass used in pharmaceutical packaging was an inert receptacle with little potential interaction with the product. With the advent of plastics, there is much more scope for interactions between the product and the package. With more and more tailor made packages, the use of plastics is on an ever increase. They, however, pose problems such as extraction of material from the plastic. This is where the regulatory authorities become much more interested in the selection, composition and performance of the package. To withstand the ever-increasing cost of research and development, the need for becoming a global player in pharmaceutical marketing is increasing. The regulatory agencies for various countries may have different requirements.

FDA packaging guidelines

This guideline defines the types of containers to be used, dividing them into parenteral (glass/plastic) or non-parenteral containers (glass, plastic and metal), pressurized containers and bulk containers for active ingredients and drug products. Also listed are closures including child-resistant and tamper-evident closures, liners, seals and elastomers when used for closure. The packaging components are discussed for physical, chemical and biological characteristics, specifications and tests to be applied, stability and compatibility. The various tests mentioned have been discussed separately under containers testing.

According to FDA guidelines, for submitting document for packaging for human drugs and biologicals the following are required:

- Purpose
  (a) Package must maintain standards, identity, strength, quality and purity of drug for intended shelf-life.
  (b) Full information needed.
  (c) USP provides guidance.
- Type of container/closure.
- Suitability for intended use.
- IND (investigational new drug) needs.
- NDA (new drug application) needs.
- Submission of packaging information and data (Table 15.28).

Table 15.28. Information to be supplied along with original form of any drug

Description

- General description of container with closure
- Name, product code, physical description, manufacturer, raw material, any additional treatment

Suitability

- Protection against light, oxygen, moisture leakage, microbes, dirt, etc.
- Safety – chemical composition extractable material test as per pharmacopoeia or any other relevant test
- Compatibility – test reports for packaging interacting with product or vice versa
- Performance – suitability for its intended use e.g. Metered Dose Inhalers (MDI)

Quality control

- Various tests and acceptance limits
- Dimensional check
- Performance
- Consistency in composition
- Manufacturer's protocol for release and manufacturer's process of component

Stability

Environmental concerns

With increased environmental concern there has been a considerable pressure to minimize contamination of the environment, with particular concern on amount of packaging and its disposal. Ozone depletion is also of concern with the use of pressurized containers. Regarding this aspect, the increase in concern has led to the EEC packaging waste directive, which requires:

1. Reduction in quantity of waste.
2. Reduction in harmfulness of waste.
3. Increase in reuse of packaging.
4. Recycling and recovery of packaging waste.
5. Reduction of the total packaging to be disposed of.

SUMMARY AND CONCLUSION

The packaging materials account for about one third of cost of medicine. For many years the role of packaging was undermined, but now the importance of pharmaceutical packaging has been duly recognized. Packaging not only provides the protection to the product from contamination, external influences and physical damage but also helps in identification of the product and display of correct information. The packaging material and product must be compatible. More care should be exercised in pharmaceutical packaging because any failure could result in contamination or loss of potency of the drug leading to failure of therapy, to adverse effects, to injury or even death of the patient. Maintenance of shelf-life of product is of foremost requirement.

Glass, plastics, metal and paper are the most commonly used packaging material in pharmaceutical technology. Each one has its own pros and cons. The selection of the packaging material of the drug is mainly dependent on the nature of the product, level of protection required, stability, cost, machinability, shipment requirement and dispensing of the dosage form. Basically the pharmaceutical packaging is classified as primary packaging (bottles, strips, blisters, jars, cans, etc.), secondary packaging (cartons, corrugated boxes, etc.) and accessories (labels, caps and closures). Further, these packagings need to be child-resistant, tamper-resistant and geriatric-friendly. Stringent quality control test should be practised to check the quality of not only the raw packaging material but also the finished products. Such growth will lead to the development of value-added containers and accessories. Development of patient-friendly packaging, anticipation and preparation of future legislative direction will be the need of coming years.

Importance of drug delivery systems has been recognized and it is capturing a good market share, which will grow further in future. Packaging requirement of novel drug delivery systems are different from those of the conventional dosage forms. The innovations and developments in packaging of such product should be foresighted and will be a key factor in successful marketing of these products.

SUGGESTIVE BIBLIOGRAPHY FOR FURTHER STUDIES

- Aulton, M.E. (2013). **Packs and Packaging in Pharmaceuticals: The Science of Dosage Form Design**, 4th ed., Churchill Livingstone, London, 811–824.
- Bauer E.J. (2009). **Pharmaceutical Packaging Handbook**, Informa Healthcare.
- **Bentley's Text Book of Pharmaceutics** (2012). Ed. of original edition-E.A. Rawlins, 8th ed., Bailliere Tindall London & All India Traveler Book Seller, pp. 711–735.
- **British Pharmacopoeia** (2016), Containers. Volume V. HMSO, London, Appendix XIX, pp. A556–A571.
- Croce, C.P., Fisher, A., Thomas, R.H. (1991). Packaging Material Science. *In:* **The Theory and Practice of Industrial Pharmacy**, Lachman, L. et al. (Eds.), 3rd ed., Varghese Publishing House, Mumbai, India, pp. 711–732.
- Dean, D.A., Evans, E.R., Hall, I.H. (Eds.) 2000. **Pharmaceutical Packaging Technology**, Taylor & Francis, London and New York Press.
- Guidance for Industry: Container closure systems for packaging human drugs and biologicals (May, 1995) US. Department of health & human services, food and drug administration, center for drug evaluation and research, center for biological evaluation and research. www.fda.gov/cber/guidelines.htm
- Guidance on packaging for pharmaceutical products (2002), World Health Organization Technical Report Series, www.who.int/medicines/organization/qsm/strategy_quality_safety/trs902ann9.pdf.
- Harburn, K. (1991). **Quality Control of Packaging Material in Pharmaceutical Industry**, Marcel Dekker, Inc., New York.
- **Indian Pharmacopoeia** (2014). Containers. Government of India, Ministry of Health & Family Welfare, New Delhi, Volume I, pp. 889-903.
- Kit L. Yan (ed.), John Wiley & Sons Inc. USA; **The Wiley Encyclopedia of Packaging Technology**, 3rd edition, 2009.
- Primary Plastic Packaging Materials. pharmacos.eudra.org/F2/eudralex/vol-3/pdfs-en/3aq10aen.pdf.
- United States Pharmacopoeia 37 and National Formulary 32 (2014), United States Pharmacopoeial Convention Inc., Volume I, pp. 318–333.

16

Pharmaceutical Pilot-Plant and Scale-Up in Product Development

O.P. Katare, Bhupinder Singh,
Pradip Nirbhavane and Rajiv Kumar

INTRODUCTION

Development of a pharmaceutical product of any drug invariably begins in a formulation research laboratory. Subsequent to establishing the proof-of-concept in terms of its efficacy, safety and stability at small-scale, the developed product is required to be produced at much larger scale to meet the commercial and clinical requirements. And this is to be accomplished in such a meticulous manner that the desired quality attributes inherent in a "laboratory product" are well preserved in the "manufactory product" too.

On the other hand, extensive differences tend to prevail between a small-scale research laboratory and large scale manufactory for commercial production. Such differences primarily arise owing to differences in various factors including the nature of equipment, environmental conditions and the available facilities. In a research laboratory, the product development is carried out employing standardized equipment of limited capacity. The latter, in no way, can serve for large scale manufacturing at the shop-floor. Customarily, the equipment (and their principles of operation) used in a research laboratory are quite different from those employed during commercial manufacturing. Further, sometimes the product has to face entirely newer kind of mechanized operations at the manufacturing plant or shop-floor, hitherto not envisioned at the development stage. Fig. 16.1 outlines some salient differences.

Also, the product development scientist many a time is not conversant with the facilities and processes of the production area. Therefore, he lacks thorough understanding of the kind of operations and machinery employed there. For all of these reasons, a research scientist, while developing the product, may not consider all those factors which may influence its large scale processing or manufacturing. Hence, a lot of problems tend to be encountered while transferring the product directly from laboratory to the production scale. Often, there is significant alteration in the product attributes, which may affect the efficacy, safety, stability and reproducibility of the product. The changes are more likely and unbearable, especially when the formulation design is highly specialized, e.g., novel drug delivery systems such as nano-particles, liposomes, products based on hot-melt extrusion, etc.

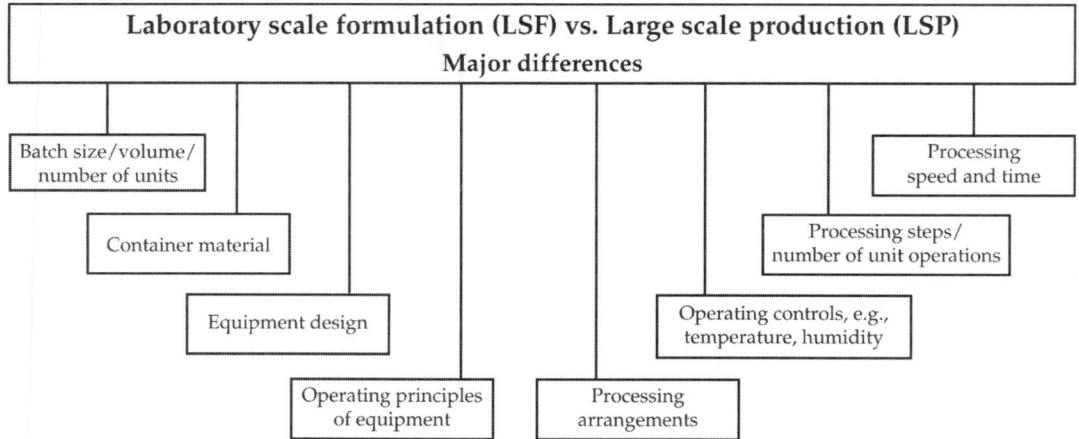

Fig. 16.1. Lab-scale and large-scale production: Key differences.

In an attempt to study and tackle the above product-transfer related problems, the concept of "pilot-plant facility" comes to rescue. It pertains to the kind of systems and arrangements, wherein the efforts are made to simulate large-scale manufacturing employing equipment and facilities of intermediate capacity. The use of pilot-plant facility allows the development scientist to experiment with relatively smaller size batches. This facilitates making necessary changes both at the product and process level so that the product can bear multiple (i.e., physical, chemical and mechanical) perturbations to maintain its originality. Consequently, the pilot-plant studies achieve the successful transfer of the results from the experimental formulation prepared in laboratory (i.e., small scale) to the production shop floor (i.e., bulk scale). The photographs in Fig. 16.2 (A, B & C) illustrate the key differences between small scale and commercial scale equipment employed in an industrial house.

Functions of pilot-plant

1. Review of the product formula to evaluate and determine its ability to withstand large scale modifications.
2. Selection, approval and validation of raw material specifications.
3. Selection and validation of appropriate processing equipment.
4. Pilot scale-up and validation studies at commercial scale.
5. Evaluation and validation of process as well as production controls.
6. Transfer of developed process/technology to the shop-floor for commercial manufacturing.

The current book chapter presents a comprehensive account of the various aspects of pilot-plant operations and scale-up techniques under the following different sections:

1. 'Quality-by-Design' (QbD) in the overall product development and key role of pilot-plant scale up.
2. Design and overall layout of a pilot-plant facility.
3. Organizational structure of a pilot-plant.
4. Pilot-plant operations.
5. Scale-up techniques for different dosage forms including newer drug delivery systems.

QUALITY BY DESIGN (QbD) IN PHARMACEUTICAL PRODUCT DEVELOPMENT: ROLE OF PILOT-PLANT SCALE-UP

The concept of pharmaceutical product development is now-a-days changing from an empirical,

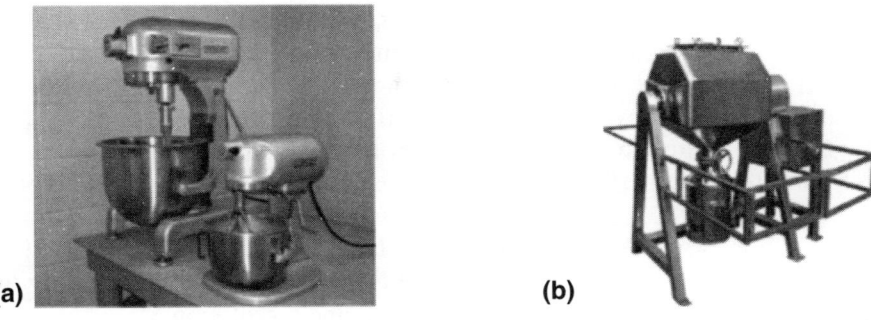

(a)   **(b)**

Fig. 16.2A. (a) Lab-scale double cone blender; and (b) commercial-scale blender.

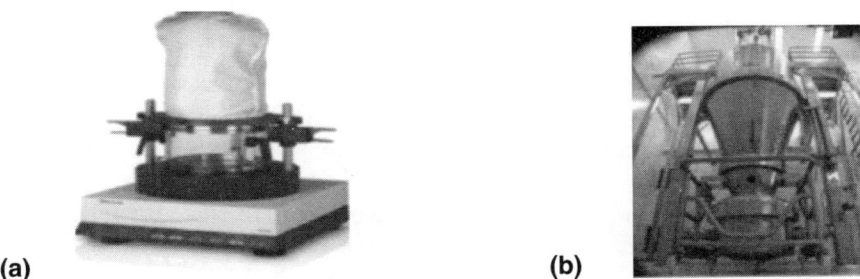

(a)   **(b)**

Fig. 16.2B. (a) Lab-scale granule dryer; and (b) commercial-scale fluid-bed dryer.

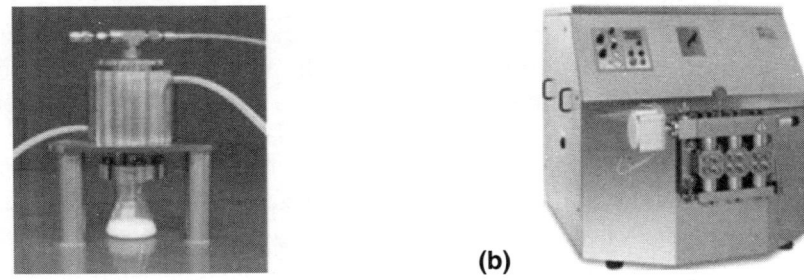

(a)   **(b)**

Fig. 16.2C. (a) Lab-scale liposome extruder; and (b) commercial-scale liposome homogenizer.

data-driven approach of development to a more systematic, knowledge-driven one. Various international regulatory authorities, especially Food and Drug Administration of United States (USFDA) and European Medicines Agency (EMEA) are emphasizing on 'Built-in-Quality' attitude rather than testing some quality parameters at the end of product development and manufacturing.

Strong emphasis is being laid down on adoption of QbD principles to achieve this goal. 'QbD' is a systematic approach to pharmaceutical development that begins with predefined objectives. It emphasizes on product and process understanding and process control, based on sound science and quality risk management. The objective is to design and develop formulations and manufacturing processes ensuring a predefined quality. And it has been strongly recommended to employ modern approaches based on 'Design of Experiment' (DoE) and 'Process Analytical Technology' (PAT) to accomplish these QbD objectives. Beginning with the introduction of the PAT Guidance in 2003, various QbD initiatives have been reported. One of the core components of this

QbD approach is the understanding of the influence of formulation and process variables upon product quality. Implementation of statistical DoE techniques further allows gaining the required understanding of how formulation and process factors impact product performance.

Benefits of QbD

1. Regulatory relief throughout the product life cycle, because post-approval changes don't require prior approval.
2. Potential reduction in the volume of data submitted; empirical data replaced by knowledge-based submissions.
3. Facilitation of continuous process improvement, because these process improvements don't require pre-approval.
4. Elimination of a need for a current model of process validation.

Quality Target Product Profile (QTPP)

It is "a prospective summary of the quality characteristics of a drug product that ideally will be achieved to ensure the desired quality, taking into account safety and efficacy of the drug product." The QTPP is an essential element of a QbD approach and forms the basis of design for the development of the product. For ANDAs, the target should be defined early in development based on the properties of the drug substance (DS), characterization of the Reference Listed Drug (RLD) product and consideration of the

RLD label and intended patient population. By beginning with the end in mind, the result of development is a robust formulation and manufacturing process with an acceptable control strategy that ensures the performance of the drug product. For example, a typical QTPP of an immediate release solid oral dosage form would include tablet characteristics, tablet identity, assay and uniformity, purity/impurity, stability, and dissolution.

Critical Quality Attribute (CQA)

It is "a physical, chemical, biological, or microbiological property or characteristic that should be within an appropriate limit, range, or distribution to ensure the desired product quality." The identification of a CQA from the QTPP is based on the severity of harm to a patient should the product fall outside the acceptable range for that attribute.

Critical Process Parameter (CPP)

It is a parameter in which a realistic change can cause the product to fail to meet the QTPP. Thus, whether a parameter is critical or not depends on how large of a change one is willing to consider. A simple example is that an impeller speed of zero will always fail. Thus, the first step in classifying parameters is to define the range of interest which we call the Potential Operating Space (POS). The POS is the region between the maximum and minimum value of interest to

Table 16.1. Current paradigm compared to Quality by Design paradigm

Current paradigm	Quality by design paradigm
Quality is tested into the product.	Quality is designed into the product.
Product specifications are based on batch testing results.	Real-time quality control, based on process analytical technology, is used.
Validation freezes the process.	Product specifications are based on fitness for use and process capability.
Process improvements require pre-approval.	Process changes within the established design space do not require pre-approval. Process validation is redundant.
Focus on reproducibility – often avoiding or ignoring variation.	Focus on robustness – understanding and controlling variation.

the sponsor for each process parameter. The POS can also be considered as the extent of the sponsor's quality system with respect to these parameters. This definition is at the discretion of the application that sponsor.

Design of Experiments (DoE)

It is a structured and organized method to determine the relationship among factors that influence outputs of a process. For applying DoE to pharmaceutical process, factors that play major role are the raw material attributes (e.g., particle size) and process parameters (e.g., speed and time), while outputs are the Critical Quality Attributes (CQA) such as blend uniformity, tablet hardness, thickness, and friability. As it is impossible to experimentally investigate all the process parameters, and variables, scientists have to use prior knowledge and risk management to identify key input and output variables. When considering scale-up, additional experimental work may be required to confirm that the model generated at the small scale is predictive at the large scale. This is because some Critical Process Parameters (CPPs) are scale dependent while others do not. The operating range of scale dependent critical process parameters will have to change because of scale-up. Prior knowledge can play a very significant role in this regard as most pharmaceutical companies use the same technologies as well as excipients on a regular basis.

Risk Assessment

Risk assessment is a valuable science-based process used in Quality Risk Management (QRM) (ICH Q9) that aided in identifying which material attributes and process parameters potentially had an effect on product CQAs. Performing a risk assessment before pharmaceutical development helps manufacturers decide which studies to conduct. Study results determine which variables are critical and which are not, which then guide the establishment of control strategy for in-process, raw material, and final testing.

Design Space

ICH Q8 (R1) defines design space as, the multidimensional combination and interaction of input variables (e.g., material attributes) and process parameters that have been demonstrated to provide assurance of quality. So, to avoid any change in final product, working within the design space is recommended. Movement out of the design space is considered to be a change and would normally initiate a regulatory post-approval change process. Design space is potentially scale- and equipment-dependent. The design space determined at the laboratory scale may not be relevant to the process at the commercial scale. Therefore, design-space verification at the commercial scale becomes essential unless it is demonstrated that the design space is scale-independent. There is always a misconception that design space and QbD are interchangeable terms. This is incorrect. For generic-drug applications, design space is optional. QbD can be implemented without a design space because product and process understanding can be established without a formal design space. It should be pointed out that implementation of QbD is strongly encouraged by FDA. For some complex drug substances or drug products, implementation of QbD is considered a required component of the application.

It can be achieved effectively through well-planned and systematically executed pilot-plant set-up only, as elaborated in the next sections of this chapter.

CASE STUDIES

QbD APPROACH IN THE DEVELOPMENT OF SOLID ORAL DOSAGE FORMS

1. QbD in the development of IR tablet

FDA in 2012 published the pharmaceutical development report summarizing the development of Immediate Release (IR) Tablets, Generic Acetriptan Tablets, 20 mg (a generic version of the reference listed drug (RLD), Brand Acetriptan Tablets, 20 mg) by using QbD approach, that are therapeutically equivalent to the RLD.

- Acetriptan is a poorly soluble, highly permeable, Biopharmaceutics Classification System (BCS) Class II compound. As such, initial efforts focused on developing a dissolution method that would be able to predict an *in vivo* performance. The developed in-house dissolution method uses 900 mL of 0.1 N HCl with 1.0% w/v sodium lauryl sulfate (SLS). This method is capable of differentiating between formulations manufactured using different acetriptan particle size distributions (PSD) and predicting *in vivo* performance in the pilot bioequivalence (BE) study.
- The CQAs included assay, content uniformity, dissolution and degradation products.
- Risk assessment was used throughout development to identify potentially high risk formulation and process variables.
- For formulation development, an *in silico* simulation was conducted to evaluate the potential effect of acetriptan PSD on *in vivo* performance and a diameter of 30 μ or less was selected. Roller compaction (RC) was selected as the granulation method due to the potential for thermal degradation of acetriptan during the drying step of a wet granulation process.
- Two Design of Experiments (DoE) were conducted. The first DoE investigated the impact of acetriptan PSD and levels of intragranular lactose, microcrystalline cellulose and croscarmellose sodium on drug product CQAs. The second DoE studied the levels of extragranular talc and magnesium stearate on drug product CQAs. The formulation composition was finalized based on the knowledge gained from these two DoE studies. Experimental studies were defined and executed in order to establish additional

scientific knowledge and understanding, to allow appropriate controls to be developed and implemented, and to reduce the risk to an acceptable level.

2. QbD in the development of MR tablet dosage form

FDA in 2011 published the pharmaceutical development report summarizing the development of modified release (MR) tablets, 10 mg [a generic version of reference listed drug (RLD), Brand MR tablets], using the QbD approach, that are therapeutically equivalent to RLD drug.

- The example MR tablet includes Z drug substance, a chemically stable BCS class I compound. As such initial reports focused on preparing IR granules and extended release (ER) coated beads with extra-granular cushioning agents and other excipients, all compressed into scored tablets, to match the RLD. Kollicoat SR 30 D was selected as the release rate controlling polymer and the formulation was optimized using design of experiments (DoE). Two grades of microcrystalline cellulose (MCC) were used in an optimized ratio to prevent segregation of the IR granules and ER coated beads. The appropriate levels of disintegrants (sodium starch glycolate) and lubricant (magnesium stearate) were used. Dissolution method was developed using USP apparatus 3 at 10 dpm in 250 mL of pH 6.8 phosphate buffer by performing an extensive evaluation of dissolution conditions.
- CPPs were (i) drug layering, (ii) ER polymer coating, (iii) blending and lubrication, and (iv) compression.
- Risk assessment was used throughout development to identify potentially high risk formulation and process variables. Each risk assessment was then updated to capture the reduced level of risk based on improved product and process understanding.

- Bottom spray fluid bed process was used for both drug layering and polymer coating of the ER beads. Diffusive mixing method was utilized for the final blend before compressing the blend into scored tablets. For each unit operation, risk assessment was conducted and then utilized DoE to investigate the identified high risk variables to determine the Critical Material Attributes (CMAs) and Critical Process Parameters (CPPs).

- First verification batch at commercial scale level failed in dissolution testing. Subsequent investigation showed that film coat thickness increased on the beads manufactured at commercial scale versus beads manufactured at pilot scale due to a difference in process efficiency. A second verification batch was manufactured by decreasing the theoretical polymer coating level from 30% to 28% to account for improved processing efficiency at commercial scale. The formulation change resulted in drug product that met with the predefined CQA targets.

3. QbD in the development of Solid Dispersion (SD) using Fluidized Bed Process (FBP)

Mukharya et al. (of Cadila Pharmaceuticals) reported the development and scale-up of novel SD formulation of Lacidipine, a poorly water-soluble, antihypertensive drug (Ca channel blocker) with Fluidized bed process (Mukharya et al., 2013). They used QbD approach for developing this solid oral dosage form.

- The fluid bed agglomeration process is a combination of three steps: dry mixing, spray agglomeration and drying to a desired moisture level or to a desired granule size. The Critical Process Parameters were rate of binder addition, degree of atomization of the binder liquid, process-air temperature and height of the spray nozzle from the bed.

- Risk assessment tools were used to identify and rank parameters with potential to have an impact on In Process/Drug Product Critical Quality Attributes (IP/DP CQAs), based on prior knowledge and initial experimental data.

- Solvent evaporation by Fluidized Bed Process (FBP) was selected as a method of choice for formulation by Solid Dispersion (SD), as it improves wettability with simultaneous increase in porosity of granules and uniform distribution of drug particles within formulation to achieve content uniformity.

- LCDP was first dissolved in ethanol (99.6% v/v). In this solution, PVP-K29/32 was slowly added with continuous stirring until a clear yellow-colored solution was obtained. Lactose Monohydrate (Pharmatose-200M) was loaded in fluidized bed processor and granulated by spraying of drug carrier solution for moistening of lactose powder substrate using top spray mechanics.

- Depending on IRMA (Initial Risk-based Matrix Analysis) & FMEA (Failure Mode Effective Analysis) results, process understanding experiments [DoE and Multi-Variate Data Analysis (MVDA)] were developed for FBP.

- Spray agglomeration stage was the most critical phase to monitor. During this phase, dynamic granule growth and breakdown takes place, along with solvent evaporation. By QbD, risk associated with scale-up was considered in Control Strategy of pilot scale development itself to maximize the probability of effectiveness at larger scale with utilized QRM tools to guide activities.

- Thus, the scale up of SD of Lacidipine was successfully done, with results showing insignificant variations between laboratory batch results and scale-up batch results.

4. QbD for freeze dried product/ lyophilization

For a freeze-dried product, the CQAs are typically things like reconstitution time, appearance, shrinkage, collapse, viability of product and shelf-life. The next step is to use analytical methods to determine the behaviour of the product during the freezing and drying process. A risk assessment technique, such as FMEA, determines which factors in the process can be expected to impact the quality of the final product. In a freeze-drying process these would typically be:

- Impact of freezing rate on the ice structure.
- Final freezing temperature.
- Ice temperature/critical temperature for collapse/micro-collapse.
- Impact of crystal structure on both the reconstitution rate and the drying rate.
- Impact of any annealing step on the pressure drop in the cake.
- Effects of drying rate on shrinkage.
- The rate of freezing may also impact the viability for live vaccines.

Process requirements may also impact the design of the freeze dryer, such as performance of cooling and vapour velocities. The basis of QbD is to make sure that the level of knowledge regarding product and how product quality varies with changes in raw materials or variability in process conditions ensures that the process is fully capable of producing a product that meets specification.

PHARMACEUTICAL PILOT-PLANT FACILITY

In order to fulfil various key objectives as well as for smooth and efficient working of a pilot-plant, its design and layout are very important twin considerations. Various factors which influence the design of a pilot-plant include (i) type of dosage forms to be manufactured, (ii) size and volume of the batches, and (iii) the nature of production process. All these aspects must be thoroughly studied before finalizing the structure of a pilot-plant facility. Sound professional expertise in this regard is mandatory. A team is made up of qualified professionals, who are experienced to plan, decide and take decisions on the final design and layout of the facility.

1. Product type

The process of scale-up widely differs from product to product. It needs to take into consideration the specifications involved in the type and technology of the product. The most commonly produced drug products and their design requirements are given in Table 16.2.

2. Product quantity (batch size and volume)

A pilot-plant is supposed to be designed to manufacture wide array of batch sizes meant for different purposes such as product development, analytical development, stability testing, formulation optimization, feasibility and scale-up batches, process development batches, etc. The type of batches to be manufactured determines the quantities to be produced of a particular product, which, in turn, influences the capacity requirements of the pilot-plant.

Quite often, a few laboratory-scale batches, for instance, are also manufactured in pilot-plant facility as a part of the product development. This type of experimental manufacturing is usually carried out employing very small batch sizes. At times, the batches need to be produced several times with minor variation(s) and modification(s). Fabrication of these types of batches demands some special provisions and necessary facilities while designing the facility. The equipment and facility, for example, should be of such type that it could be easily used for many runs in as little time as possible.

Another type of batches that are manufactured in a pilot-plant facility are developmental batches, which are typically a few kilograms or litres in size, and are used for different purposes as mentioned above. Fabrication of these types of batches requires the equipment and facilities, which are replica of that in the production shop floor.

Fabrication of batches for clinical studies is also an integral part of the product development process. As the clinical requirements increase,

Table 16.2. Pilot-plant design considerations for different dosage forms

S. No.	Dosage form	Design requirements
1	Oral solid dosage forms (tablets/hard gelatin capsules)	• Mixing, granulation and drying area and facility. • Compression/encapsulation area and facility. • Coating area and facility, etc.
2	Soft gelatin capsules	• Gelatin mass preparation area and facility. • Gelatin mass storage area and facility. • Encapsulation area and facility. • Drying area with controlled temperature and humidity, etc.
3	Liquid and semisolids	• Mixing, high shear stirring and homogenization area and facility. • Bottle filling, tube filling area and facility, etc.
4	Parenterals and biologicals	• Sterile and aseptic area for mixing, high shear stirring and homogenization area with specialized air handling equipments. • Large volume and small volume parenterals filling area and facility, etc.
5	Multi-particulate drug delivery systems	• Mixing, granulation, extrusion and spheronization and drying area and facility. • Multi-particle coating area and facility. • Encapsulation area and facility, etc.
6	Novel drug delivery systems	• High shear mixtures and homogenization area and facility. • Facility to handle requirement of inert gases, organic solvents, hot and chilled water requirement, etc.

batch size increases. And this increased clinical trial demand needs to be met by increased manufacturing capacity of the pilot-plant facility. A pilot-plant facility must be operated under the guidelines of current Good Manufacturing Practices (cGMP). Hence, cGMP compliance considerations must be included at the time of finalizing various design features of the pilot-plant. The design features should also take into account various other safety and environmental facility requirements such as handling compounds, for which only marginal information is available regarding potential toxicity, potency and physicochemical properties.

3. Activity-based considerations in the design of pilot-plant facility

Two vital activities carried out in a pilot-plant are: (i) scale-up studies as a part of product and process development, and (ii) the process validation and subsequent transfer of the process or technology to the shop floor. Scale-up studies are performed to obtain critical formulation and process performance information, which contributes towards smooth and efficient production transfer. After completion of the studies, the process is transferred to shop floor for routine or commercial manufacturing. Invariably, the fabrication of large-scale batches, viz. pre-validation batches, validation batches and full-scale production batches, is also carried out in a pilot-plant facility. Thus, for smooth execution of both these activities, the equipment of a pilot-plant must be of same operating principles as that of the production plant. In general, closer the pilot-plant equipment resemble the production equipment (with respect to design and scale), fewer are the trials necessary when transferring the process to production. Ideally, large scale equipment in the pilot-plant should approach 25–100% of the capacity of full-scale equipment; however, a minimum of 10% capacity level is mandatory.

Sometimes, the new technology that offers advantages has to be accommodated in the existing pilot-plant facility. Therefore, the design of a pilot-plant should be flexible enough to accommodate changes as well as additions or expansions. In addition, the site location factors require proximity to production, clinical packaging, and warehouse, as well as support facilities such as quality assurance (QA), quality control (QC), validation, maintenance, calibration, microbiology, etc.

PILOT-PLANT: ORGANIZATIONAL AND OPERATIONAL ASPECTS

Although a pilot-plant must simulate the manufacturing environment wherein the product will ultimately be produced yet there are many differences in their operations because of the specific objectives of the two types of facilities. While a pilot-plant supports product development activities, the manufacturing plant is meant for fabrication of large volume of a product for the market place.

Various unique organizations and functional features of a pilot-plant establishment can be elaborated as under:

A. Type of organizational structure

The effective functioning of a pilot-plant depends on a number of factors. For instance, in a small- or medium-scale pharmaceutical company, there might not be provision for separate pilot-plant facility due to economic and other reasons. In such situations the product development scientist, besides achieving success in lab-scale product development, might have to ensure the successful scale-up of the developed product at a commercial scale too. In large organization, however, it demands a team effort for pilot scale-up, process development and subsequent transfer of technology to the shop floor for commercial manufacturing. Various types of organizational arrangements for pilot-plant activities can be divided as follows:

1. Research personnel responsible for initial scale-up and production runs

In such an organizational structure, responsibility rests with the research and development (R&D) department. The product development scientist (or a team of scientists) is responsible for the scale-up and technology transfer to the production. The advantage that accrues to the production division is that a scientist who has developed the product formula and knows the most about the developed product is directly involved with the production personnel. This system carries the advantage of continuity of the product history that comes along with the persons who have developed the product and is then associated with its scale-up. The major drawback, however, of this type of system is that a person from R&D background is generally not thoroughly familiar with the equipment, facilities and operations of a commercial production area and may thus land up with many manufacturing problems. Another disadvantage associated with this type of arrangement is that significant amount of time of the research scientist/team is consumed in the product scale-up and technology transfer activities, thus affecting the of R&D program(s) of the company.

2. Pharmaceutical pilot-plant controlled by pharmaceutical research

In such an organizational structure, the different pilot-plant functions can be part of a R&D group, but with a separate set of research personnel. This type of arrangement provides the research scientist(s) with a responsibility to scale-up the formulations that have been developed by other formulator/scientist within the R&D set-up, thereby providing an opportunity for critique of formula/process. The specific advantage associated with this type of organogram is that the scheduling of scale-up runs is under the direct control of the research department. The corrective measures, such as dosage form modifications, can also be taken up immediately, if some problems are encountered during fabrication of clinical supply batches or during routine scale-up studies.

3. Production-controlled pilot-plant

The pilot scale-development, and technology transfer of a dosage form, under such an organizational set-up, is carried out by the pilot-plant personnel reporting administratively to the production division. In this kind of set-up, the responsibility of the product scientist is only to establish the practicality of formula and manufacturing procedure in a pilot-plant facility. The subsequent process development and technology transfer to the production is the responsibility of the pilot-plant personnel. In this kind of system, the direct interaction of the product scientists with the production personnel is reduced. However, this approach is advantageous, as the manufacturing problems arising at the shop floors will be directed to the pilot-plant personnel, thus initiating any troubleshooting, if required expeditiously.

Some companies prefer to have the pilot-plant and technical service group, organizationally separate from research and reporting instead to the operations side of the business. This kind of system results in operations-oriented, pragmatic and operation-receptive priorities. Some companies have adopted a composite of both the approaches in order to achieve the best attributes of R&D and the 'operations-oriented' systems. The effectiveness of the pilot-plant is determined by the ease with which new products or processes are brought into routine production. This can best be achieved if a good relationship exists between the pilot-plant group and the other interface groups with whom they interact, viz. R&D, processing, and packaging, QA/QC, engineering, regulatory and marketing, as shown in Fig. 16.3.

B. Pilot-plant personnel and training requirements

1. Qualifications & educational background

The major prerequisite for a person to work effectively in a pilot-plant organization is vast knowledge of various fundamentals of pharmaceutics coupled with practical experience in

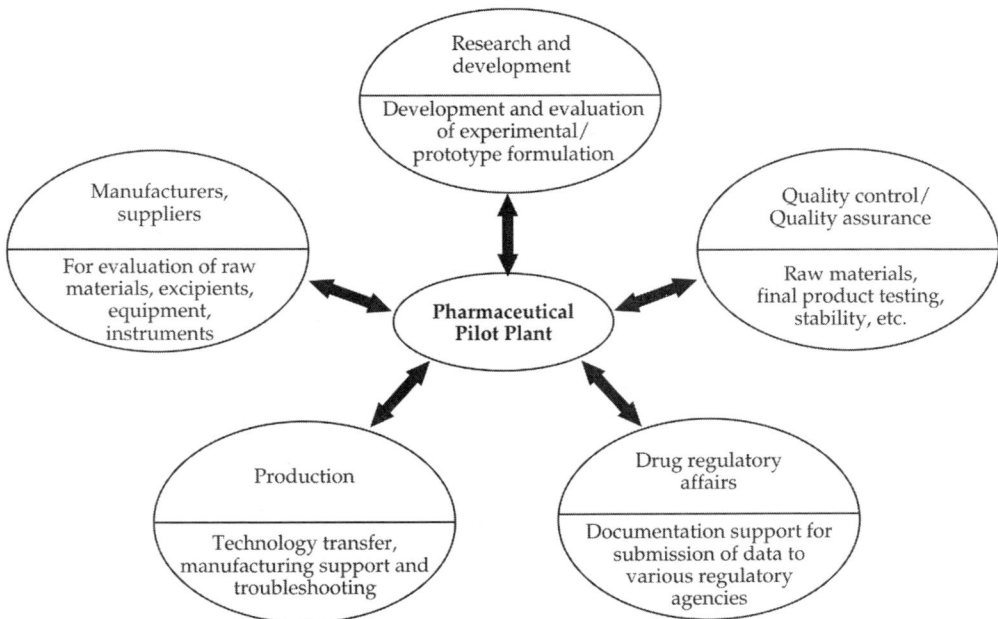

Fig. 16.3. Interdisciplinary interactions in a pilot-plant network.

pharmaceutical industry. In addition, the ability to communicate well, both in spoken and written language, and the ability to develop good relationships with other people are equally important. Experience within the group should encompass formulation aspects as well as process and equipment handling in the actual production environment. For these reasons, successful pilot-plant organizations frequently include scientists with experience in both the areas.

2. Training of pilot-plant personnel

A pilot-plant must be robust enough to prepare a variety of dosage forms in response to a wide range of product development programs. For this reason, a basic and dynamic training program for every pilot-plant person should be given. Initial training must be strengthened on regular time intervals with the current and up-to-date programs that address all the necessary changes in job requirement and performance expectations.

The basic and dynamic training program for pilot-plant personnel, therefore, is generally divided into 'initial', 'reinforcement', and 'remedial-training'. 'Initial' or entry-level training is targeted for a new or prospective employee and should provide assurance that a certain skill level has been attained. 'Reinforcement-level' training is intended for an employee who has already been trained in a certain area. This training is intended to fortify already acquired skills. The 'remedial' training, however, is intended to fulfil the identified skill deficiencies.

C. Pilot-plant activities

Key pilot-plant activities include formulation and process development/scale-up studies, and technology evaluation and transfer to the shop floor for routine manufacturing. Packaging for stability and clinical studies may also be carried out in the pilot-plant. However, these activities are often performed in separate, well-defined facilities. Fig. 16.4 represents the outline of the different pilot-plant activities.

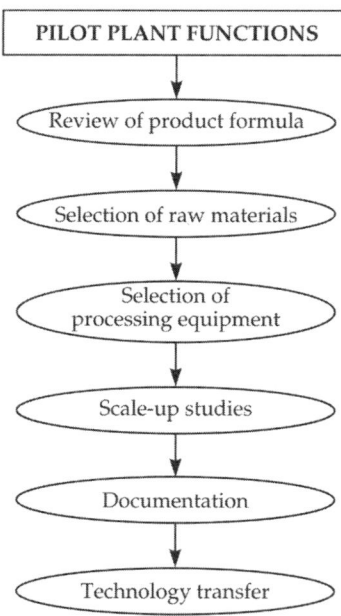

Fig. 16.4. Functions of a pharmaceutical pilot-plant.

(a) Formulation and process scale-up studies

Four key technical aspects that must be addressed during scale-up studies in a pilot-plant include identification and control of critical component and formulation variables, selection of equipment, development and optimization of the suitable process by identifying critical process parameters and operating ranges using pilot-plant equipment, and collection of product and process data to adequately characterize each unit operation, as outlined below:

(i) Analysis and review of the product formula

Thorough review of each aspect of the formulation is the first critical step carried out early during the scale-up process of a particular product formula. Significance of each ingredient and its contribution to the final product is understood. Besides the chemical properties of the active ingredient and other functional excipients, the physicochemical behavior (e.g., micromeritics, rheology, surface chemistry, solubility and phase-phenomenon) is also thoroughly reviewed, as any of these properties may prove to be critical in the overall processing of the product.

(ii) Selection and approval of raw materials

This is necessary because the raw materials used during small-scale formulation trials may not be representative of the large-volume shipments of materials used during commercial-scale production. Similarly, the active ingredient(s), which may only have been prepared on laboratory scale, are also being subjected to scale-up to meet the rising needs of the product. Albeit all the analytical specifications are met, these larger lots of active ingredients may differ in particle size, shape, or morphology, leading ultimately to differences in bulk density, static charges, rate of solubility, flow properties, color, etc. Hence, having alternate suppliers/vendors is highly desirable for companies who purchase the active ingredients. For selection and evaluation of alternate suppliers of active ingredient, several batches of product are manufactured using active ingredient from different suppliers and the performance of formulation and the stability of finished products is evaluated relative to the standard product. Thereafter, the active material specifications are finalized and every lot of active ingredient supplied by the vendor has to conform to these specifications. The process is also called as vendor validation, and also holds true for other raw materials or functional excipients as well.

(iii) Selection of equipment

Formulation development work at laboratory scale is carried out on standardized and relatively simpler equipment. During subsequent scale-up, alternative manufacturing equipment is considered. Based on the known processing characteristics of the product, the equipment that promises to be the most economical, operator-friendly, efficient, and capable of producing product consistently within the proposed specifications, is evaluated. The size of the selected equipment should be appropriate so that the different experimental trials conducted to evaluate the scalability of the product should be meaningful and relevant to the production-size batches. If the selected pilot-plant equipment is too small, the process developed may not be reliable and robust. If the equipment is too large, excessive costs will be incurred, especially if the product involves the use of a large quantity of any new and expensive active ingredient.

(iv) Product and process scale-up

In general, various unit operations of the process such as milling, mixing, heating, cooling, drying, sterilizing, compacting, and filling, which may cause tangible change in the state of the material being processed, need to be evaluated. In case of scale-up of a tablet dosage form, for instance, the following unit operations are critically monitored:

1. Order of addition of components, including adjustment of their amounts
2. Mixing speed
3. Mixing time
4. Rate of addition of granulating agents, solvents, solutions of drugs, slurries, etc.
5. Heating and cooling rates
6. Screen sizes
7. Drying temperatures
8. Drying time

Based on the effects of critical process parameters on in-process and finished product quality, the process is then optimized and validated to ensure that the selected manufacturing procedure maintains the quality of the product during various critical stages in the process as well as in the finished form. This is accomplished by monitoring the within-batch variation of different measurable parameters of the product and process, like content uniformity, moisture content and compressibility. The data, thus generated, indicate whether the process is performing as intended, and where can the problem areas be found.

Such scale-up data collected for a series of batches using particular equipment configuration in a well-documented format is termed scale-up feasibility report. If the data show that the process performs consistently at the critical steps, to produce a product falling within product specifications, the developed process can be considered validated.

(b) Pilot-plant scale-up studies: Scale-Up and Post-Approval Changes (SUPAC) guidelines

The process of scaling up an approved generic version of previously marketed drug product may require a number of changes. Besides the inevitable increase in the batch size, certain changes in the product formula composition, manufacturing process, equipment and/or manufacturing site may be necessary as well. The scale-up process and the changes thus made after product approval are better known as Scale-Up and Post-Approval Changes, or SUPAC. The USFDA has issued various types of guidelines for SUPAC changes, designated as SUPAC-IR (for immediate-release solid oral dosage forms), SUPAC-MR (for modified-release solid oral dosage forms) and SUPAC-SS (for non-sterile semisolid dosage forms including creams, ointments, gels and lotions).

The major effect of SUPAC is significant reduction in the time required to implement changes. In fact, SUPAC is a means of decreasing regulatory burden by empowering industry to make regulatory decisions.

Broadly, the SUPAC Guidelines encompass the following:

(a) The type of study information that must be generated to support changes at each level.

(b) The FDA-recommended manufacturing and control tests to support each level of change.

(c) The type of *in vitro* or *in vivo* testing required supporting various levels of change in terms of its net impact on the product quality.

(c) Documentation and technology transfer

After carrying out the process scale-up activity and obtaining the necessary data, the next responsibility of the pilot-plant personnel is to compile various product and process related data. Some of the documents and reports, which are prepared in a pilot-plant, comprise the following:

1. **Lab notebooks:** For recording initial developmental batches fabricated in the pilot-plant.

2. **Scale-up report:** Information collected during scale-up runs of the product.

3. **Validation protocol and report:** It comprises of the systematically documented tests, parameters to be evaluated during the product validation exercise and the results obtained therein.

4. **Master manufacturing instructions:** It is the most important document prepared by pilot-plant personnel. A typical master manufacturing document contains the following:

(a) Weighment sheet which indicates batch size and the exact quantities of each material of the product formula.

(b) Manufacturing instructions (step-wise) for each unit operation of the process such as specifications and appropriate ranges for addition rates, mixing times, mixing speeds, heating and cooling rates, and temperature. The actual times, temperatures, speeds, etc. at which the process is carried out are recorded and documented. The master manufacturing document, thus prepared, is called as the **batch production record (BPR)**.

(c) Clearly specified time points, stages and manner in which the in-process and finished product samples are to be taken during fabrication of the batch.

In addition, the pilot-plant personnel also prepare both in-process and finished product specifications. These are the set of standards by which a product is evaluated. The 'in-process specifications' for the product are usually narrower than the 'finished product specifications'.

Subsequent to completion of the scale-up activity, the pilot-plant transfers the technology to the shop floor for routine manufacturing of the product at commercial or production scale. The activities include the preparation of documentation required for the transfer process, i.e., related to technical aspects of process development and scale-up, and demonstration of product manufacturing techniques to production personnel at the shop floor.

(d) Engineering, maintenance and calibration support

Since pilot-plant facilities and operations become more complex and technically diverse, the need for support groups viz. engineering, maintenance and calibration, is indispensable to perform planned activities in a cGMP-compliant environment.

1. Engineering support

The primary objective of the engineering staff is to provide timely support to ensure efficient implementation of the pilot-plant operations and activities. Support provided by the engineering staff in a pilot-plant facility may include:

(a) Equipment acquisition, installation, and repair.

(b) Engineering documentation and control for new systems and equipment.

(c) Management of the facility to ensure that critical systems, e.g., environmental controls, utilities, etc., are operational for compliance with cGMP.

(d) Coordinating and scheduling equipment set-up and related activities for development projects.

(e) Ensuring a controlled inventory of critical spare parts, e.g., tablet tooling.

(f) Budgeting for equipment, technology upgrades and operating supplies.

(g) Directing housekeeping activities.

2. Maintenance and calibration support

A maintenance program is necessary within the pilot-plant to meet the cGMP requirements, and to ensure data integrity and equipment reliability during the development process. The detailed maintenance program for all the pieces of equipment, systems and utilities of the pilot-plant facility are documented. Written and approved procedures are established to carry out the maintenance activity at the prescheduled time intervals. Routine calibration of critical instruments and equipment is required for cGMP compliance as well as for maintaining the integrity of data generated during the development process.

PILOT-PLANT SCALE-UP OF VARIOUS DOSAGE FORMS

In general, after developing and testing a proto-type formulation at laboratory scale, the manu-facturing process is evaluated and scaled up to provide sufficient volume of the product to meet commercial needs. Very often, the batch size enhancement may translate into large quantities of the product. At the same time, however, it may not be reproducible in terms of quality attributes of the finished product as well as the manu-facturing process. A well-defined process may generate a perfect product in the laboratory, but may fail during quality assurance tests in production. Moreover, a process using the same type of equipment performs quite differently when the size of the equipment or the amount of material involved is increased significantly. For instance, even simple operation such as loading a mixer can become a complicated operation, when sophisticated equipment or large volumes are involved. In some cases, scale-up may involve a major process change that utilizes processing techniques and equipment, which erstwhile were either unsuitable or unavailable on a laboratory scale.

Although in certain situations, i.e., where processing is predictable and directly scalable, the scale-up studies are avoided and the full scale manufacturing and testing using production equipment is directly carried out. However, the same is not feasible in every situation or with every kind of dosage form. Moreover, the expense associated with full scale testing is usually phenomenal, as it involves large amounts of material, labour and the costly commercial scale machines to operate. Additionally, during initial phases of product development, the drug substance is usually available only in small quantities, requiring some form of manufacturing simulation on intermediate scale. In this regard, process scale-up studies, involving relatively appropriate scale-up ratios and proper identification and monitoring of process variables, is always a reasonable alternative to full-scale testing.

All these factors necessitate the need of inserting an intermediate step of pilot-plant scale-up, between laboratory and production scales, to guarantee smoother transition of the developed product. During scale-up of a pharmaceutical process, each stage of the operation is carefully considered, as each unit operation may be scalable in accordance with a specific ratio. Besides the successful technology transfer and large scale manufacturing, cost-effectiveness in terms of men, money and machines, is an additional advantage associated with pilot-plant testing and scale-up of the product.

Some scale-up errors affecting the overall process development
1. Incorrect unit operation mechanisms as the basis of scaling.
2. Incompletely characterized equipment.
3. Insufficient knowledge of the process.
4. Difference in types of equipment at different level(s) of scale-up.
5. Unrealistic expectations.
6. Incomplete recording of changes in composition or process during scale-up runs.

A. PILOT SCALE-UP OF SOLID ORAL DOSAGE FORMS – TABLETS

Oral solid dosage forms, especially tablets and capsules, constitute the most preferred class of dosage forms till date. Design and manufacture of tablet dosage form is quite challenging as it involves multiple complicated operations to help in attaining many competing objectives of this dosage form. The first set of objectives is that the tablets should have a smooth surface, good appearance and surface gloss. And the tablets should be adequately cohesive and compact too, so that these do not undergo capping, friability, powdering and chipping problems during shipping and handling. Whatever product or process modifications are undertaken to achieve these objectives, like using more binder, increasing compression pressure, applying pre-compression and increasing "dwell time" (i.e., the time for which the blend is subjected to compression forces), these are likely to affect another set of objectives viz. disintegration time, rate of dissolution and ultimate bioavailability. Therefore, to design and manufacture the quality product, a number of product and process variables need to be optimized. Typical processes and unit operations involved in production of solid dosage forms involve mixing or blending, wet granulation, drying, particle size reduction, direct compression, slugging (i.e., dry granulation), compression, and coating.

1. Mixing and blending

The dry particle mixing remains the most crucial unit operation with the final objective of producing a homogeneous mixture, as inadequate blending can result in discrete portions of the batch being either high or low in potency. This could result in variation in drug content uniformity, especially if the tablet or capsule is small and the drug concentration is relatively low in the blend. Various important factors which need to be considered during pilot-plant scale-up of mixing operations are enumerated as follows:

(a) Design and type of equipment

For optimal scale-up of mixing operation, the choice of equipment of the right design is very crucial. Amongst many design related factors viz. shape and size of the blender, baffle type, etc., the symmetry of the vessel plays significant role in achieving optimum mixing efficiency. The symmetry of the mixer (e.g., in case of tumbling blenders) is known to be the greatest impediment in achieving a homogeneous mixture, because the mixing rate often becomes limited by the amount of material that can cross from one side of the symmetry plane to the other. On the other hand, some blenders are built asymmetrically (e.g., slant cone, offset V-blender, etc.), to result in greater mixing efficiency. Nevertheless, asymmetry can also be induced through intelligent placement of baffles. The latter approach has been successfully tested on small-scale equipment. But if the equipment is symmetrical and baffles are also not available, then careful attention should be paid to the loading procedure as well as other process variables to optimize mixing efficiency.

(b) Process and formulation variables

For successful process scale-up with optimized mixing, thorough understanding of the mechanistic aspects of blending as well as the material characteristics is very important.

- **Dynamics of mixing or blending:** Mixing in blenders takes place as the result of particle motions in a thin, cascading layer at the surface of the material, while the remainder of the material below rotates with the vessel as a rigid body. Blending takes place by three essentially independent mechanisms viz. convection, dispersion and shear. Convection causes large groups of particles to move in the direction of flow (i.e., orthogonal to the axis of rotation), as a result of vessel rotation. Dispersion is the random motion of particles as a result of collisions or inter-particle motion, usually orthogonal to the direction of flow (i.e., parallel to the axis of rotation). And shear

separates the particles that have joined together as agglomerates due to cohesion, and require high force. Thus, to attain a favorable dynamics of powder mixing, various parameters need to be optimized, the most critical being blending loads, blending speed and time of blending.

- **Powder characteristics:** A critical insight into the characteristics of the material to be blended viz. particle size, shape, surface properties, hardness, bulk and tapped density, cohesive strength, etc., helps in minimizing the scale-up problems associated with blending process. For instance, a product with fragile particles or agglomerates is more readily abraded during blending operation, resulting eventually in an excessive amount of fines. These fines may mix improperly and cause problems of flow, "fill-weight" or "content uniformity".

  The presence of agglomerates could cause problems in flow and consequently irreproducible compression or encapsulation, leading ultimately to poor content uniformity in the finished product. This problem may be avoided by screening and/or milling of the ingredients prior to dry mixing.

- **Selection of optimum blender load:** Another critical variable is the maximum quantity of powders or granules to be blended using a specific mixer. Utmost care must be exercised to select the appropriate batch size, usually based on the working capacities (instead of absolute capacities) of the mixer. The necessary precautions should always be taken

---

Some vital factors for mixing operations
1. Particle size distribution.
2. Bulk density of powder.
3. Cohesiveness of powder.
4. Loading procedure.
5. Amount of loaded material.
6. Geometry and size of the mixing vessel.
7. Use of baffles in mixing vessel.
8. Wall friction.

to avoid overfilling of the mixer, which tends to affect the blending efficiency. The latter may result in improper mixing, poor lubrication of the granulation, poor content uniformity and improper color dispersion in the finished product. As a general criterion, any mixer should not be used beyond 70–75% of the capacity utilization level.

- **Handling of blended material:** The degree of mixing at the end of a blending operation is not always a good indicator of the homogeneity in the final product. Many granular mixtures can spontaneously segregate into regions of unlike composition, when perturbed by flow, vibration, shear, etc. during handling of the blends. Therefore, once a good blend is achieved, the mixture still must be handled carefully to avoid any "de-mixing".

2. Wet granulation

The major objectives for production of pharmaceutical granulation are following:

1. To impart good flow properties to cohesive or sticky materials.
2. To provide compressibility to the total mass of solids so that the final product of desired hardness can be produced without losing its ability to disintegrate in the dissolution medium.
3. To change the particle size distribution in order to improve the adhesive properties of the poorly compressible materials.

4. To disperse a small amount of potent active pharmaceutical ingredient (API) effectively and homogeneously in a carrier granulation.

Critical granule characteristics to be monitored during scale-up of granule size distribution include bulk and tapped density, final moisture content, friability and compressibility. Scale-up of a granulation process in the pilot-plant, though complicated, is yet influenced by a number of formulation and process parameters. Some of the key factors influencing the scale-up of granulation process are discussed below:

(a) Type of granulating equipment

During scale-up, the choice of appropriate equipment for granulation is also very important, as it significantly influences the development and characteristics of granules. For instance, some granulations, when prepared in production-sized equipment, yield a dough-like consistency because of the insufficiency of the desired mechanical forces, leading to the lack of powder subdivision. The latter necessitates the changes in the process, as it is to be subdivided to a more granular and porous mass to facilitate drying. In this kind of situation, the prepared granulation is further processed using an oscillating type granulator or a hammer mill. A wide variety of granulating machines are now available for pilot-plant and large scale manufacturing, Table 16.3 lists some of the commonly used granulating equipment with their specific features and advantages.

Factors to prevent de-mixing during scale-up of blending process	
Change the particle size distribution of the powder or granules	• A homogeneous blend with uniform particle size has lesser tendency to segregate.
Make the granule particle size sufficiently large	• Results in reduction in fluidization and hence reduction in segregation.
Change the cohesiveness of powder or granulate the powder	• Improves the particle surface characters and hence minimize de-mixing.
Adjust the process or equipment parameters	• Minimization of material transfer steps. • Minimization of powder drop height. • Control on generation of fines. • Reduction in flow rate. • Alteration in the design of hoppers and flow valves.

(b) Type of binder

Binders are usually added in the dry state to impart adhesive properties when exposed to the granulating fluid. They can also be dissolved or dispersed in the granulating fluid and get homogenously dispersed during the granulation process. In some instances, the binding agent imparts considerable viscosity to the granulating solution and, thus, the transfer of the fluid by either pumping or pouring becomes difficult. The problem is more evident during scale-up of such a process, while addition of the granulating agent to the powders is processed in enclosed granulation equipment. If the problem is anticipated during the formulation stage, the viscosity of the granulating solution can be adjusted to avoid this type of scale-up problems. However, during scale-up batches, this problem can be resolved by dispersing a part or the entire amount of binding agent in the dry powder prior to granulating. The granulating liquid containing the remaining binder, if any, can then be easily incorporated into the batch during granulation.

(c) Type of solvent

Occasionally, the non-aqueous solvents, or solutions that are composed of water and water-miscible solvents, are used to improve the granulating properties of a formulation or to disperse poorly soluble drugs. These are also used to dissolve the binder, to prepare the granulating fluid, as a reduced amount of energy is required to remove the more volatile solvent(s) from the granulation. But the use of organic solvents during large scale manufacturing demands selection of appropriately designed equipment as well as manufacturing area. For example, proper ventilation provisions and additional safety precautions against fire, toxicity and explosion, etc. are required.

3. Drying

(a) Oven drying

It is the most common method of drying granulation in pilot-plant or shop floor. The granules to be dried are spread on paper-lined trays, which are then kept on a rack and moved into the oven. The important factors to consider as part of scale-up of an oven drying operation are airflow rates, drying time and drying temperature. Additionally, the depth of granulation layer on paper-lined trays also affects the efficiency of drying process. For example, if the granulation bed is too deep or too dense, the drying process will be inefficient. And if soluble dyes are involved, migration of the dye to the surface of

Table 16.3. Some commonly employed granulating equipment during large scale manufacturing

Type of granulator	Features/Advantages
1. Non-shear granulators	
(a) Sigma blade mixers or heavy-duty planetary mixers	Suitable for carrying out granulation process for large scale batches, and can process 100 to 200 kg of material.
(b) Tumble blenders equipped with high-speed chopper blades	More effective in densification of light powders, but require large amounts of energy and can process limited batch sizes.
2. Shear granulators	
High-shear mixers with choppers	Often used for good densification with the advantages of high-speed choppers, which break up agglomerates and ensure uniform distribution of the granulating fluid and more controlled granule size.
3. Novel approaches	
Multifunctional continuous processors (MCP) or Quasi-continuous granulation and drying (QCGDP) process	This automated composite unit with specific design is capable of performing all the functions required to prepare finished granulation, such as dry blending, wet granulation, drying, sizing, and lubrication, as continuous process in a single piece of equipment.

the granule(s) may occur. Therefore, during scale-up and full scale production batches, the granulation bed depth should be carefully controlled.

(b) Fluidized-bed drying

On large scale manufacturing, fluidized-bed drying, however, is a time saving alternative in comparison to the circulating hot air ovens. The scale-up of fluidized bed drying process from laboratory to production size units is more complicated than scale-up of a process based on circulating hot air drying (Fig. 16.5).

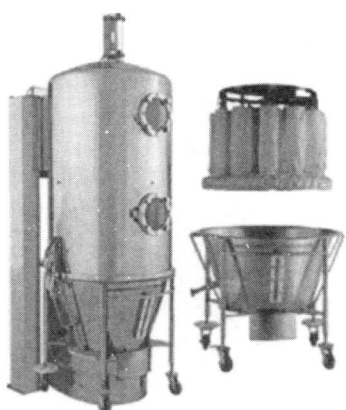

Fig. 16.5. A large-scale fluid-bed dryer along with drying bowl and filter bag.

Some general considerations for an efficient fluidized bed drying are:

1. Establishment of optimum batch loads is very critical to minimize scale-up problems as well as to optimize the efficiency of drying process.
2. The temperature of the drying air should be carefully monitored. In general, higher the drying air temperature, greater is the vapor holding capacity of the air.
3. Similarly, the outlet temperature, i.e., the difference between temperature of incoming air and the granule bed, should be higher for achieving faster drying rate.
4. The rate of airflow as well as the humidity of the incoming air must be established, since

both the parameters significantly influence drying time.
5. Prior conditioning of the air, if drawn from outside the plant, is also necessary, as large seasonal variation(s) in temperature and humidity, can alter the drying process.

4. Particle sizing

Particle size plays a pivotal role in attaining the desired quality attributes in the finished product (tablet or capsule) such as weight uniformity, content uniformity, color distribution, etc. For instance, the content uniformity in tablets is affected by oversized as well as undersized granulations. The granulation, with too large particles and insufficient fines is unable to fill the die cavities uniformly during compression, causing the weight of the tablets to fluctuate considerably. On the other hand, if too many fines are present, tablet weight variation occurs owing to flow problems. Similarly, for colored granulations, the coarser the granulation, more mottled the final tablet appearance is. A few important aspects related to pilot-plant studies and scale-up of size reduction process are discussed below:

(a) Particle size distribution comparisons

During pilot-plant studies, the first step in scaling-up the milling process is to determine the particle size distribution of the granulation. The most commonly employed approach is "sieve analysis", using a series of "stacked" sieves of decreasing mesh openings. A known amount (~100–200 g) of representative blend sample is taken and placed on the top most sieves, with maximum pore size or mesh opening in the stack. The stack of sieves is then mechanically shaken for a fixed time interval. The amount (or percentage) of pre-weighed sample, which is retained on individual screen, yields a distribution profile of unmilled granulation. The latter is used as a reference or base line for comparison of various milled samples generated by different trials, to optimize the type of equipment or process (milling) conditions such as mill type, milling speed and screen size.

(b) Selection of milling or comminution equipment

Particle size reduction of the dried granulation of production-size batches can be carried out by a variety of milling equipment such as oscillating granulator, hammer mill or multimill, and mechanical sieving devices such as vibro-sifter or turbo-sifter. Selection of milling equipment to reduce granule particle size can only be made by first determining the characteristics of the unmilled granulation. Some commonly used milling devices in a pilot-plant facility or production shop floor, along with brief details of their operational features and advantages, are discussed below:

- **Oscillating granulator:** This equipment has been in use since long in the pilot-plant and shop floors, for screening dried granulation. It is suitable for milling those granulations where the oversized portion of the granulation including agglomerates is not too hard. The ease of operation and cleaning make this equipment worth using for intermediate or large scale batches. However, while in use, necessary precautions must be taken to avoid overfeeding of the oscillating granulator, which may otherwise generate excessive number of fines and hence affect the flow. Owing to the specific design of this milling device, sometimes the wearing action of metallic screens may introduce a small amount of fines or large particles of potentially hazardous metallic material into the batch. This problem can be resolved using ferrous metal screens, so that the metallic particles can be removed by passing the granulation or compressed tablets through special magnetic devices.
- **Hammer mill:** This equipment also finds place in pilot-plant facilities and shop floors for milling the dried granulations to a specified

size range with fairly rapid throughput. Herein, the particle size distribution can be controlled by varying feed rate, screen size, milling speed and the type or number of hammer blades. This equipment is advantageous in the sense that the hammers or knives do not come in contact with the screen, thus reducing the chances of any metal abrasion or contamination.

- **Vibro-sifter:** Many of the newer granulation equipments, available now-a-days can produce the material with desired particle size range. In those circumstances, the objective of sizing operation is only to mill some agglomerates present in the sized blend. For this type of operation, the material can be subjected to simple mechanical screening equipment such as vibro-sifter. The advantage of using this equipment is no metal-to-metal contact during the screening process and hence minimum possibility of metal contamination. Since there is negligible milling action, the initial particle size range is not significantly reduced. In addition, the throughput is rapid too. Little dust is created because of the enclosed nature of the equipment, thus, minimizing the material losses and exposure of personnel.

(c) Addition of lubricants and glidants

Another important aspect of the scale-up of a milling or sieving operation is the addition of lubricants and glidants. In the laboratory, these are usually added directly to the final blend. But during large-scale manufacturing, these are usually added to the dried granulation during the sizing operation. This is done as some of these additives, such as magnesium stearate, tend to agglomerate when added in large quantities at the time of final blending. To assure adequate distribution of these dry additives, preliminary dispersion of these materials is often made during the sizing operation. This part of the process must be carefully optimized so that the lubricants are not over-mixed or under-mixed during screening and the subsequent blending operations.

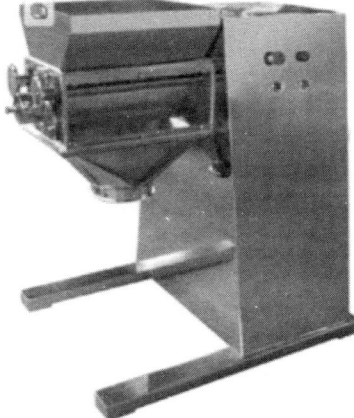

Oscillating type granulator

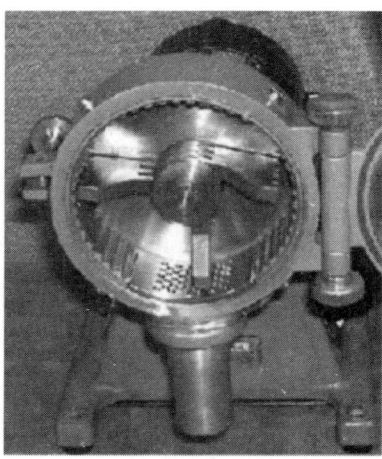

Hammer mill

Fig. 16.6. Two frequently used milling machines for solid dosage forms.

5. Direct compression

By virtue of the availability of directly compressible forms of various excipients and active drugs possessing excellent flow properties, direct compression process has considerably simplified the process of manufacturing tablet dosage forms. This process yields free-flowing granulation without the aid of granulating solutions and, hence, saves both time and energy necessary for the processing involved in conventional wet granulation procedures.

Factors affecting uniformity of drug distribution during direct compression process

1. Particle characteristics influence mixing and segregation
  (a) Particle size
  (b) Particle size distribution
  (c) Particle shape
  (d) Particle static charge
  (e) Packing arrangement
  (f) Bulk and tapped density
  (g) Powder rheology
2. Blender design
3. Blender load
4. Optimum blending speed
5. Blending time

The major requirement in case of a directly compressible formula is batch-to-batch reproducibility in drug distribution. Thus, the scale-up of direct compression process primarily depends upon thorough monitoring and evaluation of dry blending operation. The following factors are important for optimizing the process of dry blending in the pilot-plant and routine production processing.

- **Addition of components:** The order of addition of various ingredients to the blender is crucial for achieving a homogeneous blend. Various methods are adopted to facilitate uniform mixing. For instance, a low-dose active ingredient may be "sandwiched" between two portions of directly compressible excipients in the blender, to improve dispersion and/or to avoid loss to the surface of the blender. Similarly, "geometric mixing" can also be employed for efficient blending of a very low amount of active substance or any other critical ingredient of the formulation.

- **Blender load:** The amount of material volume to total mixer volume affects the efficiency of the blender. Each blender has an optimum working volume and a normal working range. Overloading a blender tends to retard the free flow of granulation and, thus, reduce the efficiency of a blender. The resulting localized concentrations of the drug cause content uniformity problems in the finished dosage form. Conversely, if the load is too small, the particles sliding (instead of rolling) behavior in a blender leads either to improper mixing, or to increase in process time for proper mixing of the powders.

- **Mixing time:** The mixing time can be decreased, if the available data show the consistency and uniformity in mixing patterns, in lesser time than originally directed. Alternatively, the time of mixing may need to be increased if the mixing time is shown to produce material with borderline uniformity. Mixing time is also important for the optimal compressibility of the finished blend, as excessive mixing may fracture brittle excipients, thus affecting their compressibility adversely.

- **Mixing action:** Mixing action is determined by the mechanics of the blender, which can only be changed by switching over to the other blender. Modifying the blender through addition of baffles or plates to alter the mixing characteristics is also a commonly employed approach.

- **Use of auxiliary equipment:** In some cases, additional piece of equipment is used to increase the efficiency of dispersion of solid or liquid ingredients. This also reduces the tendency, if any, to form agglomerates and improves the efficiency of dispersion.

6. Slugging or compaction (Dry granulation)

Compaction is a pharmaceutical unit operation to apply pressure to the powder to densify it and generate physical bonds amongst the powder particles to impart adequate strength to them. In certain situations, wet granulation process cannot be used for the dry powder blend. At the same time, a dry blend cannot be directly compressed because of the unfavorable characteristics of the raw materials such as poor compressibility, heterogeneous particle size distribution, poor flow, low density and poor cohesiveness.

In these instances, the dry powder blend is processed using compaction or slugging. Two major techniques can be employed for slugging operation. One is the conventional slugging using tablet machines and the other is roller compaction. For the effective scale-up of a dry granulation (slugging) process, the role of pilot-plant personnel is to select an appropriate compaction procedure to produce optimal granulation with the desired tableting or encapsulation properties. A few general aspects of both the processes are outlined below:

(a) Slugging by compaction

In this technique, the dry powder blend is processed using a tablet machine with some specific design features. The latter operates at very high pressures compared to a normal tablet press. Usually, extra-large tablet punches are used to fabricate compressed slugs of the powdered material. This procedure is usually slow, because the inherently poor compressibility of the powders requires slower press speeds to provide extended compression dwell time that holds the compacted material together. Depending upon the compressibility of material(s) being slugged, slugs of different size range can be prepared to yield satisfactory compacts.

Critical formulation and process variables affecting particle size distribution during compaction process

(a) Material properties of the particles being compacted viz. particle size, density, powder porosity, powder flow, percentage of fines, cohesive strength and compressibility, bulk density, lubrication

(b) Equipment (tablet press) used for compaction operation

(c) Force(s) used for the slugging operation

(d) Diameter of the punches

(e) Subsequent sizing and screening operations

(b) Roller compaction

Granulation by dry compaction can also be achieved by passing the powder blend between two rollers that compact the material at very high pressures. Because of the similarity in application, processes developed in the laboratory using a slugging operation can be directly scaled-up using a tablet machine for compaction or in some cases for roller compaction process. Materials of very low density require roller compaction to achieve a bulk density sufficient to allow encapsulation or compression.

Following compaction, the slugs are broken down using either a hammer mill or an oscillating granulator to obtain granulation with an optimum particle size distribution. If an excessive amount of fine powders is generated during milling operation, the material must be screened and the "fines" recycled through the slugging operation.

For effective scale-up of such an operation, a pilot-plant scientist should pay particular attention to the following critical aspects:

- **Tablet machine speed:** During compaction, owing to the use of certain materials which exhibit plastic deformation, higher machine speeds may pose problem(s) in achieving sufficient hardness of slugs.
- **Effect of lubricants:** Lubrication is a function of amount of lubricant(s) as well the blending time. An excessive amount or over-mixing tends to coat the lubricant onto the powder particles and impart hydrophobicity to them, thus affecting the hardness of the slugs and dissolution of the final product.

- **Length of compaction process:** The length of compaction run influences the heat build-up during the process, which may accelerate degradation or softening of the active compound or any other thermolabile ingredient(s).
- **Use of abrasive materials:** It can also produce a heat build-up due to longer process times during scale-up runs or during manufacturing of large scale batches, thus affecting the product quality as described above.

7. Compression

The major objective of the scale-up of a tableting process is to achieve reproducible compression on high speed tablet machines without affecting the quality of end product. A compression machine invariably performs different operations during the compression process viz. filling of empty die cavity with granulation, pre-compression and compression of granulation, and finally, ejection of the tablet from the die cavity. Compression of lubricated granules is basically the result of an event wherein the heads of tablet punches move in conjunction with the lower and upper pressure rollers of the tablet machine. This causes the punches to penetrate the die cavity to a preset depth, leading to compaction of the granulation to a thickness equal to the gap set between the punch surfaces. The ultimate event in the compression process is the ejection of a compressed tablet from the die cavity. This involves separation of upper punch from the upper surface of the tablet and withdrawal from the die cavity. The lower punch

Table 16.4. Different parameters to be monitored during compaction process

1. **Instrument parameters**	Dwell time, compression force, ejection force, roller pressure, roller speed, etc.
2. **Formulation parameters**	
Tablet dissolution	Gives an idea about the granules' hardness and extent of lubrication.
Tablet weight uniformity	Provides a measure of the efficiency of the granule flow.
Tablet hardness uniformity	Provides information about matched or unmatched punches during slugging by the use of tablet press, since the unmatched punches would not produce tablet slugs with uniform hardness. Furnishes an idea about lamination and capping of tablet slugs.

face then moves up through the die cavity, breaking the tablet free from the die wall and forcing it out of the die cavity. As the die table rotates, a take-off bar positioned just above the table forces the tablet to separate from the lower punch face and sweeps the tablet off the press table into a collection chute. To accomplish these functions, the following formulation and process variables need to be considered:

(a) Raw material characteristics
(b) Type and level of lubricants
(c) Machine design
(d) Machine type
(e) Machine speed
(f) Tooling design
(g) Use of feed frame
(h) Effect of other equipment items

(a) Raw material characteristics

The APIs as well as excipients should be well characterized for their physical (e.g., particle size, bulk and tapped density and surface area), chemical (e.g., solubility, stability and reactivity) and functional (e.g., compactibility and flow) attributes. Various other properties of the raw materials such as polymorphism, hygroscopicity and wettability should also be taken into account to attain effective process scale-up. For instance, a change in the particle size of the active material during scale-up batches can affect weight uniformity, flow behavior, compressibility and wetting characteristics, especially if the drug is present in high amounts. Similarly, if the API has a mean particle diameter quite different from that of the excipients, there are all possible chances of segregation upon scale-up.

(b) Type and level of lubricants

The scale-up of compression process very frequently exhibits some lubrication-dependent tablet defects, most common being picking and sticking. Evaluation of the effect of lubrication, therefore, is highly significant in pilot-plant studies pertaining to compression process. A good internal lubricant system is always

necessary to prevent sticking of the tablet to the metal surface of punches or dies. If the granulation is adequately and properly lubricated, the tendency for sticking and picking of the tablet to the punch face can be eliminated. The level at which the lubricants should be employed and the degree to which they need to be blended with the granulation must be determined experimentally during the pilot scale-up studies. Too high levels of a lubricant or its overblending, for instance, can result in softer tablets, decreased powder wettability of the powders, and extended dissolution time.

(c) Machine design

With the recent advances in tablet machine technology, different machine variables, such as granule feeder mechanisms, pre-compression and compression forces, can be easily controlled. Thus, many granulation problems or inadequacies can be easily overcome by making minor and appropriate adjustments to the press. However, the selection of a compression machine for scale-up of the compression process is very vital, which depends on many factors. Apart from output (i.e., machine speed), the ease of machine handling, ease of operation, and compression controls are some of the important criteria that must be considered in the selection of a tablet press. The size of rollers of a compression machine is another important parameter, as it determines the speed and dwell time of a compression event. Larger the compression roller, more gradually the compression force is applied and released. For instance, the tendency towards capping in a tablet formulation can often be reduced using presses with larger compression rollers, or by slowing down the press speed. Similarly, granulations that are difficult to compress or have a tendency to cap can often be compressed more effectively on a press with a series of pressure rollers. The latter tends to impart a stepwise increase in pressure, thus allowing entrapped air to escape gradually rather than as an abrupt event at the end of single-step compression.

(d) Machine type

Very often, the difference(s) between tablet machines, employed during laboratory and pilot-plant operation, may significantly affect the tablet characteristics. Picking, lamination, chipping and cracking are the most commonly observed tablet defects during scale-up studies. The change of compression machine results in altered compression times and tablet ejection forces, leading eventually to such defects. However, sometimes, these problems may arise after several hours of compression, even after using same machine with no difference in compression or ejection forces. This problem can be rectified using chrome-plated punches, controlling the machine speed and optimizing other process or formulation variables. For instance, modification in the product formula, to optimize the lubricant levels, tends to reduce the ejection force and minimizes such problems.

(e) Machine speed

Typically, the development of a tablet formulation on laboratory scale takes place on compact tablet presses, which operate at much lower speeds as compared to the tablet machines employed during the pilot-plant and shop floor operations. The use of machines with higher speed and thus higher tableting rate, necessitate the incorporation of die-induced feed frame for faster filling of die cavities. The use of the latter can result in over-mixing of the blend and, thus, can affect the process of compression and/or the tablet characteristics. In addition, the tableting rate also affects the dwell time. The dwell times differ considerably between laboratory scale and process scale-up, and therefore, result in tablet defects such as capping or lamination. For instance, sometimes a particular product cannot be successfully compressed at the upper speed range of a press. The most common remedy in this kind of situation is to reduce the speed and increase the dwell time of tablet machine. A slower machine can also be employed to allow more time for the dies to fill and to extend the dwell time of compression.

(f) Tooling design

The design and condition of the punches can also be responsible for causing problems during tablet compression. The type of embossing on the punch faces often causes the problem of sticking. This tends to happen during high embossing of letters, numbers, or symbols on the punch faces, steep angle of embossing, too sharp corners of embossing; or at times, the microscopic nicks or pits on the punch faces. To rectify the same before starting the actual fabrication of a pilot-plant or large scale batch, the new punches are often "run in" over a 4 to 8 hr period on a tablet machine, before they can run cleanly. The process is known as "seasoning" of punches. If the problem still persists, either polishing or plating of the punches needs to be carried out. Else, the embossing specifications need to be suitably altered.

(g) Use of feed frame

During compression process, after the die cavities have been filled with lubricated granulation, the excess is removed by the feed frame to the center of the die table. If the feed frame is overfilled and excess granulation is not moved towards the center of the die table, this excess may be thrown out by the centrifugal force of the rotating die table. For this reason, the clearance between the scraper blade and the die table must be carefully set. Too large a gap results in substantial granulation losses, especially if the granulation contains a lot of fines. Too close a setting causes scoring of the die table and metal contamination of the product.

(h) Effect of other equipment items

Usually, mixing and milling equipment used in production area are much more efficient than the corresponding ones employed in the laboratory. The most common problem, observed due to added efficiency of blenders, is over-lubrication of the blend to be compressed. This results in adverse effects on tablet hardness, capping and dissolution. Sometimes, the greater efficiency of

Pre-requisites for efficient scale-up of compression process
• The granulation must have good flow properties, optimal particle size distribution and relatively small mean particle size to facilitate rapid but uniform fill of the die cavities.
• The granulation delivery must not be interrupted and should be delivered to the die feed system at an adequate flow rate.
• The blend delivery system must neither cause segregation of coarse and fine particles nor should it induce static charges, which could retard the flow of the granulation and cause the active ingredient to become segregated.
• The die feed system must be able to fill the die cavities adequately in the short period of time that the die is passing under the feed frame.

large mixers can also have an untoward effect on wet granulation process such as over-wetting of granulation or difference in granule size. This, in turn, is manifested during compression as an altered compressibility or the poor dissolution of the tablets.

8. Tablet coating

Although the most common objective of tablet coating is to improve the aesthetic appeal of the tablets, in terms of color, flavor, surface gloss, etc., yet it has important role in improving the product stability and robustness, enhancing flavor attributes, facilitating ingestion and modifying drug release characteristics too. Because of newer developments in coating technology as well as amendments in safety and environmental regulations, there has been a steady transition in the pharmaceutical industry from sugar coating to non-aqueous film coating, and finally to aqueous film coating.

Although film coating systems can be efficiently developed on laboratory scale yet the final coating process always needs to be defined on production scale equipment. Irrespective of the process used, the potential process changes that commonly occur during scale-up of the coating process include increase in batch sizes, attrition rate, spray rate, type of spray guns (from single to multiple-head nozzle), drying air volumes and increase in processing times. In basic terms, the following three components of the film coating process contribute in a very interactive manner to the overall success of the scale-up of coating process.

(a) Properties of the core tablet

There is a strong need to ensure that the initial product (i.e., core tablet) is sufficiently robust to meet the needs of the operation, in terms of increased stress associated with both the environmental conditions within the process, and the attritional effects to which the product being coated is subjected. Some of the essential elements of the core tablets for optimizing the coating process are listed below:

• The core tablets must be sufficiently hard to withstand tumbling that may be encountered in the coating pan.
• Certain designs of the core tablet such as sharp edges or flat surfaces should be avoided, as these are difficult to coat.
• Engraved surfaces also make the tablet coating more difficult. This problem can be minimized, however, if the engravings are kept shallow and the cuts are angled to avoid sharp edges.
• Some tablet core materials are naturally hydrophobic. In this case, film coating with

Table 16.5. Essential attributes of the coated product and coating process	
Aesthetics	Smooth coating, gloss, absence of edge chipping, absence of cracking, logo bridging, picking
Functional attributes	Stability, drug release, taste masking, tensile strength of the film
Process characteristics	High and reproducible coating efficiency, high uniformity of coating material distribution, high yield

an aqueous system may require formulation modification(s) in the tablet core and/or the coating solution.

(b) Nature of the coating material

The materials employed in tablet coating also tend to influence the scale-up and production scale coating operation, and thus need to be optimized. Examples include coating ingredients, solvents, coating solutions and their rheological properties, tackiness, etc.

(c) Coating process

In general, during the film coating process, it is ensured that the:

- rate of application of coating fluid and the drying rate are carefully controlled;
- coating material is uniformly applied onto the surface of the substrate; and
- quality and functionality of the applied coating are maximized and reproducible.

In order to accomplish these objectives, the following critical elements of the coating process should be suitably controlled:

Design of the coating pan

Chipping and abrasion of tablets are very frequent problems during large scale coating process due to the increased attritional stress. Moreover, the debris formed adheres to other tablets in the coating pan and tends to affect the whole batch in the coating pan. Besides increasing the tablet hardness in this case, the use of appropriate baffles in the coating pan can significantly reduce chipping and abrasion of tablets. These baffles prevent the tablet bed from sliding instead of rolling. They also redistribute the weight of the tablet load uniformly over the entire tablet bed.

Operating conditions

A film coating solution may work well with a particular core tablet in a small laboratory coating pan or column, but may be totally unacceptable on a production scale. This difference in performance may be due to the increased pressure and abrasion to which the tablets are subjected when the batch size is large. Also, the differences in temperature and humidity environment, to which the individual tablets are exposed during the coating and drying cycles, affect the process efficiency. Different process variables and/or operating conditions, which need to be monitored as a part of pilot-plant evaluation of the coating process, are enumerated as follows:

1. Nozzle type

Generally, two types of high-pressure atomizing nozzles, i.e., air-less or air-atomizing, are used for pharmaceutical coating applications. For air-atomized sprayers, the atomizing air pressure and the liquid flow rate are the crucial factors in establishing proper spraying characteristics. On the other hand, the size and shape of the nozzle aperture are important for optimizing spray conditions in airless sprayers.

2. Airflow

A high airflow yields a fine spray but it also causes more turbulence and spray drying effect. Additionally, the spraying pattern i.e., continuous or intermittent, also influences the efficiency of a coating process. For instance, in case of intermittent spraying pattern, the coating cycles must be timed to prevent the rotation of dry, uncoated or partially coated tablets, which would result in abrasion and edge chipping of the tablets and a poor quality coating.

3. Number of spray guns

Selection of the number of spray gun is critical to maximize the tablet bed coverage and coating efficiency and to minimize the process time and losses of the coating material.

4. Gun to tablet bed distance

Positioning of spray guns is also important to ensure entire tablet bed coverage, to facilitate maximum surface drying time and to achieve reproducibility.

In addition to the above parameters, the spray rate, drying air volume, pan speed and pan load also affect the uniformity of distribution of applied coating, process performance and yield of the process.

B. SCALE-UP OF HARD GELATIN CAPSULES

Tablets and capsules, both are produced from ingredients that may either be dry-blended or wet-granulated to produce a dry powder or granule mix with a uniformly dispersed active ingredient. To produce capsules using modern high-speed equipment, the processed powder blend must have the desired particle size distribution, bulk density, compressibility and flow characteristics. These parameters significantly govern the formation of compacts of the right size and of sufficient cohesiveness to be filled into the capsule shells. The following factors need to be considered during pilot-plant evaluation of any encapsulation process:

(a) Granule characteristics

The poor flow characteristics of the granules may cause weight variation in the filled capsules, which, in turn, may be due to the altered bulk density or particle size distribution of the granules during scale-up trials. The moisture content of granulation is also important, as uncontrolled moisture may lead to flow problems and sticking during material transfer and filling stages. Moisture content also tends to influence the chemical or physical stability of the finished product.

(b) Effect of lubricants

Inadequate lubrication of granulation or dry powder blend may lead to sticking of plugs to the dosator, plunger surfaces or die walls and, thus, result in weight variation. Over-lubrication of the granules may also result in weight variation problems, because the softer plugs would be formed which may not be completely transferred to the capsule body. Over-lubricated capsule granules are also accountable for delaying capsule disintegration and dissolution, and consequently delayed bioavailability. As in the case of compression process, prolonged trials of many hours using multiple batches are required before a process can be adjudged as acceptable for routine production.

(c) Encapsulation equipment

Equipment used in capsule filling operations involves two types of filling systems. Some encapsulation machines work upon the principle of slug formation in a dosator, while others are based on formation of compacts in a die plate using tamping pins to form a compact. Because of differences in operating principles, selection of encapsulating equipment is invariably governed by the properties of the powder blend viz. particle size distribution, compressibility and flow behavior.

(d) Controlled environment conditions

Many encapsulation processes are less reliable than anticipated because humidity in the processing and encapsulation rooms is not adequately controlled. For instance, carrying encapsulation at higher humidity levels may cause swelling of the capsule shells, owing to the moisture absorbed. This may make separation of the capsule parts more difficult and interfere with the transport of the capsule throughout the encapsulation process. The recommended storage conditions for empty capsule shells include storage temperature between 15 and 25°C, and a relative humidity between 35 to 65%. This condition is designed to minimize moisture absorption or loss, and the resultant changes in physical dimensions during the encapsulation operation. On the other hand, low humidity conditions make the capsules brittle and increase their static charge, thereby seriously interfering with the encapsulation operation.

C. SCALE-UP OF LIQUID FORMULATIONS

(a) Non-parenteral liquids (solutions, suspensions, emulsions)

(i) Solutions

Scale-up of different non-sterile liquid pharmaceuticals, including solutions, suspensions or emulsions, presents a different set of processing concerns. A clue to the resolution of the scale-up problems for liquids resides in recognizing that their processing invariably involves the unit operation of mixing. Closer examination of this core unit operation reveals that the liquid flow conditions and viscosities during scale-up process can vary widely by several orders of magnitude on both microscopic (i.e., molecular) or macroscopic (i.e., bulk) scale. Therefore, the key to effective scale-up processing is understanding the liquid transport phenomenon at microscopic and/or macroscopic scale(s). Critical process and formulation variables for process scale-up of solutions include (i) design of mixing vessel, (ii) size of mixer, (iii) size of impeller(s), (iv) extent of mixing, and (v) liquid flow properties.

Wide arrays of mixing equipment are currently available for pilot-plant and large scale manufacturing. Herein, the selection of impeller is very vital as the dynamic part of the mixing equipment. Depending upon the mixing requirements, the impellers of different types and shapes such as blades, propellers, turbines, paddles and helical ribbons may be used for efficient mixing. Another critical variable is the location of the impeller in the mixing vessel, which affects the mixing efficiency or the mixer performance to an appreciable extent. Nevertheless, despite the availability of a variety of liquid mixers, the critical evaluation of the rate and extent of mixing as well as the flow properties of the solution dosage form(s) is also required. Each unit operation of the process such as mixing, material transfer, filtration, filling and packaging should be carefully monitored. Some other general considerations for process scale-up of solution dosage forms are as follows:

(a) Special attention must be paid to ensure adequate liquid transfer systems.
(b) The functioning of filtration equipment during pilot-plant studies and large scale manufacturing should be closely monitored to ensure selective removal of active or adjuvant ingredients.
(c) All the liquid pharmaceutical processing tanks, kettles, pipes and mills should be fabricated from suitable, non-reactive, sanitary materials and be designed and constructed to facilitate easy cleaning.

(ii) Suspensions

Unlike simple solutions, the process scale-up of suspension or emulsion dosage forms needs thorough monitoring and optimization of all the additional processing steps. The scale-up implications of mixing-related issues in case of these disperse systems, such as impeller design and placement, mixing tank characteristics, and mixing of particulate solids, demand special attention owing to their multiphasic character. The factors that control the efficient scale-up of the process encompass:

(a) Selection of equipment

In preparing large batches of pharmaceutical suspensions, the type of mixers, mills and pumps tend to significantly contribute towards the scale-up of a mixing process. The selection of type and size of the mixer is made according to the batch size and product properties such as maximum viscosity of the product during the manufacturing process. Use of an undersized mixer, for instance, results in inadequate distribution or excessive production times.

(b) Addition and dispersion of suspending agents

On laboratory scale, addition of a suspending agent may merely involve sprinkling of the material into the liquid vortex. However, when the batches are involved on production scale, it may require use of a vibrating feed system or any other novel approach.

(c) Addition and dispersion of sticky materials

Addition of a material that tends to clump during the process or that is difficult to disperse can also pose problems while handling large volumes. This problem may be resolved by employing some specially designed powder feeding mechanisms such as powder eductor. If the suspending agent is difficult to disperse, it can be successfully incorporated by preparing a slurry of the suspending agent with a portion of the vehicle. The latter facilitates rapid and complete hydration of the suspending agent, when added to the larger portion of the vehicle.

(d) Addition and dispersion of a drug

Uniformity of drug dispersion in a suspension product is relatively difficult to achieve in production scale vis-à-vis laboratory scale batches. In production scale processing, selection of dispersion procedure depends on the API's physical characteristics. If the API is easily wettable and dispersible as well as non-agglomerating in nature, simple addition of the same at a convenient stage in the manufacturing process is appropriate. However, if the API is difficult to wet or has the tendency to agglomerate, other methods for adding these ingredients must be sought. One approach to surmount this problem is to use suitable wetting agent(s) in the slurry and to employ high-shear mixing equipment. Another method is to pre-treat the hydrophobic material by blending it in a high-shear powder blender with one or some of the liquid ingredients, possibly with a surfactant included. This converts a bulky material, which erstwhile is difficult to handle at large scale due to static charges, to a dense and readily wettable powder that is much easier to handle.

(e) Removal of entrapped air

Very often, mixing at too high a speed may lead to incorporation of an excessive amount of air into the product. Air entrapped in the product as very small bubbles is difficult and time-consuming to remove. But, if not removed, it can affect the physical and chemical stability of the product and/or the reproducibility of the filling operation. The problem of air entrapment can be alleviated by making certain process or equipment modifications like optimizing mixing speeds and modifying the design of mixing vessel. Air can also be removed using specially designed vacuum equipment. Herein, the product is drawn into a vacuum chamber through an inlet line, where it is spread onto the center of a high-speed rotating disc. The centrifugal force produced by the rotation of the disc causes the product to form a thin film on the disc surface. As the film thins and moves towards the outer edge of the vacuum chamber, the entrapped air is drawn off and the deaerated product is collected from the outer edge of the vacuum chamber.

(f) Removal of particulate matter

The most common source of the particulate matter is the raw material itself or the bags, cases and drums in which the raw materials are supplied. Besides all the necessary precautions, some unwanted material is always present in the product during manufacturing. The latter necessitates the incorporation of filtration as a batch processing step. The finished suspension is filtered through an appropriate size screen before filling and packaging. Hence, the selection of a filter/screen with optimum mesh size also becomes extremely important for the process development of suspensions. Selection of a sieve or filter is based on the production batch size, or the characteristics of API and raw materials. For instance, most active ingredients have particles less than 10 microns with almost none over 25 microns. Therefore, when dealing with particulates, screens of 150 mesh having openings of around 100 microns tend to remove the unwanted suspended particles that are below the easily visible range, without retaining the suspended active ingredient(s).

(g) Filling operation

Transfer and filling processes of a finished suspension also need careful monitoring. For example, if suspensions were not constantly mixed or recirculated during transfer processes, the sedimentation of the suspended active and/or the other materials would adversely affect the uniform distribution of the active ingredient and/or suspending agent.

(iii) Emulsions

Emulsions are disperse systems similar to suspensions except that the dispersed phase is a finely divided immiscible liquid instead of a solid. The dispersed phase is usually made up of oils or waxes, which may be either in liquid or quasi-solid state. The degree to which the emulsion is refined by the reduction of the globule size of the internal phase affects the physical properties of the emulsion product, such as appearance, viscosity and physical stability. Manufacturing of liquid emulsion products entails specialized procedures like homogenization. As a result, scale-up using production equipment involves extensive process development and validation. The pivotal processing parameters and procedures that must be controlled to optimize the scale-up of emulsions are enlisted as under:

1. Mixing equipment
2. Homogenizing equipment
3. Process controls
4. In-process or final product filters
5. Material transfer pumps
6. Filling equipment

(b) Parenteral products

Since the administration of injectable products requires circumventing highly protective barriers of the human body like skin and the mucous membranes, the dosage form must conform to exceptional purity. This is generally accomplished by strict adherence to the prescribed guidelines for sterile products and good manufacturing practices. The basic principles employed in the formulation development of parenteral products do not vary from those widely used in other sterile and non-sterile liquid preparations. However, it is imperative that all the calculations be accurate and precise. Therefore, the scale-up of parenteral solutions essentially becomes a scale-up of liquid pharmaceuticals with high degree of accuracy. Some of the essential requirements are explained below:

(i) Weighing and dispensing of raw materials

The compliance to quality considerations and full adherence to GMP guidelines is very vital at every stage of producing parenteral products. The first and foremost responsibility of the pilot-plant scientist is to ensure proper compounding and dispensing of the actives and excipients for parenteral products.

(ii) Liquid mixing

For liquids, mixing is defined as a transport process that occurs simultaneously on three different scales, during which one substance (solute) achieves a uniform concentration in another substance (solvent). On a visible macroscopic scale, mixing occurs by bulk diffusion, in which the elements are blended by the pumping action of the mixer's impeller. On the microscopic scale, however, the elements that are in proximity are blended by eddy currents, creating a drag where local velocity and shear stress differences act on the fluid. On the smallest scale, final blending occurs via molecular diffusion, with the rate of diffusion being unaffected by the mechanical mixing action. Thus, in case of large-scale production of parenterals, mixing depends primarily on flow within the vessel. Therefore, it needs to be carefully monitored while optimizing the process.

(iii) Other requirements

Various other equipment used for fabrication of pilot-plant and large-scale batches of parenteral products such as sterilization equipment, filtration systems and liquid transfer pumps, as well as the packaging process, must be scalable and should be rationally selected from the wide variety available.

D. SCALE-UP OF SEMISOLID PRODUCTS

An array of semisolid class of dosage forms represents multiple types of preparations viz. pastes, gels, ointments and creams. The manufacturing of these products at shop floor i.e. production plant is subjected to a wide range of parameters, so the scale-up of these products is not an easy task. These systems most of the times are heterogeneous in nature, which contribute to their rheological status and the involvement of several variables. Hence, maintenance of uniformity, consistency and other rheological properties like thixotropic behaviour are the key concerns. The nature of materials, mechanical operations, micromeritic properties, types of operations, equipments, environmental conditions like temperature, humidity are some factors to influence the quality. The major considerations in the large scale production of semisolids are as follows:

1. Selection of mixing equipments

The mixing requirements of semisolid products are entirely different from that of the liquid suspensions or non-viscous emulsion products because of their anomalous viscosity characteristics, and further complications like the unpredictable behaviour in response to the changing environment and interactions. The mixing equipments for these products must be of appropriate design, which help to effectively and continuously move the semisolid mass from the outside walls of the mixing kettle to the center and from the bottom to the top of the kettle. This action is required both for uniform distribution of the ingredients as well as for rapid and efficient heat transfer to and from the product during the heating and cooling steps.

Similarly, the power required to carry out the mixing operation varies greatly during the manufacturing sequence and is directly related to changes in the viscosity of the product. Thus, the motors used to drive the mixing system of semisolid manufacturing equipment must be sized to handle the product at its most viscous stage. However, at very initial stages of mixing, i.e., when product viscosity is low, a mixer may be required to operate at a slower speed to prevent splashing of the intermediate phases. For this reason, most semisolid machines are designed to provide variable speed mixing.

An emulsion may be mixed by various impellers mounted on shafts, which are placed directly into the system, if the viscosity of the system is low. If high shear is required i.e. if the viscosity of the system is more, then turbine type of mixers can be employed. Similarly other types of mixers such as rotating blade mixers, planetary mixers can also be employed according to the need of the system.

However, aeration problem may occur in large scale manufacturing plant, if these mixers are used, as the high speed agitation may introduce the air into the product and low speed may not provide satisfactory emulsion.

Aeration problem can be avoided if one phase is introduced into the other in such a way that splashing and streaming are avoided. This can be done by introducing incoming liquid below the surface of other liquid in the mixing kettle, as well as careful adjustment of mixing conditions and liquid flow pattern.

For the production of semisolids, which tend to aerate excessively, completely enclosed kettles can be employed. These vessels can be operated under vacuum, thus mixing and emulsification can be performed without the involvement of air.

2. Selection of emulsifying equipment

Selection of the equipment for efficient emulsification and homogenization of the emulsion phases and dispersion of suspended active ingredients is very important.

Various types of high-shear mixers, homogenizers and colloid mills are available for large scale manufacturing of semisolid products. The most common approaches are use of colloid mill and sonic homogenization, because of simplicity and ease of operation and cleaning. A colloid mill consists of a fixed stator plate and a high-speed rotating rotor plate. Material drawn or pumped through an adjustable gap set between the rotor and stator is milled or homogenized by the physical action, and centrifugal force is created by the high-speed rotation of the rotor, which operates within 0.005 to 0.010 inch (i.e., 0.127 to 0.254 mm) of a stator. In sonic homogenization, emulsification is accomplished by imparting sufficient energy to the material through rapidly vibrating vanes that break up a liquid stream into small, discrete droplets. In high pressure homogenizer, the emulsion of two immiscible liquids is achieved by forcing their mixture through a small inlet orifice at high pressure. High pressure is achieved by the pump, which raises the pressure of the dispersion between 500–5000 psi and an orifice through which the fluid is bombarded on the homogenizing valve held in place on the valve seat by a strong spring. The spring is compressed as the pressure builds up and some of the emulsion moves between valve and valve seat. The energy, that has been stored in the liquid, is released instantaneously at this point, and subjects the product to intense turbulence and hydraulic shear. It is possible to recycle the emulsion through the homogenizer for a number of times to get a nano-sized emulsion.

3. Selection of material transfer facilities

The transfer pumps for semisolid products must be able to move large quantities of viscous material without applying excessive shear and incorporating air. Selection of the size and type of pump depends on various factors viz. viscosity of the product, desired pumping rate, product compatibility with the pump surface(s), and the pumping pressure required for transferring the material from one place to another. For instance, many cream formulations and some gel products are shear-sensitive. Changes in measured viscosity are frequently seen when these viscous products are pumped through long transfer lines or are filtered to remove unwanted particulates. Handling such products, during transfer from manufacturing kettle to holding tanks or to filling lines, requires attention to the amount of shear that such products will encounter. In other words, the relationship between shear stress and the measured viscosity values of the product must be understood for optimizing the scale-up of semisolid manufacturing process.

4. Impact of temperature

Carefully pre-determined temperatures are required to carry out many processing steps such as mixing of oil and water phases during emulsification processing, component homogenization, addition of active ingredient and product transfer. The working temperature ranges at which these operations are carried out are usually critical to the quality of the final product. For instance, during the formation of a cream, the aqueous phase and oil phase must be heated to a temperature above the solidification point of the oil phase, and then emulsified. Failure to maintain both phases at the correct temperature

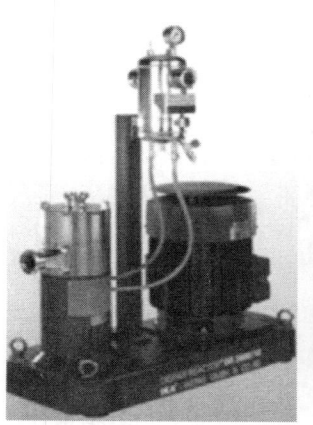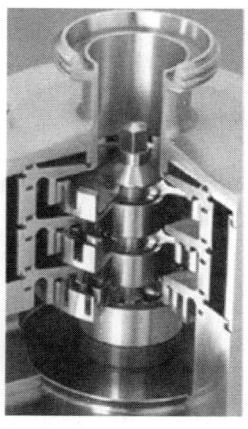

Fig. 16.7. Homogenizer: Lab scale (L), Pilot scale (R).

tends to result in a poor quality product with improperly dispersed wax. Other frequent problem is unacceptably wide ranges of product viscosity as a result of inadequate temperature control during the critical emulsification steps. Similarly, improper temperature control can have an adverse effect on the particle size and crystalline character of poorly soluble active ingredients. Addition of these ingredients at relatively high temperatures may increase the solubility, thus creating a metastable product. On subsequent cooling, crystal growth or recrystallization may occur from a saturated solution. This recrystallized material may be a different polymorphic form or a different crystal type or size, thus leading to alteration of particle size distribution. This may eventually yield a gritty and less elegant product, or one with poor stability or even biologic activity.

Concept of mixing/emulsification dynamics in semi-solid dosage forms

To be able to understand the problems associated with the scale-up of semisolids it is important to know that the processing invariably involves the unit operation of mixing. The flow conditions and viscosities during processing of this unit operation can vary by several orders of magnitude when seen at a microscopic (i.e., molecular) or a macroscopic (i.e., bulk) scale. The phenomenon operating at microscale enacts as diffusion whilst at macroscale, it is bulk flow to influence the process and product characteristics, as well. The flow of properties like mass, heat, momentum and electromagnetic energy from a region of high concentration to a region of low concentration as a result of the microscopic motion of electrons, atoms, and molecules, etc. is essentially transport by diffusion. The flow of a property as a result of bulk motion, which is induced artificially by mechanical agitation or naturally by density variations, involves either convection or advection.

Mixing operation

Mixing is a unit operation that involves manipulation of a heterogeneous physical system with the intent to make it more homogeneous. The type of operations and equipments used during mixing depends on the state of materials being mixed (liquid, semisolid, or solid) and the miscibility of the materials being processed.

Mixing in the multiphase/single phase emulsion vehicles made with hot and cold process

In multiphase emulsion vehicle systems two or more immiscible phases are mixed to form the final vehicle; these are also liquid-solid or liquid-liquid systems. In single-phase emulsion vehicle systems, two or more miscible/soluble phases are mixed to form the final vehicle; these are generally liquid-solid or liquid-liquid systems. Heating is employed in hot process type of systems because some of the components are

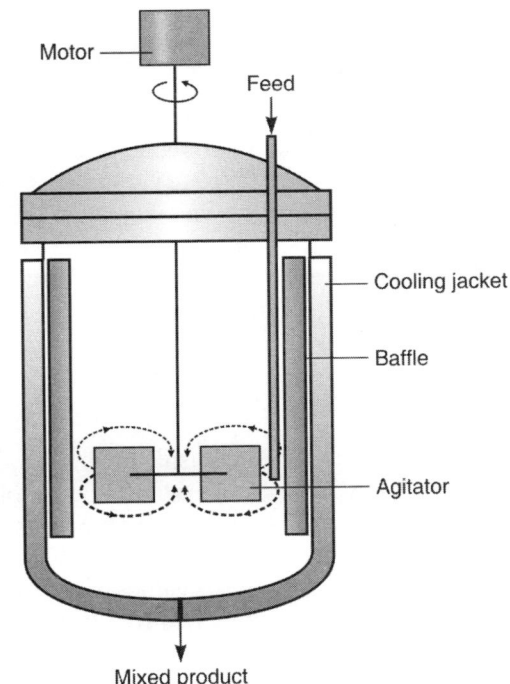

Fig. 16.8. Illustration of mixing process inside a plant scale mixer.

solid at room temperature and the two immiscible phases are required to acquire same state of form to ensure proper mixing. The heating temperature is generally selected based on the highest melting point of the component of solid phase and the temperature of mixing is kept above this temperature.

Multiphase liquid-solid or liquid-liquid emulsion systems have oil, water and surfactants. In addition to this, energy is needed to prepare an emulsion as emulsion formation is a non-spontaneous activity in these systems. This energy is needed to expand the interface.

In emulsion systems, the target size of the emulsified droplet is a matter of concern. The formation of large droplets of few microns can be achieved by the use of high speed mixers and is easy. However, the formation of small drops of submicron level requires a large amount of energy and is difficult. This high energy required for the formation of submicron level droplets can be understood from a consideration of the Laplace pressure.

Laplace pressure

The Laplace pressure is the pressure difference between the inside and the outside of a curved surface. The pressure difference is caused by the surface tension of the interface between liquid and gas.

The Laplace pressure is determined from the Young–Laplace equation given as

$$\Delta P = P_{inside} - P_{outside} = \Upsilon \left(\frac{1}{R_1} + \frac{1}{R_2} \right)$$

where P_{inside} is the pressure inside the bubble or droplet, $P_{outside}$ is the pressure outside the bubble or droplet, γ (also denoted as σ) is the surface tension, and R_1 and R_2 are the radii of curvature.

Although signs for these values vary, sign convention usually dictates positive curvature when convex and negative when concave. The Laplace pressure is commonly used to determine the pressure difference in spherical shapes such as bubbles or droplets. In this case the radii of

curvature are equal ($R_1 = R_2$) and the equation simplifies to

$$\Delta P = \frac{2\gamma}{R}$$

As ΔP and R are inversely proportional, a smaller radius will result in a larger inward force.

A common example of use is finding the pressure inside an air bubble in pure water, where $\gamma = 72$ mN/m at 25 °C (298 K). The extra pressure inside the bubble is given here for three bubble sizes:

Bubble diameter ($2r$) (μm)	ΔP (Pa)	ΔP (atm)
1000	288	0.00284
3.0	96000	0.947
0.3	960000	9.474

A 1 mm bubble has negligible extra pressure. Yet when the diameter is ~3 μ, the bubble has an extra atmosphere inside than outside. When the bubble is only several hundred nanometers, the pressure inside can be several atmospheres. One should bear in mind that the surface tension in the numerator can be much smaller in the presence of surfactants or contaminants. The same calculation can be done for small oil droplets in water, where even in the presence of surfactants and a fairly low interfacial tension = 5–10 mN/m. Interestingly the pressure inside 100 nm diameter droplets can reach several atmospheres. Such nanoemulsions can be antibacterial because the large pressure inside the oil droplets can cause them to attach to bacteria, and simply merge with them, swell them, and "pop" them.

Laplace pressure works against the stability of simple emulsions. The addition of a small quantity of electrolyte to the disperse phase was found to have a stabilizing effect in w/o emulsion, which is a consequence of counteracting the Laplace pressure effect, while in multiple emulsion (w/o/w emulsions), the osmotic pressure generated by the presence of electrolytes in the inner dispersed water phase can cause swelling and ultimately bursting of the inner dispersed droplets. So the impact of electrolyte on multiple emulsion stability is negative. In order to balance these two effects, the concentration of electrolytes has to be high enough to counteract the Laplace pressure but sufficiently low to avoid osmotic effects.

The size of the macroemulsions typically depends on how much energy was used to mix the phases; e.g. higher-energy mixing methods result into smaller emulsion particles. The energy required for this can be approximated using the following equation:

$$\Delta G_{em} = 3\frac{\gamma V}{R_f}$$

where ΔG_{em} is the energy input, γ is the interfacial tension between the two phases, V is the total volume of the mixture, and R_f is the average radius of the newly created emulsions.

This equation gives the energy requirement just to separate the particles. The input of mechanical energy by stirrers is most important case. The stirrers generate macro eddies or macro turbulence. These macro eddies decompose into micro eddies, which are finally responsible for the energy transfer and hence the breakage of the macroscopic phase. As soon as the shear exerted by the turbulent micro eddies on the droplet interface exceeds the Laplace pressure of the droplets, they split up to smaller units.

This process continues as long as a balance between the external stress and the internal stress is reached.

In practice, the energy cost is much higher, as most of the mechanical energy is simply converted to heat rather than mixing the phases.

Laplace pressure in the process of emulsification promotes an emulsion to become thermodynamically inefficient. For an emulsion to form the small, highly curved droplets, extra energy is required to overcome the large pressure that exists in the droplets. Fig. 16.9 illustrates the relationship between Laplace pressure, energy applied and the changes in dispersed phase over time period.

Weber number (N_{We})

An important parameter that describes droplet deformation is the "Weber number" (which gives the ratio of the external stress over the Laplace pressure). The Weber number represents the ratio of the driving force causing partial disruption to the resistance due to interfacial tension. Increased Weber numbers are associated with a greater tendency for droplet deformation (and consequent splitting into still smaller droplets) to occur at higher shear, i.e., with more intense mixing.

$$N_{We} = \frac{D_i^3 N^2 \rho_{cont.}}{\sigma}$$

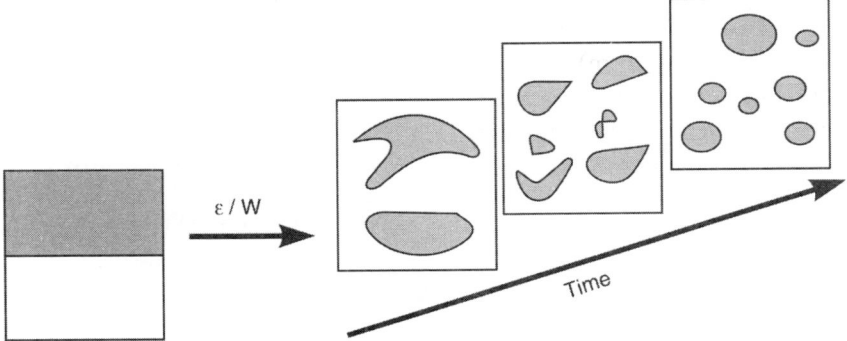

Fig. 16.9. Relationship between Laplace pressure, energy and changes in dispersed phase.

where, D_i is the diameter of the impeller, N is the rotational speed of the impeller, and ρ_{cont} is the density of the continuous phase. For a given system, droplet size reduction begins above a specific critical Weber number; above the critical N_{We}, average droplet size varies with $N^{-1.2}D_i^{-0.8}$ or, as an approximation, with the reciprocal of the impeller tip speed. In addition, a better dispersion is achieved, for the same power input, with a smaller impeller rotating at high speed.

Tip speed

Tip speed is the speed of rotor at the periphery of the rotor and is calculated by the formula:

$$\text{Tip speed} = \pi D \text{ (m/s)}$$

where D is the diameter of the rotor or impeller, m/s= meter/second

Mixing operation of multiphase emulsion vehicles is generally done using rotor-stator type of homogenizer.

For scaling-up of the processes of semisolids, prepared using in-line rotor-stator mixers, tip speed of rotor-stator gives reasonable fit between scales and Weber number is the most appropriate scaling parameter.

$$\frac{d_{3,2}}{D} = C_2 We^{-3/5}$$

where $d_{3,2}$ is the volume surface mean diameter (Sauter mean drop diameter) (m), C_2 is the dimensionless empirical constant, We is the Weber number, and D is the characteristic diameter (outer rotor diameter in m).

S. Hall et al. (Hall et al., 1999) applied above equation, which is frequently used for scaling-up of emulsification process in stirred vessels, in in-line rotor-stator mixers and studied the relationship between Weber number and dimensionless Sauter mean drop diameter and found best fit of these. However, in all of the experiments the interfacial tension was constant, hence validity of this hypothesis is limited.

E. SCALE-UP TECHNIQUES FOR NANOPHARMACEUTICAL DRUG DELIVERY SYSTEMS: CHALLENGES AND SOLUTIONS

Accurate targeting of a therapeutic compound to the desired site of action is the current interest of research scientist. To accomplish this objective several kinds of drug delivery carriers have been introduced in the last two decades. These are colloidal or vesicular carriers (e.g., liposomes, micellar systems, nanoemulsions, etc.), particulate nano-carriers (e.g., solid-lipid nanoparticles, polymeric nanoparticles, nanosuspensions, nano-drug crystals), and the supramolecular nano-carriers (e.g., dendrimers, etc.). These nanocarriers can provide superior drug delivery systems for better management and treatment of diseases. Various unique features and potential benefits of these carrier systems have enabled their use in a wide variety of specific drug delivery applications with high degree of success. So, it will be beneficial for the human beings that more and more nanopharmaceuticals should emerge in the market. However, there are some challenges to happen this. For drugs to be marketable, their production has to be planned and designed from the outset of research. Unfortunately, many nanomedicine researchers do not know exactly how to develop a drug. Although a translational advisory organization would be highly desirable, it does not exist and, in its absence, each research group is strongly advised to come up with a strategy to access this largely unpublished information. The European Technology Platform for Nanomedicine in its various reports has made some suggestions about how to do this. At the moment the lack of commercial translatability of publicly funded healthcare research is a more important issue than the level of funding. Among other areas, expertise is needed and should be sought in:

1. Process scale-up and standards

2. Specialized characterization tools and techniques
3. Analytical methods
4. Regulatory considerations
5. Packaging
6. Market analysis
7. Soft information, competitor intelligence, and patents.

The challenge of research and development (R&D) of nanomaterials for drug delivery is its large-scale production with a high degree of reproducibility. There is always a need to scale-up laboratory or pilot-technologies for eventual commercialization. For instance, a number of nano-drug delivery technologies may not be scalable due to the method and process of production and high cost of materials employed. The challenges of scaling up include low concentration of nanomaterials, agglomeration and the chemistry process. Thus, it seems easier to modify nanomaterials at laboratory scale for improved performance than at large scale. Maintaining the size and composition of nanomaterials at large scale is also a challenge. The identification of some of these potential scale-up issues forces the formulator to consider commercialization of the drug delivery system.

1. Scale-up of vesicular nano-carrier systems

In general, it has been recognized that the process of developing an effective scale-up method for large-scale production of diverse vesicular carrier systems is associated with numerous specific problems and technical restrictions. For instance, to ensure reproducible clinical performance of a liposomal drug product (LDP) produced on a large-scale, a stricter control on different quality control parameters like liposome size, drug-lipid ratio and encapsulation efficiency is required. It assumes greater significance as the global regulatory agencies like USFDA or EMEA have not issued any concrete guidelines for acceptable variations in the key quality characteristics of LDPs.

Therefore, the developed and validated scale-up manufacturing process for a LDP should be able to demonstrate that the variation in any of the quality control parameter is within the permissible limits and, thus, does not affect the pharmacodynamic profile of the manufactured product. Moreover, the developed manufacturing technique should allow economic scale-up, and evasion of hazardous solvents (e.g., chloroform, methylene chloride, etc.) and expensive detergents (e.g., bile acids, *N*-ethylglucoside, etc.) too.

Several preparatory techniques for large-scale production of LDPs or other vesicular carrier systems have been reported in the literature, viz. sonication, detergent removal, thin-film hydration, solvent injection, bubbling and extrusion. Ethanol injection, the first technique to be employed for the manufacture of liposomes on a large scale, is still in vogue round the globe. It involves injection of lipids containing solution in a water-miscible solvent (e.g., ethanol and DMSO) into an aqueous phase. Another widely used technique for large scale production of liposomes involves hydration of a lipid film formed in a multi-tubular system. The process is a modified approach of the classical Bangham method (i.e., thin-film technique), in which a thin lipid film is adsorbed on the inner surface of the glass tubes. Continuous adsorption of the lipids is achieved by feeding lipid dispersion in ethanol at the bottom of the tubes through a peristaltic pump and circulating the dispersion for fixed time and elevated temperature. Subsequently, the excess of lipids is drained and the film is dried under vacuum. The dried film is hydrated using a buffered solution in order to produce liposomes.

A relatively recent technique with a very high potential of process scale-up is the bubbling technique. Employing this method, liposome dispersions of varying size range can be produced. Liposomal dispersions with an average diameter of about 300 nm have been reported to be prepared by bubbling a stream of nitrogen through a dispersion of lipid materials. An evaluation of the scale-up feasibility of this process has also yielded promising results. A unique advantage of this technique is the remote possibilities of contamination of the prepared liposomal dispersions with the eroded metal particles, since the manufacturing can be carried out in "all glass' conditions.

Nanomedicines that are to be utilized by a route of administration that requires a sterile product will face particular challenges dependent on their particle size and composition. Nano-materials are known to be at increased risk for being damaged by sterilization techniques such as gamma irradiation or autoclaving, especially when biological materials are involved. If the structure of the particles is flexible or malleable, such as in case of some liposomal preparations, then sterilization through conventional sterile filters may not be problematic especially if the starting particle size is well below 220 nm (0.22 μ). If the mean particle size is not well below 220 nm, then substantial amounts of the active ingredient could be lost on filtration. While aseptic manufacturing is always an option, this can be quite complicated, in particular for a multiple step process that involves handling and transfer. Removal of unentrapped free drug from the liposomal dispersions prepared at large scale is another vital issue. Many available techniques, like gel-permeation chromatography (i.e., Sephadex mini-column technique), ion-exchange, protamine aggregation, ultracentri-fugation and dialysis, have one or more associated problems. Amongst these, ultracentri-fugation and dialysis technique are preferred techniques for large scale preparation of liposomes.

2. Scale-up of nanoparticulate drug delivery systems

Some of the widely used techniques for manu-facturing of nanoparticles include hot-homo-genization, high pressure homogenization, microemulsification, ultrasonication, micro-fluidization, combination of micro-precipitation and homogenization, and super-critical fluid (S-CF) technology. A recently introduced innovative technique for formation of nanoparticles is 'micro-fluidic lab-on-chip' technology, based on the application of well-controlled forces, which control fluid movements and other processing conditions in the micro-fluidizer. The technique offers many potential benefits for the production of nanoparticles such as miniaturization, integration and automation.

For large scale manufacturing of nano-particles, high-pressure homogenization and micro-emulsification are considered as most promising techniques, owing to the associated benefits of ease of manufacturing, repro-ducibility of quality control parameters, ease of production without organic solvents, etc. For large-scale preparation of nanosuspensions, the most preferred method is Media milling (bead-milling) technique. The latter is an attrition-based technique, which involves preparation of nanosuspensions using high-shear media mills. The milling chamber, charged with milling media (i.e., beads of specific size; composed of glass, zirconium oxide or highly cross-linked polystyrene resin), water, drug and stabilizer, is rotated at a very high shear rate under controlled temperatures for a specified period. The high energy shear forces are generated as a conse-quence of impaction of the milling media with the drug, resulting in the subdivision of the erst-while microparticulates to nanoparticles.

The potential benefits of this technique accrued in large-scale manufacturing include high efficiency to generate finer particle sizes, short process time, provision for continuous operation, reproducible particle size, particle stability and cost- effectiveness. Further optimi-zation and improvisation of this technique, however, is obligatory to address the issues like mill wearing, material and engineering modifications in milling beads, adaptability for thermo-sensitive drug substances, efficiency improvement, etc.

3. Scale-up of drug nanocrystals

Drug nanocrystals can be produced by the following processes:

(i) Wet ball milling

It comminutes material loaded into milling chamber with an agitator (milling media). The milling material, the drug to be nanosized, is normally provided as a treated (micronized) or untreated solid dispersed in a liquid medium (usually water) with the aid of surfactants as stabilizers. The comminution principle involved is the mechanical attrition and shear that arises due to collision between milling media and drug particles or between two drug particles or also between a drug particle and the walls of the milling chamber. The milling media are small beads or pearls made of ceramic (e.g., yttrium stabilized zirconium dioxide) or highly crosslinked polystyrene resin or stainless steel or glass having different sizes (0.3 mm or higher). However, the first two ensure minimal contamination to the product. The size reduction effectiveness could be further determined by the concentration of drug and surfactant, viscosity of the dispersion medium, temperature conditions and by the initial particle size and hardness of the drug.

(ii) High pressure homogenization

It is another process wherein the particle size reduction is brought about by shear forces. The steps involved in producing nanosuspensions by means of High pressure homogenization are similar and as simple as for Wet ball milling. Normally, a premix of the coarse drug and the dispersion medium is prepared using high speed stirrers. The dispersion medium contains normally similar surfactant and/or stabilizer systems used for the Wet ball milling approach. Subsequently, this coarse suspension (the so called "macro-suspension") is passed several times through the high pressure homogenizer. Typically, the applied pressure is increased step-wise from 10% to 100% in order to avoid

clogging of the narrow homogenization gap. At production pressure, which spans between 1000 and 2000 bar, the gap has an opening of only a few micrometer. This explains the importance of the pre-mixing procedure for de-agglomeration and wetting purposes, especially when relatively coarse material is processed. The particle size reduction itself is caused by cavitation forces, shear forces and collision. In general, several homogenization cycles are needed to reach the minimal particle size.

(iii) Supercritical Fluid Technology (SCF)

The different SCF formulation processes comprise three main steps for which scale-up is difficult: particle generation, particle collection, and fluid purification and recycle (when recycled).

A. **Atomization:** Microparticles are generated by atomization through a nozzle in most SCF formulation processes. Ideally, scale-up should be made in maintaining all parameters constant by replacing one nozzle by several similar nozzles of the same design and dimension through which the fluid or liquid velocity and pressure drop should be kept identical with those through the sole nozzle.

B. **Particle collection:** Four mechanisms are currently used to collect particles from a gas flow: (i) inertia (gravity settler, impact chambers, and cyclones), (ii) electrostatic forces, liquid scrubbing, and filtering through porous media. In fact, very fine particles can only be collected either by filtration for obtaining dry particles or by liquid scrubbing for obtaining a suspension. Despite its great efficiency, filtration has several main inconveniences because it is a batch process with conditions that may vary with time, especially the particle residence time on the filter with possible morphology changes (crystal pattern) and nonhomo-geneous properties; the worst case happens when the particles are collected before they are completely dried by the fluid (antisolvent or drying processes), leading to particle agglomeration and "sintering" inside the filter cake paper or fiber mats chosen in materials (like polytetrafluoroethylene or polyamides fibers) both compatible with the processed fluids and acceptable for drug.

C. **Fluid purification process and recycle:** For some SCF formulation processes (Rapid Expansion of Supercritical Solution (RESS), antisolvent, Depressurization of an Expanded Liquid Organic Solution (DELOS), impregnation, etc.), solvent recycle is mandatory at large scale, either with carbon dioxide, or with another fluid with better solvent properties such as propane or dimethyl ether, leading to a lower ratio. In RESS processes, recycle is difficult and expensive because the fluid must be recompressed from the atomization pressure to the dissolution pressure. In processes using an organic solvent (antisolvent, DELOS, and emulsion drying), carbon dioxide is generally used and the particle formation and collection is operated at high pressure, permitting an "easy" recycle of the fluid after purification. For the anti-solvent precipitation itself, the fluid can be recycled as it is, at the condition that the solvent concentration is perfectly constant. For solvent stripping from the collected particles, pure carbon dioxide is required and can be recycled only after the classical solvent collection by fluid depressurization followed by carbon bed adsorption.

PHARMACEUTICAL PROCESS SCALE-UP AND ROLE OF DIMENSIONAL ANALYSIS: AN OVERVIEW

Many times a specific process may generate a quality product in both the laboratory and the pilot-plant but fail quality assurance tests in production. For every process, when moving from small-scale to large-scale, there has to be some physical similarity. Once the understanding is developed as to what makes these processes similar, many scale-up issues can be addressed. A rational approach to scale-up has been used in physical sciences, viz. fluid dynamics and chemical engineering, for quite some time. This approach is based on process similarities between different scales and employs dimensional analysis that was developed a century ago and has since gained wide recognition in many industries, especially in chemical engineering.

A dimension is a purely qualitative description of a perception of a physical entity or a natural appearance. They are used to represent physical quantities. Physical quantities such as force or speed have the basic dimensional qualities of length (L), mass (M), time (T), and so forth. A dimensional system consists of all the primary and secondary dimensions and corresponding measuring units.

Dimensional analysis is based upon the recognition that a mathematical formulation of a physicotechnological problem can be of general validity only when the process equation is dimensionally homogeneous, which means that it must be valid in any system of dimensions. Dimensional analysis is a method for producing dimensionless numbers that completely characterize the process. The analysis can be applied even when the equations governing the process are not known.

According to the theory of models, two processes may be considered completely similar if they take place in similar geometrical space and if all the dimensionless numbers necessary to describe the process have the same numerical value. Two processes are considered similar if there is a geometrical, kinematic, and dynamic similarity. Two systems are called geometrically similar if they have the same ratio of characteristic linear dimensions. For example, two cylindrical mixing vessels are geometrically similar if they have the same ratio of height to diameter. Two geometrically similar systems are called kinematically similar if they have the same ratio of velocities between corresponding points. Two kinematically similar systems are dynamically similar when they have the same ratio of forces between corresponding points. For any two dynamically similar systems, all the dimensionless numbers necessary to describe the process have the same numerical value. Lack of geometrical similarity is often the main obstacle when applying dimensional analysis to solve scale-up problems.

The scale-up procedure, then, is simple: the process is expressed using a complete set of dimensionless numbers, and attempt is made to match them at different scales. This dimensionless space in which the measurements are presented or measured will make the process scale invariant. Dimensionless numbers, such as *Reynolds* and *Froude numbers*, are frequently used to describe mixing processes. This approach has been applied to pharmaceutical granulation since the early work of Hans Leuenberger in 1982. Dimensional analytical procedure was first systematically applied to fluid flow 90 years ago by Lord Rayleigh, on the basis of the principle of similitude.

Pi theorem

The fundamental theorem of the dimensional analysis, the 'Pi theorem' states that every physical relationship between n dimensional variables and constants can be reduced to a relationship between $m = n - r$ mutually independent dimensionless groups, in which r is the number of dimensions; that is, fundamental dimensional units (rank of the dimensional matrix).

The aim of dimensional analysis is to check whether or not the physical content under examination can be formulated in a dimensionally homogeneous manner. Dimensional analysis starts with a relevance list, which is a list of all variables thought to be crucial for the process being analyzed. To set up a relevance list for a process, one needs to compile a complete set of all dimensional relevant and mutually independent variables and constants that affect the process. All entries in the list can be further subdivided as geometric, physical, or operational. Each relevance list should include only one target (i.e., dependent "response") variable.

Dimensional analysis can be simplified by arranging all relevant variables from the relevance list into a matrix, with a subsequent transformation yielding the required dimensionless numbers. The 'dimensional matrix' therefore will consist of a square core matrix and a residual matrix. The rows of the matrix consist of the basic dimensions, whereas the columns represent the physical quantities from the relevance list. The most important physical properties and process-related parameters, as well as the target variable (i.e., the one we would like to predict on the basis of other variables) are placed in one of the columns of the residual matrix.

The core matrix is linearly transformed into a matrix of unity in which the main diagonal consists only of ones and the remaining elements are all zero. The dimensionless numbers are then created as a ratio of columns in the residual matrix and the core matrix, with the exponents indicated in the residual matrix.

Dimensionless numbers, such as Reynolds, Froude numbers, **Newton (power) number**, etc. are frequently used to describe pharmaceutical processes and successfully implemented for process scale-ups. For instance, Newton (power) number, which relates the drag force acting on a unit area of the impeller and the inertial stress, represents a measure of power requirement to overcome friction in fluid flow in a stirred reactor. In mixer-granulation applications, this number can be calculated from the power consumption of the impeller or estimated from the power consumption of the motor. Equation 1 describes the Newton number.

$$\mathrm{Np} = \frac{\Delta P}{\rho n^3 d^5} \qquad \ldots \text{Eqn. 1}$$

where, Np is Newton number or power number, ΔP is power required by the impeller or motor (W = J/s), dimensional units $[ML^2T^{-5}]$; ρ is specific density of particles (kg/m^3), dimensional units $[ML^{-3}]$; n is impeller speed (revolutions/s), dimensional units $[T^{-1}]$; d is impeller (blade) diameter or radius (m), dimensional units [L].

Froude number has been described for powder blending and was suggested as a criterion for dynamic similarity and a scale-up parameter in wet granulation. The mechanics of the phenomenon was described as interplay of the centrifugal force (pushing the particles against the mixer wall) and the centripetal force produced by the wall, creating a "compaction zone". Equation 2 describes Froude number.

$$Fr = \frac{n^2 d}{g} \qquad \text{... Eqn. 2}$$

where, Fr is Froude number, n is impeller speed (revolutions/s), dimensional units $[T^{-1}]$; d is impeller (blade) diameter or radius (m), dimensional units [L]; g is gravitational constant (m/s^2), dimensional units $[LT^{-2}]$.

Reynolds numbers relate the inertial force to the viscous force. They are frequently used to describe mixing processes and viscous flow (Zlokarnik, 1991). Equation 3 describes Reynolds number.

$$Re = \frac{d^2 n \rho}{\eta} \qquad \text{... Eqn. 3}$$

where, Re is Reynolds number, d is impeller (blade) diameter or radius (m), dimensional units [L]; n is impeller speed (revolutions/s), dimensional units $[T^{-1}]$; ρ is specific density of particles (kg/m^3), dimensional units $[ML^{-3}]$; η is dynamic viscosity (Pa*s), dimensional units $[ML^{-1}T^{-1}]$.

Pitfalls of dimensional analysis often relate to selecting the reference list, target variable, or measurement errors (e.g., friction losses of the same order of magnitude as the power consumption of a motor). The larger the scale-up factor, the more precise the measurements of the small-scale must be.

Advantages of the use of dimensional analysis

1. Reduction of the number of parameters required to define the problem.
2. Reliable scale-up of the desired operating conditions from lab-scale/pilot-plant to commercial scale
3. A deeper understanding of the physical nature of the process.
4. Flexibility in the choice of parameters and their reliable extrapolation within the range covered by the dimensionless numbers.

In nutshell, the scale up of a desired process condition from a laboratory scale to production scale can be accomplished reliably only if the problem is formulated and dealt with using the concept of dimensional analysis.

Dimensional analysis of tablet scale-up

Dimensional analysis can provide a solid scientific basis for tableting scale up. The analysis should be carried out before the measurements are made, because dimensionless numbers essentially condense the frame in which the measurements are performed and evaluated. It can be applied even when the equations governing the process are not known.

Dimensional analysis – Relevance list

With the basic dimensions of mass, length, and time denoted as [M], [L], and [T], respectively, the relevance list for the target quantity H $[ML^{-1}T^{-2}]$ (mechanical tensile strength of the tablet) included:

- Depth of fill, or loading depth of the powder bed $\quad h$ [L]
- Final (out-of-die) tablet thickness $\quad h_t$ [L]
- Compression roll diameter $\quad D_{cr}$ [L]
- Maximum applied compression pressure $\quad P_m$ $[ML^{-1}T^{-2}]$
- Compression rate $\quad n$ $[T^{-1}]$
- Geometric dwell time $\quad$ [T]

Geometric dwell time is an indicator of a linear speed, sort of a yardstick that allows one to compare speeds of different tablet presses. It is defined here as the time required for a punch to traverse a horizontal distance of 9.5 mm (when the flat portion of the IPT Type B punch head is in contact with the compression wheel).

Dimensional analysis – Dimensional matrix

The dimensional matrix consists of a (square) core matrix and a residual matrix. Based on our relevance list, the dimensional matrix representing a tableting process can be written as shown in Table 16.6.

Table 16.6. Core and residual matrices

Dimension	Core matrix			Residual matrix				
	K	h_t	n	H	h	D_{cr}	P_m	n
Mass [M]	–1	0	0	1	0	0	1	0
Length [L]	1	0	0	–1	1	1	–1	0
Time [T]	2	0	–1	–2	0	0	–2	1

By a simple linear transformation, the core matrix becomes a unity matrix (Table 16.6).

The dimensionless numbers are formed as fractions, where each physical quantity indicated in the residual matrix represents the numerator, while a product of all quantities of the core matrix (with the exponents indicated in the residual matrix) constitutes the denominator.

This standard procedure yielded the following set (Table 16.7).

Table 16.7. Core and residual matrices

Dimension	Core matrix			Residual matrix				
	K	h_t	n	H	h	D_{cr}	P_m	n
Mass [M]	–1	0	0	1	0	0	1	0
Length [L]	1	0	0	–1	1	1	–1	0
Time [T]	2	0	–1	–2	0	0	–2	1

CONCLUSIONS

Following its conception in the productive 'gray matter' of a research scientist, a pharmaceutical product finds its destination after travelling through various developmental stages in an industrial milieu. The sojourn that a product undertakes from research laboratory to the production floor via scaling up process is both long and tedious. Known popularly as "Pilot-Plant Scale-up", it is composed of diverse domains and dimensions. The implementation needs to host a wide variety of well-synchronized activities, under a well-knitted managerial structure, in an organized manner. Beyond doubt, stringent controls and measures are of high importance to monitor the entire system as often the drug product is quite sensitive as well as vulnerable.

With the vast advancements in the "knowledge" and "know-how" of newer technologies, it is now feasible to facilitate the process of scale-up in a more systematic and cost-effective manner. But, at the same time, the nascent innovations in pharmaceutical research keep on bringing more sophistication, diversification and subtle intricacies in the formulation design. The scale-up of a product development idea into a reality product for the masses, accordingly, is no more a cake walk today. In fact, the execution of this herculean task requires a holistic approach with proper vision and surveillance, coupled up with continued improvisation and upgradation.

Federal agencies like USFDA have made GLP and GMP guidelines as mandatory to be implemented during pilot-plant operations as well as during manufacturing. Also, the Government of India has made the compliance to GLP practices mandatory under the schedule "L-1" with effect from 1st November 2010. The basic purpose of GLP is to assure quality, integrity and reliability of the laboratory data, so that there is always a mutual recognition of the results among laboratories.

Similarly, for pharmaceutical industry in India, the requirements specified under the upgraded Schedule 'M' for GMP have become mandatory w.e.f. July 1, 2005. Schedule M protocols have been revised to harmonize it along the lines of WHO and USFDA protocols.

These revised protocols include detailed specifications on infrastructure and premises, environmental safety and health measures, production and operation controls, quality control and assurance and stability and validation studies. A fully validated pilot-plant, in this regard, can not only ensure compliance with cGMPs, but would also guarantee data integrity and data reliability during product development. Adoption of these cGMPs objectives at pilot-plants will undoubtedly result in better products meeting the desired specifications and standards.

The topic of pilot-plant and scale-up studies, accordingly, assumes immense significance in the light of the federal enforcement of pharmaceutical cGMPs guidelines to accomplish the goals of robust manufacturing, improved product quality, and harmonization both at national and international levels.

ACKNOWLEDGEMENTS

Sagacious advice by Prof. Arvind Bansal, NIPER, SAS Nagar, Panjab, is gratefully acknowledged. We also appreciate valuable advice and inputs from Lupin Limited (Research Park), Lifecare Innovations Pvt Ltd, Gurgaon; IPCA Laboratories, Mumbai; UGC Center of Excellence in Nanoapplications (Biomedical Applications), Panjab University, Chandigarh; University Institute of Pharmaceutical Sciences (UIPS), Panjab University, Chandigarh; in compiling the current manuscript.

SUGGESTED FURTHER READING

- B. Trivedi. Quality by Design (QbD) in pharmaceutical sciences. *Int. J. Pharm. Pharm. Sci.*, 4 (2012) 17–29.
- P.K. Basu, J. Quaadgras, J.E. Holleman, R.A. Mack, A.R. Noren. Pharmaceutical pilot plants are different!, *Chem. Engg. Prog.*, 93 (1997) 66–75.
- H. Benameur, A. Moes. Liposomes preparation method and plant. *In:* USPTO (Ed.), 2001, pp. 1-6.
- L.H. Block. Process scale-up for pharmaceutical liquids and semisolids. *Am. Pharm. Rev.*, 3 (2000) 14–15.
- F.J. Carleton, J.P. Agalloco. *In:* **Validation of Pharmaceutical Processes: Sterile Products**, 2nd ed., New York: Marcel Dekker, 1999.
- M.S. DeSaavedra, I.S. Cuadra. Application of a mixed optimization strategy in the design of a pharmaceutical solid formulation at laboratory scale. *Drug. Dev. Ind. Pharm.*, 27 (2001) 675–685.
- S. Gnoth, M. Jenzsch, R. Simutis, A. Lubbert. Process Analytical Technology (PAT): batch-to-batch reproducibility of fermentation processes by robust process operational design and control. *J. Biotechnol.*, 132 (2007) 180–186.
- S.H. Gohla, A. Dingler. Scaling up feasibility of the production of solid lipid nanoparticles (SLN). *Pharmazie*, 56 (2001) 61–63.
- U.S. FDA. Human Pharmacokinetics and Bioavailability; and Labeling Documentation. *In:* CDER (Ed.), 2002.
- S. Harder, G.V. Buskirk. Pilot-plant scale-up techniques. *In:* L. Lachman, H.A. Lieberman, J.L. Kanig (Eds.). **The Theory and Practice of Industrial Pharmacy**, Varghese Publishing House, Mumbai, 2002, pp. 681–710.
- T. Hlinak. Granulation and scale-up issues in solid dosage form development. *Am. Pharm. Rev.*, 3 (2000) 33–36.
- J. Huang, G. Kaul, C. Cai, R. Chatlapalli, Hernandez-Abad., P.K. Ghosh, A. Nagi. Quality by design case study: an integrated multivariate approach to drug product and process development. *Int. J. Pharm.*, 382 (2009) 23–32.
- P.D. Marcato, N. Duran. New aspects of nano-pharmaceutical delivery systems. *J. Nanosci. Nanotechnol.*, 8 (2008) 2216–2229.
- R.A. Nash, A.H. Wachter (ed.) *In:* **Pharmaceutical Process Validation**, Marcel Dekker, 129, 2003.
- H.M.S. Patel. **Good Manufacturing Practice Applied to Pilot Plants**, Special Publications of the Royal Society of Chemistry, 1997, pp. 159–190.
- E.J. Russo. Typical scale-up problems and experiences. *Pharm. Tech.*, 8 (1984) 45–56.
- N.E. Sever, M. Warman, S. Mackey, W. Dziki, M. Jiang. Process Analytical Technology in Solid Dosage Development and Manufacturing. *In:* Y. Qiu, Y. Chen, G.Z. Zhang, L. Liu, W.R. Porter

- (Eds.). **Developing Solid Oral Dosage Forms: Pharmaceutical Theory and Practice**, Academic Press, 2009, pp. 827–841.
- R.B. Shah, M.A. Khan. Nanopharmaceuticals: Challenges and Regulatory Perspective. *In:* M.M. de villiers, P. Aramwit, G.S. Kwon (Eds.). **Nanotechnology in Drug Delivery: Biotechnology: Pharmaceutical Aspects**, Springer, New York, 2009, pp. 621–646.
- SUPAC-IIVMR: Immediate Release and Modified Release Solid Oral Dosage Forms. *In:* Food and Drug Administration, U.S.D.o.H.a.H. Services (Eds.), Center for Drug Evaluation and Research (CDER), 1999, pp. 1–40.
- M.L. Wells, S.B. Balik, R.B. Caricofe, W. Charles, C.W. Crew, R.A. Sanftleben, A.W. Wood. Pilot Plant Design. *In:* **Encyclopedia of Pharmaceutical Technology**. Informa Healthcare, 2006, pp. 2875–2890.
- S.H. Willig. **Good Manufacturing Practices for Pharmaceuticals**, 5th ed., Marcel Dekker, Inc., New York, 2001.
- M. Eaton. How do we develop nanopharmaceuticals under open innovation?, *Nanomedicine*, 7 (2011) 371–375.
- M. Perrut, J.V. Clavier. Supercritical fluid formulation: Process choice and scale up. *Ind. Eng. Chem. Res.*, 42 (2003) 6375–6383.
- M. Zlokarnik. **Dimensional Analysis and Scale-Up in Chemical Engineering**, Springer-Verlag New York, 1991.
- M. Zlokarnik. Problems in the application of dimensional analysis and scale-up of mixing operations. *Chem. Eng. Sci.*, 53 (1998) 3023–3030.
- G.J.B. Horsthuis, J.A.H. van Laarhoven, R.C.B.M. van Rooij, H. Vromans. Studies on upscaling parameters of the Gral high shear granulation process. *Int. J. Pharm.*, 92 (1993) 143–150.
- J.A. Searles, S.L. Nail. Elements of Quality by Design in Development and Scale-Up of Freeze-Dried Parenterals. *Biopharm International*, 21 (2008), 1–6.
- FDA, 2012. Quality by Design for ANDAs: An Example for Immediate-Release Dosage Forms, Example QbD IR Tablet. Module 3: Quality 3.2.P.2 Pharmaceutical Development.
- FDA, 2011, Quality by Design for ANDAs: An Example for Modified Release Dosage Forms, Example QbD MR Tablet. Module 3: Quality 3.2.P.2 Pharmaceutical Development.
- I. Gorsky. Parenteral Drug Scale-Up. *In:* **Pharmaceutical Process Scale-Up**, M. Levin, Ed., Marcel Dekker, New York, NY, 1st ed., 2002, pp. 43–56.
- L.H. Block, Scale Up of Liquid and Semisolid Manufacturing Processes, Pharmaceutical Technology scaling up manufacturing, 2005. S26–S33.
- S. Hall, M. Cooke, A.W. Pacek, A.J. Kowalski, D. Rothman. Scaling up of Silverson rotor-stator mixers, *The Canadian Journal of Chemical Engineering*, 89 (2011), 1040–1050.
- A. Mukharya, P. Patel, D. Shinoy, S. Choudhary. Quality risk management of top spray fluidized bed process for antihypertensive drug formulation with control strategy engendered by Box-Behnken experimental design space. *Int. J. Pharm. Investig.*, 3(2013), 15–28.

17

Controlled and Novel Drug Delivery Systems

Manoj Nahar and N.K. Jain

FUNDAMENTALS OF CONTROLLED DRUG DELIVERY

Controlled and novel drug delivery systems aim at optimization of drug delivery meaning that the therapeutic efficacy of a drug is maximized while its toxicity (side and/or undesirable effects) is minimized and yet the delivery system is available at an affordable cost. The newer drug delivery systems are being investigated so as to alter the body distribution of drug(s) with a view to reduce the toxicity of drug and/or deliver them more efficiently to their site of action. There are a number of reasons for the intense interest in development of such novel drug delivery systems.

1. Possibility of repatenting existing drug(s) by applying the concepts and techniques of controlled drug delivery, coupled with almost prohibitively high cost of bringing new drug entities to market.
2. New systems are needed to deliver peptides, pharmacogenomics, hormones, vaccines and other proteins to their specific sites of action without incurring significant immunogenicity or biological inactivation.
3. Therapeutic efficacy and safety profile of drugs can be improved by more precise spatial and temporal placement within the body compartment, thereby reducing both the quantity and number of doses.
4. There is urgent need to develop such delivery systems for anticancer drugs, which are inherently highly toxic, so as to improve their therapeutic efficacy and side effects to a greater extent.

However, in generalized way the controlled release systems are intended to exercise control on drug release in the body, whether this be of a temporal or spatial nature or both. In other words, the system attempts to regulate drug concentrations within the tissue or cells. Such system provides the constant drug concentration in plasma after single dose administration in comparison with conventional dosage form where peak and valley type plasma concentration results after repeated dosing (Fig. 17.1).

The controlled delivery attempts to achieve the following:

1. Sustain drug action at predetermined rate by maintaining a relatively constant, effective drug level in the body with concomitant minimization of undesirable side effects associated with a saw-tooth kinetic pattern.

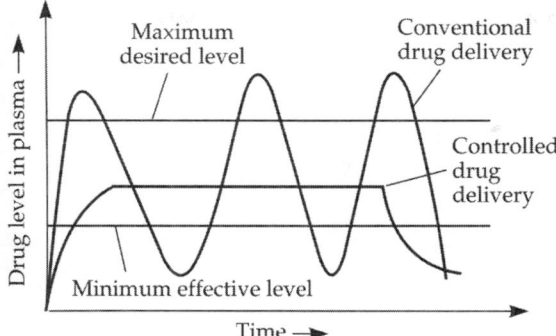

Fig. 17.1. Representative plot of controlled and conventional drug delivery.

2. Localize drug action by spatial placement of a controlled release system (usually rate controlled) adjacent to or in the diseased tissue or organ.
3. Target drug action by using carriers or chemical derivatives to deliver the drug to a particular target cell type.
4. Provide a physiologically/therapeutically based drug delivery system. The amount and the rate of drug release are determined by the physiological/therapeutic needs of the body.

Idealistically, to maintain a constant drug level in either plasma or target tissue, release rate from a controlled release system should be equal to the elimination rate from plasma or target tissue. The basic rationale for controlled drug delivery is to alter the pharmacokinetics and pharmacodynamics of therapeutically active moieties by using either polymer or by modifying parameters inherent in a selected route of administration. Recently, several technical advancements have been made. They have resulted in the development of new techniques for drug delivery. These techniques are capable of controlling the rate of drug delivery, sustaining the duration of therapeutic activity, and/or targeting the delivery of drug to a tissue. The term **sustained release** is known to have existed in the medical and pharmaceutical literature for many decades. It has been constantly used to describe a pharmaceutical dosage form formulated to retard the release of a therapeutic agent such that its appearance in the systemic circulation is delayed and/or prolonged and its plasma profile is sustained in duration. The onset of its pharmacologic action is often delayed, and the duration of its therapeutic effect is sustained. The term **controlled release** implies a predictability and reproducibility in the drug release kinetics, which means that the release of drug from a controlled-release drug delivery system proceeds at a rate profile that is not only predictable kinetically, but also reproducible from one unit to another.

Classification of modified-release delivery systems

A. **Delayed release systems** are those that use repetitive, intermittent dosing of a drug from one or more immediate-release units incorporated into a single dosage form e.g. delayed-release systems include repeat action tablets/capsules, enteric-coated tablets- where timed release is achieved by a carrier coating

B. **Sustained release systems** include any drug delivery system that achieves slow release of drug over an extended period of time. If the systems can provide some control, whether this be of a temporal or spatial nature, or both, of drug release in the body, or, in other words, the system is successful at maintaining constant drug levels in the organs tissue or cells, it is considered a controlled-release system.

C. **Site-specific and receptor targeting** refer to targeting of a drug directly to a certain biological location. In the case of site-specific release, the target is adjacent to or in the diseased organ or tissue for receptor release; the target is the particular receptor for a drug within an organ or tissue. Both of these systems satisfy the spatial aspect of drug delivery and are also considered as controlled drug delivery systems.

Advantages and disadvantages of controlled drug delivery

Advantages

1. Employ less total drug, optimize therapy and improve patient compliance.
2. Minimize or eliminate local side effects, systemic side effects and drug accumulation with chronic dosing.
3. Obtain less potentiation or reduction in drug activity with chronic use.
4. Improve control of condition i.e. reduce fluctuation in drug level; improve bio-availability and treatment efficiency of some drugs.
5. Make use of special effects, e.g. sustained-release aspirin for morning relief of arthritis by dosing before.
6. Maintenance of optimum therapeutic drug concentration in the blood with minimum fluctuations.
7. Predictable and reproducible release rates for extended duration.
8. Enhancement of activity duration for short half-life drugs.
9. Elimination of frequent dosing and wastage of drug, inconvenience of night time administration of drug.
10. Reduction of the incidences and degree of toxic and side effects and irritation of GI tract caused by some orally administrated drugs.
11. Cure or control condition more promptly.
12. Economy.

Disadvantages

1. Removal of the drug product from the system is difficult in case of adverse effects or toxicity.
2. Failure of the dosage form might lead to dose dumping and toxicity.
3. Drugs having a very high dose (>500 mg) cannot be formulated into controlled release products.

Factors influencing the design and performance of sustained or controlled release products

Drug properties

The physicochemical properties of a drug include stability, solubility, partitioning characteristics, charge and protein binding; these play a dominant role in the design and performance of controlled release systems. The design of controlled-release delivery systems is subject to several variables of considerable importance. These include the route of drug delivery, the type of delivery system, the disease being treated, the patient, the length of therapy, and the properties of the drug. Each of these variables is inter-related, and this imposes certain constraints upon choices for the route of delivery, the design of the delivery system, and the length of therapy.

The biological properties of a drug are a function of its physicochemical properties. Those attributes that can be determined from *in vitro* experiments can be considered physicochemical properties. Biological properties include those that result from typical pharmacokinetic studies on the absorption, distribution, metabolism and excretion (ADME) characteristics of a drug as well as those resulting from pharmacological studies.

Physicochemical properties

A. Partition coefficient

Ideally, the release of an ionizable drug from a controlled-release system should be programmed in accordance with the variation in pH of the different segments of the GI tract so that the amount of preferentially absorbed species, and thus the plasma level of drug, will be approximately constant throughout the time course of drug action.

Between the time that a drug is administered and the time it is eliminated from the body, it must diffuse through a variety of biological membranes that act primarily as a lipid-like barrier. A major criterion in evaluation of the ability of a drug to penetrate these lipid membranes is its apparent oil/water partition coefficient (*K*), defined as

$$K = C_0/C_w \qquad \ldots 17.1$$

where C_0 is the equilibrium concentration of all forms of the drug, e.g., ionized and un-ionized, in an organic phase at equilibrium, and C_w is the equilibrium concentration of all forms in an aqueous phase. In general, drugs with extremely large values of *K* are very oil-soluble and will partition into membranes quite readily. The relationship between tissue permeation and partition coefficient for the drug generally is known as the **Hansch correlation**. It describes a parabolic relationship between the logarithm of the activity of a drug or its ability to be absorbed. The more effectively a drug crosses membranes, the greater its activity.

B. Drug stability

Drug stability of importance for oral dosage forms is the loss of drug through acid hydrolysis and/or metabolism in the GI tract. Since a drug in the solid state undergoes degradation at a much slower rate than a drug in suspension or solution, it would seem possible to improve significantly the relative bioavailability of a drug that is unstable in the GI tract by placing it in a slowly available controlled-release form. For those drugs that are unstable in the stomach, the most appropriate controlling unit would be one that releases its contents only in the intestine.

C. Protein binding

Distribution of a drug into the extravascular space is governed by the equilibrium process of dissociation of the drug from the protein. The drug-protein complex can serve therefore as a reservoir in the vascular space for controlled drug release to extravascular tissues, but only for those drugs that exhibit a high degree of binding. Thus the protein-binding characteristics of a drug can play a significant role in its therapeutic effect, regardless of the type of dosage form. Extensive binding to plasma proteins will be evidenced by a long half-life of elimination for the drug, and

such drugs generally do not require a controlled-release dosage form. However, drugs that exhibit a high degree of binding to plasma proteins also might bind to biopolymers in the GI tract, which could have an influence on controlled-drug delivery.

The main forces of attraction responsible for binding are van der Waals forces, hydrogen bonding, and electrostatic forces. In general, charged compounds have a greater tendency to bind a protein than uncharged compounds, because of electrostatic effects. The presence of a hydrophobic moiety on the drug molecule also increases its binding potential.

D. Molecular size and diffusivity

A drug must diffuse through a variety of biological membranes during its time course in the body. In addition to diffusion through these biological membranes, drugs in many controlled-release systems must diffuse through a rate controlling membrane or matrix. The ability of a drug to diffuse through membranes, its so-called diffusivity (diffusion coefficient), is a function of its molecular size (or molecular weight).

Biological properties

A. Absorption

The rate, extent, and uniformity of absorption of a drug are important factors when considering its formulation into a controlled-release system. Since the rate-limiting step in drug delivery from a controlled-release system is its release from a dosage form, rather than absorption, a rapid rate of absorption of the drug relative to its release is essential if the system is to be successful. This becomes most critical in the case of oral administration. Slowly absorbed drugs will be difficult to formulate into controlled release systems.

The extent and uniformity of the absorption of a drug, as reflected by its bioavailability and the fraction of the total dose absorbed, may be quite low for a variety of reasons. This is usually not a prohibitive factor in its formulation into a controlled-release system. Some possible reasons for a low extent of absorption are poor water solubility, low partition coefficient, acid hydrolysis and metabolism, or site-specific absorption. The latter reason is also responsible for non-uniformity of absorption. Many of these problems can be overcome by an appropriately designed controlled-release system, as exemplified by the discussion under advantages of controlled drug therapy.

The distribution of a drug into vascular and extravascular spaces in the body is an important factor in its overall elimination kinetics. This, in turn, influences the formulation of that drug into a controlled-release system, primarily by restricting the immediate elimination of the drug and the dose size that can be employed.

Two parameters that are used to describe the distribution characteristics of a drug are its apparent volume of distribution (V_d) and the ratio of drug concentration in tissue (T) to that in plasma at the steady state (P), known as **T/P ratio**. The apparent volume of distribution is merely a proportionality constant that relates drug *concentration* in the blood or plasma to the total *amount* of drug in the body. The magnitude of the apparent volume of distribution can be used as a guide for additional studies and as a predictor for a drug-dosing regimen and hence the need to employ a controlled-release system. For drugs that obey a one-compartment model, the apparent volume of distribution (V_d) is

$$V_d = dose/C_0 \qquad \ldots 17.2$$

where C_0 is the initial drug concentration immediately after an intravenous bolus injection, but before any drug has been eliminated. The application of this equation is based upon the assumption that the distribution of a drug between plasma and tissues takes place instantaneously.

In the case of a two-compartment model, the apparent volume of distribution at steady state gives the best estimate of total volume of drug distribution

$$V_{ss} = (1 + K_{12}/K_{21}) \, V_1 \qquad \ldots 17.3$$

where V_1 is the volume of the central compartment, K_{12} is the rate constant of distribution of drug from the central to the peripheral compartment, and K_{21} is that from the peripheral to the central compartment. As its name implies, V_{ss} relates drug concentration in the blood or plasma at steady-state to the total amount of drug in the body during repetitive dosing or constant-rate infusion.

B. Metabolism

The metabolic conversion of a drug to another chemical form usually can be considered in the design of a controlled-release system for that drug. As long as the location, rate, and extent of metabolism are known and the rate constant(s) for the process(es) are not too large, successful controlled-release products can be developed.

There are some metabolic factors that present problems for their use in controlled release systems. For example, ability of the drug to induce or inhibit enzyme synthesis; this may result in a fluctuating drug blood level due to intestinal (or other tissue) metabolism or through a hepatic first pass effect.

C. Elimination and biological half-life

The rate of elimination of a drug is described quantitatively by its biological half-life, $t_{1/2}$. The half-life of a drug is related to its apparent volume of distribution V_d and its systemic clearance:

$$t_{1/2} = 0.693 V_d/Cl_s = 0.693 V_d \, AUC/dose \ldots 17.4$$

The systemic clearance, Cl_s, is equal to the ratio of an intravenously administered dose to the total area under the drug blood level versus time curve (AUC). A drug with a short half-life requires frequent dosing, and this makes it a desirable candidate for a controlled-release formulation. On the other hand, a drug with a long half-life is dosed at greater time intervals, and thus there is less need for a controlled-release system. A drug with a half-life of less than 2 hr probably should not be used, since such systems will require unacceptably large release rates and large doses. At the other extreme, a drug with a half-life greater than 8 hr also probably should not be used.

D. Dose size

Since a controlled-release system is designed to minimize repetitive dosing, it naturally will contain a greater amount of drug than a corresponding conventional form. The typical administered dose of a drug in the conventional dosage forms will give some indication of the total amount needed in the controlled-release preparation. For those drugs requiring large conventional doses, the volume of the sustained dose may be so large as to be impractical or unacceptable, depending on the route of administration. The same may be true of drugs that require a large release rate from the controlled-release system, e.g., drugs with short half-lives. For the oral route, the volume of the product is limited by patient acceptance. For the intramuscular, intravenous, or subcutaneous routes, the limitation is tolerance of the drug at the injection site.

E. Route of drug delivery

The area of the body in which drugs will be applied or administered can be restrictive on the basis of technological achievement of a suitable controlled release mechanism or device. At times, the drug delivery systems, in certain routes of administration, can exert a negative influence on drug efficacy, particularly during chronic administration, and hence other routes of administration should be considered. Performance of the controlled release systems may also be influenced by physiological constraints imposed by the particular route, such as first-pass metabolism, gastrointestinal motility, blood supply and sequestration of small foreign particle by the liver and spleen.

F. Target sites

In order to minimize unwanted side effects, it is desirable to maximize the fraction of applied dose reaching the target organ or tissue. This can be partially achieved by local administration or by the use of carriers. However, the absorptive surfaces of most routes are impermeable to macromolecules or other targeted delivery systems, thereby necessitating either intravascular or intraarterial administration.

G. Acute or chronic therapy

Consideration of whether one expects to achieve cure or control of a condition and the expected length of drug therapy are important factors in designing controlled release systems. Attempts to generate a one-year contraceptive implant present significantly different problems in design than does an antibiotic for acute infection. Moreover, long-term toxicity of rate controlled drug delivery systems is usually different from that of conventional dosage forms.

H. The disease

Pathological changes during the course of a disease can play a significant role in the design of a suitable drug delivery system. For example, in attempting to design an ocular controlled-release product for an external inflammation, the time course of changes in protein content in ocular fluids and in the integrity of the ocular barriers would have to be taken into consideration. Sometimes, one can take advantage of the unique manifestations of the disease state. For example, the higher plasmogen activator levels in some tumor cells can lead to preferential bioconversion of peptidyl prodrugs in these cells.

I. The patient

The design of a controlled-release product is influenced if the patient is ambulatory or bedridden, young or old, obese or gaunt, etc. The main objective of any drug delivery system is to provide a therapeutic amount of drug at the proper site in the body to achieve promptly and then maintain the desired drug concentration over a desired period of time. That is, the drug delivery systems should deliver drug at the rate dictated by the needs of the body over a specified period of treatment. This idealized objective points to the two aspects most important to drug delivery, namely, spatial placement and temporal delivery of a drug. **Spatial** placement relates to targeting a drug to a specific organ or tissue, while **temporal** delivery refers to controlling the rate of drug delivery to the target tissue. The term drug blood level refers to the concentration of drug in blood or plasma, but the concentration in any tissue could be plotted on the ordinate. Administration of a drug by either IV injection or an extravascular route, e.g. orally, intramuscularly, or rectally, does not maintain drug blood levels within the therapeutic range for extended period of time. The short duration of action is due to the inability of conventional dosage forms to control temporal delivery. If an attempt is made to maintain drug blood levels in the therapeutic range for longer periods by increasing the initial dose of an IV injection, toxic levels may be produced at early times. An alternative approach is to administer the drug repetitively using a constant dosing interval, as in multiple dose therapy. In this case, the drug blood level and the time required for reaching that level depend on the dose and the dosing interval.

If the dosing interval is not appropriate for the biological half-life of the drug, large peaks and troughs in the drug blood level may result. The drug blood level may not be within the therapeutic range at sufficiently early times, an important consideration for certain disease states. Patient noncompliance with the multiple-dosing regimen can result in failure of this approach.

Basic Kinetics of Controlled Drug Delivery

The influence of drug properties and the route of administration on controlled drug delivery may be better explained with the help of following mechanisms:

- Behavior of drug within its delivery systems, and
- Behavior of the drug and its delivery system together in the body.

The first of the two elements basically deals with the inherent properties of drug molecules, which influence its release from the delivery system. For conventional systems, the rate-limiting step in drug availability is usually absorption of drug across a biological membrane such as the gastrointestinal wall; the process appears, as shown below:

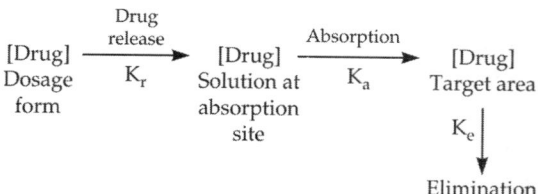

where, K_r, K_a and K_e are release, absorption and elimination rate constants, respectively.

However, in sustained/controlled release product, the release of drug from the dosage form is the rate-limiting step; thus, drug availability is controlled by the kinetics of drug release than by absorption. Consequently, the associated rate constants for drug release from the dosage form are smaller than the absorption rate constant and kinetically the process appears as shown below:

$$[Drug] \text{ Dosage form} \xrightarrow[K_r]{\text{Drug release}} [Drug] \text{ Target area} \xrightarrow{K_e} \text{Elimination}$$

Various approaches, like dissolution, diffusion, swelling, osmotic pressure, complexation, ion exchange and magnetic field can be utilized for preparing a controlled-release system of a drug.

The second element, the behavior of the drug and its delivery system in the body, is extremely complex involving the fate of drug during transit to the target site as well as its fate while in the biomedia. Availability of drug to its target generally will depend almost on its pharmacokinetics as well as the carrier. In case of drug targeting the carrier alters the pharmacokinetics of drug in the body. The influence of physiological constraints on the fate of the delivery system in the body is usually negative, for example oral absorption is usually limited by gastrointestinal transit time of the delivery system.

Oral Controlled Drug Delivery

For controlled-release systems, the oral route of administration has, by far, emerged as the most important. This is because there is more flexibility in dosage form dosing for the oral route than there is for the parenteral route. Patient acceptance of the oral route is quite high. It is relatively safe route of administration, compared with most parenteral routes, and the constraints of sterility and potential damage at the site of administration are minimal. The more common methods used to achieve sustained-release of orally administered drugs are discussed below.

Oral ingestion has long been the most convenient and commonly employed route of drug delivery. Nevertheless, current knowledge on mechanisms of drug absorption, gastrointestinal transit and the microenvironment of the GI tract is still incomplete. Oral administration is also challenged by inherent physiological constraints such as chemical degradation in the stomach, gastric emptying, intestinal motility, mucosal surface area, specific absorption sites and metabolic degradation during passage through the mucosa and subsequently the liver, with inter-subject variability. However, it is perhaps difficult to control these factors, further limiting the design of an oral drug delivery system.

The duration of a drug after oral administration is mainly a function of drug related properties such as rate of absorption and clearance as well as residence time of the delivery systems at absorption site. Gastric emptying is influenced by autonomic, hormonal activity, volume, composition, viscosity, osmolality, pH and temperature of stomach contents as well as by many drugs.

Therapeutic needs addressed by oral controlled release dosage form design

A. Systemic treatment

- Reduction in dosing frequency.
- Maintenance of therapeutic activity for full dosing interval.
- Minimization of systemic side effects, potential for local irritation and first-pass effect.
- Concomitant delivery of agents with complementary therapeutic actions.

B. Local treatment of GI tract

- Maximization of drug availability within the area of the treatment.
- Reduction in dosing frequency.
- Minimization of local irritation, systemic absorption and side effects.
- Concomitant delivery of agents with complementary therapeutic actions.

Design and fabrication of controlled drug delivery systems

The majority of the oral controlled-release systems are either tablets or capsules although a few liquid products are also available. The paucity of liquid sustained-release products is due to the nature of the sustained-release mechanisms employed. Sustained-release tablet and capsule dosage forms usually consist of two parts: an immediately available dose to establish the blood level quickly; and a sustained part that contains several times the therapeutic dose for protracted drug levels.

Several approaches are available to add the immediately available portion to the sustaining part. Simple addition of a non-sustained dose of drug to capsule or tablet is the most direct method; placement of the initial dose in the tablet coat with the sustaining portion in the core represents an alternate approach.

The majority of oral controlled-release systems rely on dissolution, diffusion or a combination of both mechanisms, to generate slow release of drug to the GI tract. Starting with limited data on a drug candidate for sustained release, such as dose, rate constants for absorption and elimination, some elements of metabolism and some physical and chemical properties of the drug, one can estimate a desired release rate for the dosage form, the quantity of drug needed and a preliminary strategy for the dosage form to be utilized.

A. Diffusion systems

In these systems, the release rate of drug is determined by its diffusion through a water-insoluble polymer. There are basically two types of diffusion devices: reservoir devices, in which a core of drug is surrounded by a polymeric membrane, and matrix devices, in which dissolved or dispersed drug is distributed uniformly in an inert polymeric matrix.

1. **Reservoir devices:** The release of drug from a reservoir device is governed by Fick's first law of diffusion

$$J = D \, dC_m/dx \qquad \ldots 17.5$$

where J is the flux of drug across a membrane in the direction of decreasing concentration (amount/area-time), D is the diffusion coefficient of the drug (area/time), and dC_m/dx is the change in concentration of drug in the membrane over a distance x, if it is assumed that the drug on either side of the membrane is in equilibrium with the respective surface layer of the membrane. The schematic of reservoir device is presented in Fig. 17.2.

2. **Matrix devices:** The rate of release of a drug dispersed as a solid in an inert matrix was described by Higuchi as shown in Fig. 17.3. In this model, it is assumed that solid drug dissolves from the surface layer of the device first; when this layer becomes exhausted of drug, the next layer begins to be depleted by dissolution and diffusion through the matrix to the external solution. In this fashion, the interface between the region containing dissolved drug and that containing dispersed drug moves into the interior as a front.

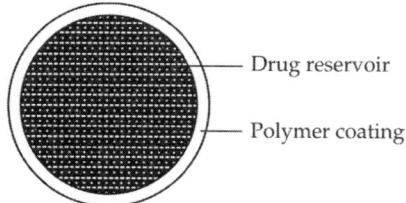

Fig. 17.2. Reservoir device for controlled drug delivery.

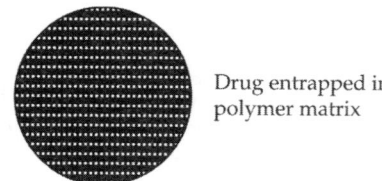

Fig. 17.3. Matrix device for controlled drug delivery.

The matrix types of materials used in the preparation of matrix devices are insoluble plastics, hydrophilic polymers, and fatty compounds. Commonly investigated plastic matrices include methyl acrylate-methyl methacrylate, polyvinyl chloride and polyethylene. An example of a dosage form using a wax matrix is the Lontab tablet (Ciba). The Graduten tablet (Abbott) was an example of a dosage form using a plastic matrix. Hydrophilic polymers include methyl cellulose, hydroxy propylmethyl cellulose, sodium carboxymethyl cellulose, and Carbopol 934. Fatty compounds include various waxes such as carnauba wax and glyceryl tristearate.

The most common method of preparation is to mix the drug with the matrix material and then compress the mixture into tablets. In the case of wax matrices, generally the drug is dispersed in molten wax, which are then congealed, granulated and compressed into cores. In any sustained-release system it is necessary for a portion of a drug to be available immediately as a priming dose and the remainder to release in a sustained fashion. This is easily accomplished in a matrix tablet by placing the priming dose in a coat of the tablet. The coat can be applied by press coating or by conventional pan or air suspension coating.

B. Dissolution systems

A drug with a slow dissolution rate will yield an inherently sustained blood level. Thus, it should be possible to prepare controlled-release products by controlling the dissolution rate of drugs that are highly water-soluble. This can be done by preparing an appropriate salt or derivative, or by coating the drug with a slowly soluble material, or by incorporating it into a tablet with a slowly soluble carrier. Ideally, the surface area available for dissolution must remain constant to achieve a constant release rate.

The dissolution process can be considered diffusion-layer controlled, where the rate of diffusion from the solid surface to the bulk solution through an unstirred liquid film is the rate-determining step. In this case the dissolution process at steady state is described by the Noyes-Whitney equation,

$$dC/dt = K_D A(C_s - C) = (D/h)A(C_s - C) \ldots 17.6$$

where dC/dt is the dissolution rate, K_D is the dissolution rate constant, A is the total surface area, C_s is the saturation solubility of the solid, and C is the concentration of solute in the bulk solution. The dissolution-rate constant, K_D, is equal to the diffusion coefficient (D) divided by the thickness of the diffusion layer thickness (h). However, as dissolution proceeds, all of these parameters, especially surface area, may change. For spherical particles, the change in area can be related to the weight of the particle, and under the assumption of sink conditions most of the products fall into two categories: encapsulated dissolution systems and matrix dissolution systems.

Encapsulated dissolution systems can be prepared either by coating particles or granules of drug with varying thickness of slowly soluble polymers or by microencapsulation. **Micro-encapsulation** can be accomplished by using phase separation, interfacial polymerization, heat-fusion, or the solvent evaporation method. The coating materials may be selected from a wide variety of natural and synthetic polymers, depending on the drug to be coated and the release characteristics desired. The most commonly used coating materials include gelatin, carnauba wax, shellac, ethyl cellulose, cellulose acetate phthalate, or cellulose acetate butyrate. Drug release from microcapsules is a mass-transport phenomenon and can be controlled adjusting the size of microcapsules, thickness of coating materials, and the diffusivity of core materials. The coating of microcapsules is normally very thin, and for a given coat : core ratio, it decreases rapidly as the microcapsule size decreases. The thickness can be varied from less than 1 μm to 200 μm by changing the amount of coating material from 3 to 30% of the total weight. If only a few different thicknesses are used, usually three or four, drugs will be released at different, predetermined times to give delayed release effect, i.e., repeat-action. If a spectrum of different thickness is employed, a more uniform blood level of the drug can be obtained. Microcapsules commonly are filled into capsules and rarely are tabulated, as their coatings tend to disrupt during compression.

Matrix dissolution devices are prepared by compressing the drug with a slowly soluble polymer carrier into a tablet form. There are two general methods of preparing drug particles: congealing and aqueous dispersion methods. In the congealing method, drug mixed with a wax material is either spray-congealed or congealed and screened. In the aqueous dispersion method, the drug-wax mixture is simply sprayed or placed in water, and the resulting particles are collected. Matrix tablets are also made by direct compression of a mixture of drug, polymer, and excipients. A list of controlled and modified release formulations currently available in market is shown in Table 17.1.

Table 17.1. Controlled and modified release formulations currently available in market

Product (Trade Name)	Drug	Type
Entocort EC	Budesonide capsule 3 mg	Controlled-release capsules for colon-specific drug delivery
Cifran OD	Ciprofloxacin tablets 500 mg/1 g	Effervescent matrix type floating tablets
Roliten OD	Tolterodine tartrate extended-release capsules 2/4 mg	Reservoir type controlled-release beads encapsulated in empty gelatin shells
Co-amoxiclav ER tablets	Amoxycillin and potassium clavulanate tablets	Matrix type controlled-release bilayer tablets
Desval ER tablets	Divalproex sodium extended-release tablets 250/500 mg/1 g	Matrix type diffusion and dissolution controlled ER tablets
Contiflo OD	Tamsulosin controlled-release beads	Diffusion and dissolution controlled beads

Classification of rate-controlled drug delivery systems

Based on their technical sophistication controlled-release drug delivery systems, that have recently been marketed, may be classified as:
1. Rate-preprogrammed drug delivery systems
2. Activation-modulated drug delivery systems
3. Feedback-regulated drug delivery systems
4. Site-targeted drug delivery systems

Rate-preprogrammed drug delivery systems

In this group of controlled-release drug delivery systems, the release of drug molecules from the delivery systems has been preprogrammed at specific rate profiles. This was accomplished by system design, which controls the molecular diffusion of drug molecules in and/or across the barrier medium within or surrounding the delivery system.

A. Polymer membrane permeation-controlled drug delivery systems

In this type of preprogrammed drug delivery systems, a drug formulation is totally or partially encapsulated within a drug reservoir compartment. A rate-controlling polymeric membrane having a specific permeability covers its drug release surface. This drug reservoir may exist in solid, suspension, or solution form. The polymeric membrane can be fabricated from a nonporous (homogeneous or heterogeneous) polymeric material or a microporous (or semi-permeable) membrane. Injection molding, spray coating, capsulation, microencapsulation, or other techniques accomplish the encapsulation of drug formulation inside the reservoir compartment. Different shapes and sizes of drug delivery systems can be fabricated.

B. Polymer matrix diffusion-controlled drug delivery systems

In this type of preprogrammed drug delivery system the drug reservoir is prepared by homo-geneously dispersing drug particles in a rate-controlling polymer matrix fabricated from either a lipophilic or a hydrophilic polymer. The drug dispersion in the polymer matrix is accomplished by either (1) blending a therapeutic dose of finely ground drug particles with a liquid polymer or a highly viscous base polymer, foiled by cross-linking of the polymer chains, or (2) mixing drug solids with a rubbery polymer at an elevated temperature. The resultant drug-polymer dispersion is then molded or extruded to form a drug delivery device of various shapes and sizes designed for specific application. It can also be fabricated by dissolving the drug and the polymer in a common solvent, followed by solvent evaporation at an elevated temperature and/or under a vacuum. The release of drug molecules from this type of controlled release drug delivery systems at a preprogrammed rate is controlled by the loading dose, polymer solubility of the drug, and its diffusivity in the polymer matrix.

C. Microreservoir partition-controlled drug delivery systems

In this type of preprogrammed drug delivery systems the drug reservoir is fabricated by micro-dispersion of an aqueous suspension of drug using a high-energy dispersion technique in a biocompatible polymer, such as silicone elasto-mers, to form a homogeneous dispersion of many discrete, unleachable, microscopic drug reservoirs. Different shapes and sizes of drug delivery devices can be fabricated from this microreservoir drug delivery system by molding or extrusion. Depending upon the physico-chemical properties of drugs, and the desired rate of drug release, the device can be further coated with a layer of biocompatible polymer to modify the mechanism and the rate of drug release.

Activation-modulated drug delivery systems

In this group of controlled-release drug delivery systems the release of drug molecules from the delivery system is activated by some physical, chemical, or biochemical processes and/or facilitated by the energy supplied externally. Regulating the process applied or energy input then controls the rate of drug release. Based on the nature of the process applied or the type of energy used, these activation-modulated drug delivery systems (DDS) can be classified into the following categories:

1. Physical means
    A. Osmotic pressure-activated DDS
    B. Hydrodynamic pressure-activated DDS
    C. Vapor pressure-activated DDS
    D. Mechanically activated DDS
    E. Magnetically activated DDS
    F. Sonophoresis-activated DDS
    G. Iontophoresis-activated DDS
    H. Hydration-activated DDS
2. Chemical means
    A. pH-activated DDS
    B. Ion-activated DDS
    C. Hydrolysis-activated DDS
3. Biochemical means
    A. Enzyme-activated DDS
Site-specific or targeted DDS

A. Osmotic pressure-activated DDS

This type of activation-controlled drug delivery system depends on osmotic pressure to activate the release of drug. In this system the drug reservoir, which can be either a solution or a solid formulation, is contained within a semiperme-able housing with controlled water permeability. The drug is activated to release in solution form at a constant rate through a special delivery orifice. Controlling the gradient of osmotic pressure modulates the rate of drug release. The release of drug molecules from this type of controlled-release drug delivery system is activated by osmotic pressure and controlled at a rate determined by the water permeability and the effective surface area of the semipermeable housing as well as the osmotic pressure gradient.

B. Hydrodynamic pressure-activated drug delivery systems

Hydrodynamic pressure has also been explored as the possible source of energy to activate the delivery of therapeutic agents. A hydrodynamic pressure-activated drug delivery system can be fabricated by enclosing a collapsible, imperme-able container, which contains a liquid drug formulation, to form a drug reservoir compart-ment inside rigid shape-retaining housing. A composite laminate of an absorbent layer and swellable, hydrophilic polymer layer is sand-wiched between the drug reservoir compartment and the housing. In the GI tract the laminate absorbs the gastrointestinal fluid through the annular openings at the lower end of the housing and becomes increasingly swollen, which generates hydrodynamic pressure in the system. The hydrodynamic pressure thus created forces the drug reservoir compartment to reduce in volume and causes the liquid drug formulation to release through the delivery orifice at a rate (Q/T) defined by

$$Q/T = P_f A_m / h_m \ (\theta_s - \theta_e) \qquad \ldots 17.7$$

where P_f, A_m and h_m are the fluid permeability, the effective surface area, and the thickness of the wall with annular openings, respectively; and $\theta_s - \theta_e$ is the difference in hydrodynamic pressure between the drug delivery system (θ_s) and the environment (θ_e). The release of drug molecules from this type of controlled-release drug delivery system is activated by hydrodynamic pressure and controlled at a rate determined by the fluid permeability and effective surface area of the wall with annular openings as well as by the hydrodynamic pressure gradient.

C. Vapor pressure-activated drug delivery systems

Vapor pressure has also been employed as a potential energy source to activate the delivery of therapeutic agents. The release of drug from this type of controlled-release drug delivery system is activated by vapor pressure and controlled at a rate determined by the differential vapor pressure, the formulation viscosity and the size of the delivery canula. In this type of drug delivery system the drug reservoir, which also exists as a solution formulation, is contained inside the infusion compartment. It is physically separated from the pumping compartment by a freely movable partition. The pumping compartment contains a fluorocarbon fluid that vaporizes at body temperature at the implantation site and creates a vapor pressure. Under the vapor pressure created the partition moves upward. This forces the drug solution in the infusion compartment to be delivered through a series of flow regulator and delivery canula into the blood circulation at a constant flow rate.

D. Mechanically-activated drug delivery systems

In this type of activation-controlled drug delivery system the drug reservoir is a solution formulation retained in a container equipped with a mechanically activated pumping system. A measured dose of drug formulation is reproducibly delivered into a body cavity, for example the nose, through the spray head, upon manual activation of the drug delivery pumping system. The volume of solution delivered is controllable, as small as 10-100 µl, and is independent of the force and duration of activation applied as well as the solution volume in the container.

E. Magnetically-activated drug delivery systems

In this type of activation-controlled drug delivery system the drug reservoir is a dispersion of peptide or protein powders in a polymer matrix from which macromolecular drug can be delivered only at a relatively slow rate. The flow rate of delivery can be improved by incorporating an electromagnetically triggered vibration mechanism into the polymeric delivery device. Combined with a hemispherical design, a zero-order drug delivery profile is achieved. A sub-dermally implantable, magnetically activated drug delivery device is fabricated by first positioning a tiny magnet ring in the core of a hemispherical drug-dispersing polymer matrix and then coating its external surface with a drug-impermeable polymer, such as ethylene-vinyl acetate copolymer or silicone elastomers, except cavity at the centre of the flat surface. This uncoated cavity is positioned directly above the magnet ring, which permits a peptide drug to be released.

F. Sonophoresis-activated drug delivery systems

This type of activation-controlled drug delivery system utilizes ultrasonic energy to activate or trigger the delivery of drug from a polymeric drug delivery device. The system can be fabricated from either a non-degradable polymer, such as ethylene-vinyl acetate copolymer, or a bioerodible polymer, such as poly[bis(p-carboxyphenoxy)alkane anhydride].

G. Iontophoresis-activated drug delivery systems

This type of activation-controlled drug delivery system uses electrical current to activate and modulate the diffusion of a charged drug molecule across a biological membrane, like the skin, in a manner similar to passive diffusion under a concentration gradient, but at a much facilitated rate. A typical example of this type of activation-controlled drug delivery system is the development of an iontophoretic drug delivery system to facilitate the percutaneous penetration of anti-inflammatory drugs, such as dexamethasone. Further development of the iontophoretic-activated drug delivery technique has recently yielded a new design of iontophoretic drug delivery system, the transdermal periodic ion therapeutic system. This new system is capable of delivering a physiologically acceptable pulsed direct current in a periodic manner with a special combination of waveform, intensity frequency, and on/off ratio, for programmed duration. It has significantly improved the efficiency of transdermal delivery of peptides and protein drugs.

H. Hydration-activated drug delivery systems

This type of activation-controlled drug delivery system depends on the hydration-induced swelling process to activate the release of drug. In this system the drug reservoir is homogeneously dispersed in a swellable polymer matrix fabricated from a hydrophilic polymer. The release of drug is controlled by the rate of swelling of the polymer matrix. The Syncro-mate B implant is fabricated by dissolving norgesterol, a potent progestin, in the alcoholic solution of a linear ethylene glycomethacrylate polymer, Hydron S. The polymer chain is then cross-linked with ethylene dimethacrylate, a cross-

linking agent, to form a solid cylindrical drug-dispersed Hydron implant.

I. pH-dependent formulations

The variable nature of chemical environment throughout the length of the GI tract is a further constraint on dosage form design. Indeed, drug administered orally would encounter a spectrum of pH ranging from 7 in the mouth, 1 to 4 in the stomach, and 5 to 7 in the small intestine. Most of the drugs being weak acids or weak bases, their release from sustained-release formulation is pH-dependent.

J. Altered density formulations

These types of formulations are designed for controlled release of drug on the basis of relationship between density of formulation and GI transit time. The approach is to alter the formulation's density by using either high or low-density pellets.

High-density approach: The density of the pellets much exceeds that of normal stomach content and should therefore be at least 1.4. The drug can be coated on a heavy core or mixed with heavy inert material such as barium sulphate, titanium dioxide, iron powder and zinc oxide. The weighted pellet can then be covered with a diffusion-controlled membrane.

Low-density approach: Globular shells, which have an apparent density lower than that of gastric fluid, can be used as a carrier of drug for sustained-release purposes. The surface of these empty shells is undercoated with sugar or with a polymeric material such as methacrylic polymer and cellulose acetate phthalate. A mixture of drug then coats the undercoated shell with polymers such as ethyl cellulose and hydroxypropyl cellulose. The final product floats on the gastric fluid for a prolonged period, while slowly releasing drug. This principle can be applied to formulate buoyant tablets or capsules.

K. Ion-activated DDS

In this system, drug release characteristics rely only on the ionic environment of the resin-containing drug and should therefore be less susceptible to environmental conditions, such as enzyme content and pH, at the site of absorption. The subcutaneous and intramuscular routes, where the pool of available ions is more controlled, would appear better suited for the approach.

When a high concentration of an appropriately charged ion is in contact with the ion-exchange group, the drug molecule is exchanged and diffuses out of the resin to the bulk solution according to the following scheme:

$$\text{Resin } [N(CH_3)]^+ X^- + Z^- \rightarrow$$
$$\text{Resin } [N(CH_3)]^+ Z + X^- \quad \dots 17.8$$

or,

$$\text{Resin } [SO_3^-] A^+ + B^+ \rightarrow$$
$$\text{Resin } (SO_3^-) B^+ + A^+ \quad \dots 17.9$$

where, X^- and A^+ are drug ions.

L. Hydrolysis-activated DDS

In this system, drug delivery system made up of polymer that can deliver the drug upon hydrolysis of the polymer. This hydrolysis leads to the polymer degradation and subsequent drug delivery from polymer matrix, e.g., polyanhydrides (poly lactide-co-glycolide) based microspheres.

M. Enzyme activated DDS

In this type, drug delivery system is made up of polymer, which can be degraded by the enzymes present in biological system (e.g. guar gum based dosage form, which can deliver the drug specifically at colon site). Moreover some enzymes which make the drug delivery system sensitive to the molecules present in biological systems (e.g. glucose oxidase enzyme loaded insulin system, which is sensitive to blood glucose level) are incorporated.

N. Site-specific or targeted DDS

The rationale of site-specific targeted delivery may be appreciated as a set of desirable events including an exclusive delivery to specific compartments with maximal potential intrinsic activity of drugs and concomitantly reduced access of drug to irrelevant non-target cells. The targeted delivery to previously inaccessible domains, e.g. intracellular sites, virus, bacteria and parasites offer distinctive therapeutic potential. The controlled rate and mode of drug delivery of pharmacological receptor and specific binding with target cells as well as bioenvironmental protection of the drug en route to the site of action are specific features of targeting. Invariably every event stated leads to higher drug concentration at the site of action combined with lower concentration of non-target tissue where toxicity might occur. The high concentration in the target site is a result of the relative cellular uptake of the drug vehicle, thus minimizing toxic effects and maximizing therapeutic index.

CONTROLLED AND NOVEL DRUG DELIVERY SYSTEMS

Novel controlled drug systems also known as Novel Drug Delivery Systems (NDDS) include any drug delivery system that tends to alter the release of the drug, rate or site of absorption of the drug or delivers the drug at its site of action. Table 17.2 describes the market status of some approved novel delivery systems. These systems are broadly categorized as described below:

Osmotic drug delivery

Numerous technologies have been used to control the systemic delivery of drugs. One of the most interesting employs osmotic pressure as a source of energy. Osmotic pressure has been used extensively in the fabrication of drug delivery systems.

Osmotic pressure created due to imbibition of fluid from external environment regulates the delivery of drug from the osmotic device. There are various factors that govern a particular pattern of drug delivery like nature and surface area of semipermeable membrane, diameter of

Table 17.2. Market status of some approved novel delivery systems

Delivery systems	Product	Candidate bioactive/Description	Indication	Market Status
Polymer micelles	NK911	PEG-aspartic acid-doxorubicin micelle	Cancer	Phase I
Liposome	Daunoxome®	Daunorubicin	Cancer	Market
	Doxil®/Caelyx®	Daunorubicin	Cancer	Market
	AmBisome®	Amphotericin	Fungal infections	Market
Nanoparticles	Endorem®	Superparamagnetic iron oxide nanoparticles	MRI agent	Market
	Abraxane®	Albumin nanoparticles containing paclitaxel	Breast cancer	Market
	Nanoss®	Engineered calcium phosphate microparticles	Composition and performance of human bone	Market
Dendrimer	Gadomer®	Dendrimer-based MRI agent (Gd-DTPA Dimeglumine)	MRI agent	Market
Microparticles	Lupron Depot	Leuprolide acetate	Prostate cancer	Market
	Sandostatin LAR	Octreotide acetate	Prostate cancer	Market
	Nutropin Depot	Somatropin	Hormone therapy	Market
	Trelstar Depot	Triptorelin	Prostate cancer	Market
	Risperdal consta	Risperidone	Schizophrenia	Market
Implant products	Ozurdex	Dexamethasone	Macular edema	Market
Long-acting injectable suspension	Zoladex	Octreotide acetate	Prostate cancer	Market
	Viadur	Leuprolide	Prostate cancer	Market
	Invega Sustenna	Paliperiodone palmitate	Schizophrenia	Market
	Zyprexa relprevv	Olanzapine	Schizophrenia	Market
	Depo-Provera	Medroxyprogesterone acetate	Hormone therapy	Market

delivery orifice, pH and electrolyte concentration in external fluid, nature and concentration of osmotic agent, etc.

Apart from general advantage of controlled drug delivery system, osmotic drug delivery systems have some unique advantages such as drug release from osmotic pump is independent of the gastric pH and hydrodynamic conditions of the body. Higher release rates are possible from osmotic systems than with conventional diffusion-based drug delivery systems. Delivery of drug from osmotic pumps can be designed to follow true zero-order kinetics. The delivery rate of drug(s) from these systems is highly predict-

able and programmable by modulating the release control parameters. A high degree of *in vitro/in vivo* correlation can be obtained from osmotic pumps. Drug release from the osmotic systems is minimally affected by the presence of food. Further, osmotic pumps are inexpensive and their production scale-up is easy. A wide spectrum of osmotic devices is in existence; out of them osmotic pump is unique, dynamic and widely employed in practice. However, their wide utility is concealed by some serious drawbacks like toxicity due to dose dumping, rapid development of tolerance, additional patient education and counselling requirement, hypersensitivity reaction occurrence after implantation and stability problems. Nevertheless these drawbacks are overpowered by more potential merits that make osmotic pumps reliable controlled drug delivery systems with reproducible results. Several different types of osmotic pumps are already available in the market and this proves their therapeutic efficacy.

This system is fabricated by applying a semipermeable membrane around a core of an osmotically active drug or a core of an osmotically inactive drug in combination with an osmotically active salt. A delivery orifice is drilled in each system by laser or by a high-speed mechanical drill.

In principle, this delivery system dispenses drug continuously at a zero order rate until the concentration of the osmotically active salt in the system falls below saturation solubility, whereupon a non-zero order release pattern results.

Elementary osmotic pump

Elementary osmotic pump invented by Theeuwes in 1974 essentially contains an active agent having a suitable osmotic pressure, formed into a tablet coated with semipermeable membrane, usually cellulose acetate. A small orifice is drilled through the membrane coating. This pump eliminates the separate salt chamber unlike in earlier versions of osmotic pump (Fig. 17.4).

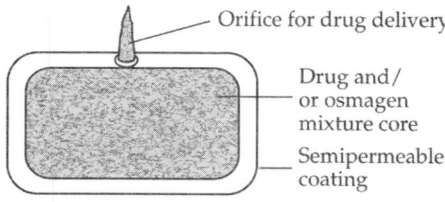

Fig. 17.4. Elementary osmotic pump.

The device, in fact, represents a coated tablet with a hole and perhaps represents ultimate simplification of the original Rose-Nelson pump. When this coated tablet is exposed to an aqueous environment, the osmotic pressure of the soluble drug inside the tablet draws water through the semipermeable coating, resulting in the formation of a saturated aqueous solution inside the device. The membrane is non-extensible and the increase in volume due to imbibition of water raises the hydrostatic pressure inside the tablet, eventually leading to flow of saturated solution of active agent out of the device through small orifice. Solubility of drug in water plays a critical role in functioning of osmotic pump. Typically the solubility of drug delivered by these pumps is at least 10 to 15% w/w. Example of drugs with this property are indomethacin sodium, potassium chloride, metoprolol and acetazolamide.

Alza Corporation is the leading manufacturer, which developed the elementary osmotic pump under the trade name OROS®, for oral controlled release.

Several coated tablets, otherwise called as controlled porosity osmotic pumps, have been reported in which pores are formed following leaching of water soluble components, such as lactose or polyethylene glycol from the coating material and drug release occurs through the pores. Once the tablet has been swallowed, water-soluble component dissolves in external fluid, resulting in initiation of pumping system.

Push-pull osmotic pumps

Pumps with two chambers separated by an elastic or movable barrier are particularly interesting and valuable because they allow delivery of drugs with limited solubility. This class of osmotic pumps can further be classified into two groups, one with internal film that moves from a rest to an expanded state leading to change in volume of chamber while the second group has fixed volume chamber communicating through opening provided in between (Fig. 17.5).

In this system, water is simultaneously drawn into both the chambers proportionate to the osmotic gradient, eventually causing the increase in volume of the osmotic agent chamber and

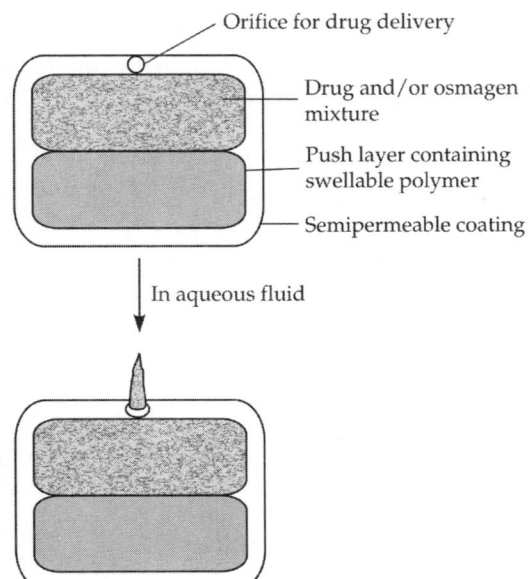

Orifice for drug delivery

Drug and/or osmagen mixture

Push layer containing swellable polymer

Semipermeable coating

In aqueous fluid

Fig. 17.5. Push-pull osmotic system.

subsequently forcing the drug out from the drug chamber. In these devices, the semipermeable membrane forms the entire shell, and water is drawn simultaneously into both the chambers. The matrix should have a sufficient osmotic pressure to draw water through the membrane into the drug chamber. Under hydrated conditions matrix has to be fluid enough to be pushed easily through a small hole by the little pressure generated by the elastic diaphragm.

Among the successful approaches, incorporation of finely dispersed drug in hydrogel presents a most valuable alternative. Many of the useful hydrogel polymers are ionic materials such as sodium carboxymethyl cellulose, which contains ionizable groups that provide most of the osmotic pressure required to draw water through the semipermeable membrane. Some FDA approved osmotic drug delivery systems, which work on either push-pull or elementary osmotic pump, are listed in Table 17.3.

Gastroretentive drug delivery

Over the past three decades there has been a tremendous advance in devices designed to be retained in the upper part of the GI tract consistently in terms of technology and diversity, encompassing a variety of systems and devices exemplified by floating systems, raft systems, expanding systems, swelling systems, bioadhesive systems and low-density systems.

Gastric retention provides advantages such as the delivery of drug(s) with narrow absorption windows in the small intestinal region. Also, longer residence time in the stomach could be advantageous for local action in the upper part of the small intestine, for example treatment of peptic ulcer disease. Furthermore, improved bioavailability is expected for drugs that are absorbed readily upon release in the GI tract.

Table 17.3. Some FDA approved osmotic delivery systems in market

Product Name	Chemical	Indication	Company Name
Calan SR	Verapamil	Hypertension	Alza/GD Searle & Co., Division of Pfizer, Inc., USA
Alpress LP	Prazosin	Hypertension	Alza/Pfizer (France)
Cardura XL	Doxazosin mesylate	Hypertension	Alza/Pfizer (Germany)
Teczem	Enalapril and Diltiazem	Hypertension	Merck/Aventis (USA)
Minipress XL	Prazosin	Hypertension	Alza/Pfizer (USA)
Procardia XL	Nifedipine	Hypertension/angina	Alza/Pfizer (USA)
DynaCirc CR	Isradipine	Hypertension	Alza/Novartis (USA)
Glucotrol XL	Glipizide	Anti-diabetic	Alza/Pfizer (USA)
Acutrim	Phenylpropanolamine	Appetite suppression	Alza/Heritage (USA)

These drugs can be delivered ideally by slow release from the stomach.

Many drugs categorized as once-a-day delivery have been demonstrated to have suboptimal absorption due to dependence on the transit time of the dosage form, making traditional extended release development challenging. Therefore, a system designed for longer gastric retention will extend the time within which drug absorption can occur in the small intestine. There are certain situations where gastric retention is not desirable. Aspirin and non-steroidal anti-inflammatory drugs are known to cause gastric lesions, and slow release of such drugs in the stomach is undesirable. Thus, drugs that may irritate the stomach lining or are unstable in its acidic environment should not be formulated in gastroretentive systems. Furthermore, other drugs, such as isosorbide dinitrate, that are absorbed equally well throughout the GI tract will not benefit from incorporation into a gastric retention system. The potential drug candidates for gastroretentive devices include:

1. Drugs absorbed rapidly from the GI tract.
2. Drugs with a narrow window of absorption.
3. Drugs acting locally in the stomach.
4. Drugs that are primarily absorbed in the stomach.
5. Drugs that are poorly soluble at an alkaline pH.
6. Drugs that degrade in the colon.

A list of various types of colon drug delivery systems is summarized in Table 17.4.

Requirements for gastric retention

To achieve gastric retention, the dosage form must satisfy certain requirements. One of the key issues is that the dosage form must be able to withstand the forces caused by peristaltic waves in the stomach and the constant contractions and grinding and churning mechanisms. To function as a gastric retention device, it must resist premature gastric emptying. Furthermore, once its purpose has been served, the device should be easily eliminated from the stomach.

Approaches to gastric retention

Various approaches have been followed to encourage gastric retention of an oral dosage form. Floating systems have low bulk density so that they can float on the gastric juice in the stomach. The problem arises when the stomach is completely emptied of gastric fluid, a situation where there is nothing to float on. Floating systems can be based on the following:

1. Hydrodynamically balanced systems (HBS): In which buoyant materials are incorporated and enable the device to float.
2. Low-density systems have a density lower than that of the gastric fluid so they are buoyant.

Table 17.4. Different types of colon drug delivery systems

Type of system	Mechanism
Microbially-controlled delivery system	Degradation and fermentation of polysaccharides to component monomers in the presence of enzymes produced by various colonic microbial species.
Timed-release systems	Transit time through the small intestine is relatively constant. Delivery systems, which release drug at a predetermined time, can be used to provide colon delivery.
pH-dependent delayed release system	pH-dependent enteric-coated systems. Site of disintegration depends on the rate of intestinal transit and the amount of coating polymer employed.
Prodrugs	Active drug is cleaved from the carrier molecules via the action of microbial enzymes or the redox potential of the colon.
Redox-sensitive polymers	Azo-polymer and disulphide polymers, which selectively respond to the redox potential of the colon.

3. Effervescent systems: Gas-generating materials such as carbonates are incorporated. These materials react with gastric acid and produce carbon dioxide, which allows them to float.
4. Bioadhesive or mucoadhesive systems: These systems permit a given drug delivery system (DDS) to be incorporated with bio/mucoadhesive agents, enabling the device to adhere to the stomach (or other GI) walls, thus resisting gastric emptying. However, the mucus on the walls of the stomach is in a state of constant renewal, resulting in unpredictable adherence.
5. Raft systems incorporating alginate gels: These have a carbonate component and, upon reaction with gastric acid, bubbles form in the gel, enabling floating.

The stomach is a size-filtering system and so it would seem ideally suited to retaining a DDS that is larger than the pylorus. The drawback is that the DDS is not small enough to be taken orally if sizes larger than the pylorus are required. Several systems have been investigated to encourage gastric retention using increasing size of DDS. Systems have been based on expansion due to gases and swelling due to intake of external liquids.

A. The use of passage-delaying excipients

The use of passage-delaying excipients has been proposed as an attempt to develop a form that exerts some influence on its own transit. Preliminary *in vivo* results depict a major problem related to the highly variable inter-subject reactions. Another analogous approach consists of using passage-delaying drugs, for example propantheline, which is generally considered undesirable because of potential side effects.

B. Heavy pellets

The use of dosage forms of high density that might remain in the stomach longer when positioned in the lower part of the antrum has been proposed as a means to increase the GI transit duration.

There may be a threshold density in the order of 2.4–2.6 g/cm^3, above which gastric and small intestine residence times of pellets are prolonged. This threshold value is much higher than density values used in previous studies (~ 1.5 g/cm^3).

If these results are confirmed by clinical studies, the technical difficulty will be the formulation of real pellets containing significant amounts of drug and with a density greater than 2.6 g/cm^3. Barium sulphate can be used as a diluent (density $= 4.9$ g/cm^3).

C. The use of large single unit forms

Delivery devices have been prepared in such a way that their size increases after ingestion to such an extent that gastric emptying is totally inhibited, even when the pyloric sphincter is in its non-contracted state. Unfolding stratified medicated polymer sheets or swelling balloon hydrogels are examples of such delivery systems.

Erodible gastric retention devices fabricated from various polymeric blends were also examined for assessment of their gastric retention potential. The passage of much smaller conventional single units can already be impeded in patients with narrow gastroduodenal lumen. This might lead to serious life-threatening effects if multiple dosing is prescribed.

D. Bioadhesive drug delivery systems

The original concept of bioadhesive polymers as platforms for oral controlled drug delivery was to use these polymers to control and to prolong the GI transit of oral controlled delivery systems for all kinds of drugs. Such systems however have failed to show any clinical outcome. Several *in vitro* and *ex vivo* methods to test the bioadhesive properties of polymers and/or of coated microparticles have been described.

E. Floating dosage forms

The floating sustained-release dosage forms present most of the characteristics of hydrophilic matrices and are known as **hydrodynamically**

balanced systems (HBS) since they are able to maintain their low apparent density while the polymer hydrates and builds a gelled barrier at the outer surface. The drug is released progressively from the swollen matrix, as in the case of conventional hydrophilic matrices. These forms are expected to remain buoyant for 3 to 4 hr on the gastric contents without affecting the intrinsic rate of emptying because their bulk density is lower than that of the gastric contents. The validity of the concept of buoyancy in terms of prolonged GRT of the floating forms, improved bioavailability of drugs and improved clinical situations is already demonstrated. These results also demonstrate that the presence of gastric content is needed to allow the proper achievement of the buoyancy retention principle (for example Prolopa® HBS hard gelatin capsules).

Among the different hydrocolloids recommended for floating formulations, cellulose ether polymers are most popular, especially hydroxypropylmethyl cellulose. Fatty material with a bulk density lower than one may be added to the formulation to decrease the water intake rate and increase buoyancy.

When a floating capsule is administered to the subjects with a fat and protein meal, it can be observed that it remains buoyant at the surface of the gastric content in the upper part of the stomach and moves down progressively while the meal empties. The reported gastric retention times range from 4 to 10 hours.

Marketed Gastric-Retention Technologies

There are a few companies that have focused efforts on the design of gastric-retention technologies. The fact that these companies are working on such platform devices highlights the need for gastric retention to improve delivery of successful 24-hour release dosage forms considering the effects of transit time. Merck & Co., Inc., has patents describing technologies using various unfolding shapes to encourage gastric retention.

Madopar® is an HBS floating system that contains 200 mg levodopa and 50 mg benserazide. The formulation consists of a capsule designed to float on the stomach contents. Following dissolution of the gelatin shell, a matrix body is formed consisting of the active drug and other substances. The drug diffuses as successively hydrated boundary layers of the matrix dissipate. Valrelease® is a floating capsule containing diazepam. The formulation is an HBS system, also prolonging gastric retention, and is used as an o.d. dosage form comparable to the previous t.i.d. non-floating dosage form. Gaviscon® preparations designed for the suppression of gastro-oesophageal reflux consist of alginate that gels in the gastric environment due to the carbonate or bicarbonate content. These systems are called 'rafts' as the viscous layer can 'ride' the stomach waves.

Another technology is based on superporous, superabsorbent hydrogels. Superporous hydrogels contain densely concentrated small pores that produce capillary channels that absorb water quickly. This rapid absorption results in dramatic swelling that is much faster than a conventional hydrogel. This expanded hydrogel cannot pass the pylorus for extended period of time and hence retained in the stomach. By modification of the hydrogel synthesis, in terms of monomers, cross-links and other additives and components, the physical/mechanical properties of the super-porous hydrogel can be controlled (Fig. 17.6).

This technology can be envisioned as playing a major role in revolutionizing the future of gastric retention in the pharmaceutical industry.

Multiple emulsion

Multiple emulsion system is a novel development in the field of emulsion technology. It is a polydispersed system where the dispersed phase contains the droplets of the continuous phase. It may be called "emulsion of emulsions", "double or triple emulsions", since the internal phase contains dispersed globules, which are miscible

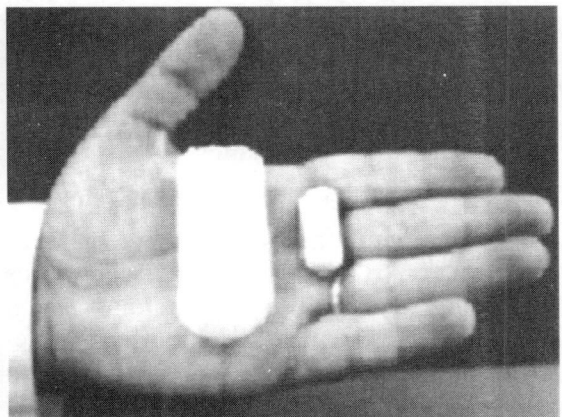

Fig. 17.6. An expandable gastroretentive drug delivery system: A superporous hydrogel in its dry (right) and water-swollen (left) state.

with the continuous phase. This leads to water-in-oil-in-water (w/o/w) or oil-in-water-in-oil (o/w/o) type. Here two miscible phases are separated by an immiscible phase; this phase is sometimes called a **liquid membrane**, which acts as semipermeable membrane through which a solute may diffuse from one phase to another. The nature of liquid membrane may be hydrophilic or hydrophobic, hence in some disciplines, multiple emulsions are also called as liquid membrane systems. These systems are characterized by their low thermodynamic stability.

In most cases, the two aqueous phases are identical and therefore a $w_1/o/w_1$ emulsion is a two component second order system and an $o_1/w/o_2$ emulsion is a three component second order system. In this manner ternary, quaternary and even higher order emulsion can be envisioned. In principle, n order emulsion can be prepared by re-micellization of an $n-1$ phase into another continuous phase. The ability to incorporate liquid crystals into emulsions leads to the development of new multiple phase system encompassing both liquid crystal and multiple emulsion technology. A few commercial preparations of multiple emulsions are available in the market put in trade by Lancaster, Bioderma, Estee Lauder and Rubinstein

Laboratories. These double emulsions are of two types:

In w/o/w type multiple emulsions small water droplets are dispersed in bigger oil droplets and these oil droplets are again dispersed in a continuous aqueous phase. It possesses many of the advantages of w/o emulsions but, in addition, due to the lower viscosity of the aqueous external phase it makes them more convenient to handle and use, especially to inject. In o/w/o type multiple emulsion small oil droplets are dispersed in larger aqueous droplet and these aqueous droplets are again dispersed in a continuous oil phase. The basic rationale for the use of w/o/w and o/w/o type multiple emulsions as a means of prolonged delivery of drugs is that the drug contained in the innermost phase is forced to partition itself through several phases prior to release at the absorption site. Thus, the partition and diffusion coefficient of the drug and the strength of the middle membrane phase, which is a multimolecular layer of oil, water and emulsifier molecules at both the interfaces of multiple emulsion system, control the drug release from these systems.

Methods of preparation

A. Double emulsification method

A two-step procedure is the most common method for preparation of multiple emulsions. In this method, the primary emulsion is prepared in a usual manner in the first step. Re-emulsification of primary emulsion in the second step leads to the formation of multiple emulsion. The w/o or o/w primary emulsion is prepared by employing lipophilic or hydrophilic surfactant, respectively. For the production of w/o/w multiple emulsion, primary w/o emulsion is emulsified in aqueous phase containing hydrophilic surfactant with the aid of stirrer. In case of o/w/o emulsion, o/w primary emulsion is emulsified in second step using a hydrophobic surfactant in oily phase. The second emulsification step is critical, as excess mixing can fracture the drops, resulting in a simple o/w or w/o emulsion. For this reason, high-shear mixers and sonication are usually unsuitable for re-emulsification of primary emulsion.

The phase inversion of the emulsion occurs when the concentration of dispersed globules in the dispersion medium is quite high i.e. the globules are packed very closely in the suspending fluid. The concentrated o/w emulsion is thermally induced to produce w/o/w emulsion in which molar ratio of the hydrophobic and hydrophilic emulsifiers should be optimized.

When an aqueous solution of hydrophilic emulsifier (Tween 80/sodium dodecyl sulphate/cetyl trimethyl ammonium salt) is introduced into an oil containing lipophilic surfactant (Span 80), the w/o/w emulsion is obtained due to phase inversion of w/o emulsion. Phase inversion technique can be exploited to produce emulsion characterized by their fine droplet size.

B. Membrane emulsification technique

In this method a w/o emulsion (dispersed phase) is extruded into an external aqueous phase (continuous phase) with a constant pressure through a porous glass membrane. The particle size of the resulting emulsion can be controlled with proper selection of porous glass membrane as the droplet size depends upon the pore size of the membrane. The relation between membrane pore size and particle size of w/o/w emulsion exhibits good correlation as described by the following equation:

$$y = 5.03x + 0.19 \qquad \ldots 17.10$$

where y is the mean particle size of the multiple emulsion prepared using membrane emulsification technique and x is the pore size.

A modified two step emulsification technique for the preparation of w/o/w emulsion is different from the conventional double emulsification technique in two points: (i) sonication and stirring are used to obtain fine, homogeneous, stable w/o emulsion, and (ii) a continuous phase is poured into a dispersed phase for preparing w/o/w emulsion (in contrast to conventional

method in which a dispersed phase is poured into a continuous phase). Moreover the composition of internal aqueous phase-oil phase-external aqueous phase is fixed at 1 : 4 : 5, which produces more stable w/o/w formulation.

C. Sphere-in-oil-in-water emulsion (s/o/w)

These emulsions are specialized forms of multiple emulsions where microspheres containing the drug form the innermost phase. Such emulsions are made by emulsifying (pre-formed) microspheres with an oil phase to produce a sphere-in-oil emulsion, which is again emulsified with an external aqueous phase to produce s/o/w emulsion.

Routes of administration

Multiple emulsions have been administered by oral, parenteral (i.v., i.p., s.c., i.m.) and topical (nasal, ocular, transdermal) routes. The fate of multiple emulsions after oral and parenteral administration requires insight from the stability and pharmacokinetic point of view. After oral administration, emulsions are absorbed almost entirely through lymphatic pathway in association with intestinal lipoproteins namely chylomicrons, produced by enterocytes. They may directly be absorbed through the intestinal macrophage system and Payer's patches to gain access into mesenteric lymph from where they are drained into circulation through thoracic lymph duct. Thus, they are able to carry bioactive within them avoiding degradation in intestine as well as liver (first pass effect). After parenteral administration, the emulsions are readily taken up by circulatory macrophage system to lymphatics as well as liver into fat metabolism pathway. Through other parenteral routes, the emulsion droplets gain access to nearby lymphatic node through interstitial spaces of lymphatic vessels, which are relatively porous as compared to blood capillaries, which have tight intracellular junctions. Thus, the system has an intrinsic lymphotropic characteristic. Therefore, it is envisaged for the delivery of therapeutic agents for the treatment of cancer metastases and bacterial infections involving lymphatic.

Applications

Multiple emulsions offer interesting advantages as drug delivery system:

1. They protect bioactive from degradation.
2. They are easy to administer via oral, parenteral, nasal, and ocular or any other route.
3. They offer encapsulating compartments for both hydrophilic and lipophilic compounds with very high efficiency.
4. The drug may be encapsulated as solution or suspension.
5. The drug release pattern may be prolonged or controlled.
6. They may be targeted by both passive and active means by surface modification.
7. They utilize pharmaceutically acceptable components, which are non-toxic, non-immunogenic and biocompatible/biodegradable.
8. The components of formulation are economical and manufacturing equipment are easily accessible; there is no special requirement.
9. They are easy to produce and scale-up.

Ion-exchange resins-based drug delivery systems

One of the attractive methods for modified drug delivery systems, preferably controlled type, is ion-exchange resins as carriers for such systems. As drug release characteristics rely on the ionic environment of the resin-containing drug, they are less susceptible to environmental conditions, such as enzyme content and pH at the site of absorption. These systems can satisfactorily achieve zero-order release kinetics in drug delivery pattern. Ion-exchange resins have specific properties like available capacity, acid base strength, particle size, porosity and swelling, on which the release characteristics of drug resonates are dependent. The large pore size, the enormous surface area, the number of exchange sites and their hydrophilic nature are the favorable characteristics, which make the drug and ion-exchange complexes as superior materials for processing certain macromolecules e.g. dextran, polyacrylamide ion-exchange gels. In these favorable surroundings, macromolecules have little tendency to become de-structured. Drug resonates, in general, are prepared with purified resins and appropriate drugs.

Ion-exchange systems are advantageous for drugs that are highly susceptible to degradation by enzymatic processes, since they offer a protective mechanism by temporarily altering the substrate. This approach to sustained release, however, has the limitation that the release rate is proportional to the concentration of the ions present in the area of administration. Although the ionic concentration of the GI tract remains rather constant with limits, the release rate of drug can be affected by variability in diet, water intake and individual intestinal content.

There are two major classes of ion-exchange polymers: cation-exchangers, whose functional groups can undergo reaction with the cations of a surrounding solution; and anion-exchangers, whose functional groups can undergo reaction with the anions of a surrounding solution. A typical cation-exchange resin is prepared by the co-polymerization of styrene and divinylbenzene. During the polymerization reaction, linear chains of polystyrene are formed first and these, in turn, become covalently bonded to each other, at intermittent point, by divinylbenzene cross links; the result is a three-dimensional insoluble hydrocarbon network. If sulfuric acid is then allowed to react with this copolymer, sulfonic acid groups ($-SO_3H^+$) are introduced into most of the benzene rings of the styrene-divinylbenzene polymer, and the final substance formed is a cation-exchange resin. A typical anion-exchange resin is prepared by first chloromethylating the benzene rings of the three-dimensional styrene-divinyl benzene copolymer to attach –CH$_2$Cl groups and then causing these to react with a tertiary amine, such as trimethylamine. This gives the chloride salt of a strong-base exchanger.

The most important step in the preparation of drug resonates is to purify the resins carefully. Purification is generally done by cycling repeatedly between the sodium and hydrogen forms with a cation-exchanger or between the chloride and hydroxide forms in the case of anionic-exchanger. After thoroughly washing with water and subsequent air-drying, the resin is sieved to get a series of fractions.

Loading of drug is done in two ways: (a) column process: a highly concentrated drug solution is eluted through a bed or column of the resin, until equilibrium is established, and (b) batch process: the resin particles are stirred with a large volume of concentrated drug solution.

Drugs that are to be formulated into resonate should satisfy the following conditions:

- Drugs should have acidic or basic groups in their chemical structure.
- The biological half-life should be between 2–6 hr; drugs with $t_{1/2} < 1$ hr or > 8 hr are difficult to formulate into this category.
- The drug is to be absorbed from all regions of the GI tract. In the case of limited absorption zone, the bioavailability will be insufficient.
- Drugs should be sufficiently stable in the gastric juice.

Advantages and applications

Ion-exchange resonates of drugs can help in reducing the dose. Reduced fluctuations in blood and tissue concentrations, fewer administrations and maintenance of drug concentration below toxic level can be achieved. Resinate formulations offer an additional advantage that certain factors influencing the rate of release of drugs from ion-exchange matrixes such as competing ions, ionic strength, pH, etc. are relatively fixed by the conditions within the GI tract. Proper

choice of resin characteristics such as acid or base strength, porosity, degree of cross-linking and particle size can help to accomplish the intended purpose. However, there are quite a few negative factors associated viz., drug accumulation, if the rate of excretion and release are not balanced. In addition, long-acting preparation may not be suitable when short time treatment is needed. Synthetic as well as natural polysaccharides based on ion-exchange resins have been used with good results for diagnostic determinations. They have also found applications as adsorbents of toxins, as antacids, and as bile acid binding agents. Therapeutic applications include the treatment of liver diseases, renal insufficiency, urologic disease and occupational skin diseases.

Transdermal drug delivery

Throughout the past two decades, the transdermal patch has become a proven technology that offers a variety of significant clinical benefits over other dosage forms. Because transdermal drug delivery offers controlled release of the drug into the patient, it enables a steady blood-level profile, resulting in reduced systemic side effects and, sometimes, improved efficacy over other dosage forms. In addition, because transdermal patches are user-friendly, convenient, painless, and offer multi-day dosing, it is generally accepted that they offer improved patient compliance.

Although transdermal drug delivery patches have a relatively short regulatory history compared to other, more traditional dosage forms, the technology has a proven record of FDA approval. Since the first transdermal patch was approved in 1981 to prevent the nausea and vomiting associated with motion sickness, the FDA has approved more than 3 dozen transdermal patch products. The US transdermal market approached $1.2 billion in 2001 and was based on 11 drug molecules. The clinical benefits, industry interest, strong market, and regulatory precedence clearly establish that transdermal drug delivery has become a successful and viable dosage form.

Transdermal patches have been useful in developing new applications for existing therapeutics and for reducing first-pass drug-degradation effects. Patches can also reduce side effects; for example, oestradiol patches are used by more than a million patients annually and, in contrast to oral formulations, do not cause liver damage. Similarly, transdermal clonidine, nitroglycerin and fentanyl patches exhibit fewer adverse effects than conventional oral dosage forms. As another example, nicotine patches have helped people quit smoking and thereby increase lifespan. A schematic of marketed transdermal product is shown in Fig. 17.7.

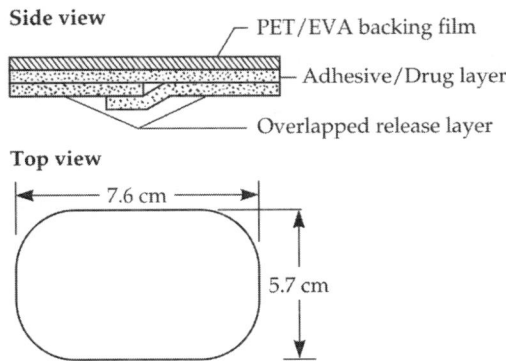

Fig. 17.7. Side and top view of a commercial transdermal product.

Classification of transdermal drug delivery systems

Presently available transdermal patches can be classified into two categories on the basis of their design: reservoir-type and matrix-type patches. A **reservoir-type patch** holds the drug in a solution or gel, from which drug delivery can be governed by a rate-controlling membrane positioned between the drug reservoir and skin. Reservoir-type patches offer an advantage over matrix-type patches in terms of formulation flexibility and tighter control over delivery rates, although they can have an initial burst of drug release. Reservoir-type patches usually involve

greater design complexity. By contrast, **matrix-type patches**, which were introduced after reservoir-type patches, combine the drug, adhesive and mechanical backbone of the patch into a simpler design that does not involve a rate-controlling membrane; skin permeability usually governs the rate of drug delivery. Although these patches are easier to fabricate, they have limited flexibility in their design compared with reservoir-type patches.

Despite these successes, the number of drugs that can be administered using conventional patches is very limited. As evidence of this, all of the drugs presently administered across skin share three characteristics: low molecular mass (< 500 Da), high lipophilicity (oil soluble), and small required dose (up to milligrams). The smallest drug presently formulated in a patch is nicotine (162 Da) and the largest is oxybutinin (359 Da). Opening the transdermal route to large hydrophilic drugs is one of the major challenges in the field of transdermal drug delivery.

Because the skin provides such a formidable barrier to the delivery of most drugs, a broad range of different chemical additives have been tested to enhance transdermal penetration. In contrast to physically enhanced delivery methods discussed below, chemical **penetration enhancers** provide certain advantages, including design flexibility with formulation chemistry and an easier possibility of patch application over a large area (> 10 cm^2). Extensive research during the past three decades has led to the formulation of several different classes of penetration enhancers, including surfactants (e.g., Tween), fatty acids/esters (e.g., oleic acid), terpenes (e.g., limonene), and solvents (e.g., dimethyl sulphoxide and ethanol). However, only a small number of chemical enhancers have been shown to induce significant therapeutic enhancement of drug transport. Enhanced delivery of high-molecular mass drugs is even more limited.

As an additional limitation, potent chemical enhancers are usually potent irritants to the skin at concentrations required for achieving useful levels of penetration enhancement and are therefore physiologically incompatible. With limited success, attempts have been made to synthesize novel chemical penetration enhancers (e.g., lauracapram, Azone) that safely achieve therapeutic transport enhancement. Some of the newer 'speciality' penetration enhancers, such as 2-*n*-nonyl-1,3-dioxolane (SEPA) also attempt to enhance skin permeation without irritation and are being evaluated for clinical applications.

Various approaches for transdermal drug delivery

A. Iontophoresis

Rates of transdermal transport can also be increased through iontophoresis, which uses an electric field to move both charged and uncharged species across the skin. Transdermal iontophoresis has been most extensively applied to the delivery of anti-inflammatory agents and other compounds for local effects in the context of physical therapy. Other FDA-approved uses include pilocarpine delivery to induce sweating as part of a cystic fibrosis diagnostic test, tap-water delivery to treat hyperhidrosis, lidocaine delivery for local anaesthesia, especially before venipuncture, and extraction of interstitial fluid for monitoring glucose levels in diabetics. Typically, a few milliamperes of current are applied to a few square centimetres of skin, which generally causes no pain or irritation other than mild erythema. In addition to the few existing FDA-approved products based on iontophoresis a number of companies are actively developing new systems for the delivery of pain medications and other drugs. The long-term promise of iontophoresis is the prospect of delivering hydrophilic drugs and even macromolecules across the skin with a user-friendly, possibly disposable system designed for home use.

B. Electroporation

Another approach to increase transdermal transport using electric field involves the application of short, high voltage pulses to the skin to transiently increase skin permeability by a mechanism related to electroporation. Transdermal transport has been shown to increase by orders of magnitude using electroporation, with partial reversibility within seconds; and full reversibility, in some cases, within minutes to hours. The largest fluxes have been observed for synthetic molecules and small macromolecules (<10 kDa), including a clinical study of lidocaine delivery in humans. Larger macromolecules have also been delivered, including heparin, insulin, vaccines, oligonucleotides, DNA and microparticles, in which electroporation combined with chemical-enhancement methods have been most effective. In addition, transdermal transport lag times can be reduced to seconds portrays opportunities for rapid-response drug delivery systems.

C. Acoustical methods

Ultrasonic waves, as well as short-duration shock waves, have been used to facilitate transdermal drug delivery. Ultrasound at various frequencies in the range of 20 kHz–16 MHz has been used to enhance skin permeability by a method called sonophoresis. Traditionally, ultrasound at high frequencies ($f > 1$ MHz, therapeutic ultrasound) was a popular choice for sonophoresis. However, transdermal transport enhancement induced by low-frequency ultrasound ($f < 100$ kHz) is significantly greater than that induced by therapeutic ultrasound. Low-frequency ultrasound has been shown to quickly permeabilize human skin and maintain it in a state of high permeabilization for a number of hours, thereby opening a window for drug delivery using a simple patch.

D. Microneedles

Recently, arrays of microscopic needles have been used for transdermal drug delivery. Needles of micron dimensions can pierce into the skin surface to create holes large enough for molecules to enter, but small enough to avoid pain or significant damage. *In vitro* experiments

Table 17.5. Commercially available transdermal drug delivery systems

Drug	Product name	Indication	Marketed by
Nitroglycerin	Nitrodisc	Angina pectoris	Robert Pharmaceutical, USA
	Nitrodur	Angina pectoris	Key Pharmaceutical, USA
	Transderm nitro	Angina pectoris	Novartis, USA
	Minitran	Angina pectoris	3M Pharmaceuticals, USA
	Deponit	Angina pectoris	UCB, Belgium
Estradiol	Alora	Postmenopausal syndrome	Thera Tech/Procter & Gamble/Watson Inc., USA
	Climaderm	Postmenopausal syndrome	Ethical Holding
	Estraderm	Postmenopausal syndrome	Alza/Novartis, USA
	Fempatch	Postmenopausal syndrome	Parke-Davis, USA
	Vivelle	Postmenopausal syndrome	Noven Pharmaceuticals/Novartis, USA
Nicotine	Habitraol	Smoking cessation	Novartis, USA
	Nicoderm	Smoking cessation	Alza, USA/GlaxoSmithKline, UK
	Nictrol	Smoking cessation	Cygnus Inc./McNeil Consumer Product Ltd., USA
	Prostep	Smoking cessation	Elan Corp., Ireland/Lederle, USA

have shown that inserting microneedles into skin can increase permeability by orders of magnitude for small drugs, large macromolecules and nano-particles. Large increases in transdermal delivery of compounds including oligonucleotides, insulin, desmopressin and human growth hormone are possible. Microneedle-based delivery of vaccines, including proteins and DNA, is of special interest, in part to target Langerhans' cells in the skin's epidermis. In human studies microneedles are shown to be painless when inserted into the skin of human subjects. A number of Fortune 500 corporations, as well as startup companies, are actively developing microneedles for transdermal drug delivery.

A number of other methods for delivering drugs across skin have also been studied. Similar to microneedles that pierce holes into the surface of the skin, thermal methods have also been used to locally heat and ablate holes in stratum corneum, thereby increasing skin permeability. This thermal poration approach has been used to deliver conventional drugs and DNA vaccines to animals, and to extract interstitial fluid glucose from human subjects. These applications are being actively pursued by a number of companies.

Microspheres

The term microcapsule is defined as a spherical particle with size varying from 50 nm to 2 mm, containing a core substance. Microspheres are, in strict sense, spherical empty particles (Fig. 17.8). The microspheres are characteristically

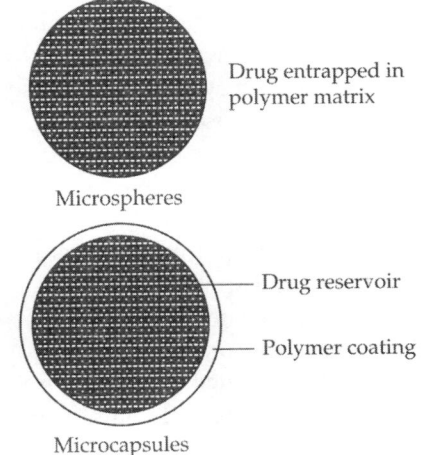

Fig. 17.8. Difference between microspheres and microcapsules.

Table 17.6. Some FDA-approved microparticles in the market

Product	Drug	Indication	Distributor
Lupron Depot	Lurprolide acetate	Prostate cancer	Abbott
Nutropin Depot	Growth hormone	Pediatric growth hormone	Genentech
Suprecur MP	Buserelin acetate	Prostate cancer	Aventis
Decapeptyl	Triptorelin pamoate	Prostate cancer	Ferring
Sandostatin LAR	Octeoride acetate	Acromegaly	Novartis
Somatuline LA	Lanerotide	Prostate cancer	Ipsen
Trelsatar Depot	Triptorelin pamoate	Schizophrenia	Watson
Resperidal consta	Risperidone	Prostate cancer	J&J/Alkermes

free flowing powders consisting of proteins or synthetic polymers, which are biodegradable in nature, and ideally having a particle size less than 200 μm. Microspheres incorporating a drug dispersed or dissolved throughout particle matrix have the potential for the controlled release of drug. These carriers received much attention not only for prolonged release but also for targeting of the drugs to the particular site.

There are various approaches in delivering a therapeutic substance to the target site in a sustained or controlled release fashion. One such approach is using polymeric microspheres as carriers for drugs. Microspheres of biodegradable and non-biodegradable polymers have been investigated for sustained release depending on the final application. In case of non-biodegradable drug carriers, when administered parenterally, the carrier remaining in the body after drug is completely released, poses the possibility of carrier toxicity over a long period of time. Biodegradable carriers that degrade in the body to non-toxic degradation products do not pose the problem of carrier toxicity and are more suited for parenteral application.

Advantages associated with microspheres are that they provide constant and prolonged therapeutic effect; reduce the dosing frequency and thereby improve patient compliance, could be injected IM/SC due to spherical shape, and their morphology allow a controlled variability in degradation and drug release.

Biodegradable carrier matrices can be designed to deliver the therapeutic agent for periods ranging from a few days to a few years. Natural polymers such as proteins and polysaccharides undergo enzymatic degradation in the body. Most synthetic biodegradable polymers contain hydrolysable linkages like amide, esters and urethanes. Polypeptides undergo enzymatic degradation while synthetic polyesters such as poly(lactic acid) and poly(glycolic acid) degrade mostly by simple hydrolysis. Since enzyme action is site-specific, enzymatic degradation can be increased by incorporating enzyme-specific moieties in the polymer chain. Biodegradation can take place by heterogeneous or homogeneous erosion of the implant depending on the chemistry of the implant. Homogeneous degradation or bulk degradation involves the cleavage of the bonds at a uniform rate throughout the matrix. Degradation in this case is independent of the surface area. In heterogeneous or surface degradation, the rate of degradation is constant with time.

Various methods are employed for the preparation of the microspheres from polymers. The microspheres can be prepared by using any of the several techniques but the choice of the technique mainly depends on the nature of the polymer used, the drug, the intended use and the duration of therapy. Moreover, the method of preparation and its choice are equivocally determined by some formulation and technology related factors. Different types of methods are employed for the preparation of microspheres. These include *in situ* polymerization, solvent evaporation, coacervation phase separation, spray drying and spray congealing, etc. Microsphere in the finished product are in a dry powder form, which is produced either as the end product of manufacturing process or by the removal of the solvent/dispersion liquid medium after the formation of microspheres by lyophilization or filtration, with final drying. Prior to administration, a microsphere product is reconstitution in liquid diluents which can be supplied in separate container or in the liquid compartment of a dual chamber prefilled syringe. While the size and size distribution of microsphere product are two key factors that control the drug release rate and resultant duration of sustained release, they also affect the syringeability and injectibiltiy of the product with respect to specific size or gauge of needle.

Nanoparticles

Nanoparticles are sub-nanosized colloidal structures composed of synthetic or semi-synthetic polymers. Nanospheres may be defined as solid core spherical particulates, which are nanometric in size. They contain drug embedded within the matrix or adsorbed onto surface; nanocapsules are vesicular system in which drug is essentially encapsulated within the central volume surrounded by an embryonic continuous polymeric sheath. The materials used in the manufacture of nanoparticles are given in Table 17.7.

The selection of the appropriate method for the preparation of nanoparticles depends on the physicochemical characteristics of the polymer and the drug to be loaded. On the contrary, the preparation techniques largely determine the inner structure, *in vitro* release profile and the biological fate of these polymeric delivery systems. Two types of systems with different inner structures are apparently possible including (a) a matrix type system consisting of an entanglement of oligomer of polymer units (nanoparticles/nanospheres), and (b) a reservoir type of system consisting of an oily core surrounded by an embryonic polymeric shell (nanocapsules).

The drug can either be entrapped within the reservoir or the matrix or otherwise adsorbed on the surface of these particulate systems. The polymers are strictly structured to a nanometric particle size range using appropriate methodologies. However, polymeric nanoparticle have several techno-commercial limitations such as toxicity due to residual solvent, aggregation/stabilization issue and scale-up issues etc., which lead to restrict market entry. S lipid nanoparticles have been investigated to counter these challenges.

Solid lipid nanoparticles

Solid lipid nanoparticles (SLNs) dispersions have been proposed as a new type of colloidal drug carrier system suitable for intravenous administration. The system consists of spherical solid lipid particles in the nanometer range, which is dispersed in water or in aqueous

Table 17.7. Various materials used for the preparation of nanoparticles

Proteins	Polysaccharides	Polymers	
		Prepolymerized	Polymerized in process
Gelatin	Alginate	Poly(ε-caprolactone) (PECL)	Poly(isobutyl cyanoacrylates) (PLCA)
Albumin	Dextran	Poly lactic acid (PLA)	Poly(butyl cyanoacrylates) (PBCA)
Lectins	Chitosan	Poly(lactide-coglycolide) (PLGA)	Polymethyl methacrylate (PMMA)
Legumin	Agarose	Polystyrene	Copolymer of aminoalkyl methacrylate methyl methacrylate
Vicilin	Pullulan		

surfactant solution. Generally, they are made of solid hydrophobic core having a monolayer of phospholipid coating. The solid core contains the drug dissolved or dispersed in the solid high melting fat matrix. The hydrophobic chains of phospholipid are embedded in the fat matrix. They have potential to carry lipophilic or hydrophilic drugs or diagnostics.

A. Advantages of solid lipid nanoparticles

SLNs include advantages of polymeric nano-particles, fat emulsion and liposomes but simultaneously preclude some of their dis-advantages. They are biodegradable and non-toxic; stable against coalescence, drug leakage, hydrolysis, particle growth; often observed in lipid emulsions and liposomes. Unlike lipid emulsions, which have a fluid core, they possess a solid matrix, which has the potential for allowing drug release over prolonged period. Other advantages include low cost of ingredients, ease of preparation and scale-up, high dispersi-bility in an aqueous medium, high entrapment of hydrophobic drug, controlled particle size and extended release of entrapped drug after single injection from few hours to several days. Multiple emulsions have inherent instabilities due to coalescence of the internal aqueous droplets within the oil phase, coalescence of the oil droplets and rupture of the oil layer on the surface of the internal droplets. In case of SLNs production, they have to be stable for few minutes, the time between the preparation of the clear multiple microemulsions and its quenching in cold aqueous medium, which is possible to achieve.

B. Methods of preparation

Various methods have been developed for the preparation of aqueous dispersions of lipid nano-particles. The different production methods use biocompatible lipids. The essential excipients of SLNs are solid lipids as matrix material and amphipathic lipids as surface stabilizer. Solid lipids such as saturated monoacid triglycerides (tristearin, tripalmitin, trilaurin, etc.), hard fat, cetyl palmitate, fatty acids (stearic acid, behenic acid, etc.) and cholesteryl acetate are recommen-ded to be used as matrix for SLN. Physiologically compatible emulsifiers such as phospholipids and bile salts are preferred as stabilizers.

1. **Melt-homogenization technique:** SLNs can be produced by melt-homogenization technique comprising of two steps. First, the lipids are heated at least 10°C above their melting point. The melted lipids are then dispersed in hot aqueous medium using a suitable dispersing agent. Dispersion is accomplished using mechanical stirring or by ultrasonication. The pre-mix formed is then passed through a thermostabilized high-pressure homogenizer under optimum homogenization conditions. The second step involves the solidification of oil droplets by cooling the hot dispersion to room temperature. For drug-loaded SLNs, the drug is dissolved either in melted lipid or in hot aqueous phase prior to emulsification. The technique uses high-pressure homogenizer that reduces efficiently the number of large particles and produces particle dispersion suitable for IV injections. A combination of shear, turbulence, collision, cavitation forces and intense mixing are among the factors responsible for the production of fine droplets with a narrow size distribution.

2. **Microemulsification-solidification:** SLNs can be produced by microemulsification of molten lipids, as the internal phase, and subsequent dispersion of the microemulsion in aqueous medium under mechanical stirring. Microemulsions are clear, thermodynamically stable, microheterogeneous dispersions usually obtained by mixing oil, water, surfactant and co-surfactant. The diameter of the disperse phase droplet is always below 100 nm. Moreover, their preparation does not require energy. Rapid crystallization of oil droplet on dispersion in cold aqueous medium produces lipid nanoparticles with solid matrix.

The microemulsion can be prepared using stearic acid internal phase, purified egg lecithin as surfactant, taurodeoxycholate sodium as co-surfactant and distilled water as continuous phase. Drug-loaded SLNs are prepared by adding drug to melted stearic acid at about 65-70°C. Surfactant, warm water, and the co-surfactant are successively added to the melted mixture. A clear microemulsion is easily obtained under stirring at about 65–70°C. SLNs are then obtained by dispersing the warm microemulsion in distilled cold water (2–3°C) under mechanical stirring; the dispersion is washed twice with distilled water by ultrafiltration. After washing, the suspension is freeze-dried. The micro-emulsions require presence of a co-surfactant for their production. When lecithin alone is used as a single surfactant it will not produce balanced microemulsion. It favors the formation of reverse microemulsion over a very limited range of concentration. This is because the lecithin molecule is too lipophilic.

3. **Multiple microemulsification solidification:** In this technique the warm w/o/w multiple microemulsions can be prepared in two steps. Firstly, w/o microemulsion is prepared by adding an aqueous solution containing drug to a mixture of melted lipid, surfactant and co-surfactant at a temperature slightly above the melting point of lipid to obtain a clear system. In second step the formed w/o microemulsion is added to a mixture of water, surfactant and co-surfactant, to obtain a clear w/o/w system. SLNs can be obtained by dispersing the warm micro multiple emulsions in cold aqueous medium in a fixed ratio, under mechanical stirring. The suspension of lipid particles is then washed with dispersion medium by ultrafiltration.

In contrast to SLN being produced from solid lipids, a modified version which is known as **nanostructured lipid carrier (NLC)** are produced by controlled mixing of solid lipids with spatially incompatible liquid lipids leading to special nanostructures with improved drug incorporation and release properties.

Based on the chemical nature of the lipid molecules, the inner structure of NLC is different from that of SLN because the former is composed of mixtures of solid and liquid lipids (oils). The solubility of active ingredients in oils is generally much higher than in solid lipids. For that reason, the higher loading capacity could be achieved by the development of NLC. With this approach, drug expulsion during the storage time is also minimized. Admixture of liquid with solid lipids leads to the creation of a less ordered inner structure. Thus, the drug molecules can be accommodated in between lipid layers and/or fatty acid chains

NLC can be produced by blending solid lipid with liquid lipid (oils). The resulting matrix shows a melting point depression compared to original solid lipid but matrix is still solid at body temperature.

Depending on the method of production and composition of the lipid blend, different types of NLC may be obtained. Fig. 17.9 shows three different types of NLC compared to the more or less highly ordered matrix of SLN. Depending on the order of matrix NLC can be of three types viz. (i) imperfect type, (ii) amorphous type, and (iii) multiple type.

In the imperfect type, the drug is randomly incorporated in the system within the lipid matrix, consisting of two or more structurally different lipids. However, in spite of having lesser crystalline matrix than SLN, drug expulsion during storage or cooling is very common. Also, the amount of drug incorporated is lesser than the other two types of NLC. The thought that the drug might be better soluble in the liquid oils is utilized as the modifications of type I. In the II type e.g. mixing of isopropyl-myristate with hydroxyoctacosanyl hydroxy-stearate, the blend of solid and liquid lipid is heated and cooled to room temperature to form solid particles. The solid character has been proved by nuclear magnetic resonance spectro-

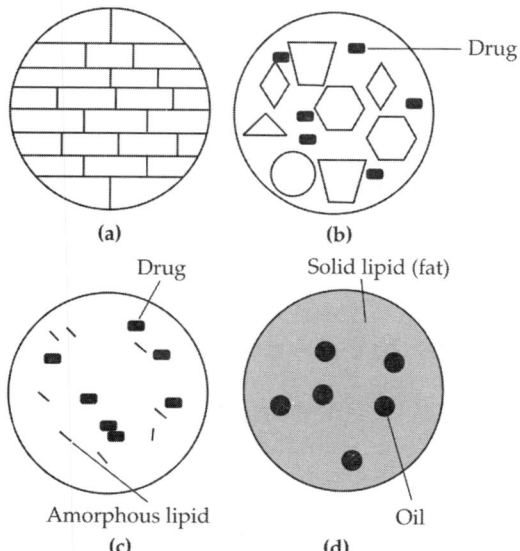

Fig. 17.9. The three types of NLC compared to the relatively ordered matrix of SLN (a). NLC types: imperfect type (b), amorphous type (c), and multiple type (d).

scopy and lack of crystallinity by differential scanning colorimetry. This is the case where oil is in low concentration. At relatively high concentration of oil, there occurs miscibility gap between the two lipid states during cooling and leads to phase separation. Thus, this type contains oil nano-compartments within the lipid particle matrix forming an oil/fat/water system. This cannot be achieved by mere mechanical means so the technique called as lipid-lipid precipitation is used. Nano-compartments are formed only when the lipid is used at such a high concentration that it is well above its solubility in the solid lipid at room temperature. In the multiple type of NLC, lipids are mixed in a way to be in the highly amorphous form maintaining its solid matrix. Preservation of the amorphous state is of utmost importance.

Resealed erythrocytes

The developing RBC has the capacity to synthesize hemoglobin; the adult erythrocytes however lose this capacity and serve only to carry hemoglobin. The membrane mainly encloses cytoplasm and a red pigment called hemoglobin. Some of the hemoglobin is lost and other cellular constituents are retained, the cells on resealing lose some of the properties of normal erythrocytes and referred to as resealed erythrocytes or engineered erythrocytes.

When erythrocytes are suspended in a hypotonic medium, they swell to about one and a half times their normal size and the membrane ruptures, resulting in the formation of pores with diameters of 200 to 500 Å. The pores allow equilibration of the intracellular and extracellular solutions. If the ionic strength of the medium then is adjusted to isotonicitiy and the cells are incubated at 37°C, the pores will close and cause the erythrocytes to "reseal". Using this technique with a drug present in the extracellular solution, it is possible to entrap up to 40% of the drug inside the resealed erythrocytes and to use this system for targeted delivery via intravenous injection. Methods of drug entrapment in erythrocytes include (i) hypo-osmotic lysis, (ii) electrical breakdown, (iii) endocytosis, (iv) membrane perturbation, (v) normal lipid transport, and (vi) lipid fusion. However, hypo-osmotic lysis method, first described in 1977, is used most commonly where the intracellular and extracellular solutes of erythrocytes are exchanged by osmotic lysis and resealing. The drug encapsulation within the erythrocyte's membrane is simply achieved by dialysis through dialysis tubing.

The advantages of using resealed erythrocytes as drug carriers are that they are biodegradable, fully biocompatible, and non-immunogenic; they exhibit flexibility in circulation time depending on their physicochemical properties; the entrapped drug is shielded from immunological detection; and chemical modification of drug is not required.

The assessment of resealed erythrocytes for use in targeted delivery has been facilitated by studies on the behavior of normal and modified reinfused erythrocytes. In general, normal aging erythrocytes, slightly damaged erythrocytes, and those coated lightly with antibodies are sequestered in the spleen after intravenous reinfusion but heavily damaged or modified erythrocytes are removed from the circulation by the liver. This suggests that resealed erythrocytes can be targeted selectively to either the liver or spleen, depending on their membrane characteristics. In addition to coating with antibodies, removal of portions of cell-surface carbohydrates reduces the circulating half-life.

Nanoerythrosomes

Nanoerythrosomes are patented nano-vesicles derived from red blood cell membranes through a process of hemodialysis through filters of defined pore size. These vesicles have the ability to be loaded with a diverse array of biologically active agents including proteins. The nanoerythrosome membrane is a most versatile natural membrane structure, which is composed of proteins, phospholipids and cholesterol. The presence of membrane is particularly advantageous since it permits the conjugation, using simple and well-known molecules polyethylene glycols and proteins, for example, monoclonal antibodies. Additionally, natural membrane stability allows the insertion of recombinant ligands providing another method for incorporating targeting moieties into the nanoerythrosomes.

Liposomes

Liposomes are made of amphiphile molecules (principally phospholipids and mixtures of lipids containing phospholipids) capable of self-organization properties. These molecules are able to form a lipidic bilayer, and this bilayer encapsulates a small internal aqueous volume (Fig. 17.10.). Hydrophilic molecules can be encapsulated in the internal aqueous volume whereas amphiphilic molecules can be incorporated in the bilayer. Liposomes are formed when thin lipid films or lipid cakes are hydrated and stacks of liquid crystalline bilayers

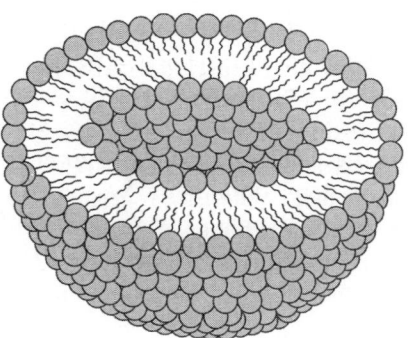

Fig. 17.10. Liposome structure formed by phospholipids.

become fluid and swell. The hydrated lipid sheets detach during agitation and self-close to form large, multilamellar vesicles (LMV) which prevents interaction of water with the hydrocarbon core of the bilayer at the edges. Once these particles have formed, reducing the size of the particle requires energy input in the form of sonic energy (sonication) or mechanical energy (extrusion).

Properties of lipid formulations can vary depending on the composition (cationic, anionic, neutral lipid species), however, the same preparation method can be used for all lipid vesicles regardless of composition. The general elements of the procedure involve preparation of the lipid for hydration, hydration with agitation, and sizing to a homogeneous distribution of vesicles.

Classification

One way of their classification relies upon the number of bilayers formed and diameters of the resultant vesicles. Liposomes are classified into small unilamellar vesicles (SUV, single bilayer, 10–100 nm), large unilamellar vesicles (LUVs, single bilayered 100 nm–1 µm), multilamellar vesicles (MLVs, several bilayers, 100 nm–20 µm), oligolamellar vesicles (OLVs, more than one but not as many as MLVs, 0.1–1 µm), and intermediate-sized unilamellar vesicles (IUVs, ~100 nm). Based on the method of manufacture, liposomes are classified into multivesicular vesicles (MUVs, 100 nm–20 µm), dried-reconstituted vesicles (DRVs, uni- or oligo-lamellar, < 1 µm), reverse-phase evaporation vesicles (REVs, unilamellar, ~0.5 µm), micro-emulsification liposomes (MEL, multilayered, 0.1–0.2 µm), large unilamellar vesicles prepared by extrusion (VET, single bilayer, 100 nm–1 µm) and stable plurilamellar vesicles (SPLVs, multilayered, 100 nm–2 µm).

Methods of preparation

The lipid soluble (lipophilic) materials are solubilized in the organic solution of the constitutive lipid(s) and then evaporated to a dry, drug-containing lipid film followed by its hydration. These methods involve the loading of the entrapped agents before or during the manufacturing procedure (passive loading). However, certain types of compounds with ionizable groups, and those which display both lipid and water solubility, can be introduced into the liposomes after the formation of intact vesicles (remote loading) (Fig. 17.11).

Characterization

The characterization of liposomes can be focused on different aspects: (i) the morphological aspects, i.e. size, shape, number of lamellae (bilayers) and stability, (ii) the structural aspect, i.e. structural organization of the lipids and derivative properties of the membrane (permeability, fluidity), and (iii) the encapsulation efficiency and stability. These three different aspects are considered and appropriate methods and techniques are selected.

Applications

Liposomes are used in cancer chemotherapy and neoplasia; as carriers for vaccines, immunological adjuvants, antigens; drugs in oral treatment; for topical applications and in pulmonary delivery, leishmaniasis, lysosomal storage diseases. Liposomes are used for the following range of therapeutic and pharmaceutical applications:

- Liposomes as drug/protein delivery vehicles.
- Controlled and sustained drug release *in situ*.
- Altered pharmacokinetics and biodistribution.
- Enzyme replacement therapy and lysosomal storage disorders.
- In antimicrobial, antifungal (lung therapeutics) and antiviral (anti-HIV) therapy.
- As biological response modifiers.
- In tumour therapy.

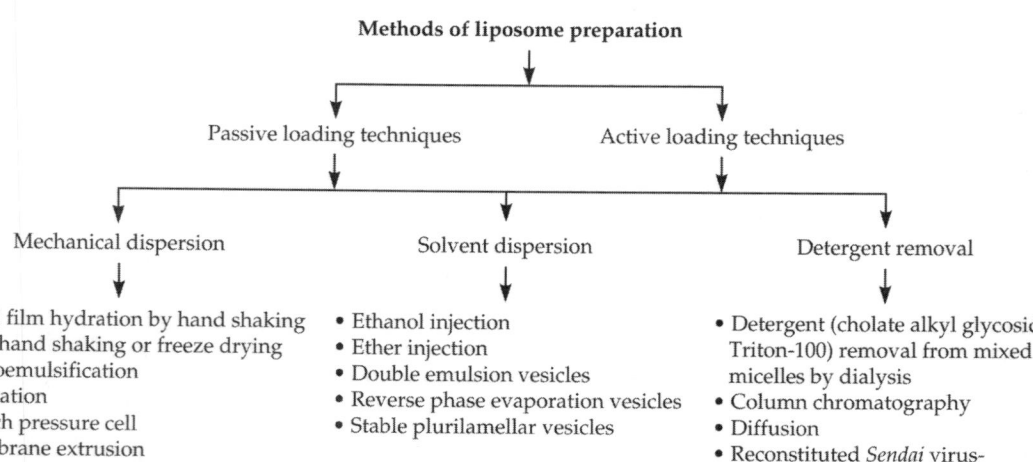

Fig. 17.11. Schematic representation of methods of preparation of liposomes.

Table 17.8. List of some marketed liposomal formulations

Product Name	Drug Name	Dosage form/ shelf life (months)	Indication	Company Name
Ambisome	Amphotericin B	Powder/36	Fungal infection	Gilead Science, USA
Myocet	Doxorubicin	Powder/18	Combination therapy with cyclophosphamide in metastatic breast cancer	Teva Pharma, UK
Doxil	Doxorubicin	Suspension/20	Kaposi's sarcoma, ovarian and breast cancer	Janseen (mfg. by Ben Venue Laboratories, USA)
Lipodox	Doxorubicin	Suspension/36	Kaposi's sarcoma, ovarian and breast cancer	Sun Pharma, India
Depocyt	Cytarabin	Suspension/18	Neoplastic meningitis and lymphomatous meningitis	Sigma-Tau Pharmaceuticals, Inc., USA (mfg. by Pacira Pharmaceuticals, USA)
Depodur	Morphine sulphate	Suspension/24	Pain management	Pacira Pharmaceuticals, USA
Epaxal	Inactivated hepatitis A virus	Suspension/36	Hepatitis A	Berna Biotech Ltd., Switzerland

- Carrier of small cytotoxic molecules.
- Vehicle for macromolecules as cytokines or genes.
- In gene delivery (gene and antisense therapy and genetic (DNA) vaccination).
- In immunology (immunoadjuvant, immuno-modulator and immunodiagnosis).
- As artificial blood surrogates.
- As radiopharmaceutical and radiodiagnostic carriers.
- In cosmetics and dermatology.
- In enzyme immobilization and bioreactor technology.

Niosomes and Discosomes

Niosomes are essentially non-ionic surfactant based multilamellar or unilamellar vesicles in which an aqueous solution of solute(s) is entirely enclosed by a membrane resulting from the organization of surfactant macromolecules as bilayers. Niosomes are formed on hydration of non-ionic surfactant film, which eventually hydrates imbibing or encapsulating the hydrating aqueous solution. Compared to phospholipids used in liposomes, the synthetic non-ionic

surfactants used in the preparation of niosomes are chemically stable, precise in chemical composition and cheaper in cost. Discosomes have disc-like destructured based on non-ionic surfactants during niosomes to mixed micelles transitions. Discosomes, in addition to their many advantages, seem to have a special advantage for ocular route wherein their large size may prevent their drainage into the systemic pool as well as the disc shape could provide for better fit in the cul-de-sac of the eye.

Aquasomes

The carriers like prodrugs, macromolecules and liposomes have served to attain the intended purpose. However, all these are prone to have biophysical constraints. The destructive inter-actions between the drug carrier and the drug are often inevitable and these always bring limitation to the drug delivery system. In such a circumstance, the aquasomes are promising carrier, which are comprised of solid carriers whose surface has been treated with a film of carbohydrate to prevent destructive denaturing drug interactions.

Aquasomes are carbohydrate stabilized nanoparticles of ceramics/calcium phosphate. Aquasomes are like "bodies of water" and their water-like properties help to protect and preserve the fragile biological molecules. It is comprised of a solid phase nanocrystalline core coated with oligomeric film to which the drug moieties or biochemically active molecules are adsorbed with or without modification. These three-layered structures are self-assembled by non-covalent and ionic bonds.

Method of preparation

By using the principle of self-assembly, the aquasomes are incorporated in three steps, i.e., (i) preparation of core, (ii) coating of core, and (iii) immobilization of drug molecules. It is well known that the aquasome is an aqueous colloid comprised of small solids formed from relatively few atoms clustered in solid crystals to which glassy carbohydrates are then applied as surface coating. The carbohydrate coated core serves as non-denaturing solid phase for the subsequent attachment of the active drug candidate, which then individually confers the final properties of colloids. The three-layered solid phase of the colloid (aquasomes), is fully self-assembling and is maintained through both ionic and non-covalent bonds, van der Waals forces and entropic forces.

The first step of aquasome preparation is the fabrication of the ceramic core. The process of ceramic core preparation depends on the selection of materials for core. These ceramic cores can be fabricated by colloidal precipitation and sonication, inverted magnetron sputtering, plasma condensation and other processes. For the core, ceramic materials were widely used because ceramics are structurally the most regular materials known. Being crystalline, the high degree of order in ceramics ensures that any surface modification will have only a limited effect on the nature of the atoms below the surface layer and thus the bulk properties of the ceramic will be preserved. The high degree of

order also ensures that the surface will exhibit high level of surface energy that will favor the binding of polyhydroxy oligomeric surface film. Two ceramic cores that are most often used are diamond and calcium phosphate. The freshly prepared particles have good properties to adsorb environmental molecules within fraction of a second (approximately 10^{-6} second).

The second step involves coating by carbohydrate on the surface of ceramic cores. There are number of processes to enable the carbohydrate (polyhydroxy oligomers) coating to adsorb epitaxially onto the surface of the nano-crystalline ceramic cores. The processes generally entail the addition of polyhydroxy oligomer to a dispersion of meticulously cleaned ceramics in ultrapure water, sonication and then lyophilization to promote the largely irreversible adsorption of carbohydrates onto the ceramic surfaces. Excess and readily desorbing carbo-hydrate is removed by stir cell ultrafiltration. The commonly used coating materials are cellobiose, citrate, pridoxal-5-phosphate, sucrose and trehalose. The applications of aquasomes are summarized in Table 17.9.

Transfersomes

Transfersomes were developed in order to take the advantage of phospholipid vesicles as transdermal drug carrier. These self-optimized aggregates, with the ultra flexible membrane, are able to deliver the drug reproducibly either into or through the skin, depending on the choice of administration or application, with high efficiency. These vesicular transfersomes are several orders of magnitude more elastic than the standard liposomes and thus well suited for the skin penetration. Transfersomes overcome the skin penetration difficulty by squeezing themselves along the intracellular sealing lipids of the stratum corneum because of the high vesicle deformability which permits the entry, due to the mechanical stress of surrounding, in a self-adapting manner. Flexibility of transfer-some membrane is achieved by mixing suitable

Table 17.9. Applications of aquasomes

Use of Aquasomes	Protein/surface	Rationale
Vaccines	Antigenic envelope	To be effective, antibodies must be raised against conformationally specific target molecules
Blood substitutes	Hemoglobin	Physiological binding and release of O_2 by hemoglobin is conformationally sensitive
Pharmaceuticals/pigments/dyes	Active drug/dye agent	Drug activity is conformationally specific wavelength
Enzymes	Polypeptide	Activity fluctuates with molecular conformation; gene therapy; genetic targeted intracellular material delivery

surface-active components in proper ratios. The resulting flexibility of transfersome membrane minimizes the risk of complete vesicle rupture in the skin and allows transfersomes to follow the natural water gradient across the epidermis, when applied under non-occlusive condition.

The high and self-optimizing deformability of typical composite transfersome membrane, which is adaptable to ambient stress, allows the ultradeformable transfersome to change its membrane composition locally and reversibly when it is pressed against or attracted into a narrow pore. The transfersome components that sustain strong membrane deformation preferentially accumulate, while the less adaptable molecules are diluted at sites of great stress. This dramatically lowers the energetic cost of membrane deformation and permits the resulting, highly flexible particles first to enter and then to pass through the pores rapidly and efficiently. This behaviour is not limited to one type of pore and has been observed in natural barriers such as an intact skin.

Methods of preparation of transfersomes

The method is simple. The mixture of vesicle-forming ingredients (phospholipid and surfactant) are dissolved in volatile organic solvent (chloroform-methanol), organic solvent is evaporated above the lipid transition temperature (room temperature, for pure PC vesicles or 50°C for di-palmitoyl phosphatidyl choline) using a rotary evaporator. Final traces of solvent can be removed under vacuum for overnight. The deposited lipid films are hydrated with buffer (pH 6.5) by rotation at 60 rpm for 1 hr at the corresponding temperature. The resulting vesicles are swollen for 2 hr at room temperature. To prepare small vesicles, resulting LMVs are sonicated at room temperature or 50°C for 30 min using a B-12 FTZ bath sonicator or probe sonicated at 4°C for 30 min. The sonicated vesicles are homogenized by manual extrusion 10 times through a sandwich of 200 and 100 nm polycarbonate membrane.

Salient features of transfersomes

1. Transfersomes possess an infrastructure consisting of hydrophobic and hydrophilic moieties together and as a result can accommodate drug molecules with a wide range of solubility.
2. Transfersomes can deform and pass through narrow constriction (from 5 to 10 times less than their own diameter) without measurable loss. This high deformability gives better penetration of intact vesicles.
3. They can act as a carrier for low as well as high molecular weight drugs e.g. analgesic, anesthetic, corticosteroids, sex hormone, anticancer, insulin, gap junction protein and albumin.
4. Being composed of natural phospholipids, similar to liposomes, they are biocompatible and biodegradable.
5. They have high entrapment efficiency, near to 90% in case of lipophilic drugs.

6. They protect the encapsulated drug from metabolic degradation.
7. They act as depot, releasing their contents slowly and gradually.
8. They can be used for both systemic as well as topical delivery of drugs.
9. They are easy to scale up, as procedure is simple, do not involve lengthy procedure and unnecessary use of pharmaceutically unacceptable additives.

Limitations of transfersomes

The limitations of transfersomes include (i) chemically unstable because of their predisposition to oxidative degradation; (ii) purity of natural phospholipids, another criteria militating against adoption of transfersomes as drug delivery vehicles, and (iii) transfersome formulations are expensive.

Applications

Transfersomes have been proposed for a variety of applications in humans, particularly as carriers for proteins including insulin and interferon, as a means of transdermal immunization, as a carrier for corticosteroids, topical analgesic and anesthetic agents, non-steroidal anti-inflammatory drugs and anticancer drugs.

Ethosomes

Ethosomes are interesting and innovative vesicular carriers that have appeared in the fields of pharmaceutical technology and drug delivery in recent years. These ethanol-containing liposomes present an ample opportunity to transport active substances more efficaciously through the stratum corneum into the deeper layers of the skin than conventional liposomes. Ethosomes are soft, malleable vesicles tailored for enhanced delivery of active agents. Due to the interdigitation effect of ethanol on lipid bilayers, it was believed that high concentrations of ethanol are detrimental to liposomal formulations. However, ethosomes which are novel permeation-enhancing lipid vesicles embodying high concentration (20–45%) of ethanol have been developed.

Because of their unique characteristics these vesicles may deliver active substances efficiently through the stratum corneum into the deeper layers of the skin than conventional liposomes. These are noninvasive delivery carriers that can be used for topical as well as for systemic administration. Enhanced delivery of bioactive molecules through the skin and cells by means of ethosomal carriers opens numerous challenges and opportunities for the research and future development of novel improved therapies. Some drugs used for transdermal application by ethosome are listed in Table 17.10.

Salient features of ethosomes

1. Ethosomes provide a mode for passive non-invasive delivery.
2. These carriers are suitable for hydrophilic, lipophilic molecules, peptides and other macromolecules.
3. They can act as a carrier for low as well as high molecular weight substances e.g. analgesic, corticosteroids, sex hormone, insulin, etc.
4. They are biocompatible and biodegradable.
5. Due to high ethanol content, they possess high entrapment efficiency.
6. They possess high cell transfection efficiency.
7. They may act as depot formulation hence sustained release is obtained.
8. They can be applicable for topical as well as systemic delivery.
9. Easy to scale up, as procedure is simple, does not involve lengthy procedure and unnecessary use of pharmaceutically unacceptable additives.

Mechanism of penetration of ethosomes

The stratum corneum is built like a wall with protein bricks and lipid mortar with intercellular lipids playing an important role in controlling the percutaneous absorption. In the case of liposomes, the phospholipids mix with the

Table 17.10. Drugs used and results from ethosomes for transdermal application

Drug	Result
Acyclovir	High transdermal flux; provides non-invasive means of therapeutic use
Minoxidil	High entrapment efficiency; improved transdermal flux; pilosebaceous targeting
Testosterone	High entrapment efficiency; greater transdermal delivery as compared to marketed patch
Trihexyphenidyl HCl	High transdermal flux; provides non-invasive means of therapeutic use
Cannabinols	Improved transdermal flux
Bacitracin	Efficient delivery to deep skin strata
Zidovudine	Reduced side effects.
Azelaic acid	High entrapment efficiency
Minoxidil	Higher transdermal delivery via cholesterol incorporated ethosomes
Ammonium glycyrrhizinate	Better anti-inflammatory activity
Melatonin	Enhanced transdermal delivery

intercellular lipids and thereby cause the swelling of intercellular lipids without altering the multiple bilayer structure of the stratum corneum. These swollen lipids may cause accumulation of the drug and thereby act as intra-cutaneous depot. In case of ethosomal system, though the exact mechanism of drug delivery still remains a speculation, a combination of processes contributes to this enhancing effect.

Ethanol is believed to affect the stratum corneum lipid multilayers, which are densely packed and highly ordered at physiological temperature. Ethanol interacts with lipid molecules in the polar head group region, resulting in the reduction in Tm of the SC lipids, thus increasing their fluidity. Once ethanol disturbs the stratum corneum's lipid bilayer organization, interdigitated, malleable etho-somes can forge a pathway in the disturbed stratum corneum.

Ethanol is a well-known penetration enhancer and is commonly believed to act by affecting the intercellular region of the stratum corneum, thus enhancing permeation. This penetration enhancing effect of ethanol could be attributed to (a) increase in thermodynamic activity due to evaporation of ethanol known as "push effect", and (b) "pull effect" in which penetration of drug molecule is increased due to reduction in barrier property of SC by ethanol. Ethanol embodied in lipid vesicles in the form of ethosomes provides fluidity to the ethosomal bilayers and on application on the skin fluidizes the SC lipids.

Pharmacosomes

Pharmacosomes are defined as colloidal dispersions of drugs covalently bound to lipids, and may exist as ultrafine vesicular, micellar or hexagonal aggregates depending on the chemical structure of the drug-lipid complex. The term 'pharmacosome' is derived from pharmacon, the active principle, and soma, the carrier. The idea for the development of vesicular pharmacosomes is based on surface and bulk interactions of lipids with water. Any drug possessing an active hydrogen atom ($-COOH$, $-OH$, $-NH_2$, etc.) can be esterified to the lipid with or without spacer chain. Synthesis of such a compound may be guided in such a way that strongly amphiphilic compound results, which will facilitate membrane, tissue or cell wall transfer in the organism. The limitations of liposomes and niosomes can be overcome by pharmacosome's approach.

Specific advantages of pharmacosomes

1. Entrapment efficiency is high and moreover predetermined because drug itself in

conjugation with lipids is forming the vesicles.

2. Unlike liposomes, there is no need of following the tedious, time-consuming step for removing unentrapped drug from the formulation.

3. Leakage of drug during storage does not occur in pharmacosomes because drug is covalently linked, however, loss may occur by hydrolysis.

4. No problem of drug incorporation.

5. The entrapment efficiency of drug molecule in liposomes depends upon encaptured volume and drug-bilayer interactions; however, it is irrelevant in pharmacosomes.

6. The lipid composition in liposomes decides its membrane fluidity, which, in turn, influences the rate of drug release and physical stability of the system. However, in pharmacosomes membrane fluidity depends upon the phase transition temperature of the drug-lipid complex, but it does not affect release rate since the drug is covalently bound.

7. The drug is released from pharmacosomes by hydrolysis (including enzymatic).

8. The physicochemical stability of pharmacosome depends upon the physicochemical properties of the drug-lipid complex.

9. Phospholipid transfer/exchange is reduced and solubilisation by HDL is low.

10. Due to amphiphilic behavior such systems allow, after medication, a multiple transfer through lipophilic membrane system or tissue through cellular walls piggyback endocytosis and exocytosis.

11. Following absorption their degradation velocity into active drug molecule depends to a great extent on the size and functional groups of drug molecule, the chain length of the lipids and the spacer. These can be varied relatively precisely for optimized *in vivo* pharmacokinetics.

12. They can be given orally, topically, extra- or intravascularly.

Pharmacosomes are usually self-vesiculating, well established procedures of hand-shaking method and ether injection method have been utilized for preparing vesicles. In hand-shaking method, the dried film of drug-lipid complex deposited in a round bottom flask, when hydrated with aqueous medium, readily gives vesicular suspension. In ether injection method, organic solution of drug-lipid complex is injected slowly into the hot aqueous medium, wherein the vesicles are readily formed.

Polymersome

If the core of the vesicle is an aqueous phase and the surrounding coating is a polymer bilayer, the particle is referred to as a polymersome. These vesicles are analogous to liposomes and find utility in the encapsulation and delivery of water-soluble drugs which can been trapped in their aqueous reservoir but they differ from liposomes in that the external bilayer is composed of amphiphilic copolymers. Polymersomes generally possess a greater PEG surface density and longer circulation times compared to PEGylated liposomes. Polymersomes have shown tendency toward greater drug loading and entrapment of water-soluble drug in their hydrophilic core.

All methods reported for liposome preparation are, in general, also valid for polymersomes. Preparation methods can be divided in two groups: solvent-free techniques and techniques with the aid of organic solvents. In the first group, the amphiphile is brought in contact with the aqueous medium in its dry state and is subsequently hydrated to yield vesicles. This approach offers the advantage that no organic solvent is present any more in the system, which can be mandatory for certain applications. In the second group of preparative methods, the block copolymer is first dissolved in an appropriate organic solvent and then mixed with water. The organic phase is subsequently excluded with an appropriate technique. This leads only to virtually solvent-free conditions, since it is not possible to completely remove all solvent.

Dendrimers

Currently the two common drug delivery systems are liposomes and polymeric systems. These both have limited applications, as liposome-based systems have poor stability and difficulty targeting specific tissues, and linear polymers are polydisperse. Dendrimers offer advantages including a lower polydispersity index, multiple sites of attachment, and a controllable, well-defined size and structure that can be easily modified to change the chemical properties of the system. In addition, macro-molecules such as dendrimers have an enhanced permeability and retention effect (EPR) that allows them to target tumor cells more effectively than small molecules. Dendrimers have applications in gene and antisense therapy, magnetic resonance imaging, and in boron neutron capture therapy. Advances in dendrimer delivery systems, biodegradable dendrimers, and release from dendrimers can be applied to drug delivery in addition to other applications. The basic structure of dendrimer is shown in Fig. 17.12.

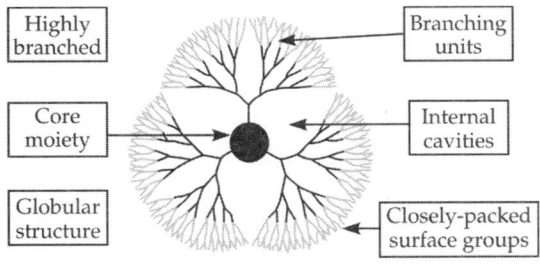

Fig. 17.12. Structure of dendrimers.

Two methods of dendrimer drug delivery are encapsulation of drugs and dendrimer-drug conjugates. Encapsulation of drugs uses the steric bulk of the exterior of the dendrimer or interactions between the dendrimer and the drug to trap the drug inside the dendrimer. Dendrimer-drug conjugates have the drug attached to the exterior of the dendrimer. Most of these conjugates are prodrugs and are inactive or have decreased activity relative to the free drug.

In 1994, Meijer and co-workers reported the first encapsulation of a molecule inside a dendrimer, the so-called "dendritic box". They were able to encapsulate three dyes: eriochrome black T, tetracyanoquinodimethane, and Rose Bengal in a fifth generation diaminobutane-based poly(propyleneimine) (PPI) dendrimer capped with N-tBOC-L-phenylalanine. Encapsulation of each dye in PPI was supported by UV spectroscopy and differences in solubilities between the dye and the dye in the box.

In addition to dyes, research began to focus on anti-cancer drugs for encapsulation. Kono and co-workers used G3 and G4 ethylenediamine based polyamidoamine (PAMAM) dendrimers with poly(ethyleneglycol) monomethyl ether (m-PEG) grafts to encapsulate the anticancer drugs methotrexate (MTX) and doxorubicin (DOX). Using higher generations or longer PEG chains resulted in more encapsulated drug molecules per mole of dendrimer.

The chemical and physical properties of a dendrimer can be optimized by systematically changing the monomer(s). By optimizing the monomer(s), dendrimers can be made to degrade into biodendrimers, which degrade to bio-compatible building blocks *in vivo*. Suitable monomers for biodendrimers include α-hydroxy acids, sugars, amino acids, fatty acids, poly (ethylene glycol) (PEG), poly(caproic acid) (PCL), and poly(trimethylene carbonate). Factors affecting the degradation rate include (1) the strength of the chemical bond between the monomers, (2) the hydrophobicity of the dendrimer, (3) the generation and molecular weight of the dendrimer, and (4) the chemical reactivity of the macromolecule.

Dendrimer carriers have progressed from merely carrying dyes, which are easily monitored by UV spectroscopy, to carrying anti-cancer drugs. Both encapsulation and dendrimer drug conjugates can be used as drug carriers; sustained release is favored by encapsulation, and targeted release is favored by dendrimer-drug conjugates. The area of dendrimers for drug delivery is continuing to grow with the recent reports of cascade release dendrimers and additional ways to release drugs. Further data are needed to determine the toxicity of the dendrimers and the ability to trigger drug release *in vivo*.

IN VITRO RELEASE EVALUATION FROM CONTROLLED-RELEASE FORMULATION

The release patterns of controlled-release formulations can be divided into those that release drug at a slow zero or first order rate and those that provide an initial rapid dose, followed by slow zero or first order release of sustained component. There are number of kinetic models, which describe the overall release of drug from the dosage forms. Because qualitative and quantitative changes in a formulation may alter drug release and *in vivo* performance, developing tools that facilitate product development by reducing the necessity of bio-studies is always desirable. In this regard, the use of *in vitro* drug dissolution data to predict *in vivo* bio-performance can be considered as the rational development of controlled-release formulations.

The development of a suitable dissolution test method should be based on the physicochemical *in vitro* and *in vivo* characteristics of the active ingredient and the drug product considering the mechanism of release. The purpose of dissolution testing in extended-release product is to discriminate between batches with respect to critical manufacturing variables which may have testing for batch to batch consistency of pivotal clinical, bioavailability and routine production batches and to determine stability of the relevant release characteristics of the product over the proposed shelf life and storage conditions.

The extended-release formulation should therefore be tested *in vitro* under various conditions [media, pH (normally pH range 1–7.5; in cases where it is considered necessary pH 1–8), apparatus, agitation, etc.]. Testing conditions, including sampling time points and frequency providing the most suitable discrimination should be chosen. If media with a low buffering capacity are used, the pH should be controlled during the dissolution test to be sure that there is no influence of dissolved active ingredients and/or excipients on the dissolution conditions during the test period. If a surfactant is used in the dissolution medium, the amount needed should be justified. The choice of the surfactant should be discussed and its consistent batch to batch quality should be ensured. The inclusion of enzymes in the media is acceptable, and even encouraged, when justified (e.g., colonic delivery). If enzymes are added to the dissolution media, a rationale should be given for the type and concentration of enzymes added. Further, consistency of the batch to batch quality of the enzymes should be ensured including activity (IU/mg or IU/ml) or concentration (mg/ml) as appropriate. Justified enzyme concentrations should be used when the enzymes constitute part of the dissolution control mechanism. The use of biorelevant media may improve the correlation to *in vivo* data and may detect a potential food effect. The volume of medium should preferably ensure sink conditions.

For formulations having a zero order release kinetics (with or without lag time) a specification of the dissolution rate over time (per cent of label claim per hour) for a given interval may be suitable instead of the cumulative amount dissolved at a given time point. For this type of product, a graphical presentation of the dissolution rate versus time should be additionally presented in order to justify that the product can be regarded as a zero-order release formulation. For additional details with respect to the choice of apparatus, testing conditions, validation/qualification and acceptance criteria, reference is made to the relevant pharmacopeia.

Special attention should be paid to the importance of any variation in the active substance (e.g. particle size, polymorphism), release controlling excipient(s) (e.g. particle size, gelling properties) or manufacturing process. The assay method of the active ingredient in dissolution samples should be validated according to the relevant ICH guidelines "Validation of analytical procedures" and "Validation of analytical procedures: Methodology", with special attention to the stability of the active ingredient dissolved in the medium and effects from the excipients.

The specification of dissolution for extended-release product should be defined .The purpose of establishing dissolution specifications is to ensure batch-to-batch consistency within a range, which guarantees acceptable biopharmaceutical performance *in vivo* and to distinguish between 'good' and 'bad' batches. Specification limits therefore have to be defined based on experience gained during the drug development stage, especially regarding clinical development and/ or bioavailability/bioequivalence studies. The capability of the manufacturing process and the commonly accepted range of 95% to 105% of stated amount for average content of drug substance have to be taken into consideration.

For pharmaceutical development, especially of extended-release formulations, the relation between *in vitro* drug release and the bio-pharmaceutical performance *in vivo* needs to be established as a valid and therapeutically relevant acceptance criteria. Therefore, the deduction of specification limits requires *in vitro-in vivo* comparison studies. Relevant guidances demonstrate increasing consensus on *in vitro-in vivo* comparison techniques, however, some approaches are still significantly different. Agreement exists that any *in vitro* test system is developed to distinguish between 'good' and 'bad' batches. The test specimen/batches need not be full production scale. For Controlled/ Modified Release (C/MR)-formulations with a Level A correlation (independent drug release)

at least 1 batch has to be tested. All other cases need at least 3 batches to be tested with the following conditions: Profiles of at least 12 individual dosage units from each lot with a coefficient of variation of not more than 10 % are required by the FDA. The number of volunteers to be included in the bioavailability study should be at least 12 according to the FIP guidelines, whereas 6 to 36 are accepted by the FDA. The specification should be established based on average data. A minimum of three time points (early, middle and late stages of the dissolution profile) are required with a dissolution > 80% at the last time point.

Another approach for defining dissolution specifications (non-level A cases) for batches, which have been manufactured and experi-mentally tested *in vitro* and *in vivo*, is the side batch approach. 'Side batches' represent batches, which are created by modification of manu-facturing variables (e g. during process validation studies) in a range expected to represent maximum variability during routine production. These batches are supposed to show differences in the biopharmaceutical characteristics and to represent the upper and lower limits of the dissolution range, an approach which is required for level B and C correlations by USP. According to USP it must be demonstrated that these batches are acceptable by performing a bioavailability/ bioequivalence study but it is not ultimately required that the batches should be strictly bio-equivalent. Bioequivalence is not strictly required between the 'side batches' but is required between the target profile and the profiles representing the upper and the lower specification limits.

Without an IVIVC the recommended range at any dissolution time point specification is ±10% related to the mean dissolution profile obtained from the clinical/bioavailability lots. In certain cases deviations from the ±10% range may be accepted. The maximum deviation then would be 25% under the condition that bio-equivalence of the side batches is proven.

REGULATORY REQUIREMENTS OF CONTROLLED AND NOVEL DRUG DELIVERY

FDA has provided the guideline for controlled drug related products about 30 years ago and most such products are regulated as combination product or modified-release products. A modified-release dosage form of a drug, where conventional release dosage form is available in the market, needs to prove its safety and efficacy prior to its approval by FDA. Such formulations are usually treated as New Drug Applications (NDA) and must comply with the FDA guidelines for NDA submission. Bioavailability studies should be performed with enough subjects to characterize adequately the performance of the drug product under study. Although crossover studies are preferred, parallel studies or cross study analysis may be acceptable. The latter may involve normalization with a common reference treatment. The reference product may be intravenous solution, aqueous oral or an immediate-release product. While USFDA recommends bioavailability data of modified-release dose form preferably in fasted state, European Union (EU) Guidelines clearly states that the bioavailability and bioequivalence studies are to be carried out both in fasting as well as in fed state. Effect of food on bio-availability of drugs formulated as modified release dosage form is an additional study, which is to be carried out for EU filing.

FDA now-a-days provides specific guideline for complex generic products like liposome nanoparticles and other depot products.

Generic liposome or other nanoparticle injection must be same qualitatively and quantitatively as the RLD or reference standard, except differences in buffers, preservatives and antioxidants provided that the applicant identifies and characterizes these differences and demonstrates that the differences do not impact the safety/efficacy profile of the drug product. Currently, FDA has no recommendations for the type of studies that would be needed to demonstrate that differences in buffers, preservatives and antioxidants do not impact the safety/efficacy profile of the drug product.

Lipid excipients are critical in the liposome formulation. ANDA sponsors should obtain lipids from the same category of synthesis route (natural or synthetic) as found in the RLD or reference standard. Information concerning the chemistry, manufacturing and control of the lipid components should be provided at the same level of detail expected for a drug substance as suggested in the liposome drug products draft guidance. ANDA sponsors should have specification on lipid excipients that are similar to those used to produce the RLD or reference standard. Additional comparative characterization (beyond meeting specifications) of lipid excipients including the distribution of the molecular species should be provided.

As with other locally acting products with complex bioequivalence requirements (such as nasal sprays and inhalation products), *in vitro* liposome/nanoparticle characterization should be conducted on at least three batches of the ANDA and the RLD or reference standard products (at least one ANDA batch should be produced by

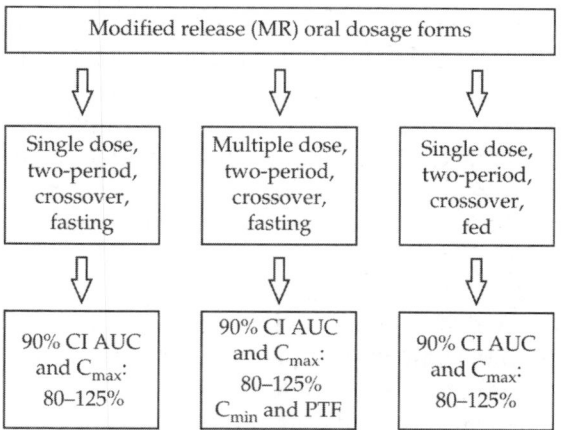

Fig. 17.13. A schematic overview of regulatory requirement for bioequivalence of modified release dosage form.

the commercial scale process and used in the *in vivo* bioequivalence study). Attributes that should be included in the characterization of liposome ANDAs claiming equivalence to the RLD or reference standard are:

1. Liposome composition
2. State of encapsulated drug
3. Internal environment (volume, pH, sulfate and ammonium ion concentration)
4. Liposome morphology and number of lamellae
5. Lipid bilayer phase transitions
6. Liposome size distribution

Grafted PEG at the liposome surface

(a) Electrical surface potential or charge, and
(b) *In vitro* leakage under multiple conditions.

SUGGESTED READINGS

- Jain, N.K. **Introduction to Novel Drug Delivery**, Vallabh Prakashan, New Delhi, 2010.
- Jain, N.K. **Controlled and Novel Drug Delivery**, CBS Publishers & Distributors, New Delhi, 1997.
- Jain, N.K. **Advances in Controlled and Novel Drug Delivery**, CBS Publishers & Distributors, New Delhi, 2001.
- Jain, N.K. **Progress in Controlled and Novel Drug Delivery**, CBS Publishers & Distributors, New Delhi, 2004.
- Chien, Y.W. **Novel Drug Delivery Systems**, Marcel Dekker, New York, 1982.
- Robinson, J.R., Lee, V.H. **Controlled Drug Delivery**, Marcel Dekker, New York, 1987.
- Verma, R.K., Krishna, D.M., Garg, S. (2001). *J. Control Release*, 79: 7–27.

18

Drug Regulatory Affairs

Harvinder Popli

INTRODUCTION

The Indian pharmaceutical industry is large and rapidly growing. Since independence, the Indian pharmaceutical industry has shown momentous growth, progressing from the multinational companies (MNCs) monopoly stages to the present R&D revolution. With the foundation laid by the Government of India in 1960, the pharma sector has indeed come a long way to achieve the current status of being the extremely lucrative strategic option for foreign counterparts.

Pharmaceuticals are among the most highly regulated commodities. Imminent regulatory changes and by signing WTO agreements, India committed itself to granting Intellectual Property Rights by amending its patent laws to recognise product and not just process patents after 2005. After this year, Indian pharmaceutical companies will lose their primary advantage over MNCs operating in India, the freedom to produce drugs developed and patented by other companies, so long as the process is modified. Regulating the pharmaceutical sector has been a constant effort of national governments, undertaken in order to 'promote the protection of human health and of

consumers of medicinal products' and trying to preserve a balance between conflicts of divergent interests: those of industry (driven by a logic of commercial productivity) and those of consumers[1].

Once pharmaceutical industry has expanded its operations beyond national borders, policies of global harmonisation of regulatory requirements have been put forward, particularly by industrialised countries. In the pharmaceutical sector, the milestones are the *International Conference on Harmonisation of Technical Requirements for Registration of Pharmaceuticals for Human Use* (ICH) during the 1990s, coordinated by pharmaceutical trade associations and the DRAs of the EU, Japan and the USA[2].

The driving force behind this has been the increase in global trade in medicinal products, the increasing complexity of country-based technical regulations related to drug safety, efficacy and quality, and above all, the need for the pharmaceutical industry to bring new chemical entities (NCEs) to market faster, in a wider market, and at a reduced cost in order to achieve an acceptable return on R&D investments. This current trend towards industry self-regulation or co-regulation with drug regulatory affairs (DRAs) is now regarded as a more pragmatic and realistic way than promulgating binding international regulations.

Marketing authorisation is the responsibility and one of the main tasks of DRAs. DRAs are operated directly by the government (e.g., department of pharmaceutical service within the ministry of health) or an autonomous agency (e.g., EMEA, FDA). Some DRAs maintain an inventory of the products available on the market; evaluate new products and issue a market authorisation on completion of the assessment process of the quality, safety and efficacy part of the dossier (most countries charge fees for the assessment of applications as a contribution to regulatory activities funding); evaluate applications to make changes to product information; establish meaningful mechanisms and initiatives for the promotion of rational drug use and performance of drug utilisation studies; and establish post-marketing activities (review of applications, pharmacovigilance, GMP inspections of manufacturers, wholesalers and pharmacies, quality control). Drug pricing being a complex and politicized issue, it is usually considered separately from the technical and scientific assessment of the pharmaceutical dossier.

This chapter attempts to shed some light on a framework of international regulation, by reviewing the various processes of harmonization, and the general impact of the globalization of regulatory and technical standards on the development and availability of medicinal products; which helped to provide an infrastructure conducive to research and development (R&D), and the marketing of an average of 55 new chemical entities (NCEs) a year. Between 1975 and 1999 the private R&D-based pharmaceutical industry worldwide marketed 1393 NCEs, whose pharmaceutical dossiers – based on criteria of quality, safety and efficacy – were approved by Western drug regulatory authorities (DRAs)

HISTORY OF REGULATION

In the United States (US) regulation started with the 1906 US Pure Food and Drugs Act (PDF), which had provisions against misbranding. In 1927 the *Food, Drug and Insecticide Administration* was created. In 1930 the title was amended to delete 'Insecticide', becoming the *Food and Drug Administration* (FDA). In 1938, FDC Act was passed by the Congress, thereby giving authority to FDA to oversee safety of Food, Drugs and Cosmetics. It was a comprehensive Act and laid the foundation of USA's current regulatory landscape. The Act requires a Manufacturer to test the medicinal product for safety and efficacy prior to gaining marketing approval through a 'New Drug Application' (NDA). Since then the Act has been amended many times (as per the experiences with mistakes and loopholes in the system) to bring different products in the ambit of FDA, to ensure their safety and at the same time expediting the process of Marketing Authorization, thereby avoiding the drying of product pipeline. The FDA now regulates the Pharmaceutical industry using the Federal Food, Drug and Cosmetic Act (as amended), 1989.

In the United Kingdom (UK), some regulatory controls were applied to vaccines, antigens, arsphenamines, insulin, pituitary hormone and catgut sutures by the 1925 Therapeutic Substances Act. After the thalidomide disaster in the 1950's a voluntary product registration scheme was begun in 1962, and this was followed in 1968 by the introduction of the Medicines Act. After the thalidomide tragedy, action was taken in other *European Community* (EC) countries to institute a regulatory control system or to strengthen existing institutions and legal requirements. For example, in The Netherlands the college *ter Beordeling van genees-middelen* was established in 1963, and in 1961 the first German Drug Law (AMG 1961) set up the *Medicines Institute of the Federal German Health Office* (Bundesgesundheitsamt or BGA). In 1965 the first of the EC Pharmaceutical

Directives (65/65/EEC) was adopted by the then members of the EC (France, Federal Republic of Germany, Italy, Belgium, The Netherlands, and Luxembourg). By 1975 the membership of the EC had increased, and Directive 75/319/EEC was adopted. This established a new committee (the *'Committee on Proprietary Medicinal Products'* – CPMP) to consider questions referred to it relating to approval, refusal, suspension, or revocation of marketing authorizations. Inevitably, the CPMP has since become concerned with European harmonization of the technical and legal requirements for marketing authorization applications, and has issued several volumes of technical guidelines as guidance[3] to the industry and to establish a common approach in assessment.

In Japan, the first law relating to pharmaceuticals was enacted in 1874, but it only covered Tokyo, Osaka and Kyoto. The Pharmaceutical Marketing and Handling Regulations in 1890 covered the nation as a whole. The *Pharmaceutical Affairs Law* (PAL) was enacted in 1943 and in 1948 it was extended to include regulations for medical devices and cosmetics. The new *Pharmaceutical Affairs Law* which was enacted in February 1961 (Law No. 145 which was announced on 10th August 1960) defined the term '*drug*', established the *Central Pharmaceutical Affairs Council* of the Ministry of Health and Welfare (MHW), and created manufacturing and import licences, etc. In 1979, because of pharmaceutical damages, the *Pharmaceutical Affairs Law* was revised to incorporate previous administrative guidance and to codify the purpose of the law as assuring the quality, safety and efficacy of drugs and related products.

HARMONISATION OF REGULATORY REQUIREMENTS AND STANDARDS

To overcome diverging national, technical and scientific requirements, which were barriers to the trade, were deliberated.

In 1985 discussions between the US and Japan on requirements began (the MOSS negotiations). The effect of these has been to accelerate the change made in Japanese technical requirements wherein these were rationalized so as to reduce the time lag and the cost of the product

In September 1988 bilateral technical discussion began between representatives of the EC and Koseisho (*The Pharmaceutical Affairs Bureau* of the Ministry of Health and Welfare in Japan), and further regular discussion then took place in Brussels and Tokyo in subsequent years. Again these discussions helped to accelerate changes in Japanese requirements, and also improved communications and allowed for increased consultation whenever new draft guidelines were issued for formal consultation. A six-month period was allowed for comment to include the time needed for the translation of the draft Japanese texts into English before circulation to the industry associations and the national regional authorities.

In 1990 and subsequent years regular biannual technical discussions took place between EC experts and officials and those of the FDA. These resulted in improvement in understanding, in a facility for formal consultation on draft guidelines, and a rapid communication facility for pharmacovigilance updates and decisions on products already registered in both US and European markets.

Road to the European Medicines Evaluation Agency (EMEA, 2004)

The world's second largest pharmaceutical market is Europe. Almost all drug companies try to get their products in this market, but must undergo a different set of regulations. The European Medicine Agency (EMEA) is equivalent to the U.S. FDA. The EMEA, funded by the European Union, is attempting to reduce the massive cost each company must incur when they need to get approval for their drugs from each nation. Now they will receive approval from the centralized EMEA.

Thalidomide and its associated human tragedy gave rise to legislation both complex and internationally varied for drug regulatory control. Although unfortunate, it is understandable that sovereign states did not see fit to act in concert with each other on the politically sensitive issue of public health protection. From the early days of the European Community, the national pharmaceutical marketing authorisation procedures within the individual Member States constituted a barrier to the free movement of medicinal products due to differences in procedures, data requirements, standards and the time taken to reach decisions on registration applications. In an attempt to remove such barriers, European Community Directives were adopted establishing:

- The requirements for pharmaceutical product marketing[4].
- The Committee for Proprietary Medicinal Products (CPMP) consisting of experts from each of the national registration agencies[5].
- The multistate procedure, a non-mandatory process of mutual recognition of pharmaceutical product licences issued by the individual agencies[6].

The procedure for gaining drug approval is as follows. A pharmaceutical company submits an application for marketing approval for authorization by the EMEA. The Committee for Medicinal Products for Human Use (CHMP) submits an evaluation. If proven safe, the European Commission gives marketing authorization and approval for the entire EU.

Once a company had received a marketing authorisation in one of the European Community countries, it was hoped that other member States, so requested, would speedily recognize this approval and authorise the product to be licensed in their respective countries. In the unlikely event of disagreement, the case could be referred to the CPMP for the final decision. In reality, however, almost every case using this multistate procedure was referred to the CPMP. In 1987, another procedure, the concentration procedure[7], was introduced to facilitate obtaining marketing authorisation for biotechnology and high technology products within Europe. The barrier to market integration resulting from the desperate decisions of the national regulatory authorities was recognised by the European Commission[8], which asked interested parties to come forward with recommendations for the removal of barriers to the free movement of pharmaceutical products within the Community. Extensive debate took place, some member States arguing strongly for continuing with mutual recognition[9] with the incorporation of a binding appeals procedure. Although it was suggested that such problems could be avoided by the creation of supranational agency to assess and issue European marketing authorisations, this option seemed to generate little enthusiasm[10]. Other options, involving aspects of both mutual recognition and supranational European agency, were also discussed[11,12,13]. The eventual outcome of the deliberations was the creation of the European Agency for the Evaluation of Medicinal Products (EMEA), in which a new CPMP was included, and two new procedures for the registration of pharmaceutical products, the centralised procedure and the mutual recognition (decentralised) procedure.

The Centralised Procedure

The *Centralised Procedure* is mandatory for all the biotechnology products using one of the manufacturing methods listed in Part A (scope of Centralized Procedure compulsorily extends up to NCEs to treat HIV-AIDS, Cancer, Diabetes, Neurodegenerative Disorders, Auto-immune and other immune dysfunctions, Viral Diseases, orphan drugs and advance therapies such as gene therapy, somatic cell therapy or tissue engineering therapy and Orphan Drugs) of the Annex to Council Regulation 2309/93[14], even if marketing is proposed in only one Member State. This procedure is optional for a number of innovative products as defined in Part

B of the above Annex. The intent of requiring that biotechnology products be approved through the centralised procedure was to encourage the development of biotechnology in the EU. Since there was limited expertise available in the individual Member States for the evaluation of biotechnology products, it was hoped that the combined EU expertise in this area would achieve a prompt, consistent and scientific assessment of such products. The initial scientific assessment takes a maximum of 120 days, excluding time when the clock stops to permit the company to answer any questions that the CPMP has posed. Once questions have been answered, the clock restarts, and the second assessment period is completed in an additional 90 days, unless unresolved issues remain. To permit the applicant enough time for a hearing, the clock may be stopped yet again. If the CPMP opinion is negative, the applicant has the right to appeal the opinion. If the decision is to grant an authorization, then the CPMP's opinion must be submitted to the Commission to be made legally binding. To date, industry has had little hands-on experience with the centralised procedure.

The Mutual Recognition Procedure

Under this procedure, a national registration may be mutually recognised by other Member States following a request by the applicant and the submission of an identical file to the Member States concerned. It is open to all types of product except for biotechnology products. If the Member States mutually recognise the first approval, with or without negotiation, then the CPMP is not involved in the procedure. This route may be used for all products not covered by Part A of the Annex to Council Regulation 2309/93[14]. When agreement cannot be reached by Day 90 in spite of negotiations, the case is referred to the CPMP for arbitration. The recommendation of CPMP is binding on all Member States involved in the *Mutual Recognition Procedure*. Decentralized Procedure

– a medicine that has not yet been authorized in the EU can be simultaneously authorized in several EU Member States.

Regulatory harmonization

Separate and different reviews in different Member States within EU signified an unnecessary duplication of efforts, with resultant waste of scarce regulatory resources and delays in the delivery of important new medicines to physicians and their patients. The correction of such extravagance becomes even more compelling at a global level. European exercise can be viewed as a pilot study and stimulus for global harmonisation.

A number of other countries have demonstrated a desire to eliminate the duplication of effort involved in multiple reviews of applications, and to bring new medications rapidly to those who need them, while at the same time reducing possible public health risk. An example of this effort is the pharmaceutical evaluation reports (PER) scheme set up by the countries of the *European Free Trade Association* (EFTA), an organisation whose membership grew and overlapped with that of the EU. This scheme promoted the concept of harmonisation through the exchange of national evaluations[15]. Additionally, in 1988, it established an expert group on pharmaceuticals and charged them with finding ways of harmonizing regulations with those of the EU. The Swedish government, a member of EFTA, signed a memorandum of understanding with the Australian government by which it periodically exchanges regulatory drug evaluations with Australia[16]. Australia and Canada have also agreed to exchange pharmaceutical evaluation reports[17]. In 1992, Iceland, Norway and Sweden (joined later by Finland) initiated the Nordic registration project, a variant of the EU multistate procedure, covering abridged applications requiring only pharmaceutical and bioequivalence data (new dosage strengths and forms and generic products) for registration. Subsequently, on January 1,

1995, Sweden and Finland joined the EU, at which time the Nordic registration project was officially concluded.

The *Council for International Organisation of Medical Sciences* (CIOMS), established under the auspices of the *World Health Organisation* (WHO) and the *United Nations Educational, Scientific and Cultural Organisation* (UNESCO), has made recommendations to standardise the format and content of the expedited reporting of serious and unexpected post-marketing adverse events to the regulatory agencies[18]. CIOMS-I working group (1990) represents the first industry/regulators collaborative effort to harmonise adverse drug event reporting on an international basis that culminated in formulation of ICH-E2A guideline (Clinical Safety Data Management) in October 1994.

The International Conference on Harmonization (ICH) Genesis

The ICH movement is bringing many of the above initiatives together and taking them a step forward in the harmonization process.

As can be seen, many of these harmonization activities occurred in, or had significant participation from, Europe. When the EU, already deeply committed to harmonization, was joined by the United States and Japan in the creation of the ICH movement, most of the world's expertise in drug development and regulators of the three regions and the regulated industry working together to achieve scientifically-based, harmonized technical data requirement and registration. These activities were intended to reduce differences in the technical requirements for drug approval among the three regions.

There are six ICH sponsors: The *European Commission*, the *European Federation of Pharmaceutical Industry Associations* (EFPIA), the U.S. *Food and Drug Administration* (FDA), the U.S. *Pharmaceutical Research and Manufacturers Association* (PhRMA), the *Japanese Ministry of Health and Welfare* (MHW) and the *Japanese Pharmaceutical Manufacturers Association* (JPMA). A Secretariat is provided by the *International Federation of Pharmaceutical Manufacturers Association* (IFPMA).

There are five steps defined in the ICH path to harmonization. Once selected for harmonization, a topic is discussed by the appropriate Expert Working Group (Step 1). These groups have representatives from all six sponsors and their deliberations are sent to the ICH Steering Committee (Step 2). This Committee, in addition to representatives from the six sponsors and IFPMA, has a number of observers. The Steering Committee then consults the participating regulatory bodies (Step 3). Final recommendations are submitted to the three sponsoring Regulatory Agencies (Step 4) for incorporation into their regulations (Step 5)[19].

The bilateral discussions lead to an increased relation on the part of the industry and the authorities that real progress could be achieved in international harmonization. Preliminary discussions were held in 1990 and 1991 between representatives of the six co-sponsors of ICH.

The first ICH conference took place in Brussels during 5–7 November 1991. The conference included three workshops (on safety, quality and efficacy), and the final plenary session was able to announce significant progress toward harmonization in a number of areas – particularly in the areas of Pre-clinical safety, testing and quality of medicines. The proceedings of the conference have been published (1992). ICH is viewed as a process of harmonization of standards.

This ultimate goal, the official adoption of the harmonised ICH guidelines by the local authorities, corresponds to step 5 of the ICH *modus operandi* commonly defined by the 6 original sponsors of ICH.

Pharmacopoeial Harmonisation

Separately from the ICH process, regular six monthly tripartite discussions between the representatives of the *United States Pharma-*

copeia (USP), the *Japanese Pharmacopeia* (JP) and the *European Pharmacopeia* (Ph Eur) have been taking place over the last several years. Particular areas of activity have included the exchange of information on work programmes, a work programme for general test method harmonization (e.g. Dissolution Test Methods), and a programme of work excipient monographs. An examination of the way in which the revision work is done in each of the three regions has also been carried out to try to obviate delays in adopting common agreed standards. The JP has introduced a new journal to allow for consultation on draft texts (an equivalent to *Pharmacopeia Forum* (PF) of the *United States Pharmacopeia* and *Pharma Europa* of the *European Pharmacopoeia*, and has started production of an annual addendum rather than wait for the five yearly cycle of publication of new additions of the JP.

In relation to excipients, the programme has targeted a first list of ten commonly used excipients (e.g. lactose, magnesium stearate, starch) for the first work programme and now a further list has been produced for the future programme. The programme is organized to give the work of elaborating a particular monograph to a 'lead' pharmacopoeia authority, which is then responsible for taking forward the task of revision. Draft tests are then published in the *Pharmacopeia Forum*, *Pharmacopeia* and the *Japanese Pharmacopoeia* Forum for consultation and comment. Revised texts are submitted to the normal processes of adoption and implementation in the three regions. The first harmonized monographs were adopted in 1993 for lactose and magnesium stearate.

Harmonisation of Regulatory and Technical Standards

The first countries to tackle harmonisation in the pharmaceutical sector were European, with the Nordic countries creating the Nordic Pharmacopoeia (1963), followed by an agreement to develop a European Pharma-

copoeia (Council of Europe). But the real kick-off of the harmonisation process occurred with the development of a single market and free movement of pharmaceuticals within the *European Economic Community* (EEC). A first European Directive on the marketing authorisation for medicinal products was issued in 1965 (European Council directive 65/65/EEC). Thirty-five years later the *European Agency for the Evaluation of Medicinal Products* (EMEA) was created, leading to a single authorisation system for the 15 European Union countries (1996). Other regional efforts in harmonisation, though less fulfilled and integrated, were the creation of the Pharmaceutical Inspection Convention (PIC) which provided for mutual recognition of pharmaceutical inspections regarding GMP requirements within the European Free Trade Association (EFTA); and the association of South East Asian Nations technical cooperation in pharmaceuticals (ASEAN-TCP), implemented since 1982. This lower degree of integration also holds true with regard to the bilateral mutual recognition agreements, such as those between the EU and Australia, New Zealand, Canada and Japan on GMPs, and the expected MRA between the EU and the US.

Table 18.1. Harmonisation in the pharmaceutical sector: affected domains

- Marketing authorisation procedures: pharmaceutical dossier (quality, efficacy, safety)
- Pharmacological standards: accepted indications, dosage and administration, dosage forms, prescribing status, adverse drug reactions
- GMPs: contents, inspection
- Intellectual property rights: product and process patent, medical indication exclusivity

Apart from the EU example, possibly the most successful effort in harmonising a regulatory requirement for pharmaceuticals has taken place within the framework of the ICH. Since the beginning of the 1990s the regulatory agencies and industry trade associations of the

EU, Japan and USA have met regularly and become "co-responsible" for the drawing-up of harmonised technical guidelines for all aspects of the pharmaceutical dossier of new chemical entities (pre-clinical and clinical testing, quality testing and safety issues of medicines). ICH, a group coordinated by the International Federation of Pharmaceutical Manufacturers Associations (IFPMA), has so far produced 45 technical guidelines on efficacy testing (e.g., clinical trial design, clinical safety, good clinical practice, clinical study reports), quality testing (e.g., stability testing, impurities, harmonisation of the EU, Japan and US pharmacopoeia) and safety testing (carcinogenicity and genotoxicity studies, toxicokinetics and pharmacokinetics). The result is that it has become possible to shorten the time needed for regulatory assessment, leading to more rapid access to new medicines. The mean time for the total development phase tripled from the 1960s to the 1980s, declined slightly from 9.0 years to 8.6 years for the 1990s and more significantly to 7.7 years for the 1997–99 approvals. Measures such as fast-track registration shortened the mean approval time from an average of 11.8 months for normal medicines down to 4.6 months for health-priority medicines (e.g., AIDS antiretrovirals), leading some to raise questions about the haste in approving new drugs that have later to be possibly withdrawn

Most of the guidelines commonly agreed between Western DRAs and pharmaceutical trade associations are at present included in the ICH countries' national regulations, giving the guidelines a legislative and regulatory nature. Since 1999, with the creation of the ICH Global Co-operation Group within the ICH Steering Committee, ICH participants aim at expanding and proselytizing the use of ICH guidelines to all non-ICH countries and progressively to the generic drugs sector. Originating in a regional approach, the initiative has become global, and may be regarded as a "test-bed" for other economic sectors.

When considering product development and marketing from a standardization perspective, the technical and regulatory aspects have to be taken into account. Pharmaceutical R&D and manufacturing consists, as is the case in many industrial activities, in using materials and products (e.g., raw materials, active ingredients, excipients), processes (e.g., manufacturing processes, chemical or biological synthesis, combinatorial chemistry) and services. To ensure that all these ingredients are fit for their purpose (i.e., human use for a given medical indication), manufacturers specify and use standards. Standards are defined as documented agreements containing technical specifications or other criteria to be used consistently as rules, guidelines, or definitions of characteristics. Adhering to the standards means that manufactured products (e.g., medicines, vaccines, medical devices) can be used with the benefit of relevant technical knowledge. This also avoids technical barriers to trade, especially if the standards are internationally recognised. These standards are usually worked out by common consent and published by private firms and members of a profession (e.g., ISO standards). However, a broad consensus is not always possible or desirable (for technical, economical or political reasons). Instead of a clear standard, guidelines are then drafted which guide the resolution of technical processes or give rules about how to proceed (e.g., WHO guidelines on registration requirements of multisource pharmaceutical products to establish interchangeability, ICH guidelines).

The pharmaceutical sector has traditionally been under the control of DRAs because of its repercussions on health and the limited capacity that consumers have to evaluate the characteristics of products they use. National governments make use of their legislative and regulatory prerogatives to lay down laws, regulations and administrative procedures protecting consumers and public health interests (e.g., health codes, marketing authorisations, guide-

Table 18.2. Examples of norms and guidelines in the R&D and marketing process of medicinal products

	Preclinical research	Clinical studies	Review and approval	Post-marketing
Scope of application	• Synthesis and purification (pharmaceutical active ingredients, excipients) Animal testing	• Phase I • Phase II • Phase III	• Pharmaceutical dossier Marketing authorization	• ADR surveillance, Product defect, reporting, Survey sampling testing, Post-approval inspections
Public norms (Quality, Effectiveness, Safety)				
National level	• National Pharmacopoeias (Q) e.g., BP, USP • National GMP, GLP • Patent law (product and process)	• National GCP, GLP (E) (S)	• Criteria for drug approval (national marketing authorization)	• Laws and regulations on labelling requirements, marketing restrictions, prescription rules, advertising
Regional or international level	• WHO International Pharmacopoeia (Q) • European Pharmacopoeia (Q) • Nordic Pharmacopoeia (Q) • WHO Certification Scheme (Q) • INN (Q) • International law on intellectual property	• EU Directive 2001/83/EC on the Community Code relating to medicinal products • Mutual recognition agreements	• EU Directive 2001/83/EC on the Community Code relating to medicinal products	
Guidelines (Q, E, S)				
National level	• National standards (Q)	• National GCP, GLP		
Regional or international level	• WHO GMP guidelines (Q) • WHO guidelines for stability testing (Q) • WHO guidelines on validation of analytical procedures (Q) • WHO guidelines on sampling of pharmaceuticals (Q) • WHO good practices for national pharmaceutical control laboratories (Q)(S)	• WHO GCP, GLP guidelines (E)(S) • ICH Efficacy guidelines E1 to E11	• WHO guidelines on pre-approval inspection • WHO Adverse reaction terminology (WHOART) • ICH M4 Common Technical document	• WHO Model list of essential medicines • WHO guidelines for inspection of drug distribution channels • WHO guidelines for the establishment of basic tests for drugs

(Contd.)

Preclinical research	Clinical studies	Review and approval	Post-marketing
• WHO guidelines for the establishment and distribution of chemical reference substances (Q) • ICH Quality guidelines Q1 to Q6 (stability testing, validation of analytical procedures, impurities guidelines, Pharmacopoeia harmonisation, quality of biotechnology products, GMP for active pharmaceutical ingredients) (Q) • ICH Safety guidelines (safety guidelines for carcinogenicity, genotoxicity, toxicity studies, and reproductive toxicology) (S) • Arab GMP guidelines (Q) • ISO standards (manufacturing process, raw materials) (Q)		• ICH M1 Medical Terminology (MedDRA)	• ICH E2C related to the PSUR for marketed drugs

lines, good practices). These normative prescriptions or public norms are, according to a hierarchical system, compulsory for all the parties involved in economic life. They are implemented in the pharmaceutical sector through the DRAs (e.g., the British Medicines Control Agency – MCA, the German Federal Institute for Medicinal Products and Devices – BfArM, or the US Food and Drug Administration – FDA). These different texts can eventually refer to technical specifications and industrial standards defined by manufacturers, making them compulsory (e.g., good manufacturing practices – GMP). Sometimes, different countries can agree on a set of common laws and regulations (e.g., EU Directives and Regulations). On the other hand, at the international level, WHO is the only authority within the United Nations system that is allowed to develop and promote international health norms which are in theory compulsory to all its Member States (e.g., international non-proprietary nomenclature for pharmaceutical substances, international biological standards, International Pharmacopoeia, WHO certification scheme on the quality of pharmaceuticals moving in international commerce).

Whichever authority is involved at the national, regional or international levels, the process of drafting a standard usually includes the following steps: identification of needs, technical drafting of the standard by an expert committee, validation of the draft standard, and approval. The regulatory process will inherently rely on a subtle balance between the different sources of political, technical and economic initiatives. The balance differs from one country to another: the public authority can exert its power either directly (e.g., Portugal, United Kingdom) or delegate it to private institutions under the control of a public authority (e.g., France with the AFNOR, EU with the European CE mark for medical devices) or leave it to independent and private institutions (e.g., Switzerland, USA). At the international level, apart from the EU example (geographically restricted) and the existing WHO monopoly to issue international health norms, there are no public institutions legally entitled to issue norms or standards.

REGULATORY REQUIREMENTS

Over the years, regulatory bodies issued numerous guidelines to assist in the development of new drug candidates. Not surprisingly, cultural characteristics and differing medical practices have led to some degree of disparity among these published guidelines. This is particularly apparent when comparing and contrasting guidelines derived in the United States with those from Europe. Unlike guidelines issued in United States, European guidelines tend to be more general in nature and do not provide detailed instructions on such matters as study design. Companies are expected to have the expertise necessary to design appropriate development programs for their products.

European community requirements of Pharmaceutical development

The requirements for data on development pharmaceutics in an EC marketing authorization dossier emanate from Directive 75/318/EEC, as amended by directive 91/507/EEC.

Part 2 A 4.1 of the Annex to Directive 91/507/EEC calls for an explanation of the choice of composition, constituents, and containers and the intended function of the excipients in finished medical product, supported by scientific data on development pharmaceutics, and the formulation and container proposed, are satisfactory for the intended use of the medicinal products specified in the application. The studies further aim to identify aspects of the formulation and the method of processing which are crucial for batch reproducibility, and which therefore must be routinely controlled[20].

The formal requirement of the EC Directive is expended in the *Notice to Applicants*[20], which lays down the format and content of applications for marketing authorizations, as accepted by all EC Member States. There is additional advice presented for those responsible for preparing the *'Pharmaceutical Experts Report'*, which forms an intrinsic part of the EU application format.

This focuses on bioavailability of solid dose forms and contents of key excipients, and also links in with information required in other parts of the dossier relating to chiral active ingredients. Although the expert in his pharmaceutical report may give an overview of pharmaceutical development studies, the provision of appropriate data in the body of the dossier is considered essential. Given the format of an EC marketing authorization application (MAA), the presentation of data at the beginning of the pharmaceutical file is very useful in presenting reviewers with a clear overview of the rationale for the development of the formulation.

With this in mind an expanded note for guidance on the subject was prepared in 1988 as an aid to MAA application[21]. Guidelines are divided into five main areas covering constituents, compositions of liquid, semi-solid and solid dose forms and containers. As the first such specific guidelines in this area, the framework has already been used above as a means of introducing the scientific principles, which lie behind pharmaceutical development studies. Nevertheless, the guidelines can be described under these five main headings insofar as it provides an agreed format for use within the EC.

The compatibility of the active constituent with inactive excipients, and in the case of combination products with other actives should be addressed. The appropriate physicochemical properties of the active substances and key excipients will be addressed in the preformulation studies, and it is expected that where particular features are of critical importance this should be reflected in the routine controls applied to these substances.

The guideline repeats the reference in both *Notice to Applicants* and Directive 91/507/EEC, that overages of active substances in a formulation must be properly explained and justified. The reason for inclusion of such overages is to cover losses during manufacture (manufacturing overage) or losses on storage (storage overages). The routine inclusion of overages by manufacturers of certain products without adequate justification cannot therefore be permitted. Similarly, the use of overages should not be an excuse for poor manufacturing, formulation and analytical procedures. For inactive constituents, their presence in a formulation should be explained and justified. Compatibility of the excipients with other excipients as well as with the active substances should be established. The guideline reminds the applicant that a new excipient proposed for medicinal usage for the first time, or for a new route of administration, needs to be fully described and its safety should be established by proper investigation where necessary. Excipients already approved in food use will require no further qualification, provided they are being administered by the oral route – additional routes may require additional studies.[22] An EC guideline on quality of excipients was updated in the year 2003.

For liquid formulations, evidence that the effect of various physical parameters on the dose form has been thoroughly investigated should be presented. The extremes of key variables proposed in the specification must not adversely affect the formulation characteristics, in particular the activity of the drug substance or added antimicrobial preservatives. Such preservatives should be shown by various studies to be of optimal concentration for their intended purpose. The guidance requires the demonstration of antimicrobial preservative efficacy by an appropriately validated test procedure, and since 1990 there has been an agreed *European Pharmacopoeia* (Ph Eur) preservative efficacy test. The Ph Eur test allows two levels of compliance, but applicants should demonstrate compliance at the higher level in all cases unless the lower level can be justified. These requirements apply also to semi-solid dose forms, and the guideline stresses that the preservative test should address both antibacterial and antifungal activity.

In the case of solid dose forms, dissolution testing, as an indicator of product's performance,

is of paramount importance, and should always be carried out by official Ph Eur methodology. Where this is not practical, dissolution test equipment described in a national pharmacopoeia of a Member State can be used, or failing this an appropriate non-compendial method, provided that appropriate justification is provided. For conventional release products, investigations at the development phase will determine whether routine finished product testing is necessary. For prolonged release preparation, however, the dissolution test would be routinely required. Finally, the demonstration of the product homogeneity, in addition to that required in the uniformity of contest test of Ph Eur where the amount of active substance present in the formulation is less than 2 mg per dose or 2% of the total mass, should also be addressed.

Development pharmaceutics guideline address contains aspects of the container, some of which are described above in relation to liquid, semi-solid or finely powered solid formulations, and the capacity for interaction with the container. Basically, such interactions are of two types – sorption and leaching. In the former case sorption of the drug or a key excipient such as an antimicrobial preservative onto the container surface might take place leading to loss in product potency or safety. These phenomenons are known to occur with rubber closures, plastic containers and with administration sets during use. The converse relates to leaching of some component from the packaging material especially in the case of plastic packaging materials into the formulation during storage or processing of the product. Leaching could be of the container material itself or additives, the closures, or even in certain cases labelling adhesive following migration through the container wall. Recently, work has been carried out on the development of a specialized guideline on plastic packaging materials which addresses many of these points in more detail.[23]

Finally, the packaging material must be examined from the point of view of integrity of the construction of the container and closure in order to reassure the regulatory authorities of the effective protection of the container containing the product. Where a dose delivery device is included with the product, e.g., metered dose of aerosol, pen injection device, liquid or powder scoop, etc., the ability to reproducibly and accurately deliver the desired dose should be demonstrated.

However, there is an EC guideline laying down requirements for assessing the quality requirements for oral solid dose prolonged-release preparation. This EC guideline focuses on specific requirements in all parts of an MAA dossier for prolonged-release preparations, which are defined as products in which the rate of release of active substance from the formulation after administration has been reduced for various therapeutic purposes. Such products must be distinguished from delayed-release preparations in which the modification is in the sight of release, both product types are, however, covered by the general Ph Eur definition of 'modified release', although only prolonged-release preparations are covered by EC guideline.

Terminology is critical in describing these types of products, since different definitions appear to be used in different territories to describe the same product behavior pattern while certain terms are unclear or even misleading. The therapeutic objectives and rationale for developing the formulation should be provided, and the physicochemical and pharmacokinetic characteristics described. The manner and mechanism of release should also be explained.

As far as *in vitro* testing is concerned a discriminatory dissolution test procedure is required, as explained earlier. The dissolution apparatus should preferably be one of those described in the Ph Eur, and other methods should be properly justified. It should also be remembered that a continuous flow-through method is now also described in the Ph Eur and this is of particular value for poorly soluble drug substances. The guideline cautions against the use of organic solvents when testing poorly soluble drugs, since the use of such media inevitably leads to a loss in discriminatory power. However, the addition of small amounts of surfactants is envisaged in order to improve the solubility of such substances. The volume of dissolution medium needs also to be controlled to ensure that sink conditions are met, equated in the guideline with an amount of drug in solution not exceeding 30% of saturation concentration.

In the development phase, it is expected that dissolution profiles will be produced for each strength of each prolonged-release preparation for which marketing authorization is sought. Where it is proposed that tablets may be halved for administration purpose then this should be fully justified. Clearly in the case of coated tablets or other preparations for which maintenance of physical integrity prior to administration is required in order to retain *in vivo* performance characteristics, tablets halving cannot be accepted. However, certain systems, e.g. multi-pelleted, can be halved without loss of prolonged-release characteristics. For these, dissolution profiling of the half tablet is additionally required. Changes in the preparation during the development phase will require repetition of the dissolution profile studies. From these profiles a definitive specification for routine testing can be established. The contents of any key excipient, which determine release rate of active substance, may need to be controlled additionally if performance cannot be guaranteed solely by dissolution behavior.

Attempts should be made to correlate the *in vitro* release characteristics with the *in vivo* bio-availability characteristic. Various techniques are proposed in the guidelines in decreasing order of predictive power as to how such correlation can be achieved. However, the choice of method is left to the applicant who must justify the correlation obtained as part of the validation of the dissolution test procedure. It is also stressed that bioavailability testing should be carried out on production scale batches where possible since performance equivalence cannot always be maintained upon scale up. This link between the development phase and production phase is made via process validation for such products whose performance is critical in particular for all products. For this reason process validation principles are presented together with development pharmaceutics in the EC guideline. Similarly, all test procedures, whether they relate to developmental or production tests require validation and a separate guideline on analytical validation (2002) addresses these concerns in all areas of the marketing authorization dossier. In this way the principles of the development pharmaceutics are inextricably linked with those of process and analytical validation.

United States Requirements of Pharmaceutical Development

Similar basic principles apply to pharmaceutical development, process and methods validation in the United States (US) as in the EC. However, although there is extensive guidance on methods validation, no FDA guideline on development pharmaceutics has been produced. The General Guideline on the chemistry, manufacturing and controls apply to the manufacture of drug substance and drug products (1989) imply a similar approach to that undertaken by the EC note for guidance. This guideline stresses the importance of physicochemical control of drug and product, insofar as this affects quality, safety and efficacy considerations.

For the drug substance, physicochemical properties such as solubility profile, solid-state form, melting point, pH, specific rotation and refractive index should be addressed. The solid-state properties, which might affect bioavailability, such as polymorphism, solvate and amorphous forms, and particle size should be examined and carefully controlled. Similarly, inactive substances should be controlled where appropriate.

For the drug product, further detail is spelled out in the Guideline on manufacture and control of the drug product (1989), intended for the submission of INDs, NDAs and ANDAs. This guideline calls for a complete statement of the formulation with alternatives justified in terms of bioavailability. In the section on specification it is clear that these must be chosen carefully to reflect the desired characteristics, which will therefore need proper justification. This approach is therefore analogous to the EC situation.

A further extremely detailed Guideline on packaging materials (1987) has also been produced by the FDA to supplement the data on drug substance and product. Throughout this document the themes of integrity and compatibility with products are repeatedly stressed, and cross-reference is made to the requirements of the *United States Pharmacopeia* (USP). Detailed requirements for containers of different materials for the various types of dose forms are laid down in this document, from the most stringent such as parenterals to the least of stringent containers. Similarly, the emphasis on closures is to ensure compatibility and effective sealing to ensure maintenance of the quality of the product. Aerosols are singled out for special mention, when it is stressed that the valve mechanism forms the most critical part and evidence to demonstrate accuracy and precision of the dose delivered together with maintenance of the correct article size is accordingly sought. For dosage forms requiring unique component systems, special data concerning suitability for intended use might be requested and the examples of medicine's dropper and intravenous administration sets are given. The measure difference between the FDA and EC systems in this regard, however, is that in the former case no formal requirement for a 'development package' is mentioned and there is no distinction made between routine testing and developmental work.

More recently, in order to verify more carefully the data supplied in support of a marketing authorization application, the FDA have introduced the concept of the pre-approval inspection, for specific NDAs/ANDAs (2004). In its Guide to Foreign Inspections (1992), the FDA has highlighted the specific documentations and operations to be covered in such inspections. In addition to demonstration of GMP, GCP, and validation data a Development Report is now called for to provide documentation based on pilot or development batches to support the proposed manufacturing process.

For oral and topical dose forms the development report should cover the formulation, equipment, manufacturing procedures, in-process test data, final dose form test results, conclusions and formal certifications. In the case of sterile products this information should be supplemented by data on certain physical factors (such as extrusion force or particulate controls), sensitivity studies to light or heavy metals, filter compatibility and integrity, oxygen sensitivity, container requirements, preservative efficacy testing and heat sensitivity (autoclaving), where appropriate (FDA 1992).

It is clear that this development report covers much of the same ground as the corresponding EC guideline, although the FDA document strays into areas covered separately under the EC system. Nevertheless the FDA approach described reinforces the close connection between development pharmaceutics, process and methods validation and therefore more closely ties the development laboratory to the production and quality control facility from the regulatory perspective.

In the area of controlled-release preparations the FDA again have requirements which closely parallel those of the EC, although terminology may differ slightly. Thus the terms "controlled release" and "modified release" appear to be used almost interchangeably by FDA[24]. USP and Ph Eur, official in their respective territories, are more or less in agreement in their usage of modified-release to define alteration in place or time of release of active substance. As far as subdivisions of the terms, again USP and FDA appear to agree on the concept of delayed release, in line with Ph Eur, and in fact USP has specific monograph for at least three products, including, aspirin and erythromycin. However, it is in the definition of 'prolonged release' preparations (EC) where divergence appears since such products are referred to in the USP as 'extended release', while FDA do not appear to have focused on a particular term and refer to prolonged release, sustained release or controlled release almost interchangeably[25]. It is therefore important to have clear understanding of different terminology when moving between the US and EC markets, and hence the desire of EC authorities to restrict the number of terms used.

As far as US requirements for such products are concerned there are number of similarities to the EC in terms of the types of development studies, which need to be undertaken. Thus, dissolution profiling at range of pH values (1–7) should be carried out, and the choice and volume of medium, and apparatus justified as outlined in *Pharmacopeial Forum (1991)*. Helpful advice is always given about which apparatus may be best suited for specific dose forms, example Apparatus 3 for 'bead-type', and Apparatus 7 for non-disintegrating oral modified-release forms.

Japanese Requirements of Pharmaceutical Development

As is the case with the Ph Eur and USP, the *Japanese Pharmacopoeia* (JP) lays down certain standards for physical parameters for the substance described. These and additional parameters may need to be taken into consideration in the specification of active substances for incorporation into appropriate products. As with the US regulatory system no separate guideline for development pharmaceutics exists but the general guidelines for preparation of new drug approval applications (NDAs) have an implicit concern for physicochemical properties of new drug substances (Draft 1992). Physicochemical properties of new active substances are covered in section B2, and parallels requirements in other territories, including solubility, hygroscopicity, melting point and thermal analysis, solution pH and pKa, partition coefficient, polymorphism and crystal properties.

Advice issued by the *Ministry of Health and Welfare* (MHW) to Japanese Industry (2002) calls for documents concerning the background to discovery and the development process including names and dates. In this way the choice of specification parameters should be including reasons for selection of the formulation excipients and their concentrations and the selection of manufacturing procedures. Where necessary, the relationship between formulation design and bioavailability should be discussed (Draft 2002). General test requirements for dose forms are laid down in the JP. In addition the draft guideline (2002) indicates for new and established substance a tabular presentation of the necessary testing protocol, although no differentiation between routine testing and developmental testing is given. Drug release tests are routinely required for solid dose forms while certain forms require particle size measurement, e.g. powders and suspensions used as aerosols, ophthalmic and parenteral preparations.

Compatibility studies of liquid preparations (injections, syrups, etc.) with diluents should be conducted and discussed in the stability section (Section C, 1992). Justification for omission of any of the tests described above should be made with any supporting data. Japanese requirements also exist for oral prolonged release dosage forms (1998), which describe testing protocols to be followed. The results of such tests together with those of evaluation tests performed during the course of final formulation development should be presented as of the NDA application (1992).

Requirements of Pharmaceutical Development in other territories

Of the three major marketing territories described above, only the EC has formal guideline for development pharmaceutics packages. Since the requirements of the principal territories apply also in other parts of the world, for example EC requirements are accepted in EFTA and most other European countries, US and Canadian requirements are becoming harmonized following the setting up of the NAFTA agreement, it is clear that there are no other major guideline operating on this subject. However, individual countries may have some specific requirements in this general area.

For example, the *Canadian Health Protection Branch* (HPB) has written extensively on the bioavailability of oral dosage formulations. Thus, Canadian Regulation C.01.012 requires manufacturers of products claiming release of drug to the body over an extended period of time to carry out appropriate investigations to demonstrate such release (1991). The *in vivo* testing requirements for modified-release dosage formulation were examined in a report prepared by the HPB Expert Advisory Committee on Bioavailability (1990). Modified-release dosage forms are defined as those, which differ in the rate of release of drug from that of conventional formulations. This definition is intended to encompass not only the 'prolonged release' approach but also the 'delayed release' type, such as enteric-coated preparations and is, therefore, in accord with the EC definition. However, the introduction of a definition for 'conventional formulation' as 'a formulation compounded in a conventional manner for rapid disintegration and/or dissolution and systemic absorption' is a useful addition.

Regulatory Requirements of Manufacturing

It is interesting to reflect that in the first of the European Community (EC) pharmaceutical Directives, 65/65/EEC, applicants for marketing authorisation were required to provide only a 'brief description of the method of preparation' of the drug product. Subsequently, in the Annex to Directive 75/318/EEC, this was qualified to ensure that 'an adequate synopsis of the nature of the operations' should be submitted. This was to include at least the following points:

- A mention of the various stages of manufacture, sufficient to enable an assessment to be made of whether the processes employed might have produced an adverse change in the constituents.
- Demonstration of batch homogeneity in the case of continuous manufacture.
- The actual manufacturing formula, including any substance which may disappear in the course of manufacture.
- An indication at which stages of the manufacture in-process control tests are carried out only where these are necessary for the Quality Control of the proprietary medicinal product.
- Experimental studies validating the manufacturing process, only in the case of non-standard methods of manufacture or where the methods employed are deemed to be critical for the product.

With respect to the last of the items, cited above, it was almost immediately accepted that sterilisation was such a critical process upon which full information was automatically required in all marketing authorisation applications. Indeed, in 1991 the text of Directive 75/318/EEC was formally amended to include an explicit reference to sterilisation and or aseptic procedures. By 1986, the EC requirements had been slightly reinterpreted[26] to require validation of the manufacturing process, and in particular the provision of data showing that 'using starting material of the stated quality and the types of manufacturing equipment specified, is suitable and will consistently yield a product of the desired quality'. Eventually, the inference was that all standard and non-standard manufacturing processes should be validated, and all the equipment utilised should be specified in the marketing authorisation application. The explicit differentiation between critical and non-critical manufacturing processes had become somewhat blurred by this interpretation.

In the United States, the situation appears to be somewhat less complicated as far as the provision of manufacturing information on drug products is concerned. The need to provide a description of the manufacturing and packaging procedures is clearly stated in the Title 21 *Code of the Federal Regulations* (CFR) 314.5, with no additional qualification regarding validation of the manufacturing process. This should not be interpreted to mean that the US *Food and Drug Administration* (FDA) is not concerned with process validation, since this is obviously not the case; however, the validation of the manufacturing process remains very much within the realms of cGMP. The consequence of this approach is that manufacturing validation data would normally be examined on site during pre-licensing and ongoing inspections. In recent years, the FDA have responded to inadequate manufacturing validation data not by requiring their submission at the marketing authorisation application stage, but by aggressively stepping up the pre-licensing inspection programme. This response clearly indicates that the FDA philosophy of regarding process validation as primarily a GMP matter is likely to continue.

There is no doubt that there has been a tendency by licensing authorities throughout the world to require an increasing amount of detailed information on the manufacturing processes for drug products. Indeed, many of the issues, which formerly could have been regarded as a matter of GMP, are now being addressed at the marketing authorisation stage.

Harmonized and internationally recognized GMP standards/regulations followed by EMEA/FDA/Japan

International Standards and Influential Regulatory Authorities

The European Medicines Agency (EMEA), the US Food and Drug Administration (FDA) and the Japan Ministry of Health, Labour and Welfare (MHLW), arguably the three most globally influential pharmaceutical regulatory authorities, have different approaches to ensure the quality of both domestic and outsourced pharmaceutical manufacturing.

Europe

The EMEA has adopted a risk assessment-based approach laying primary responsibility on drug manufacturers (or market authorization holders [MAHs]) to ensure quality compliance among their suppliers by specifying the requirements for using starting materials manufactured according to EU GMP standards.

Currently, inspections facilitated by the EMEA outside of the European Economic Area (EEA) are restricted to suppliers who are considered suspicious or who may pose possible threats to patient safety. The EU Directive 2004/27 stipulates that a GMP certificate issued by a foreign health authority is insufficient evidence for compliance with EU GMP standards.

The MAHs are responsible for assessing their suppliers and providing the results to regulators. In this way, the EMEA promotes self-inspection by second parties (manufacturers), third parties (contractors for the manufacturers) or joint audits combining the services of second and third parties.

US

The FDA now performs GMP inspections on selected pharmaceutical enterprises, regardless of location. However, there has been recent criticism of this approach, citing that the number of pharmaceutical enterprises the FDA has been able to inspect is not nearly representative of the total number of foreign suppliers exporting pharmaceutical ingredients to the US.

The FDA has started to establish more affiliates in the main exporting countries. It recently opened affiliates in Chinese cities such as Beijing, Shanghai and Guangzhou to strengthen its global presence. FDA inspections in exporting countries are expected to increase primarily in China and India.

Japan

The MHLW regulates the pharmaceutical industry with the Japan Pharmaceutical Manufacturers Association (JPMA) and the Pharmaceutical and Medical Devices Agency (PMDA) in Japan. According to a Lead Discovery report entitled The Japanese Pharmaceutical Market 2008–2023, as the world's second largest drug market, Japan is thought to have some of the most stringent standards in the world on quality and cleanliness of pharmaceutical manufacturing.

Although it has adopted the standards of the International Conference on Harmonisation of Technical Requirements for Registration of Pharmaceuticals for Human Use (ICH), Japan has yet to mutually agree on GMP inspections with the FDA or the EMEA. It had in the past restricted outsourcing and importation, keeping pharmaceutical activities within its borders.

However, this is changing rapidly and the globalization of the Japanese market is expected, as seen in a recent outsourcing of pharmaceutical activities to Taiwanese manufacturers who have undergone inspections by Japanese regulators over the past two years.

Regulators worldwide are now taking more measures to control the quality of pharmaceutical products imported from Asia, with an increased frequency of inspections in addition to those carried out by the MAHs. The largest exporters in the region, China and India, will be subjected to most of these inspections.

Appropriate training and evaluation for deficiencies will be essential to prepare Chinese and Indian pharmaceutical manufacturers for such inspections. Training, education and outsourced inspections services will be top priorities for MAHs as they work with their suppliers throughout Asia.

India

The pharmaceutical sector in India has been one of the fastest growing sectors of its economy over the past several years and it is forecast to continue growing. Similar to China, India is now one of the most important healthcare markets in the world having its own domestic market as well as a huge pool of clients for exports.

However, India is considered to be ahead of China in terms of its control of quality over pharmaceutical manufacturing. It provides economical contract research and manufacturing services, which attracts long-term agreements for outsourcing from global pharmaceutical companies.

In order to attract more investment from international pharmaceutical companies, India introduced the "Product Patent Regime" in 2005. Many Indian manufacturers have also upgraded their manufacturing plants making it one of the countries with the highest number of plants inspected by the FDA, the European Directorate for the Quality of Medicines & HealthCare (EDQM) and other regulatory agencies.

Singapore

Singapore's commitment and investment in the pharmaceutical sector has made the country perhaps the second most advanced country, behind Japan, in Asia. Singapore is well known for being a strategic manufacturing base for global pharmaceutical companies and its ability to comply with global regulations. Its domestic market has also grown healthily in the past few years.

Malaysia

In March 2001, Malaysia was subjected to an assessment by the Pharmaceutical Inspection Convention and Pharmaceutical Inspection Cooperation Scheme (jointly referred to as PIC/S) on the system of GMP inspection and licensing managed by the Malaysian National Pharmaceutical Control Bureau (NPCB).

The assessment showed that Malaysia's system was almost comparable to the requirements of a PIC/S member as it attempted to align itself with international standards. However, the depth of GMP audits was found to be insufficient

due to lack of expertise. The NPCB has since become committed to training GMP auditors in specialized areas and inspection.

It became a member of the PIC/S in 2002 and issues licences to pharmaceutical manufacturers who are deemed to be in full compliance with the code of GMP based on the current PIC/S regulated by the World Health Organization (WHO) Collaborating Centre for Regulatory Control of Pharmaceuticals.

A drug registered in Malaysia carries a registration number on its label or package starting with either PBKD or MAL to indicate satisfactory results on quality, safety and efficacy.

Taiwan

The Bureau of Pharmaceutical Affairs (BPA), established by the Department of Health, handles pharmaceutical regulation in Taiwan. GMP requirements were first established in the 1980s followed by several revisions and additions to tighten the standards. GMP pharmaceutical facilities are subject to inspection every two years by the regulatory body.

In 2007, the Taiwanese strategic review board decided to revise regulations on drug registration in order to make the country's pharmaceutical activities more appealing to international pharmaceutical companies. The Department of Health is now implementing revised regulations requiring Taiwanese pharmaceutical manufacturers to comply with EU's PIC/S standards by 2009.

South Korea

Having signed a free trade agreement with the US and given its rapid economic growth, South Korea's pharmaceutical market is considered as one of the most attractive in the Asia Pacific region after Japan, China and India.

Vietnam, the Philippines and Thailand

These three countries, all members of the Association of South East Asian Nations

(ASEAN), adhere to the ASEAN GMP codes. However, with a lack of consistent inspection standards, the degrees of success are marginal compared to the EU and US standards compliant nations.

The development of the Vietnam's pharmaceutical sector is still in the early stages. The Vietnamese Ministry of Health is investing in pharmaceutical GMP compliance in order to compete in the international market.

Thailand continues to be one of the most challenging environments for pharmaceutical development in Asia with global firms subjected to mandatory licensing by the Thai government.

Regulatory Requirements of Control Test on the Finished Product

The European Community (EC) Guide to Good Manufacturing Practice for Medicinal Products (GMP) defines 'the finished product' as 'a medicinal product which has undergone all stages of production, including packaging in its final container'. This means that, at this point in production, the medicine is potentially in the form in which it will be supplied to the patient. It should be of a quality that ensures that it will have all the safety and efficacy characteristics it was designed to have. These characteristics are guaranteed by the holder of the licensing authorization and by the manufacturer: if the product is found to be lacking with respect to these characteristics, the authorization will be withdrawn or suspended, and public health and the industrial economy will suffer the consequences.

Control tests on the finished product make it possible to assess the quality of a medicine proposed for a therapeutic indication and to establish a quality standard which the medicine must comply with throughout the existence of each batch (stability studies) and throughout its commercial lifetime; however, any changes which occur over the years will have to be taken into account (changes in the size of the batches,

in supplier of raw materials, in the manufacturing site, etc.)

The specifications should be chosen so that:

- They constitute a quality standard that guarantees that the characteristics of the product are consistently the same from one batch to another for many years in thousands of patients.
- At the same time they allow for a certain margin of variation which does not affect the chosen level of quality, and which corresponds to the unforeseeable events, which in practice can occur every day.

The principal characteristics of the dossier should be coherence (order and consistency):

- Coherence between the scientific data collected during the development of the product and the choice of specifications for the finished product.
- Coherence of the acceptable limits and how they relate to the safety and efficacy of the medicine for the patient.
- Coherence of the distribution of quality data between the licensing dossier and the GMP quality assurance dossier.
- Coherence between the specifications for batch release and the quality characteristics, which the product must comply with until the expiry date stated on the packaging selected for the product.
- Coherence between the rigor of regulatory requirements and the flexibility of adaptation to technological and industrial advances.

Whether in Europe, Japan or the United States, the philosophy on testing of the finished product in licensing dossiers is based on these common principles.

Food, Drug and Cosmetic Act provides that FDA may approve a NDA/ANDA 'only if the methods used in, the facilities and controls used for, the manufacture and testing of the drug are found adequate to ensure and preserve its identity, strength, quality and purity'. Pre-approval inspection programs are designed to provide close inspection and analytical attention to the authenticity of and accuracy of reporting of data in applications and provide information regarding facilities. Before FDA approves any application a determination will be made whether all facilities that will participate in the manufacture, packaging and testing of the finished product are in compliance with cGMP and application commitments. Inspection teams may consist of investigators, analysts (if possible, the analyst who is involved in laboratory validation of the product under review), engineers and /or computer experts, as appropriate. The inspection team reviews in detail all the data (including the R&D data) used by the manufacturer to establish its procedure and also reviews production and testing. In this way it verifies the data collected on the batches used during the clinical and/or bioavailability studies.

However, the presentation of the data varies considerably from one continent to another. It does not seem possible to harmonize this aspect of the dossier immediately since it depends on the administrative organization, the habits and the culture of each country and its regulatory authority. More specifically in the US, it seems that close contacts with FDA assessors are necessary in the early stages of work on each dossier, which will progressively become better defined as the dialogue progresses between the partners. In Japan, it is essential to follow detailed procedures; however, the most recent texts and practices emphasize the rationale for the specifications and testing methods that may deviate from the basic plan, which involves a very analytical approach. In the EC, the need to avoid differences in evaluation between national authorities within the framework of procedures for marketing authorization has led to a detailed approach for constituting and presenting a dossier. This should in future avoid wasted time and difficulties in preparing and evaluating data in a uniform manner.

Regulatory Requirements of Stability Testing

The purpose of stability testing of medicinal products is to enable information to be generated which permits well-considered proposals to be made for shelf-life of the products and the recommended storage conditions.

The function of stability testing programme is to ascertain how the quantity of a medicinal product in its proposed marketing packaging varies as a function of time and under the influence of a variety of environmental factors simulating those to which the product will be exposed during storage at the manufacturer and the subsequent shipping, distribution, sale and use.

The different requirements for stability testing in Japan, the EC and the US led to their discussion in a series of bilateral meetings between officials and experts of the three regions in 1989 and 1990. Eventually these led to the creation of an international forum for discussion on requirement for stability, quality and efficacy – the *International Conference on Harmonisation* (ICH).

The proposals for harmonization of stability testing in the EC, which led in 1988 to the CPMP guidance, were based on the concepts of climatic zones. Haynes[27], in his seminal paper in 1971, had suggested the use of a concept he called the 'virtual temperature' to reflect annual temperature variations in various locations of the world, and which could then be used as a basis for standardization of stability testing. Using the concept developed by Haynes, Grimm[28] (1980) has followed Schuster's classification of the world into zones for practical purposes as follows:

Zone I   Temperate zone
Zone II   Mediterranean zone
Zone III Hot dry zone
Zone IV   Hot humid/tropical

In the EC, the Northern European countries (Belgium, Denmark, Netherlands and Luxem-

Table 18.3. World Climatic Zones

Climatic conditions	Zone I	Zone II	Zone III	Zone IV
Mean annual temperature	20.5°C	20.5–24°C	> 24°C	> 24°C
Kinetic mean temperature	21°C	26°C	31°C	31°C
Mean annual relative humidity	45%	60%	40%	70%

bourg) all fall into Zone I. Southern European countries (Greece, Spain and Portugal) fall partly or wholly into Zone II. For the future 'Single European market' it is essential that labelling and storage conditions and shelf-life estimates reflect the worst conditions to which the product is likely to be subjected. The EC stability guidelines stipulate storage testing under test conditions simulating Zone II storage (25°C/60% RH) for long-term real time testing.

In continental North America, Canada and the northern states of the US fall into zone I, whereas parts of the southern US fall into zone II. Puerto Rico falls into Zone III. Most of Japan falls into Zone II. Since approximately 85% of all of the developed world major market comprises sales in the three regions of continental North America, Europe and Japan, it is clear that data generated under storage test conditions simulating Zone II storage would provide data suitable for most of the sales of the product.

Six stages in the development and marketing of a product require stability testing data to be provided have been identified by Mollica and Cohen (1986)[29].

1. Preformulation
2. Formulation development
3. Proposed product
4. New product
5. Established product
6. Revised product

The 'proposed product' stage would include the stage of manufacture and testing of clinical trial material (e.g. IND in the US, CTX in the UK) before its use in trial material in patients.

Stability testing is one of the most important and most expensive areas of product development. It starts with testing of feed or solution dosed to animals as part of the preclinical testing, and then proceeds to studies on the clinical trial material (often a different formulation to the finished product). The definitive studies are then carried out on the final product in its proposed marketing pack, but any substantive changes to the product or pack usually have to be monitored. It truly may be said that stability studies last from the cradle to the grave for a major product.

The gradual development of internationally harmonized testing requirements provides a framework for the industry, which enables considerable potential cost savings to be made. At the first International Conference on Harmonisation in 1991, Zahn estimated that an internationally agreed protocol for testing at defined temperatures and humidity to allow registration in Japan, the EC and the US, together with the use of stability designing that enable sample reduction (bracketing and matrixing) would reduce costs to 33% of the full cost of current testing.

Many of the changes to requirements are already clearly foreshadowed in the ICH guideline on new drug substances and products:

- The need to use the results of the stress test on the drug substance and the preformulation studies on the dosage form to design rational formulations, choose suitable packaging and design analytical methods;
- The need for control of both temperature and relative humidity in long-term real-time testing, in particular the use of 25°C/60% RH as a test condition for the EC, US and Japan;

- The use of 40°C/75% RH as an accelerated test;
- The need for similar pattern of testing of the drug substance and the dosage form;
- The need of packs to simulate the bulk container for the drug substance;
- The need for re-test dating of the drug substance;
- The acceptance of the use of reduced sampling designs for product testing (bracketing and matrixing);
- The need for a minimum of 12 months' testing on a minimum of three batches for a major new active substance product;
- The need to use batches in stability testing that will meaningfully simulate production scale batches (or use actual production scale batches);
- The need for statistical analysis of the stability data (where meaningful) to derive the shelf-life and storage requirements; and
- The need for well-defined storage warnings that avoid meaningless descriptors such as 'room temperature'.

Regulatory Requirements of Biopharmaceutics

Biopharmaceutics is the bridge discipline between formulation description usually assessed by chemistry and manufacturing divisions of chemists in regulatory agencies and pharmacology/clinical data, assessed by pharmacologists, medical and clinical scientists.

Development of a new active substance or new molecular or chemical entity as a medicinal product (or products) for use in man and/or animals follows several stages for which regulations and guidelines are common in most jurisdictions. In the US the CFR requires full documentation of all raw materials including new active substance. The preclinical and development stage examines the pharmacology and toxicology in various animal species for early risk to benefit assessment.

The next IND stage is defined in the Title 21 CFR part 312 as a new drug that is used in a clinical investigation and in humans is categorized in three phases of investigation:

- *Phase I:* Initial introduction of the drug in normal volunteers or patients to determine the pharmacokinetics, pharmacologic actions and side effects with increasing doses and if possible early evidence of effectiveness. Phase I also includes studies of drug metabolism, structure-activity relationships, mechanism of action as well as use of the drug as a tool to explore biological phenomena or disease processes.
- *Phase II:* Includes controlled clinical studies in relatively few patients to examine the risks (side effects) and benefits (effectiveness of the drug for a particular indication in patients).
- *Phase III:* Involves extended controlled and uncontrolled clinical trials to obtain additional information about safety and efficacy, to evaluate the risk/benefit of the drug in a wider context and to provide information for adequate labelling to guide physicians.

The FDA guidelines for preparation of an IND (1991) make it clear that before human use the drug must be prepared and tested in accordance with the Good Manufacturing Practice (GMP) regulation, Title 21 CFR parts 210 and 211. However, drugs will be examined on a case-by-case basis, as it is clear that manufacturing procedures and specifications will change as clinical trials advance and as research nears completion methods will become well established. This guideline also states that the GMP requirements do not apply to new drug products at the preclinical stage. However, it is important to process materials under conditions to assure their integrity and to maintain adequate records. For the IND there are thus requirements for control of components, production and process controls, equipment, package and labelling and reserve samples.

In the European Community similar requirements are noted in the *Guidelines for Good Clinical Practice for Trials on Medicinal Products in the European Community* (1990) which are conducted in the light of Directives 65/65/EEC and 75/318/EEC as amended by Directive 91/507/EEC. As with the US preclinical the Directive does not relate to preclinical 'medicinal products intended for research and development trials'. However, in Directive 91/507/EEC Annex part 3 'Toxicological and pharmacological tests', there are indications that the active substance should be prepared according to the requirements of part 2 of the Annex. The note of guidance for safety evaluation studies in animals (1991) states 'specification of the chemical and physical chemical properties of the drug substance must be given and the stability of the preparation should be provided'. In any of the clinical trials, Phase I, II or III (as in the US), the guidance states that chemical, pharmaceutical, animal pharmacological and toxicological data must be available and evaluated before a new pharmaceutical product is subjected to clinical trials.

The EC documents provide more detail on development pharmaceutics in the Annex part 2A, paragraph 4 of Directive 91/507/EEC and the supporting notes for guidance 'Development pharmaceutics and process validation' (1991) which states the important criteria for assessing active ingredients and excipients including their compatibility. Such features as crystal form, moisture content, and particle size are mentioned. Having identified a parameter as being critical, its control should be reflected in the active ingredient specification.

For each type of product formulation (liquid, semi-solid or solid dosage forms) physico-chemical parameters are to be assessed and depending on the nature of the particular formulation, 'such factors as ease of dissolution and re-dispersion, particle size, aggregation, biological properties, etc. should be considered during pharmaceutical development'.

The Commissioner strongly recommends that to avoid the conduct of an improper study and unnecessary human research, persons planning a bioavailability or bioequivalence study submit the protocol for review prior to initiation of the study.

FDA may review protocols and offer advice concerning appropriate design reference, analytical and statistical methods proposed.

Applications for FDA approval to market a new drug or antibiotic drug are termed New Drug Applications (NDAs). A full NDA requires sections on chemistry/manufacturing, non-clinical pharmacology and toxicology, human pharmacokinetics and bioavailability, a clinical section and a concluding discussion of risk benefit consideration. Additional data may be provided at FDA's request.

The regulations for abbreviations (ANDAs) were revised in 1992 (part 314 and 320) and are suitable for drug products that are the same as a listed drug, drug products that are duplicates of, or that meet the monograph for, an antibiotic drug for which FDA has approved an application.

Amendments to NDAs may be made after the NDA is filed and before approval. This usually involves a new study or re-analysis of an old one. Depending on the nature, the review period may or may not be extended from the original NDA.

International requirements for biopharmaceutic dossiers in marketing authorization application indicate the importance of this aspect in bridging the *in vitro* physicochemical/pharmaceutical aspects with the animal and human pharmacokinetics.

For bioavailability of conventional oral dose forms although, as with all science, several challenging developments are on the horizon such as matrices of rate, there has been some encouraging harmonization of requirements. There are still major problems with modified release (including nomenclature) and adequate biopharmaceutical criteria are lacking for several routes of administration including topical, some parenteral, percutaneous, vaginal, rectal and pulmonary. Regulations for bioequivalence of generic (essentially similar) formulations have been relatively well developed.

Single-dose and repeat-dose toxicity studies

Single-dose and repeat-dose toxicity studies are an essential element of the preclinical safety evaluation of all candidate drugs for the European Community (EC), United States (US) and Japan. Written guidelines of the requirements to support a marketing authorization application or clinical trial for a candidate drug are available.

Single-dose (acute) toxicity studies involve a single administration of the drug followed by a period of observation. All three territories require these studies both for clinical trials and marketing[30] (Table 18.4). The objective of such studies is to characterize the toxicity of the drug, both qualitatively and quantitatively, following the administration of single-dose.

Table 18.4. International recommendations for single-dose studies for clinical trials and marketing

EC	Two mammalian species
Japan	Two species (both rodents, or one rodent)
US	Three species (including one non-rodent)

The broad objectives of the preclinical safety evaluation process are:

- To establish the profile of the biological response of animals to the drug.
- To establish how the effects (both pharmacological and toxicological) seen in the animal models are related to the pharmacokinetic properties and metabolism of the drug.
- To define any likely primary and/or irreversible cellular damage associated with drug administration.

Repeat dose toxicity studies are a central and essential element in this process. The incidence and severity of drug-induced effects frequently increases with the dose and duration of administration. This generalization is consistent with the assumption that biological effects are related to the concentration of the 'active' moiety at the receptor (pharmacological or toxicological) site and that this is proportional to the dose administered in each species. Repeat dose toxicity studies have evolved on an empirical basis and the details of protocol content expected by EC, US and Japan are broadly similar. In reality, the repeat dose toxicity studies are 'screening' test, which are designed to alert the investigator to a wide and undefined range of possible adverse effects.

Pharmacokinetic Data

Pharmacokinetic data provide a scientific basis for interpreting clinical data on safety and efficacy by relating them to the dose, dosage regimen and dose form. For example, a given dose of a drug does not produce the same effect in different individuals; part of this variability can be explained by difference in the absorption, distribution, metabolism and excretion between individuals. Understanding processes is the goal of pharmacokinetics. Pharmacokinetic information can be obtained by measuring drug concentrations in plasma over time following a dose of drug. Another significant source of variability between individuals is the different response observed for a given plasma concentration. The response may be a surrogate pharmacodynamic endpoint or a direct measure of safety or efficacy. For pharmacokinetic data to be useful in understanding the variability in dose response there should be a predictable relationship between the measured plasma drug concentration and the effect. Without establishing a link between the pharmacokinetics and the pharmacodynamics false conclusion can be obtained about the response based solely on the pharmacokinetic information.

It is understandable and commendable that regulatory agencies do not wish to be dogmatic on such issues as pharmacokinetics since the work necessary is dependent on each drug and the results obtained. Another reason for the lack of precision is to be found within the United States system, whereby if a guideline is carefully followed then the agency must accept the information generated and cannot necessarily ask for more work to be done.

In Europe, the basic guideline for kinetics studies can be found in an EC Council Recommendation originally produced in 1983 (CPMP 1983) but updated six years later. In the US the main guideline, albeit brief, can be found in pharmacology and toxicology guidelines published by the FDA in 1985, 1987 and 1988. However, a number of employees from the FDA have over the years published their views on what could be expected in a kinetic submission [31,32,33] and these together with comments from the Pharmaceutical Manufacturers Association (PMA 1980) have helped to clarify the requirements for the US.

Preclinical Safety Data

Examination of the AUC_t or C_{max} data will allow two key questions to be answered:

- What are the plasma concentrations of drug present in each test species?
- How do the concentrations relate to dose size?

Simple graphical examination of the AUC_t or C_{max} values against dose allows consideration of the relationship between plasma concentration and dose size. Two basic relationships should be considered:

A. Drug present with linear increases in AUC_t and C_{max} with dose (dose proportionality) or super-proportional increases in AUC_t or C_{max} with dose (non-linear kinetics).

B. Drug absent or sub-proportional increases in AUC_t or C_{max} with dose (poor absorption of test drug at higher dose levels or auto-induction of metabolism).

Situations where sub-proportional increases in AUC_t occur indicate that great caution should be placed on interpreting the data from the higher dose levels when setting safe dose limits for humans. Often the problem with decreasing absorption with dose will have been foreseen from proper consideration of the physico-chemical nature of the compound (e.g. solubility). When super-proportional increases in AUC_t or C_{max} occur rapid onset of pharmaco-dynamic or toxic effects may occur. Thus, the dose response curve of the compound is exaggerated and narrower separation may exist between undesirable and desirable effects.

GOOD CLINICAL PRACTICE

Good Clinical Practice (GCP) is a code of conduct for those involved in clinical research. The terms Good Clinical Practice or Good Clinical Trial Practice better describe their purpose and scope. However in the US, Japan and the European Community (EC), GCP is now established as the name for this code, devised to ensure the accuracy of the record and that subject's rights are fully protected.

As a code of conduct, GCP is often seen to be a professional concern rather than a regulatory initiative. Certainly important ethical principles are basic to the operation of GCP. Processes such as informing patients about trial procedures and risks, obtaining their consent and ensuring their protection by having a thorough review made of trial procedures and practices by an independent Ethics Committee were conceived and developed as professional initiatives. The Nuremberg Code, devised by an international group of jurists, made an excellent definition of the principles of informed consent in 1949. These principles were developed by the *World Medical Association* in the Helsinki Declaration and its revisions.

Basics of Good Clinical Practice

The basic concepts of GCP are:

- Protection of the safety and rights of the human research subject, involving informed consent procedures and Ethics Committee consultation.

- Standardization of activities within the sponsor company, achieved by the use of good management systems and written Standard Operating Procedures (SOPs).
- Documentation and archiving to a standard that provides an intact paper trial, which will confirm all events occurring during the study.
- Monitoring and audit of investigator procedures and documentation by the sponsor (in Japan, the chief investigator stands between the company and the physician in charge to perform this function).
- In principle, verification of trial documentation by regulatory authority audit, though these procedures are developed to a different extent in the various systems.

All clinical research should, in principle, conform to the same standard but currently the full impact of GCP is upon research intended for regulatory review, that is, research on new drugs or new indications for established ones. It requires that there should be a formal approval step in which the regulatory authorities are involved to ensure that adherence to guidelines, currently the basis for GCP in most territories, can be enforced. Therefore, GCP is applied to research sponsored by pharmaceutical companies as part of the regulatory system controlling access of a medicine to the market. Other research conducted by the same investigators at the same centre may be less well documented simply because there is no financial provision for an independent monitor. It does not necessarily follow that this research will be of a lower overall standard, but monitors find few centres in which there are no errors to be corrected. Therefore, the precision of non-GCP studies can be expected to be lower than of those checked and monitored by GCP procedures.

PHASES OF DRUG DEVELOPMENT AND THE FDA

In the US, all food, drugs, cosmetics, and medical devices for both humans and animals are regulated under the authority of the FDA. The FDA and all of its regulations were created by the government in response to the pressing need to address the safety of the public with respect to its foods and medicinals.

A drug is a substance that exerts an action on the structure or function of the body by chemical action or metabolism and is intended for use in the diagnosis, cure, mitigation, treatment or prevention of disease[34]. The concept of "new drug" stems from the Kefauver-Harris Amendments to the *Federal Food, Drug and Cosmetic Act* of 1938 (FDCA). A new drug is defined as one that is not generally recognised as safe and effective for the indications proposed. However, this definition has much greater reach than simply a new chemical entity. The term new drug also refers to a drug product already in existence though never approved by the FDA for marketing in the US; new therapeutic indications; a new dosage form; a new route of administration; a new dosing schedule or any other significant clinical differences than those approved[35]. Therefore, any chemical substance intended for use in humans or animals for medicinal purposes or any existing chemical substance that has some significant change associated with it is considered not safe or effective and a "new drug" until proper testing and FDA approval is met.

FDA approval can be a fairly lengthy and expensive process. In order for a pharmaceutical manufacturer to place a product on the market for human use, a multiphasic procedure must be followed. It must be remembered that the mission of the FDA is to protect the public and they take that charge very seriously. Hence, all drug products must at least follow the stepwise process.

Preclinical Investigation

Human testing of new drugs cannot begin until there is solid evidence that the drug product can be used with reasonable safety in humans. This phase is called the *preclinical investigation*. The basic goal of preclinical investigation is to assess potential therapeutic effects of the substance on living organisms and to gather sufficient data to determine reasonable safety of the substance in humans through laboratory experimentation and animal investigation[36]. FDA requires no prior approval for investigation or pharmaceutical industry sponsors to begin a preclinical investigation on a potential drug substance. Investigators and Sponsors are, however, required to follow Good Laboratory Practices (GLP) regulations[37]. GLPs govern laboratory facilities, personnel, equipment and operations. Compliance with GLPs requires procedures and documentation of training, study schedules, processes and status reports that are submitted to facility management and included in the final study report to FDA.

It takes 12 years on average for an experimental drug to travel from lab to medicine chest. Only five in 5,000 compounds that enter preclinical testing make it to human testing. One of these five tested in people is approved. Given the attrition rate of compounds in early development it is clearly important to minimize lost opportunity costs when a compound is evaluated in the clinic and thus rationally designed clinical trials are a vital and integral part of the assessment of a drug's potential.

Investigational New Drug Application (INDA)

Unlike the preclinical investigational stage, the INDA phase has much more direct FDA activity throughout. Since a preclinical investigation is designed to gather significant evidence of reasonable safety and efficacy of the compound in live organisms, the IND phase is the clinical phase where all activity is used to gather significant evidence of reasonable safety and efficacy data about the potential drug compound in humans. Clinical trials in humans are carefully scrutinized and regulated by the FDA to protect the health and safety of human test subjects and to ensure the integrity and usefulness of the clinical study data[38]. Numerous meetings

between both the agency and sponsor will occur during this time. As a result, the clinical investigation phase may take as many as 12 years to complete. Only 1 in 5 compounds may actually demonstrate clinical effectiveness and safety and reach the US marketplace.

The Sponsor will submit the INDA Application (with Form 1571) to the FDA. The INDA must contain information on the compound itself and information of the study. All INDAs must have the same basic components: a detailed cover sheet, a table of contents, an introductory statement and basic investigative plan, an investigator's brochure, comprehensive investigation protocols, the compound's actual or proposed chemistry, manufacturing and controls, any pharmacology and toxicology information, any previous human experience with the compound and any other pertinent information the FDA deems necessary. After submission, the sponsor company must wait 30 days to commence clinical trials. If FDA does not object within that period, the trials may begin.

Prior to the actual commencement of the clinical investigations, however, a few ground rules must be established. For example, a clinical study protocol must be developed, proposed by the sponsor and reviewed by an Institutional Review Board (IRB). An IRB is required by regulations[39] and is a committee of medical and ethical experts designed by an institution such as a university medical center in which the clinical trial will take place. The charge of the IRB is to oversee the research to ensure that the rights of human test subjects are protected and that rigorous medical and scientific standards are maintained[38]. IRBs must approve the proposed clinical study and monitor the research as it progresses. It must develop written procedures of its own regarding its study review process and its reporting of any changes to the ongoing study as they occur. In addition, an IRB must also review and approve clinical study. Regulations require that potential participants are informed adequately about the risks, benefits and treatment alternatives before participating in experimental research[40]. An IRB's membership must be sufficiently diverse in order to review the study in terms of the specific research issue; community and legal standards, professional conduct and practice norms. All of its activities must be well documented and open to FDA inspection at any time.

Once the IRB is satisfied that the proposed trial is ethical and proper, it will begin. The clinical trial has three steps or phases. Each has a purpose, requires numerous patients and can take longer than 1 year to complete.

Therefore, there are essentially four phases in the development process as defined by FDA regulations in the United States. The first phase, pre-clinical research, involves laboratory and animal testing of the compound that is primarily aimed at establishing safety and efficacy. If successful, the innovator can then file an Investigational New Drug Application (INDA) with the FDA, seeking approval to move the compound into a three-phase process of human testing.

The nature of the studies conducted in each phase and their purpose are summarized in Table 18.5.

New Drug Application (NDA)

An NDA is regulatory mechanism that is designed to give the FDA sufficient information to make a meaningful evaluation of a new drug[41]. All NDAs must contain the following information: preclinical laboratory and animal data, human pharmacokinetic and bioavailability data, clinical data, methods of manufacturing, processing and packaging, a description of the drug product and substance, a list of relevant patents for the drug, its manufacture or claims and any proposed labelling. In addition, an NDA must provide a summary of the application's contents and a presentation of the risks and benefits of the new drug[42]. The NDA must be submitted complete in the proper form and with all critical data. If the FDA considers it 'acceptable', it will then determine the application's completeness. If 'complete', the agency considers the application 'filed' and will begin the review process within 60 days[42]. The purpose of an NDA from the FDA's perspective is to ensure that the new drug meets the criteria to be 'safe and effective'. The FDA is required to review an application within 180 days of filing. At the end of that, the agency is required to respond with an 'action letter'. There are three

	Preclinical testing		Phase 1	Phase 2	Phase 3		FDA	Phase 4
Years	3.5		1	2	3		2.5	Additional post-marketing testing required by FDA
Test population	Lab and animal studies	File INDA at FDA	20–80 healthy volunteers	100–300 patient volunteers	1000–3000 patient volunteers	File NDA at FDA	Review process approval	
Purpose	Assess safety and biological activity		Determine safety and dosage	Evaluate effectiveness and look for side effects	Verify effectiveness, monitor adverse reaction from long-term use			
Success rate	5000 compounds evaluated		5 enter trials				1 approved	

Table 18.5. Phases of clinical trials

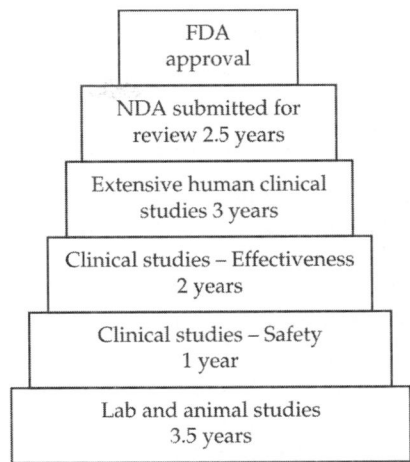

Fig. 18.1. NDA approval process by FDA.

kinds of action letters. An Approval Letter signifies that all substantive requirements for approval are met with and that the sponsor company can begin marketing the drug as of the date on the letter. An Approvable Letter signifies that the application substantially complies with the requirements but has some minor deficiencies that must be addressed before an approval letter is sent. Generally, these deficiencies are minor in nature and the product sponsor must respond within 10 days of receipt. At this point, the sponsor may amend the application and address the agency's concerns, request a hearing with the agency or withdraw the application entirely. A Non-Approvable Letter signifies that FDA has a major concern with the application and will not approve the proposed drug product for marketing as submitted. The remedies a sponsor can take for this type of action letter are similar to those as in the Approvable letter.

Therefore, the applicant, after completion of a sufficient amount of clinical work to demonstrate the safety, efficacy and effectiveness of the new drug for the use or uses for which it is intended, may then submit a new drug application (NDA) to the FDA. Material previously submitted to the FDA in the INDA or in periodic reports must be included in the NDA.

Generic drug approval

The generic pharmaceutical company, seeking to market an equivalent to an innovator's product (once the market exclusivity on the innovator's product has expired), uses a significantly less costly and faster process, the Abbreviated New Drug Application (ANDA) process. Under this process, the generic manufacturer relies on the safety and efficacy data supplied by the innovator, and only has to prove to the FDA that its product is equivalent to the branded product. When processing an ANDA, the FDA waives the requirement for conducting complete clinical studies as the innovator company has already established safety and efficacy. However, it requires the generic manufacturer to conduct bioavailability and/or bioequivalence studies of its version of the branded drug.

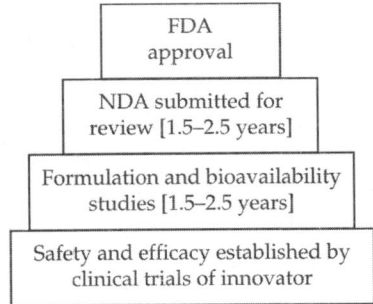

Fig. 18.2. Generic drug approval process.

Abbreviated New Drug Application (ANDA)

The generic pharmaceutical company, seeking to market an equivalent to an innovator's product (once the market exclusivity on the innovator's product has expired), uses a significantly less costly and faster process, the Abbreviated New Drug Application (ANDA) process. Under this process, the generic manufacturer relies on the safety and efficacy data supplied by the innovator, and only has to prove to the FDA that its product is equivalent to the branded product. When processing an ANDA, the FDA waives the requirement for conducting complete clinical

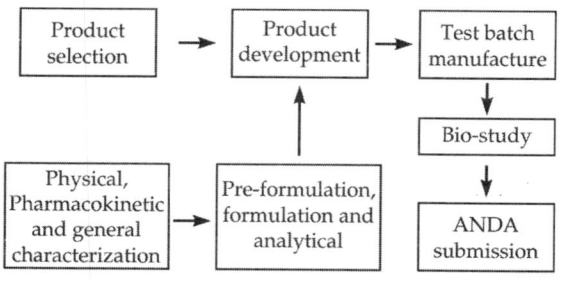

Fig. 18.3. ANDA submission process.

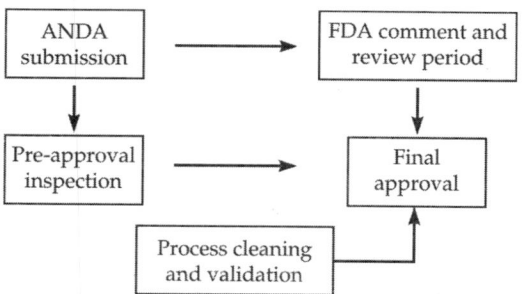

Fig. 18.4. ANDA approval process by FDA.

studies as the innovator company has already established safety and efficacy. However, it requires the generic manufacturer to conduct bioavailability and/or bioequivalence studies of its version of the branded drug.

Bioavailability studies assess the rate and extent of absorption and levels of concentration of a drug in the blood stream needed to produce a therapeutic effect. Bioequivalence studies compare the bioavailability of one drug product with another, in this case the innovator's product. When bioequivalence is established, it indicates that the rate of absorption and the levels of concentration of a generic product are substantially equivalent to the branded product. The ANDA process eliminates the lengthy and costly clinical research phase of development. As a result, generic pharmaceutical product development takes approximately 3 years. The FDA also requires that a company's manufacturing methods conform to current Good Manufacturing Practices (cGMP), as defined in the U.S. *Code of Federal Regulations*. The company must follow the cGMPs in all phases

of the manufacturing process, and must continually monitor compliance and measure quality control.

Phase IV – Post-marketing surveillance

Pharmaceutical companies that successfully gain marketing approval for their products are not exempt from further regulatory requirements. Many products are approved for market on the basis of a continued submission of clinical research data to the FDA. This data may be required to further validate efficacy or safety, detect new uses or abuses for the product or to determine its effectiveness per labelled indications under conditions of widespread usage[43]. Any changes to the approved product's indications, active ingredients, manufacture and labelling require the manufacturer to submit a supplemental NDA for agency approval. "Adverse drug events" are required to be reported to the agency. All reports must be reviewed by the manufacturer promptly and if found to be serious, life-threatening or unexpected, the manufacturer is required to submit an 'alert report' within 15 working days (15 days for serious adverse drug reactions and up to 30 days for non-serious adverse drug reactions) of receipt of the information. All adverse reactions thought not to be serious or unexpected must be reported quarterly for 3 years (these reports are called Periodic Safety Update Reports (PSURs) described format in ICH E2C guideline) after the application is approved and annually thereafter[43]. While covering the aspects of US regulations it might be beneficial to make a brief mention of Orphan Drug Act as well.

Over-the-counter (OTC) regulations

The principles used to establish OTC status are: a wide margin of safety, method of use, benefit-to-risk ratio and adequacy of labelling for self-medication. OTC market entry is less restrictive than that for prescription drugs and does not require premarket clearance. This poses fewer safety hazards than prescription drugs because they are designed to alleviate symptoms than disease. OTC drugs would be examined only by active ingredients within a therapeutic category. This review of active ingredients would result in the promulgation of a regulation or a "monograph" which is a "recipe" or set of guidelines applicable to all OTC products within a therapeutic category. OTC monographs are general and require that OTC products show "general recognition of the safety and effectiveness of the active ingredients". OTC products do not fall under prescription status if their ingredients are deemed by FDA to be " Generally Recognized as Safe and Effective" (GRASE). The monograph system is a public system with a public comment component included after each phase of the process. There are four phases in the OTC monograph system. In Phase I, an expert panel is selected to review data for each active ingredient in each therapeutic category for safety, efficacy and labelling. Their recommendations are noted in the *Federal Register*. A public comment period of 30 to 60 days was permitted and supporting or contesting data was accepted for review. Then the panel reevaluated the data and published a "proposed monograph" in the Federal Register, which publicly announced the conditions for which the panel believed that OTC products in a particular therapeutic class were GRASE. After public comment, the final monograph was established and published with the FDA's final criteria for which all drug products in a therapeutic class become GRASE.

Introduction

On January 24, 2006, FDA published a final rule that amended the requirements for the content and format of labelling for human prescription drug and biological products. The rule is commonly referred to as the *Physician Labelling Rule* (PLR) because it addresses prescription drug labelling that is used by prescribers and other health care practitioners. The rule was designed to make information in prescription drug labelling easier for health care practitioners

to access, read, and use to facilitate practitioners' use of labelling to make prescribing decisions. Labelling includes three sections: Highlights of Prescribing Information (Highlights), a Table of Contents (Contents), and the Full Prescribing Information (FPI). The final rule also reordered and reorganized the FPI, made minor changes to the content of the FPI, and set minimum graphic requirements for the format of the labelling.

Prescription drugs that are not subject to §§ 201.56(d) and 201.57 are subject to the labelling requirements under §§ 201.56(e) and 201.80. The final rule also made minor changes to these regulations. The term *PLR format* refers to labelling that meets the content and format requirements at §§ 201.56(d) and 201.57. The term *old format* refers to labelling that meets the requirements at §§ 201.56(e) and 201.80.

CONSIDERATIONS FOR REVISING LABELLING

The FPI in the PLR format contains substantially the same information as labelling in the old format, typically with reordering and reorganization of the information. For example, new labelling sections (e.g., DRUG INTERACTIONS, USE IN SPECIFIC POPULATIONS, PATIENT COUNSELLING INFORMATION). Therefore, although labelling in the old format for approved products does not contain the new section headings, most of the content already is included in the labelling under different headings or subheadings. For example, information from the old WARNINGS section and old PRECAUTIONS section is consolidated into a single new section (WARNINGS AND PRECAUTIONS) and information in certain old PRECAUTIONS subsections (e.g., *Information for Patients, Drug Interactions, Pregnancy, Labor and Delivery, Nursing Mothers, Pediatric Use, Geriatric Use*) is relocated to new labelling sections (e.g., PATIENT COUNSELLING INFORMATION, DRUG INTERACTIONS, USE IN SPECIFIC POPULATIONS).

A. Developing new sections

FDA expects that most sections or subsections from labelling in the old format can be moved, with little or no modification, to corresponding sections in the PLR format. However, the labelling in the old format may not include the information specified by the new regulations, or the content of a section may not adequately reflect scientific information needed for safe and effective use of the drug. In this case, the labelling must be updated (§ 201.56(a)). If the labelling in the old format lacks an entire section that is required in the PLR format, the section must be developed unless it is clearly inapplicable (§ 201.56(d)).

B. Data analyses or new studies

FDA recognizes that revising labelling to comply with the PLR regulations is an excellent opportunity to update labelling content to ensure that it accurately reflects current knowledge. FDA expects that, in most cases, the revisions will involve limited rewriting aimed at clarifying text, eliminating redundancies, and updating outdated terminology. Generally, no new data analyses of the information in the old format are required if the labelling is truthful and accurate. However, if new information is available that causes the labelling to be inaccurate, the labelling must be updated to incorporate the new information (§ 201.56(a)(2)). Furthermore, if essential information is missing from the labelling (e.g., new information about a class drug interaction), this information must be included (§ 201.56(a)(2)).

C. Updating information in labelling

By regulation, all express or implied claims in labelling must be supported by substantial evidence.[4] If unsubstantiated claims currently exist in labelling, the applicant must revise the labelling to remove such claims (§ 201.56(a)(3)). Consider the ADVERSE REACTIONS section. For the purposes of prescription drug labelling,

the definition of adverse reaction in § 201.57(c)(7) was revised to clarify that it does not include all adverse events observed during use of a drug, only those adverse events for which there is some basis to believe there is a causal relationship between the drug and the occurrence of the adverse event. When updating labelling, the applicant should review the ADVERSE REACTIONS section to ensure all events appropriately fall under that section and delete those events unlikely to have been caused by the drug.

DISTRIBUTING INFORMATION AMONG SECTIONS

When creating labelling in PLR format or converting labelling in the old format to the PLR format, applicants face many difficulties about how to distribute information among labelling sections. Often sections or subsections can be moved with little or no modification (see Appendix C). In some cases, it will be more appropriate to move certain information from a labelling section in the old format to a different labelling section in the PLR format or to consolidate similar issues in one place.

A. Organizing information to avoid redundancy

Clinical information pertinent to prescribing decisions should be identified, prioritized, and located in the labelling section that most appropriately communicates the type of information. Other sections of labelling may more briefly describe or refer to the topic, but not repeat the same content or level of detail. For example, information about a drug interaction that rises to the level of a warning will be described in the WARNINGS AND PRECAUTIONS section, with supporting detail in the DRUG INTERACTIONS section and other sections as appropriate (e.g., DOSAGE AND ADMINISTRATION section if a dosage modification is necessary). In some instances, information discussed in multiple sections of labelling in the old format can be consolidated in the PLR format. For example, if the old WARNINGS and old PRECAUTIONS sections each contained information about a similar topic, this information should now be consolidated under one subsection in the new WARNINGS AND PRECAUTIONS section. When consolidating information, subsections can be created and should be put in an order that reflects the content's importance and relative public health significance.

B. Using cross-references

When a topic is discussed in more than one section of labelling, the section containing the most important information relevant to prescribing should typically include a succinct description and should cross-reference sections that contain additional detail. If the detailed information is divided appropriately into more than one section, those sections should cross-reference each other. Cross-references from the more detailed discussion to the less detailed discussion should generally not be necessary (e.g., a succinct BOXED WARNING should reference the fuller discussion of the risk in WARNINGS AND PRECAUTIONS, but the WARNINGS AND PRECAUTIONS section should not refer back to the BOXED WARNING).

C. Example of the distribution of information among labelling sections

- Drug interaction information should typically appear in the DRUG INTERACTIONS and CLINICAL PHARMACOLOGY sections. If there is a subset of information that is essential for prescribing decisions, that subset of information can be distributed among several sections, including the BOXED WARNING, CONTRAINDICATIONS, WARNINGS AND PRECAUTIONS, and DOSAGE AND ADMINISTRATION sections.

- The DRUG INTERACTIONS section contains clinically relevant information, such as the need to modify a dose or regimen. FDA recommends using a descriptive header of summary concepts preceding a discussion of specific information (e.g., CYP3A Inhibitors).
- More detail about drug interaction studies, including those demonstrating no drug interaction (i.e., pertinent negatives), and any clinically relevant, nonclinical data should be included in the CLINICAL PHARMACOLOGY section.

HIGHLIGHTS

The purpose of Highlights is to provide immediate access to the information to which practitioners most commonly refer and regard as most important.

General principles

Highlights should be a concise, informative summary of crucial prescribing information, not a verbatim repetition of selected material from the FPI, or a repetition of the Contents. Rarely, it may be appropriate to repeat content verbatim from the FPI (e.g., a succinct boxed warning statement or short indication statement), but in most cases, the information should be summarized and presented in an easily accessible format (e.g., bulleted, tabular).

When information about a risk appears in more than one section of the FPI, the information should typically be presented once in Highlights under the most appropriate heading. For example, if a drug interaction is described under Warnings and Precautions in Highlights, it should not be repeated under Drug Interactions in Highlights.

Summarized information should be presented in clear language that is succinct and imparts the most relevant and complete information. For example, under Warnings and Precautions, the statement in Highlights should, as appropriate, identify the risk, its consequences, and the actions to take to prevent or mitigate it. Directive language is preferable, because it conveys explicit information most concisely (e.g., "Discontinue," as opposed to "You should discontinue"). Each summarized statement should be located under the appropriate Highlights heading and must cross-reference the section(s) or subsection(s) of the FPI that contains more detailed information (§ 201.56(d)(3)). If new information is to be added to Highlights, the existing information should be evaluated and combined so that the new information can be added while maintaining the required half page length.

Information in Highlights

Highlights were designed to enhance readability and accessibility of labelling information.

1. Highlights Title and Limitation Statement

The title **HIGHLIGHTS OF PRESCRIBING INFORMATION** must be presented at the beginning of Highlights (§ 201.56(d)(1)). On the first line under the title, the following Highlights Limitation Statement must be presented verbatim in bold: *These highlights do not include all the information needed to use (insert name of drug product) safely and effectively. See full prescribing information for (insert name of drug product)* (§§ 201.57(a)(1) and 201.57(d)(5)).

2. Product Title: Drug Names, Dosage Form, Route of Administration, and Controlled Substance Symbol (§ 201.57(a)(2))

The bolded product title consisting of the proprietary name and the established name of the drug, if any, or, for biological products, the proper name must be presented,[5] followed by the dosage form, and route of administration

3. Initial U.S. Approval (§ 201.57(a)(3))

On the line immediately beneath the product title line, the verbatim statement: **Initial U.S. Approval** must be presented, followed by the bolded four-digit year in which FDA initially

approved a new molecular entity, new biological product, or new combination of active ingredients (§§ 201.57(a)(3) and 201.57(d)(5)), regardless of dosage form or Indication.

4. Boxed Warning (§ 201.57(a)(4))

The Boxed Warning in Highlights must contain a concise summary of all of the risks described in the BOXED WARNING in the FPI (§ 201.57(a)(4)) and is limited in length to 20 lines, not including the title and required reference to the complete boxed warning in the FPI. The title of the Boxed Warning must appear after the word **WARNING**: and must identify the subject(s) of the warning contained in the box (e.g., **WARNING: ACUTE HEPATIC FAILURE and INFUSION REACTIONS)** (§ 201.57(a)(4)). The italicized verbatim statement: *See full prescribing information for complete boxed warning* must be placed immediately following the title of the boxed warning (§ 201.57(a)(4)). FDA recommends that both the title and the verbatim statement be centred within the box, and all text within the box must be in bold (§ 201.57(d)(5)).

The information summarized under the Boxed Warning heading in Highlights should emphasize the information contained in the BOXED WARNING section of the FPI and direct attention to the complete box and to the sections in the FPI that contain more detailed information. There should be only one box in the FPI and one summarized box in Highlights, even when multiple topics are presented. FDA recommends that the information under the Boxed Warning heading in Highlights be summarized in a bulleted format. Each bullet should communicate a discrete warning, clinical indication, or contraindication.

5. Recent Major Changes

When substantive labelling changes have been made to any of the following sections of the FPI within the preceding 12 months, the heading(s) of the changed section(s) must be listed in

Highlights under the heading Recent Major Changes

- Boxed Warning
- Indications and Usage
- Dosage and Administration
- Contraindications
- Warnings and Precautions

Changes that must not be listed in Recent Major Changes include:

- Changes to sections other than the five listed above
- Changes that are not substantive (i.e., minor revisions such as correcting typographical errors or grammatical changes)
- Changes resulting from converting to the PLR format alone
  a. What must be included: Each listing must include the section heading, the subsection heading (if appropriate), identifying number of the corresponding changed section or subsection, and the date on which the change was incorporated in the labelling
  b. Multiple labelling changes: If there is more than one change in the same labelling section or subsection in the preceding 12 months, only the newest date should be listed. For example, if a new indication (hypertension) was added to the labelling in March 2011, and a limitation to the hypertension indication was added in June 2011, the change under the Recent Major Changes heading should be listed as:

    Indications and Usage, Hypertension (1.2) 6/2011

    Only when space in Highlights permits, if there are changes within a section to more than one subsection during the 1-year period listed, each section heading, sub-section heading, identifying number, and date should be listed separately. For example:

Indications and Usage, Hypertension (1.2) 6/2011

Indications and Usage, Heart Failure (1.3) 9/2011

If there are changes within a section to more than one subsection during the 1-year period listed and listing subsection headings separately as above would cause Highlights to be greater than one-half page in length, only the main section heading should be listed, with the date of the most recent change. For example:

Indications and Usage (1) 9/2011

  c. Listing related information from different FPI sections: When a drug product is approved for a new indication, new information is often added to other sections of labelling If there are changes to any of the five applicable sections, each changed section must be listed under the Recent Major Changes heading (§ 201.57(a)(5)). For example:

    Indications and Usage, Hypertension (1.2) 6/2011

    Dosage and Administration, Hypertension (2.2) 6/2011

  d. Marking text in the FPI with a vertical line: The corresponding new or modified text in the FPI sections listed under Recent Major Changes must be marked with a vertical line on the left edge (§ 201.57(d)(9)) to alert the reader to the new information.

  e. Deletions from labelling: Although it is unusual for information to be completely deleted from labelling (e.g., removing a warning as opposed to revising it or moving the discussion to a different section), if such a situation occurs, the applicant should propose labelling that identifies the change in both Recent Major Changes in Highlights and in the FPI.

f. Removing a listing from Recent Major Changes: A changed section must be listed under Recent Major Changes for at least 1 year after the date the labelling change was approved and can continue to be listed until the labelling is reprinted for the first time after the 1-year period expires (§ 201.57(a)(5)).

g. Listing Recent Major Changes for Changes Being Effected (CBE) Supplements[6]: The change must be listed under Recent Major Changes for at least 1 year after the date the labelling change is made and can continue to be listed until the labelling is reprinted for the first time after the 1-year period expires (§ 201.57(a)(5)).

6. Indications and Usage

Information under the Indications and Usage heading in Highlights must include a concise statement of each of the drug's indications from the FPI, briefly noting any major limitations of use (§ 201.57(a)(6)). FDA recommends that the information be presented in a bulleted format if multiple indications exist. If the FPI includes any limitations of use, the presentation in Highlights needs to be clear as to whether the limitation applies to all indications or only certain indications. For a product with limitations of use that are applicable to all of the product's indications, it is appropriate to list those limitations or concerns together, under an appropriately titled subheading (e.g., Limitations of Use). If the drug is a member of an established pharmacologic class, the information under Indications and Usage must include the statement "(*Drug*) is a (*name of class*) indicated for (*indication(s)*)" (§ 201.57(a)(6)). If the drug is not a member of an established pharmacologic class, the applicant should propose one.[7] The FDA will then determine whether to assign a new or existing pharmacologic class to the drug or to omit a pharmacologic class entirely.

7. Dosage and Administration

Information under the Dosage and Administration heading must contain a concise summary of the recommended dosage regimen (e.g., starting dose, dose range, titration regimens, route of administration), critical differences among population subsets, monitoring recommendations FDA recommends a tabular format to enhance accessibility of information as appropriate

In general, every attempt should be made to include the critical dosing and administration information in Highlights. However, there may be instances when a cross-reference to the FPI for detailed information may be necessary for a product with complex dosing and administration information.

8. Dosage Forms and Strengths

Information under the Dosage Forms and Strengths heading must include all available dosage forms and strengths (see § 201.57(a)(8)) to assist the prescriber in product selection. If a solid oral dosage form is functionally scored, such information must be included[8] (§ 201.57(a)(8)). If a drug product has numerous dosage forms, bulleted subheadings (e.g., capsules, suspension, and injection) or tabular presentations are recommended. For some products, including limited information on packaging can facilitate prescribing (e.g., noting that a 0.5% topical cream is available in both 15 g and 30 g tubes). Because of space constraints in Highlights, multiple strengths for a dosage form should be listed on one line (e.g., Tablets: 25 mg, 50 mg, 100 mg, and 200 mg). Descriptors of the product appearance (e.g., tablet color, shape, embossing) that appear in DOSAGE FORMS AND STRENGTHS in the FPI should not appear in Highlights.

9. Contraindications

Information under the Contraindications heading must include a list of all the contraindicated situations described in the FPI or the word "None" if no contraindicated situations have been identified (§ 201.57(a)(9)). As in the FPI, *theoretical* contraindications should not be included in Highlights. For example, some labelling has included a contraindication in patients with hypersensitivity to any of the drug product's components, despite there being no such reports and no basis upon which to believe such a risk exists. For labelling being converted to PLR format, these *theoretical* contra-indications should be removed.

10. Warnings and Precautions

Information under the Warnings and Precautions heading must include a concise summary of the most clinically significant safety concerns from the FPI that affect decisions about whether to prescribe the drug, recommendations for patient monitoring to ensure safe use of the drug, and measures that can be taken to prevent or mitigate harm (§ 201.57(a)(10)). Individual risk topics should be presented in a bulleted format, with each imparting a complete piece of information.

The presentation should not merely be a list of subsection headings from Contents. Ambiguous and uninformative information (e.g., use with caution) and terminology that describes a contraindication (e.g., "do not use…") should be avoided. The order of the information should be the same as that of the FPI WARNINGS AND PRECAUTIONS section, reflecting the nature and severity of the risks.

11. Adverse Reactions

a. Most frequently occurring adverse reactions: Information under the Adverse Reactions heading must include (1) a listing of the most frequently occurring adverse reactions, even if one or more are included elsewhere in Highlights (e.g., under the Warnings and Precautions heading) and (2) the criteria used to determine inclusion (e.g., frequency cutoff rate) (§ 201.57(a)(11)(i)). The listing should be concise, not lengthy or comprehensive, and reactions should be presented in decreasing order of frequency.

Rates of most common adverse reactions vary, but should be appropriate to the nature of a drug's adverse reactions profile and the size and composition of the safety database. If adverse reaction profiles vary significantly for different indications, the most common adverse reactions should be presented separately for each indication.

b. Adverse reaction reporting contact information: Highlights must also contain adverse reaction reporting contact information, in bold type, that includes the following (§§ 201.57(a)(11)(ii), (iii), (iv) and 201.57(d)(5)):

- The verbatim statement "**To report SUSPECTED ADVERSE REACTIONS, contact**" followed by the manufacturer's name and phone number for adverse reaction reporting.
- The address of a manufacturer's web site for voluntary reporting of adverse reactions (only if such a web site exists).
- FDA's phone number and web address for voluntary reporting of adverse reactions (see below).

FDA's phone numbers and web addresses for voluntary reporting of adverse reactions:

For drug and biological products (other than vaccines) Med Watch Phone number: 1-800-FDA-1088 Web address: *www.fda.gov/medwatch*

For example, the completed adverse reaction reporting contact information statement for a drug product would read:

To report SUSPECTED ADVERSE REACTIONS, contact [name of manufacturer] at [manufacturer's phone number] or FDA at 1-800-FDA-1088 or www.fda.gov/medwatch.

If more than one entity is responsible for the product (e.g., the product is manufactured by one company and marketed by another, or the product is co-marketed), only one contact should be listed (e.g., the name of the entity identified by agreement between the companies as the recipient of safety information).

12. Drug Interactions

Information under the Drug Interactions heading must include a concise summary of those drugs (or classes of drugs) or foods that interact or are predicted to interact in clinically significant ways with the subject drug, and practical instructions for preventing or managing the interaction. Descriptive subheadings of summary concepts (e.g., CYP3A inhibitors) can precede specific information. Rarely, it may be appropriate to include pertinent negative findings of drug interaction studies under this heading if the interaction would otherwise be anticipated or is of special concern. If there are no clinically significant drug interactions, the heading should be omitted from Highlights. Information about lack of drug interactions or drug interactions that are not clinically relevant should not be included in Highlights. Interactions with serious clinical consequences that are summarized elsewhere in Highlights (e.g., in the Boxed Warning or under the Contraindications or Warnings and Precautions heading) should be described in greater detail in the DRUG INTERACTIONS section in the FPI and need not be repeated under the Drug Interactions heading in Highlights. Because some drugs have numerous clinically significant drug interactions, it may not be possible to concisely summarize all the critical information in Highlights. In these instances, a statement can be included under the Drug Interactions heading in Highlights that alerts the prescriber to the presence and significance of the drug interaction information in the FPI.

13. Use in Specific Populations

Information under the Use in Specific Populations heading must include a concise summary of any clinically important differences in response or recommendations for use of the drug in specific populations from the FPI (e.g., differences between adult and pediatric responses, need for specific monitoring in patients with hepatic impairment) (§ 201.57(a)(13)). If multiple populations are described under this heading, they should be presented in the same order in which they appear in the FPI. If there are no clinically important differences in response or recommendations for use of the drug in specific populations, the heading should be omitted from Highlights. Ordinarily, the absence of information about the safety and effectiveness of a drug in a specific population (e.g., pregnant women, children) should not be included under this heading. In unusual circumstances, if describing the absence of data provides important information for the prescriber, the heading should be retained. The pregnancy category designation is not appropriate for inclusion in Highlights because, in isolation, it tends to oversimplify the risks of drugs in pregnancy and, as a result, may be confusing. Decisions about use of a drug in pregnancy should be based on careful consideration of available data, not simply on a reference to the pregnancy category.

14. Patient Counselling Information Statement

Highlights must contain the statement **See 17 for PATIENT COUNSELLING INFORMATION** in bold or, if the product has FDA-approved patient labelling, **See 17 for PATIENT COUNSELLING INFORMATION and FDA-approved patient labelling**, or if the product has a Medication Guide, **See 17 for PATIENT COUNSELLING INFORMATION and Medication Guide** (§§ 201.57(a)(14) and 201.57(d)(5)). If the product has both a Medication Guide and another type of FDA-approved patient labelling (e.g., Instructions for Use); the statement should refer only to the Medication Guide. If the product has more than one type of FDA-approved patient labelling other than a Medication Guide

15. Revision Date

At the end of Highlights, the date of the most recent revision of the labelling must be presented (§ 201.57(a)(15)). The preferred format is **Revised: Month Year or Revised: Month/Year** in bold type (i.e., **Revised: Apr 2011** or **Revised:**

4/2011). In PLR format, this statement replaces the revision date that appears at the end of labelling in the old format (§ 201.56(e)(5)). A new approval or changes to the approved labelling will trigger a new revision date.

PROCEDURAL INFORMATION

Applications covered by the Final Rule

Section 201.56(b)(1) provides that the final rule applies to prescription drug products with a new drug application (NDA), biologics licence application (BLA), or efficacy supplement that
- is submitted on or after June 30, 2006 (the effective date of the final rule),
- is pending with the Agency on June 30, 2006, or
- was approved in the 5 years prior to June 30, 2006.

1. New NDAs, BLAs, and Efficacy Supplements

The following efficacy supplements trigger the requirement to revise labelling to the PLR format:

- Adding or modifying an indication or claim.
- Revising the dose or dose regimen.
- Providing for a new route of administration.
- Making a comparative efficacy claim naming another product.
- Significantly altering the intended patient population.
- Providing for, or providing evidence of effectiveness necessary for, the traditional approval of a product originally approved under subpart H of part 314 or part 601.
- Incorporating other information based on at least one adequate and well controlled clinical study.
- Pediatric supplements in response to written requests and the pediatric research equity act of 2007.

2. Approved Applications

When more than one approval for the same product occurred in the 5 years prior to the effective date of the final rule (e.g., NDA and efficacy supplement), the date of the most recent approval determines the timing of submission of labelling in the PLR format according to the implementation plan.

3. Submitting Draft Labelling to FDA for Review

To facilitate FDA's review of labelling, when a significant amount of new information is being added to the labelling at the same time that the labelling is being converted to the PLR format (e.g., an efficacy supplement that also converts labelling to the PLR format), we recommend that the following versions of labelling be submitted as appropriate:

Labelling in the old format

Annotated labelling in the old format explaining how existing text was incorporated into the PLR format.

A *clean* version (no red line/strike out) in the PLR format *without* the new information.

The above *clean* version in the PLR format *with* the new information (in red line/strike out).

Changes to the regulations for applications not covered by the final rule

FDA has also made minor amendments to the labelling regulations for prescription drugs and biological products not subject to the PLR content and format requirements (see §§ 201.56(e) and 201.80). Section 201.80 remains largely unchanged from previous labelling regulations, except for minor revisions to the REFERENCES section and the requirement to append FDA-approved patient labelling to the prescribing information by June 30, 2007. As always, labelling must be informative and accurate and neither promotional in tone nor false or misleading in any particular (§ 201.56(a)(3)). Therefore, the applicant should review the labelling at least annually for outdated information. Removing outdated references could be submitted in the Annual Report.

Implementation Plan for PLR Format	
Applications (NDAs, BLAs, and Efficacy Supplements) Required to Conform to PLR Labelling Requirements	**Time by Which Conforming Labelling Must Be Submitted to the Agency for Approval**
Applications submitted on or after June 30, 2006	Time of submission
Applications pending on June 30, 2006, and applications approved any time from June 30, 2005, up to and including June 30, 2006	June 30, 2009
Applications approved any time from June 30, 2004, up to and including June 29, 2005	June 30, 2010
Applications approved any time from June 30, 2003, up to and including June 29, 2004	June 30, 2011
Applications approved any time from June 30, 2002, up to and including June 29, 2003	June 30, 2012
Applications approved any time from June 30, 2001, up to and including June 29, 2002	June 30, 2013
Applications approved prior to June 30, 2001	Voluntarily at any time

Appending FDA-Approved Patient Labelling

The final rule required that by June 30, 2007, any FDA-approved patient labelling either accompany the labelling or be reprinted immediately following the last section of the labelling (§§ 201.56(e)(6), 201.57(c)(18) and 201.80(f)(2))[14]. This requirement applies to the labelling of all drugs, not just those subject to the PLR format requirements. The final rule provides the option of either reprinting the FDA-approved patient labelling (including Medication Guides) immediately following the last section of labelling or having the FDA-approved patient labelling accompany the labelling as a separate document (e.g., included in the carton with the drug).

The FDA-approved patient labelling should not be a numbered subsection under the PATIENT COUNSELLING INFORMATION section in the FPI or listed in Contents, but appended or reprinted after the last section of labelling. The PATIENT COUNSELLING INFORMATION section of the FPI is written for health care professionals and contains the information that is important to convey to patients when the drug is being prescribed, dispensed, or administered. The FDA-approved patient labelling is written for patients to provide them with information about the drug that has been prescribed. FDA believes that both of these are important tools for providing information to patients.

Submitting electronic versions of labelling

For information about submitting labelling electronically, applicants should consult the information and Guidances for industry on FDA's web site on Structured Product Labelling Resources.

Files required to be submitted to USFDA

Following these files are required to be submitted in Module one of Common Technical Document:

1.14

1.14.1

1.14.1.1 – Draft carton and container labels – 4 copies of draft for paper submissions only 9 each strength and container).

1.14.1.2 – Annotated draft labelling text 21CFR 314.94(a)(8)(iv) – Side-by-side labelling

Old Format*	PLR Format**
Description	**HIGHLIGHTS OF PRESCRIBING INFORMATION**
Clinical Pharmacology	Product Names, Other Required Information
Indications and Usage	Boxed Warning
	Recent Major Changes
Contraindications	Indications and Usage
Warnings	Dosage and Administration
	Dosage Forms and Strengths
Precautions	Contraindications
Adverse Reactions	Warnings and Precautions
	Adverse Reactions
Drug Abuse and Dependence	Drug Interactions
Overdosage	Use in Specific Populations
Dosage and Administration	**FULL PRESCRIBING INFORMATION: CONTENTS**
How Supplied	**FULL PRESCRIBING INFORMATION**
Optional sections:	Boxed Warning
Animal Pharmacology and/or	1. Indications and Usage
Animal Toxicology Clinical Studies	2. Dosage and Administration
	3. Dosage Forms and Strengths
References	4. Contraindications
	5. Warnings and Precautions
	6. Adverse Reactions
	7. Drug Interactions
	8. Use in Specific Populations
	9. Drug Abuse and Dependence
	10. Overdosage
	11. Description
	12. Clinical Pharmacology
	13. Nonclinical Toxicology
	14. Clinical Studies
	15. References
	16. How Supplied/Storage and Handling
	17. Patient Counselling Information

* As required by 21 CFR 201.56(e) and 201.80
** As required by 21 CFR 201.56(d) and 201.57

comparison of containers and carton for each strength with all differences visually highlighted and annotated.

1.14.1.3 – Draft labelling text – package insert (content of labelling) in PDF and word format, and SPL submitted electronically.

1.14.1.4 – Labelling comprehension studies – refer to pharmacy bulk package sterility assurance table (for PBS only).

1.14.3

1.14.3.1 – Annotated comparison with listed drug 21CFR 314.94(a)(8)(iv)-1 Side-by-side labelling (package and patient insert) comparison with all differences visually highlighted and annotated.

1.14.3.3 – Labelling text for reference listed drug – RLD package insert, 1 RLD container label, and if applicable 1 RLD outer container label.

Type Size Requirements for Labelling and FDA-Approved Patient Labelling Included with Labelling

	Type Size Requirements for Labelling	FDA-Approved Patient Labelling Included with Labelling	Type Size Requirements for FDA-Approved Patient Labelling
PLR Format (21 CFR 201.57)			
Trade Labelling (i.e., labelling on or within the package from which the drug is to be dispensed)	Minimum 6-point type	FDA-approved patient labelling that is not for distribution to patients	Minimum 6-point type
		Any FDA-approved patient labelling (except a Medication Guide) that is for distribution to patients	Minimum 6-point type
		Medication Guide that is for distribution to patients	Minimum 10-point type
Other Labelling (e.g., labelling accompanying promotional materials)	Minimum 8-point type	FDA-approved patient labelling that is not for distribution to patients	Minimum 8-point type
		Any FDA-approved patient labelling (except a Medication Guide) that is for distribution to patients	Minimum 8-point type*
		Medication Guide that is for distribution to patients	Minimum 10-point type
Old Format (21 CFR 201.80)			
Trade Labelling and Other Labelling	No minimum requirement	FDA-approved patient labelling that is not for distribution to patients	No minimum requirement
		Any FDA-approved patient labelling (except a Medication Guide) that is for distribution to patients	No minimum requirement
		Medication Guide that is for distribution to patients	Minimum 10-point type

* FDA does not require, but encourages a minimum type size of 10 points for this information.

Regulations pertaining to labelling

- Regulations for drugs – 21CFR 201.56
- Regulations for biologics – 21CFR 201.57.
- Labelling that meet the content and format requirements of 21CFR 201.56(d) and 21CFR 201.57 is termed "PLR format".
- FR notice volume 71, No. 15, Jan. 24, 2006.

- New and recently approved drugs required to comply with PLR format {21 CFER 201.56 and 21CFR201.57}

Those products for which NDA, BLA or efficacy supplement was approved from June 30,2001 or was pending on June 2006 there is a staged implementation schedule.

APPENDIX E – HIGHLIGHTS AND CONTENTS FORMAT SAMPLE

HIGHLIGHTS OF PRESCRIBING INFORMATION

These highlights do not include all the information needed to use [DRUG NAME] safely and effectively. See full prescribing information on [DRUG NAME].

[DRUG NAME (nonproprietary name), dosage form, route of administration, controlled substance symbol] Initial U.S. Approval: [year]

> **WARNING: [SUBJECT OF WARNING]**
>
> *See full prescribing information for complete boxed warning.*
> - [text]
> - [text]

RECENT MAJOR CHANGES

[section (X.X)]   [m/year]
[section (X.X)]   [m/year]

INDICATIONS AND USAGE

[DRUG NAME] is a [name of pharmacologic class] indicated for:
- [text]
- [text]

DOSAGE AND ADMINISTRATION

- [text]
- [text]

DOSAGE FORMS AND STRENGTHS

- [text]

CONTRAINDICATIONS

- [text]
- [text]

WARNINGS AND PRECAUTIONS

- [text]
- [text]

ADVERSE REACTIONS

Most common adverse reactions (incidence > x%) are [text].

To report SUSPECTED ADVERSE REACTIONS, contact [name of manufacturer] at [phone #] or FDA at 1-800-FDA-1088 or www.fda.gov/medwatch.

DRUG INTERACTIONS

- [text]
- [text]

USE IN SPECIFIC POPULATIONS

- [text]
- [text]

See 17 for PATIENT COUNSELLING INFORMATION [and FDA - approved patient labelling OR and Medication Guide].

Revised:[m/year]

FULL PRESCRIBING INFORMATION: CONTENTS*

WARNING: [SUBJECT OF WARNING]

1 INDICATIONS AND USAGE
1.1 [text]
1.2 [text]

2 DOSAGE AND ADMINISTRATION
2.1 [text]
2.2 [text]

3 DOSAGE FORMS AND STRENGTHS

4 CONTRAINDICATIONS

5 WARNINGS AND PRECAUTIONS
5.1 [text]
5.2 [text]

6 ADVERSE REACTIONS
6.1 [text]
6.2 [text]

7 DRUG INTERACTIONS
7.1 [text]
7.2 [text]

(Contd.)

STRUCTURE OF PHARMACEUTICAL INDUSTRY IN INDIA

The pharmaceutical industry in India is highly fragmented both in terms of number of manufacturers as well as the variety of products. Government policies as well as the regulatory framework have been the primary reason for the fragmentation. The combined effect of the IPA and the DPCO resulted in a highly fragmented structure. The lack of product patents enabled manufacturers to produce existing drugs through alternate processes.

Now compliance with TRIPS would mean introducing product patents in India for pharmaceuticals for a uniform duration of 20 years for all products. India is entitled to a 10-year transitional period, making product patents applicable by January 1st 2005. However companies, which have filed patent applications from January 1st, 1995, will enjoy exclusive marketing rights.

The impact of the prospective transition from the current process patent regime to a product patent regime in 2005 is likely to be felt only gradually over the next few years and in a substantive measure only after 2010. Till the new TRIPS compliant patent regime comes into force, Indian firms are free to manufacture drugs patented prior to January 1st, 1995. Moreover the patent laws will protect only a small proportion of drugs as the patented drugs form only 10 to 12 percent of the domestic drug turnover.

Another significant development is that many existing patented drugs will go off patent in next few years, opening up large generic markets for Indian manufacturers. The worldwide pharmaceutical market is worth US $400 billion. Out of this about 70 percent comes from non-patented drugs. In the next five years with the expiry of several patents, the non-patented segment is expected to grow to 75 percent. This would also keep the drug prices from rising steeply.

In the long run, new patent regime, and introduction of new patented products, would encourage domestic companies to invest substantially in R&D to take advantage of the abundant pool of scientific and technical resources available here. Even MNCs have recognized the opportunities of cost effective R&D in India and are planning to outsource R&D to India. Few of the MNCs like Novartis A.G., Astra Zeneca, Pfizer Inc. and Merck, have already set up 100 percent subsidiaries in India to support new research activities. Another long-term strategy that can be adopted by Indian companies would be to manufacture cost-effective intermediates for foreign companies. Joint ventures, technology collaborations and cross licensing arrangements can also be examined.

Forms for NDA

- Form 45 – Finished Formulation
- Form 45A – Bulk Substance
- Form 46 – Manufacturing
- Form 41 – Registration
- Form 10 – Import Licence

Timeline and fee for NDA

- Approx. 1 year.
- TR Challan of Rs. 50000/15000, fresh/sub-sequent application.

Post-marketing surveillance

- Procedures for distribution of records.
- Complaint handling.
- Adverse incident reporting.
- Procedure for product recall.
- Corrective action taken.

Regulatory process in India

In India, three types of permission are actually required for commercial use of imported formu-lations/in-house developments:

1. New drug permission (issued in Form 45).
2. Registration certificate (issued in Form 41).
3. Import licence (issued in Form 10).

Task 1: First application would be made for new drug permission

Data required:

- Chemical and Pharmaceutical Information.
- Pre-clinical Data.
- Clinical Data – Phase I, II, III and IV if available (or PSURs).
- Other Published Literature.
- Marketing Information.
- Any other studies conducted with the product (as per Sch Y).

Task 2: Second application would be for registration of the drug and its manufacturing site

Data required:

- Drug Master File.
- Plant Master File.
- COPP/Free Sale Certificate/CE Certification.
- WHO GMP of the Manufacturing Site.
- Power of Attorney.
- Other Data/documents mentioned in the Schedule DI & DII.

Task 3: Third application would be file for grant of Import Licence

Data required:

- Form 9.

SUMMARY

Over the past decades, new international trade and investment rules coupled with changes in business practices and political organisation have resulted in significant transformation of economic and social policy around the world. These new arrangements, often-labelled 'economic globalisation' has driven states and manufacturers to work more closely and to harmonise their practices and reference points through equivalency and mutual recognition agreements (e.g., General Agreement on Tariffs and Trade – GATT). The driving logic behind this is that harmonisation can improve economic efficiency in cross-border trade, thereby allowing the pharmaceutical sector to get new drugs onto the global market as quickly as possible. All over the world – and not only in the pharmaceutical field – we have witnessed various processes of harmonisation, all of which tend towards the creation of truly common areas for economic development. In the case of pharmaceuticals, these processes usually take into account scientific and technical aspects (e.g., chemical and pharmaceutical data, pre-clinical tests, clinical studies) as well as administrative aspects (e.g., procedures and practices required for registration) of harmonisation.

ACKNOWLEDGEMENT

The author is thankful to Mr. Rohin Sethi, Research Scholar, Drug Regulatory Affairs, Delhi Institute of Pharmaceutical Sciences and Research (DIPSAR), New Delhi for review of this script.

REFERENCES

1. Garattini S, Bertele S. Adjusting Europe's drug regulation to public health needs. *Lancet* 2001; 358: 64–7.

2. International Conference on Harmonisation of Technical Requirements for Registration of Pharmaceuticals for Human Use. Available at: *http://www.ifpma.org/ich1.html* (accessed January 2001).

3. European Community (EC). *Rules governing medicinal products in the European Community Volume III, Guidelines on the quality, safety and efficacy of medicinal products for human use.*

4. Council Directives 65/65/EEC, *Official Journal of the European Communities*, 369/65 (1965).

5. Council Directives 83/570/EEC, Article 8 amendment to Directive 75/319/EEC, *Official Journal of the European Communities*, No. L332/1 (1983).

6. Council Directives 83/570/EEC, Article 3, *Official Journal of the European Communities*, No. L332/1 (1983).

7. Council Directive 87/22/EEC, *Official Journal of the European Communities*, No. L15/38.

8. Commission of the European Communities (1988). Report from the commission on the activities of the committee for proprietary medicinal products. Com. 88:143 (1988).

9. "Un entretien bilan avec le directeur de la Pharmacie et du medicament," *LeQuatidien du Medecin*, 4 May, 1988, pp 7–8.

10. Sauer F. and Hawkin, R., "Rules governing pharmaceuticals in the European Community," *Journal of Clinical Pharmacology*, 27:639–646, 1987.

11. EFPIA Comments to the Commission of the European Communities. Completion of the internal market: Future marketing authorisation system, September 1988.

12. The Association of the British Pharmaceutical Industry. Blueprint for Europe 1988.

13. Currie, W.J.C., "Is There the Will for There to be a Way?" *J. Clin. Pharmaco.*, 29:770–774,1989.

14. Council Regulation 2309/93EEC, *Official Journal of the European Communities*, No. L214/1 (1993).

15. The Scheme for the Mutual Recognition of Evaluation Reports on Pharmaceutical Products, 1979 (Revised 1986). Published by the Secretariat of the European Free Trade Association.

16. Sandlund, M.B. and Nicholson, I.E., Memorandum of Understanding Between the National Board of Health and Welfare of Sweden and the Department of Community Services and Health of Australia on Cooperation in the field of Drug Regulation. Signed at Uppsala on 01 Feb. 1989.

17. Agreement between the Drug Directorate, Health and Welfare Canada and Therapeutic Goods Administration, Department of Community Services and Health, Australia for the Exchange of Pharmaceutical Evaluation Reports. Signed 16 March 1990.

18. International Reporting of Adverse Drug Reactions. Final Report of the CIOMS Working Group, World Health Organisation, Geneva, 1990.

19. Second International Conference on Harmonization, 1993, Plenary Session: Background to the Conference, P4.

20. European Community (EC). *Rules governing medicinal products in the European Community* (1989). Vol. I, *Guidelines on the quality, safety and efficacy of medicinal products for human use.*

21. European Community (EC). *Rules governing*

medicinal products in the European Community (1989). Vol. III, *Guidelines on the quality, safety and efficacy of medicinal products for human use.*

22. European Community (EC), *Draft note for guidance* (1993). *Excipients in the marketing authorisation dossier*, III/3196/91.

23. European Community (EC), *Draft note for guidance* (1993). *Containers and packaging material – plastic materials*. III/9090/93.

24. Skelly, J.P. and Barr, W (1987). Regulatory assessment. *In:* Controlled drug delivery, (2nd edn), (Ed., J. Robinson and V.H. Lee), Marcel Dekker, New York, p. 294.

25. Dighe, S.V. & Adams, W.P.(1988). Bio-availability and bioequivalence of oral controlled release products: a regulatory perspective. *In:* Pharmaceutics: Regulatory, Industrial and Academic Perspectives (Ed., P.G. Welling and F.L.S. Tse), Marcel Dekker. New York, p. 307.

26. Medicines Act 1968. *Guidance notes on application for product licences* (MAL 2) (1968). HMSO, London.

27. Haynes, J.D. (1971). Worldwide virtual temperatures for product stability testing. *J. Pharm. Sci.* 60.

28. Grimm, W. (1992). Harmonisation of guidelines on stability testing in the EC, Japan and the US on the move. The APV symposium brought the successful start. *Eur. J. Pharm. Biopharm.*, 38(4), 154–155.

29. Mollica, J. & Cohen, J. (1986). Follow-up stability. *STP Pharma* 2 (17), 570-576.

30. CPMP 1990; D'Arcy and Harron 1991; Pharmaceutical Manufacturers' Association 1977; *Rules governing medicinal products in the European Community*, Volume III.

31. Peck, C.C. Barr, W.H., Benet, L.Z., et al. (1992). Opportunities for integration of pharmacokinetics, pharmacodynamics and toxicokinetics in rational drug development. *Pharma. Res.*, 9,826–833.

32. Glocklin V.C. (1982). General consideration for the study of the metabolism of drugs and other chemicals. *Drug Metab. Rev.* **13**, 929-939.

33. Scheuplein, R.J., Shoaf, S.E., Brown, R.N. (1990). Role of pharmacokinetics in safety evaluation and regulatory considerations. *Ann. Rev. Pharmacol. Toxicol.* **30**,197-218.

GLOSSARY

The Code of Federal Regulations (CFR)

The Code of Federal Regulations are the codified regulations borne of the laws of the United States Federal Government. Comprised of over fifty titles, Title 21 is entitled Food and Drugs, and prescribes the procedures to be followed by companies and individuals in the food and drug business.

Preclinical Testing

A pharmaceutical company conducts laboratory and animal studies to show biological activity of the compound against the targeted disease, and the compound is evaluated for safety. These tests take approximately three and one-half years.

Investigational New Drug Application (INDA)

After completing preclinical testing, the company files an INDA with FDA to begin to test the drug in people. The INDA becomes effective if FDA does not disapprove it within 30 days. The INDA shows results of previous experiments, how, where and by whom the new studies will be conducted; the chemical structure of the compound; how it is thought to work in the body; any toxic effects found in the animal studies; and how the compound is manufactured. In addition, the INDA must be reviewed and approved by the Institutional Review Board where the studies will be conducted, and progress reports on clinical trials must be submitted at least annually to FDA

New Drug Application (NDA)

Following the completion of all three phases of clinical trials, the company analyzes all of the data and files an NDA with FDA if the data successfully demonstrate safety and effectiveness. The NDA must contain all of the scientific information that the company has gathered. NDAs typically run 100,000 pages or more. By law, FDA is allowed six months to review an

NDA. In almost all cases, the period between the first submission of an NDA and final FDA approval exceeds that limit; the average NDA review time for new molecular entities approved in 1992 was 29.9 months.

Abbreviated New Drug Application (ANDA)

An Abbreviated New Drug Application (ANDA) contains data which when submitted to FDA's Center for Drug Evaluation and Research, Office of Generic Drugs, provides for the review and ultimate approval of a generic drug product. Once approved, an applicant may manufacture and market the generic drug product to provide a safe, effective, low cost drug.

Generic drug applications are termed "abbreviated" because they are generally not required to include preclinical (animal) and clinical (human) data to establish safety and effectiveness. Instead, generic applicants must scientifically demonstrate that their product is bioequivalent.

Good Manufacturing Practice (GMP)

Good manufacturing practice (GMP) is a system for ensuring that products are consistently produced and controlled according to quality standards. It is designed to minimize the risks involved in any pharmaceutical production that cannot be eliminated through testing the final product. The main risks are: unexpected contamination of products, causing damage to health or even death; incorrect labels on containers, which could mean that patients receive the wrong medicine; insufficient or too much active ingredient, resulting in ineffective treatment or adverse effects.

GMP covers all aspects of production; from the starting materials, premises and equipment to the training and personal hygiene of staff. Detailed, written procedures are essential for each process that could affect the quality of the finished product. There must be systems to provide documented proof that correct procedures are consistently followed at each step in the manufacturing process – every time a product is made.

WHO has established detailed guidelines for good manufacturing practice. Many countries have formulated their own requirements for GMP based on WHO GMP. Others have harmonized their requirements, for example, in the Association of South-East Asian Nations (ASEAN), in the European Union and through the Pharmaceutical Inspection Convention.

Drug Master File (DMF)

A Drug Master File (DMF) is a submission to the Food and Drug Administration (FDA) that may be used to provide confidential detailed information about facilities, processes, or articles used in the manufacturing, processing, packaging, and storing of one or more human drugs. Law or FDA regulation does not require the submission of a DMF. A DMF is submitted solely at the discretion of the holder. The information contained in the DMF may be used to support an Investigational New Drug Application (INDA), a New Drug Application (NDA), an Abbreviated New Drug Application (ANDA), another DMF, an Export Application, or amendments and supplements to any of these.

Good Clinical Practice (GCP)

Good Clinical Practice (GCP) is an international ethical and scientific quality standard for designing, conducting, recording and reporting trials that involve the participation of human subjects. Compliance with this standard provides public assurance that the rights, safety and well being of trial subjects are protected, consistent with the principles that have their origin in the Declaration of Helsinki, and that the clinical trial data are credible.

International Conference on Harmonization of Technical Requirements (ICH)

International Conference on Harmonization of Technical Requirements for Registration of

Pharmaceuticals for Human Use – Members are from industry and regulatory agencies. Provides a forum for a constructive dialogue between regulatory authorities and the pharmaceutical industry on the real and perceived differences in the technical requirements for product registration in the EU, USA and Japan. Identifies areas where modifications in technical requirements or greater mutual acceptance of research and development procedures could lead to a more economical use of human, animal and material resources, without compromising safety. Makes recommendations on practical ways to achieve greater harmonization in the interpretation and application of technical requirements for registration.

Food and Drug Administration (FDA)

FDA is the Federal agency responsible for ensuring that foods are safe, wholesome and sanitary; human and veterinary drugs, biological products, and medical devices are safe and effective; cosmetics are safe; and electronic products that emit radiation are safe. FDA also ensures that these products are honestly, accurately and informatively represented to the public.

Therapeutic Goods Administration (TGA)

The Therapeutic Goods Administration (TGA) is a unit of the Australian Government Department of Health and Ageing. The TGA carries out a range of assessment and monitoring activities to ensure that therapeutic goods available in Australia are of an acceptable standard with the aim of ensuring that the Australian community has access, within a reasonable time, to therapeutic advances.

General Agreement on Tariffs and Trade (GATT)

The General Agreement on Tariffs and Trade (GATT) was first signed in 1947. The agreement was designed to provide an international forum that encouraged free trade between member states by regulating and reducing tariffs on traded goods and by providing a common mechanism for resolving trade disputes. GATT membership now includes more than 110 countries

World Trade Organization (WTO)

The World Trade Organization (WTO) is the only global international organization dealing with the rules of trade between nations. At its heart are the WTO agreements, negotiated and signed by the bulk of the world's trading nations and ratified in their parliaments. The goal is to help producers of goods and services, exporters, and importers conduct their business.

Trade Related Aspects of Intellectual Property Rights (TRIPS)

The WTO's Agreement on Trade-Related Aspects of Intellectual Property Rights (TRIPS), negotiated in the 1986-94 Uruguay Round, introduced intellectual property rules into the multilateral trading system for the first time.

Investigational New Drug Application (INDA)

Based on Preclinical dossier submission containing data from animal studies we approach FDA to get permission to conduct clinical trials (Phase I). Within 30 days, if FDA doesn't respond or interrogate the applicant, it is considered as approved.

Phase I: First time NCE tested in human volunteers.

ANDA for Formulations

Requirement for getting approval of the **Generic version of branded drug** in USA.

- Establish bioequivalence (to the reference/innovator product) criteria as per US FDA guidelines.
- For the ANDAs the patentability of development strategy is not required. But should be non-infringing.

- Rate of absorption, determined by C_{max}. This is the rate at which the drug is entering our body.
- Extent of absorption, determined by AUC (area under curve). How much drug enters into our body.
- Product is considered bioequivalent if 90% confidence interval falls within 80–125 for both C_{max} and AUC (not mandatory for NDA).

Three bioequivalence studies are required to prove the product is bioequivalent.

- Single dose fasting
- Single dose food effect studies
- Multiple dose studies.

For immediate-release products normally only first two studies are required but multiple-dose studies normally at highest strength is required for controlled-release product.

There is a biowaiver for the lower strengths, provided the higher strength is bioequivalent in all the three studies and all strengths are inter-convertible.

In food effect studies, 90% confidence interval (CI) is not applicable.

There is no need to do PD studies, as we only need to show that the C_{max} and AUC are in the 80–125% range.

For ANDAs, the same dosage form, same strength, same drug salt, same route of administration and same indication are required.

Paragraph IV

Certification to be given to FDA and Innovator that the proposed product is not infringing or the patent is invalid. Normally it involves litigation process. Only ANDAs approved under paragraph IV can get 180 days exclusivity if we are first to file such application.

Orange Book

Official listing of the FDA approved drug products with their therapeutic evaluation ratings. This also gives the list of the patents and exclusivity data relevant to the product. Only these listed patents can be targeted for Paragraph IV filings.

NDA for Formulations

- Apart from matching the T/R ratios both of C_{max} and AUC (PK), the limited clinical trials are required to support the application.
- All NDDS products should essentially be patentable to prevent others from copying the concept.
- NDAs are submitted under the 505(b) 2 and 505(b) 1. All NDDS NDAs are to be submitted under section 505(b) 2 of Federal Food, Drugs and Cosmetic Act in US.
- Applications submitted fewer than 505(b) 2 (also known as Paper NDAs) will auto-matically get all the approved indications granted without conducting trials for each indication separately.
- Full NDAs are submitted under 505 (b) 1 and are approved under section 505 (c), this involves the premarketing approval and normally NCEs are submitted under this section. Sometimes FDA asks for the post-marketing surveillance reports to be submitted as Phase IV studies.
- AUC must be above MIC or other defined parameter. The ratio of T/R for this measure-ment should be between 70–150% (this is not mandatory, may vary depending on the purpose of the controlled release).
- The applications of NDA under 505(b) 2 may be eligible for the exclusivity of three years in certain cases and similar to Para IV ANDA it involves the cost of litigation.
- PK and PD for the test product (once daily sustained-release) should be comparable to the conventional product (two times daily imme-diate-release) (IR) for a single day therapy to prove the controlled-release claim.
- No need for bioequivalence but if similar product is available then bioavailability studies are required.

19

Good Manufacturing and Laboratory Practices

Vure Prasad, Jitender Madan and P.R. Mishra

INTRODUCTION

The Food and Drug Administration strives to ensure that the regulated industries comply with a total quality conceptquality concept through its factory inspection programs, and through participation in voluntary compliance seminars and workshops sponsored jointly with the industries or with educational institutions. That a total quality assurance approach is necessary to prevent a drug product from being deemed adulterated under section of the Food, Drug, and Cosmetic Act is indicated by 21 CFR 133.1. Good Manufacturing Practice in the Manufacture, Processing, Packing, and Holding of Drugs is no where mentioned in the government documents, however, there is a comprehensive collection of specific measures to realize this concept. The concept of a total quality control system is not limited in scope in terms of analytical methods of assay, control charts, product inspection made during the manufacturing processes and prior to finished dosage form distribution nor to the statistical techniques utilized in these discrete operations, but also includes all control measures contributing to the completed market dosage form (FDA Guidance for Industry, 2004).

The main principles of GMP are outlined in Fig. 19.1. A basic tenet of GMP is that quality cannot be tested into a batch of product but must be built into each batch of product during all stages of the manufacturing process. It is designed to minimize the risks involved in any pharmaceutical production that cannot be eliminated through testing the final product.

In this chapter an attempt is made to provide specific guidelines and concepts, which can serve as checks for critical operations within the entire organization so that a total quality system may be achieved. Each requirement loosely generalized in Good Manufacturing Practice (GMP) regulations is enlarged upon and made more specific to include measures, which the authors believe are necessary for good control. (Division of Research and Testing (HFD-470), Center for Drug Evaluation and Research, Food and Drug Administration, 200 C St. SW., Washington, DC 20204, Office of the Federal Register, 800 North Capitol Street, NW., Suite 700, Washington, DC 20408).

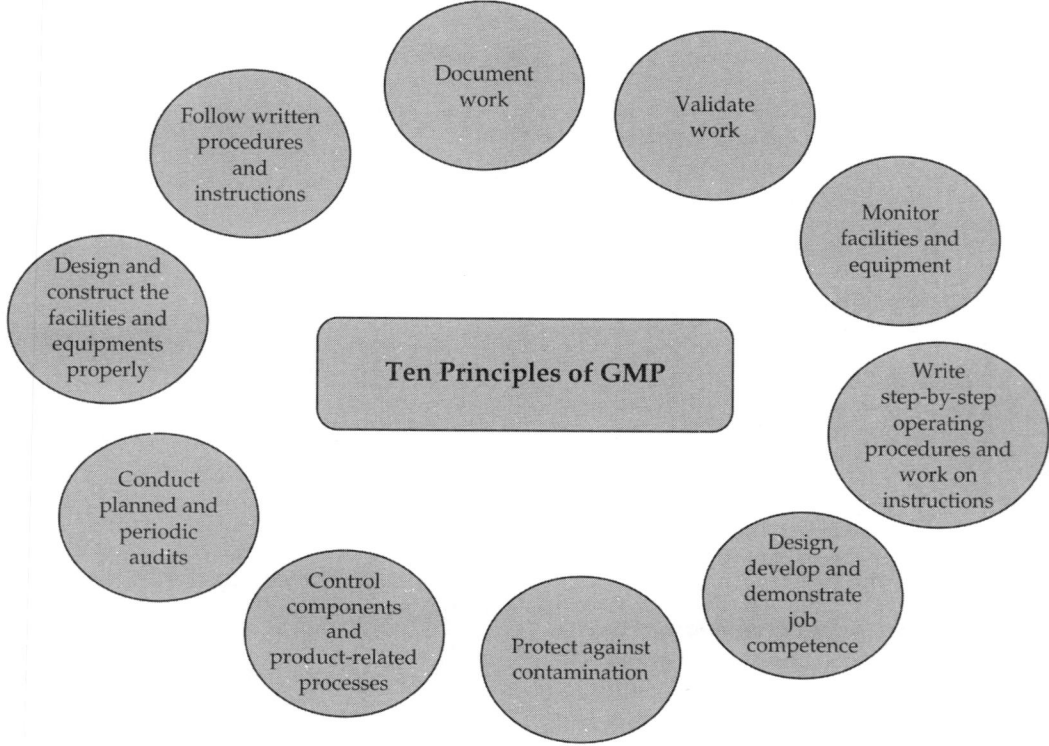

Fig. 19.1. Basic principles of cGMP.

The chapter is ordered by the subject matter of the sections of the GMP regulations

PART 210 - CURRENT GOOD MANUFACTURING PRACTICE IN MANUFACTURING, PROCESSING, PACKING, OR HOLDING OF DRUGS

General [Part 210]

Status of current good manufacturing practice regulations [210.1]

a. The regulations set forth in this part contain the minimum current good manufacturing practice for methods to be used in, and the facilities or controls to be used for, the manufacture, processing, packing, or holding of a drug to assure that such drug meets the requirements of the Act as to safety, and has the identity and strength and meets the quality and purity characteristics that it purports or is represented to possess.

b. The failure to comply with any regulation set forth in this part in the manufacture, processing, packing, or holding of a drug shall render such drug to be adulterated under section 501 (a) (2) (B) of the act and such drug, as well as the person who is responsible for the failure to comply, shall be subject to regulatory action.

Applicability of current good manufacturing practice regulations [210.2]

a. The regulations in this part and in Parts 211 through 226 pertain to a drug and in Parts 600 through 680 pertain to a biological product for human use is considered to supplement, not supersede, each other, unless the regulations explicitly provide otherwise. In the event that it is impossible to comply with all applicable regulations in these parts, the regulations specifically applicable to the drug in question shall supersede the more general.

b. If a person engages in only some operations subject to the regulations in this part and in Part 211, Part 600, and not in others, that person need only comply with those regulations applicable to the operations in which he or she is engaged.

Definitions [210.3]

Act means the Federal Food, Drug, and Cosmetic Act, as amended (21 U.S.C. 301 et seq.).

- **Batch** means a specific quantity of a drug or other material that is intended to have uniform character and quality, within specified limits, and is produced according to a single manufacturing order during the same cycle of manufacture.
- **Component** means any ingredient intended for use in the manufacture of a drug product, including those that may not appear in such drug product.
- **Drug product** means a finished dosage form, for example, tablet, capsule, solution, etc., that contains an active drug ingredient generally, but not necessarily, in association with inactive ingredients. The term also includes a finished dosage form that does not contain an active ingredient but is intended to be used as a placebo.
- **Active ingredient** means any component that is intended to furnish pharmacological activity or other direct effect in the diagnosis, cure, mitigation, treatment, or prevention of disease, or to affect the structure or any function of the body of man or other animals. The term includes those components that may undergo chemical change in the manufacture of the drug product and be present in the drug product in a modified form intended to furnish the specified activity or effect.

- **Inactive ingredient** means any component other than an active ingredient.
- **In-process material** means any material fabricated, compounded, blended, or derived by chemical reaction that is produced for, and used in, the preparation of the drug product.
- **Lot** means a batch, or a specific identified portion of a batch, having uniform character and quality within specified limits; or, in the case of a drug product produced by continuous process, it is a specific identified amount produced in a unit of time or quantity in a manner that assures its having uniform character and quality within specified limits.
- **Lot number**, **control number**, or **batch number** means any distinctive combination of letters, numbers, or symbols, or any combination of them, from which the complete history of the manufacture, processing, packing, holding, and distribution of a batch or lot of drug product or other material can be determined.
- **Manufacture, processing, packing**, or **holding of a drug product** includes packaging and labelling operations, testing, and quality control of drug products.
- **Quality control unit** means any person or organizational element designated by the firm to be responsible for the duties relating to quality control.
- **Acceptance criteria** means the product specifications and acceptance/rejection criteria, such as acceptable quality level and unacceptable quality level, with an associated sampling plan, that are necessary for making a decision to accept or reject a lot or batch (or any other convenient subgroups of manufactured units).

CURRENT GOOD MANUFACTURING PRACTICE FOR FINISHED PHARMACEUTICALS [PART 211]

A brief overview of subparts given in this section are:

A. General Provisions

Scope [211.1]

a. The regulations in this part contain the minimum current good manufacturing practice for preparation of drug products for administration to humans or animals.

b. The current good manufacturing practice regulations in this chapter, as they pertain to drug products, and in part 600, as they pertain to biological products for human use, shall be considered to supplement, not supersede, the regulations in this part unless the regulations explicitly provide otherwise. In this event it is impossible to comply with applicable regulations both in this part and in other parts of this chapter or in parts, the regulation specifically applicable to the drug product in question shall supersede the regulation in this part.

c. Pending consideration of a proposed exemption, published in the Federal Register of September 29, 1978, the requirements in this part shall not be enforced for OTC drug products if the products and all their ingredients are ordinarily marketed and consumed as human foods, and which products may also fall within the legal definition of drugs by virtue of their intended use. Therefore, until further notice, regulations under part 110 of this chapter, and where applicable, part 113, shall be applied in determining whether these OTC drug products that are also foods are manufactured, processed, packed, or held under current good manufacturing practice.

B. Organization and Personnel

Responsibilities of quality control unit [211.22]

a. There shall be a quality control unit that shall have the responsibility and authority to approve or reject all components, drug product containers, closures, in-process materials, packaging material, labelling, and drug products, and the authority to review production records to assure that no errors have occurred or, if errors have occurred, that they have been fully investigated. The quality control unit shall be responsible for approving or rejecting drug products manufactured, processed, packed, or held under contract by another company.

b. Adequate laboratory facilities for the testing and approval (or rejection) of components, drug product containers, closures, packaging materials, in-process materials, and drug products shall be available to the quality control unit.

c. The quality control unit shall have the responsibility for approving or rejecting all procedures or specifications impacting on the identity, strength, quality, and purity of the drug product.

d. The responsibilities and procedures applicable to the quality control unit shall be in writing; such written procedures shall be followed.

Personnel qualifications [211.25]

a. Each person engaged in the manufacture, processing, packing, or holding of a drug product shall have education, training, and experience, or any combination thereof, to enable that person to perform the assigned functions. Training shall be in the particular

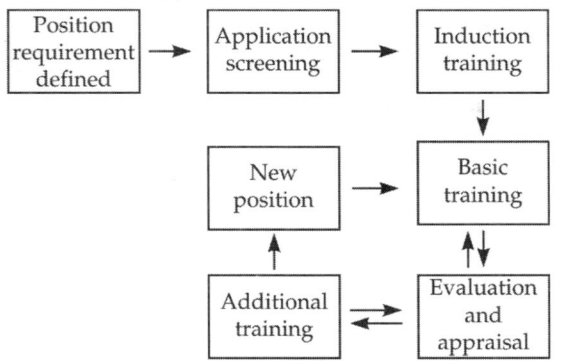

Fig. 19.2. Training and development cycle.

operations that the employee performs and in current good manufacturing practice (including the current good manufacturing practice regulations in this chapter and written procedures required by these regulations) as they relate to the employee's functions. Training in current good manufacturing practice shall be conducted by qualified individuals on a continuing basis and with sufficient frequency to assure that employees remain familiar with cGMP requirements applicable to them.

b. Each person responsible for supervising the manufacture, processing, packing, or holding of a drug product shall have the education, training, and experience, or any combination thereof, to perform assigned functions in such a manner as to provide assurance that the drug product has the safety, identity, strength, quality, and purity that it purports or is represented to possess.

c. There shall be an adequate number of qualified personnel to perform and supervise the manufacture, processing, packing, or holding of each drug product.

Personnel responsibilities [211.28]

a. Personnel engaged in the manufacture, processing, packing, or holding of a drug product shall wear clean clothing appropriate for the duties they perform. Protective apparel, such as head, face, hand, and arm coverings, shall be worn as necessary to protect drug products from contamination.

b. Personnel shall practice good sanitation and health habits.

c. Only personnel authorized by supervisory personnel shall enter those areas of the buildings and facilities designated as limited-access areas.

d. Any person shown at any time (either by medical examination or supervisory observation) to have an apparent illness or open lesions that may adversely affect the safety or quality of drug products shall be excluded from direct contact with components, drug product containers, closures, in-process materials, and drug products until the condition is corrected or determined by competent medical personnel not to jeopardize the safety or quality of drug products. All personnel shall be instructed to report to supervisory personnel any health conditions that may have an adverse effect on drug products.

Consultants [211.34]

Consultants advising on the manufacture, processing, packing, or holding of drug products shall have sufficient education, training, and experience, or any combination thereof, to advise on the subject for which they are retained. Records shall be maintained stating the name, address, and qualifications of any consultants and the type of service they provide.

C. Buildings and Facilities

211.42 Design and construction features

a. Any building or buildings used in the manufacture, processing, packing, or holding of a drug product shall be of suitable size, construction and location to facilitate cleaning, maintenance, and proper operations.

b. Any such building shall have adequate space for the orderly placement of equipment and materials to prevent mix-ups between different components, drug product containers, closures, labelling, in-process materials, or drug products, and to prevent contamination. The flow of components, drug product containers, closures, labelling, in-process materials, and drug products through the building or buildings shall be designed to prevent contamination (Fornalsaro et al., 1970).

c. Operations shall be performed within specifically defined areas of adequate size. There shall be separate or defined areas for the firm's operations to prevent contamination or mix-ups as follows: receipt, identification, storage, and withholding from use of components, drug product containers, closures, and labelling, pending the appropriate sampling, testing, or examination by the quality control unit before release for manufacturing or packaging, holding rejected components, drug product containers, closures, and labelling before disposition, storage of released components, drug product containers, closures, and labelling, storage of in-process materials, manufacturing and processing operations, packaging and labelling operations, quarantine storage before release of drug products, storage of drug products after release, control and laboratory operations, aseptic processing, which includes as appropriate: (i) floors, walls, and ceilings of smooth, hard surfaces that is easily cleanable; (ii) temperature and humidity controls; (iii) an air supply filtered through high-efficiency particulate air filters under positive pressure, regardless of whether flow is laminar or nonlaminar; (iv) a system for monitoring environmental conditions; (v) a system for cleaning and disinfecting the room and equipment to produce aseptic conditions; and (vi) a system for maintaining any equipment used to control the aseptic conditions.

d. Operations relating to the manufacture, processing, and packing of penicillin shall be performed in facilities separate from those used for other drug products for human use (60 FR 4091, 1995).

Lighting [211.44]

Adequate lighting shall be provided in all areas.

Ventilation, air filtration, air heating and cooling [211.46]

a. Adequate ventilation shall be provided.
b. Equipment for adequate control over air pressure, microorganisms, dust, humidity, and temperature shall be provided when appropriate for the manufacture, processing, packing, or holding of a drug product.
c. Air filtration systems, including prefilters and particulate matter air filters, shall be used when appropriate on air supplies to production areas. If air is recirculated to production areas, measures shall be taken to control recirculation of dust from production. In areas where air contamination occurs during production, there shall be adequate exhaust systems or other systems adequate to control contaminants.
d. Air-handling systems for the manufacture, processing, and packing of penicillin shall be completely separate from those for other drug products for human use.

Plumbing [211.48]

a. Potable water shall be supplied under continuous positive pressure in a plumbing system free of defects that could contribute contamination to any drug product. Potable water shall meet the standards prescribed in the Environmental Protection Agency's Primary Drinking Water Regulations set forth in 40 CFR parts 141. Water not meeting such standards shall not be permitted in the potable water system.
b. Drains shall be of adequate size and, where connected directly to a sewer, shall be provided with an air break or other mechanical device to prevent back-siphonage (48 FR 11426, 1983).

Sewage and refuse [211.50]

Sewage, trash, and other refuse in and from the building and immediate premises shall be disposed of in a safe and sanitary manner.

Washing and toilet facilities [211.52]

Adequate washing facilities shall be provided, including hot and cold water, soap or detergent, air driers or single-service towels, and clean toilet facilities easily accessible to working areas.

Sanitation [211.56]

a. Any building used in the manufacture, processing, packing, or holding of a drug product shall be maintained in a clean and sanitary condition, Any such building shall be free of infestation by rodents, birds, insects, and other vermin (other than laboratory animals). Trash and organic waste matter shall be held and disposed of in a timely and sanitary manner.

b. There shall be written procedures assigning responsibility for sanitation and describing in sufficient detail the cleaning schedules, methods, equipment, and materials to be used in cleaning the buildings and facilities; such written procedures shall be followed.

c. There shall be written procedures for use of suitable rodenticides, insecticides, fungicides, fumigating agents, and cleaning and sanitizing agents. Such written procedures shall be designed to prevent the contamination of equipment, components, drug product containers, closures, packaging, labelling materials, or drug products and shall be followed. Rodenticides, insecticides, and fungicides shall not be used unless registered and used in accordance with the Federal Insecticide, Fungicide, and Rodenticide Act (7 U.S.C. 135).

d. Sanitation procedures shall apply to work performed by contractors or temporary employees as well as work performed by full-time employees during the ordinary course of operations (Loughhead et al., 1969).

Maintenance [211.58]

Any building used in the manufacture, processing, packing, or holding of a drug product shall be maintained in a good state of repair.

D. Equipment

Equipment design, size, and location [211.63]

Equipment used in the manufacture, processing, packing, or holding of a drug product shall be of appropriate design, adequate size, and suitably located to facilitate operations for its intended use and for its cleaning and maintenance (Litter, 1968).

Equipment construction [211.65]

a. Equipment shall be constructed so that surfaces that contact components, in-process materials, or drug products shall not be reactive, additive, or absorptive so as to alter the safety, identity, strength, quality, or purity of the drug product beyond the official or other established requirements.

b. Any substances required for operation, such as lubricants or coolants, shall not come into contact with components, drug product containers, closures, in-process materials, or drug products so as to alter the safety, identity, strength, quality, or purity of the drug product beyond the official or other established requirements.

Equipment cleaning and maintenance [211.67]

a. Equipment and utensils shall be cleaned, maintained, and sanitized at appropriate intervals to prevent malfunctions or contamination that would alter the safety, identity, strength, quality, or purity of the drug product beyond the official or other established requirements.

b. Written procedures shall be established and followed for cleaning and maintenance of equipment, including utensils, used in the

manufacture, processing, packing, or holding of a drug product. These procedures shall include, but are not necessarily limited to, the following: (i) assignment of responsibility for cleaning and maintaining equipment, (ii) maintenance and cleaning schedules, including, where appropriate, sanitizing schedules, (iii) a description in sufficient detail of the methods, equipment, and materials used in cleaning and maintenance operations, and the methods of disassembling and reassembling equipment as necessary to assure proper cleaning and maintenance, (iv) removal or obliteration of previous batch identification, (v) protection of clean equipment from contamination prior to use, and (vi) inspection of equipment for cleanliness immediately before use.
c. Records shall be kept of maintenance, cleaning, sanitizing, and inspection as specified in 211.180 and 211.182.

Automatic, mechanical, and electronic equipment [211.68]

a. Automatic, mechanical, or electronic equipment or other types of equipment, including computers, or related systems that will perform a function satisfactorily, may be used in the manufacture, processing, packing, and holding of a drug product. If such equipment is so used, it shall be routinely calibrated, inspected, or checked according to a written program designed to assure proper performance. Written records of those calibration checks and inspections shall be maintained.
b. Appropriate controls shall be exercised over computer or related systems to assure those changes in master production and control records or other records are instituted only by authorized personnel.

Input to and output from the computer or related system of formulas or other records or data shall be checked for accuracy. The degree and frequency of input/output verification shall be based on the complexity and reliability of the computer or related system. A backup file of data entered into the computer or related system shall be maintained except where certain data, such as calculations performed in connection with laboratory analysis, are eliminated by computerization or other automated processes.

In such instances a written record of the program shall be maintained along with appropriate validation data. Hard copy or alternative systems, such as duplicates, tapes, or microfilm, designed to assure that backup data are exact and complete and that it is secure from alteration, inadvertent erasures, or loss shall be maintained (60 FR 4091, 1995).

Filters [211.72]

Filters for liquid filtration used in the manufacture, processing, or packing of injectable drug products intended for human use shall not release fibers into such products. Fiber releasing filters may not be used in the manufacture, processing, or packing of these injectables drug products unless it is not possible to manufacture such drug products without the use of such filters. If use of a fiber releasing filter is necessary, an additional non-fiber releasing filter of 0.22 μ maximum mean porosity (0.45 μ if the manufacturing conditions so dictate) shall subsequently be used to reduce the content of particles in the injectable drug product. Use of an asbestos containing filter, with or without subsequent use of a specific non-fiber releasing filter, is permissible only upon submission of proof to the appropriate bureau of the Food and Drug Administration that use of a non-fiber releasing filter will, or is likely to, compromise the safety or effectiveness of the injectable drug product.

E. Control of Components and Drug Product Containers and Closures

General requirements [211.80]

a. There shall be written procedures describing in sufficient detail the receipt, identification, storage, handling, sampling, testing, and approval or rejection of components and drug product containers and closures; such written procedures shall be followed.

b. Components and drug product containers and closures shall at all times be handled and stored in a manner to prevent contamination.

c. Bagged or boxed components of drug product containers, or closures shall be stored off the floor and suitably spaced to permit cleaning and inspection.

d. Each container or grouping of containers for components or drug product containers, or closures shall be identified with a distinctive code for each lot in each shipment received. This code shall be used in recording the disposition of each lot. Each lot shall be appropriately identified as to its status (i.e., quarantined, approved, or rejected).

Receipt and storage of untested components, drug product containers, and closures [211.82]

a. Upon receipt and before acceptance, each container or grouping of containers of components, drug product containers, and closures shall be examined visually for appropriate labelling as to contents, container damage or broken seals, and contamination.

b. Components, drug product containers, and closures shall be stored under quarantine until they have been tested or examined, as appropriate, and released. Storage within the area shall conform to the requirements of 211.80.

Testing and approval or rejection of components, drug product containers, and closures [211.84]

a. Each lot of components, drug product containers, and closures shall be withheld from use until the lot has been sampled, tested, or examined, as appropriate, and released for use by the quality control unit.

b. Representative samples of each shipment of each lot shall be collected for testing or

examination. The number of containers to be sampled, and the amount of material to be taken from each container, shall be based upon appropriate criteria such as statistical criteria for component variability, confidence levels, and degree of precision desired, the past quality history of the supplier, and the quantity needed for analysis and reserve where required by 211.170.

c. Samples shall be collected in accordance with the following procedures:

1. The containers of components selected shall be cleaned, where necessary, by appropriate means.

2. The containers shall be opened, sampled, and resealed in a manner designed to prevent contamination of their contents and contamination of other components, drug product containers, or closures.

3. Sterile equipment and aseptic sampling techniques shall be used when necessary.

4. If it is necessary to sample a component from the top, middle, and bottom of its container, such sample subdivisions shall not be composited for testing.

5. Sample containers shall be identified so that the following information can be determined: name of the material sampled the lot number, the container from which the sample was taken, the date on which the sample was taken, and the name of the person who collected the sample.

6. Containers from which samples have been taken shall be marked to show that samples have been removed from them.

d. Samples shall be examined and tested as follows:

1. At least one test shall be conducted to verify the identity of each component of a drug product. Specific identity tests, if they exist, shall be used.

2. Each component shall be tested for conformity with all appropriate written specifications for purity, strength, and

quality. In lieu of such testing by the manufacturer, a report of analysis may be accepted from the supplier of a component, provided that at least one specific identity test is conducted on such component by the manufacturer, and provided that the manufacturer establishes the reliability of the supplier's analyses through appropriate validation of the supplier's test results at appropriate intervals.

3. Containers and closures shall be tested for conformance with all appropriate written procedures. In lieu of such testing by the manufacturer, a certificate of testing may be accepted from the supplier, provided that at least a visual identification is conducted on such containers/closures by the manufacturer and provided that the manufacturer establishes the reliability of the supplier's test results through appropriate validation of the supplier's test results at appropriate intervals.

4. When appropriate, components shall be microscopically examined.

5. Each lot of a component, drug product container, or closure that is liable to contamination with filth, insect infestation, or other extraneous adulterant, shall be examined against established specifications for such contamination.

6. Each lot of a component, drug product container, or closure that is liable to microbiological contamination that is objectionable in view of its intended use shall be subjected to microbiological tests before use.

7. Any lot of components, drug product containers, or closures that meets the appropriate written specifications of identity, strength, quality, and purity and related tests under paragraph (d) of this section may be approved and released for use. Any lot of such material that does not meet such specifications shall be rejected (Delmore et al., 1969).

Use of approved components, drug product containers, and closures [211.86]

Components, drug product containers, and closures approved for use shall be rotated so that the oldest approved stock is used first. Deviation from this requirement is permitted if such deviation is temporary and appropriate.

Retesting of approved components, drug product containers, and closures [211.87]

Components, drug product containers, and closures shall be retested or re-examined, as appropriate, for identity, strength, quality, and purity and approved or rejected by the quality control unit in accordance with 211.84 as necessary, e.g., after storage for long periods or after exposure to air, heat or other conditions that might adversely affect the component, drug product container, or closure.

Rejected components, drug product containers, and closures [211.89]

Rejected components, drug product containers, and closures shall be identified and controlled under a quarantine system designed to prevent their use in manufacturing or processing operations for which they are unsuitable.

Drug product containers and closures [211.94]

a. Drug product containers and closures shall not be reactive, additive, or absorptive so as to alter the safety, identity, strength, quality, or purity of the drug beyond the official or established requirements.

b. Container closure systems shall provide adequate protection against foreseeable external factors in storage and use that can cause deterioration or contamination of the drug product.

c. Drug product containers and closures shall be clean and, where indicated by the nature of the drug, sterilized and processed to remove pyrogenic properties to assure that they are suitable for their intended use.

d. Standards or specifications, methods of testing, and, where indicated, methods of cleaning, sterilizing, and processing to remove pyrogenic properties shall be written and followed for drug product containers and closures.

F. Production and Process Controls

Written procedures; deviations [211.100]

a. There shall be written procedures for production and process control designed to assure that the drug products have the identity, strength, quality, and purity they purport or are represented to possess. Such procedures shall include all requirements in this subpart. These written procedures, including any changes, shall be drafted, reviewed, and approved by the appropriate organizational units and reviewed and approved by the quality control unit.
b. Written production and process control procedures shall be followed in the execution of the various production and process control functions and shall be documented at the time of performance. Any deviation from the written procedures shall be recorded and justified.

Charge-in of components [211.101]

Written production and control procedures shall include the following, which are designed to assure that the drug products produced have the identity, strength, quality, and purity they purport or are represented to possess:

a. The batch shall be formulated with the intent to provide not less than 100 percent of the labelled or established amount of active ingredient.
b. Components for drug product manufacturing shall be weighed, measured, or subdivided as appropriate. If a component is removed from the original container to another, the new container shall be identified with the following information: (i) component name or item code; (ii) receiving or control number; (iii) weight or measure in new container; and (iv) batch for which component was dispensed, including its product name, strength, and lot number.
c. Weighing, measuring, or subdividing operations for components shall be adequately supervised. Each container of component dispensed to manufacturing shall be examined by a second person to assure that: (i) the component was released by the quality control unit; (ii) the weight or measure is correct as stated in the batch production records; and (iii) the containers are properly identified.
d. Each component shall be added to the batch by one person and verified by a second person (Saengen et al., 1969).

Calculation of yield [211.103]

Actual yields and percentages of theoretical yield shall be determined at the conclusion of each appropriate phase of manufacturing, processing, packaging, or holding of the drug product. Such calculations shall be performed by one person and independently verified by a second person.

Equipment identification [211.105]

a. All compounding and storage containers, processing lines, and major equipment used during the production of a batch of a drug product shall be properly identified at all times to indicate their contents and, when necessary, the phase of processing of the batch.
b. Major equipment shall be identified by a distinctive identification number or code that shall be recorded in the batch production record to show the specific equipment used in the manufacture of each batch of a drug product. In cases where only one of a particular type of equipment exists in a manufacturing facility, the name of the equipment may be used in lieu of a distinctive identification number or code.

Sampling and testing of in-process materials and drug products [211.110]

a. To assure batch uniformity and integrity of drug products, written procedures shall be established and followed that describe the in-process controls, and tests, or examinations to be conducted on appropriate samples of in-process materials of each batch. Such control procedures shall be established to monitor the output and to validate the performance of those manufacturing processes that may be responsible for causing variability in the characteristics of in-process material and the drug product. Such control procedures shall include, but are not limited to, the following, where appropriate: (i) tablet or capsule weight variation; (ii) disintegration time; (iii) adequacy of mixing to assure uniformity and homogeneity; (iv) dissolution time and rate; and (v) clarity, completeness, or pH of solutions.

b. Valid in-process specifications for such characteristics shall be consistent with drug product final specifications and shall be derived from previous acceptable process average and process variability estimates where possible and determined by the application of suitable statistical procedures where appropriate. Examination and testing of samples shall assure that the drug product and in-process material conforms to specifications.

c. In-process materials shall be tested for identity, strength, quality, and purity as appropriate, and approved or rejected by the quality control unit, during the production process, e.g., at commencement or completion of significant phases or after storage for long periods.

d. Rejected in-process materials shall be identified and controlled under a quarantine system designed to prevent their use in manufacturing or processing operations for which they are unsuitable.

Time limitations on production [211.111]

When appropriate, time limits for the completion of each phase of production shall be established to assure the quality of the drug product. Deviation from established time limits may be acceptable if such deviation does not compromise the quality of the drug product. Such deviation shall be justified and documented.

Control of microbiological contamination [211.113]

a. Appropriate written procedures, designed to prevent objectionable microorganisms in drug products not required to be sterile, shall be established and followed.

b. Appropriate written procedures, designed to prevent microbiological contamination of drug products purporting to be sterile, shall be established and followed. Such procedures shall include validation of any sterilization process.

Reprocessing [211.115]

Written procedures shall be established and followed prescribing a system for reprocessing batches that do not conform to standards or specifications and the steps to be taken to insure that the reprocessed batches will conform to all established standards, specifications, and characteristics. Reprocessing shall not be performed without the review and approval of the quality control unit.

G. Packaging and Labelling Control

Materials examination and usage criteria [211.122]

There shall be written procedures describing in sufficient detail the receipt, identification, storage, handling, sampling, examination, and/or testing of labelling and packaging materials; such written procedures shall be followed. Labelling and packaging materials shall be representatively sampled, and examined or tested upon receipt and before use in packaging or labelling of a drug product. Any labelling or packaging materials meeting appropriate written specifications may be approved and released for use. Any labelling or packaging materials that do not meet such specifications shall be rejected to prevent their use in operations for which they are unsuitable. Records shall be maintained for each shipment received of each different labelling and packaging material indicating receipt, examination or testing, and whether accepted or rejected. Labels and other labelling materials for each different drug product, strength, dosage form, or quantity of contents shall be stored separately with suitable identification. Access to the storage area shall be limited to authorized personnel. Obsolete and outdated labels, labelling, and other packaging materials shall be destroyed, use of gang printing of labelling for different drug products or different strengths, or net contents of the same drug product, is prohibited unless the labelling from gang-printed sheets is adequately differentiated by size, shape, or color. If cut labelling is used, packaging and labeling operations shall include one of the following special control procedures: dedication of labelling and packaging lines to each different strength of each different drug product, use of appropriate electronic or electromechanical equipment to conduct a 100% examination for correct labelling during or after completion of finishing operations or use of visual inspection to conduct a 100% examination for correct labelling during or after completion of finishing operations for hand-applied labelling. Such examination shall be performed by one person and independently verified by a second person. Printing devices on or associated with, manufacturing lines used to imprint labeling upon the drug product unit label or case shall be monitored to assure that all imprinting conforms to the print specified in the batch production record [58 FR 41353, 1993].

Labelling issuance [211.125]

a. Strict control shall be exercised over labelling issued for use in drug product labelling operations.

b. Labelling materials issued for a batch shall be carefully examined for identity and conformity to the labelling specified in the master or batch production records.

c. Procedures shall be utilized to reconcile the quantities of labelling issued, used, and returned, and shall require evaluation of discrepancies found between the quantity of drug product finished and the quantity of labelling issued when such discrepancies are outside narrow preset limits based on historical operating data. Such discrepancies shall be investigated in accordance with 211.192. Labelling reconciliation is waived for cut or roll labelling if a 100% examination for correct labelling is performed in accordance with 211.122(g)(2).

d. All excess labelling bearing lot or control numbers shall be destroyed.

e. Returned labelling shall be maintained and stored in a manner to prevent mix-ups and provide proper identification.

f. Procedures shall be written describing in sufficient detail the control procedures employed for the issuance of labelling; such written procedures shall be followed [58 FR 41345, 1993].

Packaging and labelling operations [211.130]

There shall be written procedures designed to assure that correct labels, labelling, and packaging materials are used for drug products; such written procedures shall be followed. These procedures shall incorporate the following features:

a. Prevention of mix-ups and cross-contamination by physical or spatial separation from operations on other drug products.

b. Identification and handling of filled drug product containers that are set aside and held in unlabelled condition for future labelling operations to preclude mislabelling of individual containers, lots, or portions of lots. Identification need not be applied to each individual container but shall be sufficient to determine name, strength, quantity of contents, and lot or control number of each container.

c. Identification of the drug product with a lot or control number that permits determination of the history of the manufacture and control of the batch.

d. Examination of packaging and labelling materials for suitability and correctness before packaging operations, and documentation of such examination in the batch production record.

e. Inspection of the packaging and labelling facilities immediately before use to assure that all drug products have been removed from previous operations. Inspection shall also be made to assure that packaging and labelling materials not suitable for subsequent operations have been removed. Results of inspection shall be documented in the batch production records [58 FR 41354, 1993].

Tamper-resistant packaging requirements for OTC human drug products [211.132]

a. **General:** The FDA has the authority under the Federal Food, Drug, and Cosmetic Act to establish a uniform national requirement for tamper-resistant packaging of OTC drug products that will improve the security of OTC drug packaging and help assure the safety and effectiveness of OTC drug products. An OTC drug product (except a dermatological, dentifrice, insulin, or throat lozenge product) for retail sale that is not packaged in a tamper-resistant package or that is not properly labelled under this section is adulterated under section 501 of the Act or misbranded under section 502 of the Act, or both.

b. **Requirement for tamper-resistant package:** Each manufacturer and packer who packages an OTC drug product (except a dermatological, dentifrice, insulin, or throat lozenge product) for retail sale shall package the product in a tamper-resistant package, if this product is accessible to the public while held for sale. A tamper-resistant package is one having one or more indicators or barriers to entry which, if breached or missing, can reasonably be expected to provide visible evidence to consumers that tampering has occurred. To reduce the likelihood of successful tampering and to increase the likelihood that consumers will discover if a product has been tampered with, the package is required to be distinctive by design (e.g., an aerosol product container) or by the use of one or more indicators or barriers to entry that employ an identifying characteristic (e.g., a pattern, name, registered trademark, logo, or picture). For purposes of this section, the term 'distinctive by design" means the packaging cannot be duplicated with commonly available materials or through commonly available processes. For purposes of this section, the term "aerosol product" means a product which depends upon the power of a liquefied or compressed gas to expel the contents from the container. A tamper-resistant package may involve an immediate-container and closure system or secondary-container or carton system or any combination of systems intended to provide a visual indication of package integrity. The tamper-resistant feature shall be designed to and shall remain intact when handled in a reasonable manner during manufacture, distribution, and retail display.

1. For two-piece, hard gelatin capsule products subject to this requirement, a minimum of two tamper-resistant packaging feature is required, unless the capsules are sealed by a tamper-resistant technology.

2. For all other products subject to this requirement, including two-piece, hard gelatin capsules that are sealed by a tamper-resistant technology, a minimum of one tamper-resistant feature is required.

c. **Labelling:** Each retail package of an OTC drug product covered by this section, except ammonia inhalant in crushable glass ampoules, aerosol products as defined in paragraph (b) of this section, or containers of compressed medical oxygen, is required to bear a statement that is prominently placed so that consumers are alerted to the specific tamper-resistant feature of the package. The labelling statement is also required to be so placed that it will be unaffected if the tamper-resistant feature of the package is breached or missing. If the tamper-resistant feature chosen to meet the requirement in paragraph (b) of this section is one that uses an identifying characteristic, that characteristic is required to be referred to in the labelling statement. For example, the labelling statement on a bottle with a shrink band could say 'For your protection, this bottle has an imprinted seal around the neck'.

d. **Request for exemptions from packaging and labelling requirements:** A manufacturer or packer may request an exemption from the packaging and labelling requirements of this section. A request for an exemption is required to be submitted in the form of a citizen petition under 10.30 of this chapter and should be clearly identified on the envelope as a 'Request for Exemption from Tamper-Resistant Rule'. The petition is required to contain the following: (i) the name of the drug product or, if the petition seeks an exemption for a drug class, the name of the drug class, and a list of products within that class; (ii) the reasons that the drug product's compliance with the tamper-resistant packaging or labeling requirements of this section is unnecessary or cannot be achieved; (iii) a description of alternative steps that are available, or that the petitioner has already taken, to reduce the likelihood that the product or drug class will be the subject of malicious adulteration; and (iv) other information justifying an exemption.

e. **OTC drug products subject to approved new drug applications:** Holders of approved new drug applications for OTC drug products are required under 314.70 to provide the agency with notification of changes in packaging and labelling to comply with the requirements of this section. Changes in packaging and labelling required by this regulation may be made before FDA approval, as provided under 314.70(c). Manufacturing changes by which capsules are to be sealed require prior FDA approval under 314.70(b).

f. **Poison Prevention Packaging Act of 1970:** This section does not affect any requirement for "special packaging" as defined under 310.3(l) and required under the Poison Prevention Packaging Act of 1970 (approved by the Office of Management and Budget under OMB control number 0910-0149) [54 FR 5228, 1989].

Drug product inspection [211.134]

a. Packaged and labelled products shall be examined during finishing operations to provide assurance that containers and packages in the lot have the correct label.

b. A representative sample of units shall be collected at the completion of finishing operations and shall be visually examined for correct labelling.

c. Results of these examinations shall be recorded in the batch production or control records.

Expiration dating [211.137]

a. To assure that a drug product meets applicable standards of identity, strength, quality, and purity at the time of use, it shall bear an expiration date determined by appropriate stability testing described in 211.166.

b. Expiration dates shall be related to any storage conditions stated on the labelling, as determined by stability studies described in 211.166.

c. If the drug product is to be reconstituted at the time of dispensing, its labelling shall bear expiration information for both the reconstituted and unreconstituted drug products.

d. Expiration dates shall appear on labelling in accordance with the requirements of 201.17 of this chapter.

e. Homeopathic drug products shall be exempt from the requirements of this section.

f. Allergenic extracts that are labelled "No U.S. Standard of Potency" are exempt from the requirements of this section.

g. New drug products for investigational use are exempt from the requirements of this section, provided that they meet appropriate standards or specifications as demonstrated by stability studies during their use in clinical investigations. Where new drug products for investigational use are to be reconstituted at the time of dispensing, their labelling shall bear expiration information for the reconstituted drug product.

h. Pending consideration of a proposed exemption, published in the Federal Register of September 29, 1978, the requirements in this section shall not be enforced for human OTC drug products if their labelling does not bear dosage limitations and they are stable for at least 3 years as supported by appropriate stability data [46 FR 56412, 1981; 60 FR 4091, 1995].

H. Holding and Distribution

Warehousing procedures [211.142]

Written procedures describing the warehousing of drug products shall be established and followed. They shall include:

a. quarantine of drug products before release by the quality control unit, and

b. storage of drug products under appropriate conditions of temperature, humidity, and light so that the identity, strength, quality, and purity of the drug products are not affected.

Distribution procedures [211.150]

Written procedures shall be established, and followed, describing the distribution of drug products. They shall include:

a. a procedure whereby the oldest approved stock of a drug product is distributed first; deviation from this requirement is permitted if such deviation is temporary and appropriate, and

b. a system by which the distribution of each lot of drug product can be readily determined to facilitate its recall, if necessary.

I. Laboratory Controls

General requirements [211.160]

a. The establishment of any specifications, standards, sampling plans, test procedures, or other laboratory control mechanisms required by this subpart, including any change in such specifications, standards, sampling plans, test procedures, or other laboratory control mechanisms, shall be drafted by the appropriate organizational unit and reviewed and approved by the quality control unit. The requirements in this subpart shall be followed and shall be documented at the time of performance. Any deviation from the written specifications, standards, sampling plans, test procedures, or other laboratory control mechanisms shall be recorded and justified.

b. Laboratory controls shall include the establishment of scientifically sound and appropriate specifications, standards, sampling plans, and test procedures designed to assure that components, drug product containers, closures, in-process materials, labelling, and drug products conform to appropriate standards of identity, strength, quality, and purity. Laboratory controls shall include:

1. Determination of conformance to appropriate written specifications for the acceptance of each lot within each shipment of components, drug product

containers, closures, and labelling used in the manufacture, processing, packing, or holding of drug products. The specifications shall include a description of the sampling and testing procedures used. Samples shall be representative and adequately identified. Such procedures shall also require appropriate retesting of any component, drug product container, or closure that is subject to deterioration.

2. Determination of conformance to written specifications and a description of sampling and testing procedures for in-process materials. Such samples shall be representative and properly identified.

3. Determination of conformance to written descriptions of sampling procedures and appropriate specifications for drug products. Such samples shall be representative and properly identified.

4. The calibration of instruments, apparatus, gauges, and recording devices at suitable intervals in accordance with an established written program containing specific directions, schedules, limits for accuracy and precision, and provisions for remedial action in the event accuracy and/or precision limits are not met. Instruments, apparatus, gauges, and recording devices not meeting established specifications shall not be used.

Testing and release for distribution [211.165]

a. For each batch of drug product, there shall be appropriate laboratory determination of satisfactory conformance to final specifications for the drug product, including the identity and strength of each active ingredient, prior to release. Where sterility and/or pyrogen testing are conducted on specific batches of short-lived radiopharmaceuticals, such batches may be released prior to completion of sterility and/or pyrogen testing, provided such testing is completed as soon as possible.

b. There shall be appropriate laboratory testing, as necessary, of each batch of drug product required to be free of objectionable micro-organisms.

c. Any sampling and testing plans shall be described in written procedures that shall include the method of sampling and the number of units per batch to be tested; such written procedure shall be followed.

d. Acceptance criteria for the sampling and testing conducted by the quality control unit shall be adequate to assure that batches of drug products meet each appropriate specification and appropriate statistical quality control criteria as a condition for their approval and release. The statistical quality control criteria shall include appropriate acceptance levels and/or appropriate rejection levels.

e. The accuracy, sensitivity, specificity, and reproducibility of test methods employed by the firm shall be established and documented. Such validation and documentation may be accomplished in accordance with 211.194(a) (2).

f. Drug products failing to meet established standards or specifications and any other relevant quality control criteria shall be rejected. Reprocessing may be performed. Prior to acceptance and use, reprocessed material must meet appropriate standards, specifications, and any other relevant criteria.

Stability testing [211.166] (Haynes et al., 1971)

a. There shall be a written testing program designed to assess the stability characteristics of drug products. The results of such stability testing shall be used in determining appropriate storage conditions and expiration dates. The written program shall be followed and shall include (i) sample size and test intervals based on statistical criteria for each attribute examined to assure valid estimates of stability, (ii) storage conditions for samples retained for testing, (iii) reliable, meaningful, and specific test methods, (iv) testing of the drug product in the same container-closure system as that in which the drug product is marketed, (v) testing of drug products for reconstitution at the time of dispensing (as directed in the labelling) as well as after they are reconstituted.

b. An adequate number of batches of each drug product shall be tested to determine an appropriate expiration date and a record of such data shall be maintained. Accelerated studies, combined with basic stability information on the components, drug products, and container-closure system, may be used to support tentative expiration dates provided full shelf-life studies are not available and are being conducted. Where data from accelerated studies are used to project a tentative expiration date that is beyond a date supported by actual shelf-life studies, there must be stability studies conducted, including drug product testing at appropriate intervals, until the tentative expiration date is verified or the appropriate expiration date determined.

c. For homeopathic drug products, the requirements of this section are as follows: (i) there shall be a written assessment of stability based at least on testing or examination of the drug product for compatibility of the ingredients, and based on marketing experience with the drug product to indicate that there is no degradation of the product for the normal or expected period of use, (ii) evaluation of stability shall be based on the same container-closure system in which the drug product is being marketed.

d. Allergenic extracts that are labelled 'No U.S. Standard of Potency' are exempt from the requirements of this section [46 FR 56412, 1981].

Special testing requirements [211.167]

a. For each batch of drug product purporting to be sterile and/or pyrogen-free, there shall be appropriate laboratory testing to determine conformance to such requirements. The test procedures shall be in writing and shall be followed.

b. For each batch of ophthalmic ointment, there shall be appropriate testing to determine conformance to specifications regarding the presence of foreign particles and harsh or abrasive substances. The test procedures shall be in writing and shall be followed.

c. For each batch of controlled-release dosage form, there shall be appropriate laboratory testing to determine conformance to the specifications for the rate of release of each active ingredient. The test procedures shall be in writing and shall be followed.

Reserve samples [211.170]

a. An appropriately identified reserve sample that is representative of each lot in each shipment of each active ingredient shall be retained. The reserve sample consists of at least twice the quantity necessary for all tests required to determine whether the active ingredient meets its established specifications, except for sterility and pyrogen testing. The retention time is as follows:

1. For an active ingredient in a drug product other than those described in paragraphs (a)(2) and (3) of this section, the reserve sample shall be retained for 1 year after the expiration date of the last lot of the drug product containing the active ingredient.

2. For an active ingredient in a radioactive drug product, except for nonradioactive reagent kits, the reserve sample shall be retained for: (i) three months after the expiration date of the last lot of the drug product containing the active ingredient if the expiration dating period of the drug product is 30 days or less; or (ii) six months after the expiration date of the last lot of the drug product containing the active ingredient if the expiration dating period of the drug product is more than 30 days.

3. For an active ingredient in an OTC drug product that is exempt from bearing an expiration date under 211.137, the reserve sample shall be retained for 3 years after distribution of the last lot of the drug product containing the active ingredient.

b. An appropriately identified reserve sample that is representative of each lot or batch of drug product shall be retained and stored under conditions consistent with product labelling. The reserve sample shall be stored in the same immediate container-closure system in which the drug product is marketed or in one that has essentially the same characteristics. The reserve sample consists of at least twice the quantity necessary to perform all the required tests, except those for sterility and pyrogens. Except for those drug products described in paragraph (b)(2) of this section, reserve samples from representative sample lots or batches selected by acceptable statistical procedures shall be examined visually at least once a year for evidence of deterioration unless visual examination would affect the integrity of the reserve sample. Any evidence of reserve sample deterioration shall be investigated in accordance with 211.192. The results of examination shall be recorded and maintained with other stability data on the drug product. Reserve samples of compressed medical gases need not be retained. The retention time is as follows:

1. For a drug product other than those described in paragraphs (b)(2) and (3) of this section, the reserve sample shall be retained for 1 year after the expiration date of the drug product.

2. For a radioactive drug product, except for nonradioactive reagent kits, the reserve sample shall be retained for: (i) three months after the expiration date of the drug product if the expiration dating period of the drug product is 30 days or less; or (ii) six months after the expiration date of the

drug product if the expiration dating period of the drug product is more than 30 days.

3. For an OTC drug product that is exempt from bearing an expiration date under 211.137 the reserve sample must be retained for 3 years after the lot or batch of drug product is distributed [60 FR 4091, 1995].

Laboratory animals [211.173]

Animals used in testing components, in-process materials, or drug products for compliance with established specifications shall be maintained and controlled in a manner that assures their suitability for their intended use. They shall be identified, and adequate records shall be maintained showing the history of their use.

Penicillin contamination [211.176]

If a reasonable possibility exists that a non-penicillin drug product has been exposed to cross-contamination with penicillin, the non-penicillin drug product shall be tested for the presence of penicillin. Such drug product shall not be marketed if detectable levels are found when tested according to procedures specified in Procedures for Detecting and Measuring Penicillin Contamination in Drugs [47 FR 9396, 1982; 50 FR 8996, 1985; 55 FR 11577, 1990].

J. Records and Reports

General requirements [211.180]

a. Any production, control, or distribution record that is required to be maintained in compliance with this part and is specifically associated with a batch of a drug product shall be retained for at least 1 year after the expiration date of the batch or, in the case of certain OTC drug products lacking expiration dating because they meet the criteria for exemption under 211.137, 3 years after distribution of the batch.

b. Records shall be maintained for all components, drug product containers, closures, and labelling for at least 1 year after the expiration date or, in the case of certain

OTC drug products lacking expiration dating because they meet the criteria for exemption under 211.137, 3 years after distribution of the last lot of drug product incorporating the component or using the container, closure, or labelling.

c. All records required under this part, or copies of such records, shall be readily available for authorized inspection during the retention period at the establishment where the activities described in such records occurred. These records or copies thereof shall be subject to photocopying or other means of reproduction as part of such inspection. Records that can be immediately retrieved from another location by computer or other electronic means shall be considered as meeting the requirements of this paragraph.

d. Records required under this part may be retained either as original records or as true copies such as photocopies, microfilm, microfiche, or other accurate reproductions of the original records. Where reduction techniques, such as microfilming, are used, suitable reader and photocopying equipment shall be readily available.

e. Written records required by this part shall be maintained so that data therein can be used for evaluating, at least annually, the quality standards of each drug product to determine the need for changes in drug product specifications or manufacturing or control procedures. Written procedures shall be established and followed for such evaluations and shall include provisions for: (i) a review of a representative number of batches, whether approved or rejected, and, where applicable, records associated with the batch; and (ii) a review of complaints, recalls, returned or salvaged drug products, and investigations conducted fewer than 211.192 for each drug product.

f. Procedures shall be established to assure that the responsible officials of the firm, if they are not personally involved in or immediately aware of such actions, are notified in writing of any investigations conducted under 211.198, 211.204 or 211.208 of these regulations, any recalls, reports of inspectional observations issued by the Food and Drug Administration, or any regulatory actions relating to good manufacturing practices brought by the FDA [60 FR 4901, 1995].

Equipment cleaning and use log [211.182]

A written record of major equipment cleaning, maintenance (except routine maintenance such as lubrication and adjustments), and use shall be included in individual equipment logs that show the date, time, product, and lot number of each batch processed. If equipment is dedicated to manufacture of one product, then individual equipment logs are not required, provided that lots or batches of such product follow in numerical order and are manufactured in numerical sequence. In cases where dedicated equipment is employed, the records of cleaning, maintenance, and use shall be part of the batch record. The persons performing and double-checking the cleaning and maintenance shall date and sign or initial the log indicating that the work was performed. Entries in the log shall be in chronological order.

Component, drug product container, closure, and labelling records [211.184]

These records shall include the following:

a. The identity and quantity of each shipment of each lot of components, drug product containers, closures, and labelling; the name of the supplier; the supplier's lot number(s) if known; the receiving code as specified in 211.80 and the date of receipt. The name and location of the prime manufacturer, if different from the supplier, shall be listed if known.

b. The results of any test or examination performed (including those performed as required by 211.82(a), 211.84(d) or

211.122(a) and the conclusions derived there from.

c. An individual inventory record of each component, drug product container, and closure and, for each component, a reconciliation of the use of each lot of such component. The inventory record shall contain sufficient information to allow determination of any batch or lot of drug product associated with the use of each component, drug product container, and closure.

d. Documentation of the examination and review of labels and labelling for conformity with established specifications in accord with 211.122(c) and 211.130(c).

e. The disposition of rejected components, drug product containers, closure, and labelling (Snyder, 2003).

Master production and control records [211.186]

a. To assure uniformity from batch to batch, master production and control records for each drug product, including each batch size thereof, shall be prepared, dated, and signed (full signature, handwritten) by one person and independently checked, dated, and signed by a second person. The preparation of master production and control records shall be described in a written procedure and such written procedure shall be followed.

b. Master production and control records shall include: (i) the name and strength of the product and a description of the dosage form; (ii) the name and weight or measure of each active ingredient per dosage unit or per unit of weight or measure of the drug product and a statement of the total weight or measure of any dosage unit; (iii) a complete list of components designated by names or codes sufficiently specific to indicate any special quality characteristic; (iv) an accurate statement of the weight or measure of each component, using the same weight system (metric, avoidupois, or apothecary) for each component. Reasonable variations may be permitted, however, in the amount of components necessary for the preparation in the dosage form, provided they are justified in the master production and control records; (v) a statement concerning any calculated excess of component; (vi) a statement of theoretical weight or measure at appropriate phases of processing; (vii) a statement of theoretical yield, including the maximum and minimum percentages of theoretical yield beyond which investigation according to 211.192 is required; (viii) a description of the drug product containers, closures, and packaging materials, including a specimen or copy of each label and all other labeling signed and dated by the person or persons responsible for approval of such labeling; and (ix) complete manufacturing and control instructions, sampling and testing procedures, specifications, special notations, and precautions to be followed.

Batch production and control records [211.188]

Batch production and control records shall be prepared for each batch of drug product produced and shall include complete information relating to the production and control of each batch. These records shall include:

a. An accurate reproduction of the appropriate master production or control record, checked for accuracy, dated, and signed.

b. Documentation that each significant step in the manufacture, processing, packing, or holding of the batch was accomplished, including: (i) dates; (ii) identity of individual major equipment and lines used; (iii) specific identification of each batch of component or in-process material used; (iv) weights and measures of components used in the course of processing; (v) in-process and laboratory control results; (vi) inspection of the packaging and labelling area before and after use; (vii) a statement of the actual yield and a statement of the percentage of theoretical yield at appropriate phases of processing; (viii) complete labelling control records, including specimens or copies of all labelling used; (ix) description of drug product containers and closures; (x) any sampling performed; (xi) identification of the persons performing and directly supervising or checking each significant step in the operation; (xii) any investigation made according to 211.192; and (xiii) results of examinations made in accordance with 211.134.

Production record review [211.192]

All drug product production and control records, including those for packaging and labelling, shall be reviewed and approved by the quality control unit to determine compliance with all established, approved written procedures before a batch is released or distributed. Any unexplained discrepancy (including a percentage of theoretical yield exceeding the maximum or minimum percentages established in master production and control records) or the failure of a batch or any of its components to meet any of its specifications shall be thoroughly investigated, whether or not the batch has already been distributed. The investigation shall extend to other batches of the same drug product and other drug products that may have been associated with the specific failure or discrepancy. A written record of the investigation shall be made and shall include the conclusions and follow up (Snyder, 2003).

Laboratory records [211.194]

a. Laboratory records shall include complete data derived from all tests necessary to assure compliance with established specifications and standards, including examinations and assays, as follows: (i) a description of the sample received for testing with identification of source (that is, location from where sample was obtained), quantity, lot number or other distinctive code, date sample was taken, and date sample was received for testing; (ii) a statement of each method used in the testing of the sample. The statement shall indicate the location of data that establish that the methods used in the testing of the sample meet proper standards of accuracy and reliability as applied to the product tested. The suitability of all testing methods used shall be verified under actual conditions of use (United States Pharmocopoeia, National Formulary, Association of Official Analytical Chemists, Book of Methods); (iii) a statement of the weight or measure of sample used for each test, where appropriate; (iv) a complete record of all data secured in the course of each test, including all graphs, charts, and spectra from laboratory instrumentation, properly identified to show the specific component, drug product container, closure, in-process material, or drug product, and lot tested; (v) a record of all calculations performed in connection with the test, including units of measure, conversion factors, and equivalency factors; (vi) a statement of the results of tests and how the results compare with established standards of identity, strength, quality, and purity for the component, drug product container, closure, in-process material, or drug product tested; (vii) the initials or signature of the person who performs each test and the date(s) the tests were performed; and (viii) the initials or signature of a second person showing that the original records have been reviewed for accuracy, completeness, and compliance with established standards.

b. Complete records shall be maintained of any modification of an established method employed in testing. Such records shall include the reason for the modification and data to verify that the modification produced results that are at least as accurate and reliable for the material being tested as the established method.

c. Complete records shall be maintained of any testing and standardization of laboratory reference standards, reagents, and standard solutions.

d. Complete records shall be maintained of the periodic calibration of laboratory instruments, apparatus, gauges, and recording devices required by 211.160(b)(4).

e. Complete records shall be maintained of all stability testing performed in accordance with 211.166 [55 FR 11577, 1990].

Distribution records [211.196]

Distribution records shall contain the name and strength of the product and description of the dosage form, name and address of the consignee, date and quantity shipped, and lot or control number of the drug product. For compressed medical gas products, distribution records are not required to contain lot or control numbers (Approved by the office of Management and Budget under control No. 0910-0139) [49 FR 9865, 1984].

Complaint files [211.198]

a. Written procedures describing the handling of all written and oral complaints regarding a drug product shall be established and followed. Such procedures shall include provisions for review by the quality control unit, of any complaint involving the possible failure of a drug product to meet any of its specifications and, for such drug products, a determination as to the need for an investigation in accordance with 211.192. Such procedures shall include provisions for review to determine whether the complaint represents a serious and unexpected adverse drug experience, which is required to be reported to the FDA in accordance with 310.305 of this chapter.

b. A written record of each complaint shall be maintained in a file designated for drug product complaints. The file regarding such drug product complaints shall be maintained

at the establishment where the drug product involved was manufactured, processed, or packed, or such file may be maintained at another facility if the written records in such files are readily available for inspection at that other facility. Written records involving a drug product shall be maintained until at least 1 year after the expiration date of the drug product, or 1 year after the date that the complaint was received, whichever is longer. In the case of certain OTC drug products lacking expiration dating, because they meet the criteria for exemption under 211.137, such written records shall be maintained for 3 years after distribution of the drug product. (1) The written record shall include the following information, where known: the name and strength of the drug product, lot number, name of complainant, nature of complaint, and reply to complainant. (2) Where an investigation under 211.192 is conducted, the written record shall include the findings of the investigation and follow-up. The record or copy of the record of the investigation shall be maintained at the establishment where the investigation occurred in accordance with 211.180(c)(3) Where an investigation under 211.192 is not conducted, the written record shall include the reason that an investigation was found not to be necessary and the name of the responsible person making such a determination [51 FR 24479, 1986].

K. Returned and Salvaged Drug Products

Returned drug products [211.204]

Returned drug products shall be identified as such and held. If the conditions under which returned drug products have been held, stored, or shipped before or during their return, or if the condition of the drug product, its container, carton, or labelling, as a result of storage or shipping, casts doubt on the safety, identity, strength, quality or purity of the drug product, the returned drug product shall be destroyed unless examination, testing, or other investigations prove the drug product meets appropriate standards of safety, identity, strength, quality, or purity. A drug product may be reprocessed provided the subsequent drug product meets appropriate standards, specifications, and characteristics. Records of returned drug products shall be maintained and shall include the name and label potency of the drug product dosage form, lot number, reason for the return, quantity returned, date of disposition, and ultimate disposition of the returned drug product. If the reason for a drug product being returned implicates associated batches, an appropriate investigation shall be conducted in accordance with the requirements of 211.192. Procedures for the holding, testing, and reprocessing of returned drug products shall be in writing and shall be followed (Snyder, 2002).

Drug product salvaging [211.208]

Drug products that have been subjected to improper storage conditions including extremes in temperature, humidity, smoke, fumes, pressure, age, or radiation due to natural disasters, fires, accidents, or equipment failures shall not be salvaged and returned to the marketplace. Whenever there is a question whether drug products have been subjected to such conditions, salvaging operations may be conducted only if there is (a) evidence from laboratory tests and assays (including animal feeding studies where applicable) that the drug products meet all applicable standards of identity, strength, quality, and purity; and (b) evidence from inspection of the premises that the drug products and their associated packaging were not subjected to improper storage conditions as a result of the disaster or accident. Organoleptic examinations shall be acceptable only as supplemental evidence that the drug products meet appropriate standards of identity, strength, quality, and purity. Records including name, lot number, and disposition shall be maintained for drug products subject to this section.

B. GOOD LABORATORY PRACTICE FOR PHARMACEUTICALS

[Title 40 Code of Federal Regulations, Part 792 - Sections 792.1 through 792.195]

It is of utmost importance for government and industry to ensure quality of non-clinical health and environmental safety studies. As a result, OECD member countries have well-known criteria for the performance of these studies. To avoid different schemes of implementation that could in principle impede international trade in pharmaceuticals or chemicals, OECD member countries have pursued international harmonization of test methods and good laboratory practice. The objective of guidelines of Good Laboratory Practice is to promote the development of quality test data.

These guidelines of Good Laboratory Practice should be applied to the non-clinical safety testing of test items contained in pharmaceutical products. These test items are frequently synthetic chemicals but may also belong to natural or biological origins.

Good Laboratory Practice (GLP) is a quality system concerned with the organizational process and the conditions under which non-clinical health and environmental safety studies are planned, performed, monitored, recorded, archived and reported.

Subpart A - General Provisions

Scope [Sec. 792.1]

a. This part prescribes good laboratory practices for conducting studies relating to health effects, environmental effects, and chemical fate testing. This part is intended to ensure the quality and integrity of data submitted pursuant to testing consent agreements and test rules issued under section 4 of the Toxic Substances Control Act (TSCA) (Pub. L.94-469, 90 Stat. 2006, 15 U.S.C. 2603 et seq.).

b. This part applies to any study described by paragraph (a) of this section which any person conducts, initiates, or supports on or after September 18, 1989.

c. It is EPA's policy that all data developed under section 5 of TSCA is in accordance with provisions of this part. If data are not developed in accordance with the provisions of this part, EPA will consider such data insufficient to evaluate the health and environmental effects of the chemical substances unless the submitter provides additional information demonstrating that the data are reliable and adequate (Horowitz, 2004).

Definitions [Sec. 792.3]

- **Batch** means a specific quantity or lot of a test, control, or reference substance that has been characterized according to Sec. 792.105(a).
- **Control substance** means any chemical substance or mixture, or any other material other than a test substance feed, or water that is administered to the test system in the course of a study for the purpose of establishing a basis for comparison with the test substance for chemical or biological measurements.
- **Quality assurance unit** means any person or organizational element, except the study director, designated by testing facility management to perform the duties relating to quality assurance of the studies.
- **Raw data** means any laboratory worksheets, records, memoranda notes, or exact copies thereof, that is the result of original observations and activities of a study and is necessary for the reconstruction and evaluation of the report of that study. In the event that exact transcripts of raw data have been prepared the exact copy or exact transcript may be substituted for the original source as raw data. 'Raw data' may include photographs, microfilm or microfiche copies, computer printouts, magnetic media, including dictated observations, and recorded data from automated instruments.

- **Reference substance** means any chemical substance or mixture, or analytical standard, or material other than a test substance, feed, or water that is administered to or used in analyzing the test system in the course of a study for the purposes of establishing a basis for comparison with the test substance for known chemical or biological measurements.
- **Test substance** means a substance or mixture administered or added to a test system in a study, which substance or mixture is used to develop data to meet the requirements of a TSCA section 4(a) test rule and/or is developed under a TSCA section 4 testing consent agreement or section 5 rule or order to the extent the agreement, rule or order references this part.
- **Testing facility** means a person who actually conducts a study, i.e., actually uses the test substance in a test system. 'Testing facility' encompasses only those operational units that are being or have been used to conduct studies. TSCA means the Toxic Substances Control Act (15 U.S.C, 2601 et seq.)
- **Test site** means the location(s) at which a phase(s) of a study is conducted.
- **Study director** means the individual responsible for the overall conduct of the non-clinical health and environment safety study.
- **Standard Operating Procedures** (SOPs) means documented procedures which describe how to perform tests or activities normally not specified in detail in study plans or test guidelines.

Applicability to studies performed under grants and contracts [Sec. 792.10]

When a sponsor or other person utilizes the services of a consulting laboratory, contractor, or grantee to perform all or a part of a study to which this part applies, it shall notify the consulting laboratory, contractor, or grantee that the service is, or is part of, a study that must be conducted in compliance with the provisions of this part.

Statement of compliance or noncompliance [Sec.792.12]

Any person who submits to EPA (US Environmental Protection Agency) a test required by a testing consent agreement or a test rule issued under section 4 of TSCA shall include in the submission a true and correct statement, signed by the sponsor and the study director, of one of the following types:

a. A statement that the study was conducted in accordance with this part; or
b. A statement describing in detail all differences between the practices used in the study and those required by this part; or
c. A statement that the person was not a sponsor of the study, did not conduct the study, and does not know whether the study was conducted in accordance with this part (Title 40, CFR, Parts 160 and 792).

Inspection of a testing facility [Sec. 792.15]

A testing facility shall permit an authorized employee or duly designated representative of EPA or FDA, at reasonable times and in a reasonable manner, to inspect the facility and to inspect (and in the case of records also to copy) all records and specimens required to be maintained regarding studies to which this part applies. The records inspection and copying requirements shall not apply to quality assurance unit records of findings and problems, or to actions recommended and taken, except the EPA may seek production of these records in litigation or formal adjudicatory hearings. EPA will not consider reliable for purposes of showing that a chemical substance or mixture does not present a risk of injury to health or the environment any data developed by a testing facility or sponsor that refuses to permit inspection in accordance with this part. The determination that a study will not be considered reliable does not, however, relieve the sponsor of a required test of any obligation under any applicable statute or regulation to submit the results of the study to

EPA. Since a testing facility is a place where chemicals are stored or held, it is subject to inspection under section 11 of TSCA (*Off. J. Eur. Commu.* L 147: 1, 1975).

Effects of non-compliance [Sec. 792.17]

a. The sponsor or any other person who is conducting or has conducted a test to fulfill the requirements of a testing consent agreement or a test rule issued under section 4 of TSCA will be in violation of section 15 of TSCA if:

1. The test is not being or was not conducted in accordance with any requirement of this part;
2. Data or information submitted to EPA under this part (including the statement required by Sec. 792.12) include information or data that are false or misleading, contain significant omissions, or otherwise do not fulfill the requirements of this part; or
3. Entry in accordance with Sec. 792.15 for the purpose of auditing test data or inspecting test facilities is denied. Persons who violate the provisions of this part may be subject to civil or criminal penalties under section 16 of TSCA, legal action in United States district court under section 17 of TSCA, or criminal prosecution under 18 U.S.C. 2 or 1001.

b. EPA, at its discretion, may not consider reliable for purposes of showing that a chemical substance or mixture does not present a risk of injury to health or the environment any study, which was not conducted in accordance with this part. EPA, at its discretion, may rely upon such studies for purposes of showing adverse effects. The determination that a study will not be considered reliable does not, however, relieve the sponsor of a required test of the obligation under any applicable statute or regulation to submit the results of the study to EPA.

c. If data submitted to fulfill a requirement of a testing consent agreement or a test rule issued under section 4 of TSCA are not developed in accordance with this part, EPA may determine that the sponsor has not fulfilled its obligations under section 4 of TSCA and may require the sponsor to develop data in accordance with the requirements of this part in order to satisfy such obligations.

B. Organization and Personnel

Personnel [Sec. 792.29]

a. Each individual engaged in the conduct of, or responsible for the supervision of, a study shall have education, training, and experience, or combination thereof, to enable that individual to perform the assigned functions.

b. Each testing facility shall maintain a current summary of training and experience and job description for each individual engaged in or supervising the conduct of a study.

c. There shall be a sufficient number of personnel for the timely and proper conduct of the study according to the protocol.

d. Personnel shall take necessary personal sanitation and health precautions designed to avoid contamination of test, control, and reference substances and test systems.

e. Personnel engaged in a study shall wear clothing appropriate for the duties they perform. Such clothing shall be changed as often as necessary to prevent microbiological, radiological, or chemical contamination of test systems and test, control, and reference substances.

f. Any individual found at any time to have an illness that may adversely affect the quality and integrity of the study shall be excluded from direct contact with test systems, test, control, and reference substances and any other operation or function that may adversely affect the study until the condition is corrected. All personnel shall be instructed to report to their immediate supervisors any health or medical conditions that may

reasonably be considered to have an adverse effect on a study.

Testing facility management [Sec. 792.31]

For each study, testing facility management shall:

a. Designate a study director as described in Sec. 792.33 before the study is initiated.

b. Replace the study director promptly if it becomes necessary to do so during the conduct of a study.

c. Assure that there is a quality assurance unit as described in Sec. 792.35.

d. Assure that test, control, and reference substances or mixtures have been appropriately tested for identity, strength, purity, stability, and uniformity, as applicable.

e. Assure that personnel, resources, facilities, equipment, materials and methodologies are available as scheduled.

f. Assure that personnel clearly understand the functions they are to perform.

g. Assure that any deviations from these regulations reported by the QA unit are communicated to the study director and corrective actions are taken and documented.

Study director [Sec. 729.33]

For each study, a scientist or other professional of appropriate education, training, and experience, or combination thereof, shall be identified as the study director. The study director has overall responsibility for the technical conduct of the study, as well as for the interpretation, analysis, documentation, and reporting of results, and represents the single point of study control. The study director shall assure that:

a. The protocol, including any change, is approved as provided by Sec. 792.120 and is followed.

b. All experimental data, including observations of unanticipated responses of the test system are accurately recorded and verified.

c. Unforeseen circumstances that may affect the quality and integrity of the study are noted when they occur, and corrective action is taken and documented.

d. Test systems are as specified in the protocol.

e. All applicable good laboratory practice regulations are followed.

f. All raw data, documentation, protocols, specimens, and final reports are transferred to the archives during or at the close of the study.

Quality assurance unit [Sec. 792.35]

a. A testing facility shall have a QA unit, which shall be responsible for monitoring each study to assure management that the facilities, equipment, personnel, methods, practices, records, and controls are in conformance with the regulations in this part. For any given study, the QA unit shall be entirely separate from and independent of the personnel engaged in the direction and conduct of that study. The quality assurance unit shall conduct inspections and maintain records appropriate to the study.

b. The quality assurance unit shall: (i) maintain a copy of a master schedule sheet of all studies conducted at the testing facility indexed by test substance and containing the test system, nature of study, date study was initiated, current status of each study, identity of the sponsor, and name of the study director; (ii) maintain copies of all protocols pertaining to all studies for which the unit is responsible; (iii) inspect each study at intervals adequate to ensure the integrity of the study and maintain written and properly signed records of each periodic inspection showing the date of the inspection, the study inspected, the phase or segment of the study inspected, the person performing the inspection, findings and problems, action recommended and taken to resolve existing problems, and any scheduled date for re-inspection. Any problems which are likely to affect study integrity found during the course of an inspection shall be brought to the attention of the study director and management immediately; (iv) periodically submit to management and the study director written status reports on each study, noting any problems and the corrective actions taken; (v) determine that no deviations from approved protocols or SOPs were made without proper authorization and documentation; (vi) review the final study report to assure that such report accurately describes the methods and standard operating procedures, and that the reported results accurately reflect the raw data of the study; and (vii) prepare and sign a statement to be included with the final study report, which shall specify the date(s) inspections were made and findings reported to management and to the study director.

c. The responsibilities and procedures applicable to the QA unit, the records maintained by the QA unit, and the method of indexing such records shall be in writing and shall be maintained. These items, including inspection dates, the study inspected, the phase or segment of the study inspected, and the name of the individual performing the inspection, shall be made available for inspection to authorized employees or duly designated representatives of EPA or FDA.

d. An authorized employee or a duly designated representative of EPA or FDA shall have access to the written procedures established for the inspection and may request testing facility management to certify that inspections are being implemented, performed, documented, and followed up (QA, 4LP (98) 17).

C. Facilities

General [Sec. 792.41]

Each testing facility shall be of suitable size and construction to facilitate the proper conduct of studies. Testing facilities, which are not located within an indoor controlled environment, shall be of suitable location to facilitate the proper conduct of studies. Testing facilities shall be designed so that there is a degree of separation that will prevent any function or activity from having an adverse effect on the study.

Test system care facilities [Sec. 792.43]

a. A testing facility shall have a sufficient number of animal rooms or other test system areas, as needed, to ensure: proper separation of species or test systems, isolation of individual projects, quarantine or isolation of animals or other test systems, and routine or specialized housing of animals or other test systems.

   1. In tests with plants or aquatic animals, proper separation of species can be accomplished within a room or area by housing them separately in different chambers or aquaria. Separation of species is unnecessary where the protocol specifies the simultaneous exposure of two or more species in the same chamber, aquarium, or housing unit.

   2. Aquatic toxicity tests for individual projects shall be isolated to the extent necessary to prevent cross-contamination of different chemicals used in different tests.

b. A testing facility shall have a number of animal rooms or other test system areas separate from those described in paragraph (a) of this section to ensure isolation of studies being done with test systems or test, control, and reference substances known to be biohazardous, including volatile substances, aerosols, radioactive materials, and infectious agents.

c. Separate areas shall be provided, as appropriate, for the diagnosis, treatment, and control of laboratory test system diseases. These areas shall provide effective isolation for the housing of test systems either known or suspected of being diseased, or of being carriers of disease, from other test systems.

d. Facilities shall have proper provisions for collection and disposal of contaminated water, soil, or other spent materials. When animals are housed, facilities shall exist for the collection and disposal of all animal waste and refuse or for safe, sanitary storage of waste before removal from the testing facility. Disposal facilities shall be so provided and operated as to minimize vermin infestation, odors, disease hazards, and environmental contamination.

e. Facilities shall have provisions to regulate environmental conditions (e.g., temperature, humidity, and photoperiod) as specified in the protocol.

f. For marine test organisms, an adequate supply of clean sea water or artificial sea water (prepared from deionized or distilled water and sea salt mixture) shall be available. The ranges of composition shall be as specified in the protocol.

g. For freshwater organisms, an adequate supply of clean water of the appropriate hardness, pH, and temperature, and which is free of contaminants capable of interfering with the study, shall be available as specified in the protocol.

h. For plants, an adequate supply of soil of the appropriate composition, as specified in the protocol, shall be available as needed.

Test system supply facilities [Sec. 792.45]

There shall be storage areas, as needed, for feed, nutrients, soils, bedding, supplies, and equipment. Storage areas for feed, nutrients, soils, and bedding shall be separated from areas where the test systems are located and shall be protected against infestation or contamination. Perishable supplies shall be preserved by appropriate means. When appropriate, plant supply facilities shall be provided. These include: (i) facilities, as specified in the protocol, for holding, culturing, and maintaining algae and aquatic plants; (ii) facilities, as specified in the protocol, for plant growth, including, but not limited to, greenhouses, growth chambers, light banks, and fields; and (iii) when appropriate, facilities for aquatic animal tests shall be provided. These include but are not limited to aquaria, holding tanks, ponds, and ancillary equipment, as specified in the protocol.

Facilities for handling test, control, and reference substances [Sec. 792.47]

As necessary to prevent contamination or mix-ups, there shall be separate areas for: receipt and storage of the test, control, and reference substances; mixing of the test, control, and reference substances with a carrier, e.g., feed; storage of the test, control, and reference substance mixtures. Storage areas for test, control, and/or reference substance and for test control and/or reference mixtures shall be separate from areas housing the test systems and shall be adequate to preserve the identity, strength, purity, and stability of the substances and mixtures (Goddard, 1969).

Laboratory operation areas [Sec. 792.49]

Separate laboratory space and other space shall be provided, as needed, for the performance of the routine and specialized procedures required by studies.

Specimen and data storage facilities [Sec. 792.51]

Space shall be provided for archives, limited to access by authorized personnel only, for the storage and retrieval of all raw data and specimens from completed studies.

D. Equipment

Equipment design [Sec. 792.61]

Equipment used in the generation, measurement, or assessment of data and equipment used for facility environmental control shall be of appropriate design and adequate capacity to function according to the protocol and shall be suitably located for operation, inspection, cleaning, and maintenance.

Maintenance and calibration of equipment [Sec. 792.63]

a. Equipment shall be adequately inspected, cleaned, and maintained. Equipment used for the generation, measurement, or assessment of data shall be adequately tested, calibrated, and/or standardized.

b. The written SOPs required under Sec. 792.81(b)(11) shall set forth in sufficient detail the methods, materials, and schedules to be used in the routine inspection, cleaning, maintenance, testing, calibration, and/or standardization of equipment, and shall specify, when appropriate, remedial action to be taken in the event of failure or malfunction of equipment. The written standard operating procedures shall designate the person responsible for the performance of each operation.

c. Written records shall be maintained of all inspection, maintenance, and testing, calibrating, and/or standardizing operations. These records, containing the date of the operation, shall describe whether the maintenance operations were routine and followed the written SOPs. Written records shall be kept of nonroutine repairs performed on equipment as a result of failure and malfunction. Such records shall document the nature of the defect, how and when the defect was discovered, and any remedial action taken in response to the defect.

E. Testing Facilities Operation

Standard operating procedures (SOPs) [Sec. 792.81]

A testing facility shall have SOPs in writing, setting forth study methods which are adequate to ensure the quality and integrity of the data generated in the course of a study. All deviations in a study from SOPs shall be authorized by the study director and shall be documented in the raw data. Significant changes in established SOPs shall be properly authorized in writing by management. SOPs shall be established for, but not limited to, the following: (i) test system room preparation; (ii) test system care; (iii) receipt, identification, storage, handling, mixing, and method of sampling of the test, control, and reference substances; (iv) test system observations; (v) laboratory or other tests; (vi) handling of test systems found moribund or dead during study; (vii) necropsy of test systems or postmortem examination of test systems; (viii) collection and identification of specimens; (ix) histopathology; (x) data handling, storage and retrieval; (xi) maintenance and calibration of equipment; and (xii) transfer, proper placement, and identification of test systems. Each laboratory or other study area shall have immediately available manuals and SOPs relative to the laboratory or field procedures being performed. Published literature may be used as a supplement to SOPs. A historical file of SOPs, and all revisions thereof, including the dates of such revisions, shall be maintained.

Reagents and solutions [Sec. 792.83]

All reagents and solutions in the laboratory areas shall be labelled to indicate identity, titer or concentration, storage requirements, and expiration date. Deteriorated or outdated reagents and solutions shall not be used.

Animal and other test system care [Sec. 792.90]

a. There shall be SOPs for the housing, feeding, handling, and care of animals and other test systems.
b. All newly received test systems from outside sources shall be isolated and their health status or appropriateness for the study shall be evaluated. This evaluation shall be in accordance with EPA with acceptable veterinary medical practice or scientific methods.
c. At the initiation of a study, test systems shall be free of any disease or condition that might interfere with the purpose or conduct of the study. If during the course of the study, the test systems contract such a disease or condition, the diseased test systems should be isolated, if necessary. These test systems may be treated for disease or signs of disease provided that such treatment does not interfere with the study. The diagnosis, authorization of treatment, description of treatment, and each date of treatment shall be documented and shall be retained.

d. Warm-blooded animals, adult reptiles, and adult terrestrial amphibians used in laboratory procedures that require manipulations and observations over an extended period of time, or in studies that require these test systems to be removed from and returned to their test system-housing units for any reason (e.g., cage cleaning, treatment, etc.), shall receive appropriate identification (e.g., tattoo, color code, ear tag, ear punch, etc.). All information needed to specifically identify each test system within the test system-housing unit shall appear on the outside of that unit. Suckling mammals and juvenile birds are excluded from the requirement of individual identification unless otherwise specified in the protocol.

e. Except as specified in paragraph (e)(1) of this section, test systems of different species shall be housed in separate rooms when necessary. Test systems of the same species, but used in different studies, should not ordinarily be housed in the same room when inadvertent exposure to test, control, or reference substances or test system mix-up could affect the outcome of either study. If such mixed housing is necessary, adequate differentiation by space and identification shall be made. Plants, invertebrate animals, aquatic vertebrate animals, and organisms that may be used in multispecies tests need not be housed in separate rooms, provided that they are adequately segregated to avoid mix-up and cross contamination.

f. Cages, racks, pens, enclosures, aquaria, holding tanks, ponds, growth chambers, and other holding, rearing, and breeding areas, and accessory equipment, shall be cleaned and sanitized at appropriate intervals.

g. Feed, soil, and water used for the test systems shall be analyzed periodically to ensure that contaminants known to be capable of interfering with the study and reasonably expected to be present in such feed, soil, or water are not present at levels above those specified in the protocol. Documentation of such analyses shall be maintained as raw data.

h. Bedding used in animal cages or pens shall not interfere with the purpose or conduct of the study and shall be changed as often as necessary to keep the animals dry and clean.

i. If any pest control materials are used, the use shall be documented. Cleaning and pest control materials that interfere with the study shall not be used.

j. All plant and animal test systems shall be acclimatized to the environmental conditions of the test, prior to their use in a study.

F. Test, Control, and Reference Substances

Test, control, and reference substance characterization [Sec. 792.105]

The identity, strength, purity, and composition, or other characteristics, which will appropriately define the test, control, or reference substance, shall be determined for each batch and shall be documented before its use in a study. Methods of synthesis, fabrication, or derivation of the test, control, or reference substance shall be documented by the sponsor or the testing facility, and such location of documentation shall be specified when relevant to the conduct of the study. The solubility of each test, control, or reference substance shall be determined by the testing facility or the sponsor before the experimental start date. The stability of the test, control or reference substance shall be determined before the experimental start date or concomitantly according to written SOPs, which provide for periodic analysis of each batch. Each storage container for a test, control, or reference substance shall be labeled by name, chemical abstracts service (CAS) number or code number, batch number, expiration date, if any; and, where appropriate, storage conditions necessary to maintain the identity, strength, purity, and composition of the test, control, or reference substance. Storage containers shall be assigned to a particular test substance for the duration of the study.

a. For studies of more than 4 weeks experimental duration, reserve samples from each batch of test, control, and reference substances shall be retained for the period of time provided by Sec. 792.195.

b. The stability of test, control, and reference substances under storage conditions at the test site shall be known for all studies.

Test, control, and reference substance handling [Sec. 792.107]

Procedures shall be established for a system for the handling of the test, control, and reference substances to ensure that:

a. There is proper storage.

b. Distribution is made in a manner designed to preclude the possibility of contamination, deterioration, or damage.

c. Proper identification is maintained throughout the distribution process.

d. The receipt and distribution of each batch is documented. Such documentation shall include the date and quantity of each batch distributed or returned.

Mixtures of substances with carriers [Sec. 792.113]

For each test, control, or reference substance that is mixed with a carrier, tests by appropriate analytical methods shall be conducted: (i) to determine the uniformity of the mixture and to determine, periodically, the concentration of the test, control, or reference substance in the mixture, (ii) when relevant to the conduct of the experiment, to determine the solubility of each test, control, or reference substance in the mixture by the testing facility or the sponsor before the experimental start date, (iii) to determine the stability of the test, control or reference substance in the mixture before the experimental start date or concomitantly according to written SOPs, which provide for periodic analysis of each batch. Where any of the components of the test, control, or reference substance carrier mixture has an expiration date, that date shall be clearly shown on the container. If more than one component has an expiration date, the earliest date shall be shown. If a vehicle is used to facilitate the mixing of a test substance with a carrier, assurance shall be provided that the vehicle does not interfere with the integrity of the test.

G. Protocol for and Conduct of a Study

Protocol [Sec. 792.120]

a. Each study shall have an approved written protocol that clearly indicates the objectives and all methods for the conduct of the study. The protocol shall contain, but shall not necessarily be limited to, the following information: (i) a descriptive title and statement of the purpose of the study; (ii) identification of the test, control, and reference substance by name, chemical abstracts service (CAS) number or code number; (iii) the name and address of the sponsor and the name and address of the testing facility at which the study is being conducted; (iv) the proposed experimental start and termination dates; (v) justification for selection of the test system; (vi) where applicable, the number, body weight, sex, source of supply, species, strain, sub-strain, and age of the test system; (vii) the procedure for identification of the test system; (viii) a description of the experimental design, including methods for the control of bias; (ix) where applicable, a description and/or identification of the diet used in the study as

well as solvents, emulsifiers and/or other materials used to solubilize or suspend the test, control, or reference substances before mixing, with the carrier. The description shall include specifications for acceptable levels of contaminants that are reasonably expected to be present in the dietary materials and are known to be capable of interfering with the purpose or conduct of the study if present at levels greater than established by the specifications; (x) the route of administration and the reason for its choice; (xi) each dosage level, expressed in mg/kg of body or test system weight or other appropriate units, of the test, control, or reference substance to be administered and the method and frequency of administration; (xii) the type and frequency of tests, analyses, and measurements to be made; (xiii) the records to be maintained; (xiv) the date of approval of the protocol by the sponsor and the dated signature of the study director; and (xv) a statement of the proposed statistical method.

b. Any changes in or revisions of an approved protocol and the reasons therefor shall be documented, signed by the study director, dated, and maintained with the protocol (FDA Guidance, 1992).

Conduct of a study [Sec. 792.130]

a. The study shall be conducted in accordance with the protocol.

b. The test systems shall be monitored in conformity with the protocol.

c. Specimens shall be identified by test system, study, nature, and date of collection. This information shall be located on the specimen container or shall accompany the specimen in a manner that precludes error in the recording and storage of data.

d. In animal studies, where histopathology is required, records of gross findings for a specimen from postmortem observations shall be available to a pathologist when examining that specimen histopathologically.

e. All data generated during the conduct of a study, except those that are generated by automated data collection systems, shall be recorded directly, promptly, and legibly in ink. Data entries shall be dated on the day of entry and signed or initialed by the person entering the data. Any change in entries shall be made so as not to obscure the original entry, shall indicate the reason for such change, and shall be dated and signed or identified at the time of the change. In automated data collection systems, the individual responsible for direct data input shall be identified at the time of data input. Any change in automated data entries shall be made so as not to obscure the original entry, shall indicate the reason for change, shall be dated, and the responsible individual shall be identified.

Physical and chemical characterization studies [Sec. 792.135]

a. All provisions of the GLPs shall apply to physical and chemical characterization studies designed to determine stability, solubility, octanol-water partition coefficient, volatility, and persistence (such as biodegradation, photodegradation, and chemical degradation studies).

b. The following GLP standards shall not apply to studies designed to determine physical and chemical characteristics of a test, control, or reference substance: Section 792.31(c), (d), and (g); Section 792.35(b) and (c); Section 792.43; Section 792.45; Section 792.47; Section 792.49; Section 792.81(b) (1), (2), (6) through (9), and (12); Section 792.90; Section 792.105(a) through (d); Section 792.113; Section 792.120(a)(5) through (12), and (15); Section 792.185(a) (5) through (8), (10), (12), and (14); Section 792.195(c) and (d).

H. Reserved samples

a. An appropriately identified reserve sample that is representative of each lot in each shipment of each active ingredient shall be retained. The reserve sample consists of at least twice the quantity necessary for all tests required to determine whether the active ingredient meets its established specifications, except for sterility and pyrogen testing. The retention time is as follows:

1. For an active ingredient in a drug product other than those described in paragraphs (a) (2) and (3) of this section, the reserve sample shall be retained for 1 year after the expiration date of the last lot of the drug product containing the active ingredient.
2. For an active ingredient in a radioactive drug product, except for non-radioactive reagent kits, the reserve sample shall be retained for: (i) three months after the expiration date of the last lot of the drug product containing the active ingredient if the expiration dating period of the drug product is 30 days or less; or (ii) six months after the expiration date of the last lot of the drug product containing the active ingredient if the expiration dating period of the drug product is more than 30 days.
3. For an active ingredient in an OTC drug product that is exempt from bearing an expiration date under 211.137, the reserve sample shall be retained for 3 years after distribution of the last lot of the drug product containing the active ingredient.

b. An appropriately identified reserve sample shall be retained and stored under conditions consistent with product labelling. The reserve sample shall be stored in the same immediate container-closure system in which the drug product is marketed or in one that has essentially the same characteristics. The reserve sample consists of at least twice the quantity necessary to perform all the required tests, except those for sterility and pyrogens. Except for those drug products described in paragraph (b)(2) of this section, reserve samples from representative sample lots or batches selected by acceptable statistical procedures shall be examined visually at least once a year for evidence of deterioration unless visual examination would affect the integrity of the reserve sample. Any evidence of reserve sample deterioration shall be investigated in accordance with 211.192, the results of examination shall be recorded and maintained with other stability data on the drug product. Reserve samples of compressed medical gases need not be retained. The retention time is as follows:

1. For a drug product other than those described in paragraphs (b) (2) and (3) of this section, the reserve sample shall be retained for 1 year after the expiration date of the drug product.
2. For a radioactive drug product, except for non-radioactive reagent kits, the reserve sample shall be retained for: (i) three months after the expiration date of the drug product if the expiration dating period of the drug product is 30 days or less; or (ii) six months after the expiration date of the drug product if the expiration dating period of the drug product is more than 30 days.
3. For an OTC drug product that is exempt for bearing an expiration date under 211.137 the reserve sample must be retained for 3 years after the lot or batch of drug product is distributed.

I. On-going performance

Performance Qualification (PQ) is the process of demonstrating that an instrument consistently performs according to a specification appropriate for its routine use (Bedson and Sargent, 1996). Each laboratory should have a broad precautionary maintenance approach that is well-understood, accepted and followed by laboratory organizations, to prevent, detect and correct problems. In pharmaceutical manufacturing, results that are out of specifications (OOS) initiate a failure investigation, which can be quite time consuming.

Steps to ensure PQ can include: Preventive maintenance, Instrument calibration, Analysis of blanks, Changes of hardware, Tests of critical functions, e.g., through system suitability tests or analysis of quality control samples, firmware and software in a controlled manner, Proper error recording and handling system, Participation in proficiency testing schemes, Training programs for new employee.

PQ should be performed on a daily basis or whenever the instrument is used. The test frequency not only depends on the stability of the equipment but on everything in the system that may contribute to the analysis results. For liquid chromatography, this may be the chromatographic column or a detector's lamp.

System suitability parameters: For testing we should define the performance criteria and test procedures. We can select critical parameters as, for example, in case of liquid chromatography system this can be precision of the amounts, precision of retention times, resolution between two peaks, peak width at half height or peak tailing, limit of detection and limit of quantitation, wavelength accuracy of a UV-visible wavelength detector.

J. Records and Reports

Reporting of study results [Sec. 792.185]

a. A final report shall be prepared for each study and shall include, but not necessarily be limited to, the following:

1. Name and address of the facility performing the study and the dates on which the study was initiated and was completed, terminated, or discontinued.
2. Objectives and procedures stated in the approved protocol, including any changes in the original protocol.
3. Statistical methods employed for analyzing the data.
4. The test, control, and reference substances identified by name, CAS number or code number, strength, purity, and composition, or other appropriate characteristics.

5. Stability, and when relevant to the conduct of the study, the solubility of the test, control, and reference substances under the conditions of administration.

6. A description of the methods used.

7. A description of the test system used. Where applicable the final report shall include the number of animals or other test organisms used, sex, body weight range, source of supply, species, strain and substrain, age, and procedure used for identification.

8. A description of the dosage, dosage regimen, route of administration, and duration.

9. A description of all circumstances that may have affected the quality or integrity of the data.

10. The name of the study director, the names of other scientists or professionals and the names of all supervisory personnel, involved in the study.

11. A description of the transformations, calculations, or operations performed on the data, a summary and analysis of the data, and a statement of the conclusions drawn from the analysis.

12. The signed and dated reports of each of the individual scientists or other professionals involved in the study, including each person who, at the request or direction of the testing facility or sponsor, conducted an analysis or evaluation of data or specimens from the study after data generation was completed.

13. The locations where all specimens, raw data, and the final report are to be stored.

14. The statement prepared and signed by the quality assurance unit as described in Sec. 792.35(b)(7).

b. The final report shall be signed and dated by the study director.

c. Corrections or additions to a final report shall be in the form of an amendment by the study director. The amendment shall clearly identify that part of the final report that is being added to or corrected and the reasons for the correction or addition, and shall be signed and dated by the person responsible. Modification of a final report to comply with the submission requirements of EPA does not constitute a correction, addition, or amendment to a final report.

d. A copy of the final report and of any amendment to it shall be maintained by the sponsor and the test facility [GLP, Inspection Reports, OECD, 95, 114).

Storage and retrieval of records and data [Sec. 792.190]

a. All raw data, documentation, records, protocols, specimens, and final reports generated as a result of a study shall be retained. Specimens obtained from mutagenicity tests, specimens of soil, water, and plants, and wet specimens of blood, urine, feces, and biological fluids need not be retained after QA verification. Correspondence and other documents relating to interpretation and evaluation of data, other than those documents contained in the final report, also shall be retained.

b. There shall be archives for orderly storage and expedient retrieval of all raw data, documentation, protocols, specimens, and interim and final reports. Conditions of storage shall minimize deterioration of the documents or specimens in accordance with the requirements for the time period of their retention and the nature of the documents of specimens. A testing facility may contract with commercial archives to provide a repository for all material to be retained. Raw data and specimens may be retained elsewhere provided that the archives have specific reference to those other locations.

c. An individual shall be identified as responsible for the archives.

d. Only authorized personnel shall enter the archives.

e. Material retained or referred to in the archives shall be indexed to permit expedient retrieval.

Retention of records [Sec. 792.195]

a. Record retention requirements set forth in this section do not supersede the record retention requirements of any other regulations in this subchapter.

b. Except as provided in paragraph (c) of this section, documentation records, raw data, and specimens pertaining to a study and required to be retained by this part shall be retained in the archive(s) for a period of at least ten years following the effective date of the applicable final test rule.

1. In the case of negotiated testing agreements, each agreement will contain a provision that, except as provided in paragraph (c) of this section, documentation records, raw data, and specimens pertaining to a study and required to be retained by this part shall be retained in the archive(s) for a period of at least ten years following the publication date of the acceptance of a negotiated test agreement.

2. In the case of testing submitted under section 5, except for those items listed in paragraph (c) of this section, documentation records, raw data, and specimens pertaining to a study and required to be retained by this part shall be retained in the archive(s) for a period of at least five years following the date on which the results of the study are submitted to the agency.

c. Wet specimens, samples of test, control, or reference substances, and specially prepared material, which are relatively fragile and differ markedly in stability and quality during storage, shall be retained only as long as the quality of the preparation affords evaluation. Specimens obtained from mutagenicity tests, specimens (of soil, water, and plants, and wet specimens of blood, urine, feces, biological fluids), need not be retained after QA verification. In no case shall retention be required for longer periods than those set forth in paragraph (b) of this section.

d. The master schedule sheet, copies of protocols, and records of quality assurance inspections, as required by Sec. 792.35(c) shall be maintained by the quality assurance unit as an easily accessible system of records for the period of time specified in paragraph (b) of this section.

e. Summaries of training and experience and job descriptions required to be maintained by Sec. 792.29(b) may be retained along with all other testing facility employment records for the length of time specified in paragraph (b) of this section.

f. Records and reports of the maintenance and calibration and inspection of equipment as required by Sec. 792.63 (b) and (c), shall be retained for the length of time specified in paragraph (b) of this section.

g. If a facility conducting testing or an archive contracting facility goes out of business, all raw data, documentation, and other material specified in this section shall be transferred to the archives of the sponsor of the study. The EPA shall be notified in writing of such a transfer.

h. Specimens, samples, or other non-documentary materials need not be retained after EPA has notified in writing the sponsor or testing faculty holding the materials that retention is no longer required by EPA. Such notification normally will be furnished upon request after EPA or FDA has completed an audit of the particular study to which the materials relate and EPA has concluded that the study was conducted in accordance with this part.

i. Records required by this part may be retained either as original records or as true copies such as photocopies, microfilm, microfiche, or other accurate reproductions of the original records (Federal Register, 59: 40, 9755, 1994).

CURRENT TRENDS IN cGMP

21st Century GMPs: A Risk-based Approach

Goals of risk-based approach

These can be given as:

a. Risk management (priorities, resources allocation and setting regulatory requirements).
b. Science-based regulatory approaches (conduct scientific risk assessment and facilities technological advances).
c. Strong public health focus.
d. International cooperation.
e. Assessment and implementation of appropriate quality management systems.
f. Integrated product quality regulatory practice (review and inspection processes).

Guidelines for risk-based approach

a. The evaluation of the risk should ultimately link back to the potential risk to the patient.
b. The extent of the risk management process should be commensurate with the level of risk associated with the decision.
c. A more robust data set will lead to lower uncertainty.
d. It is essential to have a clear delineation of the risk question.
e. Risk management should be an iterative process.

People who apply risk management should have the appropriate training, skills and experience. The risk management process should be appropriately documented and verifiable. It includes:

a. Defining specifically the risk management problem or question, including the assumptions leading to the question.
b. Assembling background information and data on the hazard, harm or human health impact relevant to the assessment.
c. Identifying the necessary resources, members of the team who have the appropriate expertise, with the leader clearly identified.

d. Asking the right risk assessment questions.
e. Stating clearly the assumptions in the risk assessment.
f. Assessing the quality and sufficiency of relevant data.
g. Specifying and deliverables for the risk assessment.

Risk control describes the actions of implementing risk management decisions

- What can be done to mitigate and reduce risks?
- What options for controlling risks are available?
- What are the impacts of current risk management decisions on future options for risk management?

Risk management process is comprehensively depicted in Fig. 19.3.

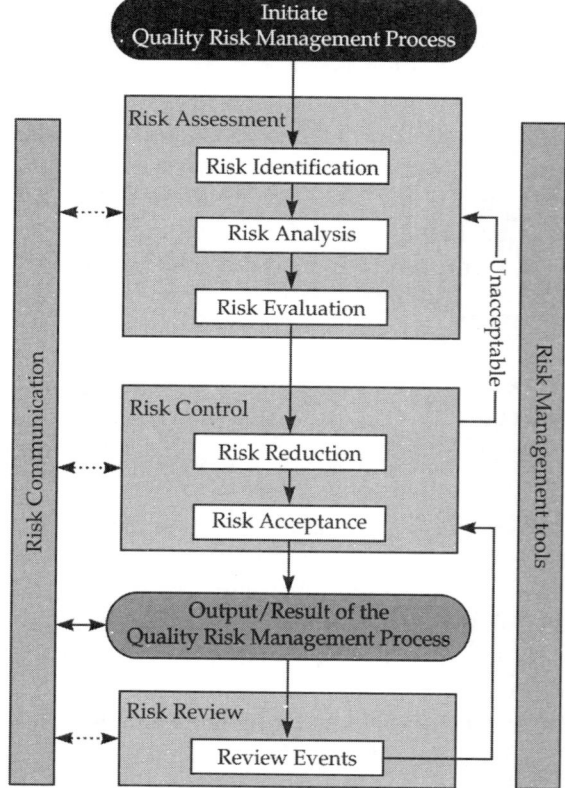

Fig. 19.3. Risk management process.

Related Terminologies

- Risk analysis is a systematic use of information to identify specific sources of harm (hazard) and to estimate the risk.
- Risk evaluation compares the estimated risk against risk criteria using a quantitative or qualitative scale to determine the significance of the risk.
- Risk management focuses on a reduction of severity of harm.
- Risk acceptance is a decision to accept risk, i.e., no additional risk control activities are necessary at that time.

Risk Assessment and Control Tools

1. Process Mapping
2. Preliminary Hazard Analysis (PHA)
3. Hazard Analysis of Critical Control Points (HACCP)
4. Fault Tree Analysis (FTA)
5. Failure Mode Effects Analysis (FMEA)
6. Failure Mode, Effects and Criticality Analysis (FMECA)
7. Risk Ranking and Filtering
8. Informal Risk Management
9. Taguchi variation Risk Management Method.

CONCLUSION

Achievement of total quality system is a prerequisite in the manufacturing organization. Total quality assurance approach is necessary to prevent a drug product from being deemed adulterated and show a uniform and consistent profile. In today's scenario we need to critically examine the parameters that would create, facilitate and activate a feedback system to establish symbiotic relationships in a continual innovation and quality stream to aid potential re-invigoration of quality processes in organizations and work for overall social good. GMP is not confined to documents only. It needs to be implemented thoroughly to meet the

standards and quality specifications of the products as per the master document. Exercising these procedures the chances of errors will be minimized and could achieve a complete control on the process parameters. This is considered as a set of criteria to be satisfied as a basis for ensuring the quality, reliability and integrity of studies, the reporting of verifiable conclusions, and the traceability of data. Its purpose is to promote the development of quality test data and to provide a managerial tool to ensure a sound approach to the management, including conduct, reporting and archiving, of laboratory studies. The GMP and GLP in India remain essentially similar in spirit as the ones described hereinabove.

BIBLIOGRAPHY

- Offic. J. Eur. Commu. L 147:1, 1975.
- Offic. J. Eur. Commu. L 240:32, 1991.
- Arling E. (2004) Biopharm. Inter. 17(6): 44–46, 48: 50–52.
- Association of Official Analytical Chemists, 2200 Wilson Blvd., Suite 400, Arlington, VA 22201-3301.
- Bedson P. and Sargent M. (1996). The development and application of guidance on equipment qualification of analytical instruments, Accreditation and Quality Assurance, 1 (6), 265/274.
- Compliance of laboratory suppliers with GLP principles, ENV/JM/MONO (99) 21.
- Compliance Program Guidance Manual (1992) Food and Drug Administration, Bioresearch Monitoring, Program 7348.808,
- Food and Drug Administration, Rockville, Maryland.
- Delmore, F. (1969) Food, Drug, Cosmetic Law J. 2411, 557–564.
- Division of Research and Testing (HFD-470), Center for Drug Evaluation and Research, Food and Drug Administration, 200.
- C St. SW., Washington, DC 20204, Office of the Federal Register, 800 North Capitol Street, NW., suite 700, Washington, DC 20408. FDA. 21 CFR 210, 211, 800, www.fda.gov.

- FDA. Draft guidance for industry: quality systems approach to pharmaceutical current good manufacturing practice regulations. www.fda/gov/cder/guidance/6452dft.htm.
- FDA. FDA announces new progress toward "21st century" regulation of pharmaceutical manufacturing. 2003.www.fda.gov/bbs/topics/NEWS/2003/NEW00936.html.
- FDA. FDA unveils new intiative to enhance pharmaceutical good manufacturing practices: a risk-based approach. 2002 www.fda.gov/bbs/topics/NEWS/2002/NEW00829.html.
- FDA. Guidance for industry, PAT – a framework for innovative pharmaceutical manufacturing and quality assurance. 2004, ww.fda.gov/cder/guidance/6419fnl. pdf.
- FDA. Milestones in US food and drug law history. www.fda.gov/opacom/backgrounders/miles.html.
- Fed. Reg. 21: 210-211, 51207,196.
- Fed. Reg. 41: 225, 51207,196.
- Fed. Reg. (1994) 59: 40, 9755.
- Fornalsaro, T. (1970) Bull. Parent. Drug Assn. 24: 110.
- Goddard, K. (1969) Bull. Parent. Drug Assn. 23: 69.
- Guidance for the preparation of GLP inspection reports, OCDE/GD (95) 114.
- Haynes, J.D. (1971) J.Pharm.Sci. 60: 927–931.
- Horowitz, D.A. (2004). Risk-based framework for GMP regulatory oversight. Presented at GMP by the Sea, Cambridge, Maryland.
- Litter, J. (1968) Organisations: Structure and Behavior, Wiley, New York.
- Loughhead, H. (1969) Bull. Parenteral Drug Assn. 23: 17.
- OECD principles of Good Laboratory Practice, ENV/MC/CHEM (98)17.
- Quality assurance and GLP, ENV/JM/MONO (99)20.
- Requesting and carrying out inspections and study audits in another country, ENV/JM/MONO (2000)3.
- Revised guidance for the conduct of laboratory inspections and study audits, OECD/GD (95)67.
- Revised guides for compliance monitoring procedures for Good Laboratory Practice, OECD/GD (95)66.
- Saengen, J. (1969) Bull. Parent. Drug Assn. 23: 179–185.
- Shewhart, W. Economic control of quality of product. Milwaukee (WI): American Society for Quality; 1989 (1931).
- Snyder, J. (2003) J. GXP Compliance, 7(3): 6–9.
- Snyder, J. (2002) J. GXP Compliance, 6(3): 29–39.
- Snyder J. Deemed and redeemed: principles of justification for deviation reviewers. Journal of GXP Compliance, 8(3):6-14. 2004.
- Snyder, J. (1999) J. GXP Compliance, 3(3): 55–59.
- Snyder, J. (2003) J. GXP Compliance, 8(2): 182–188.
- The Animal Welfare Information Center, U.S. Department of Agriculture, Agricultural Research Service, National Agricultural Library, 10301 Baltimore Ave. Beltsville, MD 20705-2351, http://www.nal.usda.gov/awic/legislat/40cfr97.
- The application of the GLP principles to field studies, ENV/JM/MONO (99)22.
- The application of the GLP principles to short-term studies, ENV/JM/MONO (99)23.
- The application of the principles of GLP to computerized systems, OECD/GD (95)115.
- The role and responsibilities of the sponsor in the application of the principles of GLP, ENV/MC/CHEM (98)16.
- The role and responsibilities of the study director in GLP studies, ENV/JM/MONO (99)24.
- Title 21, Code of Federal Regulations, Part 210 and 211.
- Title 21, Code of Federal Regulations, Part 58.3(d).
- Title 40, Code of Federal Regulations, Part 160; Fed. Reg.48:203, 1983.
- Title 40, Code of Federal Regulations, Part 792; Fed. Reg. 48:203, 53922, 1983.
- Title 40, Code of Federal Regulations, Parts 160 and 792; Fed. Reg.54:158, 34034 and 34052, 1989.
- WHO/TDR, Avenue Appia 20, 1211 Geneva 27-Switzerland.
- Woodcock, J. (2004) Keynote address, Interphex, New York. Young, J.H. (1983) Sulfanilamide and diethylene glycol, *In:* Parascandola and Whorton (Eds.) Chemistry and modern society: historical essays in honor of Aaron J. Ihde. Washington, DC: ACS.

20

Pharmaceutical Validation

Jitender Madan, Vure Prasad and P.R. Mishra

INTRODUCTION

Food and Drug Administration (FDA) proposed a concept of validation to improve the quality of pharmaceutical products. It requires careful attention to number of factors including selection of materials of quality, adequate product and process design, control of the process, and in-process and end-product testing.

The foremost priority of regulatory agencies is to ensure the safety of general public. The bio-availability of drugs is greatly influenced by the dosage form characteristics and it is imperative to ensure the consistent performance of product from batch to batch. In order to check final quality of product, a series of quality control tests has been devised. It is understood that the central role of these final stage tests is limited to measure the attributes of product produced before releasing into market. Quality control tests are tools to *ensure* not *assure* the quality of product.

The assurance of product quality is not merely an exercise of proper sampling and adequate testing of various components. It has always been known that facilities and processes involved in pharmaceutical production impact significantly on the quality of products. Quality assurance involves the establishment of control or checkpoints at various processing stages to monitor the quality of product. Each step of the manufacturing process must be controlled to maximize the probability that the finished product meets all quality and design speci-fications. Process controls are mandatory in good manufacturing practice (GMP).

The objective is to monitor on- and off-line performance of manufacturing process, and hence, validate it. Validation and end product testing are not mutually exclusive and it should be eminent that in most cases, end product testing plays a major role in ensuring that quality assurance goals are met (Traisnel & Gayot, 1995).

Validation is an integral part of the quality assurance and its simple meaning is 'action of proving' (Berry, 1988). The basic principle of quality assurance is that a drug should be produced that is fit for its intended use; this principle incorporates the understanding that the following conditions exist:

- Quality, safety, and efficacy are designed or *built* into the product.
- Quality cannot be adequately assured merely by in-process and finished-product inspection or testing.

• Each step of a manufacturing process is controlled to assure that the finished product meets all design characteristics and quality attributes including specifications.

It involves controlling the critical steps of a system, which results in output of repeatable attributes e.g. a validated tablet manufacturing process assures attributes of product consistently from batch to batch and a validated sterilization cycle assures the sterility of the product. It is neither practical nor feasible to control each and every step of a process, therefore, it is important to identify the number and relative importance of critical steps of a process that may affect the quality of a product and put control on them. Validation of a process entails demonstrating that when a process is operated within specified limits, it will consistently produce product complying with predetermined (design) requirements. Validation of a system indicates that the system has been subject to such a scrutiny, that results of a system can be practically guaranteed. Validation itself does not improve processes but confirms consistent output.

Validation protocol

A proper recorded protocol is required as to how process validation shall be conducted. It is necessary to specify the person, who is going to conduct the various tasks and to define sampling plans, testing methods, testing parameters, and specifications. It will also specify product characteristics, and equipment to be used. There must be minimum number of batches to qualify for validation studies. The protocol should specify the acceptance criteria and to designate a person who will sign/approve/disapprove the conclusions derived from such a scientific study.

The validation protocol should contain the following elements:

• Short description of the process.
• Summary of critical processing steps to be investigated.
• In process, finished product specification for release.

• Sampling plans.
• Departmental responsibility.
• Proposed time table.
• Approval of protocol.

REGULATORY BASIS OF VALIDATION

The prerequisites of validation are embodied within the scope of existing 'cGMP' regulations (Chapman, 1991, Loftus, 1993). According to U.S. Food and Drug Administration's (FDA) current good manufacturing practices (cGMP):

• **21 CFR 211.110: Control procedures** shall be established to **monitor the output** and to **validate** performance of the manufacturing processes that may be **responsible for causing variability** in the characteristics of in-process material and the drug product.
• **21 CFR 211.100:** There shall be **written procedures** for production and process **control** designed to assure that the drug products have the identity, strength, quality and purity they purport or are represented to possess.
• **21 CFR 211.113:** Appropriate **written procedures**, designed to prevent microbiological contamination of drug products purporting to be sterile, shall be established and followed. Such procedures shall include validation of any sterilization process.

Validation under the document of cGMP broadly covers overall processes of manufacturing, most of which are essentially facilities, equipment, component, procedure and process qualification. Following sections of cGMP under 21 CFR 211 refer to the validation:

• 211.68: Validation of computerized or automated processes.
• 211.84(d)(2): Validation of supplier's test results for components when these test results are accepted in lieu of in-house testing after receipt.
• 211.84(d)(3): Validation of supplier's test results for containers and closures when these

tests results are accepted in lieu of in-house testing after receipt.

- 211.110(a): Validation of manufacturing processes to ensure batch uniformity and integrity of drug products.
- 211.113(b): Validation of sterilization processes.
- 211.165(e): Validation of analytical methodologies (explicitly defines validation).
- 211.194(a)(2): Validation of analytical methodologies (implicitly defines validation).

The specific term, **process validation** should be reserved for the final stages of the product and process development sequence (Schwemer, 1990). The term process validation is not defined in cGMP regulations and the above text (in 21 CFR 211.100) implicitly refers to requirement of process validation by cGMP. The FDA in its guidelines entitled '*General Principles of Process Validation*' has presented the following definition for process validation under 21 CFR 10.90 (FDA, 1987): *Process validation is establishing documented evidence, which provides a high degree of assurance that a specific process (such as manufacture of pharmaceutical dosage forms) will consistently produce a product meeting its predetermined specifications and quality characteristics.*

The FDA has issued a number of regulatory guidelines with respect to validation, in general and specific topics.

ADVANTAGES OF VALIDATION

Though completion of process validation is a regulatory requirement to assure the safety of product, adequate validation is beneficial to manufacturer (Agalloco, 1986; Sharp, 1986; Omray, 1996), because it:

- reduces the risk of regulatory non-compliance;
- may result in reduced time to market for new products;
- reduces the chances of product recall from market;
- eliminates the scrap and reduces defect cost;
- may require less in-process control and end-product testing; parametric release of batch can be done, final release of the product batch would be expedited and freed of delays and complications caused by lengthy investigations of process or analytical related variances, and
- make process better understood; reduces the risk of preventing problems and assures the smooth running of process.

Validation, therefore, should be considered in following situations (Tetzlaff, 1992a, 1992b):

- Totally new process.
- New equipment.
- Process and equipment which have been altered to suit changing priorities.
- Process where the end product test is poor and unreliable indicator of product quality.

VALIDATION PLANNING AND ORGANIZATION

Components of a comprehensive validation program include equipment qualification/validation along with process validation. It is advantageous to assemble and organize each validation activity as individual entity as it results in flexibility and ease of management (Lingnau, 1989; Nash, 1996). Responsibilities for each individual part are clearly defined and more effectively implemented. For an example, a member of the engineering staff would be more qualified to implement an equipment qualification than validate the process. On the contrary, a process development scientist with production and quality assurance team would be best suited for process validation than equipment validation. Validation is carried out by individuals with necessary training and experiences, while GMP guide specifically identifies the responsibility of the production quality control. In practice, other departments, like engineering and research and development as well as contractors are usually involved in the programme. It is the responsibility of the pharmaceutical company to define the respective responsibilities of personnel and of external contractors in the qualification and validation programme and this should form the part of validation master plan (Nash, 1981). However, quality assurance function of a company should normally have a critical role in overseeing the whole qualification and validation protocol.

A successful validation program depends upon information and knowledge from product and process development. This knowledge and understanding is the basis for establishing an approach to control that is appropriate for the manufacturing process. Manufacturers should:

– understand the sources of variation;
– detect the presence and degree of variation;
– understand the impact of variation on the process and ultimately on product attributes; and
– control the variation in a manner commensurate with the risk it represents to the process and product.

Each manufacturer should judge whether it has gained sufficient understanding to provide a high degree of assurance in its manufacturing process to justify commercial distribution of the product. Focusing on qualification efforts without understanding the manufacturing process may not lead to adequate assurance of quality. After establishing and confirming the process, manufacturers must maintain the process in a state of control over the life of the process, even as materials, equipment, production environment, personnel, and manufacturing procedures change.

It is imperative that the most senior level of management within the company understands the personnel, time and financial resources required to execute a qualification and validation programme and commits the necessary resources to work (Tetzlaff, 1998). The responsibilities that must be carried out and the organizational structure best equipped to handle each assignment are outlined in Table 20.1. It would be wise to coordinate all documentation related to equip-

Table 20.1. Specific responsibilities of each organizational structure within the scope of process validation

Department	Responsibilities
Engineering	Installation, qualification and certification of plant, facilities, equipment, and support system
Development	Design, optimization and qualification of manufacturing process within design limits, specification and requirement (establishment of process capability information)
Manufacturing	Operation and maintenance of plant, facilities, equipment, support system, and specific manufacturing process within design limits, specification and requirements
Quality assurance	Establishment of approvable validation protocols and conducting process validation by monitoring, sampling, testing, challenging and/or auditing the specific manufacturing process for compliance with design limits, specifications, and/or requirements

ment in a validation documentation file. This file could be broken down into areas that include installation, operation and performance qualification, operating manuals, manufacturing and design specification, instrumentation, spare parts, preventive specific for that product.

EQUIPMENT VALIDATION

Equipment validation program starts from the decision to bring a piece of new equipment into organization and continues till the decommissioning of equipment at the end of useful life (Ramamurthy & Saravanakumar, 1997). It goes through three following phases (schematically shown in Fig. 20.1):

• Pre-purchase or pre-qualification phase (vendor specification, design qualification)
• Post-purchase or qualification phase (installation, operational and performance qualification)

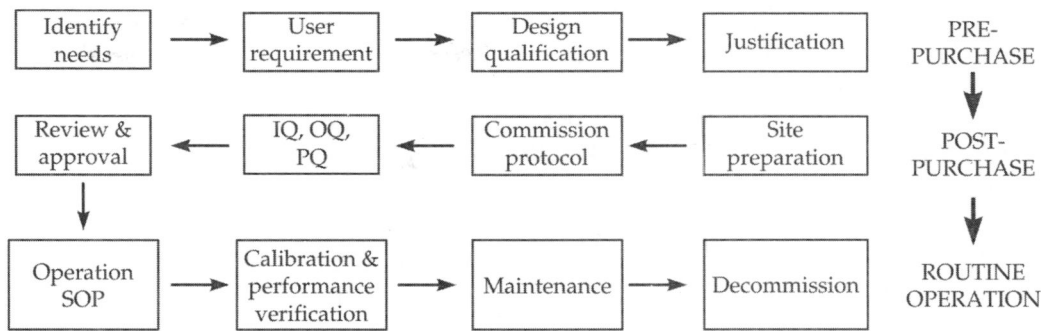

Fig. 20.1. Phases of validation.

- Maintenance, purchase order, filter program, change control program, engineering drawings, tests and inspection reports, standard operating procedures (SOPs), and cleaning and usage logbook.

Some other information related to equipment can be documented in this file. This should be in place before starting of validation.

Validation progress chart (Table 20.2) signifies that facilities and equipments are the responsibilities of engineering and manufacturing, while process and product are the responsibility of product and process development department(s). The equipment qualification is valid for processing of any number of products while the process for each product is unique and applies to one product. Therefore, process validation is routine or ongoing evaluation phase.

Pre-purchase phase

Usually an operating department will require the purchase of a piece of equipment. The rationale to bring a new piece of equipment should be well founded. The benefits of acquiring the equipment, such as increasing productivity, meeting a specific need, or enhancing the capability should outweigh the expenditure of valuable and limited resources required to acquire the equipment and support its operation. The operating department should establish requirements in order to start a project. The user should first decide on the basic functional requirement to define the type of equipment required to fulfil their needs. For example, a new HPLC system with a variable wavelength UV detector, isocratic pump is likely to be sufficient for routine analysis of main active ingredient(s) in a pharmaceutical

Key elements	Qualification stage		Validation stage
Facilities and equipment	**Installation**	**Operational prospective**	**Concurrent**
	Engineering phase	———————————————→	Manufacturing start up
		(Validation protocols) ——→	(Batch records and validation documentation)
Process and products	Developmental phase (Formula definition → and stability testing)	Scale-up phase (Process optimization → and pilot production)	QA and manufacturing phase (Full production)
	Timeline for new product introduction —————————————————————————————→		

Table 20.2. Validation progress chart

dosage form. However, if the HPLC system is intended to be used for impurity assay or multi-component mixture resolution, then a system with a gradient pump, which provides a wider choice of solvent power for better separation, and a more sensitive detector, may be required.

A more detailed operational requirement can then be defined based on the functional requirement e.g. the flow rate that an isocratic pump has to be able to achieve, the mixing mechanism for a gradient pump, the sensitivity of the detector. All these should be recorded in the user requirement document.

Vendor specification

Initially various units available in the market should be taken at a glance. The extent of resources and funds to accomplish the task should also be given due consideration. The least expensive equipment may not be the best investment. The most expensive equipment may not be the appropriate instrument for operation. Many of functionality of equipment system may not be required at all for a given organization. A consideration must also be given to the general background of the final user. Simplicity is beauty and not all users are ready to tackle very complicated operations due to time constraints and training. Although technical and economic factors have a major bearing on the selection of a vendor, no final decision should be made before analyzing each prospective vendor's capabilities in each of these areas (Tatlock et al., 1993). Below given are a number of important considerations:

- The vendor's previous experience in implementing similar projects.
- The vendor's financial stability.
- The vendor's guarantee of installation, training, start up support and after-sales support.
- The level of training offered by vendor.
- Delivery times.
- The vendor's familiarity with regulatory requirements of equipment.

- The vendor's documentation and support for testing.
- Experiences of current users.

On final selection, the vendor can be considered a team player. The vendor should offer time to assist in establishing the equipment validation plan or protocol with project team. Acceptance criteria and operational limitation shall be clearly understood by the vendor and project team.

Design qualification (DQ)

The design qualification outlines the key features of the system designed to address the user requirements, regulatory compliance and selection rationale of a particular supplier. Caution should be taken when putting together a design qualification since it will have major impact on installation, operation and performance qualifications. The more functions that are specified in the DQ, the more work has to be included in the installation, operation and performance qualification processes. The compliance of the basic design with the user requirement and regulatory requirement should be demonstrated and documented.

Post-purchase phase

Site preparation

Careful planning is required to ensure that the necessary preparations to house the new equipment in organization are completed. Insufficient site preparations cause major inconveniences and long delays in the installation process. It is the wastage of money and time to have engineer show up in premises but not able to do anything due to lack of site preparation. It is a common mistake to underestimate the effort and time required for site preparation. The following are the key considerations for the site preparation:

- *Physical dimension of the equipment and accessories:* It must be made sure that there is enough space to accommodate equipment along with accessories and the bench is strong enough to support the instrument.

- *Suitable operating environment for the instrument:* Proper temperature, humidity and vibration control must be maintained.
- *Utilities:* Some instruments will require one or more of the following utilities to operate: custom power supply, electrical plug, gases, special ventilation and enclosure and water supply, e.g. installation of LC-MS may require installation of a nitrogen generator.
- *Health and safety requirement:* For example, special licences are required to operate instruments that use radioactive substances.

Qualification

Instrument qualification is required to establish the functional capabilities and reliability of the system for its intended use. The instrument post-purchase qualification can be divided into three stages: installation, operation and performance qualification (Zutshi & Dagar, 1991).

Installation qualification (IQ)

Simply put IQ means, is it correctly installed? This is ensured through appropriate tests, related documents and records that equipment and ancillary system have been correctly commissioned, and are in conformity with installation specification, equipment manuals schematics and engineering drawing. It further consists of documented verifications that all key aspects of equipment are in working condition and have been properly installed in accordance with manufacturer's specification and placed in an environment suitable for its intended use (Auterhoff, 1996) or, in other words, IQ means: the documentary evidence to prove that the premises, supporting utilities and the equipment have been built and installed in compliance with their design specifications (Tingley et al., 1998).

The installation qualification of equipment may include, but not limited to, the following verifications:

1. **Preventive maintenance:** The IQ should document that the equipment is enrolled in a preventive maintenance program to assure that the system continues to operate properly and no component of the system becomes inoperable due to wear and tear.

2. **Equipment information and supplier instructions:** The IQ should document equipment information including the manufacturing agency, model number, and the serial number and verify that the information complies with the purchase orders and user requirement. In addition, verification of the equipment compliance with regulatory requirement should be performed. Supplier's operating and working instructions, maintenance requirements, calibration requirements and cleaning including sanitation and/or sterilization requirement for the equipment should be collected and collated.

3. **Calibration:** The IQ should document that specific devices contained with the equipment have been calibrated to traceable standards. Documentation should include date on which calibration was performed and when calibration is due. The test required to calibrate the equipment; the acceptance criteria and frequency of each test should be included in the calibration section of the SOPs. An instrument calibration record data sheet is something like shown in Fig. 20.2.

Instrument features

Description
1. Identification number:
2. Model number:
3. Serial number:
4. Capacity:
5. Location:
6. Dimensions:
7. Purpose:

Calibration information:

1. Calibration frequency:
2. Calibration number:
3. Calibration SOP No. and Title:
4. Calibration limits:
5. Utilization range
   Maximum .... Minimum ....

Compiled by .... **Date** ....

Fig. 20.2. Instrument data sheet (example format).

4. **Verification of components and equipment:** Once the equipment reaches the owner's plant, a parts list should be reviewed. This is to verify that all parts against shipping list and purchase order have been delivered and found acceptable. For the computer-assisted equipment proper communication between system components and computer control should be checked. Documentation should include operating system name and version, software name and version, location of master and backup files and CPU requirements such as processor speed, RAM capacity, hard drive specifications and requirement of any specialized hardware, etc. Each critical instrument should be tagged with an identification number, which is used for tracking purpose (Fig. 20.2).

5. **SOPs:** The IQ should document all SOPs pertaining to approved equipment and its installation place. Applicable SOPs may include preventive maintenance, calibration, operation, document archival, and equipment logbook usage. In order to give readers an idea of how an SOP looks, a typical format is shown in Fig. 20.3.

6. **Utilities and environmental conditions:** The IQ should document the manufacturer's specification for required utilities and verify that appropriate utilities are available for the system. The utilities and building service section should cover the following areas: electricity, air, lighting, plumbing, steam, vacuum, pest control, heating ventilation and air conditioning (HVAC), and cleaning. Plant engineering is responsible for providing adequate working environment. Issues that should concern this representative are equipment operation space, equipment utilities and utility capacities. After the equipment has been properly installed and all critical instruments documented and calibrated, the documentation for the equipment IQ can be completed (Fig. 20.4).

ABC Pharmaceutical Ltd. Plant Operations	Standard operating procedure
	Dept: Plant Operations
Title: Air handling system 234A-ABC-04 conditions & procedure covering the operation and preventive maintenance	**S.O.P. No.** 258-04, Revision 4
	Issue date 10/11/09
	Previous date 10/10/08
	Prepared By
	Page 1 of 5

1. Purpose:

To define the operating conditions and the standard operating procedures for the air handling system 234A-ABC-04

2. General information:

2.1 Supply Air fan

2.1.1. Fan	Manufacturer	: Narshem
2.1.2.	Model #	: 325-563-222
2.1.3.	Capacity	: 30.000 CFM
2.1.4. Motor	Manufacturer	: Khaitan Electricals.Ltd.
2.1.5.	Serial #	: 34BGH-456
2.1.6.	Horse power	: 30
2.1.7.	RPM	: 1500
2.1.8.	Power	: 440 V, 3-phase, 50 cycle

Contd.....

Operating department		Compliance			
Name	Date	Name	Date	Name	Date

Fig. 20.3. Typical standard operating procedure (SOP) format.

Operational qualification (OQ)

OQ is a series of tests that measure the performance capability of the equipment. OQ focuses on the equipment, rather than demonstrating performance capabilities relating to producing a particular product. The process should establish that the equipment or system modules operate as intended, and are capable of consistent operation within established specifications. For an HPLC system, the operation of the pump, the injector and the detector will be tested at this stage. Typical OQ tests for the HPLC system are:

- Pump – flow rate accuracy and gradient accuracy
- Detector – response, linearity, noise, drift, wavelength accuracy

```
Instrument features:
Description:
    1. Identification number:
    2. Model number:
    3. Serial number:
    4. Capacity:
    5. Location:
    6. Dimension:
    7. Purpose:
Manufacturer specifications:
    * Copy available Yes/No.
    * Location:

Purchase order (if available)
    1. Purchase order number:
    2. Location:

Materials in product/commodity contact
(Parts-material)
    1. ..................
    2. ..................
    3. ..................
    4. ..................
    5. ..................


Compiled by ........................... Date ...........................

                        Page........... of ............
```

Fig. 20.4. Equipment installation qualification.

- Injector – precision, linearity and carry over
- Column heater – temperature accuracy
- Column – resolution, height equivalent of theoretical plates (HETP)

All testing equipments must be calibrated and all the methodologies used to perform the OQ test must be validated. All documents to support the testing equipment calibration should be included in the qualification report. OQ must be performed via an established and accepted protocol. The proper operation will be verified by performing the test functions specified in the protocol. Fig. 20.5 presents a format for recording a test function summary for a test performed during OQ. The OQ testing should describe all aspects of the testing in detail. Decision should be finalized as to which parameters will be deemed critical (Tingley et al., 1998). A critical parameter is one which has

```
TEST FUNCTION SUMMARY
Equipment description
Identification number
Model number
Serial number

Test description
Test equipment/instrument needed
Test procedure
Acceptability determined by
Results
Conclusions

Compiled by ..................... Date .................

                    Page........... of ............
```

Fig. 20.5. Equipment operational qualification for both IQ and OQ.

significant impact on the equipment's ability to operate and meet process specification satisfactorily and is challenged through the use of an appropriate test function. The plans for OQ should identify the studies to be undertaken on the critical variables, the sequence of those studies and measuring equipment to be used and acceptance criteria to be met. Studies on the critical variables should include a set of conditions encompassing upper and lower processing or operating limits, circumstances commonly referred as 'worst case' conditions. Such conditions should not necessarily induce product or process failure. It is expected that during the OQ stages, manufacturer should develop draft SOPs for the equipment and services operation, cleaning activities, maintenance requirements and calibration schedules. The completion of a successful OQ should allow the finalization of operating procedures and operator instructions documentation for the equipment. This information should be used as a basis of training of operators in the requirement for satisfactory operation of equipment. Draft cleaning procedures developed at the IQ stage should be finalized after a satisfactory OQ exercise and issued as SOPs. The completion of satisfactory OQ stage should permit a formal release of equipment for the next stage of performance qualification (PQ). The release should not proceed unless calibration, cleaning, preventive maintenance and operator training requirements have been finalized and documented. The release should take the formal authorization.

Performance qualification (PQ)

PQ is defined as 'the process to verify that the system is repeatable and consistently producing a quality product' or in other words 'the process to demonstrate that the instrument can fulfil requirement outlined in the DQ'. The PQ can be demonstrated by running a typical application in DQ, which requires the system components to function together properly to deliver the expected test results. PQ should follow an authorized protocol and may include, but not limited to, the following:

1. Tests using production materials (or qualified substitutes and or simulated product) that have been developed from the specialist knowledge of the process and how the equipment or system is intended to deliver its performance characteristics.
2. Studies utilizing production materials (or qualified substitutes and/or simulated product) to include a condition or set of conditions encompassing upper and lower operating limits.

For example, integrated performance of an HPLC system in terms of resolution can be tested by injecting repeatedly a standard mixture of analytes like phenol, toluene, and naphthalene and measuring the retention time, peak area, tailing factor, peak height and width of each individual analyte when operated at given standard condition of flow rate, mobile phase and detector wavelength.

Equipment approval

After successful demonstration of equipment validation the equipment is transferred to the operating department. The validation individual circulates the completed installation, operation and process qualification documents for final comments and approvals. Once the documents are signed off (Fig. 20.6), the validation individual will transfer the document and all engineering files to the operating department for retention. The project at this point is considered complete. The operating department is responsible for organizing those files properly for controlled access.

EQUIPMENT DESCRIPTION			
Compliance		Sign.	Date
Quality assurance	☐ Acceptable ☐ Unacceptable		
Operating department	☐ Acceptable ☐ Unacceptable		
Building engineering	☐ Acceptable ☐ Unacceptable		
Validation	☐ Acceptable ☐ Unacceptable		
Remarks:			
Prepared by		Date	

Fig. 20.6. Acceptance of equipment validation.

Routine operation phase (qualification of established/in-use equipments)

After the instrument is qualified and has been transferred to the operating department, SOPs must be strictly followed for operation, maintenance and calibration of equipment.

- **Usage and service record:** Good usage and service record for the equipment must be maintained through a logbook. Such a record is required for the GMP purposes, further it facilitates the notification to the user in case of a system or calibration failure. The service records will also provide useful information about the system, which may simplify the troubleshooting effort in some instances.
- **Calibration record:** A calibration record logbook must be maintained for each equipment, stating information about date of calibration test done, name and signature of responsible person who performed the calibration and due date of next calibration test.

Instrument calibration

Calibration involves measuring and adjusting the instrument response using known standards.

The cGMP requirement dictates that the calibration of instruments should be performed at suitable intervals in accordance with an established written program. Instruments not meeting established specification must not be used. Each instrument must have calibration sticker with information related to the status of system, when the calibration was performed, who did the calibration and the next calibration date. Calibration of measuring devices is important to all kinds of process validation. It is convenient to treat calibration as a form of qualification, separately from the IQ and OQ functions, since it usually straddles both.

Systematic program is required to maintain the instrument in a state of calibration. The following points must be considered when setting up an instrument calibration and maintenance program:

- Responsibility of personnel involved in the calibration of equipment,
- Frequency of calibration for each type of instrument,
- Review and approval of calibration date,
- Procedure of issue of calibration sticker,
- Documentation requirement of the calibration and record keeping,
- Remedial action in event of calibration failure, and
- Procedure to notify users and obtain impact assessment in case of calibration failure.

Re-qualification or change control

Modification to, or relocation of, equipment should only follow satisfactory review and authorization of the documented change proposal through change control procedure. Change control is a monitoring system, which requires that a validated system remains validated by recognizing and addressing the potential impact of a change of a system (Nash, 1996). Sufficient

```
┌─────────────────────────────────────────────┐
│            OPERATING DEPARTMENT              │
│                                             │
│  Equipment No. .............. Location ......│
│  Title/Name.................................│
│  Description of change......................│
│  .............................................│
├─────────────────────────────────────────────┤
│  Purpose of change                          │
│  .............................................│
│  .............................................│
├─────────────────────────────────────────────┤
│  Originator.................... Date .........│
│                                             │
│  VALIDATION/ENGINEERING/OPERATING DEPARTMENT│
│  Results to be accomplished                 │
│  .............................................│
│  .............................................│
│  Description of tests ......................│
│  .............................................│
│  .............................................│
│  Signature................... Date..........│
│                                             │
│  Certification documents updated:           │
│  1.   □   Installation qualification        │
│  2.   □   Operation qualification           │
│  3.   □   Calibration                       │
│  4.   □   Validation                        │
│  5.   □   None                              │
│              APPROVED BY                     │
│  Departments        Signature      Date     │
├─────────────────────────────────────────────┤
│  Operating departments                      │
│  Quality assurance                          │
│  Validation                                 │
│  Engineering                                │
│  Other.................................       │
└─────────────────────────────────────────────┘
```

Fig. 20.7. Change control format.

documentation (Fig. 20.7) is necessary for each critical change in order to maintain control over the system with passage of time. Minor changes or changes having no direct impact on final or in-process product quality should be handled through documentation system of the preventive maintenance program.

PROCESS VALIDATION PHASES

Validation is required, in both general and specific terms, by the cGMP regulations in parts 210 and 211. The foundation for process validation is provided in § 211.100(a), which states that "[t]here shall be written procedures for production and process control *designed* to *assure* that the drug products have the identity, strength, quality, and purity they purport or are represented to possess" (emphasis added). This regulation requires that manufacturers design a process including operations and controls that will result in a product meeting these attributes. *Product quality* in the context of process validation means that product performance is consistent from batch-to-batch and unit-to-unit. The activities relating to process validation studies may be classified into three phases (Agalloco, 1993; Jatto & Okhamafe, 2002):

Phase 1 (Process capability design)

FDA in its process validation guidelines states that a manufacturer should evaluate all factors that affect product quality when designing and undertaking a process validation study. Not all the parameters are crucial in order to define the final product characteristics and it is therefore elemental to identify critical parameters.

Process capability is the carrying out of the studies to determine (1) the number and relative importance of critical process parameters that influence process output, and (2) the numerical values or ranges for each of the critical process parameters that result in acceptable process output (Nash, 1990).

If the process capability is properly defined, the process should result into output of consistent attributes when operated within the defined limits of critical process parameters.

Fig. 20.8 represents various processing steps of tablet manufacture and respective in-process variables that may have impact on tablet characteristics (in terms of dose uniformity and disintegration/dissolution time). In order to find critical process parameters and their relative importance each process variable is varied in a measured way within operating ranges, and its influence on final product attributes is measured (Ohm, 1997). The variables, which do not affect final product attributes, are considered non-critical while those which influence product attributes are taken as critical. Critical parameters further can be listed in order of their relative importance by measuring

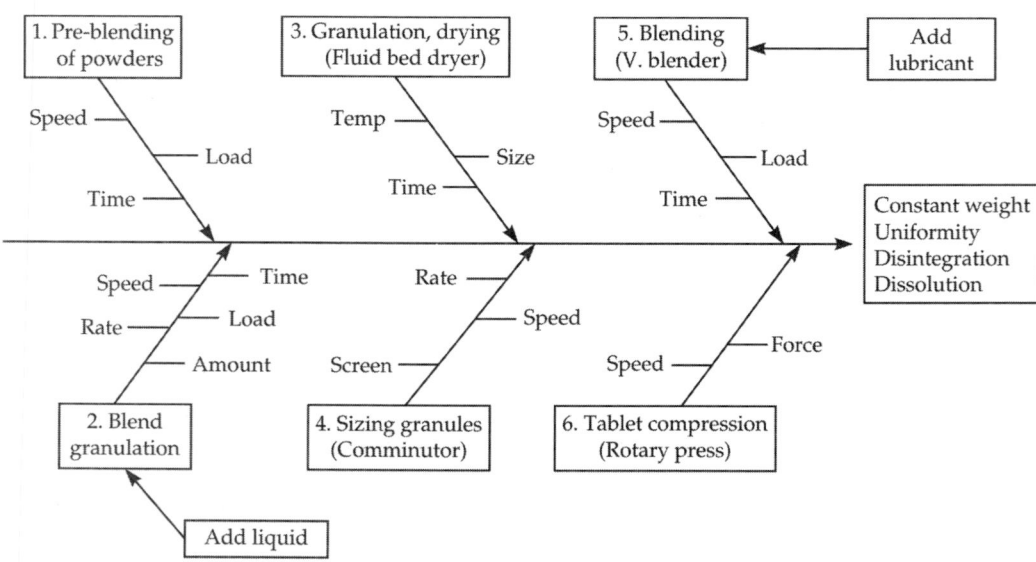

Fig. 20.8. Schematic diagram of processing steps and respective in-process variables during tablet manufacture that may influence final product attributes (dose uniformity, disintegration/dissolution time).

the extent of change in product attributes with small variation in process variables (Chow, 1997). Data to substantiate the ranges for critical process parameters generally should be obtained from laboratory- or pilot-scale batches, unless a specific parameter can only be determined from a production-scale batch (Nash, 1979).

Raw materials (active ingredients and excipients) must be clearly defined in terms of its critical quality attributes. Among the attributes that should be considered are:

- Chemical purity,
- Impurity profile (qualitative and quantitative),
- Polymorphic forms,
- Physical characterization (particle size, bulk and tap density),
- Moisture content, and
- Microbial quality (if the product is susceptible to microbial contamination).

Phase 2 (Process validation phase or Process qualification phase)

It is designed to verify that all established limits of the critical process parameters are valid and that satisfactory products can be produced even under the 'worst case' conditions (Byers, 1982). It represents the actual studies or trials conducted to show:

- that all systems, subsystems or unit operations of a manufacturing process perform as intended;
- that all critical parameters operate within their assigned control limits;
- that such studies and trials, which form the basis of process capability design and testing, are verifiable and certifiable through proper documentation.

Phase 3 (Validation maintenance phase)

It requires frequent review of all process-related documents, including validation audit reports to assure that there have been no changes, deviations, failures, modifications to the production process, and that all SOPs have been followed, including change control procedures. At this stage the validation team also assures that there have been no changes/deviations that should have resulted in re-qualification and revalidation.

Fig. 20.9 schematically represents the validation life cycle with yes/no checks. The checks at each step facilitate decision-making to complete validation exercise effectively. The product and process development usually involve following key activities:

- Process and formulation optimization based on various preliminary formulations development and designed characterization.
- Laboratory batch preparation and conducting initial accelerated stability studies.
- Pilot-scale (a scale intermediate to small laboratory scale and large full manufacturing

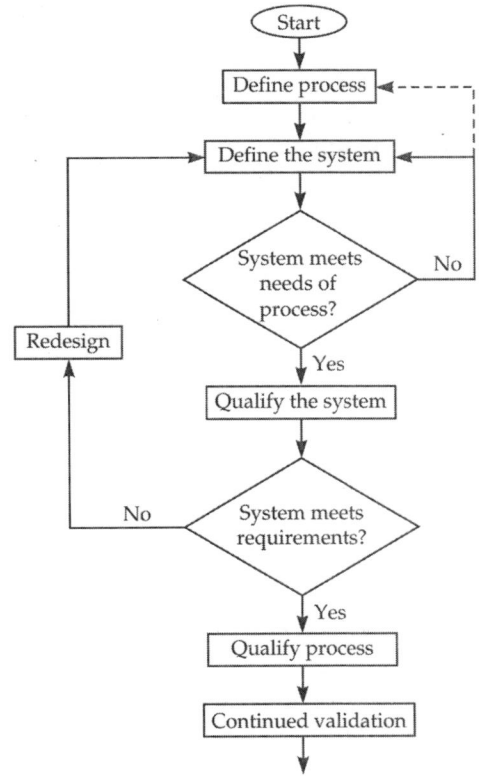

Fig. 20.9. Validation life cycle.

level production) formulation development, if formulation is deemed stable. Pilot-scale is usually gradually moved from laboratory pilot batch (10 times of laboratory scale) to manufacturing pilot production phase (usually 100 time of laboratory scale to 1/10 of intended manufacturing level).

- Full manufacturing scale production.

Process capability and qualification studies, involving process ranging, process characterization and process optimization, are usually started at laboratory pilot batch and continue until process is validated in pilot production or manufacturing production phase. Usually 3 successful completed pilot production batches are required for validation phase.

TYPES OF VALIDATION

There are three basic types of process validations. Each type represents a different pathway to concluding that a manufacturing process is in a state of control.

- **Prospective (pre-market) validation:** Validation is completed prior to the manufacture of finished product that is intended for sale.
- **Concurrent validation:** When prospective validation is not possible, it may be necessary to validate process during the routine production.
- **Retrospective validation:** Processes that have been in use for some time without any significant changes may also be validated according to an approved protocol.

There is one more type of validation apart from the three mentioned above, known as 'revalidation'.

- **Revalidation** is repetition of validation process or some specific portion of it. Revalidation of any process, equipment or facility may be performed on a periodic basis or due to some change introduced in a system.

Theoretically a validation exercise should only need to be carried out once for a given process. Practically the processes rarely remain static. Changes occur in components (raw materials, packaging materials); equipment is modified and in such cases process environment cannot be assumed to remain same as during initial validation. A documented program should exist to review the state of validation and a commitment made of the need of revalidation.

Prospective validation

Prospective validation is usually undertaken whenever a new formula, process, and/or facility need to be validated before routine pharmaceutical production starts e.g. switching to new filter medium, leak testing of lyophilizer. It is also usually employed when sufficient historical data is either unavailable or insufficient and in-process and final product testing is inadequate to ensure high degree of confidence for product quality characteristics and reproducibility, e.g. a sterile solution filled on new equipment should only be released after a media fill validation. Recently, the FDA guidelines on pre-approval inspection, associated with NDA/ANDA submission, added a new dimension to this type of validation. FDA is seeking evidence that the manufacturing process is validated before it allows a product to enter the market for sale. FDA favours prospective validation for obvious reason of higher degree of confidence and minimal risk, as it ensures process to be under control and effective prior to manufacture or release of product. Nevertheless, higher degree of confidence is also associated with higher cost of operation. Therefore, a due consideration must be given to FDA preference and cost to benefit analysis (when alternative type of validation is possible). Fig. 20.10 schematically represents the prospective validation life cycle

Concurrent validation

Concurrent validation is appropriate when:

- it is not possible to complete a validation programme before routine manufacturing starts and it is known in advance that finished

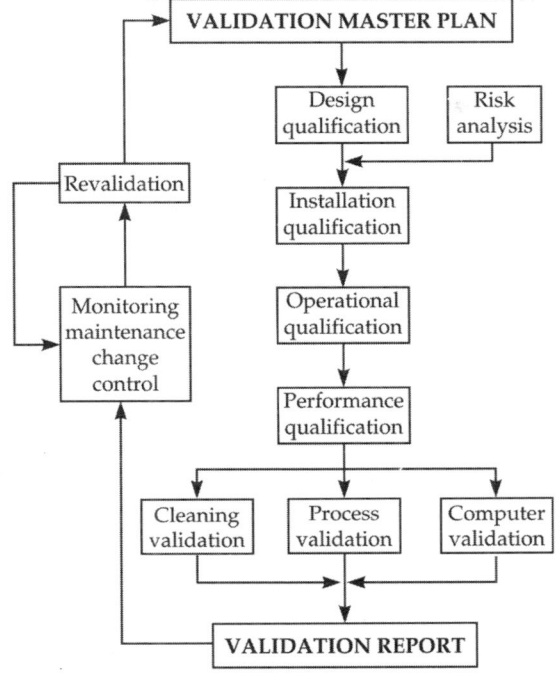

Fig. 20.10. Prospective validation life cycle.

product will be for sale e.g. during transference of process to contract manufacturer;

– it is more appropriate to validate process during routine production due to well understanding of process e.g. on change in tablet shape or strength;

– extensive testing and monitoring ensures the desired quality characteristics of product with high degree of confidence e.g. if the sufficient number of thermocouples are placed in the product throughout the load and representative samples of the products are collected from the chamber, at various intervals, for moisture analysis then it may be appropriate to validate secondary drying process for a lyophilization cycle.

FDA does not include the terminology 'concurrent validation' in its process validation guidelines and expresses its concern on reproducibility and consistency. Extensive testing and monitoring during concurrent validation may verify quality attributes of product of particular

batch, but, does not provide a high degree of assurance that subsequent batches processed under same condition and parameter will attain same quality attributes.

Nevertheless, FDA understands that in certain cases, e.g. where a product is manufactured on one time basis, prospective and retrospective validation have limited applicability and include the concept of concurrent validation under paragraph "Acceptability of Product Testing" in process validation guidelines. FDA expects evaluation of manufacturing data and test results more extensively than the usual prospective validations.

Retrospective validation

There are many processes in use in many companies that have not undergone a formally documented validation process. Validation of these processes is possible provided sufficient historical data is available to provide documentary evidence that various processes are considerably stable and are doing what they are believed to do. Retrospective validation is preferred because of cost effectiveness. Further, large historical data set available may provide higher confidence and better picture than data generated from few trial runs in prospective validation. This type of validation is acceptable only for well-established processes and where critical quality attributes and critical process parameters have been identified and documented; appropriate in-process specifications and controls have been established and documented; and there have not been excessive process/product failures attributable to causes other than operator error or equipment failure unrelated to equipment suitability. The number of batches to review will depend on the process, but, in general, data from 10 to 30 consecutive batches should be examined to assess process consistency. The review should include any batches that failed to meet specifications. However, any discrepancies or failure in the historical data may be excluded provided there is sufficient evidence that the failure was caused by isolated occurrences e.g. employee error, and were not result of process variations. The source of data for this validation may include batch documents, control charts, maintenance logbooks, records of personnel changes, process capability studies, finished product data including trend cards, and storage stability results. Whenever test data are used to demonstrate conformance to specifications, it is important that the test methodology be qualified to assure that test results are objective and accurate (Agalloco, 1983).

Appropriate personnel should evaluate data obtained, and a final validation report summarizing the results and appropriate conclusion should be prepared. This report should be reviewed and approved by the organizational units that approved the original protocol. The validation protocol should include the batch selection criteria and analytical data that will be evaluated to determine consistency of the process. Fig. 20.11 schematically represents the prospective validation life cycle

Change control/revalidation

Revalidation is the repetition of the validation process or a specific part of it. It is either performed periodically to ascertain the process or to incorporate changes in the procedure.

1. Changes to validated system

A system once validated, continues to remain validated as long as all conditions and control parameters are not changed. Therefore, a change-control quality assurance system must be established, which requires revalidation whenever there are changes in product characteristics or conditions, which can impact on product characteristics. Conditions requiring revalidation study and documentation are: changes to specifications (including formulation), test procedures, raw materials including packaging system (container/closures), facilities/plant

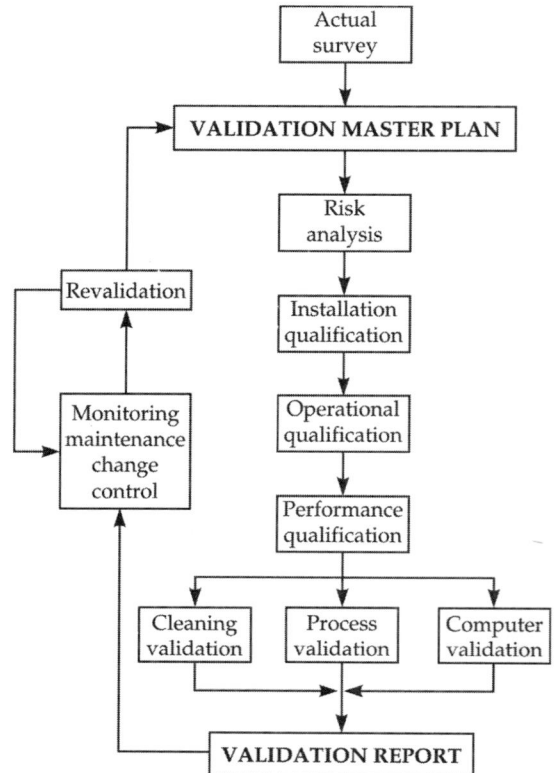

Fig. 20.11. Retrospective validation life cycle.

location or site, support systems, equipment, processing steps, batch size, packaging materials.

2. Periodic revalidation

Some manufacturers revalidate certain systems at pre-established periodic intervals, even when no change is believed to occur. The need for periodic revalidation of non-sterile processes is considered of limited usefulness than for sterile processes. In the case of standard processes on conventional equipment a review of data similar to as in retrospective validation may provide adequate assurance that process continues under control.

3. Change-control classification

The change-control program should provide a classification scheme to evaluate changes in raw/packaging materials, manufacturing site/

location, batch size, manufacturing equipment, and production processes, product attributes (changes in formulation, unit size and strength). This classification procedure should be used in determining what level of testing, validation, and documentation is needed to justify changes to a validated process. Changes should be categorized as minor or major depending on the nature and extent of the changes, and the effects these changes could impart on the product attributes. In all cases, scientific judgment should determine what additional testing and validation studies are needed to justify a change in a validated process. A minor change should be defined as one that is unlikely to have a detectable impact on the critical attributes of the product. Such changes would not shift the process in any discernible manner, and might be implemented with minimal testing and revalidation e.g. when some equipment is repaired to its initial validated state or when identical or similar equipment is introduced into the process, it is unlikely to affect the process provided it is adequately installed and qualified. A major change should be defined as one that would likely significantly affect the critical quality attributes of the product. Such changes should be justified by additional testing, and if appropriate, revalidation. FDA in its scale up and post approval changes (SUPAC) guidance classifies the various levels of changes and recommends various manufacturing, chemistry and control test and final product performance test to evaluate the impact of these changes (FDA, 1995). SUPAC guidance defines three levels of change depending upon the impact of change on quality and performance of product (Mentrup, 1997).

Level 1

Changes that are unlikely to have any detectable impact on formulation quality and performance, e.g. deletion or partial deletion of colorants or flavours or change in binder level below ± 0.5% in solid dosage forms, change to alternative equipment of the same design and operating principles of the same or of a different capacity.

Level 2

Changes that could have a significant impact on formulation quality and performance e.g. change in technical grade of excipients e.g. change of Avicel PH 102 vs. Avicel PH 200 or change in binder level between ±0.5–1.0% in solid dosage form, change in equipment to a different design and different operating principles.

Level 3

Level 3 changes are those that are likely to have a significant impact on formulation quality and performance e.g. change in binder level beyond ±1.0% in solid dosage form, change in the type of process used in the manufacture of the product, such as a change from wet granulation to direct compression of dry powder.

PROCESS VALIDATION: ORDER OF PRIORITY

It is important to know, what to validate, how much, and what are the expectations of FDA. It is not always possible to validate entire range of products of a company, simply because of resources limitations (Gold, 1996; Kieffer, 1998). It is suggested to draw up on the basis of risk potential, a list of product categories that are to be validated (Table 20.3).

The model, schematically represented in Fig. 20.12, may be useful in determining whether or not a process should be validated. The decision tree flows like this:

1. Each process should have a specification describing both the process parameters and the output desired. The manufacturer should consider whether the output could be fully verified by inspection and/or test.
2. If the answer is positive, then the consideration should be made as to whether or not verification alone is sufficient to eliminate unacceptable risk and is a cost effective solution.

Table 20.3. Categorization of various dosage forms on the basis of risk potential

Risk level	Dosage form
High risk (high priority)	Sterile products (parenterals, ophthalmics) including sterile implants, and sterile otic products
Moderate risk	Low dose or high dose tablets and capsules, oral suspensions and emulsions, reconstituted powders, transdermal delivery system, inhalation and intranasal delivery system
Low risk (low priority)	Suppositories, troches and lozenges, oral solution, topical solution/suspension/emulsions/powders

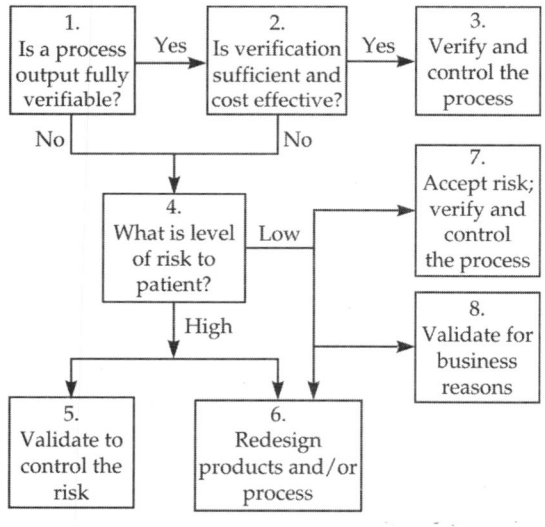

Fig. 20.12. Validation decision tree.

3. If yes, the output should be verified and the process should be appropriately controlled.
4. If the output of the process is not verifiable then the manufacturer should consider the risk to the patient of the process or the final product.
5. If the risk is high then the decision should be to validate the process.
6. It may become apparent that the product or process should be redesigned to reduce variation and improve the product or process.

7. If the risk is low, then the manufacturer may consider justifying not validating the process and accept those risks.
8. Also, if the risk is low, management may decide to validate a process even though the output of the process is verifiable. This may be because the cost of ensuring compliance with output requirements of a non-validated process is too high, or because the manufacturer may not be prepared to accept the risk-to-patient of verification only, or for other reasons. Redesigning the product or process to a point where simple verification is an acceptable decision may also reduce the risk or cost.

Table 20.4 is a list of examples of processes which normally: (1) should be validated, (2) may be satisfactorily covered by verification, and (3) processes for which the above model may be useful in determining the need for validation.

PRE-REQUISITES FOR SUCCESSFUL VALIDATION

The tool or elements required for conducting effective validations are (Neal, 2003):

Understanding and communication

Given the fact that regulated drug manufacturers must perform validations, it is very important that this understanding be shared throughout the organization. Apart from validation department only, thorough understanding of the need of validation should be understood by each department personnel (Powell-Evans, 1998). Starting from validation department, good understanding should be disseminated throughout the entire organization. Why can't the laboratory use a piece of equipment undergoing validation? Why are validations so expensive? If the entire company is fairly educated on what validation entails, less time will be required defending validation actions. The best way to improve environmental understanding is effective communication. When is the validation of unit ABC

Table 20.4. General criticality of validation for various pharmaceutical processes

1. **Processes which should be validated**
   - Sterilization
   - Clean room ambient conditions
   - Sterile packaging sealing
   - Lyophilization
   - Heat treating
   - Plating
   - Plastic injection moulding
2. **Processes which may be satisfactorily covered by verification**
   - Manual cutting
   - Testing for colour, turbidity, total pH for solutions
3. **Processes for which the above model may be useful for determining the need for validation**
   - Cleaning
   - Filling

scheduled to begin? How many resources will be required? When do the protocols have to be approved? At what sites will sampling occur? These are the typical questions that can be answered through communications like conversations, memos, periodic meetings and training sessions.

Experience

A firm's validation team must have solid validation experience in order for the validation program to be successful. The average person cannot be expected to perform open-heart surgery. Seasoned validation staff, in the midst of completing the validation, encounters a failure that will necessitate validation to be repeated completely. However, with proper coaching and consultation, some success can be realized. A solid validation requires solid background.

Cooperation and plan

Execution of a validation program is multidepartment activity such as process engineering, quality assurance, quality control, accounting, project management, or regulatory. Each department has its own set of departmental priorities and typically they may put validation as back priority.

Cooperation is essential and critical to realize department's and validation objectives, both. In order to get a team synergy all departments shall plan to get best of inputs and output.

Resources

For a successful validation it is essential to allocate the proper resources in terms of validation personnel, materials to conduct validation, equipment to be validated, laboratories to perform necessary analysis, money to pay, and time in which to perform validation.

Training

Both the personnel conducting the studies and those running the process being studied should be appropriately trained and qualified and should be suitable and competent to perform the task assigned to them.

Requirement of training goes beyond the act of mere teaching. The regulating bodies require the proper documentation that proves that key resources have undergone required training. Proper documentation should minimally include employee identification, a description of training course, and the date on which training occurred.

SOPs, instruments and methodologies

Before process validation starts the entire SOP related to equipment must be finalized, approved, trained upon and implemented for routine use. All analytical instruments must be calibrated and all validation methodologies must be validated.

Realistic completion dates

Validation is expensive affair both in terms of money and time. The time required for validation should be realistic in terms of completion of activity. If it is overly constrained, disappointment will result when the completion date is not met. Often times, commercial campaigns are planned, based upon projected completion date. These campaigns may involve contractual commitments. If the dates are not met, financial losses may occur or company may lose its reputation. If the time is too pessimistic chances are, environment will not be ready to react when validation is completed well before the projected date. In this case, campaigns may not be persuaded in a timely manner, and therefore opportunity to earn money will be lost. Either one of these extremes causes some degree of disarray.

VALIDATION MASTER PLAN

Validation, in general, requires a meticulous preparation and careful planning of the various steps in the process. Validation is a costly affair, which requires multidisciplinary team co-

operation; therefore, all such work should be carried out in a structured way. As a prerequisite, all studies should be conducted in accordance with detailed pre-established protocol, which in turn are subject to a formal change control procedure.

Protocols in context of validation is a document that gives detail of the critical parts of the manufacturing process, the parameters that should be measured, their allowable range of variability and the manner in which the system will be tested.

For example, validation of solid dosage form product protocol should include items such as:

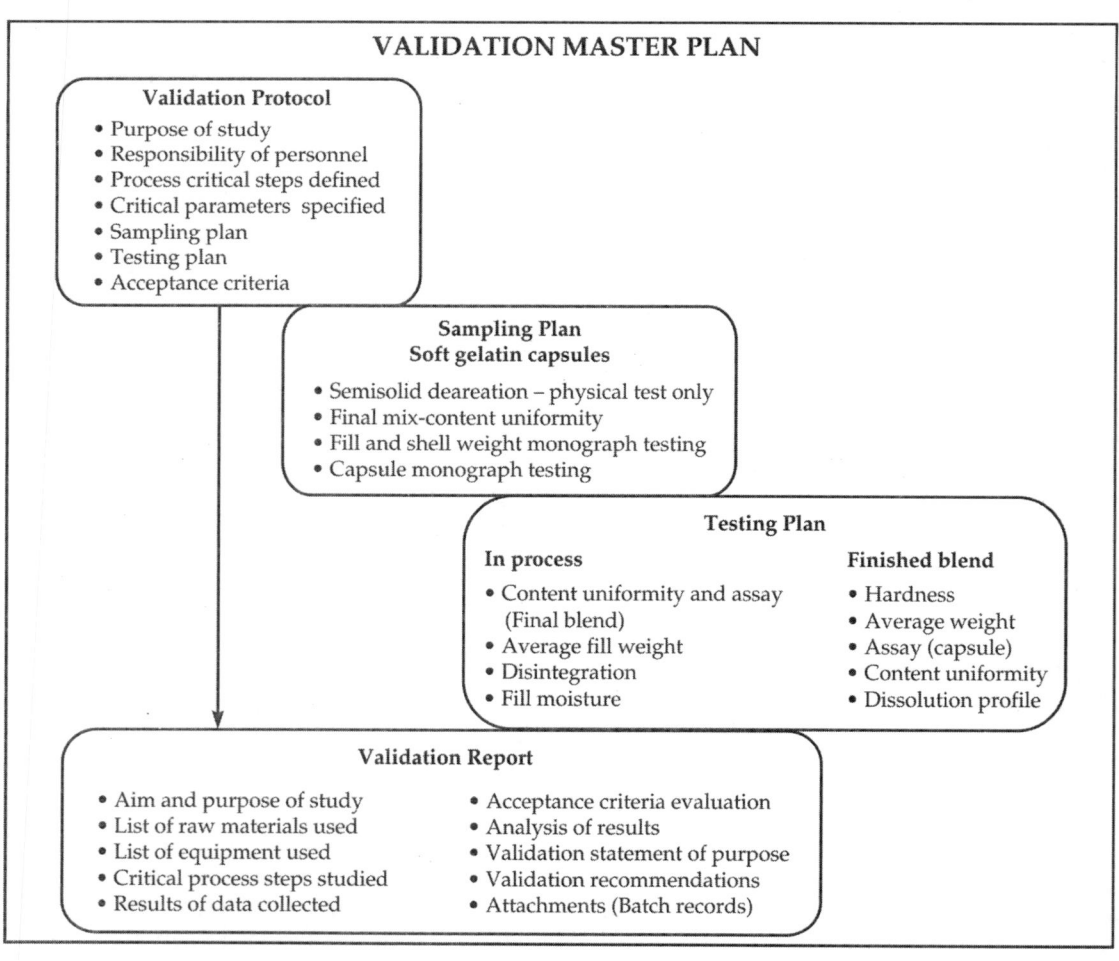

Fig. 20.13. Pictorially representation of the various elements of validation master plan.

- Acceptable limits for equipment operating parameters (e.g. feed rate in milling, blender shell and intensifier bar rpm for blending).
- Sampling procedure for granulations.
- Specification for testing the active ingredients, particle size and bulk density (if applicable).

The results of recorded parameters should be compared with the acceptance criteria set down in the testing protocol. If necessary, equipment, manufacturing procedure, and measurement methodologies may be altered to suit the intended purpose, and the reasoning behind the change must be documented.

Validation Master Plan (VMP) specifies and coordinates all qualification/validation activities to ensure the production of pharmaceutical products according to accepted international standards. It also specifies the responsibilities for validation procedures and helps to plan the necessary activities.

A validation master plan is a document, which presents overview of the entire validation operation, organizational structure, content and planning (Ramamurthy & Saravanakumar, 1997). A validation master plan (VMP) should contain data on following chapters (Maynard, 1993):

- Validation policy of company, general description of the scope of those operations covered by VMP, location and schedule.
- Organization and structure of validation activities, personnel responsibility for each activity such as VMP itself, protocols of individual projects, validation work, report and document preparation and their control, approval of validation protocols and reports in all stages of validation processes, tracking system for review, training needs in support of validation.
- Rationale behind any challenge or 'worst case' situation.
- Specific requirement of the plant/processes etc. that need extra attention may be briefly outlined.

- List of products, processes and systems to be validated.
- Installation and qualification requirement for new equipment.
- Key acceptance criteria.
- Documentation format to be used for protocols and reports.
- Planning and scheduling i.e. estimate of staffing (including training needs), equipment and specific requirements to complete the validation, time plan of project with detailed planning of subprojects.
- Change control – a statement of company's commitment to controlling critical changes to materials, facilities, equipment or processes, analytical methods.
- The VMP should be a summary document and should therefore be brief, concise and clear. It should not repeat information documented elsewhere. The core of VMP is the list/inventory of items to be validated and the planning schedule (Auterhoff, 1996).
- A VMP helps
  - Management – to know what validation programme involves with respect to time, people and money and to understand the necessity for the programme;
  - Members of validation team – to know their tasks and responsibilities; and
  - GMP inspectors – to understand company's approaches to validation and the setup an organization of all validation activities.

Data analysis

- It is the evaluation of the entire study against the protocol requirements as outlined above.
- It should be prepared and the conclusion drawn at each stage stated.
- The final conclusions should reflect whether protocol requirements were met.
- The evaluation should include an assessment of the planned calibration and maintenance programs for the equipment and instrument to maintain the validated conditions.
- All process monitoring and control procedures, required to routinely ensure the

Table 20.5. Internet links of regulatory agencies of various countries

Country and regulatory agency	Web page	Web page on validation/GMP regulations/guidelines
Australia, Therapeutic Goods Administration (TGA)	http://www.tga.gov.au	http://www.tga.gov.au/manuf/index.htm#gmp
Canada, Health Products and Food Branch Inspectorate	http://www.hc-sc.go.ca	http://www.hc-sc.go.ca/hpfb-dgpsa/inspectorate/gmp_guidelines_2002.html
Europe, European Medicines Agency (EMEA)	http://www.emea.eu.int/	http://www.emea.eu.int/Inspections/GMPhome.html
India, Ministry of Health and Family Welfare	http://www.mohfow.nic.in	Schedule 'M' on Good Manufacturing Practices under Drugs and Cosmetic Rules. Amendment notification (GCR 894(E) dated 18.11.2001) pending for final implementation and publication in Gazette of India is available at http://www.mohfow.nic.in/gr894e.htm
South Africa, Medicines Control Council (MCC)	http://www.mccza.com/	http://www.mccza.com/show document.asp
United Kingdom (UK), Medicines and Healthcare Products Regulatory Agency (MHRA)	http://www.mca.gov.uk/	http://www.mhra.gov.uk
United States (US), Food and Drug Administration (FDA)	http://www.fda.gov	
World Health Organisation (WHO)	http://www.who.int	
International Conference on Harmonisation (ICH)	http://www.ich.org	

validated conditions are maintained, should be reported.

- The analysis should be signed by authorized officers of organization, who were members of team establishing the protocol and who have appropriate expertise in the area assigned to them.
- Overall approval of the study should be authorized by the head of quality control department and head of validation team.

The validation report

A written report should be available after completion of the validation. If found acceptable, it should be approved and authorized (signed and dated). The report should include at least the following:

- Title and objective of study,
- References to protocols,
- Details of materials,
- Equipments.
- Programme and cycles used,
- Details of procedures and test methods,
- Results (compared with acceptance criteria), and
- Recommendation on the limit and criteria to be applied on future basis.

CONCLUSION

Pharmaceutical validation which includes assay validation, cleaning validation, equipment validation as well as overall process validation is crucial in stability analysis, animal studies and early phases of clinical development such as bioavailability and bioequivalence studies. After the drug is approved, pharmaceutical validation and process controls are necessary to ensure that the drug product will meet pharmaceutical standards for identity, strength, quality, purity, stability evaluation, safety and efficacy.

In conclusion, validation is 'documented common sense' i.e. documenting what and how some thing would be done and documenting how the same thing was done. Validation of a system, therefore, requires an entire set of documents, typically including a validation protocol, which is a written plan stating how the process validation will be conducted; a documentation plan that states what documents will be included and how they will be approved; functional requirements specifications that cover the technical aspects of the system; a risk analysis, which considers inherent risks of the process and potential contingency plans; executed installation, operational, and performance quali-fication protocols, traceable to the functional requirements; validation summary reports stating whether the system is fit to manufacture the product by summarizing results of validation testing and signifying that all required approval signatures have been obtained. In general, pharmaceutical validation and process controls provide a certain assurance of batch uniformity and integrity of the product manufactured.

Currently the pharmaceutical companies definitely live in an era of rapid change. There-fore it is a need of the hour to gear up for the global integration with regard to quality of the products, which eventually impinge on safety of public. To remain globally competitive, urgent attention has to be paid to augment the quality of product. The quality of the product can be ensured and assured only when each and every step of the manufacturing process is controlled, which in turn maximize the probability that the finished product meets all the mandatory speci-fications. Quality assurance involves the establishment of control or checkpoints at various processing stages to monitor the quality of product. In the post GATT era it will be onus on the manufacturer to provide consistent quality product, which could be materialized through validation processes.

Validation of a system indicates that the system has been subject to such a scrutiny that results of a system can be practically guaranteed. Validation itself does not improve processes but confirms consistent output.

ADVANCES IN PROCESS VALIDATION

Concurrent release of performance qualification batches

In most cases, the PQ protocol needs to be completed before the commercial distribution of a product. In special situations, the PQ protocol can be designed to release a PQ batch distribution before completion of the protocol. The conclusions about the manufacturing process should be made when the protocol is completed and the data is fully evaluated. FDA expects that concurrent release will be used rarely. Concurrent release might be appropriate for processes used infrequently because of limited demand for the product (e.g., orphan drugs), processes with necessarily low production volume per batch (e.g., radiopharmaceuticals, including positron emission tomography drugs), and processes manufacturing medically necessary drugs to alleviate a short supply, which should be coordinated with the Agency. When warranted and used, concurrent release should be accompanied by a system for careful oversight of the distributed batch to facilitate rapid customer feedback. For example, customer complaints and defect reports should be rapidly assessed to determine root cause and whether the process should be improved or changed. We recommend that each batch in a concurrent release program also undergo stability testing and that this test data be promptly evaluated to ensure rapid detection and correction of any problems.

NEW PROCESS VALIDATION GUIDANCE AS GIVEN BY FDA

The FDA's new process validation guidance emphasized on life-cycle approach to validation.

This actually involves to provide scientific evidence as compared to previous documented evidence. The documented evidence as is used previously is actually a late stage documentation exercise. The new definition, however, describes process validation as a continuous process of collection and evaluation of data, rather than a static event. The idea of FDA is to consider it as scientific attempt rather than documentation process (FDA, 2011).

Defining the new process-validation stages

The guidance (2011) implemented the life-cycle model as illustrated in ICH Q10 and in FDA's 2006 guidance for industry on *Quality Systems Approach to Pharmaceutical cGMP Regulations*, which states that, "quality should be built into the product, and testing alone cannot be relied on to ensure product quality" (ICH 2008; FDA 2006).

The new document illustrates validation activities in three stages using a life-cycle model. Stages have been narrated as separate entity, however they could occur either single or overlapping stages. The guidance describes these three stages as follows:

Stage 1

Process design: The commercial-manufacturing process is defined during this stage based on knowledge gained through development and scale-up activities.

Stage 2

Process qualification: During this stage, the process design is evaluated to determine whether the process is capable of reproducible commercial manufacturing.

Stage 3

Continued process verification: Ongoing assurance is gained during routine production that the process remains in a state of control.

REFERENCES

- Agalloco, J. (1993) Validation life cycle. *J. Parentr. Sci. Tech.* 47, 142–147.
- Agalloco, J.P. (1983) Practical consideration in retrospective validation. *Pharm. Tech.* 7, 88–90.
- Agalloco, J.P. (1986) Other side of process validation. *Bulletin Parentr. Drug Assoc.* 40, 251–252.
- Auterhoff, G. (1996) PIC recommendations on validation. *Drugs Made in Germany* 39, 83-86, 91–95.
- Berry, I.R. (1988) Process validation: Practical application to pharmaceutical products. *Drug Dev. Ind. Pharm.* 14, 377–389.
- Byers, T.E. (1982) Validation – burden or benefit? *Drug Cosmet. Ind.* 130, 43–44, 82, 86.
- Chapman, K.G. (1991) The history of validation in the United States. Part - I. *Pharm. Tech.* 15, 82-96.
- Chow, S. (1997) Pharmaceutical validation and process controls in drug development. *Drug Inf. J.* 31, 1195–1201.
- FDA, *Guidelines on general principles of process validation* (1987). Published by Center for Drugs and Biologics, Rockville, Maryland, USA.
- FDA, *Guidance for Industry: Process Validation: General Principles and Practices* (Rockville, MD, Jan. 2011).
- FDA, *Guidance for Industry: Quality Systems Approach to Pharmaceutical cGMP Regulations* (Rockville, MD, September 2006).
- FDA, *Guidance for industry, immediate release solid oral dosage forms scale-up and post approval changes: Chemistry, manufacturing, and controls, in vitro dissolution testing, and in vivo bio-equivalence documentation* (1995). Published by Center for Drug Evaluation and Research (CDER), Rockville, Maryland, U.S.
- Gold, D.H. (1996) Validation: Why, what, when, how much. *PDA J. Pharm. Sci. Tech.* 50, 55–60.
- Jatto, E. and Okhamafe, A.O. (2002) An overview of pharmaceutical validation and process controls in drug development. *Trop. J. Pharm. Res.* 1, 115–122.
- Kieffer, R.G. (1998) Global trends, needs, issues. *PDA J. Pharm. Sci. Tech.* 52, 151–153.
- Lingnau, J. (1989) Optimization and validation of manufacturing processes. *Drug Dev. Ind. Pharm.* 15, 1029–1046.

- Loftus, B.T. (1993) The regulatory basis of process validation. *In:* Berry, I.R. and Nash, I.R. (Eds.) **Pharmaceutical Process Validation**. Marcel Dekker Inc. New York, USA 2 ed. Vol. pp 1–8.
- Maynard, D.W. (1993) Validation master planning. *J. Parentr. Sci. Tech.* 47, 84–88.
- Mentrup, E. (1997) Handling of process changes during scale-up. *Pharm. Tech.* 9, 62–72.
- Nash, R.A. (1979) Process validation for solid dosage forms. *Pharm. Tech.* 3, 105–107.
- Nash, R.A. (1981) Process validation: Solid dosage forms. *Drug Cosmet. Ind.* 129, 38-39, 104–106.
- Nash, R.A. (1990) The essential of process validation. *In:* Lachman, L. and Schwartz, J.B. (Eds.) **Pharmaceutical Dosage Forms**. Marcel Dekker. New York 2 ed. Vol. 3, pp 417–453.
- Nash, R.A. (1996) Process validation: 17 years retrospective of solid dosage form. *Drug Dev. Ind. Pharm.* 22, 25–34.
- Neal, C. (2003) Prerequisites for successful validation. *J. Validation Tech.* 9, 240–245.
- Ohm, A. (1997) Process validation of oral solid dosage forms – semiscientific overview. *Pharm. Tech.* 9, 30–38.
- Omray, A. (1996) Validation – way of life. *Pharma Times* 28, 31–33.
- Powell-Evans, K. (1998) Validation – bad manufacturing practice? *Pharm. Tech.* 10, 29–30.
- Ramamurthy, M.S. and Saravanakumar, M.K. (1997) Validation. *Eastern Pharmacist* 40, 45–47.
- Rockville M.D. Guideline on General Principles of Process Validation. U.S. Food and Drug Administration., U.S. FDA: 2010.
- Schwemer, W.L. (1990) Validation: Foundation of GMP. *Pharm. Engg.* 10, 44–46.
- Sharp, J.R. (1986) The problems of process validation. *Pharm. J.* 1, 43–45.
- Tatlock, R.; Taylor, R.; Noble, L.; Manternach, R. and Salazar, J. (1993) Key success factors in automating a pharmaceutical process. *Pharm. Tech.* 17, 54–60.
- Tetzlaff, R.F. (1992a) Validation issues for new drug development. Part 1. Review of current FDA policies. Pharm. Tech. 16, 44–56.
- Tetzlaff, R.F. (1992b) Validation issues for new drug development. Part 2. Review of current FDA policies. *Pharm. Tech.* 16, 84–94.
- Tetzlaff, R.F. (1998) Project plans for new drug development activities. *Pharm. Tech.* 22, 46–60.
- Tingley, S.; Walker, S.; Messing, J.; Keogh, D. and Davis, P. (1998) Case study of the IQ/OQ and practical implementation of an automated water based integrity test for hydrophobic filters. *Pharm. Tech.* 22, 58–76.
- Traisnel, M. and Gayot, A.T. (1995) Practice of validation. *Drug Dev. Ind. Pharm.* 21, 79–91.
- Zutshi, R. and Dagar, V. (1991) Process validation in pharmaceutical organization. *Eastern Pharmacist* 34, 37–38.

21

Polymers in Pharmaceutical Sciences

Sanjay Jain and N.K. Jain

INTRODUCTION

Polymer science has been the key driver for the development of new therapeutic, diagnostic and theranostic formulations for the past many decades and its advances have led to the development of several novel applications in pharmaceutical sciences. The constantly changing requirements and product life-cycle of new pharmaceutical products require the new product development for various applications. A product development starts with new concepts, pre-formulation, formulation, scale-up, quality control/assurance, packaging and marketing of a wide range of new and life-cycle management of existing or generic molecules/drugs.

Due to the extraordinary range of properties accessible in polymeric materials [Roiter and Minko, 2005; Painter and Coleman, 1997], they have come to play an essential role in everyday life [McCrum et al., 1997], from plastics and elastomers on the one hand, to natural biopolymers, e.g., DNA and proteins that are essential for life, on the other. Natural polymeric materials e.g., shellac, amber, and natural rubber have been in use for centuries. A proper selection of surface and bulk properties can help in the designing of polymers for various applications in pharmacy. These are widely used as pharmaceutical aids (e.g., suspending agent, emulsifying agent, adhesives, coating agents, adjuvants, etc.), packaging materials and medical devices (e.g., in conventional and controlled drug delivery systems) as well as theranostic agents (e.g., drug and diagnostic agent loaded nanoparticles for the detection and simultaneously killing cancer cells). The pharmaceutical polymers with specific properties (e.g., stimuli sensitivity, bio-degradability, film-forming nature, etc.) offer interesting opportunities.

The polymer sciences have been the backbone of product development in the modern pharmaceutical industry. In addition to this, recent advances in polymer nanotechnology have changed the nature of diagnosis and treatment in the biomedical field.

HISTORICAL BACKGROUND

The word polymer is derived from the Greek words πολν (poly), meaning 'many'; and μεροσ (meros), meaning 'part'. It is a large molecule composed of repeating structural units typically connected by covalent chemical bonds. Henri

Braconnot (1811) did pioneering work in derivative cellulose compounds. Berzelius (1833) first used the term "polymeric" to describe the relationship of ethylene to butane. Baekeland (1907) created the first completely synthetic polymer, Bakelite, by reacting phenol and formaldehyde. Hermann Staudinger (1992) proposed that polymers consisted of long chains of atoms held together by covalent bonds. Wallace Carothers (1920s) also demonstrated that polymers could be synthesised rationally from their constituent monomers [Omidian et el., 2011].

Flory, Mark and others (1940s) were responsible for rapid expansion of polymer science [http://chem.pdx.edu]. The distinction between temporary and permanent pharmaceutical applications of polymers was made only in 1960s [Uhrich et al., 1999]. Polymeric delivery systems are mainly intended to achieve either a temporal or spatial control of drug delivery [Li and Vert, 1999]. The introduction of the first synthetic polymer-based (polyglycolic acid; PGA) drug delivery system (DDS) led to an interest in the design and synthesis of novel biodegradable polymers. Identifying that contact between a delivery system and an epithelial cell layer improves the residence time as well as the efficacy of the DDS, resulted in the design of bioadhesive polymers. Advances in polymer science led to polymeric hydrogel systems that can self-regulate the delivery of a bioactive agent in response to a specific stimulus [Pillai and Pachagnula, 2001]. Flory's (1974) work on polymers included the kinetics of step-growth polymerisation and of addition polymerisation, chain transfer, excluded volume.

Synthetic polymer materials, e.g., nylon, polyethylene, Teflon, and silicone, have formed the basis for a growing polymer industry. These are produced in high volume on appropriately scaled organic synthetic techniques. Synthetic polymers today find application in nearly every industry and area of life. Nonetheless, natural polymers are emerging and gaining popularity due to their inherent advantages.

TERMS USED IN POLYMER SCIENCES

A polymer molecule is made by linking many small units (monomers) together to form a large molecule. This can be made of a single species (homopolymer) or of several different monomers (copolymer). Polymers occur naturally (biopolymers) but are also made synthetically in large amounts. Polymers may also be categorised by physical properties, e.g., crystallinity or linearity/branching. They owe their unique properties to their size, three-dimensional shape and asymmetry. The chemical reactivity of polymers depends on the chemistry of their monomer units, but their properties depend to a large extent on the way the monomers are put together. The pharmaceutically important terms used in polymer sciences are defined below [Florence and Attwood, 1998, 2011; www.studsvik.uu.se; Omidian et al., 2011]:

- **Addition polymerisation:** This is a polymerisation reaction that occurs by addition of a monomer to a double bond between two carbon atoms. Repeated addition of ethylene in this way gives rise to a long chain polymer (polyethylene): $RCH_2=CH_2 + CH_2=CH_2 \rightarrow RCH_2-CH_2-CH_2=CH_2$.

- **Alternating copolymer:** An alternating copolymer is a polymer formed from two monomers in a regular alternating sequence, e.g., that of A and B monomers: ABABABABAB.

- **Biopolymer:** A polymer that occurs naturally (e.g., proteins and carbohydrates). Many materials including DNA, muscle tissue and some components of foods are biopolymers.

- **Block copolymer:** A copolymer in which the different components are separated into discrete regions of each individual polymer molecule. A di-block copolymer of monomers A and B would have a sequence of the type AAAAAAABBBBBBB.

- **Branched polymer:** This is a polymer with branch points in the backbone of the molecule. The physical properties, e.g., viscosity and crystallinity may depend on the extent of branching.

- **Chi parameter:** This is the Flory-Huggins parameter that describes the enthalpy of interaction of a polymer with a solvent or of interaction between two polymers.
- **Comb copolymer:** A comb copolymer is a polymer formed side chains that consist of a different monomer.
- **Concentrated polymer solution:** This is a polymer solution above the overlap concentration. The polymers are entangled with each other. Diffusion is highly hindered and the viscosity will be large as the molecules are constrained to move by reptation.
- **Condensation polymerisation:** This is a polymerisation reaction in which a small molecule (e.g., water) is released, e.g., polyesters: $RCOOH + HOR' \rightarrow RCOOR' + H_2O$.
- **Conformation:** The way polymer molecules are arranged is known as its conformation, e.g., free rotation about some bonds lead to many different possible conformations. The balance of free energy of polymer-polymer/polymer-solvent interactions determines different conformations.
- **Contour length:** A contour length is the length of the chain backbone in its fully extended state.
- **Copolymer:** The polymers formed from one or more monomers, the molecule consists of chemically heterogeneous components, arranged in different ways, e.g., block copolymers, etc.
- **Crystalline melting temperature (Tm):** This is the temperature at which a crystalline polymer is converted to a liquid, or crystalline domains of a semi-crystalline polymer melt.
- **Degree of polymerisation:** This is the number of monomers that combine together to form a polymer molecule. The molecular mass of the polymer, M, is related to the degree of polymerisation, N, and the molecular mass of the monomer, m, by $M = Nm$.

- **Good solvent:** A good solvent for a polymer is one in which the interactions with the solvent molecules are energetically favoured over interactions with other segments of the polymer in solution. In a good solvent the size of a polymer molecule (radius of gyration, R_g) varies with the degree of polymerisation, N, as $R_g \sim N^{0.6}$.
- **Graft copolymer:** The linking a polymer of one type to another polymer molecule of a different composition makes a grafted copolymer.
- **Homopolymer:** These are polymers that are formed from one type of monomer so that the molecule consists of chemically uniform components. They can be linear, star or branched.
- **Ionomer:** A polymer molecule containing ionisable subunits is known as a polyelectrolyte or ionomer.
- **Linear polymer:** This is a polymer without branch points in the molecule. The physical properties, e.g., viscosity and crystallinity, may depend on the extent of branching.
- **Mark-Houwink equation:** The Mark-Houwink equation is $[\eta] = kM^{\alpha}$, where k and α are tabulated constants. These are generally specific to each polymer/solvent pair. α is usually in the range 0.4–1.0.
- **Oligomer:** An oligomer is a molecule made from a few monomers.
- **Overlap concentration:** It is the concentration of a polymer in a solution at which the molecules begin to interpenetrate each other and become entangled leading to significant changes in properties, e.g., sharp increases of viscosity. The overlap concentration, C_o, may be crudely estimated from the molecular mass, M and the radius of gyration, R_g by $C_o \sim M/R_g^3$.
- **Phantom chain:** A model with a 'phantom' chain is one in which polymer molecules would be free to pass through each other rather than be constrained by physical entanglements or cross-links.

- **Polymerisation:** The term polymerisation describes chemical reactions that produce polymers by repeated combination of monomers to make long or large molecules. These include the physical state of reagents (e.g., emulsion polymerisation, suspension polymerisation), nature of the reaction (e.g., condensation, addition) or type of initiator or catalyst (e.g., anionic polymerisation).

- **Random copolymer:** A copolymer in which the different components are arranged randomly. A sequence of monomers (A and B) in a random copolymer might be AABABBAABBBBBABABBA.

- **Reptation:** The mechanism by which polymers move through entanglements with other polymers in melts or concentrated solutions.

- **Star polymer:** A star polymer is a molecule that has multiple branches from a single point. It is characterised by the number of arms as well as the length of the arms.

- **Thermoplastic:** Thermoplastic materials are those which become processable (flow) on heating either by melting of crystallites or by softening of a glass at the glass transition.

- **Thermoset:** Thermoset polymers are materials that become rigid on heating usually by chemical reactions leading to a rigid cross-linked network.

- **Theta solvent (θ-solvent):** This is a solvent for a polymer in which the macromolecule has the same interactions with a solvent molecule as with monomers of polymer molecules.

- **Theta temperature (θ-temperature):** This is a specific temperature at which a specified combination of polymer and solvent form a θ solution.

- **Virtual tube:** A virtual tube defines the constraints on a polymer imposed by entanglements. This can be used to explain the motion (reptation) of polymers in melts and concentrated solutions.

CLASSIFICATION OF POLYMERS

The polymers can be classified as outlined below [Florence and Attwood, 1998, 2011; Angelova and Hunkeler, 1999; Omidian et al., 2011]:

A. Polymer based on backbone structure

- **Polymers with carbon chain backbone:** Polyethylene, polypropylene, polystyrene, poly(vinyl chloride) (PCL), polytetrafluoroethylene (PTFE), polyacrylonitrile, poly(vinyl alcohol), poly(vinyl acetate), polyacrylamide, poly(methyl methacrylate) (PMA), polyvinylpyrrolidone (PVP), etc.

- **Polymers with hetero-chain backbone:** Poly (ethylene oxide) (PEO), poly(propylene oxide) (PPO), cellulose (polyglucoside, $\beta \rightarrow 1,4$), amylose (polyglucoside, $\alpha \rightarrow 1,4$) (component of starch), pectinic acid (polygalacturonoside), polyethylene glycol terephthalate (PEGT), polydimethylsiloxane (PDMS), etc.

B. Natural or synthetic polymer

Natural polymers

- **Protein-based:** Albumin, collagen, gelatin, etc.

- **Polysaccharide-based:** Agarose, alginate, carrageenan, chitosan, cyclodextrins, dextran, hyaluronic acid (HA), polysialic acid (PSA), etc.

Synthetic polymers

Biodegradable

- **Polyesters:** Poly(lactic acid) (PLA), poly (glycolic acid) (PGA), poly(hydroxy butyrate) (PHB), poly(ε-caprolactone) (PCL), poly(β-malic acid) (PMA), poly(dioxanones) (PDA), etc.

- **Polyanhydrides:** Poly(sebacic acid) (PSBA), poly(adipic acid) (PAPA), poly(terphthalic acid) (PTA), etc.

- **Polyamides:** Poly(imino carbonates) (PIC), polyamino acids (PAA), etc.

- **Phosphorous-based:** Polyphosphates, poly-phosphonates, polyphosphazenes, etc.
- **Others:** Poly(cyano acrylates) (PCA), poly-urethanes, polyortho esters, polydihydro-pyrans, poly-acetals, etc.

Non-biodegradable

- **Cellulose derivatives:** Carboxymethyl cellulose (CMC), ethylcellulose (EC), cellulose acetate (CA), cellulose acetate propionate (CAP), hydroxypropyl methyl-cellulose (HPMC), etc.
- **Silicones:** Polydimethylsiloxane (PDS), colloidal silica, etc.
- **Acrylics:** Polymethacrylates (PMA), poly (methyl methacrylate) (PMMA), poly hydro (ethyl-methacrylate) (PHEM), etc.
- **Others:** Polyvinyl pyrrolidone (PVP), ethyl vinyl acetate (EVA), poloxamers, pol-oxamines, etc.

The nomenclature of the polymers is generally based on:

- **Monomer source:** This is the most common method for naming addition polymers, e.g., polyethylene (PE), poly(vinyl chloride) (PVC), poly(methyl methacrylate) (PMMA).
- **Polymer structure:** This is the most common method for condensation polymers, since the polymer typically contains different functional groups than the monomers, e.g., poly(ethylene terphthalate) (Dacron), poly(hexamethylene adipamide) (Nylon 66).
- **Common or trade names:** This is frequently used for many polymers, e.g., Carbopols.
- **IUPAC system:** This identifies repeat unit, starting with highest priority atoms in chain and putting substituents on lowest number positions, e.g., –(OCHFCH$_2$)–, poly[oxy(1-fluoroethylene)].
- **Standardised polymer nomenclature:** There are multiple conventions for naming polymer substances. Many commonly used polymers are referred to by a trivial name. It is assigned based on historical precedent. Both the American Chemical Society (ACS) and IUPAC have proposed standardised naming conventions. In both standardised conventions, the polymers' names are intended to reflect the monomer(s) from which they are synthesised. The differences between the various naming conventions are given below: [http//www.iupac.org; http//acs.org]:

Common Name	ACS Name	IUPAC Name
Poly(ethylene-terephthalate) or (PET)	Poly(oxy-1,2-ethanediyloxy-carbonyl-1,4-phenylenecarbonyl)	Poly(oxy-ethyleneoxy-terephthaloyl)

POLYMER SYNTHESES AND THEIR PROPERTIES

The various ways of synthesis and properties of polymers are as follows [Florence and Attwood, 1998; Omidian et al., 2011]:

Synthesis

Polymerisation is the process of combining many small molecules known as monomers into a covalently bonded chain. During this process, some chemical groups may be lost from each monomer, e.g., in the polymerisation of PET polyester, the monomers are terephthalic acid (HOOC–C$_6$H$_4$–COOH) and ethylene glycol (HO–CH$_2$–CH$_2$–OH) but the repeating unit is –OC–C$_6$H$_4$–COO–CH$_2$–CH$_2$–O–, which corresponds to the combination of the two monomers with the loss of two water molecules.

- **Laboratory synthesis:** Laboratory synthetic methods are generally divided into: Chain growth polymerisation, where monomers are added to the chain one at a time only, whereas in Step-growth polymerisation chains of monomers may combine with one another directly [Sperling, 2006]. However, some newer methods, e.g., plasma polymerisation, do not fit into either category.

  Click chemistry refers to a group of reactions that are fast, simple to use, easy to purify, versatile, regiospecific, and give high product yields. It has found applications in a wide variety of research areas, including materials sciences, polymer chemistry, and pharmaceutical sciences [Hein et al., 2008].

- **Biological synthesis:** There are three main classes of biopolymers: polysaccharides, polypeptides, and polynucleotides. In living cells, they may be synthesised by enzyme-mediated processes, e.g., the formation of DNA catalysed by DNA polymerase. The synthesis of proteins involves multiple enzyme-mediated processes to transcribe genetic information from the DNA to RNA and subsequently translate that information to synthesise the specified protein from amino acids. The protein may be modified further following translation in order to provide appropriate structure and functioning.

- **Modified natural polymers:** Many commercial polymers are synthesised by chemical modification of naturally occurring polymers, e.g., the reaction of nitric acid and cellulose to form nitrocellulose.

Properties

The most basic property of a polymer is the identity of its constituent monomers. Microstructure describes the arrangement of these monomers within the polymer at the scale of a single chain. These basic structural properties play a major role in determining bulk physical properties of the polymer. Chemical properties describe how the chains interact through various physical forces.

Microstructure

The microstructure or configuration of a polymer relates to the physical arrangement of monomer residues along the backbone of the chain [Sperling, 2006]. Structure has a strong influence on the properties of a polymer, e.g., two samples of natural rubber may exhibit different durability, even though their molecules comprise the same monomers.

- **Chain length:** The physical properties of a polymer are strongly dependent on the size or length of the polymer chain, e.g., as chain length is increased, melting and boiling temperatures increase quickly [Rubinstein and Colby, 2003]. Impact resistance also tends to increase with chain length, as does the viscosity, or resistance to flow, of the polymer in its melt state. Increasing chain length furthermore tends to decrease chain mobility, increase strength and toughness, and increase the Tg. This is a result of the increase in chain interactions [McCrum et al., 1997; Painter and Coleman, 1997; Rubinstein and Colby, 2006].

Periodic copolymers have monomer residue types arranged in a repeating sequence. Statistical copolymers have monomer residues arranged according to a known statistical rule. A statistical copolymer in which the probability of finding a particular type of monomer residue at a particular point in the chain is independent of the types of surrounding monomer residue may be referred to as a truly random copolymer [Painter and Coleman, 1997; Sperling, 2006]. Block copolymers have two or more homopolymer subunits linked by covalent bonds [Painter and Coleman, 1997]. Polymers with two or three blocks of two distinct chemical species (e.g., A and B) are called diblock copolymers and triblock copolymers, respectively. Polymers with three blocks, each of a different chemical species (e.g., A, B, and C) are termed triblock terpolymers. Graft or grafted copolymers contain side chains that have a different composition or configuration than the main chain.

- **Architecture:** Branching of polymer chains affects the ability of chains to slide past one another by altering intermolecular forces, in turn, affecting bulk physical polymer properties. The architecture of the polymer is often physically determined by the functionality of the monomers from which it is formed [Campbell et al., 2006]. This property of a monomer is defined as the number of reaction sites at which it may form chemical covalent bonds. Chemical cross-linking is the formation of covalent bonds between chains. Crosslinking tends to increase Tg and increase strength and toughness, e.g., strengthen rubbers by crosslinking with sulphur [Painter and Coleman, 1997].

- **Tacticity:** Tacticity is the relative stereo-chemistry of chiral centres in neighbouring structural units within a macromolecule, which are isotactic (all substituents on the same side), atactic (random placement of substituents), and syndiotactic (alternating placement of substituents).

Morphology

Polymer morphology describes the arrangement of chains in space and microscopic ordering of polymer chains.

- **Chain conformation:** The space occupied by a polymer molecule is Rg, an average distance from the centre of mass of the chain to the chain itself or pervaded volume, a volume of solution spanned by the polymer chain and scales with the cube of the Rg [Rubinstein and Colby, 2003].
- **Crystallinity:** A synthetic polymer may be described as crystalline if it contains regions of three-dimensional (3D) ordering on atomic length scales.
- Synthetic polymers may consist of both crystalline and amorphous regions; the degree of crystallinity may be expressed in terms of a weight fraction or volume fraction of crystalline material [http://www.iupac.org]. Polymers with microcrystalline regions are generally tougher, more flexible and more impact-resistant than totally amorphous polymers. Polymers with a degree of crystallinity approaching zero or one tend to be transparent, while polymers with inter-mediate degrees of crystallinity tend to be opaque due to light scattering by crystalline or glassy regions [Allcock et al., 2003].

Mechanical properties

The bulk properties of a polymer dictate how the polymer actually behaves on a macroscopic scale.

- **Tensile strength:** The tensile strength of a material quantifies how much stress the material will endure before failing [Ashby et al, 1996; Meyers and Chawla, 1999]. This is important in applications that rely upon a polymer's physical strength or durability, e.g., a rubber band with a higher tensile strength will hold a greater weight before snapping.
- **Transport properties:** Transport properties/ e.g., diffusivity, relate to how rapidly molecules move through the polymer matrix. These are important in applications of polymers for films, etc.
- **Young's modulus of elasticity:** Young's modulus quantifies the elasticity of the polymer for small strains, as the ratio of rate of change of stress to strain. Like tensile strength, this is relevant in polymers involving the physical properties, e.g., rubbers. The modulus is dependent on temperature.

Phase behaviour

The different phase behaviour properties of polymers are as follows:

- **Boiling point:** The boiling point of a poly-meric material is strongly dependent on chain length. High polymers with a large degree of polymerisation do not exhibit a boiling point because they decompose before reaching theo-retical boiling temperatures. For oligomers, a boiling transition may be observed and will generally increase rapidly as chain length is increased.
- **Glass transition temperature (T_g):** T_g describes the temperature at which amorphous polymers undergo a second-order phase transition from a rubbery, viscous amorphous solid, or from a crystalline solid to a brittle, glassy amorphous solid. The T_g may be engineered by altering the degree of branching

or by the addition of plasticiser in the polymer [Brandup et al., 1999].

- **Inclusion of plasticisers:** Plasticisers create gaps between polymer chains for greater mobility and reduced inter-chain interactions.
- **Melting point (T_m):** The term melting point to polymers suggests not a solid-liquid phase transition but a transition from a crystalline or semi-crystalline phase to a solid amorphous phase.
- **Mixing behaviour:** Polymeric mixtures are far less miscible than mixtures of small molecule materials, since polymeric molecules are much larger and hence generally have much higher specific volumes than small molecules.

Chemical properties

Different side groups on the polymer can lend the polymer to ionic bonding or hydrogen bonding between its own chains. These stronger forces typically result in higher tensile strength and higher crystalline melting points. The intermolecular forces in polymers can be affected by dipoles in the monomer units. Polymers containing amide or carbonyl groups can form hydrogen bonds between adjacent chains; the partially positively charged hydrogen atoms in N–H groups of one chain are strongly attracted to the partially negatively charged oxygen atoms in C=O groups on another. These strong hydrogen bonds, for example, result in the high tensile strength and melting point of polymers containing urethane or urea linkages.

SELECTION OF POLYMERS

A thorough understanding of the surface and bulk properties of the polymer is required to achieve the desired chemical, interfacial, mechanical and biological functions. The choice of polymer is dependent on the need for biochemical characterisation and specific preclinical tests to prove its safety. Microstructural design and chemical composition can be used to adapt the structure-property relationship and tailor improved polymeric matrices. The manufacturing process also needs to be considered, because the additives used during polymerisation may degrade the drug. Surface properties (e.g., lubricity) govern the biocompatibility with tissues and blood, in addition to influencing physical properties [Angelova and Hunkeler, 1999]. The materials for long-term use must be water-repellent to avoid degradation processes that lead to changes in toughness and loss of mechanical strength. Bioadhesiveness need to be taken into account when DDS are targeted to mucosal tissues, whereas polymers for ocular devices have to be aqueous or lipid-soluble in addition to having good film-forming ability and mechanical stability for good retention [Colthrust et al., 2000]. Structural properties of the matrix, its micromorphology and pore size are important with respect to mass transport (of water) into and (of drug) out of the polymer. For non-biodegradable matrices, drug release in most cases is diffusion-controlled and peptide drugs with low permeability can only be released through the pores and channels created by the dissolved drug phase [Mao et al., 1999]. The various properties that need to be considered for drug delivery applications of polymers are [Florence and Attwood, 1998; Schott, 1998; Pillai and Panchagnula, 2001; Siepman and Peppas, 2001; Omidian et al., 2011]:

- **Adsorption:** The ability of some macro-molecules (e.g., gelation, acacia) to adsorb at interfaces is being exploited in suspension and emulsion stabilisation. The albumin adsorbs (non-specifically) at the glass or plastic surface and presents a more polar surface to the solution, thus reducing adsorption of the protein (e.g., insulin). The adsorption of macromolecules at interfaces, for example, those of hyaluronic acid, can act as biological lubricants in joint fluids [Weidenfield et al., 1968].
- **Bioadhesion:** Adhesion between a biological surface and a surface of a hydrophilic polymer arises from interactions between the polymer chains and the macromolecules on the mucosal

surface. The charge on the molecules is important, and for two anionic polymers maximum interaction occurs when they are not charged. Penetration and association pH must be balanced. The adhesive performance of polymers can be excellent (e.g., carboxymethylcellulose), good (Carbopol), fair (gelatin) or poor (povidone) [Liveson et al., 1994].

- **Crystallinity:** Polymers form perfect crystals only with difficulty because of the low probability of arranging the chains in regular fashion, especially at high MWs. Advantage can be taken of defects in crystals in the preparation of microcrystals. Microcrystalline cellulose, a tablet excipient and a binder-disintegrant, is prepared by disruption of larger crystals. When it is dispersed in water it forms colloidal gels, and it can be used to form heat-stable o/w emulsions.

- **Interaction with solvents:** Polymers interact with solvents in a more complex fashion than do smaller crystalline solutes. A given polymer may have no saturation solubility; it usually either dissolves completely or is only swollen by a given liquid. Swelling decreases as the degree of cross-linking increases. It is a function of the solubility parameter of the liquid phase, and if the polymer is ionic, swelling will be dependent on the ionic strength of the solution. Highly polar polymers like poly(amide), PVC and some cellulose derivatives require polar liquids as solvents, in which dipole interactions or hydrogen bonding between polymer and solvent molecules occur. Linear polysaccharides tend to form spirals in solution but in their tendency to associate they may form double helices. Under certain conditions of concentration and temperature the double helices may associate, forming gels. The firmness or strength of gels produced by such interactions will depend on the degree of interaction of the complex with water and the properties of the bridging units. The ability of carbohydrates and other macro-molecules to imbibe large quantities of water is put to use both mechanically and industrially, for example, in surgical dressings.

- **Complexes:** Polymers provide ample opportunity for the formation of complexes in solution, e.g., when an aqueous solution of high MW polyacids is mixed with polyglycols. The viscosity and pH of the solution of the equimolar mixture of polyacid and glycol remain the same with the increase in oligomer chain length up to a critical point. This occurs only when the PEG molecules have reached a certain size. Such macromolecular reactions are highly selective and strongly dependent on molecular size, conformation, heat, etc. Biological macromolecules undergo complex reactions, which are often vital to their activity. Calcium is coordinated between certain uronic acid-containing and has dietary significance.

- **Dissolution:** Unlike non-polymeric materials, polymers do not dissolve instantaneously, and the dissolution is controlled by either the disentanglement of the polymer chains or by the diffusion of the chains through a boundary layer adjacent to the polymer-solvent interface [Miller-Chou and Koenig, 2003]. Narasimhan [2001] focused on the modelling efforts to understand the physics of the drug release process from dissolving polymers, which can be classified into two broad approaches – phenomenological models and Fickian equations, and anomalous transport models and scaling law-based approaches.

- **Erosion and biodegradation:** Degradation is a chemical process, whereas erosion is a physical phenomenon dependent on dissolution and diffusion processes. Depending on the chemical structure of the polymer backbone, erosion can occur by either surface or bulk erosion. Surface erosion occurs when the rate of erosion exceeds the rate of water permeation into the bulk of the polymer and is desirable because the kinetics of erosion and rate of drug release (zero order) are highly reproducible. Bulk erosion occurs when water molecules permeate into the bulk of the matrix at a faster rate than erosion, thus exhibiting complex degradation/erosion kinetics. The erosion process can be manipulated by modifying the surface area of the DDS or by including hydrophobic monomer units in the polymer [Uhrich et al., 1999].

Most polymeric implants are biodegraded by chemical degradation mechanisms: hydrolysis, and oxidation. Hydrolytic biodegradations are often accompanied by substantial decrease of pH whilst oxidative biodegradation processes are usually very slow due to consumption of stoichiometric amounts of oxidising agents. A dramatic acceleration of the biodegradation can be expected, if the biodegradation can be initiated by catalytic amounts of oxidation agents. Poly (ethylene carbonate) is biodegraded by such catalytic oxidation processes and shows all the characteristics of surface erosion [Kost et al., 1985].

The biodegradability can be manipulated by incorporating a variety of labile groups e.g., ester, orthoester, anhydride, carbonate, amide, urea and urethane in their backbone [Langer, 2000; Mao et al., 1999]. Biodegradation can be of enzymatic, chemical or microbial origin. These may operate either separately or simultaneously and are often influenced by many other factors like adsorbed and absorbed compounds (water, lipids, ions, etc.); annealing and storage history; chemical structure and composition; configuration structure; distribution of repeat units in multimers; mechanism of degradation (enzymatic, hydrolysis, microbial, etc.); MW distribution; morphology (amorphous, semicrystalline, crystalline, microstructure, residual stress, etc.); physical factors (shape, size, chain defects, etc.); physicochemical factors (ion-exchange, ionic strength, pH, etc.); presence of low MW compounds; presence of unexpected units or chain defects; processing conditions and sterilisation

process; route of administration and site of action; and sterilisation process and storage history and shape and site of implantation [Pillai and Panchagnula, 2001; Peppas, 1997].

Polymer degradation is a change in the properties like tensile strength, colour, shape, etc. of a polymer or polymer-based product under the influence of one or more environmental factors, e.g., heat, light, chemicals and, in some cases, galvanic action. These changes may be undesirable, e.g., changes during use; or desirable, as in biodegradation, or deliberately lowering the molecular mass of a polymer. Such changes occur primarily because of the effect of these factors on the chemical composition of the polymer.

- **Solubility:** Water-soluble polymers interact with water to provide sufficient energy to remove individual polymer chains from the solid state, thus increase the viscosity of solvents at low concentrations, swell or change shape in solution, and adsorb at surfaces. On the other hand, partially soluble polymers are used to form thin films, as film-coating materials, surgical dressings, membranes for dialysis or filtration, or matrices for enveloping drugs to control their release properties, or simply as packaging materials.

- **Syneresis:** The separation of liquid from a swollen gel is known as syneresis, a form of instability in aqueous and non-aqueous gels. Separation of a solvent phase is thought to occur because of the elastic contraction of the polymeric molecules. In the swelling process during gel formation the macromolecules involved become stretched and the elastic forces increase as swelling proceeds.

- **Viscosity:** The presence in solution of large macromolecular solutes may have an appreciable effect on the viscosity of the solution. From a study of the concentration dependence of the viscosity it is possible to gain information on the shape or hydration of these polymers in solution and also their average MW. The shape of molecules is, to a large extent, the determinant of flow properties. The change in shape due to changes in polymer-solvent interactions and the binding of small molecules with the polymer may lead to significant changes in solution viscosity. The nature of the solvent is thus of prime importance in this regard. Concentrated polymer solutions frequently exhibit a very high viscosity because of the interaction of polymer chains in a three-dimensional fashion in the bulk solvent. Conventional eye medication has been modified over the years through the addition to formulations of a variety of viscosity-enhancing agents, polymers, e.g., HPMC, PVA and silicones.

CHARACTERISATION OF POLYMERS

The polymers are characterised by some of the following techniques [www.studsvik.uu.se; Schott, 1993]:

- **Confocal laser scanning microscopy:** Confocal laser scanning microscopy (CLSM) methods have been developed to exploit the imaging capabilities to study a wide range of pharmaceutical systems, e.g., phase-separated polymers, colloidal systems; to measure diffusion in gels; physical interaction of dosage forms with biological barriers, e.g., the eye, skin and intestinal epithelia, etc. [Pygall et al., 2007].

- **Differential scanning calorimetry:** The differential scanning calorimeter (DSC) makes calorimetric measurements of heat capacity and energies of phase transitions. For polymers, a glass transition can be observed as a discontinuity in the heat capacity. The degree of crystallinity of semi-crystalline polymers can be determined from the heat of melting. Melting temperatures can easily be measured and these are often found to depend on heating rates.

- **Gel permeation chromatography:** Gel permeation chromatography (GPC) involves passing a solution of polymer through a column with porous packing. The small molecules are retained longer on the column and are eluted and detected after the large molecules, a technique for determination of the MW and polydispersity (Pd) of a polymer sample alongside other parameters. The polymers can be detected as they are eluted, by measuring changes in the refractive index, infrared absorption, viscosity or light scattering detectors connected to/directed to the output stream and give a direct measure of the absolute molecular mass.

- **Light scattering:** This is an experimental method to determine the size and/or mobility of polymers. It can be divided into two different techniques: static light scattering in which the angular distribution of scattered intensity is measured to determine the size of scattering objects, and dynamic light scattering in which a correlation function of scattered photons is measured and is often used to determine mobility and to deduce a hydro-dynamic size.

- **Other techniques:** The techniques such as wide angle X-ray scattering, small angle X-ray scattering and small angle neutron scattering are used to determine the crystalline structure of polymers. FTIR, Raman and NMR can be used to determine composition. Pyrolysis followed by analysis of the fragments is another technique for determining the possible structure of the polymer. Thermo-gravimetry (TG) is a useful technique to evaluate the thermal stability of the polymer, which allows us to know about the phase segregation in polymers. Rheological properties are also commonly used to help determine molecular architecture as well as to understand how the polymer will process, through measurements of the polymer in the melt phase.

Automatic Continuous Online Monitoring of Polymerisation Reactions (ACOMP) provides real-time characterisation of polymerisation reactions. It can be used as an analytical method in research and development (R&D), as a tool for reaction optimisation at the bench and pilot plant level and, eventually, for feedback control of full-scale reactors. ACOMP measures in a model-independent fashion the evolution of average molar mass and intrinsic viscosity, monomer conversion kinetics and, in the case of copolymers, also the average composition drift and distribution. It is applicable in the areas of, e.g., free radical and controlled radical homo- and copolymerisation, polyelectrolyte synthesis, heterogeneous phase reactions [US patent 6052184 and 6653750; Florenzano et al., 1998; Alb et al., 2008].

The polymers are generally characterised for following parameters:

- **Flory-Huggins parameter:** This describes the energy of interaction of a polymer segment with other polymers or with solvent molecules. The energy is normally expressed in units of kBT where T is the absolute temperature and kB is Boltzmann constant. A negative value indicates favourable interactions and a positive value indicates an unfavourable interaction.

- **Glass transition temperature:** This is the temperature at which an amorphous polymer changes from a solid to a liquid state. Above this temperature, large scale diffusive motion of the polymer molecules becomes possible.

- **Hydrodynamic radius:** This is the radius of a particle or polymer molecule in solution that is determined from a measurement of mobility or diffusion, e.g., viscosity or dynamic light scattering experiments.

- **Isoelectric point:** The ionisation of many biopolymers depends on the pH of the solvent. Different functional groups will dissociate at different pH. If there are mixtures of acidic and basic groups there will be a pH at which there will be an average charge of zero called isoelectric point.

- **Molecular mass:** The molecular mass of a polymer is defined as the mass in grams of a

mole of molecules. Most synthetic polymers will have a distribution of molecular mass and it is often important to characterise this. It is common to distinguish various different averages of the molecular mass, e.g., the number average molecular mass (M_n), the weight average molecular mass (M_w), mass of the peak (M_p), mass of higher species (M_z), etc. This is determined by chemical analysis, osmotic pressure, viscosity, and refractive index or light scattering measurements or by combination of some of them. The universal tri-detection system is based on determination of M_w based on combination of viscosity, refractive index and light scattering data.

- **Monodispersity:** A monodisperse sample consists of polymer molecules having identical size or mass ($M_w/M_n = 1$). Monodisperse polymers are difficult to achieve by chemical synthesis except in nature. Some materials, e.g., DNA can be made with perfect uniformity.

- **Number average molecular mass (M_n):** The distribution of polymer sizes in most synthetic materials implies that different averages will give different values. The number average is defined as the sum of n_iM_i divided by the sum of n_i where n_i is the number of molecules in the distribution with mass M_i. The number average molecular mass is the quantity measured by determination of colligative properties, e.g., osmotic pressure: $M_n = \Sigma n_iM_i/\Sigma n$.

- **Persistence length:** The persistence length is a measure of the 'stiffness' of a polymer molecule. It describes the length scale for which the chain can be thought to be rigid.

- **Polydispersity:** The distribution of molecular mass of polymers is described as the polydispersity. The details of the shape of the distribution will depend on the preparation and any fractionation. A simple measure of the distribution is often quoted as M_w/M_n.

- **Radius of gyration (R_g):** This is a measure of the size of a polymer molecule and can be defined in terms of the distribution of distances of each monomer in the molecule from the centre of gravity of the molecule: $R_g^2 = \Sigma_i r_i^2$. It can be shown that a freely jointed chain of N links of length 'a' has the following formula, R_g: $R_g^2 = N a^2/6$.

- **Strain birefringence:** When a material is aligned by means of deformation, there may be induced birefringence. This phenomenon can be a tool to measure the molecular orientation in polymers.

- **Tacticity:** Tacticity describes the stereochemistry of a polymer with substituent groups on each monomer. As the polymer backbone or chain is long, a carbon atom in the chain with two different substituent groups X and Y will have a stereochemical centre. The relative orientation of the groups on successive monomers is described by the tacticity.

- **Weight average molecular weight (M_w):** The distribution of polymer sizes in most synthetic materials implies that different averages will give different values. M_w is defined as the sum of $n_i M_i^2$ divided by the sum of $n_i M_i$ where n_i is the number of molecules in the distribution with mass M_i. M_w is the quantity measured in an elastic light scattering experiment, which is biased towards larger molecules. M_w will always be bigger than M_n ($M_w > M_n$), $M_w = \Sigma n_i M_i^2 / \Sigma n_i M_i$.

- **Z-average molecular weight (M_z):** The distribution of polymer sizes in most synthetic materials implies that different averages will give different values. The *Z-average* is defined as the sum of $n_i M_i^3$ divided by the sum of $n_i M_i^2$ where n_i is the number of molecules in the distribution with mass M_i. This quantity can be compared with other averages of the molecular mass, e.g., M_w and M_n, $M_z = \Sigma n_i M_i^3 / \Sigma n_i M_i^2$.

BIOMATERIALS

Different types of biomaterials/polymers synthesised to deliver drugs, macromolecules, cells and enzymes are described below:

Polyesters

Polyester-based polymers are widely investigated for drug delivery. PLA, PGA and their copolymers PLGA are some of the well-defined biomaterials with regard to design and performance for drug-delivery applications [Li and Vert, 1999]. It is possible to modify the mechanical, thermal and biological properties of PLA by altering its stereochemistry. Further, biodegradability can be tuned by changing the proportion of PLA and PGA in the copolymer. Although PLGA represents the gold standard of biodegradable polymers, increased local acidity because of degradation can lead to irritation at the site of polymer application [Uhrich, 1999]. The increased local acidity may also be detrimental to the stability of protein drugs [Fu et al., 2000]. The physical presence of these polymers in the biological environment must be transient, and their physicochemical properties are expected to meet the in-use requirements and allow their transport or clearance from the application site when the intended efficacy is achieved. The transport or clearance of these polymers while in contact with tissues is termed bioabsorption [Shalabv et al., 1994].

- **Polyglycolic acid:** These are totally synthetic absorbable polymers. The PLGA suture was introduced in 1970. The advantages of these synthetic materials are control over uniformity and mechanical properties. Histological response to synthetic polymer is generally predictable whereas reaction to non-synthetic materials (catgut) is variable and may produce a more intense inflammatory reaction.

- **Polylactic acid:** Polylactide is prepared from the cyclic diester of lactic acid by ring opening polymerisation. Lactic acid (LA) exists as two optical isomers or enantiomers. The L-enantiomer occurs in nature, and a D,L racemic mixture results from the synthetic preparation of lactic acid. Fibres spun from 'L' polylactide (mp 170°C) have high crystallinity when drawn, whereas fibres spun from poly DL-lactide are amorphous. The rate of poly-L-lactide degradation has been increased by plasticisation with triethyl citrate, but this produced a less crystalline, more flexible material. Time required for poly-L-lactide implants to be absorbed is relatively long and depends on polymer quality, processing conditions, implant site, and physical dimensions of the implant. High MW polymer of PLA can be prepared and fibre samples with large tensile strength are available, by hot-drawing filaments spun from solution. Exposure of PLA to gamma radiation has been shown to result in a decrease in MW. Unlike PLA (absorbed slowly), PGA is absorbed within a few months post-implantation due to greater hydrolytic susceptibility. *In vitro* experiments have shown an effect on degradation by enzymes, buffer, pH, annealing treatments, and gamma irradiation. Since PGA is susceptible to degradation from moisture and gamma rays, low humidity ethylene oxide gas sterilisation procedures and moisture-proof packaging are recommended.

- **Polydioxanone:** Fibres made from polymers containing a high percentage of PGA are too stiff for monofilament suture and thus are available only in braided form above the micro-suture size range. In polydioxanone (PDS, Ethicon) the monomer p-dioxanone is analogous to glycolide but yields a poly-(ether-ester). Polydioxanone monofilament fibres retained tensile strength longer than the braided PGA and were absorbed in about six months with minimal tissue response. Polydioxanone degradation *in vitro* was affected by gamma irradiation dosage but not substantially by the presence of enzymes.

- **Polycaprolactone:** PCL is synthesised from ε-caprolactone. This semi-crystalline polymer absorbed very slowly *in vivo* and released ε-hydroxycaproic acid as the sole metabolite. Fragments are scavenged by macrophages and giant cells. Amorphous regions of the polymer are degraded prior to breakdown of the crystalline regions. Copolymers of ε-caprolactone and L-lactide are elastomeric when prepared from 25% ε-caprolactone, 75% L-lactide and rigid when prepared from 10% ε-caprolactone, 90% L-lactide.

- **Polyhydroxybutyrate:** Poly-α-hydroxybutyrate is a biodegradable polymer that both occurs in nature and can easily be synthesised *in vitro*. Synthetic PHB, however, has not shown the stereo-regularity found in the natural product. High MW, crystalline, and optically active PHB has been extracted from bacteria. This polymer is melt processable and has been proposed for use as absorbable suture. Copolymers of hydroxybutyrate and hydroxyvalerate (Biopol) have been developed to provide a wide variety of mechanical properties and more rapid degradation than can be achieved with pure PHB.

- **Other polyesters:** Synthetic absorbable polyesters suffer from loss of mechanical properties upon sterilisation with gamma irradiation. Yet poly(ethylene terphthalate), Dacron®, is a polyester that is resistant to gamma radiation induced degradation. Thus polyester analogous to Dacron containing glycolate ester linkages was synthesised as a gamma radiation resistant absorbable polymer. A similar copolymer has been prepared using dioxanone instead of glycolide to improve the gamma radiation stability of polydioxanone [Heller and Gurny, 1999]. A number of applications have been found for polyorthoesters and crosslinked polyorthoestes, e.g., delivery of 5-fluorouracil, periodontal delivery systems of tetracycline and pH-sensitive polymer systems for insulin delivery [Andrianov and Payne, 1998]. By varying the monomer ratio of aliphatic (sebacic acid) and aromatic (carboxyphenoxypropane) polyanhydrides, polymer-carmustine disks were fabricated for chemotherapy of brain cancer, which was the first US Food and Drug Administration (FDA)-approved polymer-based chemotherapy DDS [Langer, 2000].

Polymers

- **Poly(amino acids):** The use of amino acids as building blocks for synthetic absorbable polymers would seem logical. But synthesis and processing of such materials present difficulties. Attachment of methotrexate to poly-L-lysine enhanced transport into the cells where the drug was released due to degradation of the poly(amino acid) moiety by lysosomal enzymes. Enzymatically degradable synthetic peptides have also been used to form crosslinks in drug releasing synthetic hydrogels. Poly-amino acids that have good biocompatibility have been investigated for the delivery of low-MW compounds. However, their use is limited by their antigenic potentials and poor control of release because of the dependence on enzymes for biodegradation. Poly(imino carbonates), which are 'pseudo' polyamino acids, have been synthesised from tyrosine dipeptide to overcome the above-mentioned limitations [Uhrich, 1999].

Phosphorous-based polymers

- **Polyphosphazenes:** A class of biodegradable polymers belonging to polyphosphoesters has a unique backbone consisting of phosphorous atoms attached to either carbon or oxygen. The uniqueness of this class of polymer lies in the chemical reactivity of phosphorus, which enables a wide range of side chains to be attached for manipulating the biodegradation rates and the MW of the polymer [Mao et al., 1999; Gopferich, 1999].

Polysaccharides-based polymers

- **Cyclodextrins:** These are potential high-performance carrier materials that have the ability to alter physical, chemical and biological properties of guest (drug) molecules through the formation of inclusion complexes both in solution and solid state [Uekama, 1999]. The α, β and γ-cyclodextrins are the most common natural cyclodextrins consisting of six, seven and eight D-glucopyranose residues, respectively, linked by α-1,4 glycosidic bonds into a macrocycle. The cyclodextrins include hydrophilic, hydrophobic and ionic derivatives to expand the physicochemical properties and inclusion capability of natural cyclodextrin as novel drug carriers [Szente, 1999].

- **Chitosans:** These are promising natural polymers that show good absorption-enhancing, controlled-release as well as bioadhesive properties. The degree of deacetylation and derivatisation with various side chains can be a source of manipulation for specific drug-delivery applications [Dodane and Vilivalam, 1998].

- **Polysialic acid:** Molecules or materials that are inconspicuous to the innate and adaptive immune systems of the body have the best chance of surviving for long periods in the circulation. Among the hundreds of bacterial polysaccharides that exist, polysialic acid (PSA) is truly unique in being non-immunogenic. This is because PSA is also a human polymer, found in the body attached to certain cell-adhesion molecules, where it plays an anti-adhesive function. Unlike many other carbohydrate oligomers and polymers, there are no known natural receptors for PSA, which in biological terms is a fundamentally inert substance. PSAs, as nature's ultimate stealth technology, are polymers of repeating N-acetyl neuraminic acid (Neu5Ac, sialic acid), a sugar abundantly present on the surface of cells and many proteins. PSAs are highly hydrophilic and highly hydrated, which is essential in order to maintain systemic injectability. Moreover, they can be easily produced in large quantities from bacterial cultures using a non-pathogenic, adapted strain of *Escherichia coli* K1. Neuraminidases are responsible for the breakdown of PSA to non-toxic excretable products (i.e., Neu5Ac) of which intracellular (lysosomal) neuraminidases are particularly active upon (α 2-8)-linked PSAs [Jain et al., 2004; Gregoriadis et al., 2005].

Silicone-based polymers

- **Polysiloxanes:** These are non-deformable polymers possessing good low-temperature flexibility, excellent electrical properties, water repellency and remarkable bio-compatibility, features that are not common with hydrocarbon polymers [Kumar and Kumar, 2001]. Because of ease of fabrication and high permeability, polydimethyl siloxanes (PDMSs) are useful for water-soluble drugs and steroids for long-acting DDS, e.g., sub-dermal implants [Bodmeir and Siepmann, 1999]. Many silicones are hydrophobic liquid polymers, although high MW silicones exist as waxes and resins. Silicones are polymers with a structure containing alternate atoms of silicon and oxygen. The dimethicones are fluid polymers with the general formula $CH_3[Si(CH_3)_2]_nSi(CH_3)_3$ in which each unit has two methyl groups and an oxygen atom attached to the silicon atom in the chain. The viscosity range extends from 0.65 cS to 3×10^6 cS. The dimethicones 20, 200, 350 and 1000 have rheological properties that allow them to be used in ophthalmology and in rheumatoid arthritis. More common uses are as barrier substances, silicone lotions and creams acting as water-repellent applications protecting the skin against water-soluble irritants. Methylphenyl-silicone is used as a lubricant for hypodermic syringes. Glassware, which has been treated with a thin film of silicone, is rendered hydrophobic; solutions and aqueous suspensions thus drain completely from such vessels. Activated dimethicone is a mixture of liquid dimethicones containing finely divided silica to enhance the defoaming properties of the silicone. By varying the amounts of polymer in resin a variety of products can be formed, including catheters, tubing materials for reconstructive surgery and as membranes for drug reservoirs. The release of lipophilic steroids from silicone elastomer matrices is dependent partly on the crosslinking density of the polymer and the content of filler, and also on the lipophilicity of the drug. Pressure-sensitive silicone adhesives are formed from the most highly crosslinked systems.

Others polymers

- **Polyethylene oxide (PEO) and polyoxy-propylene (POP):** These copolymers are used for nanoparticulate drug delivery systems, commercially available as Polaxmers in a range of liquids, pastes and solids. Since the 1950s, they have found a wide range of applications in the pharmaceutical and bio-medical fields [Moghimi and Hunter, 2000]. Soluble block copolymers based on PEO–PLA can self-assemble into novel supramolecular structures and are being investigated for delivery of anti-cancer agents, proteins and plasmid DNA [Kuon and Okano, 1999]. They are advantageous in terms of drug targeting and safety, and they can mimic biological transport systems, lipoproteins or viruses.

- **Polyoxyethylene glycols (Macrogols):** The polyoxyethylene glycols (PEGs) are liquid over the MW range 200–700. The liquid members and semisolid members of the series are hygroscopic. Macrogol 200 has a hygroscopicity 70% that of glycerol but this decreases with MW. The comparable value for Macrogol 1540 is only 30%. They are used as solvents for drugs, e.g., hydrocortisone. The Macrogols are incompatible with phenols and can reduce the antimicrobial activity of other preservatives. Higher MW PEGs are more effective on a molecular basis as complexing agents. The semisolid and waxy members of the series may be used as suppository bases.

- **Lectins:** These are molecules of plant or microbial origin, as well as biotechnologically generated derivatives. They have interesting characteristics to control the binding, uptake and intracellular routing of macromolecules as well as colloidal carrier systems [Lehr, 2000]. In contrast to other mucoadhesive polymers, lectin binds directly to epithelial cells rather than to the mucus gel layer.

- **Polyvinylpyrrolidone:** Polyvinylpyrrolidone (PVP) is used as a suspending and dispersing agent, a tablet binding and granulating agent, and a vehicle for drugs, e.g., penicillin, cortisone, etc., to delay their absorption and prolong their action. It forms hard films, which are utilised in film-coating processes. It is available in a range of grades designated by numbers ranging from K15 to K90. The K values represent a function of the mean MW. Viscosity is essentially independent of pH over the range 0-10 and aqueous solutions exhibit a high tolerance for many inorganic salts. Its wide solubility in organic solvents is unusual. PVP forms molecular adducts with many substances. Insoluble complexes are formed when aqueous solutions of PVP are added to tannic acid, poly(acrylic acid) and methyl vinyl ether-maleic anhydride copolymer. Soluble complexes, called iodophors, are formed with iodine. The iodophor retains the germicidal properties of iodine.
- **Smart polymers:** The concept of smart polymers originated from the ability of certain synthetic polymers (hydrogels) to mimic the non-linear response of biopolymers (DNA, proteins, etc.) caused by cooperative interactions between monomers [Galaew and Mathiasson, 1999]. Because of their excellent water-absorbing capacity, hydrogels resemble natural living tissues more closely than any other class of synthetic polymeric materials [Lawman and Peppas, 1997]. Both the swelling and permeability characteristics of hydrogels and their ability to undergo structural changes in response to a variety of physical, chemical and biological stimuli have given rise to the concept of intelligent or stimuli-responsive DDSs [Kost and Langer, 1991]. They are based on chemical (formation of charge-transfer complex causes swelling and release of drug), electrical (change in charge distribution causes swelling and drug release), enzyme substrate (product of enzymatic conversion causes swelling and

release of drug), ionic strength (change in concentration of ions inside the gel causes swelling and release of drug), magnetic (applied magnetic field causes pore in gel and swelling followed by drug release), pH (pH change causes swelling and release of drug), thermal (change in polymer–polymer and polymer–water interactions cause swelling and drug release), and ultrasound (temperature increase causes release of drug irradiation) [Pillai and Panchagnula, 2001; Siepman and Peppas, 2001].

A hydrogel of polyacrylamide semi-interpenetrating networks can respond to antigen, which could find potential application for delivery of drugs in response to a specific antigen and has far-reaching implications in treatment of variety of immunological-based diseases [Miyoto et al., 1999]. Hydrogel systems responsive to microbial infection have been designed based on proteinase specific to a bacteria as a triggering mechanism for release of antibiotics, and have found application in the localised delivery of antibiotics for wound healing [Tanihara et al., 1999]. This can overcome the renal and liver toxicity problems associated with prolonged use of antibiotics, in addition to reducing the possibility of emergence of drug resistance. Interplay of 'innovative' chemistry of coating responsive hydrogel microspheres with lipid bilayer resulted in emulating the physiological secretory granules that can release the stored drugs on application of an electroporation pulse, which then allows the fusion of the hydrogel with the lipid bilayer, releasing the drug by an ion-exchange mechanism [Kiser et al., 1998].

- **Water-insoluble polymers and polymer membranes:** Crystallinity defines several features like rigidity, fluidity, the resistance to diffusion of small molecules in the polymer and solubility. In hydrogels, T_g is a measure of polymer structure, crosslinking density, solvent content and polymer-solvent interactions. The presence of flexible groups in main chain, flexible side chains, plasticiser content reduces the T_g, whereas bulky, inflexible side chains increase in main chain polarity and increase in crosslinking increases T_g of the polymer [Peppas and Khare, 1993; Florence and Attwood, 1998].

Hydrophobic polymers are used as membranes, containers or tubing material and hence their surfaces may come into contact with solutions. The interaction of drugs and preservatives with plastics depends on the structure of the polymer and on the affinity of the compound for the plastic.

Transdermal applications

Control of the rate of release of a drug when administered by oral or parenteral routes is aided by the use of polymers that function as a barrier to drug movement [Florence and Attwood, 1998; Omidian et al., 2011].

Several transdermal systems dependent ostensibly on rate-controlling membranes are available for the delivery of nitroglycerin, scopolamine, oestradiol, fentanyl, clonidine and other drugs.

FABRICATION TECHNOLOGY FOR POLYMERS

Some polymers (e.g., thermoplastic resins) are fabricated in the molten state by extrusion into films or fibres and by molding into 3D objects.

- **Extrusion:** A single-screw extruder consists of a screw, driven by a motor connected to its shaft through a gear reducer, rotating inside a cylindrical barrel. The rotating screw moves the resin pellets forward and generates by shear most of the heat required to melt the pellets, as well as the hydrostatic pressure to force the molten plastic through the die.

    Microcrystalline cellulose (MCC) is widely used to manufacture spherical particles (pellets) via extrusion-spheronisation since wetted microcrystalline cellulose has the proper rheological properties, cohesiveness and plasticity to yield strong and spherical particles. However, MCC is not universally applicable due to prolonged drug release of poorly soluble drugs, chemical incompatibility with specific drugs, drug adsorption onto MCC fibers, etc. Hence, several products have been evaluated to explore their application as extrusion-spheronisation aid, aiming to avoid the disadvantages of MCC and to provide a broad application platform for extrusion-spheronisation: powdered cellulose, starch, chitosan, kappa-carrageenan, pectinic acid, hydroxypropylmethyl cellulose, hydroxyethyl cellulose, polyethylene oxide, cross-linked polyvinylpyrrolidone, glycerol monostearate. To determine the true potential of the proposed alternatives for MCC, Dukic-Ott et al., (2009) critically discussed the properties of the different materials and the quality of the resulting pellets in relation to the properties required for an ideal extrusion-spheronisation aid.

- **Molding:** Injection molding is widely used. In this process, the thermoplastic resin, in the form of pellets, is heated, melted, and pushed into die cavity, which is filled with melt. The molten plastic cools and solidifies in the mold while under pressure. Finally, the mold is opened and the part is ejected. Molds may have several cavities for the simultaneous molding of several parts, or a single cavity [Schott, 1993].

- **Nano-emulsion templates:** The active principles and drugs encapsulated in nanoparticles can potentially be affected by nano-emulsion formulation processes. Such potential differences may include drug sensitivity to temperature, high-shear devices, or even contact with organic solvents. Likewise, nano-emulsion formulation processes must be chosen in function of the selected therapeutic goals of the nano-carrier suspension and its administration route. This requires the nanoparticle formulation processes to be more adapted to the nature of the encapsulated drugs, as well as to the chosen route of administration [Anton et al., 2008].

PHARMACEUTICAL APPLICATIONS

Salient applications of polymers are highlighted below:

- **Acrylic acid polymers for drug delivery applications:** Carbopol® polymers are polymers of acrylic acid cross-linked with polyalkenyl ethers or divinyl glycol. They are produced from primary polymer particles of about 0.2 to 6 μm average diameter. Carbopol polymers, along with Pemulen® and Noveon® polymers are all cross-linked. They swell in water up to 1000 times their original volume to form a gel when exposed to a pH environment above 4.0 to 6.0. Because the pKa of these polymers is 6.0 to 6.5, the carboxylate groups on the polymer backbone ionise, resulting in repulsion between the negative charges, which adds to the swelling of the polymer. The T_g temperature of Carbopol polymers is 105°C in powder form and it decreases significantly as the polymer comes into contact with water. The polymer chains start gyrating, and the R_g becomes increasingly larger [Guo, 1994].

- **Alginate DDS:** Alginates are natural polymers, widely used in the food industry because of their biocompatible, biodegradable character, non-toxicity and easy availability. The bioadhesive character of these polymers makes them useful in the pharmaceutical industry in the areas of DDS and these systems can be formulated as gels, matrices, membranes, nanospheres, microspheres, etc. [Jain and Bar-Shalom, 2014].

- **Biodegradable polymers and their potential use in parenteral veterinary DDS:** The most common formulation for biodegradable materials is microparticles, which have been used in oral delivery systems and, even more often, in subcutaneously injected delivery systems. Given appropriate fabrication methods, microparticles of PLGA can be prepared in a fairly uniform manner to provide essentially nonporous microspheres [Lawman and Peppas, 1991, 1997; Peppas et al., 2000; Peppas and Robinson, 1995; Winzenburg, 2004].

- **Biopolymeric wound healing systems:** When designing a wound healing system or dressing, it is pivotal that key factors e.g., optimal gaseous exchange, a moist wound environment, prevention of microbial activity and absorption of exudates are considered. Combining biopolymers that are crucial for wound healing may provide opportunities to synthesise matrices that are inductive to cells and that stimulate and trigger target cell responses crucial to the wound healing process [Mayet et al., 2014].

- **Bioresponsive polymer-based nucleic acid carriers:** Nucleic acid carriers need to possess multi-functionality for overcoming biological barriers, e.g., the stable encapsulation of nucleic acids in extracellular milieu, internalisation by target cells, controlled intracellular distribution, and release of nucleic acids at the target site of action. Bio-responsive polymers that can alter their structure responding to site-specific biological signals are highly useful. pH, redox potential, and enzymatic activities vary along with micro-environments in the body, the responsiveness to these signals enables to construct nucleic acid carriers with programmed functionalities [Takemoto et al., 2014]. Along with non-covalently formed polyplexes, the development of covalent polymer-oligonucleotide conjugates with bio-responsive linkers is also promising as nucleic acid therapeutics [Yu and Wagner, 2009].

- **Cancer immunotherapy:** Immunotherapy is a promising option for cancer treatment. The optimal engineering of nano-carriers based on the unique features of the tumour micro-environment and extra-/intracellular conditions of tumour cells can greatly tip the triangle immunobalance among host, tumour and nano-particulates in favour of anti-tumour responses [Li et al., 2014].

- **Cellulose nano-crystals in tissue engineering strategies:** Cellulose nano-crystals (CNCs) are rod-shaped nano-crystals that can be produced from a variety of highly available and renewable cellulose-rich sources. CNCs are endowed with exceptional physicochemical properties. Because of their low toxicity and eco-toxicological risk, CNC-based functional biomaterials have potential for tissue engineering (TE) applications, focusing on nano-composites obtained through different processing technologies usually employed in the fabrication of TE scaffolds into various formats, e.g., dense films and membranes, hierarchical 3D porous constructs (e.g., micro/nanofiber mats), and hydrogels [Dòmingues et al., 2014].

- **Chitin and chitosan derivatives in the pharmaceutical field:** Chitosan, a natural polymer, has received extensive attention in DDS due to its valued physicochemical and biological properties. Chitin and chitosan derivatives are used as excipients and drug carriers in the pharmaceutical field. Chitosan tablet can exhibit a sustained drug release compared to commercial products. Films prepared using chitin or chitosan have been developed as wound dressings, oral muco-adhesive and water-resisting adhesive by virtue of their release characteristics and adhesion. Intra-tumoural administration of gadopentetic acid-chitosan complex nano-particles has been more effective for gadolinium neutron-capture therapy compared with a group treated with the solution. *N*-succinyl-chitosan (Suc-Chi) has been studied for cancer chemotherapy as a drug carrier and the conjugates of mitomycin-C with Suc-Chi exhibited good anti-tumour activities against various tumours. Furthermore, trimethyl-chitosan and mono-carboxymethyl-chitosan

have been shown to be effective as intestinal absorption enhancers due to their physio-logical properties. Chitosan-thioglycolic acid conjugates have been found to be a promising candidate as scaffold material in tissue engineering due to their physicochemical properties. The application of chitin and chitosan derivatives for hospital preparations and drug carriers has been successful [Yoshinari et al., 1998; Mourya and Inamdar, 2009].

Hydrophobic moiety-conjugated glycol chitosan can form amphiphilic self-assembled glycol chitosan nanoparticles (GCNPs) and simultaneously encapsulate hydrophobic drug molecules inside their hydrophobic core as well as exhibit excellent tumour-homing efficacy, results in improved therapeutic efficiency [Lee et al., 2014]. Chitin systems (CS) are recognised and degraded by the vertebrate immune system [Koch et al., 2015]. The unique properties of CS like its capability to interact with various epithelia and its mucoadhesion potential are interesting. The mild preparation conditions of CS nano-systems offer the opportunities to load stress sensitive hydrophilic macromolecules, e.g., proteins and genetic materials. Moreover, CS are able to protect their cargo from the environ-ment (e.g., pH, enzymes). Chitosan originated nano-carriers have been prepared by mini-emulsion, chemical or ionic gelation, coacervation/precipitation, and spray-drying methods [Yang et al., 2014].

- **Collagen – biomaterial for drug delivery:** The most successful applications of collagen are shields in ophthalmology, injectable dispersions for local tumour treatment, sponges carrying antibiotics and mini-pellets loaded with protein drugs. The need is to control drug release in a sense that by tailoring the polymer, desired properties, e.g., degradation mechanism and rate, surface characteristics for cellular attachment or structural response to biological factors like glucose levels, can be adapted and custom-made. Due to interactions with cells and proteins like metalloproteases as well as the natural appearance in tissue, collagen materials are used in wound repair. In drug delivery, not only is the physiological response of the body relevant but the release mechanism is also of importance. In most cases, collagen systems are used for local drug delivery. Gels can be prepared as injectable systems loaded with drug. Dense monolithic systems can be prepared in order to further sustain drug release via diffusion as compared to collagen gels and to use collagenolytic matrix degradation as a control tool. Furthermore, porous systems are typically used with collagen, e.g., in wound healing and as haemostat. Apart from small molecule drug delivery, a newly developed system, which combines a collagen sponge with a differentiation factor, is developed. This combination provides sustained local delivery and allows cells to penetrate into the pores of the matrix, to differentiate and to form new bone [Schlapp and Friess, 2003].

- **Collagen and gelatin-based systems:** Collagen and gelatin and their hydrolysis peptides have been widely used in the food, pharmaceutical, and cosmetic industries due to their excellent biocompatibility, easy biodegradability, and weak antigenicity. In addition to their established nutritional value as a protein source, collagen and collagen-derived products may exert various potential biological activities on cells in the extracellular matrix through the corresponding food-derived peptides after ingestion for applications in dietary supplements and pharmaceutical preparations [Liu et al., 2015].

- **Controlled release from recombinant polymers:** Recombinant polymers provide a high degree of molecular definition for correlating structure with function in controlled release. The wide array of amino acids available as building blocks for these materials lend many advantages including biorecognition, biodegradability, potential biocompatibility, and control over mechanical properties among other attributes. Genetic engineering and DNA manipulation techniques enable the optimisation of structure for precise control over spatial and temporal release. Unlike the majority of chemical synthetic strategies used, recombinant DNA technology has allowed for the production of monodisperse polymers with specifically defined sequences. Recombinant polymers used for controlled drug delivery include elastin-like, silk-like, and silk-elastin-like proteins, as well as emerging cationic polymers for gene delivery [Price et al., 2014].

- **Controlled release of drugs:** Interpenetrating network (IPN) and semi-IPN polymer structures that are capable of releasing drugs in a controlled manner have gained much wider importance recently with reference to anticancer, anti-asthmatic, antibiotic, anti-inflammatory, anti-tuberculosis and anti-hypertensive drugs [Aminabhavi et al., 2014].

- **Cyclodextrin nanoparticles in drug delivery:** Cyclodextrins (CDs) have brought a revolution in the pharmaceutical field over the last decade. Natural and modified CDs have been studied and some have gained the USFDA approval or achieved 'Generally Regarded As Safe' (GRAS) status. Another characteristic of CDs is the ease with which they can be induced to form supramolecular structures for its use in drug delivery. CDs, grafted or crosslinked with polymers, are now being developed into 'smart' systems for efficient targeted drug delivery, especially for hydrophobic drugs. Amphiphilic CDs have the ability to form nanospheres or nanocapsules via a simple nano-precipitation technique [Lakkakula et al., 2014].

- **Drug release to lungs:** Drug delivery to the lungs by inhalation offers a targeted drug therapy for respiratory diseases. However, the therapeutic efficacy of inhaled drugs is limited by their rapid clearance in the lungs. Carriers providing sustained drug release in the lungs can improve therapeutic outcomes of inhaled medicines because they can retain the drug load within the lungs and progressively release the drug locally at therapeutic levels. Large and porous microparticles offer excellent aerodynamic properties. Their large geometric size reduces their uptake by alveolar macro-phages, making them a suitable carrier for sustained drug release in the lungs. Similarly, nanocarriers present significant potential for prolonged drug release in the lungs because they largely escape uptake by lung-surface macrophages and can remain in the pulmonary tissue for weeks. They can be embedded in large and porous microparticles in order to facilitate their delivery to the lungs. Conju-gation of drugs to polymers as PEG can be particularly beneficial to sustain the release of proteins in the lungs as it allows high protein loading. Drug conjugates can be readily delivered to respiratory airways by any current nebuliser device. Nonetheless, liposomes represent the formulation most advanced in clinical development. Liposomes can be prepared with lipids endogenous to the lungs and are particularly safe [Loira-Pastoriza et al., 2014].

- **Dendrimer-based polymers:** A dendrimer is a polymer, which is a large molecule comprised of many smaller ones linked together. This type of polymer is being used for solubilization, controlled release, etc. of many drugs. They have been used in the production of industrial adhesives. They are expected to serve as components in a variety of nanomachines. Dendrimers are of interest to researchers in medical technology, where they might help carry and deliver drugs in the body, or serve as replacements for plasma components. Dendrimers might also prove useful in the manufacture of nanoscale batteries and lubricants, catalysts, and herbicides [http://whatis.techtarget.com].

- **Dendrimer-nanoparticle conjugates:** Colloidal inorganic nanoparticles (NPs) have been attracting considerable interest in biomedicine, from drug and gene delivery to imaging, sensing and diagnostics. It is essential to modify the NPs surface to have enhanced biocompatibility and reach multi-functional systems for the *in vitro* and *in vivo*, especially in delivering drugs locally and recognising overexpressed biomolecules [Parat et al., 2015]. Dendrimers are emerging as potential non-viral vectors for the efficient delivery of drugs and nucleic acids to the brain and cancer cells. These polymers are highly branched, 3D macromolecules with modi-fiable surface functionalities and available internal cavities that make them attractive as delivery systems for drug and gene delivery applications [Somani and Dufès, 2014].

- **Dendrimers for enhanced drug solubi-lisation:** Approximately 40% of newly developed drugs are rejected by the pharma-ceutical industry and will never benefit a patient because of low water solubility. Another 17% of launched drugs exhibit sub-optimal performance for the same reason. Given the growing impact and need for drug delivery, a thorough understanding of delivery technologies that enhance the bioavailability of drugs is important. The high level of control over the dendritic architecture (size, branching density, surface functionality, etc.) makes dendrimers ideal excipients for enhanced solubility of poorly water-soluble drugs. Many commercial small-molecule drugs with anti-cancer, anti-inflammatory and antimicrobial activity have been formulated successfully with dendrimers, e.g., poly (amidoamine) (PAMAM), poly (propylene imine) (PPI or DAB) and poly (etherhydroxylamine) (PEHAM). Some dendrimers themselves show pharmaceutical activity in these three areas, providing the opportunity for combination therapy in which the dendrimers serve as the drug carrier and simultaneously as an active part of the therapy [Svenson and Chauhan, 2008].

- **Dextrans for targeted and sustained delivery of therapeutic and imaging agents:** Dextrans have been investigated for delivery of drugs, proteins/enzymes, and imaging agents. These highly water-soluble polymers are available commercially as different MWs with a relatively narrow MW distribution. Additionally, dextrans contain a large number of hydroxyl groups, which can be easily conjugated to drugs and proteins by either direct attachment or through a linker. In terms of PK, the intact polymer is not absorbed to a significant degree after oral administration. Therefore, most of the applications of dextrans as macromolecular carriers are through injectable routes. Pharmacodynamically, conjugation with dextrans has resulted in prolongation of the effect, alteration of toxicity profile, and a reduction in the immunogenicity of drugs and/or proteins. A substantial number of studies on dextran conjugates of therapeutic/imaging agents have reported favourable alteration of PK and pharmacodynamics (PD) of these agents [Mehvar, 2000].

- **Elastin-like polypeptides in drug delivery:** Elastin-like polypeptides (ELPs) are biopolymers inspired by human elastin. Their lower critical solution temperature phase transition behaviour and biocompatibility make them useful materials for stimulus-responsive applications in biological environments. Due to their genetically encoded design and recombinant synthesis, the sequence and size of ELPs can be exactly defined. These design parameters control the structure and function of the ELP with a precision that is unmatched by synthetic polymers. Due to these attributes, ELPs have been used extensively for drug delivery in a variety of different embodiments as soluble macromolecular carriers, self-assembled nanoparticles, cross-linked microparticles, or thermally coacervated depots. These ELP systems have been used to deliver biologic therapeutics, radionuclides, and small molecule drugs to a variety of anatomical sites for the treatment of diseases including cancer, type 2 diabetes, osteoarthritis, and neuroinflammation [MacEwan and Chilkoti, 2014].

- **Functional polymers for treatment of myocardial infarct:** The conventional medical therapy for ischemic heart disease is focused on the use of drug eluting stents, coronary-artery bypass graft surgery and anti-thrombosis. Gene therapy provides great opportunities for treatment of cardiovascular disease. In order for gene therapy to be successful, the development of proper gene delivery systems and hypoxia-regulated gene expression vectors are the most important factors. Several non-viral gene transfer methods have been developed to overcome the safety problems of viral transduction, some of which include plasmids that regulate gene expression that is controlled by environment specific promoters in the transcriptional or the translational level [Won et al., 2014].

- **Glucomannan polymers as bioactive materials:** Two plant-derived glucomannans (GMs)-Konjac glucomannan (KGM) and the polysaccharide of *Bletilla striata* (BSP) have emerged as new sources for development of biomaterials. They have been fabricated into drug delivery vehicles and wound healing dressings in varying shapes and sizes, and demonstrated strong gelling properties, high biocompatibility and remarkable convenience for processing and modification. Notably, they demonstrate bioactivities, e.g., response to enzymes produced in special biological niches and/or affinity for carbohydrate receptors on specific cells [Wang et al., 2015].

- **Hyaluronic acid family for cancer chemoprevention and therapy:** Hyaluronic acid is the most uncomplicated large polymer that regulates several normal physiological processes and, at the same time, contributes to the manifestation of a variety of chronic and acute diseases, including cancer. Members of the HA signalling pathway (HA synthases, HA receptors, and HYAL-1 hyaluronidase) have been experimentally shown to promote tumour growth, metastasis, and angiogenesis, and hence each of them is a potential target for cancer therapy. Furthermore, as these members are also overexpressed in a variety of carcinomas, targeting of the HA family is clinically relevant. A variety of targeted approaches have been developed to target various HA family members, including small-molecule inhibitors and antibody and vaccine therapies. These treatment approaches inhibit HA-mediated intracellular signalling that promotes tumour cell proliferation, motility, and invasion, as well as induction of endo-thelial cell functions. Being nontoxic, non-immunogenic, and versatile for modifications, HA has been used in nanoparticle preparations for the targeted delivery of chemotherapy drugs and other anticancer compounds to tumour cells through interaction with cell-surface HA receptors [Lokeshwar et al., 2014].

- **Hybrid nanoparticles for theranostic applications:** Hybrid nanoparticles are composed of both inorganic and organic components. They have been exploited as promising platforms for cancer imaging and therapy. This class of nanoparticles can not only retain the beneficial features of both inorganic and organic materials, but also allow systematic fine-tuning of their properties through the judicious combination of functional components. Nanoscale metal-organic frameworks and polysilsesquioxane nanoparticles have been successfully used in cancer imaging and therapy [He and Lin, 2015].

- **Hydrogel composites as tissue engineering scaffolds:** Hydrogels closely resemble the extracellular matrix (ECM) and can support cell proliferation while new tissue is formed, making them materials of choice as tissue

engineering scaffolds. However, their sometimes-poor mechanical properties can hinder their application. The addition of meshes of nano-fibres embedded in their matrix forms a composite that draws from the advantages of both components. Given that these materials are still in the early stages of development, there is a lack of uniformity across methods for characterising their mechanical properties. The fibrous constituent improves the mechanical properties of the hydrogel, while the biocompatibility and functionality of the gels are maintained or even improved [Butcher et al., 2014; Dumville et al., 2015]. Bio-derived hydrogels can be divided into single-component hydro gels (collagen, hyaluronic acid, chitosan, alginate, silk fibroin, etc.) and multi-component hydrogels [Matrigel, the extract of extracellular matrix (ECM), and decellularised ECM]. They have favorable biocompatibility and bioactivity because they are mostly extracted from the ECM of biological tissue. Among them, hydrogels derived from decellularised ECM, whose composition and structure are more in line with the require-ments of bionics, have incomparable advantages and prospects. This kind of scaffold is the closest to the natural environ-ment of the cell growth. Bio-derived hydrogels have been widely used in tissue engineering research in spite of many challenges such as poor mechanical properties, rapid degradation, the immunogenicity or safety, vascularisation, sterilisation methods [Fu and Lü, 2014].

- **Hydrogels and scaffolds for immuno-modulation:** Much of the field of biomaterial-based immunotherapy has relied on evaluating model antigens, e.g., chicken egg ovalbumin in mouse models. Nevertheless, such model antigens have provided important insights into the mechanisms of immune regulation and served as a proof-of-concept for plethora of biomaterial-based vaccines. It is only recently that an experimental scaffold vaccine implanted beneath the skin has begun to use the human model to study the immune responses to cancer vaccination by co-delivering patient-derived tumour lysates and immunomodulatory proteins. If successful, this scaffold vaccine may change the way we approached untreatable cancers, but more importantly, may allow a faster and more rational translation of therapeutic regimes to other cancers, chronic infections, and autoimmune diseases [Singh and Peppas, 2014].

- **Hydrogels for 3D cell culture:** 3D cell cultures have drawn a large amount of interest in the scientific community with their ability to closely mimic physiological conditions. Hydrogels have been used extensively in the development of extracellular matrix (ECM) mimics for 3D cell culture. Compounds, e.g., collagen and fibrin, are commonly used to synthesise natural ECM mimics; however, they suffer from batch-to-batch variation. Lowe et al. explored the synthesis route of hydrogels; how they can be altered to give different chemical and physical properties; how different biomolecules, e.g., arginyl-glycylaspartic acid (RGD) or vascular endothelial growth factor (VEGF), can be incorporated to give different biological cues; and how to create concentration gradients with UV light. They also emphasised on the types of techniques available in high-throughput processing, e.g., nozzle and droplet-based biofabrication, photoenabled biofabrication, and microfluidics. The combination of these approaches and techniques allow the preparation of hydrogels which are capable of mimicking the ECM [Lowe et al, 2014].

- **Hydrogels in pharmaceutical formulations:** Hydrogels are hydrophilic, three-dimensional networks, which are able to imbibe large amounts of water or biological fluids, and thus resemble, to a large extent, a biological tissue. These materials can be synthesised to respond to a number of physiological stimuli present in the body, e.g., pH, ionic strength and temperature. The ideal drug-delivery system should provide therapeutics in response to physiological requirements, having the capacity to 'sense' changes and alter the drug-release process accordingly. Intelligent polymers also referred as "stimuli-responsive polymers" undergo strong property changes (in shape, surface characteristics, solubility, etc.) when only small changes in their environment (changes in temperature, pH, ionic strength, light, electrical and magnetic field, etc.) take place. They have been used in several novel applications, DDS, tissue engineering scaffolds, bioseparation, bio-mimetic actuators, etc. The most popular member of these type of polymers is poly(N-isopropylacrylamide) [(poly(NIPA)], which exhibits temperature-sensitive character, in which the polymer chains change from water-soluble coils to water-insoluble globules in aqueous solution as temperature increases above the lower critical solution temperature (LCST) of the polymer. Copolymerisation of NIPA with acrylic acid (AAc) allows the synthesis of both pH and temperature-responsive copolymers [Piskin, 2004].

- **Inhaled DDS for targeting alveolar macrophages:** Most drugs do not effectively reach the macrophages at therapeutic levels. Alveolar macrophages also play an important role to initiative adaptive immunity toward combating inflammation and cancer in the lung. Lee et al. reviewed the development of micro- and nanotechnology-based DDS to target alveolar macrophages in association with intracellular infections, cancer and lung inflammation. The regulation of physico-chemical parameters of particles could be a recipe to enhance macrophage targeting and uptake. However, there is still a need to identify more target-specific receptors in order to facilitate drug targeting. Besides that, the toxicity of nanocarriers arising from prolonged residence in the lung should be taken into consideration during formulation [Lee et al., 2015].

- **Intracellular delivery of biopolymers:** Kornev et al. [2015] reported the basic methods of intracellular delivery of biopolymers; the structure and synthesis of magnetic nanoparticles, their stabilising surfactants; the interaction of nanoparticles with biopolymers, e.g., nucleic acids and proteins; and challenges with physiology and biocompatibility of magnetic nanoparticles.

- **Mechanosensing of cells in 3D gel matrices:** Cells *in vivo* typically are found in 3D matrices, the mechanical stiffness of which is important to the cell and tissue-scale biological processes. Although it is well characterised that as to how cells sense matrix stiffness in 2D substrates, the scenario in 3D matrices needs to be explored. Thus, materials that can mimic native 3D environments and possess wide, physiologically relevant elasticity are highly desirable. Natural polymer-based materials and synthetic hydrogels could provide a better 3D platform to investigate the mechano-response of cells with stiffness comparable to their native environments. However, the limited stiffness range together with interdependence of matrix stiffness and adhesive ligand density are inherent in many kinds of materials, and hinder efforts to demonstrate the true effects contributed by matrix stiffness. These problems have been addressed by the recently emerging exquisitely designed materials based on native matrix components, designer matrices, and synthetic polymers [Shan et al., 2014].

- **Micelles of block copolymers for biomedical applications:** Target drug delivery methodology is becoming increasingly important to overcome the shortcomings of conventional drug delivery absorption method. It improves the action time with uniform distribution and poses minimum side effects, but is usually difficult to design to achieve the desired results. Economically favorable, environment-friendly, multifunctional, and easy to design, hybrid nanomaterials have demonstrated their enormous potential as target drug delivery vehicles. A combination of both micelles and nanoparticles makes them fine target delivery vehicles in a variety of biological applications where precision is primarily required to achieve the desired results as in the case of cytotoxicity of cancer cells, chemotherapy, and computed tomography-guided radiation therapy [Bakshi, 2014].

- **Micro/nanomotors in drug delivery:** Nanomachines offer considerable promise for the treatment of diseases. The ability of man-made nanomotors to rapidly deliver therapeutic payloads to their target destination represents a novel nanomedicine approach. Synthetic nanomotors, based on a multitude of propulsion mechanisms, have been developed toward diverse biomedical applications. As future micro/nanomachines become more powerful and functional, these tiny devices are expected to perform more demanding biomedical tasks and benefit different drug delivery applications [Gao and Wang, 2014].

- **Molecularly imprinted particles for medical applications:** Molecular imprinting (MI) represents a strategy to introduce a 'molecular memory' in a polymeric system obtaining materials with specific recognition properties. MI particles can be used as DDS providing a targeted release and thus reducing the side effects. The introduction of molecular recognition properties on a polymeric drug carrier represents a challenge in the development of targeted delivery systems to increase their efficiency. Molecularly imprinted drug carriers can be considered interesting candidates to significantly improve the efficiency of a controlled drug treatment [Gagliardi and Mazzolai, 2015]. The potential of these sol-gel materials was well demonstrated in a few applications of critical interest for medicinal/biomedical science. The vast room left for expansion and improvement envisages a continuously growing interest by researchers in the future, eventually resulting in important medical applications able to enter the professional and consumer medical markets [Concu et al., 2015].

- **Mucoadhesive polymeric platforms for controlled drug delivery:** The attractiveness of mucosal-targeted controlled drug delivery of active pharmaceutical ingredients (APIs), has led formulation scientists to engineer numerous polymeric systems for such tasks. Formulation scientists have at their disposal a range of *in vitro* and *in vivo* mucoadhesion testing setups in order to select candidate adhesive drug delivery platforms. As such, mucoadhesive systems have found wide use throughout many mucosal covered organelles for API delivery for local or systemic effect. Evolution of such mucoadhesive formulations has transgressed from first-generation charged hydrophilic polymer networks to more specific second-generation systems based on lectin, thiol and various other adhesive functional groups [Andrews et al., 2009].

- **Multifunctional nanoparticles for theranostic applications:** Theranostics is a promising field that combines therapeutics and diagnostics into single multifunctional formulations. This field is driven by advancements in nanoparticle systems capable of providing the necessary functionalities. By utilising these powerful nanomedicines, the concept of personalised medicine can be realised by tailoring treatment strategies to the individual. Considerations when choosing a class of nanoparticle include the size, shape, charge, and surface chemistry, while classes of nanoparticles discussed are polymers, liposomes, dendrimers, and polymeric micelles. To image the interactions with disease states, contrast agents are included in the nanoparticle formulation. Imaging options include optical imaging techniques, computed tomography, nuclear-based, and magnetic resonance imaging. The interplay between all

of these components needs to be carefully considered when designing a theranostic system [Cole and Holland, 2015].

- **PCL based amphiphilic block copolymers:** Polycaprolactone (PCL) and its copolymers are a type of hydrophobic aliphatic polyester based on hydroxyalkanoic acids. They possess exceptional qualities: biocompatibility; FDA approval for clinical use; biodegradability by enzyme and hydrolysis under physiological conditions and low immunogenicity. These critical properties have facilitated their value as sutures, drug delivery vehicles and tissue engineering scaffolds in pharmaceutical and biomedical applications. However, the hydrophobicity of PCL and its copolymers remains a concern for further biological and biomedical applications. One promising approach is to design and synthesise well-controlled PCL-based amphiphilic block copolymers [Li and Tan, 2014].

- **PEGylation and its impact protein-based medicines:** PEGylation, a covalent conjugation of PEG to therapeutic molecules, is a clinically proven approach for extending the circulation half-life and reducing the immunogenicity of protein therapeutics. Most clinically used PEGylated proteins are heterogeneous mixtures of PEG positional isomers conjugated to different residues on the protein main chain. Current research is focused to reduce product heterogeneity and to preserve bioactivity. So far protein PEGylation has yielded more than 10 marketed products and in view of the lack of equally successful alternatives to extend the circulation half-life of proteins, PEGylation will still play a major role in drug delivery for many years to come [Ginn et al., 2014].

- **Peptide-nanoparticles for cancer therapy:** Polymersome vesicles and wormlike filomicelles self-assembled with amphiphilic, degradable block copolymers have recently shown promise in application to cancer therapy. In the case of filomicelles, dense, hydrophilic brushes of poly(ethylene glycol) (PEG) on these nanoparticles combine with flexibility to non-specifically delay clearance by phagocytes *in vivo*, which has motivated the development of "self" peptides that inhibit nanoparticle clearance through specific interactions. Delayed clearance, as well as robustness of polymer assemblies, opens the dosage window for delivery of increased drug loads in the polymer assemblies and increased tumour accumulation of drug(s). Antibody-targeting and combination therapies, e.g., with radiotherapy, are emerging in preclinical animal models of cancer. Such efforts are expected to combine with further advances in polymer composition, structure, and protein/peptide functionalisation to further enhance transport through the circulation and permeation into disease sites [Oltra et al., 2014].

- **Poly(lactic-co-glycolic acid) nanoparticles:** Poly(lactic-co-glycolic acid) (PLGA) has been exploited widely in the design of nanoparticles because it is biodegradable, biocompatible, protects the drug molecules from degradation, and aids in producing sustained and targeted delivery. However, certain constraints associated with PLGA nanoparticles, e.g., poor drug encapsulation, polymer degradation, and scale-up issues, have led to the development of emerging hybrid PLGA delivery systems. These hybrid nanoparticles are core-shell nanostructures comprising either a PLGA core or a PLGA shell combining multiple functionalities within one system and, thus, exhibiting the complementary characteristics of two different platforms used for the delivery of a wide range of therapeutics and imaging [Pandita et al., 2015].

- **Poly(malic acid)-based derivatives:** Poly (malic acid) (PMLA) extracted from microorganisms or synthesised from malic or aspartic acid was used to prepare water-soluble drug carriers or nanoparticles. The results obtained by several groups highlight the

interest of such polyesters in the field of drug delivery [Loyer et al., 2014].

- **Polycation-mediated integrated cell death processes:** One of the major challenges in the field of nucleic acid delivery is the design of delivery vehicles with attributes that render them safe as well as efficient in transfection. To this end, polycationic vectors have been intensely investigated with native polyethylenimines (PEIs) being the gold standard. PEIs are highly efficient transfectants, but depending on their architecture and size they induce cytotoxicity through different modes of cell death pathways [Parhamifar et al., 2014].

- **Polyester particles with specific drug targeting and drug release properties:** PLA and PLGA microspheres and nanoparticles remain the focus of intensive research effort directed to the controlled release and *in vivo* localisation of drugs. In recent years engineering approaches have been devised to create novel micro- and nanoparticles, which provide greater control over the drug release profile and present opportunities for drug targeting at the tissue and cellular levels. This has been possible with better understanding and manipulation of the fabrication and degradation processes, particularly emulsion-solvent extraction, and conjugation of polyesters with ligands or other polymers before or after particle formation. As a result, particle surface and internal porosity have been designed to meet criteria-facilitating passive targeting (e.g., for pulmonary delivery), modification of the drug release profile (e.g., attenuation of the burst release) and active targeting via ligand binding to specific cell receptors. It is now possible to envisage adventurous applications for polyester microparticles beyond their inherent role as biodegradable, controlled drug delivery vehicles. These may include drug delivery vehicles for the treatment of cerebral disease and tumour targeting, and co-delivery of drugs in a pulsatile and/or time-delayed fashion [Mohamed et al., 2008].

- **Polylactides/glycolides-excipients for injectable drug:** The choice of PLA and PLGA as polymers for sustained-release formulations originated from their use in the medical device industry to make bio-absorbable sutures. However, their unique properties, including versatile degradation kinetics, established safety, and bio-compatibility, made them ideal for drug delivery applications. Not only do they modify the PK of the encapsulated drug, but they also shield the drug from enzymatic attack. In addition, because the polymers degrade at the injection site, their safety and biocompatibility become a critical factor in the success of the product. The consistency of product performance strongly depends on the properties of the polymer, which, in turn, depend on the production process, catalysts used, and final MW as critical factors. Currently, a number of approved products in the market utilise PLA and PLGA as excipients to achieve sustained release of the active ingredient (e.g., PLA-doxycycline hyclate for periodontal disease; PLA-leuprolide acetate for prostate cancer and endometriosis; PLGA-human growth hormone for growth deficiencies; PLGA-glucose-octreotide for acromegaly; PLGA-triptorelin pamoate for prostate cancer; PLA-goserelin acetate for prostate cancer and endometriosis). Future demand for these polymers is likely to grow, as parenteral chemotherapeutics as well as modern biotechnology drugs (proteins and antibodies) become targets for reformulation and life cycle management [Chaubal, 2004].

- **Polymer carriers of epidoxorubicin and cyclophosphamide in cancer therapy:** Chemotherapy using cytostatic drugs based treatment is the main method of therapy of metastatic cancers. Cytostatics have an important role in the cancer therapy. They have particular meaning in the therapy of solid and haematological tumours. However, using cytostatic drugs is limited due to their toxic effects on healthy cells. In last years, the decrease in toxicity of cytostatic drugs and the increase in their therapeutic properties are intensively investigated [Zótowska and Sobczak, 2014].

- **Polymeric electro-spun nanofibers for drug delivery:** Electro-spinning is a simple unit operation process by which polymeric nanofibers can be fabricated using an electrostatically operated jet of polymer solution or polymer melt. Nanofibers because of their interesting features, e.g., surface-to-volume ratio, high surface area, microporosity, and nonwoven structure, provide numerous opportunities to design novel carrier systems for large commodities of therapeutics. Physicochemical properties of nanofibers depend on several process and formulation parameters, e.g., applied voltage, flow rate, polymer selection, and concentration of polymer used [Sharma et al., 2014].

- **Polymeric micelles for drug delivery in cancer:** The growing interest in polymeric micelles as drug delivery vehicle is promoted by the advantages they offer for hydrophobic anticancer agents. The size of most polymeric micelles lies within the range 10–100 nm ensuring that they can selectively leave the circulation at tumour site via the enhanced permeability and retention effect. Their unique structure allows them to solubilise hydrophobic drugs, prolong their circulatory half-life and eventually lead to enhanced therapeutic efficacy. In addition, they can undergo several structural modifications to further augment tumour cell uptake [Mohamed et al., 2014]. Drug combinations are common in cancer treatment and are rapidly evolving, moving beyond chemotherapy combinations to combinations of signal transduction inhibitors. For the delivery of drug combinations, i.e., multi-drug delivery, major considerations are synergy, dose regimen, pharmacokinetics (PK), toxicity, and safety. In concurrent drug delivery, polymeric micelles deliver multi-poorly water-soluble anticancer agents, satisfying strict requirements in solubility, stability, and safety. In sequential drug delivery, polymeric micelles participate in pre-treatment strategies that "prime" solid tumours and enhance the penetration of secondarily administered anticancer agent or nanocarrier [Cho et al., 2015].

- **Polymeric micelles for drug targeting:** Polymeric micelles are nano-delivery systems formed through self-assembly of amphiphilic block copolymers in an aqueous environment. The nanoscopic dimension, stealth properties induced by the hydrophilic polymeric brush on the micellar surface, capacity for stabilized encapsulation of hydrophobic drugs offered by the hydrophobic and rigid micellar core, and finally a possibility for the chemical manipulation of the core/shell structure have made polymeric micelles one of the most promising carriers for drug targeting. To date, three generations of polymeric micellar delivery systems, i.e., polymeric micelles for passive, active and multifunctional drug targeting, have arisen from research efforts, with each subsequent generation displaying greater specificity for the diseased tissue and/or targeting efficiency. Mahmud et al. reviewed the research efforts made for the development of each generation and provided an assessment on the overall success of polymeric micellar delivery system in drug targeting. The emphasis is placed on the design and development of ligand modified, stimuli responsive and multifunctional polymeric micelles for drug targeting [Mahmud et al., 2007].

- **Polymeric nanoparticle technologies for oral drug delivery:** Biologics increasingly are being used for the treatment of many diseases. These treatments typically require repeated doses administered by injection. Alternate routes of administration, particularly oral, are considered favourable because of improved convenience and compliance by patients, but physiological barriers, e.g., extreme pH level, enzyme degradation, and poor intestinal epithelium permeability limit absorption. Encapsulating biologics in DDS, e.g., polymeric nanoparticles, prevent inactivation and degradation caused by low pH and enzymes of the gastrointestinal tract. However, transport across the intestinal epithelium remains the most critical barrier to overcome for efficient oral delivery [Pridgen et al., 2014].

- **Polymers derived from the amino acid:** The natural amino acid L-tyrosine is a major nutrient having a phenolic hydroxyl group. This feature makes it possible to use derivatives of tyrosine dipeptide as a motif to generate diphenolic monomers, which are important building blocks for the design of biodegradable polymers. Particularly useful monomers are desaminotyrosyl-tyrosine alkyl esters (abbreviated as DTR, where R stands for the specific alkyl ester used). Using this approach, a wide variety of polymers have been synthesised. Tyrosine-derived poly-carbonates, polyarylates, and polyether are reported with special emphasis on recent developments relating to cellular and *in vivo* responses, sterilisation techniques, surface characterisation, drug delivery, and processing and fabrication techniques [Bourke and Kohn, 2003].

- **Polymers for nucleic acid transfer:** The improvements in macromolecular chemistry and the recognition of distinct biological extra- and intracellular delivery hurdles triggered several breakthrough developments, including the discovery of natural and synthetic poly-cations for compaction of nucleic acids into stable nanoparticles termed polyplexes; the incorporation of targeting ligands and surface-shielding of polyplexes to enable receptor-mediated gene delivery into defined target tissues; and strongly improved intracellular transfer efficacy by better endosomal escape of vesicle-trapped polyplexes into the cytosol. These experiences triggered the development of second-generation polymers with more dynamic properties, e.g., endosomal pH-responsive release mechanisms, or bio-degradable units for improved biocompatibility and intracellular release of the nucleic acid pay load. Despite a better biological understanding, significant challenges, e.g., efficient nuclear delivery and persistence of gene expression persist. Bioinspired multi-functional polyplexes resembling "synthetic viruses" appear as attractive opportunity, but provide additional challenges: how to identify optimum combinations of functional delivery units, and how to prepare such polyplexes reproducibly in precise form? Design of sequence-defined polymers, screening of combinatorial polymer and polyplex libraries are tools for further chemical evolution of polyplexes [Wagner, 2014].

- **Polymers for the microencapsulation of cells:** The encapsulation of living mammalian cells within a semi-permeable hydrogel matrix is an attractive procedure for many biomedical and biotechnological applications, e.g., xenotransplantation, maintenance of stem cell phenotype and bio-printing of three-dimensional scaffolds for tissue engineering and regenerative medicine. In this review, Gasperini et al. focused on naturally derived polymers that can form hydrogels under mild conditions and that are thus capable of entrapping cells within controlled volumes. The emphasis has been on polysaccharides and proteins, including agarose, alginate, carrageenan, chitosan, gellan gum, hyaluronic acid, collagen, elastin, gelatin, fibrin and silk fibroin [Gasperini et al., 2014].

- **Polysaccharides for biomedical applications:** Polysaccharides are abundant in nature – renewable, nontoxic, and intrinsically biodegradable. They possess a high level of functional groups including hydroxyl, amino, and carboxylic acid groups. These functional groups can be used for further modification of polysaccharides with small molecules, polymers, and crosslinkers; the modified polysaccharides have been used as effective building blocks in fabricating novel biomaterials for various biomedical applications, e.g., drug delivery carriers, cell-encapsulating biomaterials, and tissue engineering scaffolds [Wen and Oh, 2014]. The physicochemical properties of these materials, e.g., excellent biocompatibility, low cytotoxicity, surface charges that interact with DNA, protein and RNA, and cost effectiveness, make them exceptional base materials for nanocarrier fabrication. The mechanism for the complex formation of polysaccharides-DNA includes the electrostatic interactions between cationic polymers and anionic DNA to form polyplexes that offer unique possibilities for overcoming cellular barriers by escaping endosomal trafficking followed by cellular internalisation and, consequently, enhancing the efficacy of drug and macro-molecule delivery to targeted cells and tissue. Depending upon the cellular uptake and trafficking, nanocarriers are designed for different pharmacological and therapeutic applications [Singh et al., 2014].

- **Poly-ε-caprolactone microspheres and nanospheres:** Poly-ε-caprolactone is a biodegradable, biocompatible and semicrystalline polymer having a very low glass transition temperature. Due to its slow degradation, PCL is ideally suitable for long-term delivery extending over a period of more than one year. This has led to its application in the preparation of different delivery systems in the form of microspheres, nanospheres and implants. Various categories of drugs have been encapsulated in PCL for targeted drug delivery and for controlled drug release. Microspheres of PCL either alone or of PCL copolymers have been prepared to obtain the drug release characteristics [Sinha and Kumaria, 2004].

- **Protein and peptide delivery:** Proteins and peptides are widely indicated in many diseased states. Parenteral route is the most commonly employed method of administration for therapeutic proteins and peptides. However, requirement of frequent injections due to short *in vivo* half-life results in poor patient compliance. Non-invasive drug delivery routes, e.g., nasal, transdermal, pulmonary, and oral offer several advantages over parenteral administration. Intrinsic physicochemical properties and low permeability across biological membrane limit protein delivery via non-invasive routes. One of the strategies to improve protein and peptide absorption is by delivering through nanostructured delivery carriers. Among nanocarriers, polymeric nanoparticles (NPs) have demonstrated significant advantages over other delivery systems [Patel et al, 2014; d'Angelo et al., 2015]. Characterised by large surface area, high vascularisation and thin blood-alveolar barrier, drug delivery by the pulmonary route has benefits over other administration routes. However, most of the marketed inhalable products are short-acting formulations that require the patient to inhale several times every day, thus reducing patient compliance. Controlled pulmonary drug delivery is a promising system but the formidable airway clearance mechanisms need to be avoided. The large porous particles, swellable microparticles and porous nanoparticle-aggregate-based particles are the most promising carriers to control drug release in the lung [Liang et al., 2015].

- **Recent developments in tubulin polymerisation inhibitors:** During past few years, rapid development of the novel tubulin polymerisation inhibitors has been witnessed. Diverse classes of chemical compounds from the natural as well as from the synthetic origin have been extensively studied [Kaur et al., 2014].

- **Collagen I hydrogels for bioengineered tissue microenvironments:** Type I collagen hydrogels have been used successfully as three-dimensional substrates for cell culture and have shown promise as scaffolds for engineered tissues and tumours. A critical step in the development of collagen hydrogels as viable tissue mimics is quantitative characterisation of hydrogel properties and their correlation with fabrication parameters, which enables hydrogels to be tuned to match specific tissues or fulfil engineering requirements. A significant body of work has been devoted to characterisation of collagen I hydrogels to determine the parameter space covered by existing data and identifying key gaps in the literature so that future characterisation and use of collagen I hydrogels for research can be most efficiently conducted [Antoine et al., 2014].

- **Sequence-defined polymers for the delivery of oligonucleotides:** Short synthetic oligonucleotides (ONs) are a group of therapeutic molecules with enormous clinical potential owing to their high specificity and ability to target the expression of virtually any single or group of genes. Clinical translation of ONs is hampered by the inadequate bioavailability in the target cells due to the substantial extracellular and intracellular barriers exposed to these molecules. Different cationic polymers have been successfully deployed for the delivery of ONs [Lehto and Wagner, 2014].

- **Silicones for topical and transdermal drug delivery:** Polydimethylsiloxanes are polymers that are typically used either as an active in oral drug products or as excipients in topical and transdermal drug products. Inherent characteristics like hydrophobicity, adhesion and aesthetics allow silicones to offer function and performance to drug products. Recent technologies like swollen cross-linked silicone elastomer blend networks, sugar siloxanes, amphiphilic resin linear polymers and silicone hybrid pressure sensitive adhesives promise potential performance advantages [Aliyar and Schalau, 2015].

- **Silk-based biomaterials for sustained drug delivery:** Silk presents a rare combination of desirable properties for sustained drug delivery, including aqueous-based purification and processing options without chemical cross-linkers, compatibility with common sterilisation methods, controllable and surface-mediated biodegradation into non-inflammatory by-products, biocompatibility, utility in drug stabilisation, and robust mechanical properties. Silk-based formulations utilise silk's well-defined structural hierarchy, stimuli-responsive self-assembly pathways and crystal polymorphism, as well as sequence and genetic modification options towards targeted pharmaceutical outcomes. Furthermore, by manipulating the interactions between silk and drug molecules, near-zero order sustained release may be achieved through diffusion- and degradation-based release [Yucel et al., 2014].

- **Smart nanomaterials for biomedicals:** Multi-functional nano-devices can be fabricated using different approaches to achieve multi-directional patterning in a scaffold with the ability to alter topographical cues at scale of less than or equal to 100 nm. Smart nanomaterials are made to understand the surrounding environment and act accordingly by either protecting the drug in hostile conditions or releasing the "payload" at the intended intracellular target site. All of this is achieved by exploiting polymers for their functional groups or incorporating conducting materials into a natural biopolymer to obtain a "smart material" that can be used for detection of circulating tumour cells, detection of differences in the body analytes, or repair of damaged tissue by acting as a cell culture scaffold [Choi et al., 2014].

- **Stimuli sensitive polymers and self-regulated DDS:** Stimuli-responsive polymers are an important component for preparation of stimuli-responsive DDS with less side effects and improved efficacy, e.g., cancer treatment. There are endogenous stimuli-including redox-/pH-/enzyme-responsive polymers and exogenous stimuli including thermo-/photo- and ultrasound-responsive polymers for delivery of anti-cancer drugs which have been explored [Cheng et al., 2014]. Both open loop and closed loop systems have been successfully discussed [Siegel, 2014].

- **Strategies for targeting skin diseases:** Abdel-Mottaleb et al. reviewed the skin inflammation or dermatitis as it is one of the most common skin problems, describing the different types and causes of dermatitis, as well as the typical treatment regimens. The potential use of nanocarriers for targeting skin inflammation and the achievement of higher therapeutic effects using nanotechnology was also explored [Abdel-Mottaleb et al., 2014]. Recent advancement in nanotechnology-based nanomedicines has led to the possibility of improving the efficacy and safety of pharmacotherapeutic agents for psoriasis. Novel nanomedicines (e.g., liposomes, polymeric nanoparticles, etc.) have shown their potential in improving therapeutic benefits of antipsoriatic drugs by increasing their therapeutic efficacy with minimal toxicity [Rahman et al., 2015].

- **Sugar-based amphiphilic polymers for biomedical applications:** Sugar-based amphiphilic polymers (SBAPs) are comprised of branched, sugar-based hydrophobic segments and a hydrophilic PEG chain. Similar to many amphiphilic polymers, SBAPs self-assemble into polymeric micelles. These nanoscale micelles have extremely low critical micelle concentrations offering stability against dilution, which occurs with systemic administration. Gu et al. illustrated applications of SBAPs for anticancer drug delivery via physical encapsulation within SBAP micelles and chemical conjugation to form SBAP pro-drugs capable of micellisation. They also showed that SBAPs are excellent at stabilising liposomal delivery systems. The atherosclerotic cascade is usually triggered by the unregulated uptake of oxidised low-density lipoprotein, a cholesterol carrier, in macrophages of the blood vessel wall; SBAPs can significantly inhibit oxidised low-density lipoprotein uptake in macrophages and abrogate the atherosclerotic cascade. By modification of various functionalities (e.g., branching, stereochemistry, hydrophobicity, and charge) in the SBAP chemical structure, SBAP bioactivity was optimised, and influential structural components were identified. SBAPs are promising biomaterials for medical applications [Gu et al., 2014]. The pharmaceutical and food industries are interested in the use of heterochitooligosaccharides because of their unique properties, e.g., good water solubility; minimal toxicity; biocompatibility; the ability to penetrate cell membranes, resulting in a high degree of absorption (unlike chitin and chitosan); and their biological activity. Therefore, researchers have focused their attention on studying the relationship of the structure of oligosaccharides and their specific activity, e.g., antitumour, antimicrobial, antioxidant, immunomodulatory, and other activities [Il'ina et al., 2015].

Polymeric systems in drug delivery

- **Film coatings:** Polymer solutions allowed to evaporate produce polymeric films, which can act as protective layers for tablets or granules containing sensitive drug substances or as rate-controlling barriers to drug release. Film coats can be those that dissolve rapidly and those that behave as dialysis membranes allowing slow diffusion of solute or some delayed diffusion by acting as gel layers. Materials that have been used as film formers include shellac, zein, cellulose acetate phthalate, glyceryl stearates, paraffins and a range of anionic and cationic polymers, e.g., the Eudragit polymers, etc. Shellac has traditionally been used as an enteric coating material, as it has a pH-dependent dissolution mechanism. Newer materials used for the same purpose include cellulose acetate phthalate (CAP).

- **Matrices:** If hydrophobic water-soluble polymers are used, the mechanism of release is by the passage of drug through pores in the plastic, or by leaching or slow diffusion of drug through the polymer wall. The depot forms employing polymeric films, matrices and their mechanism include barrier coating (beeswax; diffusion), fat embedment (glycerol palmoitostearate; erosion, hydrolysis of fat, dissolution), plastic matrix (polyethylene; leaching), repeat action (cellulose acetate phthalate; dissolution of enteric coat), ion exchange (amberlite; dissociation of drug resin complex), hydrophilic matrix (CMC), epoxy resin beads (epoxy resins; dissolution of resin on swelling), microcapsules (gelatin; diffusion), soft gelatin depot capsules (shellac-PEG; diffusion), etc.

- **Microcapsules and microspheres:** Microencapsulation is a technique, which involves the encapsulation of small particles of drug, or solution of drug, in a polymer film or coat. Microspheres on the other hand are solid, but not necessarily homogeneous particles which can entrap drug. Microspheres can be prepared by a variety of techniques, e.g., coacervation, spray coating, etc. Desolvation of water-insoluble macromolecules in non-aqueous solvents would lead to the deposition of a coacervate layer around aqueous or solid disperse droplets. The various water-soluble and water-insoluble macromolecules, which have been used in coacervation processes, are arabinogalactan, cellulose acetate phthalate, carboxymethylcellulose, cellulose nitrate, gelatin, ethylcellulose, gum arabic (acacia), poly(ethylene vinylacetate), hydroxyethylcellulose, poly(methyl methacrylate), poly(acrylic acid), polyethyleneimine, poly(vinyl alcohol), polyvinylpyrrolidone, methylcellulose, starch, etc. Desolvation, and thus coacervation, can be induced thermally and this is the basis of some preparative techniques. The conditions for phase separation are best obtained using phase diagrams.

- **Eroding systems:** Release of drug by erosion of the polymeric or macromolecular matrix in which a drug is dissolved or dispersed provides another mechanism for controlling drug absorption. A typical bioerodible system would be that achieved by the molecular association of cellulose acetate phthalate (CAP) with a Poloxamer block copolymer, e.g., Pluronic L101. This interaction is between the proton-donating CAP and the proton-accepting poloxamer. By varying the ratio of CAP to Poloxamer the erosion periods can be controlled from hours to days. Computer simulation of eroding matrices can represent the process accurately and can predict the position of the erosion front and the weight of the matrix.

PRECLINICAL TESTING

The potential for adverse interactions or alterations in the way the drug is delivered to or distributed in the body, the toxicologic profile of the new dosage form could be quite different from that of the active ingredient alone. Thus, the controlled-release formulations may be considered a new entity for toxicity evaluation. The various animal toxicological tests, which are used to evaluate the toxicity of both active and inactive ingredients, as well as the combinations found in the new dosage forms, are:

1. Acute toxicity (types of animals, route of administration, vehicle, etc.).
2. Subchronic toxicity (types of animals, species, routes of administration, dose levels, observations, anatomic pathology, recovery groups, blood level data, etc.).
3. Carcinogenicity.
4. Local irritation (skin, vein and muscle, etc.).
5. Sensitisation.
6. Reproductive functions, etc.

In addition to above said factors, the pharmacokinetic parameters of the new materials are also needed. The toxicology of a new untested substance can be expensive and time-consuming. Thus, the selection of non-active components of polymer-based alternative dosing must be made carefully. Selecting previously tested materials may eliminate the necessity of reproducing extensive toxicology studies. On the other hand, development of unique and potentially useful adjuncts must not be diminished because of inadequate existing toxicology data [Majors and Friedman, 1991].

REGULATORY REQUIREMENTS

The various regulatory requirements for new polymer-based drug submission are:

1. A brief review of legislative history.
2. Content of an investigational new drug application (animal toxicity data; chemistry, manufacturing and controls information; proposed clinical plan; submitting the IND; responsibility of the sponsor; responsibility of the investigator).
3. Content of a New Drug Application (FDA authority for NDA), marketing exclusivity, FDA Drug Review Classification System (Application format); interaction with the FDA, etc. [Gustafson and Kiernan, 1991].

COMMERCIAL ASPECTS

- **Localised delivery:** The product can be implanted directly at the site where drug action is needed and hence systemic exposure of the drug can be reduced. This becomes especially important for toxic drugs, which are related to various systemic side effects (e.g., chemotherapeutic drugs).
- **Sustained delivery:** The drug encapsulated is released over extended periods and hence eliminates the need for multiple injections. This feature can improve patient compliance especially for drugs for chronic indications, requiring frequent injections (e.g., deficiency of certain proteins).

- **Stabilisation:** The polymer can protect the drug from the physiological environment and hence improve its stability *in vivo*. This particular feature makes this technology attractive for the delivery of labile drugs, e.g., proteins.

Interest in this field has increased considerably, especially after the commercial success of products, e.g., Lupron Depot®, Zoladex®, Norplant® and Gliadel®, all of which use the principles of sustained and localised drug release. The drug will be released over time either by diffusion out of the polymer matrix; by degradation of the polymer backbone; or combination of the both. This continuous release of the drug could potentially lead to a pharmacokinetic profile close to the ideal case scenario (avoiding saw tooth pattern). The polymer degradation can occur by enzymatic degradation, hydrolysis or combination of both. Further, hydrolysis can be result of bulk or surface erosion [Batycky et al., 1997]. For a given drug, the release kinetics from the polymer matrix are governed predominantly by three factors, *viz.* the polymer type, polymer morphology, and the excipients present in the system.

Morphology of the polymer matrix plays an important role in governing the release characteristics of the encapsulated drug. The polymer matrix could be formulated as either micro-/nanospheres, gel, film or an extruded shape (e.g., cylinder, rod, etc.). The shape of the extruded polymer can be important to the drug release kinetics, e.g., it has been shown that zero order drug release can be achieved using a hemispherical polymer form. Polymer microspheres are the most popular form due to manufacturing advantages as well as ease of administration (injectability by suspending in a vehicle). The type of technique used affects factors, e.g., porosity, size distribution and surface morphology of the microspheres and may subsequently affect the performance of the drug delivery product [http://www.drugdel.com/polymer.htm].

SUMMARY, CONCLUSION, AND FUTURE DIRECTIONS

Polymer science is an integral part of the product development. Polymer therapeutics include rationally designed macromolecular drugs, polymer-drug and polymer-protein conjugates, polymeric micelles containing covalently bound drug, and polyplexes for DNA delivery. The successful clinical application of polymer-protein conjugates, and promising clinical results arising from trials with polymer-anticancer-drug conjugates, bode well for the future design and development of the ever more sophisticated bio-nanotechnologies that are needed to realize the full potential of the post-genomic age [Duncan, 2003].

The most exciting opportunities in controlled drug delivery lie in the arena of responsive delivery systems, with which it will be possible to deliver drugs through implantable devices in response to a measured blood level or to deliver a drug precisely to a targeted site. Such systems include: copolymers with desirable hydrophilic/hydrophobic interactions; block or graft copolymers; complexation networks responding via hydrogen or ionic bonding; dendrimers or star polymers as nanoparticles for immobilization of enzymes, drugs, peptides, or other biological agents; and new biodegradable polymers; new blends of hydrocolloids and carbohydrate-based polymers, etc. The introduction of absorbable biopolymers demonstrates that new polymers can be created to meet the performance requirements of new devices and to displace the use of nonabsorbable polymers and metals. This trend is certain to continue. Just as the lactide-glycolide polymers are achieving greater clinical acceptance in various forms at present, other polymers are likely to emerge further to extend the utility and indications for absorbable devices [http://www.courses.ahc.umn.edu].

The field of specific drug delivery is an expanding research domain. Besides the use of liposomes formed from various lipids, natural and synthetic polymers have been developed to prepare more efficient DDS either under macromolecular prodrugs or under particulate nanovectors. To ameliorate the biocompatibility of such nanocarriers, degradable natural or synthetic polymers have attracted the interest of many researchers [Loyer et al., 2014].

The formulation and delivery of bio-pharmaceutical drugs, e.g., monoclonal antibodies and recombinant proteins, poses substantial challenges owing to their large size and susceptibility to degradation [Mitragotri et al., 2014].

Assuming that most of the materials used are biocompatible and biodegradable, the toxicity caused by them when formulated into nano-particles is required. Size, charge and surface properties will influence their PK after oral administration [Araújo et al., 2015].

In addition to applicability for carriers in drug delivery, these release methods are significant for another area directly related to pharmacology – modulation of the permeability of the membranes and thus promoting the action of drugs. Emerging technologies, including ionic current monitoring through a lipid membrane on a nanopore, are also reported [Wuytens et al., 2014].

The new biomaterials – tailor-made co-polymers with desirable functional groups – are being created by researchers who envision their use not only for innovative DDS but also as potential linings for artificial organs, as substrates for cell growth or chemical reactors, as agents in drug targeting and immunology testing, as biomedical adhesives and bio-separation membranes, and as substances able to mimic biological systems. Successfully developing these novel formulations will obviously require assimilation of a great deal of emerging information about the chemical nature and physical structure of these new materials. Considerable research is in progress to achieve biocompatibility of synthetic polymers through surface modification to prevent blood clotting, to make porous implants that permit in growth of adjoining tissue, and to search for stronger and more durable polymers. A skin substitute to cover burns has been introduced recently.

Sustained-release dosage forms are a fertile area for the application of plastics, elastomers, and film-forming polymers. Future advances in polymer science are likely to be based on modifying the chemical and physical properties of the polymer, a novel and 'creative' combination of copolymers with targeting and bioresponsive components that can deliver a wide variety of bioactive agents. Further, newer fabrication and manufacturing processes, e.g., molecular imprinting [Allender et al., 2000], supercritical fluid technology [Ghaderi et al., 2000] and nanoscale engineering are bound to revolutionize the design, development and performance of polymer-based DDSs.

Polymer conjugates are nano-sized, multi-component constructs already in the clinic as anticancer compounds, both as single agents or as elements of combinations. They have the potential to improve pharmacological therapy of a variety of solid tumours. Polymer-drug conjugation promotes passive tumour targeting by the enhanced permeability and retention (EPR) effect and allows for lysosomotropic drug delivery following endocytic capture. The experience gained on these studies provides the basis for the development of a more sophisticated second-generation of polymer conjugates. However, many challenges still lie ahead providing scope to develop and refine this field. The "technology platform" of polymer therapeutics allows the development of both new and exciting polymeric materials, the incorporation of novel bioactive agents and combinations thereof to address recent advances in drug therapy. The rational design of polymer drug conjugates is expected to realise the true potential of these "nanomedicines" [Greco et al., 2008].

Establishing the first therapeutics in a new class is never easy. However, throughout the

1990s a steady stream of polymeric drugs began to emerge. PEG has been widely used for conjugation due to its good safety profile, its hydrophilicity and the ability to mono-functionalise for protein conjugation. Many novel polymers, including biodegradable polymer backbones, dendritic architectures, block copolymer micelles and polymers containing pendant cyclodextrin are being used to prepare second-generation polymer therapeutics [Vicent et al., 2009].

Successful progression of polymer therapeutics towards clinical development requires interdisciplinary collaboration covering all the core preclinical skills (polymer chemistry, analytical techniques, biological rationale and models), and, not least, clinical input to guide both polymer therapeutic and clinical trial design. An urgent need for rapid transfer of new concepts from lab to clinic is acknowledged by all, but it is equally apparent that translational research is frequently delayed due to a lack of understanding within the academic community of industrial/clinical development needs and challenges [Vicent et al., 2009].

Polymers have already revolutionized the drug delivery and have even greater potential in future in terms of evolution of personalized as well as precisely controlled and targeted, safe and effective drug delivery. Interdisciplinary cooperation may provide most fruitful results.

REFERENCES

- Abdel-Mottaleb MM, Try C, Pellequer Y, Lamprecht A. _Nanomedicine_ (Lond). 2014 Aug; 9(11): 1727–43.
- Alakhova DY, Kabanov AV. _Mol Pharm_. 2014 Aug 4; 11(8): 2566–78.
- Alb, AM, Drenski, MF, Reed, WF (2008) Implications to industry: Perspective. Automatic continuous online monitoring of polymerisation reactions (ACOMP). _Polymer International_, 57, 390–396.
- Aliyar H, Schalau G. _Ther Deliv_. 2015 Jul; 6(7): 827–39.
- Allcock, Harry R, Lampe, Frederick W, Mark, James E. Contemporary Polymer Chemistry, Pearson Education, 3rd ed. (2003), p. 546.
- Allender, CJ, Richardson, C, Woodhouse, B, Heard, CM, Brain, KR. _Int. J. Pharm._, 2000, 195, 39–43.
- Allison, SD (2008). _Expert Opin Drug Deliv_. 5(6): 615–28.
- Aminabhavi TM, Nadagouda MN, More UA, Joshi SD, Kulkarni VH, Noolvi MN, Kulkarni PV. _Expert Opin Drug Deliv_. 2015 Apr; 12(4): 669–88.
- Andrews GP, Laverty TP, Jones DS. _Eur J Pharm Biopharm_ . 2009 Mar., 71(3): 505-18.
- Andrianov, AK, Payne, LG (1998) _Adv Drug Deliv. Rev_. 31: 185–196.
- Angelova, N, Hunkeler, D (1999) _Trends Biotechnol_. 17: 409–421.
- Antoine EE, Vlachos PP, Rylander MN. _Tissue Eng Part B Rev_. 2014 Dec; 20(6): 683–96.
- Anton, N, Benoit, JP, Saulnier, P (2008) _J Control Release_. 128(3): 185–99.
- Araújo F, Shrestha N, Granja PL, Hirvonen J, Santos HA, Sarmento B. _Expert Opin Drug Metab Toxicol_. 2015 Mar; 11(3): 381–93.
- Ashby, M and Jones, D. Engineering Materials. p. 191–195. Oxford: Butterworth-Heinemann, 1996. Ed. 2.
- Avci P, Erdem SS, Hamblin MR. _J Biomed Nanotechnol_. 2014 Sep; 10(9): 1937–52.
- Bajerová, M, Gajdziok, J, Dvorácková, K, Masteiková, R, Kollár, P (2008) _Ceska Slov Farm_. 57(2): 63–9.
- Bakshi MS. _Adv Colloid Interface Sci_. 2014 Nov; 213:1–20.
- Batycky, RP, Hanes, J, Langer, R, Edwards, DA (1997) _J. Pharm. Sci._ 86(12): 1464–1477.
- Bodmeir, R, Siepmann, S (1999) Nondegradable polymers for drug delivery. _In:_ Mathowitz, EM (ed.), Encyclopaedia of Controlled Drug Delivery 1, John Wiley and Sons, New York, pp. 664–689.
- Bourke, SL, Kohn, J (2003) _Adv. Drug Deliv. Rev_. 54(4): 447–466.
- Brandrup, J, Immergut, EH, Grulke, EA. eds. Polymer Handbook, 4th Ed. New York: Wiley-Interscience, 1999.
- Brocchini, S, Godwin, A, Balan, S, Choi, JW, Zloh, M, Shaunak, S (2008) _Adv Drug Deliv Rev_. 60(1): 3–12.

- Bromberg, L (2003) *Curr. Pharm. Biotechnol.* 4(5): 339–49.
- Bumgardner JD. *Ther Deliv.* 2015 Jul; 6(7): 855–71.
- Butcher AL, Offeddu GS, Oyen ML2. *Trends Biotechnol.* 2014 Nov; 32(11): 564–70.
- Campbell, Neil A, Brad Williamson, Robin J. Heyden (2006) Biology: Exploring Life. Boston, Massachusetts: Pearson Prentice Hall. ISBN 0132508826. http://www.phschool.com/el_marketing.html.
- Chaubal, M (2004) *Drug Dis. Today*, 15; 9(14): 603–9.
- Cheng W, Gu L, Ren W, Liu Y. *Mater Sci Eng C Mater Biol Appl.* 2014 Dec; 45: 600–8.
- Cho H, Lai TC, Tomoda K, Kwon GS. *AAPS PharmSciTech.* 2015 Feb; 16(1): 10–20.
- Choi S, Tripathi A, Singh D. *J Biomed Nanotechnol.* 2014 Oct; 10(10): 3162–88.
- Cole JT, Holland NB. *Drug Deliv Transl Res.* 2015 Jun; 5(3): 295–309.
- Colthrust, MJ, Williams, RL, Hiscott, PS, Grierson, I (2000) *Biomaterials* 21: 649–665.
- Concu R, Ornelas M, Azenha M. *Curr Top Med Chem.* 2015; 15(3): 199–222.
- Daglia M, Di Lorenzo A, Nabavi SF, Talas ZS, Nabavi SM. *Curr Pharm Biotechnol.* 2014; 15(4): 362–72.
- d'Angelo I, Conte C, Miro A, Quaglia F, Ungaro F1, *Curr Top Med Chem.* 2015; 15(4): 386–400.
- Dodane, VV, Vilivalam, D (1998) *Pharm. Sci. Tech. Today* 1: 246–253.
- Domingues RM, Gomes ME, Reis RL. *Biomacromolecules.* 2014 Jul 14; 15(7): 2327–46.
- Dukic-Ott, A, Thommes, M, Remon, JP, Kleinebudde, P.; Vervaet, C (2009) *Eur J Pharm Biopharm.* 71(1): 38–46.
- Dumville JC, Stubbs N, Keogh SJ, Walker RM, Liu Z. *Cochrane Database Syst Rev.* 2015 Feb 17; 2: CD011226.
- Duncan, R (2003) Polymer-anticancer drug conjugates, Biomedical Aspects of Drug Targeting. Muzykantov, VR, Torchilin, VP. (eds.). Kluwer Academic Publication, Boston, pp.193–209.
- Duncan, R, Dimitrijevic, S, Evagorou, EG (1996) *STP Pharma Sci.* 6(4): 237–263.
- Florence, AT, Attwood, D. (eds.) (2011) Physicochemical Principles of Pharmacy, Fifth edition, Pharmaceutical Press, London, pp. 281–330.
- Florence, AT, Attwood, D. (eds.) (1998) Physicochemical Principles of Pharmacy, Third edition, Palgrav Press, New York, pp. 308–370.
- Florenzano, FH, R Strelitzki, WF Reed. Absolute, Online Monitoring of Polymerisation Reactions. *Macromolecules* 1998, 31(21), 7226–7238.
- Fu Y, Lü Q, Zhongguo Xiu. *Fu Chong Jian Wai Ke Za Zhi.* 2014 Aug; 28(8): 1030–6.
- Fu, KD, Pack, W, Kilbanov, AM, Langer, R (2000) *Pharm.* Res. 17: 100–106.
- Gagliardi M, Mazzolai B. *Future Med Chem.* 2015; 7(2): 123–38.
- Galaew, IY, Mathiasson, B (1999) *Trends Biotechnol.* 17: 335–339.
- Gao W, Wang J. *Nanoscale.* 2014 Sep 21; 6(18): 10486–94.
- Gasperini L, Mano JF, Reis RL. *J R Soc Interface.* 2014 Nov 6; 11(100): 20140817.
- Ghaderi, R, Artursson, P, Carlfors, J (2000) *Eur. J. Pharm.* Sci. 10: 1–9.
- Gilmore, J.L, Yi, X, Quan, L, Kabanov, AV (2008) *J Neuroimmune Pharmacol.* 3(2):83-94.
- Giuvărăteanu, I (2007) *Rom J Morphol Embryol.* 48(3): 257–61.
- Ginn C, Khalili H, Lever R, Brocchini S. *Future Med Chem.* 2014; 6(16): 1829–46.
- Gopferich, A (1999) Biodegradable polymers: polyanhydrides. *In:* Mathowitz (ed.), Encyclopaedia of Controlled Drug Delivery 1, John Wiley and Sons, New York, pp.60–71.
- Greco, F, Vicent, MJ (2008) *Front Biosci.* 13: 2744–56.
- Gregoriadis, G, Jain, S, Papaioannou, I, Laing, P (2005) *International J. of Pharmaceutics*, 300: 125–130.
- Gu L, Faig A, Abdelhamid D, Uhrich K. *Acc Chem Res.* 2014 Oct 21; 47(10): 2867–77.
- Guo, JH (1994) *J. Pharm. Pharmacol.*, 46(8): 647–50.
- Gustafson, F, Kiernan, RD (1991) *In:* Polymers for controlled drug delivery, Tarcha, PJ. (ed.), CRC Press, Boston, pp. 241–264.
- Hadjiargyrou, M, Chiu, JB (2008) *Expert Opin Drug Deliv.* 5(10): 1093–106.
- Haider, M, Zaki, M, Hamidreza, G (2004) *J. Contr. Rel* 95(1): 1–26.
- He C, Lin W. *Cancer Treat Res.* 2015; 166: 173–92.
- Hein, CD, Liu, XM, Wang, D (2008) *Pharm Res.* 25(10): 2216–30.

- Heller, J, Gurny, R (1999) Poly (orthoesters). *In:* Mathowitz, E. (ed.). Encyclopaedia of Controlled Drug Delivery 2, John Wiley and Sons, New York, pp. 852–874.
- Heller, J, Pangburn, SH, Penhale, DWH (1987) Use of Bioerodible Polymers in Self-Regulated DDS. *In:* Controlled-Release Technology, Pharmaceutical Applications, Lee, PI, Good WR. (eds). Washington DC, ACS Symposium Series, pp.172–187.
- http://acs.org
- http://chem.pdx.edu
- http://en.wikipedia.org
- http://whatistechtarget.com
- http://www.courses.ahc.umn.edu
- http://www.drugdel.com/polymer.htm
- http://www.iupac.org/publications/books/pbook/PurpleBook-C4.pdf.
- Huang W, Rollett A, Kaplan DL. *Expert Opin Drug Deliv.* 2015 May; 12(5): 779–91.
- Huh, KM, Cho, YW, Park, K (2003) *Drug Del. Tech.* 3(5): 1–7.
- Il'ina AV, Varlamov VP. *Prikl Biokhim Mikrobiol.* 2015 Jan-Feb; 51(1): 5–14.
- Ivanov AN, Norkin IA, Puchin'ian DM. *Tsitologiia.* 2014; 56(8): 543–8.
- Jain D, Bar-Shalom D. *Drug Dev Ind Pharm.* 2014 Dec; 40(12): 1576–84.
- Jain, S, Hreczuk-Hirst, D, Laing, P, Gregoriadis, G (2004) *Drug Del. Sys. Sci.*, 4(1): 3–9.
- Jennings JA, Wells CM, McGraw GS, Velasquez Pulgarin DA, Whitaker MD, Pruitt RL, *Thera. Deliv.*, 2015, 61(13): 1117–1120.
- Kaur R, Kaur G, Gill RK, Soni R, Bariwal. *J. Eur J Med Chem.* 2014 Nov 24; 87: 89–124.
- Kim, SW (1996) Temperature Sensitive Polymers for Delivery of Macromolecular Drugs. *In:* Advanced Biomaterials in Biomedical Engineering and DDS, Ogata, N, Kim, SW, Feijen, J, et al. (eds). Tokyo, Springer, pp. 126–133.
- Kiser, PF, Wilson, G, Needham, D (1998) *Nature* 394: 459–462.
- Koch BE, Stougaard J, Spaink HP. *Glycobiology*, 2015 May; 25(5): 469–82.
- Kornev AA, Dubina MV. *Ross Fiziol Zh Im I M Sechenova.* 2014 Mar; 100(3): 257–73.
- Kost, J, Langer, R (1991) *Adv. Drug Deliv. Rev.* 6: 19–50.
- Kost, J, Horbett, TA, Ratner, BD (1985) *J. Biomed. Mater. Res.*, 19: 1117–1133.
- Kumar, MNV, Kumar, N (2001) *Drug Dev. Ind. Pharm.* 27: 1–30.
- Kuon, GS, Okano, T (1999) *Pharm. Res.* 16: 597–600.
- Lakkakula JR, Maçedo Krause RW. *Nanomedicine* (Lond). 2014 May; 9(6): 877–94.
- Lambkin, I, Pinilla, C, Hamashin, C, Spindler, L, Russell, S, Schink, A, Moya-Castro, R, Allicotti, G, Higgins, L, Smith, M, Dee, J, Wilson, C, Houghten, R, O'Mahony, D (2003) *Pharm. Res.* 20: 1258–1266.
- Langer, R (2000) *Acc. Chem. Res.* 33: 94–101.
- Lawman AM, Peppas, NA (1991) Hydrogels. *In:* Mathowitz, E. (Ed.). Encyclopaedia of Controlled Drug Delivery 2, John Wiley and Sons, New York (1999), pp 397–418.
- Lawman, AM, Peppas, NA (1997) *Polym. Preprints*, 38(2): 566–567.
- Lee SJ, Min HS, Ku SH, Son S, Kwon IC, Kim SH, Kim K.*Nanomedicine* (Lond). 2014 Aug; 9(11): 1697–713.
- Lee WH, Loo CY, Traini D, Young PM. *Expert Opin Drug Deliv.* 2015 Jun; 12(6): 1009–26.
- Lehr, CM (2000) *J. Contr. Rel.* 65: 19–29.
- Lehto T, Wagner E. *Nanomedicine* (Lond). 2014 Dec; 9(18): 2843–59.
- Li W, Wei H, Li H, Gao J, Feng SS, Guo Y. *Nanomedicine* (Lond). 2014 Nov; 9(16): 2587–605.
- Li Z, Tan BH. *Mater Sci Eng C Mater Biol Appl.* 2014 Dec; 45: 620–34.
- Li, S, Vert, M (1999) Biodegradable polymers: polyesters. *In:* Mathowitz, E. (Ed.), Encyclopaedia of Controlled Drug Delivery 1, John Wiley and Sons, New York (1999), pp. 71–93.
- Liang Z, Ni R, Zhou J, Mao S. *Drug Discov Today.* 2015 Mar; 20(3): 380–9.
- Lipinsky, C (1998) *American Association of Pharmaceutical Sciences*, Annual Meeting.
- Liu D, Nikoo M, Boran G, Zhou P, Regenstein JM. *Annu Rev Food Sci Technol.* 2015; 6: 527–57.
- Liveson, HL, Lehr, CM, et al. (1994) *J. Contr. Rel.* 29: 329-330.
- Loira-Pastoriza C, Todoroff J, Vanbever R. *Adv Drug Deliv Rev.* 2014 Aug; 75: 81–91.
- Lokeshwar VB, Mirza S, Jordan A. *Adv Cancer Res.* 2014; 123: 35–65.
- Lowe SB, Tan VT, Soeriyadi AH, Davis TP, Gooding JJ. *Bioconjug Chem.* 2014 Sep 17; 25(9): 1581–601.

- Loyer P, Cammas-Marion S. *J Drug Target*. 2014 Aug; 22(7): 556–75.
- MacEwan SR, Chilkoti A. *J Control Release*. 2014 Sep 28; 190: 314–30.
- Mahmud, A, Xiong, XB, Aliabadi, HM, Lavasanifar, A (2007) *J Drug Target*. 15(9): 553–84.
- Majors, KR, Friedman, MB (1991) *In:* Polymers for controlled drug delivery, Tarcha, PJ (ed.). CRC Press, Boston, pp. 231–240.
- Mao, HQ, Kdaiyala, I, Leong, KW, Zhao, Z, Dang, W (1999) Biodegradable polymers: poly (phosphoester)s. *In:* Mathowitz, E. (ed.). Encyclopaedia of Controlled Drug Delivery 1, John Wiley and Sons, New York, pp. 45–60.
- Mayet N, Choonara YE, Kumar P, Tomar LK, Tyagi C, Du Toit LC, Pillay V. *J Pharm Sci*. 2014 Aug; 103(8): 2211–30.
- McCrum NG, Buckley CP, Bucknall CB. Principles of Polymer Engineering, Oxford University Press, 1997, pp 1–37.
- Mehavar, R (2000) *J. Cont. Rel*. 69 (2000) 1–25.
- Meng, F, Zhong, Z, Feijen, J (2009) Biomacromolecules. 10(2): 197–209.
- Meyers and Chawla. Mechanical Behavior of Materials. pg. 41. Prentice Hall, Inc. 1999.
- Miller DW, Kabanov, AV (1999) *Colloids Surf. B Biointerfaces* 16: 321–330.
- Miller-Chou, BA, Koenig, JL (2003) *Progress in Polym. Sci.*, 28: 1223–1270.
- Mishima, K (2008) *Adv Drug Deliv Rev*. 60(3): 411–32.
- Mitragotri S, Burke PA, Langer R. *Nat Rev Drug Discov*. 2014 Sep; 13(9): 655–72.
- Miyoto, T, Asami, N, Uragami, T (1999) *Nature* 399: 766–769.
- Moghimi, SM, Hunter, AC (2000) *Trends Biotechnol*. 18: 412–420.
- Mohamed S, Parayath NN, Taurin S, Greish K. *Ther Deliv*. 2014 Oct; 5(10): 1101–21.
- Mohamed, F, Van der Walle, CF. (2008). *J Pharm Sci*. 97(1): 71–87.
- Mourya, VK, Inamdar, NN (2009) *J Mater Sci Mater Med*. 20(5): 1057–79.
- Munden, BJ, Kay, HDK, Banker, GS. (1964). *J. Pharm. Sci*. 53: 395–396.
- Narasimhan, B (2001) *Adv. Drug Deliv. Rev.*, 48(2–3): 195–210.
- Oltra NS, Nair P, Discher DE. *Annu Rev Chem Biomol Eng*. 2014; 5: 281–99.
- Omidian H, Park K, Sinko P. Pharmaceutical Polymers. *In:* Martin's Physical Pharmacy and Pharmaceutical Sciences (Sinco PJ, Singh Y eds) Walters Kluwer, 2011 pp 492-515
- Painter PC and Coleman MM. Fundamentals of Polymer Science, CRC Press, 1997, p 22–100.
- Pandita D, Kumar S, Lather V. *Drug Discov Today*. 2015 Jan; 20(1): 95–104.
- Parat A, Bordeianu C, Dib H, Garofalo A, Walter A, Bégin-Colin S, Felder-Flesch D. *Nanomedicine (Lond)*. 2015; 10(6): 977–92.
- Parhamifar L, Andersen H, Wu L, Hall A, Hudzech D, Moghimi SM. *Adv Genet*. 2014; 88: 353–98.
- Patel A, Patel M, Yang X, Mitra AK. *Protein Pept Lett*. 2014; 21(11): 1102–20.
- Peppas, NA (1997) *MPB*. 34–36.
- Peppas, NA, Bures, P, Leobandung, W, Ichikawa, H (2000) *Eur. J. Pharm. Biopharm*. 50(1): 27–46.
- Peppas, NA, Khare, AR (1993) *Adv. Drug. Deliv. Rev.*, 11: 1–10.
- Peppas, NA, Robinson, JR (1995) *J. Drug Target*. 3(3): 183–184.
- Pillai, O, Panchagnula, R (2001) *Curr. Opin. Chem. Biol*. 5(4): 447–451.
- Piskin, E (2004) *Int. J. Pharm*. 277(1–2): 105–118.
- Price R, Poursaid A, Ghandehari H. *J Control Release*. 2014 Sep 28; 190: 304–13.
- Pridgen EM, Alexis F, Farokhzad OC. *Clin Gastroenterol Hepatol*. 2014 Oct; 12(10): 1605–10.
- Pygall, SR, Whetstone, J, Timmins, P, Melia, CD (2007) *Adv Drug Deliv Rev*. 59(14): 1434–52.
- Rahman M, Akhter S, Ahmad J, Ahmad MZ, Beg S, Ahmad FJ. *Expert Opin Drug Deliv*. 2015 Apr; 12(4): 635–52.
- Roiter, Y, and S. Minko, AFM. Single Molecule Experiments at the Solid-Liquid Interface: In Situ Conformation of Adsorbed Flexible Polyelectrolyte Chains, *Journal of the American Chemical Society*, vol. 127, iss. 45, pp. 15688–15689 (2005)
- Rubinstein, M, Colby, R (2003) *Polymer Physics*. pp. 5–50.
- Sandri G, Bonferoni MC, Ferrari F, Rossi S, Mori M, Caramella C. *Curr Top Med Chem*. 2015; 15(4): 401–12.
- Schlapp, M, Friess W (2003) *J. Pharm. Sci*. 92(11): 2145–2151.
- Schott, H (1993) Polymer Science. *In:* Physical Pharmacy: Physical Chemical Principles in the

Pharmaceutical Sciences, Martin, A. (Ed.), 4th ed., Lea and Febiger, Philadelphia, pp. 557–601.

- Schweizer D, Serno T, Goepferich A. *Eur J Pharm Biopharm*. 2014 Oct; 88(2): 291–309.
- Sevda, S, Susan, JM (2004) *Adv. Drug Deliv. Rev.* 56: 1467–1480.
- Shalabv, SW, Ikada, Y, Langer, R, et al. (Eds.) (1994) Polymers of Biological and Biomedical Significance, Washington DC, ACS Symposium Series.
- Shan J, Chi Q, Wang H, Huang Q, Yang L, Yu G, Zou X. *Cell Biol Int*. 2014 Nov; 38(11): 1233–43.
- Sharma R, Singh H, Joshi M, Sharma A, Garg T, Goyal AK, Rath G. *Crit Rev Ther Drug Carrier Syst*. 2014; 31(3): 187–217.
- Siegel RA. *J Control Release*. 2014 Sep 28; 190: 337–51.
- Siepman, J, Peppas, NA (2001) *Adv. Drug Deliv. Rev.* 48(2-3): 137–138.
- Siepmann, F, Siepmann. J, Walther, M, MacRae, RJ, Bodmeier, R (2008) *J Control Release*; 125(1): 1–15.
- Singh A, Peppas NA. *Adv Mater*. 2014 Oct; 26(38): 6530–41.
- Singh D, Han SS, Shin EJ. *J Biomed Nanotechnol*. 2014 Sep; 10(9): 2149–72.
- Singh, I, Rehni, AK, Kalra, R, Joshi, G, Kumar, M (2008) *Pharmazie*. 63(7): 491–6.
- Singh, R, Singh, S, Lillard, JW (2008) *J Pharm Sci*. 97(7): 2497–523.
- Sinha, VR, Bansal, K, Kaushik, R, Kumria, R, Trehan, A (2004) *Int. J. Pharm*. 278 (1): 1–23.
- Sinha, VR, Kumaria, R (2004) *Eur. J. Pharm. Sci*. 18(1): 3–18.
- Sobarzo-Sánchez E, Nabavi SM, Uriarte E, Santana L. *Curr Top Med Chem*. 2015; 15(4): 282–6.
- Somani S, Dufès C. *Nanomedicine* (Lond). 2014 Oct; 9(15): 2403–14.
- Sperling LH (2006) Introduction to Physical Polymer Science, Wiley and Sons, pp. 10–47.
- Sriramoju B, Kanwar RK, Kanwar JR. *Curr Med Chem*. 2014; 21(36): 4154–68.
- Sugibayashi, K, Sakanoue, C, Morimoto, Y (1994) *J. Pharm. Pharmacol*. 46(4): 261–269.
- Svenson, S, Chauhan, AS (2008) *Nanomed*. 3(5): 679–702.
- Szente, L (1999) *Adv. Drug Deliv. Rev* 36: 17–28.
- Takemoto H, Miyata K, Nishiyama N, Kataoka K. *Adv Genet*. 2014; 88: 289–323.

- Tammam SN, Azzazy HM, Lamprecht A. *J Biomed Nanotechnol*. 2015 Apr; 11(4): 555–77.
- Tanihara, M, Suzuki, Y, Nishimura, Y, Suzuki, K, Kakimarau, Y, Fukunishi, Y (1999) *J. Pharm. Sci*. 88: 510–514.
- Uekama, K (1999) *Adv. Drug. Deliv. Rev*. 36: 1–2.
- Uhrich, KE, Cannizzaro, SM, Langer, RS, Shakesheff, KM (1999) *Chem. Rev*. 99: 3181–3198.
- Upadhyay RK. *Biomed Res Int*. 2014; 2014: 869269.
- US patent 6052184 and US Patent 6653150.
- Uskokoviæ V, Desai TA. *Expert Opin Drug Deliv*. 2014 Dec; 11(12): 1899–912.
- Vicent, MJ, Ringsdorf, H, Duncan, R (2009) *Advanced Drug Delivery Reviews* 61, 1117-20.
- Wagner E. *Adv Genet*. 2014; 88: 231–61.
- Wang Y, Liu J, Li Q, Wang Y, Wang C. *Biotechnol Lett*. 2015 Jan; 37(1): 1–8.
- Watts, P, Smith, A (2009) *Expert Opin. Drug Deliv*. 6(5): 543–52
- Weidenfield, S, et al. (1968) *Diabetes* 17: 766–768.
- Wen Y, Oh JK. *Macromol Rapid Commun*. 2014 Nov; 35(21): 1819–32.
- Wheate, NJ (2008) *J Inorg Biochem*. 102(12): 2060–6.
- Winzenburg, G, Schmidt, C, Fuchs, S, Kissel, T (2004) *Adv. Drug Deliv. Rev*. 56(10): 1453–1466.
- Won YW, Bull DA, Kim SW. *J Control Release*. 2014 Dec 10; 195: 110–9.
- Wuytens P, Parakhonskiy B, Yashchenok A, Winterhalter M, Skirtach A. *Curr Opin Pharmacol*. 2014 Oct; 18: 129–40.
- www.studsvik.uu.se
- Yang Y, Wang S, Wang Y, Wang X, Wang Q, Chen M. *Biotechnol Adv*. 2014 Nov 15; 32(7): 1301–16.
- Yeo, Y, Kohane, DS (2008) *Eur J Pharm Biopharm*. 68 (1): 57–66.
- Yi , S, Yi, MP, Harson, RE, Zabner, J, Welsh, MJ (2001) *Gene Ther*. 8: 1826–1832.
- Yoshinari, B, Naohika, M, Kohichiro, S, Yoshinobu, K (1998) *Anal. Scis*. 14: 687–688.
- Yu, H, Wagner, E (2009) *Curr .Opin. Mol. Ther*. 11(2): 165–78.
- Yucel T, Lovett ML, Kaplan DL. *J Control Release*. 2014 Sep 28; 190: 381–97.
- Zótowska K, Sobczak M. *Polim Med*. 2014 Jan-Mar; 44(1): 51–62.

Index